Live Advise
Medical Terminology

Lippincott Williams & Wilkins
offers online teaching advice and student tutoring with this textbook!

Instructors—have you ever wanted to:
…get help generating classroom activities or discussion ideas from an expert in your discipline?

…ask questions about the content of your adopted textbook or ancillary package, and have someone get back to you right away?

…have your lesson plans evaluated?

Students— have you ever needed:
…help studying for a test at a time your instructor was not available?

…questions answered outside of class?

…feedback on assignments before turning them in?

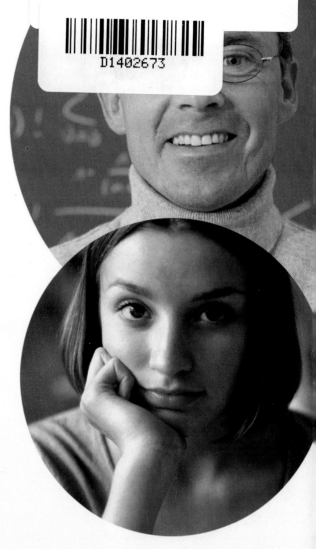

If so, **Live**Advise: Medical Terminology is the service you need!

Our tutors are handpicked educators that we train to help you. They are very familiar with the textbook you are using in class and the text's ancillary package. You can connect live to a tutor during certain hours of the week, or send e-mail style messages to which the tutor will respond quickly – often within 24 hours.

And the best part—the service is free with the purchase of your textbook!

Instructors—to use this service, please visit <u>http://connection.LWW.com/LiveAdvise</u>

Students—see the codebook inside the front cover of this book for more details.
In it you'll find instructions for using this great service, along with your own personal code to log on and get started.

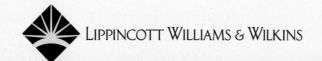

LIPPINCOTT WILLIAMS & WILKINS

Using Medical Terminology:
A Practical Approach

Using Medical Terminology

A Practical Approach

Judi Lindsley Nath, Ph.D.

Professor of Biology
Lourdes College
Sylvania, Ohio

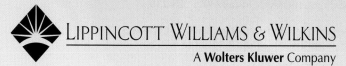
LIPPINCOTT WILLIAMS & WILKINS

A **Wolters Kluwer** Company

Philadelphia • Baltimore • New York • London
Buenos Aires • Hong Kong • Sydney • Tokyo

Acquisitions Editor: John Goucher
Development Editors: Robyn Alvarez and Tom Lochhaas
Marketing Manager: Hilary Henderson
Production Editor: Christina Remsberg
Artist: Dragonfly Media Group
Designer: Risa Clow
Compositor: Maryland Composition
Printer: RR Donnelley - Willard

Printed in the United States of America

Library of Congress Cataloging-in-Publication Data

Nath, Judi L.
Using medical terminology : a practical approach / Judi L. Nath.
p. ; cm.
Includes index.
ISBN 0-7817-4868-2
1. Medicine—Terminology—Problems, exercises, etc. I. Title.
[DNLM: 1. Terminology—Problems and Exercises. W 18.2
N274u 2006]
R123.N32 2006
610′.1′4—dc22
2005022242

To purchase additional copies of this book, call our customer service department at **(800) 638-3030** or fax orders to **(301) 223-2320**. International customers should call **(301) 223-2300**.

Visit Lippincott Williams & Wilkins on the Internet: http://www.LWW.com. Lippincott Williams & Wilkins customer service representatives are available from 8:30 am to 6:00 pm, EST.

05 06 07 08 09
1 2 3 4 5 6 7 8 9 10

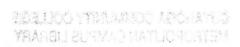

For Grandma, who always said I should write.
For Mom, who was my biggest supporter.
For Pam, who continues to inspire.
For Dad, who was ever so proud.
For Sasha, who was a loyal companion.
For Mike, who stays on the same page, yet reads them all.

Preface

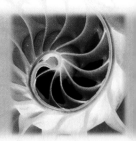

Welcome to the exciting and emerging field of medical terminology. This textbook is designed to teach you the language of your medical career in an engaging and meaningful manner. Textbooks often fail to adequately represent the real world, and students are expected to leap from the confines of a classroom to practice without being acquainted with actual application. By using medical terminology in context, you will be prepared to enter the workforce. This book's concept and practice exercises give you life-long tools to use, regardless of your chosen medical profession. Training in medical terminology is quick, yet covers a wide area of mainstream and allied health fields; and you will be amazed by how much you learn!

INNOVATIVE APPROACH

This workbook–textbook hybrid (a "worktext") teaches medical terminology within the framework of applied anatomy and physiology using a "total-immersion" approach. This means that you will learn whole terms in an anatomy and physiology context, rather than simply memorizing word parts. It is a departure from the methods employed in current medical terminology textbooks because it makes learning the origin, use, and application of terms important. Understanding whole terms enables you to better understand and remember the terms. This approach improves retention of information, enables written and verbal expression, and motivates students.

You will learn medical terminology while learning basic anatomy, physiology, and pathophysiology. This method reinforces the complementary relationship of medical terminology and anatomy, physiology, and pathophysiology. Because medical terms describe the human body in health and in disease, attaining a working knowledge of anatomy, physiology, and pathology will do much to ensure long-term memory of the language. At the end of the course, you will be astounded at the body of knowledge (or knowledge of the body) you possess.

Using the medical terms in context, rather than deconstructing the language, facilitates learning because you will be using the language from the very beginning, much like you might in a foreign-language class. In fact, grasping medical terminology is like learning a foreign language. The words sound odd and many are probably not part of your everyday vocabulary; however, just as you can learn to speak another language, you can learn another aspect of the English language. That is, medical terminology is just a variation of the language you already know!

This textbook provides a number of methods not only to encourage you but also to enable you to walk away with a thorough understanding of the words and with the ability to use them in your new career. Throughout the whole-language lessons, you will be totally immersed in the language, for it is only through reading, writing, speaking, visualizing, and hearing the words that they will become part of your vocabulary. This book follows the proven methods of natural language acquisition that many instructors use in foreign language courses.

In addition, I designed each chapter to work independently of the others. Although you may read the chapters in any order, Chapter 1, "Introduction to Medical Terminology," provides the blueprint for subsequent chapters and gives the foundation on which all other chapters are built.

FOCUS ON LEARNING STYLES

Each of us has a unique learning style. Some of us are auditory learners, others are visual learners, and still others learn through hands-on (kinesthetic) measures. This book employs several effective methods that tap into each of those learning styles. Ample opportunity will be given to learn through a variety of methods from the very beginning.

You will not be bogged down with memorizing lists. Rather, the medical terms will appear in context to reinforce learning. Each chapter follows the same template, beginning with an introduction to the relevant word parts, accompanied by several exercises to boost retention. After the introductory content, the bulk of the chapter follows a predictable pattern: read, review, and practice. Terms appear in digestible chunks of anatomy and physiology discussions, followed by a review of the key terms and a practice of those terms. Each chapter then ends with a variety of exercises, including a spelling test using audio files on the accompanying CD-ROM. Following a pattern that appeals to different learning styles reinforces comprehension and minimizes the need for memorization. Profiles of health-care professionals, interesting tidbits of information, case studies, and real medical reports will spark your interest while presenting medical terms in a variety of contexts. Concepts are best learned through experience, and this book provides you with the tools for successful learning.

TEXT FEATURES

The text is full of a wide variety of features to engage you and to reinforce learning.

Objectives

Each chapter begins with a list of learning objectives to guide you toward success in the course.

Introduction

The first section introduces the chapter and emphasizes the importance of the body system or topic to the comprehension of medical terms. Common medical problems associated with the particular system may also be presented here.

Professional Profile

Medicine and its affiliated health professions are home to an increasing variety of careers. Medical terminology not only turns up in numerous health and medical offices, undergraduate and graduate programs, and certification programs, but also is used routinely in the ever-expanding health and health-related professions. Each chapter highlights a specific career in the "Professional Profile" section by introducing you to a person working in a health-care field related to the chapter's content. That person then serves as a tour guide, leading you through the chapter by demonstrating the significance of medical terminology to his or her particular field.

Medical Term Parts

The "Medical Term Parts" section is divided into four tables. The first table consists of word parts, a list of word elements—prefixes, suffixes, and roots—that are pertinent to the content of each chapter. The "Word Etymology" table identifies medical word roots that can exist as stand-alone medical terms or serve as the base word from which combining forms are derived. For reference and reinforcement purposes, tables of prefixes and suffixes repeat some of the word parts listed earlier.

Word Grouping Exercise

To reinforce retention of the "Medical Term Parts" tables, the word grouping exercise requires you to identify the word part for each definition. This section helps you group the chapter's word parts by common meanings. For example, you will learn that there are two word parts that refer to the kidneys: *neph-* and *ren-;* thus, when you encounter the word *kidney,* you will be able to provide two word parts that refer to it. In essence, if you know that $3 + 2 = 5$, you also know that $5 - 3 = 2$. This analogy may seem elementary, but it actually begins the process of learning the language of medical terminology. You, as the student, must provide the links, and this reinforces learning.

Word Building Exercise

The word building exercise puts the chapter's medical terms in an everyday context. In this section, you immediately begin working with the word parts by identifying and listing common or familiar medical words that contain those word parts. In addition, medical terms are given to demonstrate how those word parts are used in a professional context. This exercise allows you to find medical terms or word parts that are already in your everyday vocabulary and to gain practical experience with the word parts you are learning.

System Structures

Each chapter dealing with a body system includes a list of the key anatomic parts and associated structures. Identifying key organs introduces you to some of the words you will learn in the chapter.

System Preview

A short narrative introduction to the anatomy and physiology of the body system—such as overall functions of the body system—provides a backdrop for the anatomy and physiology content of the chapter.

Key Terms

Each block of narrative contains boldface medical terms that are introduced in context. These *key terms,* their pronunciations, and their definitions appear in a table following the narrative. This whole-language method of presenting words in context—rather than breaking down each one into its word parts—allows you to attach meaning and grasp concepts instead of memorizing.

Pronunciations

In the key term tables (and sometimes within the text itself), the pronunciation of each unfamiliar term is given in parentheses. Pronunciation of each new term is purposefully omitted from the bulk of the text so that the narrative is not interrupted by the odd-looking phonetics. Chapter 1 includes a phonetic pronunciation guide that presents the words in a manner that mimics common spoken sounds. The pronunciations of everyday words are not provided. If you are unsure of the pronunciation of some of these words, they can be found in any English-language dictionary.

Key Term Practice

At the end of each section, key term practice questions reinforce your understanding of the newly introduced terms. These questions focus on contextual definitions of terms, but some of them pertain to spelling. The information appears in short, digestible blocks and is therefore readily attainable. If your response to any of the key term practice questions reveals that you did not grasp a particular concept, simply go back to the beginning of the section and reread it. In this manner, you learn by reading and doing, increasing your familiarity with the words to enhance your comprehension and memory.

Fast Facts

Short, single-sentence facts that pertain to each chapter's topic are scattered throughout the textbook. Here you will find interesting tidbits of information that allow you to have fun with the topic (yes, learning can be fun), while learning a bit of trivia.

The Clinical Dimension

The "Clinical Dimension" section of each chapter contains the pathophysiology discussion. It is divided into blocks of narrative on different disorders, which integrate terms and definitions for signs and symptoms, clinical tests and diagnostic procedures, and treatments. These terms commonly appear in medical reports or in higher-level health-related courses.

Clinical Terms

At the end of the Clinical Dimension section, a single table summarizes the disorders, signs and symptoms, clinical tests and diagnostic procedures, and treatment options for the conditions affecting the particular body system discussed in each chapter. Keep in mind that the categories in this table are not cut and dry (for example, some diagnostic procedures can also be treatments). Most of the terms listed here are from the key term tables, which allows you to put the new terms into a practical and professional context. This table also includes terms that were discussed in the chapter but that were not highlighted as "key terms." In addition, some terms in the table are newly introduced because they are commonly associated with the functional and physical alterations of the specific system or with the diagnosis and treatment of conditions associated with the chapter's topic. Thus, depending on your area of work or study, there is a good chance you will encounter these terms in your studies or professional practice.

Lifespan

The "Lifespan" section contains information on developmental anatomy and physiology and significant alterations seen throughout human life. While focusing on the chapter's topic, the discussion covers lifespan issues from the "womb to the tomb," paying special attention to key alterations that occur in utero, childhood, adolescence, adulthood, and older adulthood, and it uses terms from the chapter, which continues the immersion approach.

In the News

"In the News" takes a story from the popular media and offers another opportunity to put the chapter's medical terminology in context. It provides interesting, real-life scenarios related to the topic studied. This feature links popular science with medical terminology and provides additional application of the terms.

Common Abbreviations

This table lists the common, accepted abbreviations and acronyms introduced in the chapter. Such abbreviations provide a medical shorthand. Each table can be used as a quick reference guide.

Case Study

Case studies provide a conceptual framework for studying medical terminology, and in this textbook they also bridge the path from "Professional Profile" to "Real World Report." In this section, we follow the health-care professional introduced in the beginning of the chapter as he or she treats a patient. Each case emphasizes the relevance of medical terminology to professional practice. The clinical signs and symptoms of each patient reinforces the chapter's key terms. Each case study is followed by questions that allow you to test your comprehension of the chapter's terms. This method provides you with an opportunity to interact with the chapter's topic in a medical context.

Real Word Report

The "Real World Report" section provides you with the opportunity to see how medical terms are used in actual medical reports. This feature uses a medical report compiled for the patient introduced in the case study to demonstrate how medical terms are used in clinical practice. The questions for this section highlight the terms that appear in the report and explain/introduce new terms. Because the report is linked to both the case study and the chapter's professional, it caps a unifying theme: A professional working the field sees a patient with a particular medical history. Diagnostic testing or treatment results in a medical report, which must be understood by the health-care professionals who interact with that patient and by those who deal with that patient's records. The forms that are included in this section are factual reports, although all identifying information has been removed and every name is fictitious.

Review and Application: Three-Level Learning System

Each chapter includes a three-part set of exercises to provide opportunities for recall, concept review, and critical thinking. The questions consist of a variety of exercises and focus on anatomy and physiology, pathophysiology, and medical terminology. All three levels are designed to enhance learning and reinforce concepts.

Key Terms Spelling Test

The spelling test for each chapter requires the CD-ROM. You are asked to spell each word after hearing it pronounced.

Answers

Finally, each chapter includes the answers to all the exercises, except for the Key Terms Spelling Test (answers can be found in the key term and clinical term tables or in a dictionary). Moreover, justifications for correct answers and rationales for incorrect answers are given for the Case Study questions.

LEARNING AND TEACHING RESOURCES

Using Medical Terminology is more than a textbook; it is a package of learning resources. A suite of ancillary material is available for both faculty and students. This supplemental material was created specifically to enhance and strengthen both student learning and instructor teaching.

Learning Resources

The student resources for *Using Medical Terminology* do not end with the textbook. The CD-ROM and Smarthinking (discussed below) work with the extensive features in the textbook to provide a comprehensive learning experience.

Discovering Your Learning Style

The purchase of this textbook allows you access to a valuable tool that you can use to help you more easily learn medical terminology and that can help you throughout your professional life. "My Power Learning" is an online tool that helps you determine your learning style. Research has demonstrated that the manner in which a person gains knowledge is known as his or her learning style. This online assessment will help you discover how *you* learn, even if you think you already know, and will provide you with strategies to employ while sitting in class, with approaches to use for studying, and with tips for test taking.

As a veteran teacher committed to student learning, I not only recommend but encourage you to log onto My Power Learning to discover tools for success. You will find a link to it on the Website associated with this book (http://connection.lww.com/go/nath); your instructor will provide you with a user ID. The goal is to maximize your achievement. In fact, before beginning Chapter 1, you should determine your individual style so that you will be empowered with the knowledge to "attack" this course. Although instructors try to accommodate all students, who come to the classroom with different backgrounds and levels of preparedness, you, the student, are ultimately in command of your own education.

Student Interactive CD-ROM

The CD-ROM included with this textbook contains numerous opportunities for enhancing your learning experience. It contains the following elements:

- Learning style guidelines
- Audio spelling tests
- Labeling exercises
- Medical records exercises
- Flash cards with audio pronunciations
- Audio pronunciation glossary
- Animations of selected concepts and materials presented in the textbook
- Videos of selected medical procedures and processes

LiveAdvise

LiveAdvise: Medical Terminology, an online tutoring resource for students and an advice center for instructors (powered by Smarthinking) comes free with every text! See the ad and login information in the front of the book for details.

Teaching Resources

In addition to the ancillary material available for students, this text also comes with extensive instructor resources. This supplemental material was created specifically to enhance and strengthen both student learning and instructor teaching. The free Instructor Resource CD-ROM contains the following:

- Comprehensive lesson plans
- Brownstone test generator
- Image collection
- *PowerPoint* slides, instructor version
- *PowerPoint* slides, student version
- Learning style guidelines
- Animations of selected concepts and materials presented in the textbook
- Videos of selected medical procedures and processes

In addition, this text provides an online course and course management package powered by WebCT and Blackboard. For a demonstration of this course, visit http://connection.lww.com/nath.

Using Medical Terminology: A Practical Approach utilizes an innovative method to learning medical terminology by immersion within the framework of anatomy, physiology, and pathology. Throughout the pages, the student is exposed to the use of medical terms in a variety of contexts, and consistency among the chapters creates a pattern to ensure achievement. As the health-care system and medical fields continue to expand, this textbook will provide an invaluable resource for practitioners in all health professions.

Judi L. Nath, Ph.D.
Professor of Biology
Lourdes College
Sylvania, Ohio

Acknowledgments

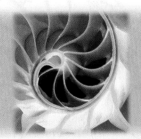

I would like to acknowledge the following people:

Cherol Wahl, a working health-care professional whose insight, knowledge base, and contacts within the medical establishment shaped the framework of this text.

Robyn Alvarez, my development editor, whose attention to detail is remarkable.

John Goucher, my acquisitions editor, who believed in the project.

Karen Gulliver, art program manager, whose services were invaluable.

David Brake and Content Connections, who were instrumental in getting this project off the ground and sustaining it throughout.

Mike and Laura Wahl who graciously supplied photographs.

Tim, Julie, and Brianna Cheek, who poured through photos for the perfect depiction.

Wendy Gaul and Matt Curtis, who opened their woodland home during the creative process.

Ruth Anne O'Keefe, MD, surgeon, photographer, and educator extraordinaire, who was always just a phone call or e-mail away throughout the writing.

Clinical psychologist Pat Bellomo, PhD, and associate professor Thomas Estrella, educators whose professional expertise was invaluable while I was writing the chapter on mental disorders.

Susan Rine, MSN, RN, CNS, a teaching professional who provided nursing tips and clarification.

Mark Tamburrino of RS Office Solutions, who was able to perform magic at the 11th hour.

Terry Wiseman, MD, the pediatrician who was always "at the ready" to answer questions.

Lori Waters, MS Ed, LPC of The Pennsylvania State University, who assisted in matters of clinical significance related to mental health.

John Waters of The Pennsylvania State University, a colleague, friend, and sounding board throughout, who willingly supplied professional expert opinion.

Sue Van Dootingh, OD, medical professional who answered questions clearly, responded rapidly, and opened her office doors readily.

Geoffrey Grubb, PhD, and Robert Helmer, PhD, JD, who provided pronunciations, clarifications, and historical perspective on term derivations.

Ben Pansky, MD, PhD, author, educator, mentor, collaborator, friend, and renown anatomist.

Cindy Hartsel, PT, PhD, whose knowledge and expertise in musculoskeletal injuries were of great assistance.

And the other members of the LWW Team: Tom Lochhaas (development editor), Regen Ness (editorial assistant), Molly Ward (ancillary editor), Hilary Henderson (marketing manager), Christina Remsberg (production editor), and Susan Katz (vice president of health professions).

REVIEWERS

The publisher and author gratefully acknowledge the many professionals who shared their expertise and assisted in developing this textbook, helping us refine our plan, appropriately targeting our marketing efforts, and setting the stage for subsequent editions. In particular, the following reviewers provided the most in-depth feedback through all phases of development:

Nancy Coffman-Kadish, MS, RHIA
Clinical Assistant Professor
School of Nursing and Health
  Professions
Indiana University Northwest
Gary, Indiana

Janice Edelstein, RN-CS, EdD
Associate Professor of Nursing
Marian College
Fond du Lac, Wisconsin

Susan Erue, RN, BSN, MEd
Instructor
Department of Nursing
Iowa Wesleyan College
Mount Pleasant, Iowa

Judith Johle, MEd
Adjunct Instructor
Medical Office Technology Program
Kingwood College
Kingwood, Texas

Merrill Landers, DPT, OCS
Assistant Professor
Department of Physical Therapy
University of Nevada—Las Vegas
Las Vegas, Nevada

Jacqueline McNair, BA, RHIT
Adjunct Faculty
Allied Health Department
Baltimore City Community College
Baltimore, Maryland

Lauren Perlstein
Associate Professor, Medical Assistant
  Coordinator
Department of Nursing and Allied
  Health
Norwalk Community College
Norwalk, Connecticut

Diane Roche, CMA, BSHCA, MSA
South Piedmont Community College
Monroe, North Carolina

Brandy Ziesemer, MA, RHIA
Health Information Program Manager
Health Information Management
Lake-Sumter Community College
Leesburg, Florida

The following reviewers were integral to the development of this text, and the publisher and author wish to thank them for their detailed and valuable feedback.

Nancy Akery
North Harris College
Houston, Texas

James Allen
Lansing Community College
Lansing, Michigan

L. Andriese
Visalia Adult School
Visalia, California

Ed Armstrong
University of Arizona
Tuscon, Arizona

Judy Aronow
Vermont Technical College
Randolph Center, Vermont

Vinita Arora
Faculty of Pharmacy, University of
  Toronto
Toronto, Ontario
Canada

Ben Atchison
Western Michigan University
Kalamazoo, Michigan

Lynn Augenstern
Ridley-Lowell Business & Technical
  Institute
Binghampton, New York

Zubin Austin
University of Toronto
Toronto, Ontario
Canada

Eleanor Ayers
Herzing College
Minneapolis, Minnesota

Lynda Baker
Wayne State University
Detroit, Michigan

Ann Barton
Riverside Community College
Riverside, California

Nina Beaman
Bryant and Stratton College
Richmond, Virginia

Liane Beckwith
Lake Washington Technical College
Kirkland, Washington

Denise Bender
University of Oklahoma Health Sciences
    Center
Oklahoma City, Oklahoma

Patti Biro
Del Mar College
Corpus Christi, Texas

Heather Bislew
University of Minnesota
Minneapolis, Minnesota

Denise Blay
Fanshawe College
London, Ontario
Canada

Julie Boles
Ithaca College
Ithaca, New York

Ada Boone Hoerl
Sacramento City College
Sacramento, California

Marie Bosscawen
The Learning Curve Plus
Cary, North Carolina

Jennifer Brach
University of Pittsburgh
Pittsburgh, Pennsylvania

Jonathon Bradshaw
George Brown College
Toronto, Ontario
Canada

John Capeheart
University of Houston—Downtown
Houston, Texas

Cathy Carlson
Indiana University—Purdue University
    Fort Wayne
Fort Wayne, Indiana

Babs Cerna
Highline Community College
Des Moines, Iowa

Jean Chenu
Genesee Community College
Batavia, New York

Douglas Clarke
Applied Career Training
Arlington, Virginia

John Clouse
Owensboro Community and Technical
    College
Owensboro, Kentucky

Candice Coffin
Briar Cliff University
Sioux City, Iowa

Kay Cook
Mississippi Gulf Coast Community
    College, Jefferson Davis Campus
Gulfport, Mississippi

Jill Cyr
Loyalist College
Belleville, Ontario
Canada

Connie Danko
Maria College
Albany, New York

Jan Davidson
Lambton College
Sarnia, Ontario
Canada

Ronald DeBellis
Massachusetts College of Pharmacy and
    Health Sciences
Worcester, Massachusetts

Terry Derting
Murray State University
Murray, Kentucky

Carol Dew
Baker College of Flint
Flint, Michigan

Mary Dey
Kalamazoo Valley Community College
Kalamazoo, Michigan

Linda Donahue
Delgado Community College
New Orleans, Louisana

Karla Duran
Butler County Community College
El Dorado, Kansas

Jean Erwin
Franklin Technology Center at Missouri
   Southern State University
Joplin, Missouri

Susan Eubank
Temple University
Philadelphia, Pennsylvania

Mary Fabick
Milligan College
Milligan College, Tennessee

Janet Falk-Kessler
Columbia University
New York, New York

Karl Fiebelkorn
University at Buffalo School of Pharmacy
   and Pharmaceutical Sciences
Buffalo, New York

Pamela Fischer
Blackhawk Technical College
Janesville, Wisconsin

Douglas Gardenhire
Georgia State University
Atlanta, Georgia

Alice Gardner
Massachusetts College of Pharmacy and
   Health Sciences
Worcester, Massachusetts

Mary Gebhardt
Georgia State University
Atlanta, Georgia

Louise Glover
College Boreal
Timmins, Ontario
Canada

Mable Gordon
SUNY Buffalo
Buffalo, New York

Cheri Goretti
Quinebaug Valley Community College
Danielson, Connecticut

Joanne Grant
Reading Hospital
West Reading, Pennsylvania

Debra Gray
Florida Community College
Jacksonville, Florida

Marilyn Greene
Draughon's Junior College
Nashville, Tennessee

Tony Greenfield
Southwest Minnesota State University
Marshall, Minnesota

Sandy Gustafson
Hibbing Community College
Hibbing, Minnesota

JoAnne Habenicht
Manhattan College
Riverdale, New York

Marilyn Halaska
Middle Georgia College
Cochran, Georgia

Evelyn Hall
Vance-Granville Community College
Henderson, North Carolina

Karen Hamill
Sisseton-Wahpeton College
Sisseton, South Dakota

Kay Hanna
Stark State College of Technology
North Canton, Ohio

Polly Hansen
National College of Business and
   Technology
Salem, Virginia

Glenda Hatcher
Southwest Georgia Technical College
Thomasville, Georgia

Bobbi Haugen
Montana State University—Billings
Billings, Montana

William Havins
Albuquerque Technical Vocational
   Institute
Albuquerque, New Mexico

Catherine Hearty
Clarkson College
Omaha, Nebraska

Carolyn Helms
Atlanta Technical College
Atlanta, Georgia

Bonnie Hemp
Owens Community College
Toledo, Ohio

Liz Hoffman
Baker College
Clinton Township, Michigan

Kimberly Hoskins
Lansing Community College
Lansing, Michigan

Julie Howe
Saint Louis University
St. Louis, Missouri

Mary Paulette Humphries
Indiana University East
Richmond, Indiana

Barbara Hundt
Madison Area Technical College
Madison, Wisconsin

Elizabeth Huss
Austin Community College
Austin, Texas

Beverlee Jackson
Central Oregon Community College
Bend, Oregon

Katherine Jenkins
Riverside School of Professional Nursing
Newport News, Virginia

Rene Johnson
Oklahoma Panhandle State University
Goodwell, Oklahoma

Geri Kale-Smith
William Rainey Harper College
Palatine, Illinois

Christine Kasinskas
Quinnipiac University
Hamden, Connecticut

Mary Keehn
University of Illinois at Chicago
Chicago, Illinois

Lynn Keenan
Traviss Technical Center
Lakeland, Florida

Angela Kennedy
Louisiana Tech University
Ruston, Louisiana

Linda King
Montgomery College
Conroe, Texas

Lori Knight
SIAST, Wascana Campus
Regina, Saskatchewan
Canada

Peggy Knittel
Eastern Wyoming College
Torrington, Wyoming

Nancy Kostin
Madonna University
Livonia, Michigan

Mary Kowalski
Cerro Coso Community College
Ridgecrest, California

Judy Kronenberger
Sinclair Community College
Dayton, Ohio

Marsha Lawrence
Albany State University
Albany, Georgia

R. Elaine Lenz
University of Kansas Medical Center
Kansas City, Kansas

Susan Lesko
Vancouver Community College
Vancouver, British Columbia
Canada

Vivian Lilly
North Harris College
Houston, Texas

Donna Lindblom
Northern Lakes College
Grande Prairie, Alberta
Canada

Rosanne Lipcius
University of Connecticut
Storrs, Connecticut

Julie Loewen
SIAST, Kelsey Campus
Saskatoon, Saskatchewan
Canada

Mary Agnes Luczak
Career Training Academy
New Kensington, Pennsylvania

Cynthia Lundgren
Houston Community College System
Houston, Texas

Donna Maher
Renton Technical College
Renton, Washington

Melissa Marchisotto
Pace University—Lenox Hill Hospital PA
   Program
New York, New York

Denise Marshall
Wor-Wic Community College
Salisbury, Maryland

Pat Martin
Pennsylvania College of Technology
Williamsport, Pennsylvania

Ruth Mason
Northwest-Shoals Community College
Muscle Shoals, Alabama

Catherine Mastroianni
Ashmead College
Seattle, Washington

Bill May
Itawamba Community College
Fulton, Mississippi

Albert McMullen
Andrews University
Barrien Springs, Michigan

Laura Menke
Southeastern Community College
Mount Pleasant, Iowa

Sharon Meyer
Spokane Community College
Spokane, Washington

Pat Moeck
El Centro College
Dallas, Texas

Barbara Moffett
Southeastern Louisiana University
Hammond, Louisiana

Elinor Monahan
Purdue University North Central
Westville, Indiana

Karen Murphy, RN, BSN
Klamath Community College
Klamath Falls, Oregon

Kevin Murray
Danville Regional Health System School
   of Radiologic Technology
Danville, Virginia

Lisa Nedlan
College of the Redwoods
Eureka, California

Cora Newcomb
Technical College of the Lowcountry
Beaufort, South Carolina

Diane Nickols
Anne Arundel Community College
Arnold, Maryland

Caryn Nobles
Lassen Community College
Susanville, California

A. Okrainec
Brandon University
Brandon, Manitoba
Canada

Mary Olsen
Rochester Community and Technical
   College
Rochester, Minnesota

Diane Pacitti
Massachusetts College of Pharmacy and
   Health Sciences
Worcester, Massachusetts

Nand Panjwani
New York Medical Career Training
   Center
Flushing, New York

Tomma Parco
Pueblo Community College
Pueblo, Colorado

Jeannie Parscal
Butler Community College
El Dorado, Kansas

David Pearce
Baker College—Cadillac
Cadillac, Michigan

Fred Pearson
Brigham Young University Idaho
Rexburg, Idaho

Elizabeth Pelham
Our Lady of the Lake College Health
   Career Institute
Baton Rouge, Louisiana

Kathleen Peterson
Santa Barbara City College
Santa Barbara, California

F. C. Piper
Truman State University
Kirksville, Missouri

Robin Ploeger
University of Tulsa
Tulsa, Oklahoma

Roberta Pohlman
Wright State University
Dayton, Ohio

Pamela B. Primrose
Ivy Tech State College
South Bend, Indiana

Elizabeth Rash
University of Central Florida
Orlando, Florida

Marilyn Reeder
GASC Technology Center
Flint, Michigan

Elaine Rejimbal
Lake Technical Center
Eustis, Florida

Pamela Reynolds
Gannon University
Erie, Pennsylvania

Andrea Robins
Daytona Beach Community College
Daytona Beach, Florida

Marie Rogers
Kalamazoo Valley Community College
Kalamazoo, Michigan

Carol Ryan
Chippewa Valley Technical College
Eau Claire, Wisconsin

Jane Ryder
Yakima Valley Community College
Yakima, Washington

Jody Seabright
West Liberty State College
West Liberty, West Virginia

Janet Sesser
High-Tech Institute
Phoenix, Arizona

Karin Sherrill
Mesa Community College
Mesa, Arizona

Gregg Shutts
Daemen College
Amherst, New York

June Skinner
Nova Scotia Community College
Halifax, Nova Scotia
Canada

Dr. Paul Slifer
MicroTech Training Center
Jersey City, New Jersey

Tammy Smith
Panola College
Carthage, Texas

LuAnn Soliah
Baylor University
Waco, Texas

Sandra Speller
Cincinnati State Technical and
    Community College
Cincinnati, Ohio

Karen Sybert
Mount Aloysius College
Cresson, Pennsylvania

James Taggart
Ogden-Weber Applied Technology
    College
Ogden, Utah

Mary Taylor
Dalton State College
Dalton, Georgia

Margaret Tice
Sharon Regional Health System
Sharon, Pennsylvania

Diuane Tomasic
West Liberty State College
West Liberty, West Virginia

Valeria Truitt
Craven Community College
New Bern, North Carolina

Jana Tucker
Salt Lake Community College
Salt Lake City, Utah

Pam Tully
Bossier Parish Community College
Bossier City, Louisiana

Sylvia van der Weg
Georgian College
Barrie, Ontario
Canada

Wally Waldron
Southwest Georgia Technical College
Thomasville, Georgia

Kathy Webb
Bucks County Community College
Newton, Pennsylvania

Greg Wellman
Ferris State University
Big Rapids, Michigan

Ryan Werenskjold
Certified Careers Institute
Salt Lake City, Utah

Lucy White
Ivy Tech State College
Columbus, Indiana

Cam Williams
Finlandia University
Hancock, Michigan

Kent Williston
Traviss Technical Center
Lakeland, Florida

Heather Worthington
Northern Alberta Institute of
   Technology
Edmonton, Alberta
Canada

Mary Young
Red River College
Winnipeg, Manitoba
Canada

User's Guide

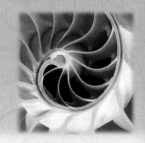

LAYING THE FOUNDATION

Learning medical terminology is just like learning a foreign language. Therefore, it makes sense to teach medical terminology like a foreign language. From the beginning of each chapter you are encouraged to use full medical terms in context. This approach gives you a greater understanding of the language that will serve as the foundation for your future career.

The features that open each chapter are an introduction to guide you through the remainder of the lesson.

OBJECTIVES

After completing this chapter, you should be able to:

1. State the meaning of word parts related to the cardiovascular system
2. Identify common arteries and veins
3. Identify anatomical features of the heart
4. Explain how blood pressure is measured
5. Define common signs, symptoms, and treatments of various cardiovascular system diseases
   ...procedures related to the cardiovascular

CHAPTER OBJECTIVES:
Clear objectives listed before each chapter help you identify learning goals.

INTRODUCTION

The cardiovascular (CV) system is composed of the heart, arteries, veins, and capillaries. The heart functions to pump blood that is low in oxygen to the lungs where it is oxygenated, and then oxygen-rich blood is pumped to the entire body. Each day, the heart pumps approximately 7,000 liters (1855 gallons) of blood throughout the body, ensuring survival.

...and capillaries make up the body's blood vessels. Capillaries are the ...... Blood courses ...... tis- ...... s for ...... and ...... logy, ... aphy, ... grams

INTRODUCTION:
A chapter introduction familiarizes you with the material covered in the chapter.

Professional Profile: Registered Nurse in a Cardiovascular Intensive Care Unit

Heidi is a registered nurse (RN) working in the cardiovascular intensive care unit (CVICU) of a public hospital where she has been employed for 5 years. The CVICU is separate from the intensive care unit (ICU) and receives only patients with cardiovascular or cardiovascular-related disorders. This hospital receives patients within a sixty-mile radius.

Heidi received her RN diploma and Associate of Arts (AA) in Natural Science degree from a hospital-based school of nursing, which has an affiliation with a local college. This RN program is a "3 + 1" program, which means that after completing the first 3 years of the program, graduates earn a diploma and an AA degree. After the initial 3-year course of study, graduates of this program may continue for one additional year to earn the Bachelor of Science in Nursing (BSN) degree.

One month after graduating, Heidi passed her National Council Licensure Examination (NCLEX) and began her full-time nursing career working on the rehabilitation floor. This exam is required to receive professional licensure in the nursing field. When the position in the CVICU opened up, she applied and was transferred. Many cardiac patients are in serious condition when they arrive on Heidi's unit. The acuity level ranges from moderate to high. Patients have often undergone medical procedures such as coronary artery bypass, valve replacement, and vascular and thoracic surgeries. Regardless of the situation, the focus remains on quality care for patients and their families.

As a cardiovascular nurse, one realizes the impact that the cardiovascular system has on every other system in the human body. Therefore, continuing education, attendance at update and conferences, and advanced training courses are mandatory. Cardiovascular nurses also have to update their advanced cardiac life support (ACLS) certification regularly.

PROFESSIONAL PROFILE:
At the beginning of each chapter, this profile introduces you to a profession in the health-care field. This profile provides a real-world context for how medical terminology is applied in a clinical setting. The individual profiled in this section also appears in the Case Study and Real World Report.

BUILDING KNOWLEDGE

Arranged in learning segments, the text introduces and explains a specific topic, then reviews your knowledge before you move on to the next topic. This learning system will ensure your success as you work through the material.

fever infection continue to attack heart tissue. Primary signs and symptoms are cough, dyspnea, and hemoptysis. The diagnosis is confirmed through the presence of a heart murmur and constriction shown by echocardiogram. Treatments include drugs to reduce the heart workload, anticoagulants, **commissurotomy** (surgical division of a stenosed valve), or valve replacement.

Key Terms

Key Terms	Definitions
rheumatic (roo MAT ick) **heart disease (RHD)**	valvular disease of heart resulting from rheumatic fever
sequela (se KWEL uh)	disorder that is caused by a preceding disease in the same individual
mitral (MIGH trul) **insufficiency**	incomplete closure of bicuspid valve causing backflow of blood into atrium from ventricle

Key Term Practice: Valvular Heart Disease

1. Name the heart disease that results from prior rheumatic fever infection.

   _____.

2. The disorder characterized by incomplete closure of the left atrioventricular valve due to an anatomical or physiological defect is _____.

APPLYING KNOWLEDGE

Once you work through the learning segments in each chapter, you are introduced to the pathology of the system at hand. In these sections, you practically apply the knowledge from previous sections.

THE CLINICAL DIMENSION: The pathology of the system being studied is introduced in these sections.

THE CLINICAL DIMENSION

Pathology of the Cardiovascular System

Pathology of the cardiovascular system falls into several broad categories. Many primary diseases have a genetic predisposition or are the result of lifestyle factors. Viral and bacterial infections are implicated in several secondary CV disorders, and congenital diseases are present at birth. Fortunately, a number of treatments are available for the numerous pathological conditions.

Congenital Heart Def

Congenital heart defects are c orders are not as common a termed **aortic coarctation**. It results in upper extremity hyp

CLINICAL TERMS TABLES: Include the terminology associated with the pathology of the system.

Term	Description
DISORDERS	
Aneurysm	Abnormal, outward bulge in an artery
Aortic coarctation	Congenital narrowing of aorta
Arteriosclerosis	Hardening of the arteries and loss of elasticity as a result of plaque formation
Atherosclerosis	Plaque formation on inner arterial wall
Atrial septal defect	Abnormal opening between atria allowing blood to shunt back and forth
Cardiac arrest	Sudden stoppage of heartbeat
Cardiac tamponade	Heart compression due to fluid accumulation in pericardial sac
Cardiomyopathy	Disease of heart muscle

Features and Boxes

Throughout each chapter, you will find a variety of elements that provide interesting facts and newsworthy stories related to the medical terminology of the chapter.

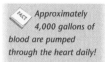

Approximately 4,000 gallons of blood are pumped through the heart daily!

FAST FACTS:
Interesting tidbits of system-related trivia.

LIFESPAN:
Discussion of the developmental anatomy and physiology throughout all stages of life.

A to Z *Lifespan*

Beginning on the fifteenth day of in utero development, angioblast cells from the mesoderm give rise to blood vessels. The next major feature is the function of the fetal heart, which begins around week four. Important fetal structures, such as the foramen ovale, ductus arteriosus, and ductus venosus, function until birth. While in utero, the foramen ovale and ductus arteriosus allow blood to bypass the non-functioning lungs, while the ductus venosus permits blood to bypass the fetal liver. At birth, the umbilical vein and two umbilical arteries, important structures that enable nutrient and waste exchange between mother and fetus, cease functioning.

As the infant devel-
Blood pres-

...ture increases, and the heart tissue grows. ...ndergoes considerable change. The average ...od, there is a gradual increase in both sys-...ent that an average BP in adulthood is ...adually increases with aging, and in the ...idered hypertensive.

In the News: Aspirin

The phrase is familiar: aspirin, the wonder drug. Is it really, or is this marketing hype? The pharmaceutical name for aspirin is acetylsalicylic acid (ASA). Aspirin is a common non-steroidal anti-inflammatory drug (NSAID). Its properties are numerous ranging from anti-inflammatory effects to acting as an analgesic, antipyretic (fever reducing), and thrombolytic.

Studies indicate that prophylactic aspirin therapy is beneficial for secondary prevention of vascular events in persons with a history of CV disease. The Food and Drug Administration (FDA) has approved aspirin use at 325 mg/day for primary myocardial infarction prevention. Aspirin used clinically at a dosage level of 81 mg/day (baby aspirin) demonstrated anti-platelet effects that last eight to ten days, the lifespan of a thrombocyte (platelet).

Other research has demonstrated that aspirin administration of 325 mg/day decreased the incidence of transient ischemic attacks (TIAs), unstable angina, coronary artery thrombosis with MI, and thrombosis after coronary artery bypass grafting (CABG). Other trials showed that aspirin administration of 325 mg every other day decreased MI incidence 40% in male physicians.

The findings appear promising in terms of disease prevention. Yet, aspirin ingestion of 500 mg/day greatly increases the incidence of gastrointestinal bleeding and may increase the occurrence of peptic ulcer. Therefore, aspirin should be used cautiously as an adjunct therapy and only under the guidance of a healthcare professional.

IN THE NEWS: Presentation of a notable news item related to the body system discussed in the chapter.

TESTING KNOWLEDGE

Each chapter includes exercises designed to engage every type of learner (auditory, visual, and kinesthetic) and provides ample opportunity to practice and master medical terminology.

Case Studies and Questions

Clinical scenarios are presented in case-study format along with related questions to help you build critical thinking skills.

Case Study

Mr. Jay Tigress, age 67, was brought to the emergency room by ambulance. Prior to arrival at the hospital, he had been suffering ~~...~~ symp-

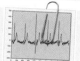

~~...~~ Tigress stated that he had ~~...~~st remembered eating some ~~...~~onfused, but stated he was a ~~...~~ days. Initial examination and

	Normal Values
60	70 – 110 mg/dL
10	3.8 – 5.0 mEq/L
4.1	1.8 – 2.6 mEq/L
3.2	0.6 – 1.2 mEq/L
100	135 – 145 mEq/L
0% - 6%	
of total	

Case Study Questions

Select the best answer to each of the following.

1. **Mr. Tigress has a BP of 90/60. BP is an abbreviation for**

   A. bicuspid pressure.
   B. blood pressure.
   C. bradycardia pressure.
   D. beating pressure.

2. **A BP of 90/60 means**

   A. the systolic pressure is 90 and the diastolic pressure is 60.
   B. the diastolic pressure is 90 and the systolic pressure is 60.

3. **An ECG was ordered to evaluate**

   A. brain function.
   B. cardiac function.
   C. liver function.
   D. kidney function.

4. **An elevated CK-MB is an indication of**

   A. renal failure.
   B. liver failure.
   C. damaged cardiac tissue.
   D. hypertension.

Real World Reports and Questions

Medical records with practice questions provide a real-world context to the terminology of the chapter.

REAL WORLD REPORT: CARDIOVASCULAR SYSTEM

Mr. Tigress was admitted to Heidi's floor, the cardiovascular intensive care unit (CVICU) because he was experiencing multiple organ failure secondary to renal failure. His heart was fragile. Here is the cardiologist's report.

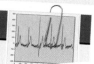

NAME: Jay Tigress
ATTENDING: J.L. Manjunata,
ORDERING: M.M. Issac, M.D

REASON FOR STUDY: Heart fa

PROCEDURE: The patient unde
1. The left ventricle demonstrat
   estimated to be no more tha
2. The right ventricle is normal i
3. Normal size atria and aortic r
4. The mitral valve is mildly thick
5. The aortic valve is not very we
6. Tricuspid valve was not very we
7. Pulmonic valve is not visualized

CONCLUSION: This is an abnorma
severe systolic dysfunction. Ejectior
sent without hemodynamics of sigr

REAL WORLD REPORT QUESTIONS

The following exercises review the medical terms in the preceding medical report. A few terms with which you may not be familiar are M-Mode and 2-D Doppler. The M-Mode is a diagnostic ultrasound utilizing Doppler sound waves in which the echoes displayed correlate to time (T) and motion (M). It is often referred to as TM-mode. The 2-D refers to the two-dimensional image.

1. The left ventricle demonstrates severe systolic dysfunction. Provide a definition for systolic dysfunction.

   _____

   _____

   _____

2. Hypokinesis is global.

   A. hypo means _____

   B. kinesis means motion or movement

   C. hypokinesis means _____

B. Provide another way of stating "trivial degree of mitral valve regurgitation."

   _____

4. Pericardial effusion is present.

   A. peri means _____

   B. cardial means _____

   C. pericardial effusion refers to _____

   _____

Review and Application: Three-Level Learning System

A wide variety of exercises focus first on recall, then move on to concept review, and finally test critical thinking abilities. These exercises are found at the end of the chapter. They are carefully designed to enhance learning while engaging a variety of learning styles.

REVIEW AND APPLICATION: 3-LEVEL LEARNING SYSTEM

LEVEL ONE: REVIEWING FACTS AND TERMS USING RECALL

Select the best response to each of the following.

1. Components of the cardiovascular system include
   A. the heart.
   B. arteries.
   C. veins.
   D. all of

2. Identify
   diac tissu
   A. atriun
   B. endoc
   C. myoc
   D. perica

B. venules; lungs
C. arteries; lungs
D. arteries; heart

8. A _____ monitor is a _____ machine.
   A. Fowler; sonogram
   B. Holter; sonogram
   C. Fowler; ECG
   CG

pacemaker is
node.
ricular node
onduction c
ricular bun

LEVEL TWO: REVIEWING CONCEPTS

14. Anatomical layers of arteries and veins are termed _____. Provide a medical term to complete a meaningful analogy.

15. Systole is to diastole as _____ is to repolarization.

16. Tunica interna is to tunica intima as tunica externa is to tunica _____.

LEVEL THREE: THINKING CRITICALLY

66. List 5 factors that can influence blood pressure.
   _____
   _____
   _____
   _____
   _____

67. Explain why there is a difference in muscle wall thickness between the left and right ventricles.
   _____
   _____
   _____

Bonus CD-ROM

Packaged with this textbook, the CD-ROM is a powerful learning tool. It includes the following features to help you reinforce and review your knowledge.

- Animations
- Guidelines to help you maximize your learning potential based on whether you are an auditory, a visual, or a kinesthetic learner
- Auditory spelling tests
- Audio pronunciation glossary
- Audio and printable flash cards

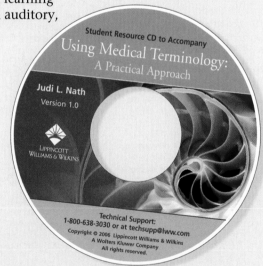

Student Resource CD to Accompany
Using Medical Terminology:
A Practical Approach
Judi L. Nath
Version 1.0

LIPPINCOTT
WILLIAMS & WILKINS

Technical Support:
1-800-638-3030 or at techsupp@lww.com
Copyright © 2006 Lippincott Williams & Wilkins
A Wolters Kluwer Company
All rights reserved.

LiveAdvise: Medical Terminology

Online teaching advice and student tutoring is available with this textbook! Our tutors are handpicked educators that are trained to help you. They are familiar with this book, and the ancillary package. You can connect live with a tutor at times listed on the Website or you can send e-mail messages to a tutor, who will quickly respond—often within 24 hours. This service is free with the purchase of the textbook!

Instructors, to use this service, please visit http://connection.LWW.com/LiveAdvise. Students, see the codebook in the front of this book for more details. In it you'll find instructions for using the service, along with your own personal code to log on and get started.

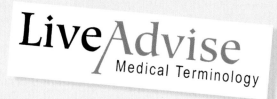

A NOTE ABOUT OUR DESIGN

In choosing an icon to give this book a unique identity, we looked to nature. The book *The Architecture and Design of Man and Woman: The Marvel of the Human Body* by Alexander Tsiaras (Doubleday Books, 2004) shows us the parallels between the human body and nature. This concept complements a medical terminology textbook, like this one, that teaches medical terminology through anatomy and physiology. The nautilus shell we chose as our icon mirrors the cochlea in the human ear; it symbolizes the auditory nature of medical terms and demonstrates the natural way of learning language.

Contents

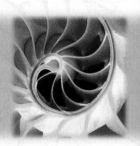

Introduction to Medical Terminology

OBJECTIVES

After completing this chapter, you should be able to:

1. Summarize how medical terms are derived.
2. Correctly write scientific names.
3. Define the terms *affix, prefix, suffix, root,* and *combining form.*
4. State the general rules for making plural forms of singular words.
5. Define the meanings of common medical prefixes, combining forms, and suffixes.
6. Correctly pronounce medical terms.
7. State the importance of coding guidelines as outlined in *Current Procedural Terminology* and *International Classification of Diseases.*
8. Identify abbreviations of common medical terms.

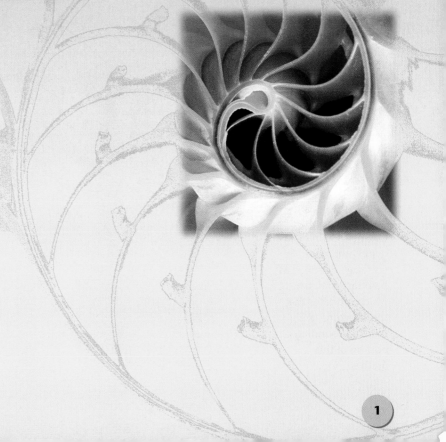

INTRODUCTION

Anatomic and physiological language is the foundation of medical terminology. The book that serves as the authority on correct anatomic nomenclature is *Terminologia Anatomica,* also called by its English title, *International Anatomical Terminology.* Its purpose is to ensure that scientists and doctors use the same name for each structure worldwide. To achieve this goal, *Terminologia Anatomica* provides standardized terms for all body parts. Despite valiant attempts, the language of medicine is not yet uniform, as is evidenced by reading medical reports and textbooks, which often refer to the same structure by two different terms.

Medical terms derived from a person's name are called eponyms. Body parts, diseases, syndromes, tests, and procedures are often named after their discoverer, the person who first described it, or a scientist who perfected or invented a particular test or procedure. Eponyms are still used, but there is a general trend toward eliminating them. It is simpler to use the correct anatomic name for a body part or disease description because that eliminates confusion and creates standardization. For example, Cowper glands are more correctly identified as bulbourethral glands. The word *Cowper* does not assist in locating these glands, whereas the word *bulbourethral* indicates that the structures are bulbs found around a portion of the urethra (Fig. 1-1). One's medical training or geographic location often dictates the prevalence of specific word usage. Thus eponyms, along with their alternate medical terms, may be cited in general medical writing.

Many medical terms are derived from the Greek and Latin languages. Therefore, when learning these terms it may seem as if you were taking a foreign-language course. Fortunately, there are guidelines and rules to assist you. Once you conquer the terms, a world of opportunity exists. The number of careers for which a knowledge of medical terminology is beneficial is growing. As the allied health fields expand, so will the job market. Some occupations and fields of study that require a solid foundation in medical terminology are given in Box 1-1.

FACT **Medical billing and related occupations are among the fastest growing careers in the United States!**

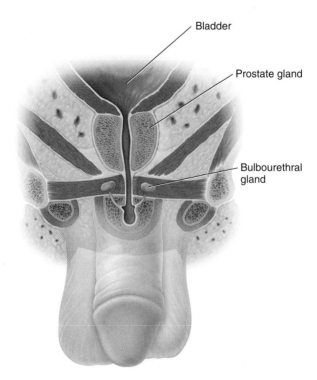

FIGURE 1-1
Cowper glands. The glands are more correctly identified as bulbourethral glands, which indicates that the structures are bulbs surrounding a portion of the urethra.

Bladder

Prostate gland

Bulbourethral gland

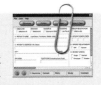

Professional Profile: Medical Assistant

Cheryl is a medical assistant in a physician's office. She notes that one needs to know anatomy to bill appropriately, document accurately, and communicate effectively within the medical field. To illustrate the significance of anatomy in her work, she reported a recent conversation pertaining to billing codes in her office.

The doctor had accessed the left femoral artery (upper leg artery), maneuvered the catheter to the right common iliac artery (extension of femoral artery), and then imaged the renal artery (kidney artery), which was anastomosed (connected) to the common iliac. A coder in her office questioned whether this should be coded as an extremity angio (vessel in the leg) or a selective renal (kidney vessel) procedure. (The code is a system of numbers that stand for medical procedures and is used for reimbursement purposes.) As it turned out, the procedure could be coded as a selective renal into the iliac with two different codes. Thus the importance of understanding medical terminology and anatomy is underscored (Fig. 1-2)!

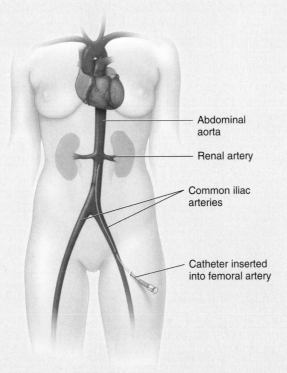

Abdominal aorta

Renal artery

Common iliac arteries

Catheter inserted into femoral artery

FIGURE 1-2
Is this procedure an "extremity angio" or a "selective renal"? It is important to understand anatomy even for a simple billing procedure in a medical office.

If inappropriate codes for a procedure are assigned, reimbursement from third-party payers, such as insurance companies, is in jeopardy. In addition, clear communication with patients and physicians and understanding written health records both require a working knowledge of medical terminology.

Cheryl has taken an array of courses pertaining to health careers. She most recently completed the medical assisting program, which enabled her to sit for the certification examination. The Commission on Accreditation of Allied Health Education Programs (CAAHEP) accredited her program. Coursework included computers, basic science, ethical/legal concerns, clinical procedures, medical billing and coding, medical transcription, medical office procedures, basic anatomy and physiology, and medical terminology.

BOX 1-1.   *Professional Fields That Require Knowledge of Medical Terminology*

- Allied health
- Biology
- Chemistry
- Cytotechnology
- Dentistry
- Dietetics
- Engineering
- Epidemiology
- General technology
- Genetics/genetic counseling
- Health education
- Health services
- Law
- Massage therapy
- Medical assisting
- Medical billing
- Medical coding

- Medical editing
- Medical illustration
- Medical transcription
- Medicine
- Microbiology
- Nursing
- Occupational therapy
- Optometry
- Pharmacy
- Phlebotomy
- Physical therapy
- Psychiatry
- Psychology
- Radiology technology
- Respiratory therapy
- Stenography
- Technical writing

THE MEDICAL RECORD

People over age 60 years see an average of three doctors on a regular basis!

A patient's medical record provides the person's physical, emotional, nutritional, and social history. The personal medical history form identifies individual information along with current and past medical conditions. It also lists prescription and nonprescription drug use, drug sensitivities, and allergies.

Patient medical record information is used to assess previous treatment, to enhance the continuity of care, and to avoid unnecessary tests and/or procedures. Because it is an invaluable tool for health-care providers, it is a working document that needs to be as complete as possible. To that end, knowledge of medical terminology is essential. The person documenting the information must be skilled in recording the data accurately, making sure the terms are spelled correctly, and ensuring that the facts supplied by the patient make sense within the context of the conversation. As a primary means of communication, this collection of facts and data is read and scrutinized by all clinicians treating the patient or office personnel servicing the person. A thorough understanding of medical terminology is necessary for adequately documenting, describing, and relaying pertinent health information.

The aim of the questions on typical history and physical (H&P) examination forms is to obtain a complete representation of the patient. The history (Hx) portion is generally categorized into the following headings: medical/surgical history, family history (FH), social history (SH), occupational history (OH), diet/exercise history, and review of systems (ROS). Females also answer questions pertaining to menstrual, gynecologic, pregnancy, contraceptive, and sexual history. Males answer questions of contraception, sexual history, and performance.

Once the personal medical history has been obtained, practitioners typically evaluate the patient through a physical examination (PE or Px). The physical examination includes assessment of general appearance; vital signs; head, eyes, ears, nose, and throat (HEENT); neck; lungs; heart; rectopelvis; extremities; neurologic condition; laboratory data; general impression (Imp), or general view of patient's condition; and plan (P).

Through conversation, written documentation, and a cursory examination, more information is obtained for the H&P form. Commonly used terms and phrases (with their abbreviations) to document findings include chief complaint (CC) or complains of (c/o); diagnosis (Dx); family members living and well (L&W); no acute distress (NAD); no known allergies (NKA); no known drug allergies (NKDA); pupils equal, round, and reactive to light and accommodation (PERRLA); rule out (R/O); symptom (Sx); usual childhood diseases (UCHD); and within normal limits (WNL).

Progress notes, often using the SOAP method, are made in a patient's medical record after the H&P has been finished. SOAP is an acronym for subjective, objective, assessment, plan. The subjective portion identifies the patient's symptoms, and the objective section lists the signs. Symptoms are experienced by the patient and may include such things as pain and dizziness. Signs include functions that can be measured, such as blood pressure, respiration rate, temperature, height, and weight. The assessment is the professional judgment made of the patient's progress. Finally, the plan is the outline for treatment.

Federal law mandates that patient health information be treated with respect and confidentiality. Public Law 104-191—Health Insurance Portability & Accountability Act (HIPAA) of 1996—is a set of national standards to protect the privacy and personal health information of Americans. This applies to all medical information that is conveyed orally, in written form, or by electronic means. The law provides standards for security, transactions, and coding. It further serves as a guide for privacy, research, and public health.

In addition to the history and physical reports and progress notes of individual patients, many health-care professionals must be acquainted with two important general references: *Current Procedural Terminology* (*CPT*) and *International Classification of Diseases* (*ICD*). The *CPT* lists codes for working clinical nomenclature. The codes describe procedures and services performed in health-care settings that are used for reporting medical services. These HIPAA-mandated procedure codes are used in all medical billing. The *CPT* provides a means of communication among physicians, patients, and third parties (insurance companies, Medicare, and Medicaid). The *ICD* is similar to the *CPT,* but its focus is on coding related to human disease. The code sets are necessary for statistical purposes, medical documentation, and reimbursement. At the writing of this text, the preliminary form of the 10th edition (*ICD*-10) of the reference was available. Regardless of edition, these manuals will be referred to as *CPT* and *ICD* in this textbook. Accurate coding is essential to the reimbursement process.

> **FACT** *Approximately 43% of people in the U.S. do not have copies of their own medical records!*

A BRIEF LESSON IN LANGUAGE

The purpose of language is to communicate effectively and accurately, thus spelling counts! This is particularly true for medical terms, for which an incision in the *ilium* or the *ileum* could be the difference between cutting a hip bone (ilium) or a segment of the small intestine (ileum) (Fig. 1-3)!

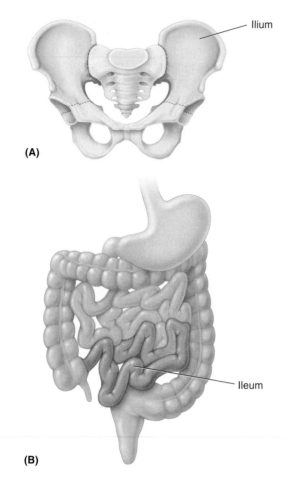

FIGURE 1-3
Correct spelling is important for medical terms, when an incision in the ilium **(A)** or the ileum **(B)** could mean the difference between surgery on the hipbone or a segment of the small intestine.

Linguists are devoted to the study of language. They have identified four basic systems of language: lexicon, grammar, semantics, and phonology. Although these systems are quite structured, humans can easily speak, read, and write understandable words.

We will concern ourselves primarily with lexicon (vocabulary) and secondarily with phonetics (pronunciation). The lexicon is governed by rules for word formation. Meaningful units of sound are called phonemes, and approximately 40 different phonemes have been identified in the English language. However, written and spoken language is dynamic—for example, our language is constantly changing as terms are created for new technology and new knowledge. Medicine is a field in which these changes are rapidly occurring, and keeping pace can be challenging.

Word Parts

Word parts is the general phrase used in this text to identify prefixes, suffixes, and combining forms. Memorizing the definition of a word root and its combining form will help you break down the meaning of new medical terms. In the word part tables, hyphens are used to signify prefixes, suffixes, and combining forms. The hyphen indicates that a particular word element forms part of a compound and indicates the placement of the word part when used to form a medical term. For example, a hyphen placed after the word part, as in hypo-, means the part is a prefix or a combining form; a hyphen placed before the word part means the part is a suffix.

Many medical terms are made by combining word parts. To illustrate, the word *cardiology*, which means "the study of the heart and its functions," is made by joining the word part *cardio-*, which means "heart" with *-logy*, which means "study of."

Prefixes and suffixes are linguistic elements that are not independent words but that modify the word root's meaning. Prefixes are word parts that appear at the beginning of the medical word or base. Not all medical terms have prefixes; but when present, prefixes make the meaning more specific. For example, the word *sphere* means "round." Adding the prefix *hemi-* creates the word *hemisphere* (*hemi-* is the prefix), meaning "half of a sphere," as in the sentence "The brain has two hemispheres" (Fig. 1-4).

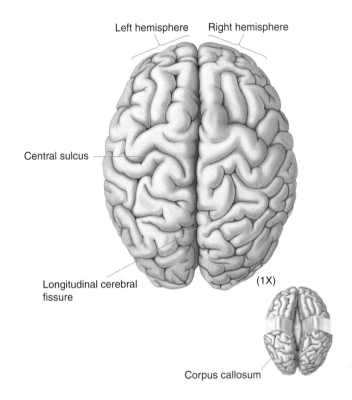

Left hemisphere   Right hemisphere

Central sulcus

Longitudinal cerebral fissure

(1X)

Corpus callosum

FIGURE 1-4
The brain is made up of two *hemi*spheres. The prefix *hemi-*.

Suffixes appear at the end of the word or base. In medical words, a suffix may describe a body condition. For example, *-itis* means "inflammation," so *prostatitis* refers to an "inflamed prostate." Because a whole-language approach to learning medical terminology can be used, word dissection skills are not a prerequisite for success; however, if you learn the meaning of the word parts, you will be able to figure out many of the new medical terms you read.

Word Etymology

Etymology is the study of the origins of words or word parts and their evolution to their current form and meaning. Medical terms in particular have historical roots that can be traced to Greek and Latin origins. A word root is the basis of a medical term and conveys its main meaning. Think of the root as the word form without any affixes (neither a prefix nor a suffix). Other terms that mean the same thing as "root" are *base, stem, theme,* and *radical.* It is important to note that language is always evolving and changing as new terms are coined for novel discoveries, inventions, techniques, procedures, processes, and therapies. Furthermore, new words often develop through everyday oral or written use before they appear in publications; remember dictionaries include words that have a history of use, and thus newer words may not be listed.

Combining Vowels

To make medical terms easier to pronounce, the combining vowels *o* and *i* are frequently used between word parts. These combining vowels are added to word roots when attaching a suffix that begins with a consonant or another root. The term *combining form* describes the word root with its associated combining vowel. A combining form cannot stand alone in a sentence and makes sense only when it occurs in combination with affixes or other words to form compounds. For example, *viscer* means "organ." The combining vowel *o* makes the word part *viscero-*. An example term is *visceroskeleton,* "the bony framework surrounding an organ." Another example is *hepatorenal,* which refers to the liver and kidney. Without the combining vowel, it would be "hepatrenal", which is more difficult to pronounce. Again, if you know the meaning of a medical term's prefix, suffix, and root, you can figure out what the term means.

Biologic Systematics

Medical reports may cite names of various types of biologic organisms, ranging from plants and worms to viruses and bacteria. Technical notation of such names follows a scheme referred to as biologic systematics, which is the accepted standard for naming organisms. The names of organisms are set in italics (or when written by hand, underlined), with the genus name capitalized and the species name beginning with a lower-case letter. This is the accepted international classification system, or taxonomy. For example, the common bacterium found in yogurt is *Lactobacillus acidophilus* (or <u>Lactobacillus acidophilus</u>). The genus name is *Lactobacillus,* and the species name is *acidophilus.* After it has been spelled out once, genus names are often abbreviated; for example the yogurt bacterium is abbreviated *L. acidophilus.* When writing out or typing genus and species names (instead of using a computer), be sure to underline the names. Names of microbes often appear on laboratory reports and are mentioned in everyday life as well.

PRONUNCIATION KEY

Complete uniformity in pronunciation of medical terms, like other words in any language, is not possible. Correctly pronouncing medical terms is necessary for good communication. For example, in spoken language, renin (REE nin) is often mispronounced as rennin (REN in). The difference in meaning is profound because renin is an enzyme in the kidney that converts one compound to another and plays a role in blood pressure, whereas rennin is an enzyme found in gastric (stomach) juice. Geography, training, and common practice all influence phonetics, hence medical dictionaries commonly give variant pronunciations. For that reason, any pronunciation key should be used only as a guide. Table 1-1 is the pronunciation guide for the terms in this book. In parentheses, after most terms in the key term tables, the words are spelled just as they sound, or phonetically. The syllables are separated by a single space and individual words are separated by a double space within the parentheses. Stressed, or accented, syllables are designated by capital letters. Alternate spelling and singular/plural forms are given when appropriate.

RULES FOR PLURALS

It is important to follow the general rules for making plural forms of singular words. Table 1-2 lists the rules for common endings.

TABLE 1-1   Pronunciation Key

Letters	Phonetics	Examples	Pronunciation
Long vowel sounds			
a	ay	bay	BAY
		fatal	FAY tul
e	ee	bee	BEE
		fetal	FEE tul
i	eye	eye	EYE
		island	EYE lund
i	igh	arthritis	ahr THRIGH tis
o	oh	post	POHST
		low	LOH
u	yoo	union	YOON yun
u	ue	supine	SUE pine
		superficial	sue per FISH ul
u	ew	mute	mewt
*In-between vowel sounds*ᵃ			
a, e, i, o, u, y	uh	anatomy	uh NAT uh mee
Short vowel sounds			
a	a	fat	FAT
e	e	get	GET
i	i	bit	BIT
o	o	not	NOT
u	u	but	BUT
Combination vowels			
ae	ee	bursae	BER see
oe	e	roentgen	RENT gen
oi	oi	void	VOID
eu at the beginning of a word	yoo	eupnea	yoop NEE uh
Hard and Soft Sounds			
c before e, i, and y	soft s	cerebrum	se REE brum
		cicatrix	SIK uh triks
		cystic	SIS tick
c before a, o, and u	hard k	cava	KAY vuh
		colon	KOH lun
		culture	KUL chur
g before e, i, and y	soft j	gene	JEEN
		gingivitis	jin ji VYE tis
		gyrus	JYE rus
g before a, o, and u	hard g	galactometer	gal ack TOM e tur
		goiter	GOY tur
		gustation	gus TAY shun

TABLE 1-1 Pronunciation Key *(continued)*

Letters	Phonetics	Examples	Pronunciation
Other consonant/vowel sounds			
ch at the beginning of a word	sometimes k	cholesterol	koh LES tur ol
		chronic	KRON ick
dys at the beginning of a word	dis	dystrophy	DIS truh fee
i at the end of a word	eye	nuclei	NEW klee eye
gn at the beginning of a word	n	gnathic	NATH ick
pn at the beginning of a word	n	pneumonia	new MOH nyuh
pn in the middle of a word	hard p, hard n	apnea	AP nee uh
ps at the beginning of a word	s	psychosis	sigh KOH sis
ph at the beginning of a word	f	pharmacology	fahr muh KOL uh jee
pt at the beginning of a word	t	pterygoid	TERR i goid
rh at the beginning of a word	r	rheumatoid	ROO muh toid
x at the beginning of a word	z	xiphoid	ZYE foid

Note: This sound is referred to as a *schwa,* which is a neutral or unstressed vowel sound. It is the most common sound in the American English language and can be found in words such as *about* (uh BOWT), *synthesis* (SIN thuh sis), *harmony* (HAR muh nee), *medium* (MEE dee uhm), and *syringe* (suh RINJ).

TABLE 1-2 Rules for Plurals

Singular Ending	Rule	Plural Ending	Examples
-a	keep the -a and add -e	-ae	vertebra → vertebrae
-ax	drop -ax and add -aces	-aces	thorax → thoraces
-en	drop -en and add -ina	-ina	foramen → foramina
-ex	drop -ex and add -ices	-ices	pollex → polices
-ion	drop -ion and add -ia	-ia	ganglion → ganglia
-is	drop -is and add -es	-es	axis → axes
-itis	drop -itis and add -itides	-itides	dermatitis → dermatitides
-ium	drop -ium and add -ia	-ia	epithelium → epithelia
-ix	drop -ix and add -ices	-ices	appendix → appendices
-oma	keep -oma and add -ta	-omata	hematoma → hematomata
	keep -ma and add -s	-omas	hematoma → hematomas
-sis	drop -sis and add -ses	-ses	diagnosis → diagnoses
-um	drop -um and add -a	-a	ovum → ova
-us	drop -us and add -i	-i	embolus → emboli
-x	drop -x and add -ges	-ges	phalanx → phalanges
-y	drop -y and add -ies	-ies	biopsy → biopsies

MEDICAL TERM PARTS

COMMON PREFIXES

Commonly used medical term prefixes, suffixes, and combining forms are introduced in this section. Note that some combining forms are also used as prefixes.

Word Part	Meaning
a-	without
ab-	away from
ad-	toward
ambi-	both sides
an-	without
ana-	up
ante-	before, in front of
anti-	against
auto-	self
brady-	slow
caud-, caudo-	tail
cephal-, cephalo-	head
chrom-, chromo-	color, colored
circum-	around
contra-	against
cry-, cryo-	cold, freezing
cyst-, cysti-, cysto-	bladder
de-	away from, without
dextr-, dextro-	right, toward the right
dist-, disto-	distant, distal
dys-	painful, difficult
ec-	out, out of
encephal-, encephalo-	brain
end-, endo-	within, inner
epi-	upon, following
equi-	equal, equally
eu-	true, normal
ex-, exo-	out, outside
extra-	outside
heter-, hetero-	other, different

Word Parts	Meaning
homo-	same
hydro-	water
hyper-	above, beyond, over
hypo-	below, under
im-	not
in-	not, into
infra-	beneath, under
inter-	among, between
intra-	within, inside
juxta-	near
mal-	abnormal, bad, ill
mes-, meso-	middle
meta-	change, between
mid-	middle
ne-, neo-	new, newly formed
pan-	all
par-, para-	adjacent to, near
per-	through
peri-	around
post-	after, behind
pre-	before
pro-	supporting, in front of, before
pseudo-	false
re-	back
retro-	behind, backward
sinist-, sinistro-	left, toward the left
sub-	below, under
super-	above
supra-	above, upon
sym-	together, with
syn-	together, with
tachy-	rapid
trans-	through, across
ultra-	beyond, excess

WORD GROUPING

Using the table of common prefixes, identify the prefix form for each of the following definitions. The first one has been done as an example.

Definition	Word Part
away from	*ab-*
abnormal, bad, ill	
above	
above, beyond, over	
above, upon	
adjacent to, near	
after, behind	
against	A. B.
all	
among, between	
around	A. B.
away from, without	
back	
before	
before, in front of	
behind, backward	
below, under	A. B.
beneath, under	
beyond, excess	
bladder	
both sides	
brain	
change, between	
cold, freezing	
color, colored	
distant, distal	
equal, equally	
false	
head	

Definition	Word Part
left, toward the left	
middle	A. B.
near	
new, newly formed	
not	
not, into	
other, different	
out, out of	
out, outside	
outside	
painful, difficult	
rapid	
right, toward the right	
same	
self	
slow	
supporting, in front of, before	
tail	
through	
through, across	
together, with	A. B.
toward	
true, normal	
up	
upon, following	
water	
within, inner	
within, inside	
without	A. B.

WORD BUILDING

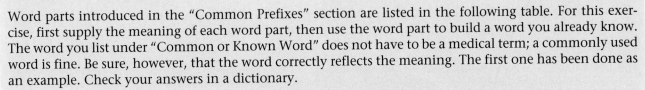

Word parts introduced in the "Common Prefixes" section are listed in the following table. For this exercise, first supply the meaning of each word part, then use the word part to build a word you already know. The word you list under "Common or Known Word" does not have to be a medical term; a commonly used word is fine. Be sure, however, that the word correctly reflects the meaning. The first one has been done as an example. Check your answers in a dictionary.

Word Part	Meaning	Common or Known Word	Example Medical Term
ab-	away from	abduct	abduction
ad-			adduction
ante-			anterior
anti-			antibody
auto-			autoimmune
circum-			circumcision
contra-			contraceptive
dys-			dysuria
ex-, exo-			exhale
heter-, hetero-			heterozygous
homo-			homozygous
hyper-			hypertension
hypo-			hypotonic
inter-			interosseous
intra-			intramuscular
juxta-			juxtaglomerular
meta-			metaphysis
ne-, neo-			neoplasm
post-			postpartum
retro-			retroperitoneal
sub-			subdural

PREFIXES RELATED TO NUMBER AND SIZE

Commonly used medical prefixes and combining forms pertaining to number or size are introduced in this section. The use of two prefixes relating to numbers is shown in Figure 1-5.

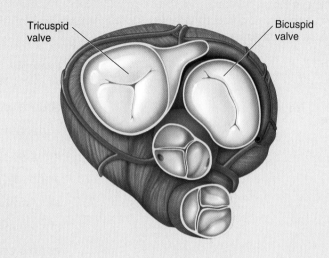

Tricuspid valve

Bicuspid valve

FIGURE 1-5
The heart has a bicuspid valve and a tricuspid valve. The prefixes *bi-* and *tri-* indicate number.

Word Part	Meaning
bi-	two
di-	two
diplo-	double
hemi-	half
hex-, hexa—	six
macr-, macro-	large
maxi-	extra large
mega-	big, large, great
micro-	small
mini-	small, miniature
mono-	one
multi-	many
noni-	nine
oct-, octa-, octo-	eight
pent-, penta-	five
poly-	many, much
quadri-, quadru-	four
semi-	half, partial
sept-, septi-	seven
sex-, sexi-	six
tetra-	four
tri-	three
uni-	one

WORD GROUPING

Using the table of prefixes related to number and size, identify the prefix or combining form for each of the following definitions. The first one has been done as an example.

Definition	Word Part
two	A. bi- B. di-
big, large, great	
double	
eight	
extra large	
five	
four	A. B.
half	
half, partial	
large	
many	
many, much	
nine	
one	A. B.
seven	
six	A. B.
small	
small, miniature	
three	

WORD BUILDING

Word parts introduced in the "Prefixes Related to Number and Size" section are listed in the following table. For this exercise, first supply the meaning of each word part, then use the word part to build a word you already know. The word you list under "Common or Known Word" does not have to be a medical term; a commonly used word is fine. Be sure, however, that the word correctly reflects the intended meaning. The first one has been done as an example. Check your answers in a dictionary.

Word Part	Meaning	Common or Known Word	Example Medical Term
bi-	two	bicycle	bicuspid
di-			diotic
hemi-			hemisphere

Word Part	Meaning	Common or Known Word	Example Medical Term
macr-, macro-			macromastia
micro-			microorganism
mono-			monozygous
multi-			multicellular
poly-			polyuria
quadri-, quadru-			quadrigemina
semi-			semicomatose
tri-			tricuspid

PREFIXES RELATING TO MEASUREMENT

Commonly used medical term prefixes relating to measurement are introduced in this section. Laboratory reports often include measurements, which may be reported in terms that use the following prefixes.

Word Part	Meaning
centi-	one hundredth
dec-, deca-	ten
deci-	one tenth
giga-	billion
hect-, hecto-	one hundred
kilo-	thousand
meg-, mega-	million
micro-	one millionth
milli-	one thousandth
nano-	one billionth

WORD GROUPING

Using the table of prefixes relating to measurement, identify the prefix or combining form for each of the following definitions. The first one has been done as an example.

Definition	Word Part
ten	*dec-, deca-*
billion	
million	
one billionth	
one hundred	
one hundredth	

Definition	Word Part
one millionth	
one tenth	
one thousandth	
thousand	

WORD BUILDING

Word parts introduced in the "Prefixes Relating to Measurement" section are listed in the following table. For this exercise, first supply the meaning of each word part, then use the word part to build a word you already know. The word you list under "Common or Known Word" does not have to be a medical term; a commonly used word is fine. Be sure, however, that the word correctly reflects the intended meaning. The first one has been done as an example. Check your answers in a dictionary.

Word Part	Meaning	Common or Known Word	Example Medical Term
centi-	one hundredth	centiliter	centimeter
dec-, deca-			decagram
deci-			deciliter
kilo-			kilogram
micro-			micrometer
milli-			milliliter

MEDICAL TERM PARTS USED AS SUFFIXES

Commonly used medical term suffixes are introduced in this section. Table 1-3 lists several subcategories of these word parts.

Word Part	Meaning
-ac	pertaining or relating to
-ad	toward
-al	pertaining or relating to
-algia	pain
-ase	enzyme
-blast	immature precursor cell
-cele	swelling, hernia
-centesis	surgical puncture to remove fluid
-cide	kill
-cise	cut
-clast	something that breaks; to break
-cyte	cell

TABLE 1-3 Subcategories of Suffixes

Category	Suffix	Example Medical Term
Condition of	-ia	myalgia
	-iac	cardiac
	-id	invalid
	-osis	cirrhosis
Pertaining to	-ac	iliac
	-al	brachial
	-eal	peroneal
	-ia	insomnia
	-iac	cardiac
	-ic	cephalic
Medical specialty	-logy	physiology
	-ist	dentist
	-ian	pediatrician
	-iatrics	geriatrics
	-iatry	podiatry

Word Part	Meaning
-desia	surgical fixation, fusion
-eal	pertaining to
-ectasis	expansion, dilation
-ectomy	surgical removal
-emia	condition of the blood
-esis	condition, action, process
-genesis	origination
-genic	produced by
-gram	written record or picture
-graph	record or picture
-graphy	a writing, description
-ia; -iac	condition of, pertaining to
-iasis	presence of
-ic	pertaining to
-id	condition of
-ior	pertaining to
-ism	process
-it is	inflammation
-lith	stone
-logia, -logy	study of
-lysis	breakdown, destruction

Word Part	Meaning
-malacia	abnormal softening
-megaly	large, enlargement
-oid	resembling
-ology	study of
-oma	tumor or neoplasm
-osis	condition
-parous	giving birth
-pathy	disease
-penia	few, deficiency
-pexy	fixation
-phasia	speech
-phil-, -phile, -philia	attraction for
-phobia	abnormal fear
-plasia	growth
-plasty	surgical repair
-plegia	paralysis
-pnea	breathing
-poiesis	production, formation
-praxia	movement
-rrhage, -rrhagia	excessive, abnormal flow
-rrhaphy	to stitch or suture
-rrhea	fluid discharge or flow
-rrhexis	rupture
-scope	an instrument for viewing
-scopy	to visualize
-sect	to cut
-sis	state of
-spasm	twitch, involuntary muscle contraction
-stalsis	constriction, contraction
-stenosis	abnormal narrowing, stricture
-stomy	artificial or surgical opening
-taxis	movement toward a stimulus
-tome	part or section; instrument or cutting
-tomy	incision, cutting
-tripsy	crushing
-trophy	growth, nourishment
-uria	pertaining to the urine

WORD GROUPING

Using the table of medical term parts used as suffixes, identify the suffix form for each of the following definitions. The first one has been done as an example (Fig. 1-6).

Definition	Word Part
swelling, hernia	-cele
abnormal fear	
abnormal narrowing, stricture	
abnormal softening	
artificial or surgical opening	
attraction for	
breakdown, destruction	
breathing	
cell	
condition	
condition, action, process	
condition of	
condition of, pertaining to	
condition of the blood	
constriction, contraction	
cut	
cut, to	
crushing	
disease	
enzyme	
excessive, abnormal flow	
expansion, dilation	
few, deficiency	
fixation	
fluid discharge or flow	
giving birth	
growth	
growth, nourishment	
immature precursor cell	
incision, cutting	
inflammation	
instrument for viewing, a	
kill	

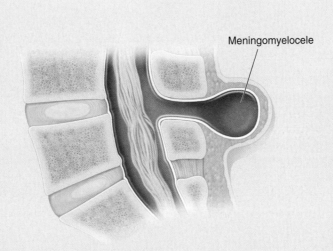

Meningomyelocele

FIGURE 1-6
The suffix -*cele* means swelling. This is a meningomyelocele, or a swelling of the spinal cord.

Definition	Word Part
large, enlargement	
movement	
movement toward a stimulus	
origination	
pain	
paralysis	
part or section; instrument for cutting	
pertaining to	A. B. C.
pertaining to or relating to	A. B.
pertaining to the urine	
presence of	
process	
produced by	
production, formation	
record or picture	
resembling	
rupture	
something that breaks; to break	
speech	
state of	
stitch or suture, to	
stone	

Definition	Word Part
study of	A. B.
surgical fixation, fusion	
surgical puncture to remove fluid	
surgical removal	
surgical repair	
toward	
tumor or neoplasm	
twitch, involuntary muscle contraction	
visualize, to	
writing, description, a	
written record or picture	

WORD BUILDING

Word parts introduced in the "Medical Term Parts Used as Suffixes" section are listed in the following table. For this exercise, first supply the meaning of each word part, then use the word part to build a word you already know. The word you list under "Common or Known Word" does not have to be a medical term; a commonly used word is fine. Be sure, however, that the word choice correctly reflects the intended meaning. The first one has been done as an example. Check your answers in a dictionary.

Word Part	Meaning	Common or Known Word	Example Medical Term
-ac	pertaining to	cardiac	cardiac
-ad			cephalad
-gram			angiogram
-graph			radiograph
-ic			pelvic
-ology			histology
-phobia			claustrophobia
-scope			otoscope

COMMON ABBREVIATIONS

Abbreviation	Term
CAAHEP	Commission on Accreditation of Allied Health Education Programs
CC	chief complaint
c/o	complains of
CPT	*Current Procedural Terminology*
Dx	diagnosis
FH	family history
HEENT	head, eyes, ears, nose, and throat
H&P	history and physical
HIPAA	Health Insurance Portability & Accountability Act
Hx	history
ICD	*International Classification of Diseases*
Imp	impression
L&W	living and well
NAD	no acute distress
NCHS	National Center for Health Statistics
NKA	no known allergies
NKDA	no known drug allergies
OH	occupational history
P	plan
PE	physical examination
PERRLA	pupils equal, round, and reactive to light and accommodation
Px	physical examination
R/O	rule out
ROS	review of systems
SH	social history
SOAP	subjective, objective, assessment, plan
Sx	symptom
UCHD	usual childhood diseases
WHO	World Health Organization
WNL	within normal limits

REVIEW AND APPLICATION: THREE-LEVEL LEARNING SYSTEM

LEVEL ONE: REVIEWING FACTS AND TERMS USING RECALL

Select the best response to each of the following questions.

1. An eponym is a medical term derived from _____.

    a. a person's name

    b. Latin roots

    c. Greek roots

    d. its anatomic location

2. Standardized anatomic nomenclature is determined by _____.

    a. your instructor

    b. the text book industry

    c. *Terminologia Anatomica*

    d. *Index Medicus*

3. Commonly used combining vowels are _____.

    a. *a* and *e*

    b. *o* and *i*

    c. *i* and *u*

    d. *i* and *y*

4. A combining form is defined as a _____.

    a. word root plus a prefix

    b. prefix plus a suffix

    c. word root plus a vowel

    d. word root plus a suffix

5. A word root _____.

    a. is another term for *affix*

    b. is the main part of a word

    c. conveys the primary meaning of the word

    d. B and C are correct

6. A suffix _____.

    a. occurs at the beginning of the term

    b. occurs in the middle of the term

    c. occurs at the end of the term

    d. conveys the main meaning of the term

7. Medical term suffixes _____.

    a. can describe a body condition

    b. can serve as verbs

    c. usually do not affect the root meaning

    d. usually end in *s*

8. If a word is spelled phonetically, it is written _____.

    a. in consonants only

    b. just as it sounds

    c. in vowels only

    d. using the Greek alphabet

LEVEL TWO: REVIEWING CONCEPTS

Select the best response to each of the following questions.

9. If a suffix begins with a consonant, a combining _____ is needed.

    a. vowel

    b. consonant

    c. affix

    d. prefix

10. Which of the following terms is an eponym?

    a. calcaneal tendon

    b. Langerhans cells

    c. phalanx

    d. biceps

What is the plural form for each given term?

11. phalanx _____

12. nucleolus _____

13. mitochondrion _____

14. cervix _____

15. sclerosis _____

16. epithelium _____

What is the singular form for each given term?

17. fungi _____

18. ganglia _____

19. fractures _____

20. atria _____

21. sarcomata _____

Match the prefix with its correct meaning.

_____ 22. hyper-   a. within

_____ 23. endo-   b. above, beyond

_____ 24. mal-   c. below, under

_____ 25. hypo-   d. abnormal, bad

_____ 26. par-, para-   e. adjacent to

Match the meaning with its correct prefix.

_____ 27. four   a. sex-, sexi-

_____ 28. seven   b. sept-, septi-

_____ 29. six   c. noni-

_____ 30. nine   d. quadri-, quadru-

Match the suffix with its correct meaning.

_____ 31. -al   a. condition of the blood

_____ 32. -emia   b. breathing

_____ 33. -poiesis   c. pertaining to

_____ 34. -taxis   d. formation, production

_____ 35. -pnea   e. movement toward a stimulus

What is the prefix for each of the following terms?

36. one hundred _____

37. ten _____

38. one tenth _____

39. one hundredth _____

40. million _____

Define the following word parts.

41. -itis _____

42. -cyte _____

43. -osis _____

44. -pathy _____

45. hypo- _____

Define the following terms.

46. hemiplegia _____

47. polyuria _____

48. lithotripsy _____

49. hypertrophy _____

50. apraxia _____

Identify the correctly spelled term in each set.

51. _____

   a. epponym

   b. aponym

   c. eponym

   d. eponim

52. _____

  a. diarrea

  b. diarrhea

  c. diarhea

  d. diarrhia

53. _____

  a. myalgia

  b. myoalgia

  c. myialgia

  d. mylgia

Identify the correctly styled biological name in each set.

54. _____

  a. mycobacterium tuberculosis

  b. Mycobacterium Tuberculosis

  c. *Mycobacterium Tuberculosis*

  d. *Mycobacterium tuberculosis*

55. _____

  a. escherichia coli

  b. escherichia Coli

  c. <u>Escherichia coli</u>

  d. <u>Escherichia Coli</u>

56. _____

  a. *Clostridium* botulinum

  b. *clostridium Botulinum*

  c. *C. botulinum*

  d. *clostridium botulinum*

LEVEL THREE: THINKING CRITICALLY

Write a short answer to the following question.

57. Tina works in a medical office, where she files medical records and answers the telephone. One afternoon, she received a phone call from an irate parent requesting sensitive medical information about her 20-year-old daughter. Tina told the mother she was unable to divulge any information contained in any patient's medical record. Did Tina act appropriately under these circumstances? Why?

_____

_____

_____

ANSWERS

WORD GROUPING (COMMON PREFIXES)

Definition	Word Part
away from	ab-
abnormal, bad, ill	mal-
above	super-
above, beyond, over	hyper-
above, upon	supra-
adjacent to, near	par-, para-
after, behind	post-
against	A. anti-
	B. contra-
all	pan-
among, between	inter-
around	A. circum-
	B. peri-
away from, without	de-
back	re-
before	pre-
before, in front of	ante-
behind, backward	retro-
below, under	A. hypo-
	B. sub-
beneath, under	infra-
beyond, excess	ultra-
bladder	cyst-, cysti-, cysto-
both sides	ambi-
brain	encephal-, encephalo-
change, between	meta-
cold, freezing	cry-, cryo-
color, colored	chrom-, chromo-
distant, distal	dist-, disto-
equal, equally	equi-
false	pseudo-
head	cephal-, cephalo-
left, toward the left	sinist-, sinistro-
middle	A. mes-, meso-
	B. mid-
near	juxta-
new, newly formed	ne-, eno-
not	im-
not, into	in-
other, different	heter-, hetero-
out, out of	ec-
out, outside	ex-, exo-
outside	extra-
painful, difficult	dys-
rapid	tachy-
right, toward the right	dextr-, dextro-
same	homo-
self	auto-
slow	brady-
supporting, in front of, before	pro-
tail	caud-, caudo-
through	per-
through, across	trans-
together, with	A. sym-
	B. syn-
toward	ad-
true, normal	eu-
up	ana-
upon, following	epi-
water	hydro-

Definition	Word Part
within, inner	end-, endo-
within, inside	intra-
without	A. a-
	B. an-

WORD BUILDING (COMMON MEDICAL PREFIXES)

Word Part	Meaning	Common or Known Word	Example Medical Term
ab-	away from	abduction	abduct
ad-	toward	adduct	adduct
ante-	before, in front of	anteroom	anterior
anti-	against	antibacterial	antibody
auto-	self	automobile	autoimmune
circum-	around	circumvent	circumcision
contra-	against	contraband	contraceptive
dys-	painful, difficult	dysfunction	dysuria
ex-, exo-	out, outside	exit	exhale
heter-, hetero-	other, different	heterogenous	heterozygous
homo-	same	homosexual	homozygous
hyper-	above, beyond, over	hyperextend	hypertension
hypo-	below, under	hypodermic	hypotonic
inter-	among, between	interstate	interosseous
intra-	within, inside	intramural	intramuscular
juxta-	near	juxtaposition	juxtaglomerular
meta-	change, between	metabolism	metaphysis
ne-, neo-	new, newly formed	neoimpressionism	neoplasm
post-	after, behind	postgraduate	postpartum
retro-	behind, backward	retrofit	retroperitoneal
sub-	below, under	submarine	subdural

WORD GROUPING (PREFIXES RELATED TO NUMBER AND SIZE)

Definition	Word Part
two	A. bi-
	B. di-
big, large, great	mega-
double	diplo-
eight	oct-, octa-, octo-
extra large	maxi-
five	pent-, penta-
four	A. quadri-, quadru-
	B. tetra-
half	hemi-
half, partial	semi-
large	macr-, macro-
many, much	A. multi-
	B. poly-
nine	noni-
one	A. mono-
	B. uni-
seven	sept-, septi-
six	A. hex-, hexa-
	B. sex-, sexi-
small	micro-
small, miniature	mini-
three	tri-

WORD BUILDING (PREFIXES RELATED TO NUMBER AND SIZE)

Word Part	Meaning	Common or Known Word	Example Medical Term
bi-	two	bicycle	bicuspid
di-	two	diameter	diotic
hemi-	half	hemisphere	hemisphere
macr-, macro-	large	macrobiotic	macromastia
micro-	small	microbiology	microorganism
mono-	one	monogram	monozygous
multi-	many	multicolor	multicellular
poly-	many, much	polyester	polyuria
quadri-, quadru-	four	quadruple	quadrigemina
semi-	half, partial	semicircle	semicomatose
tri-	three	triathlete	tricuspid

WORD GROUPING (PREFIXES RELATED TO MEASUREMENT)

Definition	Word Part
ten	dec-, deca-
billion	giga-
million	meg-, mega-
one billionth	nano-
one hundred	hect-, hecto-
one hundredth	centi-
one millionth	micro-
one tenth	deci-
one thousandth	milli-
thousand	kilo-

WORD BUILDING (PREFIXES RELATED TO MEASUREMENT)

Word Part	Meaning	Common or Known Word	Example Medical Term
centi-	one hundredth	centiliter	centimeter
dec-, deca-	ten	decagram	decagram
deci-	one tenth	deciliter	deciliter
kilo-	thousand	kilogram	kilogram
micro-	one millionth	microbiology	micrometer
milli-	one thousandth	millipede	milliliter

WORD GROUPING (MEDICAL TERM PARTS USED AS SUFFIXES)

Definition	Word Part
swelling, hernia	-cele
abnormal fear	-phobia
abnormal narrowing, stricture	-stenosis
abnormal softening	-malacia
artificial or surgical opening	-stomy
attraction for	-phil, -phile, -philia
breakdown, destruction	-lysis
breathing	-pnea
cell	-cyte
condition	-osis
condition, action, process	-esis

Definition	Word Part
condition of	-id
condition of, pertaining to	-ia, iac
condition of the blood	-emia
constriction, contraction	-stalsis
cut	-cise
cut, to	-sect
crushing	-tripsy
disease	-pathy
enzyme	-ase
excessive, abnormal flow	-rrhage, -rrhagia
expansion, dilation	-ectasis
few, deficiency	-penia
fixation	-pexy
fluid discharge or flow	-rrhea
giving birth	-parous
growth	-plasia
growth, nourishment	-trophy
immature precursor cell	-blast
incision, cutting	-tomy
inflammation	-itis
instrument for viewing, an	-scope
kill	-cide
large, enlargement	-megaly
movement	-praxia
movement toward a stimulus	-taxis
origination	-genesis
pain	-algia
paralysis	-plegia
part or section; instrument for cutting	-tome
pertaining to	A. -eal
	B. -ic
	C. -ior
pertaining to or relating to	A. -ac
	B. -al
pertaining to the urine	-uria
presence of	-iasis
process	-ism
produced by	-genic
production, formation	-poiesis
record or picture	-graph
resembling	-oid
rupture	-rrhexis
something that breaks; to break	-clast
speech	-phasia
state of	-sis
stitch or suture, to	-rrhaphy
stone	-lith
study of	A. -logia, -logy
	B. -ology
surgical fixation, fusion	-desia
surgical puncture to remove fluid	-centesis
surgical removal	-ectomy
surgical repair	-plasty
toward	-ad
tumor or neoplasm	-oma
twitch, involuntary muscle contraction	-spasm
visualize, to	-scopy
writing, description, a	-graphy
written record or picture	-gram

WORD BUILDING (MEDICAL TERM PARTS USED AS SUFFIXES)

Word Part	Meaning	Common or Known Word	Example Medical Term
-ac	pertaining or relating to	cardiac	cardiac
-ad	toward	caudad	cephalad
-gram	written record or picture	telegram	angiogram
-graph	record or picture	telegraph	radiograph
-ic	pertaining to	psychic	pelvic
-ology	study of	biology	histology
-phobia	abnormal fear	arachnophobia	claustrophobia
-scope	an instrument for viewing	telescope	otoscope

REVIEW AND APPLICATION: THREE-LEVEL LEARNING SYSTEM

Level One: Reviewing Facts and Terms Using Recall

1. a
2. c
3. b
4. c
5. d
6. c
7. a
8. b

Level Two: Reviewing Concepts

9. a
10. b
11. phalanges
12. nucleoli
13. mitochondria
14. cervices
15. scleroses
16. epithelia
17. fungus
18. ganglion
19. fracture
20. atrium
21. sarcoma
22. b
23. a
24. d
25. c
26. e
27. d
28. b
29. a
30. c
31. c
32. a
33. d
34. e
35. b
36. hect-, hecto-
37. dec-, deca-
38. deci-
39. centi-
40. meg-, mega-
41. inflammation
42. cell
43. condition
44. disease
45. below
46. paralysis on half of the body
47. excessive urination
48. stone crushing
49. excessive growth
50. without movement
51. c
52. b
53. a
54. d
55. c
56. c

Level Three: Thinking Critically

57. Yes, Tina acted appropriately. Medical information is private information and cannot be divulged without patient consent.

chapter 2

Anatomical and Physiological Terminology

OBJECTIVES

After completing this chapter, you should be able to:

1. Explain the difference between anatomy and physiology.
2. List the levels of organization within the human body.
3. Identify key cellular organelles and give a key function of each.
4. Describe the anatomic position.
5. Identify the body cavities, quadrants, and regions.
6. Use directional terms to describe body planes.
7. Define word parts used for describing the human body.
8. Provide definitions for key terms.
9. Explain various signs, symptoms, treatments, clinical tests, and procedures.
10. Cite anatomical and physiological alterations throughout the lifespan.
11. Identify common abbreviations related to anatomy and physiology.
12. Correctly define, spell, and pronounce the chapter's medical terms.

INTRODUCTION

Not only is knowledge of anatomy and physiology critical in any health-care profession but also fundamental appreciation is important for understanding our own bodies. No book can do justice to describing the intricacies of the living organism called the human body. Yet we can learn a great deal about its structure (anatomy) and its function (physiology) by studying medical terminology. Furthermore, we can synthesize a vast amount of information about medical terminology and the language of medicine by studying anatomy and physiology. There are no clearly defined borders among the health sciences, thus overlapping concepts are commonplace. Terms associated with anatomy and physiology are, therefore, prevalent in other aspects of human biology, disease, medicine, and allied health fields. This chapter is devoted to introducing you to general terms associated with the body, its structure, function, and position.

Throughout early history, the belief that humans could understand natural processes grew in popularity. This in turn stimulated people to think about physiology and anatomy. Anatomic form is based on its function; and the purpose depends on the construction, otherwise noted as "function follows form." For example, the arrangement of parts in the hand, with long, jointed fingers is related to the function of grasping objects. Individuals studying body structure are called anatomists, and physiologists are people who focus on body function.

A prevailing theme within physiology is that of homeostasis, the tendency to maintain a stable internal environment in relationship to the external arena. When the body is in homeostatic balance, it remains relatively constant in terms of chemical composition, temperature, and pressure for optimum function. All body systems attempt to maintain homeostasis; therefore, this is a fundamental concept in physiology. The nervous and endocrine systems play key roles in preserving homeostasis. Common examples of homeostasis include preserving blood glucose parameters, regulating temperature, and controlling blood gas concentrations.

Body parts function most efficiently when the concentration of water, food substances, oxygen, heat, and pressure remains within specified narrow limits. This delicate balance is accomplished partly by a process called metabolism. Metabolism refers to the physical and chemical changes occurring in the body that are necessary for life.

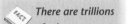
There are trillions of microorganisms living on the body!

This chapter focuses on the body as a whole. It provides an overview of anatomic and physiological disciplines, outlines the various body systems, and describes the various terms used for anatomical orientation.

MEDICAL TERM PARTS

WORD PARTS

Medical term prefixes, suffixes, and combining forms related to anatomical and physiological terminology are introduced in this section.

Word Parts	Meaning
abdomin-, abdomino-	abdomen, abdominal
acr-, acro-	extremity, end
ante-	before, in front of
antero-	anterior, front

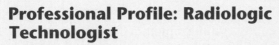
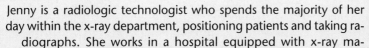

Professional Profile: Radiologic Technologist

Jenny is a radiologic technologist who spends the majority of her day within the x-ray department, positioning patients and taking radiographs. She works in a hospital equipped with x-ray machines, a computerized tomography (CT) scanner, and magnetic resonance imaging (MRI) equipment.

One aspect of her job that is particularly appealing is patient interaction. Before performing any imaging procedure, she explains it thoroughly to the person in an effort to alleviate fears and anxieties. This is especially important for a patient about to undergo an MRI study, during which he or she may feel claustrophobic because the individual is passed through a close-fitting cylindrical tube.

In addition to situating the patient, radiologic technologists oversee the operation of the machinery. This includes keying commands into the computer, setting exposure time and distance, and documenting scan sequences. Working with radiation requires that health precautions are met to ensure the safety of all those in the area. Furthermore, measures are taken to ensure compliance with government regulations.

After the CT scan, x-ray, or MRI pictures are taken, radiologic technologists review them for technical quality. If the image is substandard, the procedure must be repeated. Experience teaches the technologist how best to position a given individual, based on his or her somatotype, on the examination table to achieve the highest quality images. However, less-than-ideal conditions may make it difficult to obtain usable images on the first try—for example, if the technologist must use a mobile unit in the emergency department or the patient's room.

Once good-quality images are obtained, they are forwarded to the radiology division, where radiologists interpret the images and provide detailed reports. These reports are of diagnostic value for identifying pathology, confirming the presence of an abnormality, or indicating if follow-up tests are necessary.

To become a certified radiologic technologist, one must complete a two-year radiology technician program and pass a qualification test. The only entrance requirement for typical programs is a high school diploma. Programs range in length from one to four years and lead to a certificate plus an associate degree or a bachelor's degree. The two-year programs are the most popular and currently exist in 35 states and Puerto Rico.

Word Parts	Meaning
brachi-, brachio-	arm
bucco-	cheek
calcane-, calcaneo-	heel, calcaneus
cardi-, cardio-	heart
cephal-, cephalo-	head
carvic-, cervico-	neck, cervix
chem-, chemo-	chemistry
cost-, costi-, costo-	rib

Word Parts	Meaning
crani-, cranio-	skull, cranium
cyt-, cyto-	cell
embry-, embryo-	embryo
etio-	cause
facio-	face
-genesis	origin, beginning process
histio-, histo-	tissue
homeo-	same, steady
ili-, ilio-	ilium, hip bone
latero-	lateral, to one side
mamm-, mammo-	breasts
morph-, morpho-	form, shape
nas-, naso-	nose
nucl-, nucleo-	nucleus
occipit-, occipito-	occiput, back part of head
oro-	mouth
ot-, oto-	ear
parieto-	body wall or parietal bone
path-, patho-, -pathy	disease
ped-, pedi-, pedo-	foot or child
pelv-, pelvio-, pelvo-	pelvis
peritoneo-	peritoneum
pleur-, pleura-, pleuro-	lung membrane, side
postero-	posterior, at the back
physi-, physio-	physiological
prox-, proxi-, proximo-	proximal
pubo-	pubic
retro-	back, backward, behind
sacr-, sacro-	sacrum
somat-, somatico-, somato-	body
spin-, spino-	spine
stern-, sterno-	sternum
tars-, tarso-	tarsus (root of foot)
thorac-, thoracico-, thoraco-	chest (thorax)
vertebr-, vertebro-	vertebra (backbone)
viscero-	viscera (internal organs)

WORD ETYMOLOGY

Some words have Greek or Latin roots but are not true word parts. This section lists those that are used as medical terms.

Word	Definition
cauda	tail
distalis	distal
dorsum	back
inguen	groin
karpos	wrist
lumbus	loin
mentum	chin
stasis	standing still
systema	organized whole
typus	type
umbilicus	navel

MEDICAL TERM PARTS USED AS PREFIXES

Prefix	Definition
ante-	before, in front of
antero-	anterior, front
bucco-	cheek
etio-	cause
facio-	face
homeo-	same, steady
latero-	lateral, to one side
oro-	mouth
parieto-	body wall or parietal bone
peritoneo-	peritoneum
postero-	posterior, at the back
pubo-	pubic
retro-	back, backward, behind
viscero-	viscera (internal organs)

MEDICAL TERM PARTS USED AS SUFFIXES

Suffix	Definition
-genesis	origin, beginning process

WORD GROUPING

Using the "Medical Term Parts" tables, identify the prefix, suffix, or combining form for each of the following definitions. The first one has been done as an example.

Definition	Word Part
body wall or parietal bone	parieto-
abdomen, abdominal	
anterior, front	
arm	
back, backward, behind	
before, in front of	
body	
breasts	
cause	
cell	
cheek	
chemistry	
chest (thorax)	
disease	
ear	
embryo	
extremity, end	
face	
foot or child	
form, shape	
head	
heart	
heel, calcaneus	
ilium, hip bone	
lateral, to one side	
lung membrane, side	
mouth	
neck, cervix	
nose	
nucleus	
occiput, back part of head	
origin, beginning process	
pelvis	

Definition	Word Part
peritoneum	
physiological	
posterior, at the back	
proximal	
pubic	
rib	
sacrum	
same, steady	
skull, cranium	
spine	
sternum	
tarsus (root of foot)	
tissue	
vertebra (backbone)	
viscera (internal organs)	

WORD BUILDING

Word parts, introduced in the "Medical Term Parts" section, are listed in the following table. For this exercise, first supply the meaning of each word part, then use the word part to build a word you already know. The word you list under "Common or Known Word" does not have to be a medical term; a commonly used word is fine. Be sure, however, that the word correctly reflects the meaning. The first one has been done as an example. Check your answers in a dictionary.

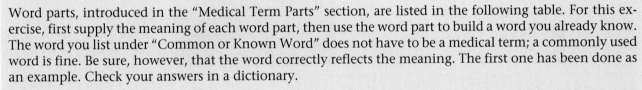

Word Part	Meaning	Common or Known Word	Example Medical Term
antero-	anterior, front	anterior	anterior
cardi-, cardio-			pericardium
chem- chemo-			chemotherapy
embry-, embryo-			embryo
-genesis			osteogenesis
homeo-			homeostasis
latero-			lateral
mamm-, mammo-			mammary gland
nas-, naso-			nasopharynx
nucl-, nucleo-			nucleus
retro-			retroperitoneal
vertebr-, vertebro-			vertebral column

ANATOMY AND PHYSIOLOGY DEFINED

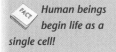

Human beings begin life as a single cell!

Anatomy (anat.) is the study of the physical structure of the human body. The shape of a specific anatomic structure is referred to as its **morphology.** For instance, the patella (kneecap) is an anatomic structure whose morphology is round. The study of the form and structure of something is also called morphology. A full description of all the possible fields of anatomic study is beyond this text's scope; however, a few examples—cytology, embryology, gross anatomy, histology, and pathology—are described here.

The word part *cyto-* refers to "cell" and *-ology* means "study of." Hence, **cytology** is the study of cells. It is a microscopic anatomy and requires special slide preparation and staining techniques before the cells can be seen under the microscope. Much study of the human body is done using a microscope. It is interesting that the tiny human egg cell, ovum, is the only cell in the body that can be seen with the naked eye.

Embryology is the study of development from the fertilized egg through the 8th week in utero, meaning in the mother's womb, or uterus. While in the uterus, the developing human is termed an embryo until the end of the 8th gestational week (Fig. 2-1). Thereafter, it is called a fetus.

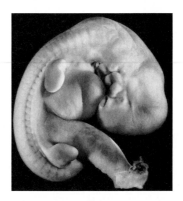

FIGURE 2-1
Embryo at the 5th gestational week. The developing human is termed an embryo until the end of the 8th gestational week. (Reprinted with permission from Blechmidt E. The stages of human development before birth. Philadelphia: Saunders, 1961.)

Gross anatomy is the study of surface anatomy. It is macroscopic; meaning it can be seen with the naked eye. Courses in gross anatomy generally involve cadaver dissection. **Histology** is a form of microscopic anatomy that studies the cells, tissues, and organs in relation to their function.

The study of diseased body structures is referred to as **pathology** because the prefix *path-* indicates "disease." A pathologist is a physician with special training who studies diseased anatomy.

Physiology is the study of the function of body structures. Think of it in terms of "what the body parts do and how they do it." It is difficult to separate anatomy from physiology because the structures of body parts are so closely related to their functions. As with anatomy, there are several disciplines within the broader field of physiology that focusing on different aspects of how an organism functions. An **organism** is a living thing, such as a plant, animal, or bacterium, composed of all of the body parts functioning together. Hence, a human organism is a collection of structurally and functionally integrated systems.

Key Term	Definition
anatomy (uh NAT uh mee)	study of the physical body structure
morphology (mor FOL uh jee)	form of a body part or study of the structure of something
cytology (si TOL uh jee)	branch of biology that studies cells
embryology (em bree OL uh jee)	study of the embryo and its development
gross anatomy (GROCE uh NAT uh mee)	study of the body that does not require magnification
histology (his TOL uh jee)	study of tissues, including cells and organs
pathology (pa THOL uh jee)	scientific study of disease
physiology (fiz ee OL uh jee)	study of body function
organism (OR guh NIZ um)	living individual

Key Term Practice: Anatomy and Physiology Defined

1. If *-ology* refers to the "study of," and *hist-* refers to "tissue," what is the medical term that means the study of body tissues? _____

2. The study of bodily disease is known as _____.

3. Anatomy is the study of human form. What is the word that describes the study of human function? _____

Cells and Organizational Structure

Larger body structures are made up of smaller parts, which are composed of yet smaller structures. Figure 2-2 presents the structural organizational levels of the human body, beginning with the smallest and building up to include the following levels: chemical, organelle, cell, tissue, organ, system, and organism. At the chemical level of organization, atoms are bound together to form molecules. The molecules are then joined to form organelles.

Cells are the basic structural and functional components of life and are the smallest living units of structure. The major portions of a cell are the membrane, organelles, and cytoplasm. The **cell membrane**, composed of lipids, proteins, and some carbohydrates, is an extremely thin, yet flexible bilayer that controls the movement of particles into and out of the cell. It is said to be selectively permeable because it allows the passage of some substances but restricts others. The surface of the membrane is **hydrophilic** (water loving), and thus water soluble. The **hydrophobic** (water fearing) interior of the membrane is water insoluble. The interior consists largely of fatty acids that give it its oily characteristics.

Structures found within the cytoplasm, fluid contained by a cellular membrane, include **organelles**, which are living parts of the cells that perform specialized functions. Approximately two dozen human cellular organelles have been identified. Examples of organelles filling the cytoplasm are the ribosomes, mitochondria, and nucleus. **Ribosomes** are clusters of proteins and ribonucleic acid (RNA) that manufacture proteins. **Mitochondria** are membranous sacs with inner partitions that

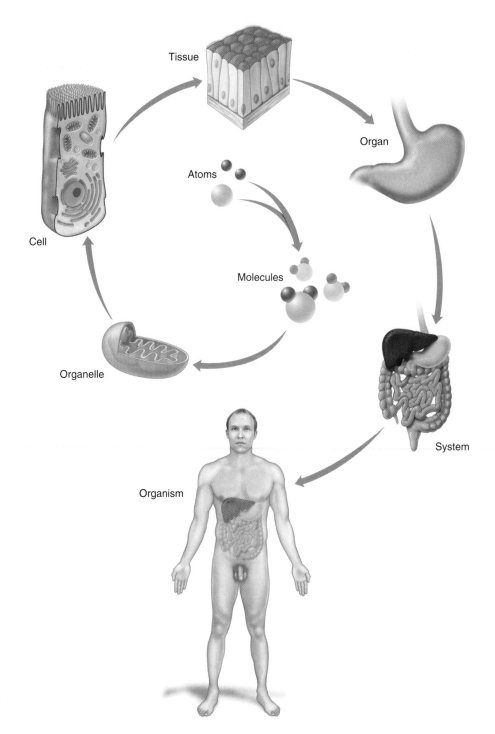

FIGURE 2-2
The structural organizational levels of the human body, beginning with the smallest (the atom).

release energy from food and transform that energy into a usable form called adenosine triphosphate (ATP). Mitochondria are commonly referred to as the cell's "power house."

The **nucleus** is a relatively large, spherical structure that directs activities of the cell. It contains the cell's deoxyribonucleic acid (DNA), nucleolus, and chromatin. The **nucleolus** is a dense, nonmembranous body located within the nucleus; it is composed of protein and RNA, which ultimately forms ribosomes. The nucleus is the innermost part and is enclosed by a nuclear envelope. A typical cell is shown in Figure 2-3.

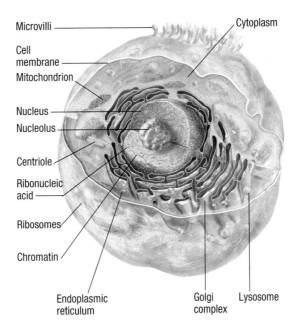

Microvilli —
Cytoplasm

Cell membrane —

Mitochondrion —

Nucleus —

Nucleolus —

Centriole —

Ribonucleic acid —

Ribosomes —

Chromatin —

Endoplasmic reticulum

Golgi complex

Lysosome

FIGURE 2-3
A typical human cell. (Image provided by Anatomical Chart Co.)

Cells must undergo a series of chemical and physical changes through a process called metabolism to survive. On the cellular level, specialization is necessary for optimal organism functioning, thus cells differentiate into various types that perform specific jobs. For example, nerve cells have long, thread-like extensions that transmit nerve impulses; epithelial cells are thin, flattened, tightly packed structures designed to protect underlying cells; and muscle cells, which pull parts closer together, are slender and rod-like.

Tissues are the next level of organization. A **tissue** is defined as a grouping of comparable cells that perform a specific function. Thus tissues consist of groups of similarly specialized cells. There are four basic types of tissues in the human: epithelial, connective, muscular, and nervous. Each of these tissue types has various divisions. Epithelium is the type of tissue that covers body surfaces and lines internal organs. The *-al* ending in "epithelial" indicates the adjective form, whereas the *-um* ending is the noun form. Connective tissue, such as adipose (fat) and cartilage, supports and protects. Muscle tissue produces movement, and nervous tissue conducts impulses.

An aggregation (grouping) of two or more tissues that are integrated to perform a particular function is an **organ**. Organs vary greatly in size and have definite forms and functions. Lungs, kidneys, and hearts are examples of organs.

The next stage of organization is the systemic level. A **system** consists of various organs that have similar or related functions. The 11 major human systems are cardiovascular (circulatory), digestive, endocrine, integumentary, lymphatic/immune, muscular, nervous, reproductive, respiratory, skeletal, and urinary. The final level of organization involves the interplay of these systems to form a complete organism.

FACT *Every minute, billions of cells die and are replaced by new ones!*

Key Term	Definition
cell	smallest unit of life
cell membrane (MEM brane)	barrier that surrounds the cytoplasm
hydrophilic (high droh FIL ick)	capable of attracting water; water loving
hydrophobic (high droh FOH bick)	unable to attract water; water fearing
organelle (OR guh nel)	specialized cellular structure
ribosomes (RYE boh sohmz)	sites of protein synthesis within the cytoplasm

Key Term	Definition
mitochondria (migh toh KON dree uh)	organelles that make and store ATP
nucleus (NEW klee us)	cellular center that contains DNA and the nucleolus
nucleolus (NEW klee oh lus)	center of the nucleus that contains RNA
tissue	aggregation of similar cells
organ	body structure with a specific function
system	functional combination of organs

Key Term Practice: Cells and Organizational Structure

1. A/An _____ is the smallest unit of life.

2. The definition for a/an _____ is an aggregation of similar cells specialized for a particular function.

3. These structures are suspended within a cell's cytoplasm: _____.

Human Body Systems

The complex human has 11 different interrelated systems. The **integumentary** system serves a protective function and helps regulate body temperature. Providing the framework and protection for internal organs is the **skeletal** system, whereas the **muscular** system aids in maintaining posture and providing force for movement. Note that these are often combined as the musculoskeletal system. The **nervous** system integrates all systems by its vast communicating network. The secretion of hormone, which exert their effects on other glands or tissues, is the responsibility of the **endocrine** system. As a result of their coordinated effects, these two systems are commonly called the neuroendocrine system. The **digestive** system converts food to a usable form. The **respiratory** system exchanges gases between the blood and air, the **cardiovascular** system transports nutrients and oxygen via the bloodstream, and the **lymphatic/immune** system transports fluids from spaces within tissues back to the blood. The tenth system, **urinary**, removes waste and maintains electrolyte balance, and the **reproductive** system ensures continuation of the species by producing offspring. Figure 2-4 demonstrates the human body systems, and Table 2-1 highlights the major organs found within each system.

Key Term	Definition
integumentary (in teg yoo MEN tuh ree) **system**	system that serves a protective function
skeletal (SKEL e tul) **system**	system that functions in protection, support, and movement
muscular (MUS kew lur) **system**	system responsible for movement
nervous system	system that functions in communication, integration, and control
endocrine (EN doh krin) **system**	system that secretes hormones and interacts with the nervous system
digestive (di JES tiv) **system**	system that process and regulates food

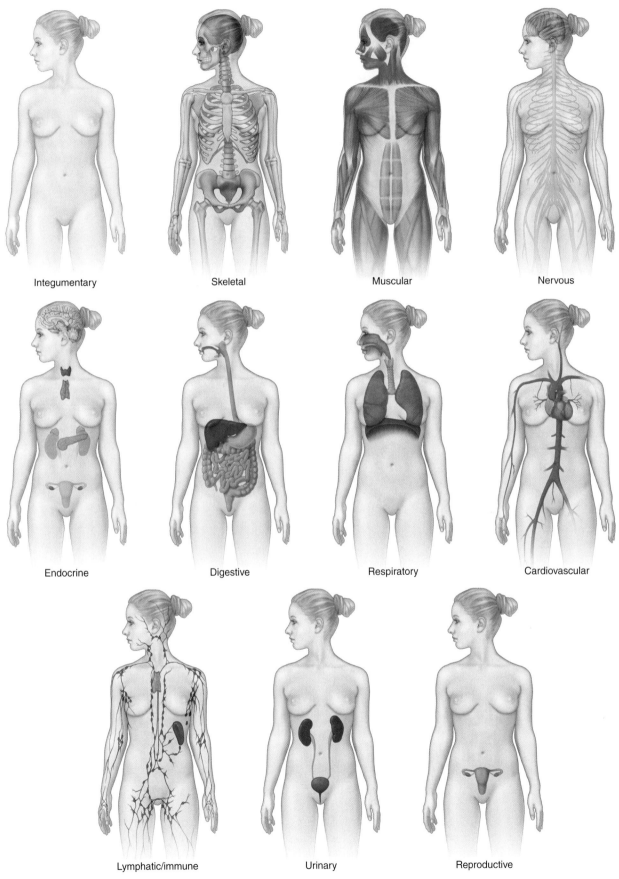

Integumentary   Skeletal   Muscular   Nervous

Endocrine   Digestive   Respiratory   Cardiovascular

Lymphatic/immune   Urinary   Reproductive

FIGURE 2-4
The 11 body systems of the human.

TABLE 2-1   Body Systems and Their Organs

System	Major Organs
integumentary	skin, hair, nails, and glands
skeletal	bones, ligaments, cartilage
muscular	muscles
nervous	brain, spinal cord, and nerves
endocrine	pituitary gland, hypothalamus, adrenal glands, thymus, thyroid, and pancreas
digestive	esophagus, stomach, intestines, and liver
respiratory	lungs and accessory structures
cardiovascular	heart, arteries, veins, and other blood vessels
lymphatic/immune	lymphatic vessels, glands, and nodes
urinary	kidneys, ureters, bladder, and urethra
reproductive	*female:* mammary glands, ovaries, oviducts, uterus, and vagina; *male:* testes and penis

Key Term	Definition
respiratory (RES pi ruh toh ree) **system**	system involved with gas exchange
cardiovascular (karr dee oh VAS kew lur) **system**	system that transports substances in the blood
lymphatic (lim FAT ik) **system**	system responsible for fluid transportation
immune system	system responsible for body defense
urinary (YOOR i nerr ee) **system**	system involved with excretion, secretion, and filtration
reproductive (ree pruh DUCK tiv) **system**	system concerned with human development and continuation

Key Term Practice: Human Body Systems

1. Identify the 11 human body systems.

   _____

   _____

   _____

2. The systems making up the neuroendocrine system are the _____ system and the _____ system.

Body Membranes

The human body has four primary membranes: the serous, pleural, pericardial, and peritoneal. A **membrane** is a thin tissue layer that surrounds a body part, separates cavities, lines cavities, or connects adjacent body structures.

Serous membranes, also called the **serosa**, line the thoracic (chest) and abdominopelvic (lower trunk) cavities. Serous membranes cover organs and secrete a watery fluid called serous fluid. Composed of connective tissue and a single layer of flattened cells (called simple squamous epithelium), serous membranes compartmentalize, protect, and lubricate organs (Fig. 2-5).

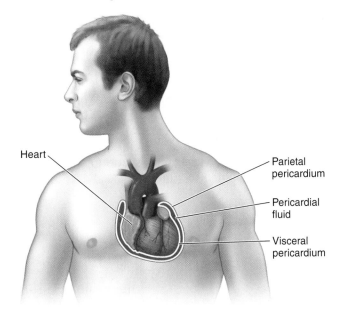

Heart

Parietal pericardium

Pericardial fluid

Visceral pericardium

A

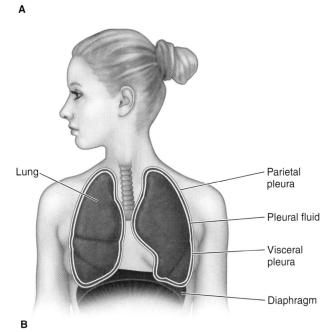

Lung

Parietal pleura

Pleural fluid

Visceral pleura

Diaphragm

B

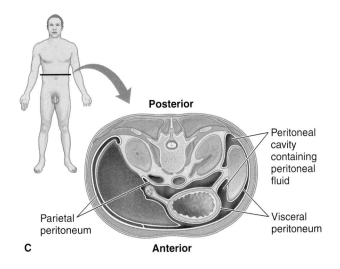

Posterior

Peritoneal cavity containing peritoneal fluid

Visceral peritoneum

Parietal peritoneum

C

Anterior

FIGURE 2-5
(A–C) The serous membrane, also called the serosa, lining the thoracic and abdominopelvic cavities.

Pleural membranes are associated with the lungs or pleural cavity. The word part *pleur-* means "lung." **Pericardial membranes** are associated with the heart and pericardial cavity, and **peritoneal membranes**, or **peritoneum**, are associated with the abdominal cavity.

Two main body linings are the parietal and visceral. **Parietal** means pertaining to the outer wall of a body cavity. **Visceral** means pertaining to an internal organ. For example, the parietal pleura is the inside lining of the thoracic cavity, and the visceral pleurae cover the lungs. Parietal membranes line body cavities and visceral membranes cover organs. Viscera refers to internal organs and the term can be used in place of the word *organ*. **Mesentery** is a double-layered membrane that attaches abdominal organs, such as the intestines, to the abdominal wall.

Key Terms	Definitions
membrane (MEM brane)	thin tissue layer surrounding a body part
serous (SEER us) **membranes**	cavity-lining membranes that secrete a watery fluid
serosa (se ROH suh)	serous membrane
pleural (PLOOR ul) **membranes**	membranes associated with the lungs
pericardial (perr i KAHR dee ul) **membranes**	membranes associated with the heart
peritoneal (perr i toh NEE ul) **membranes**	membranes associated with the abdominal cavity
peritoneum (PER i toh NEE um)	peritoneal membranes
parietal (puh RYE e tul)	forming or situated on a body wall
visceral (VIS ur al)	pertaining to the organs
mesentery (MES un terr ee; MEZ un terr ee)	peritoneal folds that attach abdominal organs to the abdominal wall

Key Term Practice: Body Membranes

1. If a membrane is associated with an organ, it is termed _____.

2. If a membrane is associated with a body wall or cavity, it is termed _____.

Somatotypes

People are of various sizes and shapes. The description of a person's morphology is termed his or her **somatotype**. The three types are I endomorph, II mesomorph, and III ectomorph. Most individuals, however, display a mixture of somatotype components.

The first type, **endomorph**, is characterized by a short neck and relatively short limbs. Smooth contours rounded out by fat deposits are common. Heavily muscled individuals, such as body builders, with large, prominent bones and well-defined shoulders have the characteristic **mesomorph** features. People with a predominance of height over fat or muscle display the typical **ectomorph** traits. Ectomorphs are generally thin individuals. See Figure 2-6 for an illustration of the three different somatotypes.

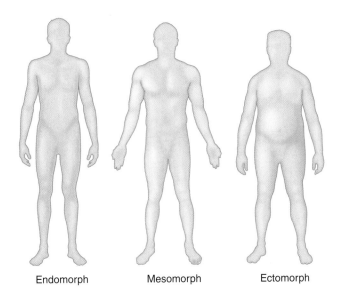

FIGURE 2-6
The three somato-types: endomorph, mesomorph, and ectomorph. Most individuals display a mixture of somato-type components.

Endomorph   Mesomorph   Ectomorph

Key Terms	Definitions
somatotype (SOH muh toh tipe)	body structure
endomorph (EN doh morf)	fat body type
mesomorph (MEZ oh morf)	heavily muscled body type
ectomorph (ECK toh morf)	thin body type

Key Term Practice: Somatotypes

1. The term used to describe one's physical stature is _____.

2. An Olympic gymnast would most likely fall into which body type category? _____

Anatomic Position and Body Cavities

Anatomic terms are used to identify direction and position. To avoid confusion, all bodily references are made in accordance with the anatomic position. Figure 2-7 demonstrates the **anatomic position**, which refers to a person standing erect, facing an observer, with the arms placed at the sides and the palms of the hands turned forward.

The human body can be divided into two major sections: axial and appendicular components. The head, neck, shoulders, and torso compose the **axial** section, whereas the appendages (arms and legs) make up the **appendicular** portion. For general orientation, specific terms describe the body while lying. The positional term **supine** refers to lying on the back, face upward, and **prone** refers to lying face downward. The word *up* is found in s*up*ine, thus the face is up while in a supine position.

Body cavities are described as anterior and posterior (Fig. 2-8). The diaphragm divides the anterior cavity into the upper thoracic cavity and the lower ab-dominopelvic cavity. The **posterior** (backside or dorsal) cavity includes the cranial

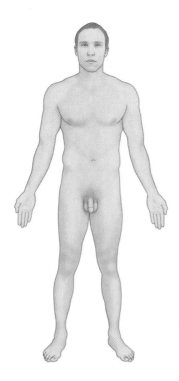

FIGURE 2-7

The anatomic position. The person is standing erect, facing the observer, with the arms placed at the sides and the palms of the hands turned forward.

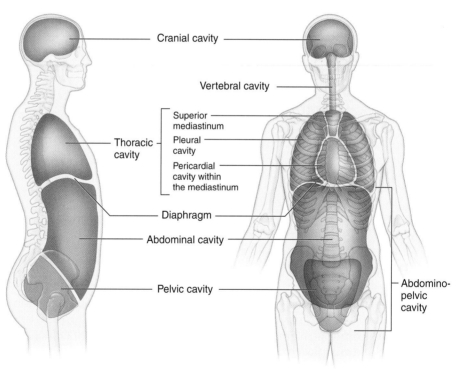

FIGURE 2-8

The body cavities in lateral (**A**) and anterior (**B**) views.

and vertebral cavities; the **anterior** cavity (front side or ventral) includes the thoracic, abdominal, and pelvic cavities. In medical charts, anteroposterior is often abbreviated AP and is frequently used to describe the perspective of x-ray images. The **cranial cavity** contains the brain, whereas the **vertebral cavity** houses the spinal cord and portions of spinal nerves.

The **thoracic cavity** (thorax) includes two pleural cavities, which hold the lungs, and the mediastinum. The **mediastinum** is the middle section of the thorax that surrounds all thoracic viscera except the lungs. Extending from the sternum to the vertebral column, it contains the esophagus, trachea, heart, and cardiac great vessels, including the superior vena cava and inferior vena cava.

The **abdominopelvic cavity** is divided into the superior (upper) abdominal and the inferior (lower) pelvic cavity by an imaginary line that extends from the symphysis pubis (where the pubic bones meet) to a specific point on the sacrum known as the sacral promontory. Be careful of the tricky spelling of this term, as you might be inclined to incorrectly call it the "abdomin*al*pelvic" cavity. Viscera of the **abdominal cavity** include the stomach, spleen, pancreas, liver, gallbladder, small intestine, and most of the large intestine. Viscera of the **pelvic cavity** include the urinary bladder, sigmoid colon, rectum, and internal male and female reproductive structures. The visceral peritoneum covers all abdominal organs.

Other body cavities are the oral cavity with the teeth and tongue, the nasal cavity within the nose including some sinuses, the orbital cavity that protects the eye and associated muscles and nerves, and the middle ear cavity, which contains the middle ear bones.

Key Terms	Definitions
anatomic (an uh TOM ick) **position**	pose in which a person is facing forward, standing erect, with the hands at the side and palms turned outward in the supine position
axial (ACK see ul)	body portion consisting of head, neck, and torso
appendicular (ap en DICK yoo lur)	body portion consisting of the arms and legs
supine (suh PINE; SUE pine)	lying face up
prone	lying face down
posterior (pos TEER ee ur)	toward the human back side
anterior (an TEER ee ur)	toward the human front side
cranial (KRAY nee ul) **cavity**	space occupied by the brain
vertebral (VUR te brul) **cavity**	space occupied by the spinal cord
thoracic (thoh RAS ick) **cavity**	space occupied by the lungs, heart, and trachea
mediastinum (mee dee as TYE num)	space in the middle of the chest
abdominopelvic (ab dom i noh PEL vick) **cavity**	combination of the abdominal and pelvic cavities
abdominal (ab DOM i nul) **cavity**	space between the diaphragm and the pelvic floor
pelvic (PEL vick) **cavity**	space within the bony pelvis

Key Term Practice: Anatomic Position and Body Cavities

1. Explain what is meant by *anatomic position*.
   _____
   _____
   _____

2. The combination of the abdominal and pelvic cavities is commonly known as the _____ cavity.

3. The body portion consisting of the arms and legs is called the _____, whereas the portion consisting of the head, neck, and chest is referred to as the _____.

Directional Terms

Directional terms are used to indicate the relationship of one body part to another (Fig. 2-9). Common terms are described in pairs with opposite meanings. For instance, the word *anterior* means near or at the front of the body, and the term *posterior* refers to a structure near or at the back of the body: The nipple is on the anterior surface, and the kidneys are posterior to the intestines. **Dorsal** and **ventral** are alternate terms for posterior and anterior, respectively. Although the terms are often used within human anatomy, ventral and dorsal are usually reserved for describing nonhuman animals.

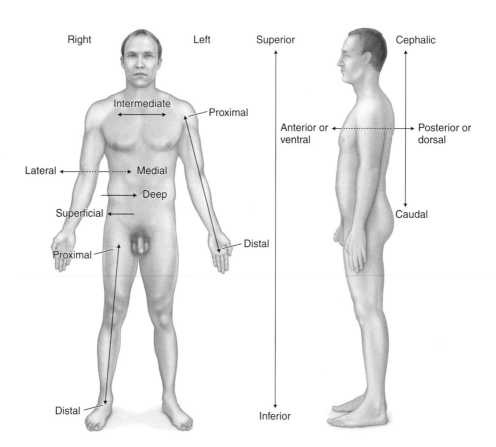

FIGURE 2-9
Directional terms are used to indicate the relationship of one body part to another.

Medical terms used to indicate the directions that can be described using the common words *up* and *down* include caudal, cephalic, inferior, and superior. **Caudal** refers to the lower portion of the spine. The word *cauda* means "tail." The opposite of caudal is **cephalic**, which indicates toward or pertaining to the head. The term that means away from the head is **inferior**, and the opposite of inferior, **superior**, means toward the head or upper part of a structure. Superior, cranial, and cephalic all mean toward the top. Caudal is a term used in human anatomy but is more appropriate for describing animals that actually have a tail, such as dogs and cats. To illustrate the correct use of these terms, the feet are inferior to the hips, whereas the thoracic region is superior to the abdominal region.

Words specifying location include deep and superficial. **Deep** means internal or away from the body surface. Deep is used in reference to an internal structure, as in "the brain is deep to the skull." **Superficial** means external, toward the surface, or on the body. This term can be used to describe a structure located on the body's exterior or to describe muscles that overlay other muscles. For example, the skin is superficial to the bones, and the pectoralis major muscle is superficial to the pectoralis minor muscle.

Proximal is used to describe a structure that is toward the attachment of an extremity to the trunk or to the point closest to the main mass of the body. For example, the knee is proximal to the foot. **Distal** means that a structure is farther from the extremity's attachment. Think of it as being toward the end or at distant point away from the origin. For example, the hand is distal to the elbow.

Lateral (lat.) means toward the side of the body. The ears are lateral to the head. **Contralateral** refers to a structure being on the opposite side of another structure. For example, the right kidney is contralateral to the left kidney. A term that means on the same side of the body is **ipsilateral.** The left arm and left leg are ipsilateral.

Medial means nearer the midline of the body or nearest to the middle of a body structure. For example, the heart is medial to the lungs. **Intermediate** suggests that a structure is located between a medial and a lateral structure. For example, the uterine tube is intermediate to the uterus and the ovary. The term **peripheral** is used to describe the position of anything around an organ or extending outward from the body trunk. The periphery of the heart is the outer border and peripheral nerves form networks extending from the spinal cord.

Key Terms	Definitions
dorsal (DOR sul)	back side
ventral (VEN trul)	anterior, belly side
caudal (KAW dul)	toward the tail
cephalic (se FAL ick)	toward or pertaining to the head
inferior (in FEER ee ur)	lower than another part
superior (sue PEER ee ur)	higher than another part
deep	away from the surface
superficial (sue pur FISH ul)	pertaining to the surface
proximal (PROCK si mul)	toward the point of origin
distal (DIS tul)	farther from the point of origin
lateral (LAT ur ul)	pertaining to the side
contralateral (kon truh LAT ur ul)	situated on opposite side
ipsilateral (ip si LAT ur ul)	situated on the same side
medial (MEE dee al)	toward the midline
intermediate	between two structures
peripheral (pe RIF e rul)	outward or near the surface

Key Term Practice: Directional Terms

1. The hand is _____ to the shoulder.

2. The head is _____ to the feet.

3. The opposite of anterior is _____.

4. The opposite of deep is _____.

Abdominopelvic Quadrants and Regions

To describe the location of body structures and provide points of reference, the abdominopelvic cavity is divided into quadrants. **Quadrants** are four regions of the abdominopelvic cavity that are used in physical examinations. Imaginary horizontal and vertical lines passing through the umbilicus (belly button) create the following four sections (Fig. 2-10): left upper quadrant (LUQ), right upper quadrant (RUQ), left lower quadrant (LLQ), and right lower quadrant (RLQ).

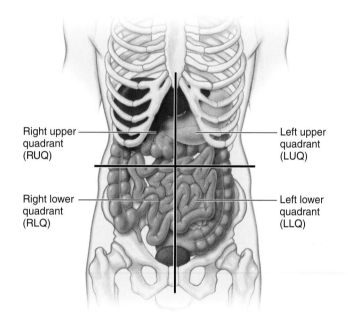

Right upper quadrant (RUQ)

Left upper quadrant (LUQ)

Right lower quadrant (RLQ)

Left lower quadrant (LLQ)

FIGURE 2-10
Abdominopelvic quadrants are four regions of the abdominopelvic cavity that are used in physical examinations.

A different approach divides the lower trunk into nine separate regions. **Regions** are abdominopelvic body divisions. The regions are arranged like a tic tac toe game, divided by two vertical lines and two horizontal lines that run through the body to create nine squares (Fig. 2-11): the **epigastric**, **left** and **right hypochondriac**, **umbilical**, **left** and **right lumbar**, **hypogastric**, and **left** and **right inguinal**. Knowing the location of specific organs in these regions is necessary because it helps clinicians isolate sources of aches and pains. For example, pain in the right hypochondriac region may indicate a gallbladder problem.

Key Terms	Definitions
quadrants (KWAH drunts)	four regions of the abdominopelvic area
regions	nine areas of the abdominopelvic cavity
epigastric (ep i GAS trick) **region**	upper middle part between the two hypochondriac regions
left hypochondriac region (high poh KON dree ack)	left upper lateral region below the lower ribs
right hypochondriac (high poh KON dree ack) **region**	right upper lateral region below the lower ribs
umbilical (um BIL i kul) **region**	middle region below the epigastric region and above the pubic region

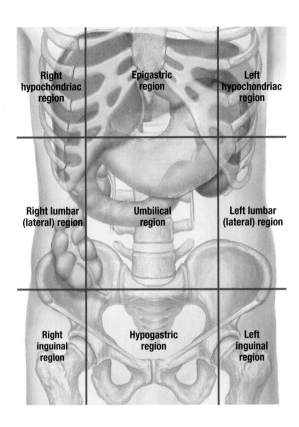

FIGURE 2-11
The nine abdominopelvic regions. (Image provided by Anatomical Chart Co.)

Key Terms	Definitions
left lumbar (LUM bahr) **region**	to the left side of the umbilical region
right lumbar (LUM bahr) **region**	to the right side of the umbilical region
hypogastric (high poh GAS trick) **region**	pubic region
left inguinal (ING gwi nul) **region**	left lower region beside the pubic region
right inguinal (ING gwi nul) **region**	right lower region beside the pubic region

Key Term Practice: Abdominopelvic Quadrants and Regions

1. The abdominopelvic cavity can be divided into nine _____.

2. The four areas of the abdominopelvic cavity are termed _____.

Anatomic Planes

The body can be diagrammed according to planes of reference. This enables one to study and visualize the structural arrangement of various organs. **Planes** are imaginary flat surfaces used to divide the body or organs into definite areas. Figure 2-12 shows the three fundamental planes of reference: sagittal, coronal, and transverse.

A **sagittal plane** divides the body into left and right sides. A specific type of sagittal plane is a midsagittal (median). A **midsagittal** or **median plane** is a vertical surface through the midline of the body that divides it into equal left and right sides. The key is *equal* because it passes through the midplane of the body.

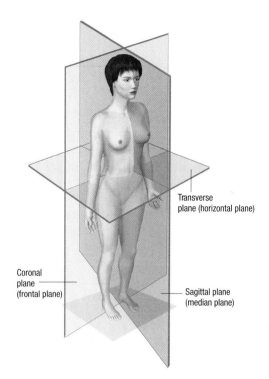

Transverse
plane (horizontal plane)

Coronal
plane
(frontal plane)

Sagittal plane
(median plane)

FIGURE 2-12
The body can be sectioned and diagrammed according to planes of reference. (Image provided by Anatomical Chart Co.)

A **coronal plane**, also called a **frontal plane**, is a plane passing lengthwise to divide the body or organs into anterior and posterior portions. In essence, the body or part is sectioned into front and back segments.

A **transverse plane**, or **horizontal plane**, is a line drawn parallel to the ground at a right angle to the sagittal and coronal planes. It divides the body or organs into superior (upper) and inferior (lower) portions.

Key Terms	Definitions
planes	imaginary lines delineating flat surfaces used to divide the body
sagittal (SAJ i tul) **plane**	line bisecting the body into left and right halves
midsagittal (mid SAJ i tul) **plane**	line bisecting the body at the median creating equal left and right halves; median plane
median (MEE dee un) **plane**	line bisecting the body or a structure into equal left and right halves; midsagittal plane
coronal (KOR oh nul) **plane**	frontal plane; line dividing the body into front and back parts
frontal plane	coronal plane; line dividing the body into front and back parts
transverse (trans VURCE) **plane**	horizontal plane; line parallel to the body's axis creating superior and inferior portions
horizontal plane	transverse plane; line parallel to the body's axis creating superior and inferior portions

Anatomic Terms

Anatomic terms are words describing superficial landmarks used for body orientation. All references are based on the person being in the anatomic position. Figure 2-13 demonstrates these landmarks, and Table 2-2 lists anatomic terms with their adjective form and common term. Many of these terms provide the foundation for the names of other anatomic structures; thus learning the terms now will make the later chapters more understandable.

THE CLINICAL DIMENSION

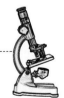

Generalized terms identifying signs and symptoms, clinical tests and diagnostic procedures, pathology, and treatments are defined in this section. Disorders affecting various body systems and chapter-specific medical terms related to those conditions will be given in the appropriate lessons to follow.

Signs and Symptoms

Disease is an indication that the body's homeostatic balance has been disrupted. Signs and symptoms indicate abnormal states. **Signs** are objective evidence of disease—that is, they can be determined by physical examination and clinical tests. Irregular pulse and respiratory rates, fever, and abnormal blood pressure are examples of signs. **Symptoms** are less obvious because they are subjective—that is, symptoms are something that the person experiences, such as dizziness, pain, and itching. Signs and symptoms (S&S) pertaining to diseases that affect particular body systems are presented in subsequent chapters.

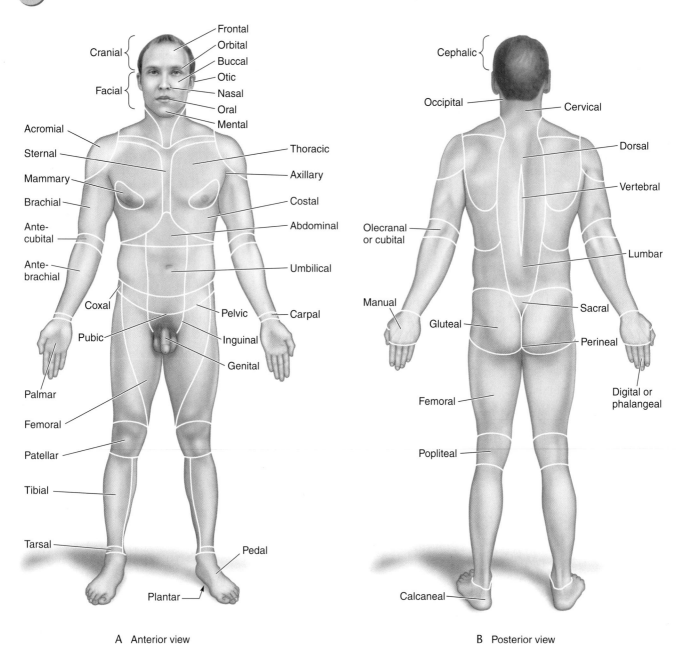

A Anterior view   **B** Posterior view

FIGURE 2-13
(A–B) Anatomical terms describing superficial landmarks used for body orientation.

Key Terms	Definitions
signs	objective evidence of disease
symptoms	subjective state of disease

Key Term Practice: Signs and Symptoms

1. Dizziness and headache are examples of _____.

2. Fever and high blood pressure are examples of _____.

TABLE 2-2 Anatomical Terms

Anatomical Term	Adjective Form	Common Name
abdomen (ab DOH mun)	abdominal (ab DOM i nul)	abdomen; inferior cavity of the trunk
acromion (a KROH mee on)	acromial (a KROH mee ul)	point of shoulder
antebrachium (an te BRAY kee um)	antebrachial (an te BRAY kee ul)	forearm
antecubitis (an te KEW bi tus)	antecubital (an te KEW bi tul)	front of elbow; inner elbow
axilla (ack SIL uh)	axillary (ACK si lerr ee)	armpit
brachium (BRAY kee um)	brachial (BRAY kee ul)	arm
bucca (BUCK uh)	buccal (BUCK ul)	cheek
calcaneus (kal KAY nee us)	calcaneal (kal KAY nee ul)	heel of foot
carpus (KAHR pus)	carpal (KAHR pul)	wrist
cephalon (SEF uh lon)	cephalic (se FAL ick)	head
cervix (SUR vicks)	cervical (SUR vi kul)	neck
costa (KOS tuh)	costal (KOS tul)	rib
coxa (KOCK suh)	coxal (KOCK sul)	hip
cranium (KRAY nee um)	cranial (KRAY nee ul)	skull
cubitus (KEW bi tus)	cubital (KEW bi tul)	elbow
digit (DIJ it)	digital (DIJ i tul)	finger or toe
dorsum (DOR sum)	dorsal (DOR sul)	back
face	facial (FAY shul)	face
femur (FEE mur)	femoral (FEM uh rul)	thigh
front	frontal	forehead
genitalia (jen i TAY lee uh)	genital (JEN i tul)	reproductive organs
gluteus (gloo TEE us)	gluteal (GLOO tee ul)	buttocks
hallux (HAL ucks)		great toe; big toe
inguen (ING gwen)	inguinal (ING gwi nul)	groin
lumbar (LUM bahr)	lumbar (LUM bahr)	lower back
mamma (MAM uh)	mammary (MAM uh ree)	breast
manus (MAN us)	manual	hand
mentum (MEN tum)	mental	chin
nasus (NAY sus)	nasal	nose
occiput (OCK si put)	occipital (ock SIP i tul)	lower back of head
olecranon (oh LECK ruh non)	olecranal (oh LECK ruh nul)	back of elbow
orbit	orbital (OR bi tul)	eye socket

(continues)

TABLE 2-2 Anatomical Terms *(continued)*

Anatomical Term	Adjective Form	Common Name
oris (OR is)	oral (OR ul)	mouth
otikus (OH ti kus)	otic (OH tick)	ear
palma (PAWL muh)	palmar (PAWL mur)	palm
patella (pa TEL uh)	patellar (pa TEL ur)	kneecap
pectus (PECK tus)	pectoral (PECK tuh rul)	chest or breast
pedis (PEE dis); pes (PES)	pedal (PED ul)	foot
pelvis (PEL vis)	pelvic (PEL vick)	pelvis
perineum (perr i NEE um)	perineal (perr i NEE ul)	between the vulva (females) or the scrotum (males) and the anus
phalanx (FAY lanks)	phalangeal (fa LAN jee ul)	finger or toe
planta (PLAN tuh); plantaris (plan TERR is)	plantar (PLAN tur)	sole of foot
pollex (POL ecks)		thumb
popliteus (pop li TEE us)	popliteal (pop LIT ee ul; pop li TEE ul)	back of knee
pubes (PEW beez); pubis (PEW bis)	pubic (PEW bick)	anterior groin
sacrum (SAY krum)	sacral (SAY krul)	lowest area of back
sternum (STUR num)	sternal (STUR nul)	middle of chest
tarsus (TAHR sus)	tarsal (TAHR sul)	top instep of foot
thoracis (THOR uh sis)	thoracic (thoh RAS ick)	chest
tibia (TIB ee uh)	tibial (TIB ee ul)	shin
umbilicus (um BIL i kus)	umbilical (um BIL i kul)	navel; bellybutton
vertebra (VER te bruh)	vertebral (VER te brul)	spinal column

Clinical Tests and Diagnostic Procedures

Disease diagnosis is based on the accumulation of information gleaned from professional experience, physical examination, visual inspection, and the results of clinical tests and investigative procedures. Despite the profession's great knowledge of physiology and the advances in technology, medicine remains an art as well as a science.

Using their fingers, clinicians often detect landmarks or attempt to isolate tender spots and sore lumps by applying firm pressure to the body surface. This procedure is termed **palpation**. When a clinician taps sharply on various body locations, this is called **percussion** (Fig. 2-14*A*). To determine fluid accumulation and organ densities, the thoracic and abdominal regions are percussed to detect resonating vibrations. Tapping over the chest determines the presence of normal air content in the lungs, and tapping over the abdomen evaluates air in the intestines and the sizes of the solid organs. Another common procedure, **auscultation**, refers to using a **stethoscope** to listen to various organs as they perform their functions (Fig. 2-14*B*). For example, one can listen to breathing sounds, heartbeats, and digestive noises.

To determine the state of certain parts of the nervous system and specific organs of innervation, reflex responses are used. A **reflex response** is the involuntary movement

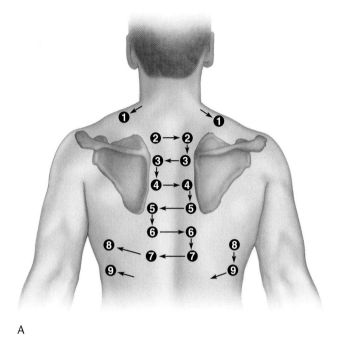

A

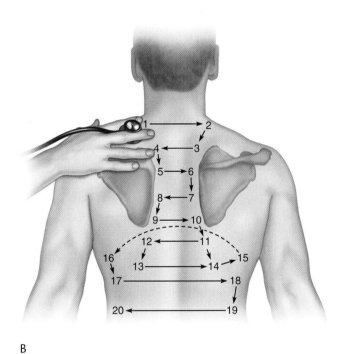

B

FIGURE 2-14
Sites of percussion
(**A**). Percussion can
determine fluid
accumulation and
organ densities. Sites
of auscultation (**B**).
During auscultation, a
clinician can listen
through a stethoscope
to various organs as
they perform their
functions.

that occurs after a stimulus has been applied. For example, a clinician uses a rubber hammer to strike the knee directly below the patella; in response to this, the lower leg kicks out (knee-jerk response).

Various anatomy scanning instruments and equipment used to visualize the internal body are available. Some of these include conventional radiography (x-ray imaging), CT, cine CT, fluoroscopy, dynamic spatial reconstructor (DSR), positron-emission tomography (PET), and MRI. These diagnostic tools are discussed in other chapters.

Key Terms	Definitions
palpation (pal PAY shun)	examination through touch
percussion (pur KUSH un)	firmly tapping to elicit sounds
auscultation (aws kul TAY shun)	listening for sounds coming from various organs
stethoscope (STETH uh skope)	instrument used to detect body sounds
reflex response	involuntary action to a stimulus

Key Term Practice: Clinical Tests and Diagnostic Procedures

1. The term _____ refers to physical examination of the body through touch.

2. Listening to heart sounds through a stethoscope is called _____.

Pathology

The mechanisms of disease are varied and numerous. Common causes of disease are related to autoimmunity, pathogens (protozoa, bacteria, and viruses), degeneration, fungi, genes, inflammation, malnutrition, physical agents, toxins, chemical agents, tumors, and neoplasms. The following chapters describe how many of these items promote the onset of disease. Other disease risk factors include genetics, age, lifestyle, stress, environment, and pre-existing conditions that lead to ill health.

Pathology is the scientific study of the nature, origin, progress, characteristics, and effects of disease. Some frequently used terms in the field of pathology are pathophysiology, epidemiology, and pathogenesis. **Pathogenesis** refers to the origin and course of disease development. It attempts to answer the **etiology**, factors that contribute to the occurrence, of the disease. If the cause cannot be determined, it is termed **idiopathic**. The study of physiological process associated with disease is termed **pathophysiology**. The study of disease occurrence, distribution, and transmission is called **epidemiology**. For example, when there is an outbreak of a particular disease, such as Ebola fever, specialists called epidemiologists track the course and development of the disease. They also try to locate the very first person, or **index case**, who exhibited signs and symptoms of the illness they are studying.

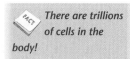

There are trillions of cells in the body!

Key Terms	Definitions
pathogenesis (path oh JEN i sis)	origin and course of disease development
etiology (ee tee OL uh jee)	study of the cause and course of disease development
idiopathic (id ee oh PATH ick)	caused by unknown origin
pathophysiology (path oh fiz ee OL uh jee)	study of body function modified by disease
epidemiology (ep i dee mee OL uh jee)	study of disease occurrence and distribution
index case	first documented person identified with a particular disease

Key Term Practice: Pathology

1. The first person identified with an outbreak of chickenpox is called the _____ case.

2. If the suffix -*gist* refers to a person who works in a particular field, then a person who studies pathology would be called a/an _____.

3. A person who studies the distribution and occurrence of disease is called a/an _____.

Treatments

Pathologic conditions may be resolved or altered through treatment. Treatment is often synonymous with therapy and involves therapeutic measures to alleviate signs and symptoms or to cure the disease. Treatment can include medication therapies, physical rehabilitation, exercise, nutrition strategies, surgery, radiation therapy, or psychological therapy.

The prevention or treatment of disease by chemical agents and medicines is termed **chemotherapy. Physical rehabilitation** is a type of therapy that helps the individual regain functional use of a particular body part or the body as a whole. The goal of physical rehabilitation is the restoration of the ability to function in a normal or near-normal manner after disease, illness, or injury. It may involve the professional services of physical therapists. Moreover, exercise is often a treatment option to preserve or restore health.

Nutrition strategies are employed to maintain and/or repair the body. Nutrition involves the ingestion of the appropriate vitamins, minerals, and nutrients (carbohydrates, fats, and proteins). There is growing evidence that good nutrition plays a large role in preventing and treating disease processes. **Surgery** is an operative procedure used to treat various conditions. In many cases, surgical intervention is used as a last resort when other treatment options fail, or it is used because research has demonstrated its superiority over the alternatives.

Radiation therapy treats disease with ionizing radiation such as x-rays, β-rays, and γ-rays. It is commonly used for cancer treatment. **Psychological therapy** is used for treating the mind. It involves counseling with a psychiatrist, psychologist, or counselor.

Key Terms	Definitions
chemotherapy	use of chemical agents to treat disease
physical rehabilitation	therapy to regain function
nutrition strategies	eating well for health
surgery	operative procedure
radiation therapy	treatment using ionizing radiation
psychological therapy	treatment for the mind

Key Term Practice: Treatments

1. _____ may be prescribed to a patient who has just had a cast removed from her arm.

2. The umbrella term describing the use of chemical agents to treat disease is _____.

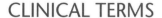

CLINICAL TERMS

Clinical Dimension	Term	Description
DISORDERS		
	epidemiology	study of disease occurrence and distribution
	etiology	study of the cause and course of disease development
	idiopathic	caused by unknown origin
	index case	first documented person identified with a particular disease
	pathogenesis	origin and course of disease development
	pathophysiology	study of body function modified by disease
SIGNS AND SYMPTOMS		
	signs	objective evidence of disease
	symptoms	subjective state of disease
CLINICAL TESTS AND DIAGNOSTIC PROCEDURES		
	auscultation	listening for sounds coming from various organs
	palpation	examination through touch
	percussion	firmly tapping to elicit sounds
	reflex response	involuntary action to a stimulus
	stethoscope	instrument used to detect body sounds
TREATMENTS		
	chemotherapy	use of chemical agents to treat disease
	nutrition strategies	eating well for health
	physical rehabilitation	therapy to regain function
	psychological therapy	treatment for the mind
	radiation therapy	treatment using ionizing radiation
	surgery	operative procedure

Lifespan

Lifespan is the maximum number of years a human is able to live. Despite available products aimed at increasing one's years on earth, the human lifespan appears to be fixed at approximately 120 years. Many have approached her, but the world's longest-lived person at 122 years was Jeanne Calment of France, who was born February 21, 1875, and died August 4, 1997.

The lifespan varies by species, ranging from 1 day for mayflies to about 13 years for medium-size dogs to 5000 years for a bristle-cone pine tree. Lifespan should not be confused with life expectancy, which is the number of years one can look forward to living under particular circumstances. For example, cigarette smoking greatly increases the risks of cardiovascular disease, which decreases one's chances of living a very long life. As of 2001 (the latest year for which the Centers for Disease Control and Prevention has data), the average life expectancy in the United States was 77.2 years.

Throughout the human lifespan, from conception to death, many changes occur within the various levels of body organization. A critical period in human development occurs during the first few weeks when embryonic membranes form and then transform into three primary germ layers: endoderm, ectoderm, and mesoderm. These germ layers differentiate into all body cells, tissues, organs, and systems.

Human life phases are marked by embryonic development, fetal stage, neonatal period, infancy, childhood, puberty and adolescence, adulthood, and senescence. Aging occurs at all levels of organization, but the manifestations may not necessarily be experienced until advanced old age. The focus of the lifespan section in subsequent chapters will be on key system-specific physiological, anatomic, and pathologic alterations that occur throughout the aging process.

In the News: Wrong-Site Surgery

Imagine the horror of waking up from anesthesia to discover that the wrong limb had been amputated. On February 20, 1995, that is exactly what happened to Willie King of Tampa, Florida. Owing to complications of diabetes, Mr. King was scheduled for a below-the-knee right-leg amputation. Surgeons had mistakenly removed his *left* leg. Two weeks later, his diseased right leg was removed, greatly affecting his quality of life.

Wrong-site surgical procedures fall into four broad categories: (1) wrong-side surgery, (2) wrong-level/wrong-part surgery, (3) correct-site/wrong-procedure surgery, and (4) wrong-patient surgery. Wrong-side surgeries are described as those procedures performed on the opposite anatomic extremity or body structure. Wrong-level and wrong-part surgeries are done in close proximity to the correct spot. Correct-site/wrong-procedure surgeries occur when the correct anatomic structure is treated but the incorrect procedure is performed. Last, the wrong-patient category includes procedures performed on the wrong person and the wrong surgery performed on the right person.

The Joint Commission on Accreditation of Healthcare Organizations (JCAHO) lists wrong-site surgery as the fourth most commonly reported event. The most commonly occurring anatomic location of wrong-site orthopedic surgery was the knee, followed by the ankle/foot, hip, leg, hand/fingers, and wrist.

Safety measures have been established to prevent wrong-site surgeries. The practice with the greatest potential seems to be the "sign your site" program. Patients undergoing a surgical procedure involving a limb sign their initials at the surgical site; physicians also endorse the site. This initial double-check system is used in conjunction with a verification checklist to ensure procedures are performed on the proper body part. Knowing correct anatomic terminology and position is crucial for preventing wrong-site amputations.

COMMON ABBREVIATIONS

Abbreviation	Term
anat.	anatomical, anatomy
ATP	adenosine triphosphate
A-P	anteroposterior

Abbreviation	Term
cine CT	cine computed tomography
CT	computed tomography
DNA	deoxyribonucleic acid
DSR	dynamic spatial reconstructor
JCAHO	Joint Commission on Accreditation of Healthcare Organizations
lat.	lateral
LLQ	left lower quadrant
LUQ	left upper quadrant
MRI	magnetic resonance imaging
PET	positron-emission tomography
RLQ	right lower quadrant
RNA	ribonucleic acid
RUQ	right upper quadrant
S&S	signs and symptoms

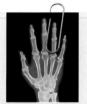

Case Study

Mr. Smythe, a 67-year-old with diabetes, arrived in the physician's office with pain in his right back. His history indicated that he has had diabetes for 30 years, takes regular insulin injections, gets no exercise, and had a right nephrectomy 1 month ago. He also had a right hip replacement several years ago. He is 6 feet 3 inches tall and weighs 145 lbs. The physical examination revealed nothing remarkable other than pain when palpating the right lumbar region. Chemical analysis of the urine was negative. Jenny, the radiologic technologist, will perform the CT scans of the abdomen and pelvis, which were ordered by the physician.

Case Study Questions

Select the best answer to each of the following questions.

1. Mr. Smythe had a right nephrectomy 1 month ago. This means that he had _____.

a. both kidneys removed
b. his right kidney removed
c. tests performed on his kidney
d. an artificial kidney operation

2. The somatotype that best represents Mr. Smythe is _____.

a. endomorph.
b. ectomorph.
c. mesomorph.
d. none of these.

3. Why might right lumbar pain be expected after a right nephrectomy?

a. That is the location of the right kidney.
b. That is the location of the bladder.
c. That is the location of the right lung.
d. That is the location of the heart.

4. CT scans of the abdomen and pelvis were ordered. CT images are created from which type of technology?

a. magnetic resonance
b. soundwaves
c. x-rays
d. fluoroscopy

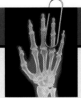

REAL WORLD REPORT

Mr. Smythe arrived at the hospital to undergo CT scanning of his abdominal and pelvic areas. The scans were performed by Jenny. The radiologist's report follows.

IMAGING DEPARTMENT: CT SCAN

NAME:	Matt Smythe
DATEORD:	August 10, 2003
ORDPHYS:	Dr. Flagg
TEST:	Abdomen CT
ATTENDING:	N/A
REFERRING:	N/A
CLINIC:	Hospital
ADDORD:	N/A
PT:	Smythe
EXAM:	N/A
ROOM:	CT
ACCT:	0010213
TYPE:	N/A
DATE:	August 20, 2003

CLINICAL INFORMATION: Status post previous right nephrectomy; follow-up.

CT ABDOMEN

CT scans of the abdomen were obtained before and after intravenous contrast administration. The enteric contrast was given before the examination. The previous examination of July 20, 2001, was compared.

The liver is of unremarkable size without focal mass or biliary dilatation. The spleen and the adrenal glands are unremarkable. There is moderate atrophy of the pancreas, which is probably an unremarkable finding.

Previous right nephrectomy is evident. There is no evidence of recurrent retroperitoneal mass or lymphadenopathy. The left kidney shows clustered perinephric cysts, which are of no clinical significance. No focal mass or hydronephrosis is demonstrated at the left kidney. No paranephric fluid collection is noted. There is no ascites.

There is a small ventral hernia in the midline of the midabdomen, a small nondilated small-bowel loop is present within the hernia without evidence of obstructive phenomenon.

There is a metallic device at the lower anterior abdominal wall to reinforce the previous anterior abdominal incision in the midline. There is also a small hernia present along the left side of the metallic device within the lower abdomen. A small nondilated small-bowel loop is present within this second ventral hernia.

CT PELVIS

CT scans of the pelvis were obtained before and after intravenous contrast administration. The enteric contrast was given before the examination.

There is no pelvic mass or lymph nodal enlargement. The anatomic details of the soft tissue structures are somewhat limited at the right lower pelvis owing to the metallic right hip prosthesis.

IMPRESSION

- Status post previous right nephrectomy; no evidence of recurrent retroperitoneal mass or lymphadenopathy.
- Peripelvic cysts at the left kidney; otherwise the left kidney is unremarkable.
- Normal appearing liver.
- Two ventral hernias within the mid and the lower abdomen.

DICTATED BY: Dr. Amy Weissen

REAL WORLD REPORT QUESTIONS

The following exercises review the medical terms used in the preceding medical report.

1. The first section of the report describes a CT scan of the abdomen.

   a. CT is the medical abbreviation for _____.

   b. Using directional terminology, describe the location of the abdomen.

   _____

   _____

   _____

2. What organs were found in the abdominal scan?

   _____

   _____

   _____

3. The report indicated a "small ventral hernia in the midline of the midabdomen.

   a. Is this hernia located toward the front or toward the back of the abdomen?

   _____.

   b. Is this hernia located in the middle of, left of center of, or right of center of the abdomen?

   _____.

4. The report cited an "anterior abdominal incision in the midline." In nonmedical terms, describe the location of the incision.

   _____

   _____

   _____

5. Describe the location of the pelvis.

   _____

   _____

   _____

6. The report states that "tissue structures are somewhat limited at the right lower pelvis." Using the medical terminology for the abdominopelvic regions and quadrants, give alternate terms for this specific area.

   a. _____

   b. _____

7. *Retroperitoneal* is a common word used in medical reports to describe structures in the abdominopelvic region.

   a. Word part *retro-* means _____.

   b. Word part *peritoneo-* means _____.

   c. What does *retroperitoneal* mean?

   _____.

8. If the prefix *nephr-* means "kidney" and the suffix *-ectomy* means "surgical removal," what word from the report means removal of a kidney?

   _____

LEVEL ONE: REVIEWING FACTS AND TERMS USING RECALL

Select the best answer to each of the following questions.

1. The study of body structure is termed _____.
   a. anatomy
   b. physiology
   c. biology
   d. pathophysiology

2. The study of body function is termed _____.
   a. anatomy
   b. physiology
   c. systemic anatomy
   d. homeostasis

3. _____ is the term used to describe an anatomic shape.
   a. Somatotype
   b. Anatomy
   c. Axial
   d. Morphology

4. Embryology is the study of _____.
   a. disease processes
   b. human development after birth
   c. human development in utero until the end of the eighth week
   d. body structures

Match the system with its primary function.

_b_ 5. nervous   a. movement

_c_ 6. endocrine   b. integration

_a_ 7. cardiovascular   c. hormone secretion

_e_ 8. muscular   d. nutrient transport

_f_ 9. urinary   e. protection

_e_ 10. skeletal   f. waste removal

Select the best answer to each of the following questions.

11. The membrane covering the lung is the _____.
    a. parietal pleura
    b. visceral pleura
    c. pericardial pleura
    d. serous pleura

12. The _____ peritoneum adheres to the abdominal wall.
    a. parietal
    b. visceral
    c. pericardial
    d. pleural

Match the somatotype with its chief characteristic(s).

____ 13. I endomorph   a. short and fat

____ 14. II mesomorph   b. tall and thin

____ 15. III ectomorph   c. heavily muscled

Select the best answer to each of the following questions.

16. Identify the word part(s) that mean(s) "head."
    a. cyt-, cyto-
    b. etio-
    c. cephal-, cephalo-
    d. bucco-

17. Identify the correct sequence, from smallest to largest, of the levels of organization.
    a. cell → organ → tissue → system → organism
    b. tissue → cell → organ → system → organism
    c. cell → molecule → organ → system → tissue
    d. cell → tissue → organ → system → organism

Define the following word parts.

18. acr-, acro- = _____

19. homeo- = _____

20. parieto- = _____

21. pelv-, pelvio-, pelvo- = _____

22. brachi-, brachio- = _____

Supply a directional term to make each statement correct.

23. The right arm is _____ to the left arm.

24. The feet are _____ to the head.

25. The elbow is _____ to the hand.

Supply a regional name to make each statement correct.

26. The neck is called the _____ region.

27. The _____ region refers to the posterior knee.

28. The upper arm is the _____ region.

LEVEL TWO: REVIEWING CONCEPTS

For each of the following terms, what term has the opposite meaning?

29. distal / _____

30. deep / _____

31. anterior / _____

32. inferior / _____

Match the body system with organs found in that system.

_____ 33. urinary   a. esophagus and stomach

_____ 34. endocrine   b. kidneys and bladder

_____ 35. digestive   c. trachea and lungs

_____ 36. respiratory   d. thyroid and thymus

Select the best answer to each of the following questions.

37. This type of plane divides the body into left and right halves.

    a. sagittal

    b. frontal

    c. coronal

    d. midsagittal

38. This type of plane divides the body into anterior and posterior portions.

    a. coronal or frontal

    b. coronal or sagittal

    c. transverse or horizontal

    d. frontal or median

39. In which region is the bladder located?

    a. lumbar region

    b. hypogastric region

    c. inguinal region

    c. epigastric region

40. The lungs are located in the _____ cavity.

    a. abdominal

    b. pelvic

    c. thoracic

    d. vertebral

41. Signs of an infection may include _____.

    a. fever

    b. tiredness

    c. sweating

    d. A and C

Match the cellular organelle with its description.

_____ 42. ribosome   a. power house of cell

_____ 43. nucleus   b. protein synthesis

_____ 44. nucleolus   c. contains DNA

_____ 45. mitochondrion   d. contains RNA

Identify the correctly spelled term in each set.

46. _____
   a. adominopelvic
   b. abdamenopelvic
   c. abdominopelvic
   d. abdomialpelvic

47. _____
   a. iliac
   b. illiac
   c. ileaic
   d. illeac

48. _____
   a. saggital
   b. sagattal
   c. saggittal
   d. sagittal

49. _____
   a. popliteal
   b. poplliteal
   c. poplitial
   d. popplitial

50. _____
   a. hypochondriak
   b. hypochondriack
   c. hypochondriac
   d. hypocondriac

Provide a medical term to complete a meaningful analogy.

51. Atoms are to molecules as cells are to _____.
   a. organelles
   b. tissues
   c. organs
   d. systems

52. Cranial is to skull as gluteal is to _____.
   a. head
   b. chest
   c. buttocks
   d. knee

53. Calcaneal is to calcaneus as sternal is to _____.
   a. sternum
   b. stern
   c. sternus
   d. sternial

What is the plural form for each given term?

54. coxa _____

55. phalanx _____

56. umbilicus _____

What is the singular form for each given term?

57. crura _____

58. buccae _____

59. pelves _____

60. mitochondria _____

LEVEL THREE: THINKING CRITICALLY

Select the best answer to each of the following questions.

61. Nursing notes indicate that sutures were placed superior to the right tarsus, inferior to the patellar region. Identify the location in common terms.
   a. right shin
   b. right thigh
   c right forearm
   d. right shoulder

62. Dr. Cutter is about to amputate a patient's left leg inferior to the patella. Standing at the foot of the patient's bed, facing the patient, the leg that is to be removed should be closest to _____ .

    a Dr. Cutter's left arm.

    b. Dr. Cutter's right arm.

63. Mikey has had abdominal aches all evening. He thought it was just gas pains from eating too many beans. Since the pain was so severe, he went to the emergency clinic. After palpating the hypogastric region, the physician concluded it was appendicitis. What probably lead to this diagnosis?

    _____

    _____

    _____

    _____

    _____

    _____

KEY TERMS SPELLING TEST FROM CD-ROM

Use the CD-ROM to test yourself on the spelling of key terms from this chapter. Listen to the terms and write them on a separate sheet of paper. Use a medical dictionary to check your answers.

ANSWERS

WORD GROUPING

Definition	Word Part
abdomen, abdominal	abdomin-, abdomino-
anterior, front	antero-
arm	brachi-, brachio-
back, backward, behind	retro-
before, in front of	ante-
body	somat-, somatico-, somato-
body wall or parietal bone	parieto-
breasts	mamm-, mammo-
cause	etio-
cell	cyt-, cyto-
cheek	bucco-
chemistry	chem-, chemo-
chest (thorax)	thorac-, thoracico-, thoraco-
disease	path-, patho-, -pathy
ear	ot-, oto-
embryo	embry-, embryo-
extremity, end	acr-, acro-
face	facio-
foot or child	ped-, pedi-, pedo-
form, shape	morph-, morpho-
head	cephal-, cephalo-
heart	cardi-, cardio-
heel, calcaneus	calcane-, calcaneo-
ilium, hip bone	ili-, ilio-
lateral, to one side	latero-
lung membrane, side	pleur-, pleura-, pleuro-
mouth	oro-
neck, cervix	cervic-, cervico-
nose	nas-, naso-
nucleus	nucl-, nucleo-
occiput, back part of head	occipit-, occipito-
origin, beginning process	-genesis
pelvis	pelv-, pelvio-, pelvo-
peritoneum	peritoneo-
physiological	physi-, physio-
posterior, at the back	postero-
proximal	prox-, proxi-, proximo-
pubic	pubo-
rib	cost-, costi-, costo-
sacrum	sacro-

Definition	Word Part
same, steady	homeo-
skull, cranium	crani-, cranio-
spine	spin-, spino-
sternum	stern-, sterno-
tarsus (root of foot)	tars-, tarso-
tissue	histio-, histo-
vertebra (backbone)	vertebr-, vertebro-
viscera (internal organs)	viscero-

WORD BUILDING

Word Part	Meaning	Common or Known Word	Example Medical Term
antero-	anterior, front	anterior	anterior
cardi-, cardio-	heart	cardiac arrest	pericardium
chem- chemo-	chemistry	chemistry	chemotherapy
embry-, embryo-	embryo	embryo	embryo
-genesis	origin, beginning process	genesis	osteogenesis
homeo-	same, steady	homeopathy	homeostasis
latero-	lateral, to one side	lateral	lateral
mamm-, mammo-	breasts	mammary	mammary gland
nas-, naso-	nose	nasal	nasopharynx
nucl-, nucleo-	nucleus	nucleus	nucleus
retro-	back, backward, behind	retrofit	retroperitoneal
vertebr-, vertebro-	vertebra (backbone)	vertebrate	vertebral column

KEY TERM PRACTICE

Anatomy and Physiology Defined
1. histology
2. pathology
3. physiology

Cells and Organizational Structure
1. cell
2. tissue
3. organelles

Human Body Systems
1. integumentary, skeletal, nervous, muscular, endocrine, digestive, urinary, reproductive, respiratory, lymphatic/immune, and cardiovascular
2. nervous; endocrine

Body Membranes
1. visceral
2. parietal

Somatotypes
1. somatotype
2. II mesomorph

Anatomic Position and Body Cavities
1. The person is standing erect, facing forward, with the arms at the sides and the palms facing forward.
2. abdominopelvic
3. appendicular; axial

Directional Terms
1. distal
2. superior
3. posterior
4. superficial

Abdominopelvic Quadrants and Regions
1. regions
2. quadrants

Anatomic Planes
1. a. transverse; b. horizontal
2. anterior; posterior
3. median; midsagittal

Anatomic Terms
1. tibial
2. antecubital
3. knee

Signs and Symptoms
1. symptoms
2. signs

Clinical Tests and Diagnostic Procedures
1. palpation
2. auscultation

Pathology
1. index
2. pathologist
3. epidemiologist

Treatments
1. physical rehabilitation
2. chemotherapy

ANSWERS TO CASE STUDY

1. b is the correct answer.
   - a is incorrect because there are two kidneys (one on the left, and one on the right), he had his right one removed.
   - c and d are incorrect because "nephrectomy" refers to a kidney removal.
2. b is the correct answer.
   - a and c are incorrect because endomorphs are typically short and plump and mesomorphs are generally well muscled.
   - d is incorrect because the endomorph somatotype is clearly characterized.
3. a is the correct answer.
   - b is incorrect because the bladder is found in the hypogastric region.
   - c is incorrect because the lungs are found in the thoracic region.
   - d is incorrect because the heart is found in the mediastinum of the chest.
4. c is the correct answer.
   - a, b, and d are all incorrect; these technologies refer to other techniques for body visualization.

ANSWERS TO REAL WORLD REPORT

1. a. computed tomography; b. The abdomen is located in the inferior cavity of the body trunk. It is bordered superiorly by the diaphragm.
2. Organs found in this CT abdominal scan were the spleen, adrenal glands, pancreas, liver, kidneys, and small bowel.
3. a. toward the front; b. middle of the abdomen
4. An incision had been made on the front of the body, along the center of the belly.
5. The pelvis is located inferiorly to the abdominal region and is bordered by the pelvic bones.
6. a. right inguinal (iliac) region; b. right lower quadrant (RLQ)
7. a. behind; b. peritoneum; c. behind the peritoneum
8. nephrectomy

ANSWERS TO REVIEW AND APPLICATION: THREE-LEVEL LEARNING SYSTEM

Level One: Reviewing Facts and Terms Using Recall

1. a
2. b
3. d
4. c
5. b
6. c
7. d
8. a
9. f
10. e
11. b
12. a
13. a
14. c
15. b
16. c
17. d
18. extremity, end
19. same, steady
20. wall, parietal
21. pelvis
22. arm
23. contralateral
24. inferior
25. proximal
26. cervical
27. popliteal
28. brachial

Level Two: Reviewing Concepts

29. proximal
30. superficial
31. posterior

32. superior
33. b
34. d
35. a
36. c
37. d
38. a
39. b
40. c
41. d
42. b
43. c
44. d
45. a
46. c
47. a
48. d
49. a
50. c
51. b
52. c
53. a
54. coxae
55. phalanges
56. umbilici
57. crus
58. bucca
59. pelvis
60. mitochondrion

Level Three: Thinking Critically

61. a
62. b
63. The appendix is found in this specific region.

3

Radiology

OBJECTIVES

After completing this chapter, you should be able to:

1. Define the meaning of word parts related to radiology.
2. Explain basic radiology terms.
3. Describe components of diagnostic radiology, ultrasound, radiation oncology, and nuclear medicine.
4. Explain clinical tests and diagnostic procedures related to diagnostic radiology, ultrasound, radiation oncology, and nuclear medicine.
5. Explain variations in diagnostic procedures throughout the lifespan.
6. Define abbreviations related to the radiology.
7. Define terms used in medical reports.
8. Correctly define, spell, and pronounce the chapter's medical terms.

INTRODUCTION

Radiology is the branch of science dealing with the medical use of imaging techniques to diagnose and treat disease. Examination of body structures is made using ionizing radiation, radionuclides, other forms of penetrating radiation, nuclear magnetic resonance, and ultrasound. This is an area of health care with broadening applicability. As technology increases and noninvasive procedures replace exploratory surgery, this field will continue to expand. Interventional radiology, in which fluoroscopy (x-ray examination using a fluoroscope), computed tomography (CT), and ultrasound are used to guide percutaneous procedures, is becoming a leading therapeutic measure for treatment of disease. Biopsies, fluid drainage, catheter insertion, and vessel stenting and dilation are all performed using interventional radiology. Furthermore, demand for skilled professionals in every aspect of this area from billing and coding to technicians and physicians is currently greater than the supply. This chapter focuses on the relationship between anatomy and physiology and the numerous clinical tests and diagnostic procedures related to radiology, including diagnostic radiology, nuclear medicine, radiation oncology, and ultrasound.

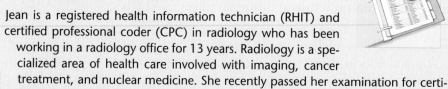

Professional Profile: Certified Professional Coder

Jean is a registered health information technician (RHIT) and certified professional coder (CPC) in radiology who has been working in a radiology office for 13 years. Radiology is a specialized area of health care involved with imaging, cancer treatment, and nuclear medicine. She recently passed her examination for certification in radiology coding. To qualify for the RHIT examination, she had to graduate from a two-year associate-degree program accredited by the Commission on Accreditation of Allied Health Education Programs (CAAHEP). The RHIT exam is offered by the American Health Information Management Association (AHIMA). The American College of Radiology (ACR) accredited the radiology coding certification.

Jean's educational background and work experience are primarily within health care. After high school, she worked in the medical records office at the hospital while she completed her associate degree in health information technology. Coursework included *International Classification of Diseases* (ICD) and *Current Procedural Terminology* (CPT) (surgical and nonsurgical) coding procedures, the diagnosis related group (DRG) system, anatomy, physiology, medical terminology, legal aspects of health information coding, and health information systems. Jean has little direct contact with patients.

Codes are assigned to each procedure performed by the physician. Coders must rely on knowledge of disease processes and anatomy and have skills in using the classification manuals to supply the appropriate code for hundreds of procedures. The DRG and CPT code determine reimbursement amounts for patients who are covered by Medicare and other insurance. Sometimes Jean needs to communicate directly with physicians to clarify diagnoses or to obtain additional information for the medical record.

Coders generally work 40 hours per week in a quiet, comfortable office spending most of the time reading medical reports and sitting at a computer monitor logging information. Paying attention to details and coding accurately are essential in this job. Jean keeps abreast of new information by attending seminars and conferences sponsored by the Society of Cardiovascular & Interventional Radiology (SCVIR), Radiology Business Management Association (RBMA), and American Healthcare Radiology Administrators (AHRA).

MEDICAL TERM PARTS

WORD PARTS

Medical term prefixes, suffixes, and combining forms related to radiology, nuclear medicine, and diagnostic ultrasound are introduced in this section.

Word Parts	Meaning
brachy-	short
cine-	motion picture
dacry-, dacryo-	tears, lacrimal apparatus
electro-	electricity
end-, endo-	internal, within
fluo-	flow
-gram	recording, usually by an instrument
-graph	something written, instrument for making a recording
grapho-, -graphy	writing, description
nucle-, nucleo-	nuclear, nucleus
onco-, oncho-	tumor
phon-, phono-	sound
porto-	portal
ptyal-, ptyalo-	salivary glands, saliva
pyr-, pyro-	fever, fire, heat
radio-	radiation
sial-, sialo-	saliva
son-, sono-	sound
spectro-	spectrum
tel-, tele-, telo-	distant
-tome	section
ultra-	beyond, excess
xer-, xero-	dry

WORD ETYMOLOGY

Some words have Greek or Latin roots but are not true word parts. This section lists those that are used as medical terms.

Word	Definition
gramma	character, mark
grapho	to write
onkos	bulk, mass

MEDICAL TERM PARTS USED AS PREFIXES

Prefix	Definition
brachy-	short
cine-	motion picture
electro-	electricity
fluo-	flow
grapho-	writing, description
porto-	portal
radio-	radiation
spectro-	spectrum
ultra-	beyond, excess

MEDICAL TERM PARTS USED AS SUFFIXES

Suffix	Definition
-gram	recording, usually by an instrument
-graph	something written, instrument for making a recording
-graphy	writing, description
-tome	section

WORD GROUPING

Using the "Medical Term Parts" tables, identify the prefix, suffix, or combining form for each of the following definitions. The first one has been done as an example.

Definition	Word Part
motion picture	cine-
beyond, excess	
distant	
dry	
electricity	
fever, fire, heat	
flow	
internal, within	
nuclear, nucleus	
portal	

Definition	Word Part
radiation	
recording, usually by an instrument	
saliva	
salivary glands, saliva	
section	
short	
something written, instrument for making a recording	
sound	A. B.
spectrum	
tears, lacrimal apparatus	
tumor	
writing, description	

WORD BUILDING

Word parts, introduced in the "Medical Term Parts" section, are listed in the following table. For this exercise, first supply the meaning of each word part, then use the word part to build a word you already know. The word you list under "Common or Known Word" does not have to be a medical term; a commonly used word is fine. Be sure, however, that the word correctly reflects the meaning. The first one has been done as an example. Check your answers in a dictionary.

Word Part	Meaning	Common or Known Word	Example Medical Term
brachy-	short	brachycephalic	brachytherapy
cine-			cineradiography
electro-			electromyography
end-, endo-			endoscopic catheterization
fluo-			fluoroscopy
-gram			sonogram
-graph			angiograph
grapho-, -graphy			arteriography
nucle-, nucleo-			nuclear medicine
onco-, oncho-			oncology
phon-, phono-			phonocardiography
pyr-, pyro-			hyperpyrexia
radio-			radiology
son-, sono-			sonography

Word Part	Meaning	Common or Known Word	Example Medical Term
tel-, tele-, telo-			teletherapy
-tome			tomography
ultra-			ultrasound
xer-, xero-			xeromammography

RADIOLOGY

Radiology Preview

Radiology is the science of radiation and radioactive substances and their application to medicine. The field has expanded to include various forms of imaging techniques that may not necessarily use radiation yet are used to view body structures. As a diagnostic tool, radiology has been in use since the early 1900s, and diagnostic imaging encompasses all imaging modalities used in radiology, such as ultrasound, magnetic resonance imaging, computed tomography, mammography, positron emission tomography, and traditional x-rays (radiographs). A **radiologist** is a physician specializing in the diagnostic and/or therapeutic use of x-rays, radionuclides, and other imaging techniques. Diagnostic radiologists assist in treatments by inserting catheters and delivering therapy through interventional methods. Radiologists are the professionals who interpret images, regardless of the modality used.

An imaging technique that uses high-frequency sound waves reflecting off internal body parts to create pictures for identifying the nature or cause of a disorder or for recognition and treatment purposes is termed **diagnostic ultrasound. Radiation oncology** is the treatment of cancer using radioactive substances. **Nuclear medicine**, the branch of medicine in which radioactive materials are used to diagnose and treat diseases, is a more recent addition to the medical arsenal. Interventional radiology, which uses guided procedures, is advancing the treatment of disease and enhancing health by providing less-invasive procedures. Various forms of radiology, nuclear medicine, diagnostic ultrasound, and radiation oncology are described in this chapter.

FACT: It takes 10–12 years of training to become a radiologist!

Key Terms	Definitions
radiology (ray dee OL uh jee)	branch of medicine that deals with radioactive substances, x-rays, and ionizing radiation for treating and diagnosing disease
radiologist (ray dee OL uh jist)	physician specializing in radiology
diagnostic (dye ug NOS tik) ultrasound	use of high-frequency sound waves in diagnosing and treating conditions
radiation oncology (ray dee AY shun ong KOL uh jee)	use of radioactive substances for treating cancer
nuclear (NEW klee ur) medicine	branch of medicine that deals with the use of radioisotopes in diagnosis and therapy

Key Term Practice: Radiology Preview

1. The use of high-frequency sound waves for diagnosing and treating disorders is termed _____.

2. _____ is the health-care branch that uses radioactive materials for treating and diagnosing disease.

Radiology Basic Terms

In 1901, German physicist Wilhelm K. Roentgen won the Nobel Prize in Physics for his discovery of x-rays in November 1895. Thus the eponym *Roentgen rays* is another term for x-rays. An x-ray is an electromagnetic radiation that penetrates various thickness of solids, ionizes tissues, and causes some substances to fluoresce (glow). A photograph taken with Roentgen rays (x-rays) is known as a radiograph or x-ray (also spelled X-ray, but always with a hyphen).

Radiographs (x-rays) are photographs made by projecting x-rays or gamma-rays through the body and onto sensitive film (Fig. 3-1). They are frequently used to diagnose musculoskeletal and lung disorders. To highlight organs and tissues during these diagnostic procedures, various media are often used. Because it absorbs radiation to a different degree than body tissues, a **contrast medium** highlights radiographic images of structures or spaces. This type of medium is **radiopaque**, impervious to light or radiation, making the outline of the body part easier to visualize on x-ray images. Commonly used contrast media are barium for the gastrointestinal tract; water-soluble iodinated compounds for blood vessels, glands, and genitourinary imaging; air for a variety of images; and paramagnetic (weakly magnetized) substances for magnetic resonance imaging.

Knowing a few basic radiology terms is essential to understanding fundamental procedures while providing the foundation for their application in medicine. Atomic nuclei that emit alpha-, beta-, or gamma-rays are termed **radioactive.** Radioactive substances give off energy in the form of streams of particles, owing to the decay of their unstable atoms. The **half-life** ($T_{1/2}$) refers to the time a radioactive substance takes to lose half its radioactivity through decay. The half-life of a particular radioactive material determines the substance's use as a radiotracer and is used to calculate appropriate dosages. A **radiotracer** is a radioactive substance introduced into the body as a detector or tag to locate diseased cells or tissue. The radiolabeled chemical is generally

> *According to the American Society of Radiologic Technologists, there are currently 30,000 job vacancies nationwide!*

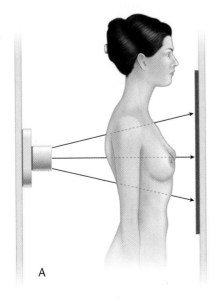

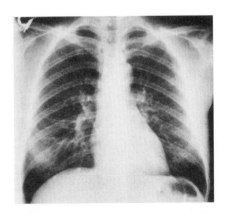

A

B

FIGURE 3-1
Radiography technique (**A**). Plain chest x-ray (**B**). (Image provided by LifeART, © 2006 Lippincott Williams & Wilkins. All rights reserved.)

a **radionuclide,** which is a radioactive isotope of artificial or natural origin. Isotopes are forms of the same element with the same atomic number but different numbers of neutrons. The absorption of the radiotracer by a tissue is known as **uptake.**

Units used to measure radioactive material are grays, millicuries, and microcuries. An internationally accepted system of units of measurement used for scientific work is known as the International System (SI or Système International d'Unités). **Gray (Gy)** is the derived SI unit for the absorbed dose of ionizing radiation. Radioactive materials are administered in units called **millicurie (mCi)** and **microcurie (μCi).**

Finally, the side effects of radiation exposure require consideration. Adverse reactions are commonly experienced by patients undergoing oncology radiation and include alopecia, mucositis, xerostomia, nausea and emesis, and myelosuppression. Alopecia is hair loss, especially from the head, and mucositis refers to inflammation of the mucous membranes. Dry mouth, **xerostomia,** often accompanies mucositis. Nausea is the unsettling feeling in the stomach that accompanies the urge to vomit; emesis refers to expelling the contents of the stomach through the mouth. Reduced development of white blood cells and platelets from the bone marrow is called myelosuppression.

Key Terms	Definitions
radiograph (RAY dee oh graf)	images produced on film by x-rays passing through a body part; another term for x-rays
x-rays	images produced on film by x-rays passing through a body part; another term for radiographs
contrast medium	substance introduced into the body that is opaque to x-rays, thereby allowing a structure's image to appear on film
radiopaque (ray dee oh PAKE)	impenetrable by light or x-rays
radioactive	atomic nuclei emitting subatomic particles
half-life	period in which the number of atoms or radioactivity of a substance decreases by 50%
radiotracer	radiolabeled chemical used as a detector in diagnostic tests
radionuclide (RAY dee oh NEW klide)	radioactive isotope of artificial or natural origin
uptake	absorption of something, such as a radionuclide, by tissue
gray	unit of measurement for radiation absorbed by and delivered to tissues
millicurie (MIL i kew ree)	amount of radioactive substance that undergoes 3.7×10^7 disintegrations per second
microcurie (MIGH kroh kew ree)	amount of radioactive substance that undergoes 3.7×10^4 disintegrations per second
xerostomia (zeer oh STOH mee uh)	dry mouth

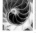
Key Term Practice: Radiology Basic Terms

1. Absorption of an introduced substance in the body is termed _____.

2. A dye or substance that cannot be penetrated by x-rays is known as a/an _____.

THE CLINICAL DIMENSION

Pathology Related to Radiology

This section is organized according to area of radiology. Diagnostic radiology, along with its subspecialty components, is described first. Diagnostic ultrasound, including its diverse applications, is discussed next. Finally, elements of radiation oncology and nuclear medicine are introduced. When appropriate, a procedure is explained in context with the specific body system for which it is used. This organization reflects real-world radiologic practice.

Diagnostic Radiology

Diagnostic radiology, also called diagnostic imaging, is the branch of medicine that determines the nature of a patient's disease through x-rays, radioactive substances, nuclear magnetic resonance, ultrasound, and other forms of ionizing radiation. In some cases, it also provides treatment for pathology. **Interventional radiology** is a subspecialty that uses fluoroscopy, computed tomography, and ultrasound to guide percutaneous procedures, such as performing biopsies, draining fluids, inserting catheters, and dilating or stenting narrowed ducts or vessels. The following text describes a number of diagnostic and interventional techniques. Box 3-1 provides a list of diagnostic radiology procedures.

BOX 3-1. *Diagnostic Radiology Procedures*

Angiocardiography	Digital subtraction angiography	Percutaneous transhepatic cholangiography (PTC; PTHC)
Angiography	Diskography	
Antegrade pyelography	Duodenography	Percutaneous transhepatic portography
Aortography	Electromyography	
Arteriography	Endoscopic catheterization	Percutaneous transluminal angioplasty (PTA)
Arthrography	Epididymography	
Barium enema, lower gastrointestinal (GI)	Hysterosalpingography	Percutaneous transluminal balloon angioplasty (PCTA)
Barium swallow, upper gastrointestinal (GI)	Intravenous pyelography (IVP)	Phonocardiography
Bronchography	Laryngography	Ptyalography
Cardiac catheterization	Lymphangiography	Pyelography
Cholangiography	Magnetic resonance angiography (MRA)	Radiography
Cholecystography		Retrograde pyelography (RP)
Cinefluoroscopy	Magnetic resonance imaging (MRI)	Shuntogram
Cineradiography		Sialography
Cisternography	Magnetic resonance spectroscopy	Splenoportography
Computed tomography (CT)	Mammary ductogram	Transcatheter biopsy
Contrast studies	Mammary galactogram	Transluminal atherectomy
Corpora cavernosography	Mammography	Urethrocystography
Cystography	Myelography	Urography
Cystourethrography	Pelvimetry	Vasography
Dacryocystography	Percutaneous needle biopsy	Venography (phlebography)
Densitometry/ photodensitometry		Vesiculography
		X-ray

Key Terms	Definitions
diagnostic radiology (dye ug NOS tik ray dee OL uh jee)	use of x-rays and other ionizing radiation forms for the diagnosis and treatment of disease
interventional radiology (in ter VEN shun ul ray dee OL uh jee)	specialty area of radiology that employs catheters, scopes, and various procedures to guide instruments for the diagnosis and treatment of pathology

Key Term Practice: Diagnostic Radiology

1. A specialty area of radiology that uses catheters and scopes for the diagnosis and treatment of diseased states is called _____.

2. What is the alternate term for *diagnostic imaging*?

_____.

Radiography

The examination of any part of the body using x-rays is termed **radiography.** A shunt is a surgically created bypass or diversion. A radiographic study to determine shunt placement is referred to as a **shuntogram.**

By the year 2008, more than 50,000 additional radiology technologists will be needed!

Joints can be imaged via arthrography or diskography. **Arthrography** is an x-ray of the joint space taken after a contrast medium has been injected into the joint capsule to enhance the image of the intra-articular structures. (An articulation is a joint.) Arthrography is used to diagnose knee and shoulder injuries. X-ray examination of intervertebral disks (pads of fibrocartilage between the vertebrae) undertaken after the direct injection of a contrast medium into the structures is termed **diskography.**

Key Terms	Definitions
radiography (ray dee OG ruh fee)	making and using radiographs (x-rays) for medical purposes
shuntogram (SHUNT oh gram)	x-ray examination of an artificially created passage to determine shunt placement
arthrography (ahr THROG ruh fee)	examination of a joint's interior after the injection of a contrast medium
diskography (disk OG ruh fee)	examination of the intervertebral disks after the direct injection of a contrast medium

Key Term Practice: Radiography

1. The word part *arthro-* means "joint"; the word part _____ means "writing, description"; therefore, the term _____ means "radiographic assessment of a joint."

2. Radiographic evaluation of intervertebral disks is termed _____.

Radiography in Motion

Organs in motion can be viewed using specialized imaging techniques. Radiography of an organ while it is moving is called **cineradiography** or **cinefluoroscopy**. The term cineradiography is derived from the word part *cine-*, which means "motion picture." A fluorescent screen of crystals excited by x-rays produces an image. This technique is commonly used to obtain views of the heart and gastrointestinal tract and to assist in catheter placement.

Key Terms	Definitions
cineradiography (sin e ray dee OG ruh fee)	radiography of an organ in motion; another term for cinefluoroscopy
cinefluoroscopy (sin e floor OS kuh pee)	radiography of an organ in motion; another term for cineradiography

Key Term Practice: Radiography in Motion

1. The word part *cine-* means _____; the word part *radio-* means _____; and the word part _____ means "description." Thus the term _____ describes the procedure of viewing an organ in motion.

2. In the term *cinefluoroscopy*, the word part *fluo-* means _____.

Tomography

The term **tomography** refers to sectional radiography that highlights structures in one selected plane at a time as the x-ray tube moves, leaving structures in other planes unfocused. **Computed tomography** (CT) is an imaging modality that uses a moving scanner and detector that encircle the patient; a computer creates cross-sectional x-ray images. This procedure is useful for diagnosing conditions of the brain, abdomen, and chest. It is known by several terms, including computer-assisted tomography (CAT), computed axial tomography (CAT), and computerized axial tomography (CAT) (Fig. 3-2). A technique combining CT with angiography to view blood or lymphatic vessels is termed **computed tomographic angiography.**

CT pelvimetry is measurement of the inlet and outlet diameters of the bony pelvis. Pelvimetry is performed to assess whether there will be any difficulty during vaginal childbirth. It is also called radiocephalpelvimetry.

Key Terms	Definitions
tomography (toh MOG ruh fee)	technique in which images in certain planes are focused while images in other planes are blurred
computed tomography (toh MOG ruh fee)	technique for producing images of body cross sections
computed tomographic angiography (toh moh GRAF ik an jee OG ruh fee)	combination CT and angiography for visualizing blood or lymphatic vessels
CT pelvimetry (pel VIM e tree)	measurement of the dimensions of the bony pelvis using CT scans; another term for radiocephalpelvimetry

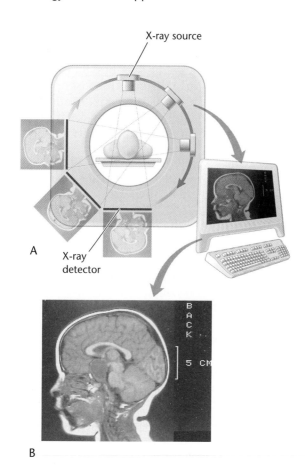

FIGURE 3-2
Computed tomography technique (**A**). CT scan of the head (**B**). The scanner takes a series of cross-sectional images one slice at a time in a full-circle rotation. A computer calculates and converts each image into a picture on a screen. (Reprinted with permission from Becker KL, Bilezikian JP, Brenner WJ, et al. Principles and practice of endocrinology and metabolism, 3rd ed. Philadelphia: Lippincott Williams & Wilkins, 2001.)

Key Term Practice: Tomography

1. A procedure that combines CT imaging with angiography is termed _____.

2. A technique for producing cross-sectional images of the body is known as _____.

Catheterization, Biopsy, and Percutaneous Radiographic Procedures

Catheter placement is an area that requires knowledge of anatomy. The clinician must understand the anatomy related to the puncture site and final catheter position as well as the pathways of the vascular systems. The **vascular family** refers to a group of vessels fed by a primary branch of the aorta or branches of the vessel punctured. With respect to the arterial system, **nonselective arterial catheter placement** means that the needle is placed directly into a vessel and is not manipulated into a branch or that the catheter is negotiated into the thoracic and/or abdominal aorta from any approach. A **selective arterial catheter placement** describes a procedure in which the needle is manipulated into another portion of the arterial system from which it was originally inserted.

Vessel ordering describes the amount of work required to position a catheter into its destination. Vessel ordering is identified as first order, second order, third order, etc., depending on the pathway taken. Placing the catheter into a primary branch is described as first order; passing the catheter into secondary or tertiary branches is labeled second or third order, respectively. The approach to the destination vessel is usually accomplished by puncturing a readily accessible vessel. The term *puncture* is commonly referred to as a "stick."

In regard to the venous system, **nonselective venous** describes the procedure in which the needle is placed directly into a vessel with no manipulation into a branch. **Selective venous** procedures require manipulation beyond the puncture site. Direct puncture sites are peripheral veins, the inferior vena cava, the superior vena cava, and the vena cava.

The removal of a living tissue sample for laboratory examination is called a biopsy. During a **transcatheter biopsy**, a tissue sample is taken via a thin, flexible tube—called a catheter—which is inserted into the body. The term *percutaneous* refers to something being administered or absorbed "through the skin." **Percutaneous needle biopsy** is excision of tissue performed with a needle through a skin incision.

A generalized procedure using an instrument called an endoscope, which transmits light and carries images of the internal body back to the observer, is termed **endoscopic catheterization.** The long tube is usually inserted through a small incision. Endoscopic catheterization is used for diagnostic examination and surgical procedures.

Another type of tissue removal is transluminal atherectomy. *Transluminal* means "across or through a lumen," which is the space inside a blood vessel, duct, or tube. A lipid deposit or atherosclerotic plaque is known as an atheroma. The surgical removal or catheterization of an atheroma is called atherectomy. Hence **transluminal atherectomy** is the removal of plaque or lipid deposits from the inner lining of a structure.

An operation that enlarges narrowed vascular lumen via a balloon on the tip of a catheter is known as **percutaneous transluminal balloon angioplasty** (PCTA) or **percutaneous transluminal angioplasty** (PTA). Once the catheter tip reaches the blockage, the balloon is enlarged to crush the obstruction, thereby restoring circulation. Figure 3-3 demonstrates this procedure.

During a **cardiac catheterization**, a tubular instrument is passed through an artery or vein to the heart for visualization. Blood samples can be withdrawn, pressures within heart and vessels can be measured, and contrast media can be injected for angiography. Images obtained by the procedure enable the physician to identify cardiac structures and possible obstructions. Cardiac catheterization is used to diagnose heart disorders, anomalies, and stenosed (narrowed, occluded) vessels.

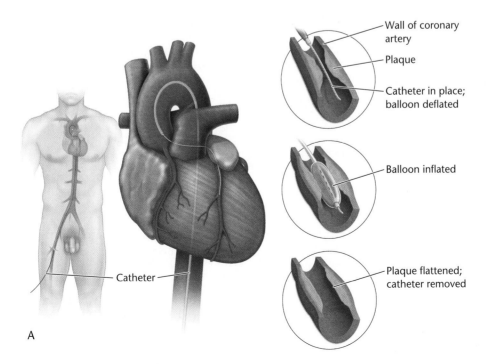

Wall of coronary artery

Plaque

Catheter in place; balloon deflated

Balloon inflated

Plaque flattened; catheter removed

Catheter

A

FIGURE 3-3
Coronary angioplasty. A guide catheter is threaded into the coronary artery (**A**). A balloon catheter is then inserted through the occluded artery, and the balloon is inflated and deflated until the plaque is flattened and the vessel is open.

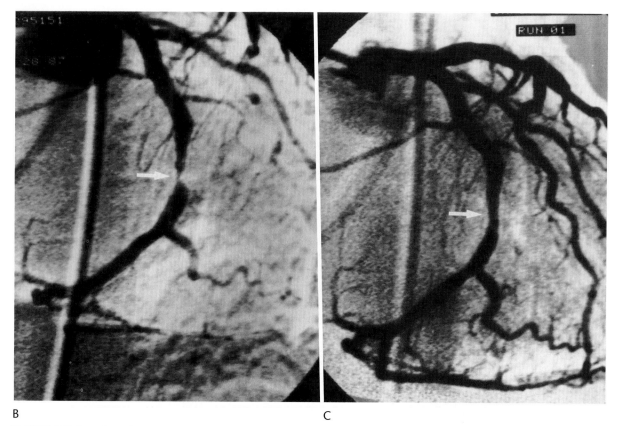

B

C

FIGURE 3-3 *(continued)*
The artery, before the balloon has been inflated, is shown (**B**). After the procedure, the vessel is open (**C**). (Reprinted with permission from Snell RS. Clinical anatomy, 7th ed. Baltimore: Lippincott Williams & Wilkins, 2003.)

Percutaneous transhepatic cholangiography (PTHC or PTC) is radiography of bile ducts via needle puncture. For this procedure, contrast radiography of the biliary system is performed by injection of radiopaque dye through a percutaneously placed needle that is inserted into an intrahepatic bile duct (Fig. 3-4).

Radiographic depiction of the hepatic (liver) portal venous system after injection of contrast medium into the spleen or portal vein is termed **percutaneous transhepatic portography.** The portal system refers to the hepatic portal vein and its tributaries found in the liver. The passage of blood from gastrointestinal (GI) capillaries and the spleen to the liver is the portal circulation. Several routes provide portal access. The catheter can be positioned into the portal vein via nearly any route using transhepatic, transvenous, or trans-splenic vessels.

Key Terms	Definitions
vascular family	group of vessels fed by a primary vessel
nonselective arterial catheter placement	catheter placed into an arterial vessel and not manipulated to another arterial site
selective arterial catheter placement	catheter placed into another portion of the arterial system from which it was originally inserted
vessel ordering	term describing the amount of work required to place a catheter at its destination
nonselective venous	catheter placed into a vein and not manipulated to another venous site

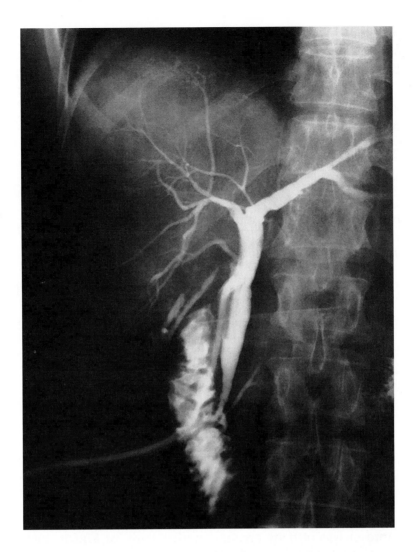

FIGURE 3-4
The percutaneous transhepatic cholangiography is contrast radiographic examination of the bile ducts via needle puncture. A percutaneously placed needle is inserted into an intrahepatic bile duct, and radiopaque dye is injected.

Key Terms	Definitions
selective venous	catheter placed into a vein and manipulated into another venous site
transcatheter biopsy (trans KATH e tur BYE op see)	tissue sample taken via a catheter
percutaneous (pur kew TAY nee us) **needle biopsy** (BYE op see)	excision of tissue by a guided needle through the skin
endoscopic catheterization (en duh SKOP cik kath e tur i ZAY shun)	procedure using an endoscope to view internal body structures
transluminal atherectomy (trans LEW mi nul ath e RECK toh me)	removal of deposits on the inner lining of a body structure
percutaneous transluminal (pur kew TAY nee us tans LEW mi nul) **balloon angioplasty** (AN jee oh plas tee)	use of a balloon catheter to widen a narrowed artery; another term for percutaneous transluminal angioplasty
percutaneous transluminal angioplasty (pur kew TAY nee us trans LEW mi nul AN jee oh plas tee)	use of a balloon catheter to widen a narrowed artery; another term for percutaneous transluminal balloon angioplasty
cardiac catheterization (kath e tur i ZAY shun)	examination of the heart after threading a catheter through a vessel into the heart for diagnostic, therapeutic, or visualization purposes

Key Terms	Definitions
percutaneous transhepatic cholangiography (pur kew TAY nee us trans he PAT ick koh lan jee OG ruh fee)	radiography of the bile ducts using contrast medium delivered via needle puncture
percutaneous transhepatic portography (pur kew TAY nee us trans he PAT ick por TOG ruh fee)	radiography of portal venous system using a contrast medium delivered via needle puncture

Key Term Practice: Catheterization, Biopsy, and Percutaneous Radiographic Procedures

1. A tissue sample obtained via a catheter is termed a/an _____.

2. A _____ venous procedure requires manipulation of the catheter to another specific site.

3. What is the alternate term for *percutaneous transluminal angioplasty*?

   _____.

4. _____ is radiography of the portal venous system via a needle stick.

Magnetic Resonance Imaging

A nonionizing diagnostic radiology tool is magnetic resonance imaging (MRI). During **magnetic resonance imaging**, the patient is placed within a tube and is surrounded by electromagnetic coils that excite hydrogen atoms in the body. Radiofrequency waves are aimed at the body, which cause internal hydrogen nuclei to change their alignment. This, in turn, causes the body to emit signals that a computer translates into images of body organs. Another term for MRI is nuclear magnetic resonance (NMR) imaging. Magnetic resonance imaging is used to determine blood flow and identify tumors of bone and fluid-filled soft tissues. Open and stand-up MRI machines have been developed to make the experience less claustrophobic for patients. Figure 3-5 illustrates the MRI technique.

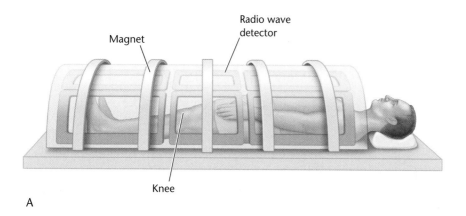
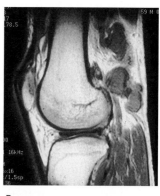

FIGURE 3-5

Magnetic resonance imaging (**A**). MRI study of the knee (**B**). MRI uses magnetic fields and radiofrequency waves to visualize anatomic structures. (Reprinted with permission from Bucholz RW, Heckman JD. Rockwood & Green's fractures in adults, 5th ed. Baltimore: Lippincott Williams & Wilkins, 2001.)

Imaging of blood vessels using magnetic resonance sequences that enhance the signal of flowing blood and suppress signals from other tissues is called **magnetic resonance angiography** (MRA). Another MRI variation is **magnetic resonance spectroscopy**, which is the detection and measurement of the resonant spectra of molecules in a tissue sample. Spectroscopy involves the measuring of absorbed light energy (spectrum) in a body structure.

> **FACT** *Radiologic technologists have the highest vacancy rate of any hospital profession!*

Key Terms	Definitions
magnetic resonance imaging	imaging technique that uses electromagnetic radiation to obtain pictures of the body's soft tissues
magnetic resonance angiography (an jee OG ruh fee)	imaging blood vessels using MRI
magnetic resonance spectroscopy (speck TROS kuh pee)	imaging structures using lightwaves

Key Term Practice: Magnetic Resonance Imaging

1. Imaging blood vessels using MRI is termed _____, which is derived from the word part *angio-*, which means "vessels," and the word part _____, which means "a description."

2. A noninvasive technique that uses lightwaves to create images is called _____.

Contrast Studies and Digestive System Radiography

Contrast studies are used for comparative purposes to highlight marked differences in the appearance of organs or tissues. Structures are made more visible when radiographs are taken after a contrast medium has been introduced. Types of GI contrast studies include the barium enema for lower GI evaluation and the barium swallow for upper GI study. **Barium sulfate** ($BaSO_4$) is a water-insoluble salt used as an opaque radiographic contrast medium. A **barium enema** study involves infusing the rectum with barium sulfate for radiographic and fluoroscopic study of the lower GI tract to identify obstructions and tumors. The oral administration of barium sulfate for radiographic study of the upper GI tract is termed a **barium swallow.** The barium swallow is used to diagnose disorders of the esophagus, stomach, and duodenum (first segment of the small intestine). A radiographic depiction of only the duodenum using a contrast medium is **duodenography.**

The salivary glands can be viewed via a unique procedure. Radiographic examination of the salivary glands and ducts after they have been injected with an opaque dye is termed **sialography** or **ptyalography.** Both terms are derived from the word parts meaning "saliva": *sialo-* and *ptyalo-*.

Examination of the bile ducts and gallbladder is accomplished through cholangiography and cholecystography, which come from the word part *chol-*, which means "bile." Radiography of the bile ducts with a contrast medium is known as **cholangiography.** It is used to diagnose tumors or stones. If no obstruction exists, the biliary structures readily empty into the intestinal tract. **Cholecystography** is radiography of the gallbladder after ingestion or intravenous (IV) injection of a radiopaque substance that is then excreted in bile. Usually, the patient swallows a tablet containing the dye the night before the x-ray examination. **Splenoportography** is radiographic examination of the splenic and portal vein system after a contrast medium has been injected into the spleen.

Key Terms	Definitions
barium (BAIR ee um) **sulfate**	compound used as a contrast medium because it is not penetrated by x-rays
barium enema (BAIR ee um EN e muh)	introduction of a barium salt suspension into the rectum and colon for x-ray examination
barium (BAIR ee um) **swallow**	ingestion of barium sulfate for x-ray examination of the upper GI tract
duodenography (dew oh de NOG ruh fee)	x-ray examination of the duodenum after introduction of a contrast medium
sialography (sigh uh LOG ruh fee)	x-ray examination of the salivary glands after administration of a contrast medium; another term for ptyalography
ptyalography (tigh uh LOG ruh fee)	x-ray examination of the salivary glands after administration of a contrast medium; another term for sialography
cholangiography (koh lan jee OG ruh fee)	examination of the bile ducts using a contrast medium
cholecystography (koh lee sis TOG ruh fee)	examination of the gallbladder after injection or ingestion of a contrast medium
splenoportography (splee noh por TOG ruh fee)	x-ray examination of the splenic and portal vein system after injection of a contrast medium

Key Term Practice: Contrast Studies and Digestive System Radiology

1. The procedure in which digestive structures are viewed after the ingestion of barium sulfate ($BaSO_4$) is known as a/an _____.

2. The radiographic examination of the duodenum using a contrast medium is termed _____.

Nervous System Radiography

Several areas of the brain and spinal cord can be visualized with x-rays. **Cisternography** is visualization of the subarachnoid cisternae (spaces) after introducing a contrast dye. **Myelography** is radiographic demonstration of the spinal cord, nerve roots, and subarachnoid space after introduction of a contrast medium or air into the space. Myelography is used to detect lesions, herniated disks, tumors, and cysts.

Diagnostic radiography particular to eye structures includes dacryocystography. **Dacryocystography** is radiography of the eye's lacrimal apparatus after injection of a contrast medium. The lacrimal apparatus secretes lubricating tears. The examination is used to determine the presence or site of obstruction.

Key Terms	Definitions
cisternography (sis tur NOG ruh fee)	visualization of the subarachnoid space after introducing a contrast medium
myelography (migh e LOG ruh fee)	radiographic examination of the spinal cord after injection of radiopaque dye
dacryocystography (dack ree oh sis TOG ruh fee)	x-ray examination of the lacrimal apparatus after injection of a contrast dye

Key Term Practice: Nervous System Radiology

1. Radiographic examination of the lacrimal apparatus after administration of a contrast dye is known as _____, a term derived from the word part _____, which means "lacrimal apparatus."

2. _____ is the x-ray examination of the spinal cord after injection of a radiopaque dye.

Heart and Vessel Radiography

Radiology techniques pertaining to the heart and vessels include angiography, digital subtraction angiography, angiocardiography, aortography, arteriography, and lymphangiography. **Angiography** is the visualization of blood or lymph vessels after injection of a radiopaque dye by capillaroscopy, fluoroscopy, or radiography. Common types of angiography are cardiac, cerebral, peripheral, and pulmonary. Presurgical vessel mapping accomplished by angiography is used for vascular surgery procedures such as creating fistulas and grafting.

Computer-assisted radiography that permits imaging of vascular structures separate from images of bone or soft tissue is termed **digital subtraction angiography** (DSA). Structures not enhanced by the contrast medium are removed from the picture to improve the visualization of the vessels. Radiographic examination of veins after the administration of a contrast medium is termed **venography** or phlebography. Incomplete vein filling indicates an obstruction.

Radiographic examination of thoracic vessels and the heart chambers after intravascular injection of radiopaque material is called **angiocardiography**. An x-ray of the aorta after intravascular injection of a radiopaque material is termed **aortography**, and x-ray examination of arteries after the intravascular injection of a dye is known as **arteriography**.

Radiographic visualization of lymph channels and nodes after the injection of a radiopaque dye into afferent lymphatic vessels is termed **lymphangiography** or lymphography. In cases of cancer, lymph node mapping by lymphangiography enables the clinician to locate the sentinel node, which is the first lymph node into which a tumor drains. This allows the surgeon to remove only those nodes likely to be cancerous rather than all nodes in an area.

Key Terms	Definitions
angiography (an jee OG ruh fee)	examination of blood vessels after introduction of a contrast dye
digital subtraction angiography (an jee OG ruh fee)	computer-assisted radiograph of vascular structures without superimposed bone or soft tissue
venography (vee NOG ruh fee)	x-ray examination of veins or vein networks after injection of a radiopaque dye
angiocardiography) (an jee oh kahr dee OG ruh fee	x-ray examination of heart and blood vessels after injection of a contrast dye
aortography (ay or TOG ruh fee)	x-ray examination of the aorta after injection of a contrast dye
arteriography (ahr teer ee OG ruh fee)	x-ray examination of arteries after injection of a contrast dye
lymphangiography (lim fan jee OG ruh fee)	x-ray examination of lymphatic vessels after introduction of a contrast medium

Key Term Practice: Heart and Vessel Radiography

1. _____ is the examination of blood vessels after intravenous administration of a radiopaque dye.

2. X-ray examination of arteries after injection of a contrast dye is termed _____.

Reproductive System Radiography

Studies of the male and female reproductive systems are possible through several diagnostic radiology procedures. **Corpora cavernosography** is radiographic examination of the parallel columns of erectile tissue in the penis.

The epididymis is a coiled tube located in the testicle that stores sperm. A radiograph of the epididymis is termed **epididymography**. Radiography of the vas deferens to determine patency (state of being freely open) is termed **vasography**. The seminal vesicles are a pair of glands that secrete fluid that includes the semen. Radiography of these structures after the injection of a contrast medium is named **vesiculography**.

Mammography is radiographic examination of breast tissue, occasionally performed with a contrast medium (Fig. 3-6). It is used to detect breast abnormalities, tumors, and cysts. Although mammography screening does not prevent or cure breast cancer, it may detect disease before signs and symptoms become apparent. Tumors can exist for 6–10 years before they are large enough to be detected by mammography. A **mammary ductogram** or **mammary galactogram** is a variant of mammography in which the breast is examined after the injection of contrast medium into the mammary ductal system.

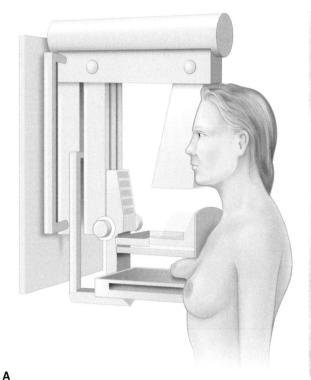

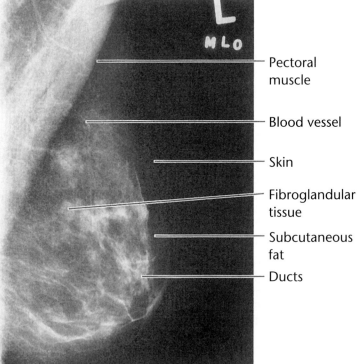

Pectoral muscle

Blood vessel

Skin

Fibroglandular tissue

Subcutaneous fat

Ducts

A

B

FIGURE 3-6
Mammography (**A**). Mammogram (**B**). Mammography is the radiologic examination of the breast by means of x-ray, ultrasound, or nuclear magnetic resonance imaging. (Image provide by LifeART, © 2006 Lippincott Williams & Wilkins. All rights reserved.)

Radiographic examination of the uterus and uterine tubes after injection of a contrast medium into the cavities is called **hysterosalpingography** (*hystero-* means "uterus"; *salpingo-* means "tube"). Hysterosalpingography is used to diagnose uterine pathology, evaluate tubal patency, and identify possible causes of infertility.

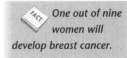

One out of nine women will develop breast cancer.

Key Terms	Definitions
corpora cavernosography (KOR poh ruh kav ur noh SOG ruh fee)	x-ray examination of the penile erectile tissue
epididymography (ep i did i MOG ruh fee)	x-ray examination of the epididymis using a contrast medium
vasography (vay ZOG ruh fee)	x-ray examination of the vas deferens using a contrast medium
vesiculography (ve sick yoo LOG ruh fee)	x-ray examination of seminal vesicles using a contrast medium
mammography (ma MOG ruh fee)	x-ray examination of the breast
mammary ductogram (MAM uh ree DUCK toh gram)	radiograph of the mammary ductal system; another term for mammary galactogram
mammary galactogram (MAM uh ree ga LACK toh gram)	radiograph of the mammary ductal system; another term for mammary ductogram
hysterosalpingography (his tur oh sal ping OG ruh fee)	x-ray examination of the uterus and oviducts using a contrast dye

Key Term Practice: Reproductive System Radiology

1. The word part mammo refers to "breast"; *-graphy* means "a description"; thus _____ is the x-ray evaluation of breast tissue.

2. Cite two terms describing a radiologic examination of the ductal system of the breast.

_____

Respiratory System Radiography

A commonly performed test to evaluate lung obstruction, such as pneumonia, or abnormalities in the heart, aorta, and bones of the thoracic area is the chest x-ray. Both an anterior (A) and a posterior (P) view are normally taken.

Radiographic visualization of the bronchial tree after the introduction of radiopaque dye through a tracheal catheter is termed **bronchography. Laryngography** is the radiographic examination of the larynx (voice box) after the mucosal surfaces have been coated with a contrast medium. The test is performed to evaluate vocal cord function.

Key Terms	Definitions
bronchography (brong KOG ruh fee)	radiographic examination of the lung bronchial tree after introduction of a contrast dye
laryngography (luh rin GOG ruh fee)	radiography of the larynx (voice box) after coating the surface with a radiopaque dye

Key Term Practice: Respiratory System Radiography

1. X-ray examination of the larynx is termed _____.

2. X-ray examination of the bronchial tree after introduction of a contrast medium is known as _____.

Urinary System Radiography

Pyelography is the branch of radiography dealing with the kidneys and surrounding tissue. Radiography of the renal pelvis, ureter, and bladder after filling with an opaque solution either directly via a catheter or percutaneously is termed **pyelography**. **Intravenous pyelography** (IVP) is the x-ray examination of the renal pelvis, ureter, and bladder after a contrast medium is administered intravenously (Fig. 3-7). During a **retrograde pyelography** (RP) procedure, a contrast medium is injected into the ureters from an endoscope placed in the bladder. It is called *retrograde* because the fluid is moving contrary to the normal direction of flow. The contrast medium is injected into the kidney, specifically the renal pelvis or renal calyces, during an **antegrade pyelography**, and the fluid flows in the normal direction of flow.

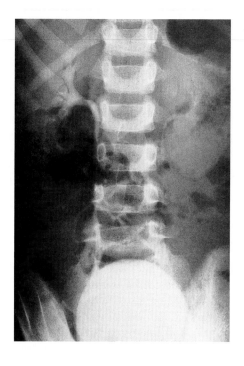

FIGURE 3-7
Intravenous pyelography reveals a contusion on the left kidney. An opaque solution is inserted in the renal pelvis, ureter, or bladder, and an x-ray is taken. (Reprinted with permission from Fleisher GR, Ludwig S, Baskin MN. Atlas of pediatric emergency medicine. Philadelphia: Lippincott Williams & Wilkins, 2004.)

A radiographic evaluation of the urinary tract, which includes the kidneys, ureters, and bladder, after introducing a contrast medium is termed **urography**. Radiography of only the urinary bladder after introduction of a contrast medium is termed **cystography**. Radiographic visualization of the urethra and bladder using a contrast medium is termed **urethrocystography** or **cystourethrography**, and this study provides images during voiding (urination). Urography, cystography, and cystourethrography identify tumors, defects, reflux (backflow), and stones. Figure 3-8 illustrates an intravenous urogram.

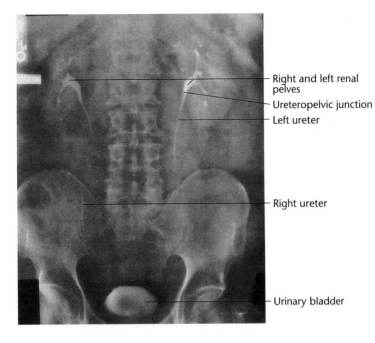

Right and left renal pelves
Ureteropelvic junction
Left ureter
Right ureter
Urinary bladder

FIGURE 3-8
Urography is radiographic evaluation of the urinary tract, including the kidneys, ureters, and bladder, after introducing a contrast medium. (Reprinted with permission from Erkonen WE, Smith WL. Radiology 101: Basics and fundamentals of imaging. Philadelphia: Lippincott Williams & Wilkins, 1998.)

Key Terms	Definitions
pyelography (pye e LOG ruh fee)	radiography of the kidneys and surrounding tissue using a contrast medium
intravenous pyelogram (pye e loh gram)	x-ray of the urine-collecting part of the kidney, ureter, and bladder using a contrast dye
retrograde pyelography (RET roh grade pye e LOG ruh fee)	radiography of the kidneys after a contrast dye is injected into the ureters, resulting in backward fluid movement
antegrade pyelography (AN te grade pye e LOG ruh fee)	radiography of the kidneys after a contrast dye is injected into the renal pelvis or renal calyces
urography (yoo ROG ruh fee)	radiography of the urinary tract
cystography (sis TOG ruh fee)	x-ray examination of the bladder using a contrast dye
urethrocystography (yoo ree throh sis TOG ruh fee)	x-ray examination of the urethra and bladder using a contrast dye; another term for cystourethrography
cystourethrography (sis toh yoo ree THROG ruh fee)	x-ray examination of the bladder and urethra using a contrast dye; another term for urethrocystography

Key Term Practice: Urinary System Radiology

1. Radiography of the kidneys is called _____.

2. What are the two terms that describe radiography of the bladder and urethra?

_____

Other Diagnostic Radiology Services

Phonocardiography is a graphic recording of heart sounds and murmurs during a cardiac cycle using an instrument with amplifiers, filters, and microphones placed over the heart. An electrocardiogram (ECG) measures the heart's electrical activity, which is simultaneously recorded for reference (Fig. 3-9).

Electromyography (EMG) is the study of the electric activity of a muscle in response to electrical stimulation. Electromyography studies are beneficial for the diagnosis of motor nerve and muscle tissue disorders.

Bone density can be measured using a densitometer, which is an instrument that measures optical density. The densitometer measures the extent to which a tissue absorbs or reflects light. **Densitometry** or **photodensitometry** is a procedure that uses a densitometer in a clinical setting. Known also as radiographic absorptiometry, it is used especially for determining bone density. Thus it is a valuable diagnostic tool for detecting osteoporosis.

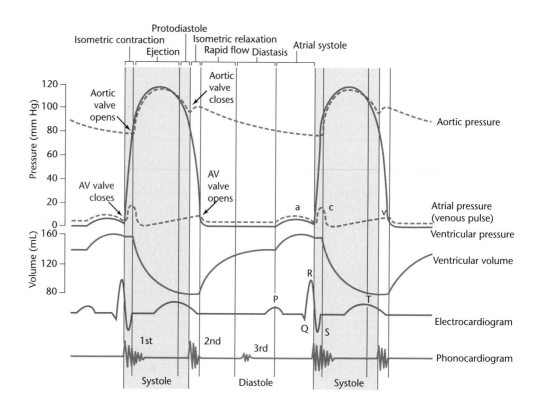

FIGURE 3-9
Phonocardiography. This technique provides a graphic recording of heart sounds and murmurs and is recorded along with an ECG.

Key Terms	Definitions
phonocardiography (foh noh kahr dee OG ruh fee)	procedure for obtaining a visual record of heart sounds and murmurs made by a phonocardiograph
electromyography (ee leck troh migh OG ruh fee)	procedure used to diagnose nerve and muscle disorders by measuring electrical activity of muscle tissue
densitometry (den si TOM uh tree)	examination of bone density using light absorption and reflection; another term for photodensitometry
photodensitometry (foh toh den si TOM uh tree)	examination of bone density using light absorption and reflection; another term for densitometry

Key Term Practice: Other Diagnostic Radiology Services

1. _____ is a graphic recording of heart sounds and is derived from the word part _____, meaning "sound," and the word part _____, meaning "writing, description."

2. Which two terms mean "examination of bone density using light absorption and reflection"?

_____

Diagnostic Ultrasound

Sound waves that have frequencies above the upper limit of the normal range of human hearing, about 20 kilohertz, are termed ultrasonic. A hertz (Hz) is a frequency equal to one cycle per second; hence a kilohertz is equal to 1000 hertz. Ultrasound is an imaging technique using high-frequency sound waves that bounce off internal body parts to create images. **Ultrasonography**, **echography**, and **sonography** are synonymous terms used to describe the procedure that uses pulse-echo techniques for providing pictorial representation of anatomic structures.

During **ultrasound**, a pulsing crystal produces energy. The reflection of high-frequency (ultrasound) sound waves is used to locate, measure, and outline deep structures. A computer determines the distance to the sound-reflecting or sound-absorbing surface and creates a two-dimensional image called an ultrasonogram. Ultrasound is used in three primary manners in medicine, depending on the power level: diagnostic, therapeutic, and treatment. Diagnostic ultrasound uses sound waves below 0.1 watt per square centimeter (W/cm^2). For example, obstetric ultrasound is used during pregnancy to assess embryonic and fetal status, and it has use in gynecology to view the vagina (Fig. 3-10). Ultrasound at 1–3 W/cm^2 is used for physiotherapy in joint and muscle disorders. Ultrasound for cancer treatment is set at 5 W/cm^2 to destroy tissue. Box 3-2 lists several diagnostic ultrasound procedures.

Johann Christian Doppler was an Austrian mathematician and physicist who defined what is now known as the Doppler effect. This principle states that when a source of

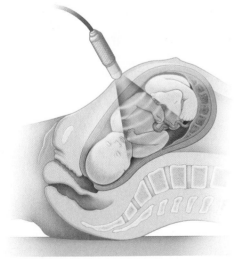

A

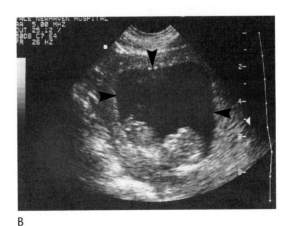

B

FIGURE 3-10
Sonography technique (**A**). A sonogram (**B**). (Photo courtesy of L. Scoutt.)

BOX 3-2. *Diagnostic Ultrasound Procedures*

Doppler echocardiography
Doppler ultrasonography
Echocardiography
Echoencephalography

Hysterosonography
Intravascular ultrasound
Ultrasound

---

light or sound is moving rapidly, the wavelength or pitch of sound appears to increase as the object approaches the observer and to decrease as the object recedes from the observer. The Doppler unit is an instrument that emits an ultrasonic beam into the body. The ultrasound reflected from moving structures has a changed frequency caused by the Doppler effect. It is used for diagnosing peripheral vascular and cardiac disease.

Pulse echoes used for diagnosis are termed **Doppler ultrasonography.** This form of ultrasonography applies the Doppler effect to detect movements of scatters (beams of particles), which are usually caused by red blood cells. Because it is noninvasive, poses no known risk to patients, is of moderate cost, and provides real-time imaging of organs, this technique has replaced radiography in many instances. It is particularly useful for viewing tissues, blood flow, heart structures, and embryos and fetuses. Figure 3-11 illustrates the Doppler ultrasonography procedure and provides an image of normal blood flow in the carotid artery.

Echocardiography is also known as ultrasonic cardiography or ultrasound cardiography. **Doppler echocardiography** uses Doppler ultrasonographic techniques to augment two-dimensional echocardiography by registering velocities within the image on a strip chart. It is used to diagnose valve and structural abnormalities in the heart (Fig. 3-12).

Echoencephalography (*cephalo-* means "head") is the study of intracranial structures and disease using pulse echoes. It is used to diagnose the midline shift of brain structures. An ultrasound of the uterine cavity is called **hysterosonography,** and an ultrasound of blood vessels or lymphatics is **intravascular ultrasound.**

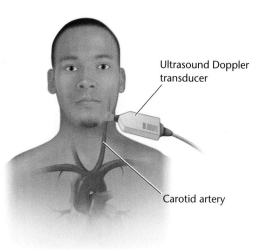

Ultrasound Doppler transducer

Carotid artery

A

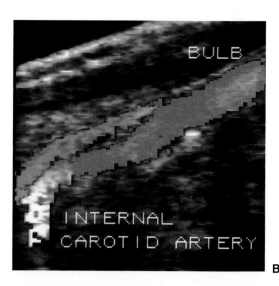

BULB

INTERNAL CAROTID ARTERY

B

FIGURE 3-11

Doppler ultrasonography. This technique is particularly useful for viewing tissues, blood flow, heart structures, embryos, and fetuses (**A**). Normal Doppler of carotid artery (**B**).

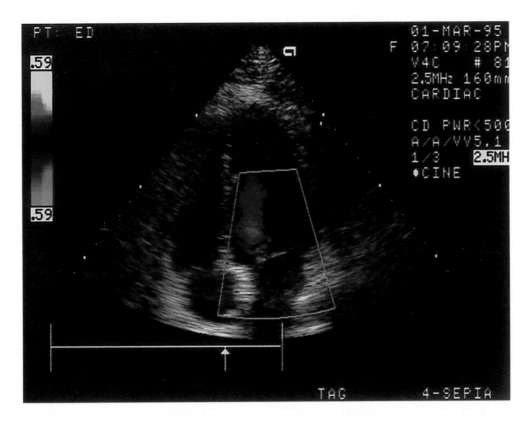

FIGURE 3-12
Echocardiography uses Doppler ultrasonic techniques to augment two-dimensional echocardiography. (Reprinted with permission from Smeltzer SC, Bare BG. Textbook of medical-surgical nursing, 9th ed. Philadelphia: Lippincott Williams & Wilkins, 2000.)

Key Terms	Definitions
ultrasonography (ul truh suh NOG ruh fee)	imaging technique using high-frequency sound waves; another term for echography or sonography
echography (ECK oh graf ee)	imaging technique using high-frequency sound waves; another term for ultrasonography or sonography
sonography (so NOG ruh fee)	imaging technique using high-frequency sound waves; another term for echography or ultrasonography
ultrasound	imaging technique using high-frequency sound waves
Doppler ultrasonography (DOP ler ul truh suh NOG ruh fee)	imaging technique applying the Doppler effect
echocardiography (eck oh kahr dee OG ruh fee)	ultrasound technique for observing and examining the heart
Doppler echocardiography (DOP ler eck oh kahr dee OG ruh fee)	ultrasound technique employing the Doppler effect to enhance two-dimensional echocardiography
echoencephalography (eck oh en sef uh LOG ruh fee)	study of intracranial structures using ultrasound
hysterosonography (his tur oh so NOG ruh fee)	ultrasound of the uterine interior
intravascular (in truh VAS kew lur) **ultrasound**	ultrasound of blood and lymphatic vessels

Key Term Practice: Diagnostic Ultrasound

1. The general term for an imaging technique using sound waves is _____.

2. An ultrasound of the uterus is termed _____, derived from the word parts *hystero-*, "meaning uterus"; _____, meaning "sound"; and *-graphy,* meaning _____.

Radiation Oncology

Radiation oncology is the branch of medicine that deals with the study and treatment of malignant tumors using ionizing radiation. This form of radiation therapy uses radiation to treat cancer and is also called **radiotherapy** or therapeutic radiology. Several procedures are described in this section, and Box 3-3 lists common radiation oncology procedures.

Irradiation is the medical use of radiation, such as x-rays, gamma-rays, and other radioactive sources. Irradiation of body tissue involves bombarding the site with ionizing radiation to destroy unwanted cells and tissues or administering radionuclides in pill form. Measuring the amount of exposure or dosage of delivered x-rays is known as **dosimetry.** The instrument used to measure the amount of radiation absorbed by the body is called a dosimeter. Calculations are necessary for the accurate determination of medicinal doses from internally administered radionuclides.

Total body irradiation exposes the whole body to ionizing radiation. This form of radiotherapy is often given in several doses before bone marrow transplantation to kill any remaining cancerous cells in the patient. If is often used in conjunction with chemotherapy. Radiotherapy in which the source of irradiation is placed close to the body surface or within a body cavity is termed **brachytherapy. Interstitial brachytherapy** is a form of radiation treatment in which radioactive needles or other sources are implanted directly into and around tissue to be irradiated.

Intracavitary therapy is disease management accomplished by administering radiation into an organ or body cavity. This form of treatment, accomplished by treating whole body cavities with radiation, is termed **endocavitary irradiation. Intraoperative cone irradiation** involves aiming a beam of x-rays directly at the target through a cylinder during a surgical procedure. The goal is to eradicate cancerous growth.

A palliative cancer therapy involving radiation to half of the body is termed **hemibody radiation.** Hemibody radiation can treat multiple disease sites simultaneously

---

BOX 3-3. *Radiation Oncology Procedures*

Brachytherapy	Intracavitary therapy
Dosimetry	Intraoperative cone irradiation
Endocavitary irradiation	Radionuclide seeds
Hemibody radiation	Teletherapy
Hyperthermia	Total body irradiation
Interstitial brachytherapy	

and is demonstrating effectiveness in treating disseminated malignancy. Some pain and symptoms are alleviated, but the cause will not be eliminated.

Prostate cancer is often treated with **radionuclide seeds**, which involves the planting of radioactive particles directly in the cancerous tissue. Treatment with radiation from a source that is far from the body is known as **teletherapy** or external radiation therapy. Teletherapy uses a beam of radiation positioned above the patient that is aimed directly at the tumor. After the initial treatment, a small ink tattoo is fixed to the skin so that during future treatments the exact location can be identified and the radiation beam can be focused on the same site. This form of radiotherapy is usually performed once a day, 5–6 days per week, for several weeks.

Treatment of disease by inducing a fever through inoculation with an infection, injection of foreign proteins, or physical means is known as **hyperthermia** or hyperpyrexia. Cancer cells are more sensitive to heat than are normal cells, and raising the body temperature by either internal or external methods has therapeutic merit in selectively destroying malignant cells. External methods include using thermal blankets, radiofrequencies, and ultrasound; internal methods involve administering pyrogens (fever-inducing agents). Some research suggests that hyperthermia combined with radiation therapy provides greater benefit than radiation treatment alone for treating cancer.

FACT One in six men is at risk of developing prostate cancer.

Key Terms	Definitions
radiotherapy (ray dee oh THERR uh pee)	treating cancer growths by radiation; another term for radiation oncology
irradiation (i ray dee AY shun)	medical use of radiation—such as x-rays, gamma-rays, or other radioactive sources—to treat cancer
dosimetry (doh SIM e tree)	measurement of exposure to radiation
total body irradiation (i ray dee AY shun)	exposing the entire body to ionizing radiation
brachytherapy (brack ee THERR uh pee)	radiotherapy in which the source is placed directly on or in close proximity to the body
interstitial brachytherapy (in tur STISH ul brack ee THERR uh pee)	radiation treatment via implanted sources
intracavitary (in truh KAV i terr ee) **therapy**	managing a disease by introducing radiation into an organ or body cavity
endocavitary irradiation (en doh KAV i terr ee i ray dee AY shun)	treating body cavities with radiation
intraoperative (in truh OP ur uh tiv) **cone irradiation** (i ray dee AY shun)	using x-rays aimed at a target to destroy cancerous cells during surgery
hemibody (HEM i bod ee) **radiation**	radiotherapy of one half of the body
radionuclide (ray dee oh NEW klide) **seeds**	radioactive particles that are implanted in the body for treating cancer
teletherapy (tel e THERR uh pee)	radiation treatment from a source distant from the body
hyperthermia (high pur THUR mee uh)	therapeutically induced fever; another term for hyperpyrexia

Key Term Practice: Radiation Oncology

1. The treatment of disease with radiation is termed _____.

2. _____ is exposure to ionizing radiation.

Nuclear Medicine

Nuclear medicine is the branch of medicine that uses radioisotopes in diagnosis and therapy. Radionuclides or radioisotopes are used for diagnostic or therapeutic measures or as tracers to be detected in the body. They are observed in contained compartments of the body such as the vascular, urinary, or lymphatic systems. Box 3-4 lists various nuclear medicine procedures.

Nuclear scan studies use radionuclides, radiopharmaceuticals, radiation detectors with imaging instruments, and computers to view internal structures. The radionuclide is administered either orally or intravenously (IV) and can then be measured by a camera that detects the amount of radiation emitted. The data are then converted into a two-dimensional image.

A **multiple-gated acquisition (MUGA) scan** images cardiac functions. It is a nuclear medicine cardiac blood pool study used for ejection fraction (the volume of blood ejected by the ventricles) and heart wall motion assessment.

Another variation of tomography has an application in nuclear medicine. **Positron emission tomography** (PET) creates images by computer analysis when low-dose radioactively tagged substances are incorporated into tissue (Fig. 3-13). PET scans assess metabolic activity and physiologic function rather than anatomic structure. It is a useful tool for performing experimental living brain investigations. Diagnostic information can be obtained for central nervous system and cardiac function and for cancer evaluation. These scans can recognize some dementias, Parkinson disease, Huntington disease, and epilepsy. Blood flow and viable myocardial tissue can also be identified. This technique is beneficial for the noninvasive assessment of tumor behavior in cancer patients.

BOX 3-4. *Nuclear Medicine Procedures*

Bone scan	Scintigraphy
Gallium scan	Single photon emission computed tomography (SPECT)
Multiple-gated acquisition (MUGA) scan	
Nuclear scan studies	Spleen imaging
Positron emission tomography (PET)	Thallium (Tl) scan
Pulmonary perfusion imaging	Thyroid imaging
Pulmonary ventilation imaging	Tomography
Radioactive iodine uptake	Urea breath test
Radioimmunoassay	Ventriculography
Radiopharmaceutical therapy	Vitamin B_{12} absorption study
Schilling test	

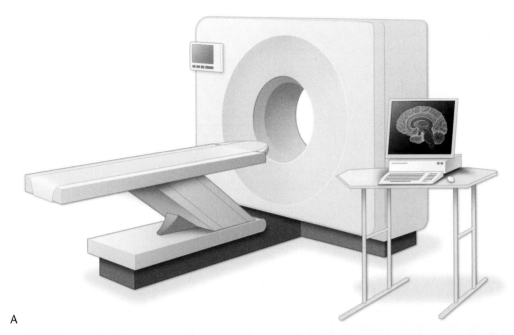

A

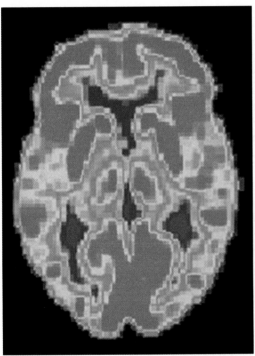

B

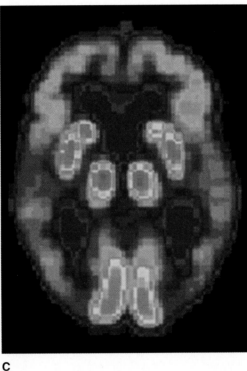

C

FIGURE 3-13
Positron emission tomography (PET) (**A**). This technique combines nuclear medicine and computed tomography to create images of body parts. PET scan of the brain of a healthy person (**B**). PET scan of the brain of a person with Alzheimer disease (**C**). The blue areas indicate reduced brain activity. (B and C Reprinted with permission from the Alzheimer's Disease Education and Referral Center, a service of the National Institute on Aging.)

Radioisotopes of iodine are used as radiopharmaceuticals for nuclear medicine studies. A **radiopharmaceutical** is a radioactive chemical or pharmaceutical preparation labeled with a tracer used as a diagnostic or therapeutic agent. Iodine-123 (^{123}I) is a radioisotope of iodine used for studies of thyroid disease and renal function; iodine-125 (^{125}I) is used as a label in immunoassay studies; iodine-131 (^{131}I) is used as a tracer in thyroid studies, as a therapy in hyperthyroidism and thyroid cancer, and as a label in immunoassay studies.

Radioimmunoassay is a method for determining and quantifying antigens or antibodies in the blood using radiolabeled reactants. The tracer-tagged antigen will

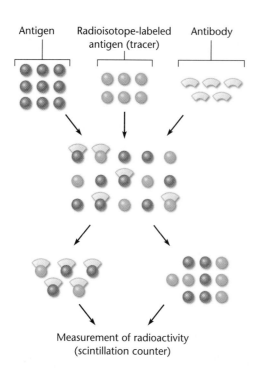

Antigen   Radioisotope-labeled   Antibody
           antigen (tracer)

Measurement of radioactivity
(scintillation counter)

FIGURE 3-14
Radioimmunoassay is a method for determining and quantifying antigens or antibodies in a blood sample using radiolabeled reactants. Antigens that have been tagged by a tracer will bind with an antigen if it exists. If the antigen-antibody complex forms, the attached tracer can easily identify it.

bind with an antibody, if one exists. If the antigen–antibody complex forms, the attached tracer allows the clinician to readily identify it (Fig. 3-14).

Scintigraphy determines the distribution of a radioactive tracer in intact tissue via an external scintillation camera placed over the area. A photo obtained by scintigraphy is also called a scintophotogram or scintiphotograph (Fig. 3-15).

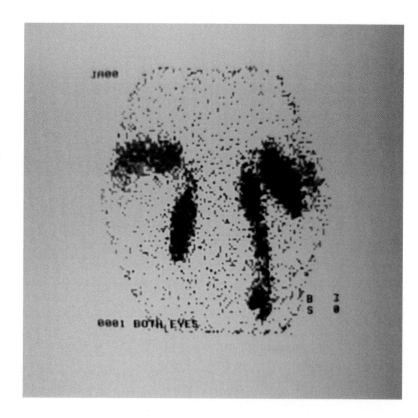

FIGURE 3-15
Scintigraphy. This technique is used to determine the distribution of a radioactive tracer in intact tissue. An external scintillation camera scans over the area. Note the obstruction of the right tear duct. (Reprinted with permission from Tasman W, Jaeger E. The Wills Eye Hospital atlas of clinical ophthalmology, 2nd ed. Baltimore: Lippincott Williams & Wilkins, 2001.)

Another imaging technique that uses radiopharmaceuticals is **single photon emission computed tomography** (SPECT). This technique provides a tomographic image of metabolic and physiologic functions in tissues after the administration of a radionuclide.

A radioisotope of thallium (TI), thallium-201 (^{201}TI), is used for myocardial nuclear **thallium scan** imaging. It is also taken up by some tumors and can be readily detected.

The **urea breath test** is used to detect the presence of *Helicobacter pylori,* the bacterium that causes gastric ulcers. Patients swallow a capsule containing carbon-14 (^{14}C), a radioisotope of carbon. If the isotope is detected in the breath, it indicates the presence of the bacterium. The **Schilling test** is a method of assessing vitamin B_{12} absorption by determining the amount excreted in the urine using cyanocobalamin tagged with a radioisotope of cobalt.

Ventriculography is a method of demonstrating brain ventricles by radiography after the cerebrospinal fluid (CSF) has been replaced by gas or an opaque medium injected directly into the ventricles. The technique is also used to demonstrate contractility of cardiac ventricles after measuring the distribution of an intravenously injected radionuclide.

Technetium (Tc) is a synthetic radioactive metallic element. Bone scans use technetium-99 (^{99}Tc). A **bone scan** is a radiograph of the entire body used to evaluate the skeletal system, connective tissue disease, fracture, and bone infection. A high dose of a radioactive substance is injected into the body and the scan reads the distribution of radioactivity. Gallium (Ga) is a rare metallic element; the isotope gallium-67 (^{67}Ga) is used as a tumor and inflammation radiotracer for a **gallium scan.**

Other organs visualized with nuclear scans are the spleen and thyroid. **Spleen imaging** is accomplished by administering a radionuclide intravenously. The spleen then absorbs the medium and an image can be made. Spleen scans are used to diagnose cysts, abscesses, tumors, ruptures, or splenomegaly. **Thyroid imaging** is a picture of the thyroid gland after it takes up radioactive iodine. Radioactive iodine is administered either orally by capsule or intravenously in the **radioactive iodine uptake** test. During this test, the thyroid traps and retains the iodine, which is used to make hormones. The ability to capture the iodine indicates thyroid function.

Two pulmonary nuclear medicine studies are pulmonary perfusion imaging and pulmonary ventilation imaging. *Perfusion* refers to a substance being spread throughout a tissue, and *ventilation* indicates that the substance has entered the gas exchange structures of the lungs (alveoli). During **pulmonary perfusion imaging**, an intravenous radiopharmaceutical is administered, and the radioactive compound is dispersed in the lung capillaries. The extent of perfusion is captured in an x-ray image. Xenon (Xe) is a heavy, colorless, odorless gas. For **pulmonary ventilation imaging**, xenon-133 (^{133}Xe) gas is inhaled, and the radiopharmaceutical is identified in lung alveoli on an x-ray image.

There are about 584 schools accredited to train "rad techs" (radiology technologists)!

Key Terms	Definitions
nuclear (NEW klee ur) **scan study**	procedures that use isotopes in the body for diagnostic purposes
multiple-gated acquisition scan	nuclear medicine study to evaluate cardiac function
positron (POZ i tron) **emission tomography** (toh MOG ruh fee)	nuclear medicine technique for assessing metabolic activity of organs, diagnosing cancer, locating brain tumors, and investigating brain function
radiopharmaceutical (ray dee oh far muh SOO ti kul)	radioactive substance used in nuclear medicine

Key Terms	Definitions
radioimmunoassay (ray dee oh im yoo noh as SAY)	technique for identifying antibodies using a radioactive tracer
scintigraphy (sin TIG ruh fee)	two-dimensional imaging technique using a radioactive tracer
single photon emission computed tomography (toh MOG ruh fee)	imaging technique that creates three-dimensional pictures by identifying a radioactive tracer absorbed by an organ or tissue
thallium (THAL ee um) **scan**	nuclear imaging technique using a radioisotope of thallium
urea (yoo REE uh) **breath test**	test using carbon-14 to determine the presence of *H. pylori*
Schilling (SHIL ing) **test**	technique for determining B_{12} absorption
ventriculography (ven trick yoo LOG ruh fee)	radiographic examination of the brain ventricles (after replacing the CSF with a gas or detectable dye) or the heart ventricles (after injecting a radionuclide)
bone scan	radiograph of the entire skeletal system using technetium-99 as a tracer
gallium (GAL ee um) **scan**	imaging technique using gallium-67 for the identification of tumors and inflammation
spleen imaging	radiograph of the spleen after administering a radionuclide
thyroid imaging	radiograph of the thyroid after administering a radionuclide such as radioactive iodine
radioactive iodine uptake	test used to determine thyroid function by assessing the amount of radioactive iodine absorbed by the thyroid gland
pulmonary perfusion (PUL muh nerr ee pur FEW zhun) **imaging**	use of a radiopharmaceutical to form an image of lung tissue by detecting it in the capillaries
pulmonary (PUL muh nerr ee) **ventilation imaging**	use of xenon-133 gas to form an image of lung tissue by identifying its presence in the alveoli

Key Term Practice: Nuclear Medicine

1. A radiograph of the entire skeletal system using ^{99}Tc is termed a/an _____.

2. _____ is an imaging technique using radioactively tagged substances, which are assessed for metabolic activity and physiologic function instead of anatomic structure.

CLINICAL TERMS

Clinical Dimension	Term	Description
CLINICAL TESTS AND DIAGNOSTIC PROCEDURES		
	angiocardiography	x-ray examination of heart and blood vessels after injection of a contrast dye
	angiography	examination of blood vessels after introduction of a contrast dye
	antegrade pyelography	radiography of the kidneys after a contrast dye is injected into the renal pelvis or renal calyces
	aortography	x-ray examination of the aorta after injection of a contrast dye
	arteriography	x-ray examination of arteries after injection of a contrast dye
	arthrography	examination of a joint's interior after the injection of a contrast medium
	barium enema	introduction of a barium salt suspension into the rectum and colon for x-ray examination
	barium swallow	ingestion of barium sulfate for x-ray examination of the upper GI tract
	bone scan	radiograph of the entire skeletal system using technetium-99 as a tracer
	bronchography	radiographic examination of the lung bronchial tree after introduction of a contrast dye
	cardiac catheterization	examination of the heart after threading a catheter through a vessel into the heart for diagnostic, therapeutic, or visualization purposes
	cholangiography	examination of the bile ducts using a contrast medium
	cholecystography	examination of the gallbladder after injection or ingestion of a contrast medium
	cinefluoroscopy	radiography of an organ in motion; another term for cineradiography
	cineradiography	radiography of an organ in motion; another term for cinefluoroscopy
	cisternography	visualization of the subarachnoid space after introducing a contrast medium
	computed tomographic angiography	combination CT and angiography for visualizing blood or lymphatic vessels
	computed tomography (CT)	technique for producing images of body cross sections

Clinical Dimension	Term	Description
	corpora cavernosography	x-ray examination of the penile erectile tissue
	CT pelvimetry	measurement of the dimensions of the bony pelvis using CT scans; another term for radiocephalpelvimetry
	cystography	x-ray examination of the bladder using a contrast dye
	cystourethrography	x-ray examination of the bladder and urethra using a contrast dye; another term for urethrocystography
	dacryocystography	x-ray examination of the lacrimal apparatus after injection of a contrast dye
	densitometry	examination of bone density using light absorption and reflection; another term for photodensitometry
	diagnostic radiology	use of x-rays and other ionizing radiation forms for the diagnosis and treatment of disease
	diagnostic ultrasound	use of high-frequency sound waves in diagnosing and treating conditions
	digital subtraction angiography (DSA)	computer-assisted radiograph of vascular structures without superimposed bone or soft tissue
	diskography	examination of the intervertebral disks after the direct injection of a contrast medium
	Doppler echocardiography	ultrasound technique employing the Doppler effect to enhance two-dimensional echocardiography
	Doppler ultrasonography	imaging technique applying the Doppler effect
	dosimetry	measurement of exposure to radiation
	duodenography	x-ray examination of the duodenum after introduction of a contrast medium
	echocardiography	ultrasound technique for observing and examining the heart
	echoencephalography	study of intracranial structures using ultrasound
	echography	imaging technique using high-frequency sound waves; another term for ultrasonography or sonography
	electromyography (EMG)	procedure used to diagnose nerve and muscle disorders by measuring electrical activity of muscle tissue
	endoscopic catheterization	procedure using an endoscope to view internal body structures

Clinical Dimension	Term	Description
	epididymography	x-ray examination of the epididymis using a contrast medium
	gallium scan	imaging technique using gallium-67 for the identification of tumors and inflammation
	hysterosalpingography	x-ray examination of the uterus and oviducts using a contrast dye
	hysterosonography	ultrasound of the uterine interior
	interventional radiology	specialty area of radiology that employs catheters, scopes, and various procedures to guide instruments for the diagnosis and treatment of pathology
	intravascular ultrasound	ultrasound of blood and lymphatic vessels
	intravenous pyelogram (IVP)	x-ray of the urine-collecting part of the kidney, ureter, and bladder using a conrast dye
	laryngography	radiography of the larynx (voice box) after coating the surface with a radiopaque dye
	lymphangiography	x-ray examination of lymphatic vessels after introduction of a contrast medium
	magnetic resonance angiography (MRA)	imaging blood vessels using MRI
	magnetic resonance imaging (MRI)	imaging technique that uses electromagnetic radiation to obtain pictures of the body's soft tissues
	magnetic resonance spectroscopy	imaging structures using light waves
	mammary ductogram	radiograph of the mammary ductal system; another term for mammary galactogram
	mammary galactogram	radiograph of the mammary ductal system; another term for mammary ductogram
	mammography	x-ray examination of the breast
	multiple-gated acquisition (MUGA) scan	nuclear medicine study to evaluate cardiac function
	myelography	radiographic examination of the spinal cord after injection of radiopaque dye
	nonselective arterial catheter placement	catheter placed into an arterial vessel and not manipulated to another arterial site
	nonselective venous	catheter placed into a vein and not manipulated to another venous site
	nuclear scan study	procedure that uses isotopes in the body for diagnostic purposes
	percutaneous needle biopsy	excision of tissue by a guided needle through the skin

Clinical Dimension	Term	Description
	percutaneous transhepatic cholangiography (PTHC or PTC)	radiography of the bile ducts using contrast medium delivered via needle puncture
	percutaneous transhepatic portography	radiography of the portal venous system using a contrast medium delivered via needle puncture
	percutaneous transluminal angioplasty (PTA)	use of a balloon catheter to widen a narrowed artery; another term for percutaneous transluminal balloon angioplasty
	percutaneous transluminal balloon angioplasty (PTCA)	use of a balloon catheter to widen a narrowed artery; another term for percutaneous transluminal angioplasty
	phonocardiography	procedure for obtaining a visual record of heart sounds and murmurs made by a phonocardiograph
	photodensitometry	examination of bone density using light absorption and reflection; another term for densitometry
	positron emission tomography (PET)	nuclear medicine technique for assessing metabolic activity of organs, diagnosing cancer, locating brain tumors, and investigating brain function
	ptyalography	x-ray examination of the salivary glands after administration of a contrast medium; another term for sialography
	pulmonary perfusion imaging	use of a radiopharmaceutical to form an image of lung tissue by detecting it in the capillaries
	pulmonary ventilation imaging	use of xenon-133 gas to form an image of lung tissue by identifying its presence in the alveoli
	pyelography	radiography of the kidneys and surrounding tissue using a contrast medium
	radioactive iodine uptake	test used to determine thyroid function by assessing the amount of radioactive iodine absorbed by the thyroid gland
	radioimmunoassay	technique for identifying antibodies using a radioactive tracer
	retrograde pyelography (RP)	radiography of the kidneys after a contrast dye is injected into the ureters, resulting in backward fluid movement
	Schilling test	technique for determining vitamin B_{12} absorption
	scintigraphy	two-dimensional imaging technique using a radioactive tracer
	selective arterial catheter placement	catheter placed into another portion of the arterial system from which it was originally inserted

Clinical Dimension	Term	Description
	selective venous	catheter placed into a vein and manipulated into another venous site
	shuntogram	x-ray examination of an artificially created passage to determine shunt placement
	sialography	x-ray examination of the salivary glands after administration of a contrast medium; another term for ptyalography
	single photon emission computed tomography (SPECT)	imaging technique that creates three-dimensional pictures by identifying a radioactive tracer absorbed by an organ or tissue
	sonography	imaging technique using high-frequency sound waves; another term for echography or ultrasonography
	spleen imaging	radiograph of the spleen after administering a radionuclide
	splenoportography	x-ray examination of the splenic and portal vein system after injection of a contrast medium
	thallium scan	nuclear imaging technique using a radioisotope of thallium
	thyroid imaging	radiograph of the thyroid after administering a radionuclide such as radioactive iodine
	tomography	technique in which images in certain planes are focused while images in other planes are blurred
	transcatheter biopsy	tissue sample taken via a catheter
	transluminal atherectomy	removal of deposits on the inner lining of a body structure
	ultrasonography	imaging technique using high-frequency sound waves; another term for echography or sonography
	ultrasound	imaging technique using high-frequency sound waves
	urea breath test	test using carbon-14 to determine the presence of *H. pylori*
	urethrocystography	x-ray examination of the urethra and bladder using a contrast dye; another term for cystourethrography
	urography	radiography of the urinary tract
	vasography	x-ray examination of the vas deferens using a contrast medium
	venography	x-ray examination of veins or vein networks after injection of a radiopaque dye

Clinical Dimension	Term	Description
	ventriculography	radiographic examination of the brain ventricles (after replacing the CSF with a gas or detectable dye) or the heart ventricles (after injecting a radionuclide)
	vesiculography	x-ray examination of the seminal vesicles using a contrast medium
TREATMENTS		
	brachytherapy	radiotherapy in which the source is placed directly on or in close proximity to the body
	endocavitary irradiation	treating body cavities with radiation
	hemibody radiation	radiotherapy of one half of the body
	hyperthermia	therapeutically induced fever; another term for hyperpyrexia
	interstitial brachytherapy	radiation treatment via implanted sources
	intracavitary therapy	managing a disease by introducing radiation into an organ or body cavity
	intraoperative cone irradiation	using x-rays aimed at a target to destroy cancerous cells during surgery
	irradiation	medical use of radiation—such as x-rays, gamma-rays, or other radioactive sources—to treat cancer
	radiation oncology	use of radioactive substances for treating cancer
	radionuclide seeds	radioactive particles that are implanted in the body for treating cancer
	radiotherapy	treating cancer growths by radiation; another term for radiation oncology
	teletherapy	radiation treatment from a source distant from the body
	total body irradiation	exposing the entire body to ionizing radiation

FACT *A patient over age 55 years requires the services of a radiologist three times more frequently than a younger patient!*

Lifespan

Many procedures identified in this chapter can be used at any point in life. Diagnostic ultrasound can detect the presence of embryonic life and can be performed as early as the 4th week of pregnancy. Although some procedures carry considerable risk, others such as ultrasound and magnetic resonance imaging have very little. Hence, the latter are deemed safe throughout the lifespan.

In the News: X-Rays Reveal Location of Live Grenade

Military doctors have chronicled the removal of explosive materials from the body since World War II. Recently, South American health-care personnel reported another case. A Colombian solider was accidentally shot in the face with a gun-launched grenade. Radiologic examination revealed the location of the live ammunition lodged in the nasal region beneath the skull.

Under the direction of x-ray technology, the surgeons were able to successfully remove the plum-size projectile. In a surgical procedure that lasted approximately 4 hours, the physicians extracted the grenade through a surgical incision within the young man's mouth. They then treated the wound and repaired the patient's facial bone fractures. Reports indicate the man has recovered with only minor scars.

COMMON ABBREVIATIONS

Abbreviation	Term
A	anterior
ACR	American College of Radiology
AHIMA	American Health Information Management Association
AHRA	American Healthcare Radiology Administrators
$BaSO_4$	barium sulfate
^{14}C	carbon-14
CAAHEP	Commission on Accreditation of Allied Health Education Programs (CAAHEP)
CAT	computerized axial tomography computer-assisted tomography computed axial tomography
CPC	certified professional coder
CPT	*Current Procedural Terminology*
CSF	cerebrospinal fluid
CT	computed tomography
DRG	diagnosis related group
DSA	digital subtraction angiography
ECG	electrocardiogram
EMG	electromyography
Ga	gallium
^{67}Ga	gallium-67
GI	gastrointestinal
Gy	gray
Hz	hertz
^{123}I	iodine-123
^{125}I	iodine-125
^{131}I	iodine-131
ICD	*International Classification of Diseases*
IV	intravenous
IVP	intravenous pyelography
mCi	millicurie
μCi	microcurie
MRA	magnetic resonance angiography

Abbreviation	Term
MRI	magnetic resonance imaging
MUGA scan	multiple-gated acquisition scan
NMR	nuclear magnetic resonance
P	posterior
PCTA	percutaneous transluminal balloon angioplasty
PET	positron emission tomography
PTA	percutaneous transluminal angioplasty
PTC	percutaneous transhepatic cholangiography
PTHC	percutaneous transhepatic cholangiography
RBMA	Radiology Business Management Association
RHIT	registered health information technician
RP	retrograde pyelography
SCVIR	Society of Cardiovascular & Interventional Radiology
SI	International System
SPECT	single photon emission computed tomography
$T_{1/2}$	half life
Tc	technetium
^{99}Tc	technetium-99
TI	thallium
^{201}TI	thallium-201
Xe	xenon
^{133}Xe	xenon-133

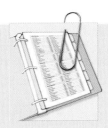

Case Study

Max Korinna's case is typical of the type seen in Jean's radiology office. The medical report indicated that a chest x-ray was performed to determine intravenous catheter placement. Clinical information stated the patient was a 67-year-old male. The test performed was a chest radiography and was marked "chest, 1 view AP."

Report Information

AP view obtained of the chest with the patient erect shows cardiac monitoring electrodes overlying the anterior chest wall. A radiopaque catheter is identified extending from the left side, the tip of which is localized to the superior vena cava. The heart is prominent in regard to size. The lungs demonstrate no evidence of acute pulmonary pathology. There is no evidence of pneumothorax.

Impression

1. Cardiomegaly exists with underlying chronic pulmonary changes.
2. The tip of the indwelling catheter is thought to reside within the superior vena cava.

Case Study Questions

Select the best answer to each of the following questions.

1. *AP view* refers to _____.
   a. anatomy and physiology.
   b. axial and proximal.
   c. anterior and posterior.
   d. appendicular and physical.

2. **The word part *cardio-* refers to _____, and the word part -*megaly* means _____; so *cardiomegaly* refers to _____.**
   a. vessel; large; large vessel
   b. heart; small; an atrophied (small, wasting) heart
   c. chest; large; enlarged chest cavity
   d. heart; large; enlarged heart

3. **Which is the correct definition for *catheter*?**
   a. A thin flexible tube inserted into a body part
   b. An artificially created passage to redirect circulation
   c. A unit of measurement for the absorbed dose of ionizing radiation
   d. A substance opaque to x-rays that is used to make the outline of a body part easier to see on radiographs

4. **The term *radiopaque* means that the catheter _____.**
   a. could be visualized on radiographic examination because it blocked the passage of x-rays
   b. could not be visualized on radiographic examination because it blocked the passage of x-rays
   c. contained radioactive material
   d. was colored

REAL WORLD REPORT

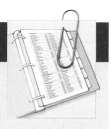

Jean's office received Max Korinna's medical report from the imaging department for coding and billing purposes.

CENTRAL IMAGING DEPARTMENT

NAME:	Max Korinna	
DATE ORDERED:	January 20, 2004	AGE:67Y
ORDPHYS:	M. R. Tambo, M.D.	EXAM DATE: 01/20/2004
DOB:	02/02/1936	TEST: ANGIO, CAR/CRBRL, BIL, RS&I
ATTENDING:	M. R. Tambo, M.D.	REFERRING: P. J. Miter, M.D.

CLINICAL INFORMATION: Follow-up for possible lesion at distal cervical segment of the right internal carotid.

NONSELECTIVE RIGHT CAROTID ANGIOGRAM

Following right brachial arterial puncture at the antecubital region, a 4 French straight catheter was placed at the innominate artery for nonselective right carotid angiogram. Frontal and oblique projections were made. The patient tolerated the procedure well and left the department in stable condition.

Comparison was made to previous cerebral and carotid angiogram of January 18, 2004.

The previously noted segmental narrowing at the distal portion of the cervical segment of the right internal carotid is no longer demonstrated on this examination; therefore, the previous finding is from spasm. There is no significant plaque formation or narrowing of the right internal or external carotid arteries. Incidentally noted is plaque formation at the origin of the left internal carotid without significant stenosis. Bilateral vertebral arteries appear unremarkable.

Refer to the previous cerebral and carotid angiogram for anatomic details of the intracranial circulation.

DICTATED BY: M. J. Manju, M.D.

REAL WORLD REPORT QUESTIONS

The following exercises review the medical terms in the preceding medical report.

1. The term *nonselective* means _____.

2. Provide a brief description of an angiogram.

3. Was this procedure performed to evaluate arteries or veins?

   _____.

4. The regions of the body through which the catheter passed include _____.

   a. arm, neck, and head

   b. leg, neck, and arm

   c. head, chest, and leg

   d. leg, neck, and head

REVIEW AND APPLICATION: THREE-LEVEL LEARNING SYSTEM

LEVEL ONE: REVIEWING FACTS AND TERMS USING RECALL

Select the best response to each of the following questions.

1. The branch of medicine that deals with radioactive substances in the diagnosis and treatment of disease is known as _____.

   a. urology

   b. radiology

   c. oncology

   d. hematology

2. A physician specializing in the diagnostic and/or therapeutic use of x-rays and radionuclides is a/an _____.

   a. radiologist

   b. urologist

   c. professional coder

   d. radiographer

3. _____ is the branch of medicine that uses radioisotopes in diagnosis and therapy.

   a. Nuclear medicine

   b. Diagnostic medicine

   c. Therapeutic medicine

   d. Mammography

4. The branch of radiology that uses guided procedures for diagnosing and treating pathology is _____ radiology.

   a. oncology

   b. nuclear

   c. interventional

   d. diagnostic

5. An x-ray of the joint space after introduction of a contrast medium is termed _____.

   a. shuntogram

   b. CT pelvimetry

   c. cineradiography

   d. arthrography

6. _____ is an imaging technique in which certain planes of the body are focused while other planes are blurred.

   a. Scintigraphy

   b. Ultrasound

   c. Radiology

   d. Tomography

7. Which of the following is a palliative therapy in which half of the body is radiated to treat multiple cancer sites simultaneously?

   a. hemibody radiation

   b. teletherapy

   c. brachytherapy

   d. interstitial brachytherapy

8. A method of imaging ventricles after injection with a gas or radiopaque medium is _____.

   a. spleen imaging

   b. ventriculography

   c. thyroid imaging

   d. pulmonary perfusion imaging

9. The branch of medicine that uses radioactive substances for cancer treatment is called _____.

   a. nuclear medicine

   b. ultrasonography

   c. diagnostic ultrasound

   d. radiation oncology

10. Examination of the intervertebral disks after direct injection of a contrast medium is known as _____.

    a. vessel ordering

    b. cineradiography

    c. diskography

    d. cinefluoroscope

11. A procedure in which a tubular instrument is passed through a blood vessel to the heart for imaging purposes is termed _____.

    a. cardiac catheterization

    b. percutaneous transluminal angioplasty

    c. percutaneous balloon angioplasty

    d. percutaneous needle biopsy

12. Imaging blood vessels using MRI is termed _____.

    a. vessel ordering

    b. CT scanning

    c. magnetic resonance angiography

    d. all of these

13. A group of vessels fed by a primary vessel is called a _____.

    a. vessel ordering

    b. vascular family

    c. millicurie

    d. rad

14. A catheter placed into an arterial vessel and not manipulated is _____, whereas a catheter placed into a vein and not manipulated to another site is _____.

    a. nonselective venous; nonselective arterial catheter placement

    b. nonselective arterial catheter placement; nonselective venous

    c. selective venous; selective arterial catheter placement

    d. selective arterial catheter placement; selective venous

15. A _____ is a radiolabeled chemical used as a detector in diagnostic tests.

    a. gray

    b. radionuclide

    c. radiotracer

    d. rad

16. A/an _____ is a unit of measurement for radiation absorbed by and delivered to tissues.

    a. radiotracer

    b. microcurie

    c. opaque

    d. gray

17. Radioactivity is measured in units called _____.

    a. radiations

    b. millicuries

    c. microcuries

    d. B and C

18. A radiograph of the entire skeletal system is a _____.

    a. gallium scan

    b. biopsy

    c. bone scan

    d. scintigraphy

19. _____ is an imaging technique that uses electromagnetic radiation.

    a. X-ray

    b. MRI

    c. CAT

    d. Ultrasound

20. Excision of tissue by a guided needle through the skin is called _____.

    a. subcutaneous needle incision

    b. percutaneous needle incision

    c. percutaneous needle biopsy

    d. percutaneous subcutaneous needle biopsy

21. Use of a balloon catheter to widen a narrowed artery is _____.

    a. percutaneous transluminal angioplasty

    b. subcutaneous transluminal angioplasty

    c. percutaneous subcutaneous angioplasty

    d. none of the above

22. Examination of bone density using light absorption and reflection is termed _____.

    a. ultrasonography

    b. photodensitometry

    c. angioplasty

    d. electromyography

23. An x-ray of the urine-collecting part of the kidney after IV administration of a dye is termed _____.

    a. antegrade pyelography

    b. retrograde pyelography

    c. anterograde pyelography

    d. intravenous pyelogram

24. An imaging technique that uses radionuclides to assess metabolic function is _____.

    a. positron emission tomography

    b. radioimmunoassay

    c. computed axial tomography

    d. ultrasound

25. _____ studies use isotopes in the body for diagnostic purposes.

    a. Ultrasound

    b. Nuclear scan

    c. Densitometry

    d. Teletherapy

LEVEL TWO: REVIEWING CONCEPTS

Select the best response to each of the following questions.

26. During a _____ catheter placement, the catheter is threaded into another artery from the original puncture site.

    a. selective arterial

    b. nonselective arterial

    c. selective venous

    d. nonselective venous

27. _____ pyelography demonstrates forward fluid movement, and _____ pyelography shows backward flow.

    a. Antegrade; retrograde

    b. Retrograde; antegrade

    c. Antegrade; anterograde

    d. Retrograde; intravenous

Provide a medical term to complete a meaningful analogy.

28. Ultrasonic cardiography and ultrasound cardiography are to _____ as _____ is to echography or sonography.

29. Urethrocystography is to _____ as _____ is to ptyalography.

30. Radiograms are to shadowgraphs as _____ are to roentgenograms.

Match the term or procedure with its description.

_____ 31. barium swallow

_____ 32. x-ray image

_____ 33. endoscopic catheterization

_____ 34. shuntogram

_____ 35. barium enema

a. x-ray examination to determine shunt placement

b. procedure using an endoscope to view internal structures

c. rectal infusion with barium sulfate for radiographic and fluoroscopic study of the lower GI tract

d. ingestion of barium sulfate for x-ray examination of the upper GI tract

e. image produced on film after roentgen rays are passed through the structure

Match the term or procedure with its description.

_____ 36. cholangiography

_____ 37. cholecystography

_____ 38. cisternography

_____ 39. sialography

_____ 40. splenoportography

a. x-ray examination of the salivary glands

b. x-ray examination of bile ducts after administration of a contrast dye

c. x-ray examination of the gallbladder after administration of a contrast dye

d. x-ray examination of the spleen and portal vein after administration of a contrast dye

e. x-ray examination of the subarachnoid space after administration of a contrast dye

Match the term or procedure with its description.

_____ 41. digital subtraction angiography

_____ 42. cardiac catheterization

_____ 43. lymphangiography

a. x-ray examination of the heart after threading a catheter from another vessel

b. radiography of an organ in motion

c. computer-assisted radiograph of vascular structures without superimposed bone or soft tissue

_____ 44. cinefluoroscopy

_____ 45. electromyography

d. procedure used to diagnose motor nerve and muscle disorders

e. x-ray examination of lymphatic vessels after administration of a contrast dye

Match the term or procedure with its description.

_____ 46. corpora cavernosography

_____ 47. hysterosalpingography

_____ 48. CT pelvimetry

_____ 49. cystography

_____ 50. urography

a. x-ray examination of the urinary tract

b. x-ray examination of the bladder after administration of a contrast medium

c. x-ray examination of the penile erectile tissue

d. measurements of pelvic dimensions

e. x-ray examination of the uterus and oviducts after administration of a contrast dye

Match the term or procedure with its description.

_____ 51. echocardiography

_____ 52. echoencephalography

a. imaging technique using high-frequency sound waves

b. imaging technique applying the Doppler effect

_____ 53. Doppler echocar-diography

    c. ultrasound technique for observing the heart

_____ 54. Doppler ultra-sonography

    d. ultrasound technique employing the Doppler effect to enhance two-dimensional echocardio-graphy

_____ 55. ultrasound

    e. ultrasound technique for studying intracranial structures

Match the term or procedure with its description.

_____ 56. brachytherapy

    a. therapeutically in duced fever

_____ 57. hemibody radiation

    b. radiotherapy in which the source is placed close to or on the body

_____ 58. hyperthermia

    c. radiation of half of the body

_____ 59. scintigraphy

    d. two-dimensional imaging technique using a radioactive tracer

_____ 60. urea breath test

    e. ^{14}C test to determine the presence of _H. pylori_

Match the term or procedure with its description.

_____ 61. gallium scan

    a. nuclear imaging technique using ^{201}TI

_____ 62. Schilling test

    b. study used in nuclear medicine to evaluate cardiac function

_____ 63. thallium scan

    c. technique used to determine absorption of vitamin B_{12}

_____ 64. pulmonary ventilation imaging

    d. imaging technique using ^{67}Ga

_____ 65. MUGA scan

    e. technique using ^{131}Xe

Using the following word parts, form a medical term for each definition. Each word part is used only once.

aorto-	-graphy	hystero-
angio-	-graphy	mammo-
arterio-	-graphy	phono-
cardio-	-graphy	sono-
cardio-	-graphy	vaso-
epididymo-	-graphy	veno-
-graphy-	-graphy	vesiculo-
-graphy	-graphy	

66. ultrasound of the uterus = _____

67. x-ray examination of the aorta after injection of a contrast medium = _____

68. x-ray examination of veins after injection of an opaque dye = _____

69. x-ray examination of the heart and blood vessels after administration of a contrast dye = _____

70. x-ray examination of arteries after injection of a contrast dye = _____

71. procedure for obtaining a visual record of heart sounds = _____

72. x-ray examination of the seminal vesicles after administration of a contrast medium = _____

73. x-ray examination of the vas deferens after introducing a contrast medium = _____

74. x-ray examination of the epididymis after introducing a contrast medium = _____

75. radiographic examination of the breast tissue = _____

Define the following terms.

76. radionuclide = _____

77. half-life = _____

78. barium sulfate ($BaSO_4$) = _____

79. intravascular ultrasound = _____

What is the term described by each of the following definitions?

80. term describing the amount of work required to position a catheter at its destination _____

81. absorption of radionuclide by tissue _____

82. radiology of bile ducts via needle puncture through the skin _____

83. introduction of a barium salt suspension into the rectum and colon for x-ray examination _____

84. aiming a beam of x-rays directly at the target tissue through a cylinder _____

85. radiographic examination of brain ventricles after replacing CSF with gas or a detectable dye _____

Identify the correctly spelled term in each set.

_____ 86. a. veinography   b. venography

c. venegraphy   d. venogrephy

_____ 87. a. galacktogram   b. glactiogram

c. galactogram   d. gelactogram

_____ 88. a. yoorography   b. uregraphy

c. urrography   d. urography

_____ 89. a. radiopaque   b. radioopaque

c. radipaque   d. radiopake

_____ 90. a. telatherapy   b. teletherapy

c. telotherapy   d. telletherpy

_____ 91. a. radinuclide   b. radionucleide

c. radionuclide   d. radionuklide

_____ 92. a. radio-   b. radio-
            farmaceutical   pharmacutical

c. radiophar-   d. radiophar-
meceutical   maceutical

Unscramble the letters in each set to create a medical term.

93. namee _____

94. diveaaoritc _____

95. mitesdryo _____

96. aaadiioommnussyr _____

97. aaeouqprdi _____

98. ridthoy _____

Define the following abbreviations.

99. μCi _____

100. PTA _____

101. PET _____

102. CT _____

103. MRI _____

104. EMG _____

LEVEL THREE: THINKING CRITICALLY

105. A physician orders a procedure that involves catheter placement through the aorta to the left common carotid artery, ending in the left external carotid artery.

a. The primary branch is the _____.

b. The secondary branch is the _____.

KEY TERMS SPELLING TEST FROM CD-ROM

Use the CD-ROM to test yourself on the spelling of the key terms from this chapter. Listen to the terms and write them on a separate sheet of paper. Use a medical dictionary to check your answers.

ANSWERS

WORD GROUPING

Definition	Word Part
motion picture	cine-
beyond, excess	ultra-
distant	tel-, tele-, telo-
dry	xer-, xero-
electricity	electro-
fever, fire, heat	pyr-, pyro-
flow	fluo-
internal, within	end-, endo-
nuclear, nucleus	nucle-, nucleo-
portal	porto-
radiation	radio-
recording, usually by an instrument	-gram
saliva	sial-, sialo-
salivary glands, saliva	ptyal-, ptyalo-
section	-tome
short	brachy-
something written, instrument for making a recording	-graph
sound	A. phon-, phono-
	B. son-, sono-
spectrum	spectro-
tears, lacrimal apparatus	dacry-, dacryo-
tumor	onco-, oncho-
writing, description	grapho-, -graphy

WORD BUILDING

Word Part	Meaning	Common or Known Word	Example Medical Term
brachy-	short	brachycephalic	brachytherapy
cine-	motion picture	cinema	cineradiography
electro-	electricity	electronics	electromyography
end-, endo-	internal, within	endothermic	endoscopic catheterization
fluo-	flow	fluorescent	fluoroscopy
-gram	recording, usually by an instrument	sonogram	sonogram
-graph	something written, instrument for making a recording	photograph	angiograph
grapho-, -graphy	writing, description	photography	arteriography
nucle-, nucleo-	nuclear, nucleus	nuclear reaction	nuclear medicine
onco-, oncho-	tumor	oncogene	oncology
phon-, phono-	sound	phonics	phonocardiography
pyr-, pyro-	fever, fire, heat	pyrotechnics	hyperpyrexia
radio-	radiation	radioactive	radiology
son-, sono-	sound	sonogram	sonography
tel-, tele-, telo-	distant	telephone	teletherapy
-tome	section	dermatome	tomography
ultra-	beyond, excess	ultraviolet	ultrasound
xer-, xero-	dry	xerox	xeromammography

KEY TERM PRACTICE

Radiology Preview

1. diagnostic ultrasound
2. Nuclear

Radiology Basic Terms

1. uptake
2. contrast medium

Diagnostic Radiology

1. interventional radiology
2. diagnostic radiology

Radiography

1. -graphy; arthrography
2. diskography

Radiography in Motion

1. motion picture; radiation; -graphy; cineradiography
2. flowing

Tomography

1. computed tomography angiography
2. computed tomography (CT); the following are also correct: computerized axial tomography (CAT), computer assisted tomography (CAT), computed axial tomography (CAT)

Catheterization, Biopsy, and Percutaneous Radiographic Procedures

1. transcatheter biopsy
2. selective
3. percutaneous transluminal balloon angioplasty
4. Percutaneous transhepatic portography

Magnetic Resonance Imaging

1. magnetic resonance angiography; -graphy
2. magnetic resonance spectroscopy

Contrast Studies and Digestive System Radiology

1. barium swallow
2. duodenography

Nervous System Radiology

1. dacryocystography; dacry-, dacryo-
2. Myelography

Heart and Blood Vessels Radiology

1. Angiography
2. arteriography

Reproductive System Radiography

1. mammography
2. mammary ductogram; mammary galactogram

Respiratory System Radiology

1. laryngography
2. bronchography

Urinary System Radiology

1. pyelography
2. cystourethrography; urethrocystography

Other Diagnostic Radiology Services

1. Phonocardiography; phono-; -graphy
2. densitometry; photodensitometry

Diagnostic Ultrasound

1. ultrasonography (ultrasound) or echography
2. hysterosonography; sono-; writing, description

Radiation Oncology

1. radiotherapy
2. Irradiation

Nuclear Medicine

1. bone scan
2. Positron emission tomography (PET)

CASE STUDY

1. c. is the correct answer.
   - a, b, and d are incorrect because in reference to radiology, AP means anterior and posterior, or anteroposterior.
2. d is the correct answer.
   - a, b, and c are incorrect because the term *cardiomegaly* is formed from the word parts meaning "heart" and "large."
3. a. is the correct answer.
   - b. is incorrect because an artificially created passage to redirect circulation is a shunt.
   - c. is incorrect because a unit of measurement for the absorbed dose of ionizing radiation is a gray (Gy).

   - d. is incorrect because a substance opaque to x-rays that is used to make the outline of a body part easier to see on radiographs is a contrast medium.
4. a. is the correct answer.
   - b. is incorrect because it could be visualized on radiographic examination.
   - c. is incorrect because the term *radioactive* indicates that an object emits energy in the form of particle streams.
   - d. is incorrect because the color of the catheter would not be evident on an x-ray.

REAL WORD REPORT

1. The term *nonselective* means that the needle is placed directly into a vessel and is not manipulated into a branch.

2. An angiogram is an x-ray of a blood vessel after introducing a contrast medium.
3. This procedure was done to evaluate arteries.
4. A is the correct answer.

REVIEW AND APPLICATION: THREE-LEVEL LEARNING SYSTEM

Level One: Reviewing Facts and Terms Using Recall

1. b
2. a
3. a
4. c
5. d
6. d
7. a
8. b
9. d
10. c
11. a
12. c
13. b
14. b
15. c
16. d
17. d
18. c
19. b
20. c
21. a
22. b
23. d
24. a
25. b

Level Two: Reviewing Concepts

26. a
27. a
28. echocardiography; ultrasonography
29. cystourethrography; sialography
30. radiographs or x-rays
31. d
32. e
33. b
34. a
35. c
36. b
37. c
38. e
39. a
40. d
41. c
42. a
43. e
44. b
45. d
46. c
47. e
48. d
49. b
50. a
51. c
52. e
53. d
54. b
55. a

56. b
57. c
58. a
59. d
60. e
61. d
62. c
63. a
64. e
65. b
66. hysterosonography
67. aortography
68. venography
69. angiocardiography
70. arteriography
71. phonocardiography
72. vesiculography
73. vasography
74. epididymography
75. mammography
76. artificial or natural isotope demonstrating radioactivity
77. period of time in which the radioactivity of a substance decreases by half (50%)
78. compound used in medicine because it cannot be penetrated by x-rays
79. ultrasound imaging technique for viewing blood and lymphatic vessels
80. vessel ordering
81. uptake
82. percutaneous transhepatic cholangiography
83. barium enema
84. intraoperative cone irradiation
85. ventriculography
86. b
87. c
88. d
89. a
90. b
91. c
92. d
93. enema
94. radioactive
95. dosimetry
96. radioimmunoassay
97. radiopaque
98. thyroid
99. microcurie
100. percutaneous transluminal angioplasty
101. positron emission tomography
102. computed tomography
103. magnetic resonance imaging
104. electromyography

Level Three: Thinking Critically

105. a. left common carotid; B. left external carotid artery

4

Integumentary System

OBJECTIVES

After completing this chapter, you should be able to:

1. Identify structures of the skin, hair, and nails.
2. Describe the primary function of each component of the skin and the integumentary system.
3. Label anatomical structures of the integumentary system.
4. Define word parts used for the integumentary system.
5. Describe common integumentary system diseases and their various signs, symptoms, clinical tests, diagnostic procedures, and treatments.
6. Summarize anatomical and physiological alterations throughout the lifespan.
7. Identify common abbreviations related to the integumentary system.
8. Define terms used in medical reports.
9. Correctly define, spell, and pronounce the chapter's medical terms.

Professional Profile: Cytotechnologist

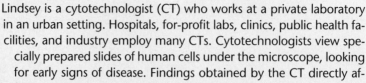

Lindsey is a cytotechnologist (CT) who works at a private laboratory in an urban setting. Hospitals, for-profit labs, clinics, public health facilities, and industry employ many CTs. Cytotechnologists view specially prepared slides of human cells under the microscope, looking for early signs of disease. Findings obtained by the CT directly affect a patient because treatments are generally designed around the test results.

Most often the cultures and tissue samples come from physician offices or small area hospitals and clinics. When viewing the slide, the skilled CT looks for cellular abnormalities in color, size, and morphology (shape) that could be clues to pathology (disease). If the slide appears normal, a final report is issued to the ordering physician. However, if there are indications of irregularity, Lindsey works with the pathologist to reach a final diagnosis. A pathologist is a physician who identifies the nature, origin, and cause of disease. Lindsey views dermatology slides daily, and much of her work is subjective. Thus this lends credence to the phrase "as much of an art as a science."

Cytotechnologists are proficient in problem solving and work independently with little supervision. Excellent verbal and written communication skills are essential because many other professionals read the reports and are involved with patient care. To become a cytotechnologist, one completes a baccalaureate degree plus one year of clinical education in an accredited cytotechnology program. The Commission on Accreditation of Allied Health Education Programs (CAAHEP) grants accreditation of a program.

This is a growing field. Students are qualified for a job immediately after they complete the program and pass the boards. The Board of Registry of the American Society for Clinical Pathology (ASCP) is responsible for the national certification examination. The job outlook for cytotechnologists is bright because there are more positions available than qualified people to fill them.

INTRODUCTION

Between 30,000 and 50,000 microscopic skin flakes are shed per minute! These make up a majority of the dust found in homes!

The skin, also called the integument, and its associated structures such as hair, nails, and glands, make up the integumentary system. Skin is the body's largest organ. Its primary functions include maintenance of body temperature and homeostasis, protection, stimuli reception, excretion, vitamin D synthesis, and melanin production. Serving as a covering for the body's internal structures, the integument is crucial to survival.

Because skin provides the first line of defense against a host of environmental insults, damage to this protective covering allows the entry of microorganisms, which can cause disease. Signs of skin disorders are usually obvious, yet at times it is necessary to obtain tissue samples for cellular analysis. Symptoms, tests, diagnostic procedures, and treatments related to integumentary disorders are discussed in the chapter. Furthermore, age-related changes that occur throughout the lifespan are also given.

MEDICAL TERM PARTS

WORD PARTS

Medical term prefixes, suffixes, and combining forms related to the integumentary system are introduced in this section.

Word Parts	Meaning
adip-, adipo-	fat
aut-, auto-	self

Word Parts	Meaning
cero-	wax
chrom-, -chrome, chromat-, chromato-, chromo-	color
cry-, cryo-	cold
cyan-, cyano-	blue
cyt-, -cyte, cyto-	cell
derm-, derma-, dermat-, dermato-, dermo-	skin
erythr-, erythro-	red or red blood cell
hidr-, hidro-[a]	sweat
histio-, histo-	tissue
ichthy-, ichthyo-	fish
kerat-, kerato-	horny tissue or cornea
leuc-, leuco-, leuk-, leuko-	white or white blood cell
lip-, lipo-	fatty
melan-, melano-	black
myc-, myco-	fungus
necr-, necro-	death
-oma	tumor
onych-, onycho-	fingernail or toenail
papulo-	pimple, circumscribed solid elevation
path-, patho-, -pathy	disease
phyt-, phyto-	plants
pil-, pilo-	hair
-plasia	formation
py-, pyo-	pus accumulation
-rrhea	flowing
scler-, sclero-	hardness
squamo-	epidermal scale
seb-, sebi-, sebo-	sebum (oil)
steato-	fat
sub-	beneath
sudor-	sweat
trich-, trichi-, tricho-	hair
vesic-, vesico-, vesiculo-	vesicle, blister
xanth-, xantho-	yellow
xer-, xero-	dry

[a]*Note:* The word parts *hidr-* and *hidro-* mean "sweat." Do not confuse them with *hydr-* and *hydro-*, which mean "water." Notice the difference in spelling.

WORD ETYMOLOGY

Some words have Greek or Latin roots but are not true word parts. This section lists those that are used as medical terms.

Word	Definition
albus	white
causa	cause
cutis	skin
diaphoresis	perspiration
epiderm, epiderma	epidermis
kauterion	branding iron
macula	spot
palpebra	eyelid
pediculus	louse
porphyra	purple
rhytis	wrinkle
squama	skin scale
unguis	nail
vita	life

MEDICAL TERM PARTS USED AS PREFIXES

Prefix	Definition
cero-	wax
papulo-	pimple, circumscribed solid elevation
squamo-	epidermal scale
steato-	fat
sub-	beneath
sudor-	sweat

MEDICAL TERM PARTS USED AS SUFFIXES

Suffix	Definition
-oma	tumor
-plasia	formation
-rrhea	flowing

WORD GROUPING

Using the "Medical Term Parts" table, identify the prefix, suffix, or combining form for each of the following definitions. The first one has been done as an example.

Definition	Word Part
beneath	sub-
black	
blue	
cell	
cold	
color	
death	
disease	
dry	
epidermal scale	
fat	A. B.
fatty	
fingernail or toenail	
fish	
flowing	
formation	
fungus	
hair	A. B.
hardness	
horny tissue or cornea	
pimple, circumscribed solid elevation	
plants	
pus accumulation	
red or red blood cell	
sebum (oil)	
self	
skin	
sweat	A. B.
tissue	
tumor	
vesicle, blister	

Definition	Word Part
wax	
white or white blood cell	
sweat	
yellow	

WORD BUILDING

Word parts, introduced in the "Medical Term Parts" section, are listed in the following table. For this exercise, first supply the meaning of each word part, then use the word part to build words you already know. The word you list under "Common or Known Word" does not have to be a medical term; a commonly used word is fine. Be sure, however, that the word correctly reflects the meaning. The first one has been done as an example. Check your answers in a dictionary.

Word Part	Meaning	Common or Known Word	Example Medical Term
adip-, adipo-	fat	adipose	adipocytes
aut-, auto-			autoimmune
cyt-, -cyte, cyto-			erythrocyte
derm-, derma-, dermat-, dermato-, dermo-			epidermis
erythr-, erythro-			erythrocyte
histio-, histo-			histology
lip-, lipo-			liposuction
melan-, melano-			melanocyte
path-, patho-, -pathy			pathophysiology
-rrhea			seborrhea
scler-, sclero-			scleroderma
sub-			subcutaneous
vesic-, vesico-, vesiculo-			vesicle

ANATOMY AND PHYSIOLOGY

Structures of the Integumentary System

- Cutaneous membrane
- Hair
- Integument
- Nails
- Sebaceous glands
- Sudoriferous glands
- Sweat glands

Integumentary System Preview

Skin is considered an organ because two or more kinds of tissues are grouped together to perform its specialized function. It is also considered a membrane and is composed of epithelial and connective tissues. The integumentary system is made of **cutaneous** (pertaining to the skin) membranes and various accessory organs. The skin, or **integument**, consists of associated structures such as **hair, nails, sudoriferous glands** (**sweat glands**), and **sebaceous** (oil) **glands**. The skin and its epidermal structures such as hair, fingernails, toenails, and glands make up the integumentary system. The study of the skin and the integumentary system is termed **dermatology**, and a physician who specializes in this field is called a **dermatologist.**

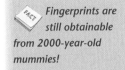

Fingerprints are still obtainable from 2000-year-old mummies!

The skin is responsible for maintaining body temperature, thus keeping homeostatic balance. When the body becomes too warm, heat is carried away from the body in the form of sweat, which is a mixture of water, salt, and organic wastes.

Hair and nails are skin derivatives. Hair is made of **keratin,** a tough, waterproof protein that develops in the membranes. Every hair has an associated sebaceous gland that secretes **sebum,** an oil, to keep the skin soft and pliable. The term **pilosebaceous** means "pertaining to hair (pilo-) follicles and sebaceous glands." Nails are made of epithelial cells that cover the distal portion of each finger and toe.

There are about 100,000 hair follicles on the scalp!

The integumentary system serves a protective function by creating a physical barrier that prevents microbes from entering. Broken skin increases the risk of infection. Additional protective features include the production of melanin and keratin. **Melanin** is a dark pigment produced by **melanocytes,** cells in the epidermal layer of the skin, that gives the skin its color. The primary purpose of melanin is to filter ultraviolet (UV) radiation, which can disrupt underlying cellular activity in a variety of tissues. The interaction of UV radiation with melanocytes is responsible for suntanned skin. Keratinocytes produce keratin, which is a protein that serves as a water repellent. About 90% of skin cells are of this type because keratin is the principal element of the outer skin. The skin also has Langerhans cells, which serve an immune function by protecting the body from disease.

Furthermore, the epidermal cells of the skin synthesize vitamin D. Vitamin D is important for normal bone development throughout life.

Key Terms	Definitions
cutaneous (kew TAY nee us)	pertaining to or involving the skin
integument (in TEG yoo munt)	term for skin
hair	keratinized filaments covering the body
nails	protective coverings on the fingers and toes
sudoriferous (sue dur IF ur us) **glands**	glands that secrete sweat
sweat glands	structures that discharge fluid to the skin surface
sebaceous (se BAY shus) **glands**	structures that secrete sebum to the skin surface
dermatology (dur muh TOL uh jee)	the study of skin
dermatologist (dur muh TOL uh jist)	physician specializing in skin and the integumentary system
keratin (KERR uh tin)	protein associated with hair and nails
sebum (SEE bum)	oily secretion
pilosebaceous (pye loh se BAY shus)	pertaining to hair follicles and sebaceous glands

melanin (MEL uh nin)	black or dark brown pigment produced by cells called melanocytes
melanocytes (me LAN oh sites)	cells that produce melanin

Key Term Practice: Integumentary System Preview

1. Identify three functions of the skin.

   _____

2. Another term for skin is _____.

3. Which gland secretes sebum?

   _____

4. The word part *dermato-* means "skin." The suffix *-ology* means "study of." What word means "the study of skin"?

   _____

Skin Layers

The principal layers of the skin are the epidermis, dermis, and subcutaneous. These layers and other structures associated with the skin are shown in Figure 4-1. The **epidermis** is the outermost layer, which is composed of stratified squamous epithelium. *Squamous* means "scale-like"; therefore, this layer appears scaly. The epidermis contains several layers, called **strata**. The epidermal layers, from deepest to most superficial are stratum basale, stratum spinosum, stratum germinativum, stratum granulosum, stratum lucidum (when present), and stratum corneum. The deeper layers of the epidermis also contain melanin-secreting melanocytes. Cells of the stratum basale undergo mitosis (cellular division) to create new skin cells. As keratinocytes (specialized cells of the epidermis) age, they harden through a process called **keratinization** (or cornification). Newer cells composed of tough keratin push the older cells toward the skin surface. Keratin is a waterproof protein that makes up the dead outer layer of the epidermis, creating the stratum corneum; this layer is extremely thick on the soles of the feet.

Mites live on eyebrows and eyelashes, making a meal of dead skin cells!

The stratum lucidum is a clear layer found in the epidermis of the skin covering the palms of the hands and the soles of the feet. This layer is 4–5 mm (0.16–0.20 in) thick and is called *thick skin*. The stratum lucidum is absent in all other body locations.

The **dermis**, or **corium**, is the middle inner layer and is composed of a variety of tissues, including fibrous connective, epithelial, smooth muscle, nerve, and blood. The dermis is thicker than the epidermis and binds the epidermis to underlying tissues. Hair, sebaceous (oil) glands, sudoriferous (sweat) glands, and blood vessels are derived from this layer. The sebum that is secreted by the sebaceous glands makes the skin soft and pliable. The sudoriferous glands allow excess body heat to escape in the form of sweat. **Collagen**, a fibrous protein, is a major component of the connective tissue; *colla* means "glue." Collagen and elastic fibers make skin tough, yet stretchable.

Turgor refers to normal skin tension as a result of its elasticity. It is often used as an assessment tool to determine signs of dehydration or connective tissue disorders. After a fold of skin is gently grasped and pulled, it should return to its normal state in about 3 seconds after release. Stretch marks, or **striae**, are linear tears in the der-

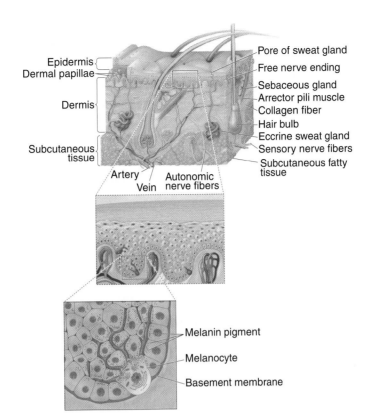

Epidermis
Dermal papillae
Dermis
Subcutaneous tissue
Artery
Vein
Autonomic nerve fibers
Pore of sweat gland
Free nerve ending
Sebaceous gland
Arrector pili muscle
Collagen fiber
Hair bulb
Eccrine sweat gland
Sensory nerve fibers
Subcutaneous fatty tissue
Melanin pigment
Melanocyte
Basement membrane

FIGURE 4-1
Anatomy of the skin. (Top image provided by Anatomical Chart Co.)

mal layer. They occur when there is rapid skin growth and stretching, such as in pregnancy or weight gain.

The **hypodermis**, commonly called the **subcutaneous** layer, is the innermost layer and connects the dermis to underlying tissues. Masses of loose connective and adipose tissue are found in the subcutaneous layer. In medical records, subcutaneous tissue may be abbreviated in a number of ways, including SC, subcu., and subq. **Adipose** (fat) tissue is formed by **lipocytes** (fat cells) within this layer. Adipose serves as an important heat insulator and organ protector.

Key Terms	Definitions
epidermis (ep i DER mis)	superficial skin layer
stratum (STRA tum)	layer(s)
keratinization (kerr uh tin i ZAY shun)	formation of keratin and the horny layer
dermis (DUR mis)	layer of skin below the epidermis
corium (KOH ree um)	dermis
collagen (KOL uh jin)	fibrous protein
turgor (TUR gur)	normal skin tension
stria (STRYE uh)	narrow band(s), stretch mark(s)
hypodermis (heye poh DER mis)	innermost skin layer
subcutaneous (sub kew TAY nee us)	connective tissue skin layer, hypodermis
adipose (AD i poce)	fat
lipocytes (LIP oh sights)	fat cells

Key Term Practice: Skin Layers

1. The outer layer of the skin is called the _____.

2. The _____ is the innermost layer of the skin.

3. The middle layer of the skin is termed the _____ layer.

4. What are the singular and plural forms of the term that means "layer"?

   A. Singular = _____

   B. Plural = _____

Skin Color and Birthmarks

> **FACT** *Fingerprints are unique per individual. No two people, including identical twins, have the same fingerprints!*

> **FACT** *Skin makes up about 15% of a person's weight!*

Human skin color is the result of genetics, environment, and physiology. In all cases, the basic determinant is the quantity of melanin produced by the melanocytes. Melanin, a dark pigment that absorbs light energy, prevents UV radiation from damaging deeper skin cells. Individuals inherit genes from both parents for melanin production, which is regulated by hormones and enzymes. Melanocyte numbers are relatively constant regardless of ethnicity; hence variations in skin coloration are the result of the amount of melanin produced, as reflected by one's genes and exposure to UV radiation. Mutant genes cause a lack of melanin production that results in **albinism.** Albinos (individuals with albinism) have the same number of melanocytes as others; however, their cells are not capable of producing melanin.

Several environmental factors affect skin color. Sunlight, UV radiation, and x-rays cause existing melanin to darken rapidly and stimulate melanocytes to produce more pigment, which is then transferred to nearby epidermal cells. In lighter-complected individuals, the pigment resides primarily in the stratum germinativum and stratum spinosum; but in darker-skinned individuals, it is also transferred into the deeper stratum granulosum, causing a more persistent coloration.

Physiology plays a role in skin coloration as well. The primary physiological factors affecting skin color are blood and disease. For example, the oxygen content in the dermal capillaries of light-skinned people affects skin color. This is accomplished because oxygen-carrying hemoglobin gives off a pinkish hue. When the blood is rich in oxygen, the skin has a characteristic red-pink color. If blood oxygen levels are low, hemoglobin is dark, and the skin may appear bluish, a condition called **cyanosis.** Various skin diseases may affect skin color as well. When a person suffers from liver disease, the skin may appear yellow from an accumulation of the bile pigment bilirubin. This is referred to as **jaundice.**

When considering skin color, it is important to mention birthmarks. Birthmarks are congenital skin **lesions** (structural or functional alterations of the anatomy) that generally fall into two categories: vascular hamartomas and pigmented nevi. A hamartoma is a developmental anomaly resulting in a mass composed of normal tissue but in an abnormal proportion. Nevi are masses of pigmented tissue. A **port wine stain** is a large, reddish birthmark that may be removed by laser surgery. The colored skin patch can occur singly or in multiples, can be raised or flat, and typically occurs on the face. A raised, reddish purple birthmark that usually dissipates without treatment around age 7 years is termed a **strawberry hemangioma.** Strawberry hemangiomas often have a lumpy, lobed appearance. Similarly, a **cherry hemangioma** is red to purple in color and is marked by a smooth, dome-shaped papule. A solid, circumscribed (enclosed by an encircling boundary) skin elevation is called a **papule.** Mosquito bite bumps are examples of papules.

Conditions of the skin and the integumentary system are frequently described in medical terms denoting color. Table 4-1 provides common word parts and terms used to describe a variety of colors associated with the skin. Examples are also given in the table.

TABLE 4-1   Word Parts Pertaining to the Color of Skin

Word Parts and Term Derivations	Color	Example
albus	white	albinism
anthraco-	black	anthracosis
chlor-, chloro-	green	chlorophyll
cyan-, cyano-	blue	cyanosis
eryth-, erytho-	red	erythematous
jaune	yellow	jaundice
kirrkos	yellow	cirrhosis
leuk-, leuko-	white	leukoderma
luteus	yellow	corpus luteum
melan-, melano-	black	melanin
polio-	gray	poliomyelitis
porphyra	purple	allergic purpura
rosaceus, roseus	rosy	roseola
ruber	red	rubeola
xanth-, xantho-	yellow	xanthoderma

Key Terms	Definitions
albinism (AL bi niz um)	hereditary absence of melanin
cyanosis (sigh uh NOH sis)	bluish skin and mucous membranes resulting from a lack of oxygen in the blood
jaundice (JAWN dis)	yellowish skin resulting from bilirubin accumulation
lesion (LEE zhun)	structural or functional alterations
port wine stain	type of birthmark
strawberry hemangioma (he man jee OH muh)	type of birthmark
cherry hemangioma (he man jee OH muh)	type of birthmark
papule (PAP yool)	solid circumscribed skin elevation

Key Term Practice: Skin Color and Birthmarks

1. What is the hereditary condition in which melanin is not produced?

   _____

2. A condition in which the skin and mucous membranes appear bluish is termed _____.

Hair

Epidermal derivatives are structures that develop from the embryonic epidermis. These derivatives include hair, nails, and skin glands. Hair is found covering all body surfaces except the palms of the hands, the soles of the feet, portions of the external genitalia, and the lips. The genes that direct the type and amount of pigment produced by epidermal melanocytes determine hair color.

Hair, composed of a root and a shaft, is found within a hair **follicle**, which is the tube-like depression extending from the surface into the dermis that contains the hair root (Fig. 4-2). The **shaft** is the visible part that extends beyond the surface. The **root** penetrates the dermis and subcutaneous layer. New hair develops at the base of the hair follicle when epidermal cells undergo cell division forcing older cells to move outward. As new cells are pushed toward the surface, they undergo keratinization. Hair goes through periods of growth, rest, and replacement. On average, head hair grows about 12.5 cm (5 inches) per year.

Bundles of smooth muscle cells, referred to as the **arrector pili muscles**, are attached to each hair follicle. When nerve impulses stimulate these muscles to contract, they create "goose bumps."

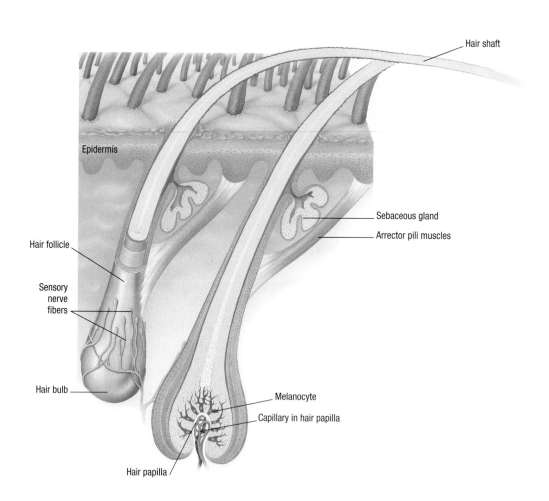

FIGURE 4-2
Cross-section of hair and accessory structures. (Image provided by Anatomical Chart Co.)

Key Terms	Definitions
follicle (FOL i kul)	space containing the hair root
shaft	visible portion of the hair

| root (hair) | hair portion attached to the dermis |
| arrector (a RECK tur PYE lye) pili muscles | involuntary muscles attached to hair follicles that cause goose bumps when contracted |

Key Term Practice: Hair

1. The principal parts of hair are _____, _____, and _____.

2. These muscles contract to create goose bumps on the flesh.

_____

Glands

Basic skin glands secrete oil, sweat, or wax. Those secreting oil are termed sebaceous, those secreting sweat are called sudoriferous, and those secreting wax are called ceruminous. Sebaceous glands are usually connected to hair follicles and secrete an oily substance called sebum. Sebum is a fatty acid that functions to keep skin soft, pliable, and relatively waterproof. Sebaceous glands are not found on the palms and soles.

Sudoriferous glands produce perspiration, which carries water, waste products (ammonia, urea, and lactic acid), and heat to the skin surface to assist in maintaining body temperature and homeostasis (Fig. 4-3). These glands are most numerous on the

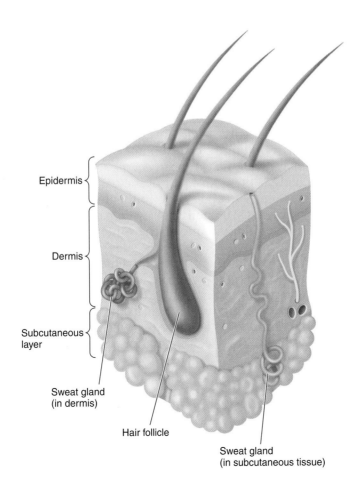

Epidermis

Dermis

Subcutaneous layer

Sweat gland (in dermis)

Hair follicle

Sweat gland (in subcutaneous tissue)

FIGURE 4-3
The sweat glands.

palms, soles, forehead, armpits, neck, and back. **Hidrosis** means sweat production and excretion. Sweat glands have an extensive distribution; ducts that terminate at **pores** (openings) on the epidermal surface allow the secretions to escape. Enlarged sebaceous or sudoriferous glands may produce blackheads, pimples, and boils. **Comedo** is the medical term for a blackhead, resulting from an enlarged pore that becomes clogged with sebum, bacteria, and pigment. The black dot at the skin surface results from the oxidation of sebum in the follicle.

Ceruminous glands are modified sudoriferous glands that secrete cerumen (ear wax). They are found in the external auditory meatus, the canal that leads from the outer ear to the tympanic membrane (ear drum). Cerumen is secreted to keep the membrane pliable. Moreover, cerumen is a water and insect repellent.

Key Terms	Definitions
hidrosis (high DROH sis)	sweat production and excretion
pores	openings
comedo (KOM ee doh)	blackhead
ceruminous (se ROO mi nus) **glands**	glands that secrete cerumen

Key Term Practice: Glands

1. A _____ is the medical term for a blackhead.

2. The medical term for sweating is _____.

Nails

Nails, or **ungues**, are hard, keratinized epidermal cells located over the dorsal surfaces of the terminal segments of fingers and toes. The principal parts of nails are the nail body, nail bed, root, lunula, eponychium, and hyponychium (Fig. 4-4). The last two terms are derived from the word part *onych-*, which means "nail."

The **nail body** is the visible part of the nail that rests on the **nail bed,** which is a layer of epithelium. The underlying epithelium that makes up the nail bed is abundant in blood vessels. The **nail root** is the part of the nail hidden by a fold of skin called the **eponychium** or **cuticle.** The white moon-shaped growth area nearest the root is called the **lunula.** The distal **free edge** (the part one clips with nail scissors) extends beyond the nail bed at the **hyponychium,** an area of thickened epithelium at the junction of the fingertip and the nail bed. The matrix is the growth layer composed of the stratum germinativum, the cells of which are undergoing mitosis. Cell division of this matrix produces new nails through the keratinization process. The average fingernail turnover is 3–5 months, whereas it may take 12–18 months for total toenail replacement. The medical term for nail biting is **onychophagia.**

The record for the longest nail is 4 feet 8 inches (1.22 meters 20.32 cm)

Key Terms	Definitions
unguis (UNG gwis)	fingernail or toenail
nail body	main part of the nail

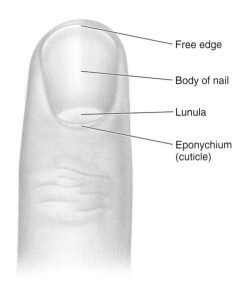

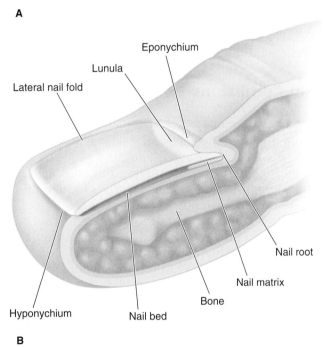

FIGURE 4-4
Surface structures of the fingernail (**A**). Cross-section of a fingertip (**B**). (Image B provided by Anatomical Chart Co.)

nail bed	vascular epithelial tissue on which the nail rests
nail root	nail part beneath the cuticle
eponychium (ep oh NICK ee um)	cuticle
cuticle (KEW ti kul)	eponychium, fold of skin near the nail root
lunula (LOO new luh)	white, semilunar area of nail near the root
free edge	portion of the nail growing beyond the phalanx tips
hyponychium (high poh NICK ee um)	epithelium of the nail bed
onychophagia (on i koh FAY jee uh)	nail biting

Key Term Practice: Nails

1. Another term for fingernails or toenails is _____.

2. The white, semilunar area of the nail is termed the _____.

3. *Eponychium* is the medical term for the _____.

THE CLINICAL DIMENSION

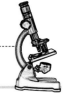

Pathology of the Integumentary System

Disorders and abnormalities of the skin range from trivial moles to serious cancers. Skin pathologies commonly result from sun exposure, diet, environment, and genetics. This section describes signs, symptoms, clinical tests, procedures, treatments, and pathologic conditions related to the skin and the integumentary system.

Skin Conditions

Skin conditions are evident in a variety of visual patterns. The noninfectious inflammatory disease of the hair follicles and associated sebaceous glands is termed **acne vulgaris.** Comedones, papules, and pustules characterize it. Skin elevations containing pus are referred to as **pustules. Nodules,** deeper boil-like structures larger than a papule, can also occur. Acne vulgaris is located primarily on the face, neck, and back and has a peak onset during adolescence. Although its cause is unknown, it is suspected that hormonal changes, stress, and endocrine disorders lead to its development. Steroid drug use is a known precipitating factor. Treatment involves the use of topical or oral antibiotics and the topical application of keratolytic agents. Keratolytic agents cause increased **exfoliation** (shedding of the skin layer) of the epidermis.

Commonly referred to as a bruise, a **contusion** is an injury to subcutaneous tissue in which the skin is not broken. An **abrasion** or **excoriation** is damaged skin caused by scraping or rubbing.

A condition that develops after a penetrating wound injury, **causalgia** is marked by severe burning pain in the hand or foot. It commonly occurs after injury to a peripheral nerve. The overlying skin appears smooth and shiny or scaly and discolored, with profuse sweat gland activity. Signs and symptoms are particularly enhanced during periods of stress.

A hereditary skin condition that gives the outward appearance of fish scales is **ichthyosis. Pemphigus** is an acute or chronic skin disorder in which bullae, burning sensations, and itching develop. **Bullae** (sing. bulla) are large blisters or blebs within or beneath the epidermis that are filled with lymph or serum.

A mass of tissue cells filled with fat found in the subcutaneous tissue is termed a **xanthoma.** Xanthomas appear yellow and often occur around tendons. **Xeroderma,** not to be confused with xanthoma, is excessively dry skin. **Xeroderma pigmentosum** (XDP or XP) is a genetic skin disease (genodermatosis) characterized by keratoses (extremely thick skin patches), the inability to repair UV damage, and both hyperpigmentation and hypopigmentation.

An abnormal thickening of subcutaneous and cutaneous tissues is known as **pachydermia.** Also called **elephantiasis,** it results from lymphatic obstruction and subsequent chronic edema (swelling). **Edema** occurs when fluid from capillaries leaks out into the tissue space. Elephantiasis is caused by the filaria (a type of worm) *Wuchereria bancrofti.*

Purpura is a condition in which purple hemorrhages occur in the skin. Signs include **petechiae** (small, rounded spot of bleeding on the skin surface), ecchymoses, and **vibices** (linear hemorrhages).

Key Terms	Definitions
acne vulgaris (ACK nee vul GAIR ris)	inflammation of the hair follicle and associated sebaceous glands
pustules (PUS tyoolz)	skin elevations containing pus
nodules (NOD yoolz)	deep, boil-like structures
exfoliation (ecks foh lee AY shun)	peeling and shedding of the epidermis
contusion (con TEW zhun)	bruise
abrasion (uh BRAY zhun)	wearing down of skin by rubbing or scraping
excoriation (ecks koh ree AY shun)	skin abrasion
causalgia (kaw SAL jee uh)	condition characterized by burning sensations
ichthyosis (ick thee OH sis)	hereditary skin condition giving the appearance of scales
pemphigus (PEM fi gus)	skin disorder with groups of bullae
bulla; pl. bullae (BULL uh; BULL ee)	blister(s), bleb(s)
xanthoma (zan THO muh)	fat-filled cells in subcutaneous tissue
xeroderma (zeer oh DUR muh)	extremely dry skin
xeroderma pigmentosum (zeer oh DUR muh pig men TOH sum)	genetic skin disease characterized by hypopigmentation and hyperpigmentation
pachydermia (pack i DUR mee uh)	abnormal skin thickening caused by filarial infection
elephantiasis (el e fan TYE uh sis)	pachyderma
edema (e DEE muh)	swelling
purpura (PUR pew ruh)	condition with purple skin hemorrhages
petechia (pee TEE kee uh)	spot of hemorrhaging
vibices (VYE bi seez)	linear hemorrhage on the skin surface

Key Term Practice: Skin Conditions

1. _____ is a condition characterized by burning sensations in the extremities.

2. The shedding of the epidermal layer of skin tissue is termed _____.

Burns

A **burn** is defined as an epithelial injury caused by contact with a thermal, radioactive, chemical, or electrical agent. Burns are classified according to the depth of damage to tissue as first degree, second degree, and third degree (Fig. 4-5).

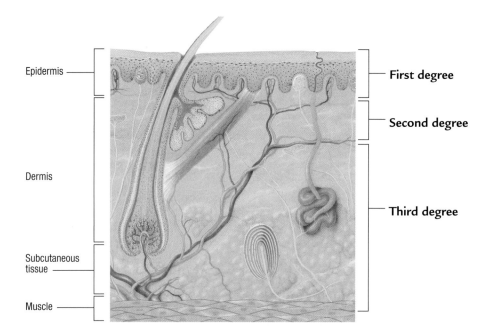

Epidermis

Dermis

Subcutaneous tissue

Muscle

First degree

Second degree

Third degree

FIGURE 4-5
Classification of burns according to the depth of damage to tissue. (Image provided by Anatomical Chart Co.)

With a **first-degree** (simple hyperemic or superficial) **burn**, the epidermal layer is affected. *Hyperemic* means that there is "an increase in blood flow" to the site. Characteristics include redness, pain, and edema. There is no blistering or scarring, but the surface layers shed within a few days. A minor sunburn is a classic example. A **second-degree** (vesicant or partial-thickness) **burn** involves both the epidermal and dermal layers. *Vesicant* means "blistering agent." Generally, there is severe pain, blistering, and edema. Recovery is usually complete but slow, and scarring is common. A **third-degree** (full-thickness) **burn** destroys the epidermal and dermal layers as well as some underlying muscle and nerves. There is no immediate pain because nerve endings are affected. Ulcerating wounds characterize this type of burn. Skin grafts are frequently required and scar tissue often results.

Burn wound healing often has specific features. One such mark is a thick scar or scab, termed an **eschar**, which forms over the severely burned tissue. Burn injuries commonly result in the dermis separating from the epidermis, a phenomenon called **epidermolysis**. After regular wound healing, a **cicatrix** forms, which is soft, red, fibrous connective tissue surrounding the site. It later develops into fibrous tissue known as a **scar**, a permanent blemish.

Key Terms	Definitions
burn	tissue reaction as a result of thermal, radioactive, chemical, or electrical insult
first-degree burn	damage to the epidermal layer
second-degree burn	damage to the epidermal and dermal layers
third-degree burn	full-thickness burn
eschar (ES kahr)	thick scar that forms over a healed burn
epidermolysis (ep i dur MOL i sis)	dermal–epidermal separation
cicatrix (SICK uh tricks)	soft, red fibrous connective tissue
scar	permanent blemish

Key Term Practice: Burns

1. Give a brief definition of the term *burn*.

   _____

   _____

   _____

2. Burns are categorized according to the extent of damage to the underlying tissue. What are the three categories of burns?

   _____

Alopecia

Alopecia, commonly known as baldness, is loss of hair. The loss is typically from the scalp and may be partial, total, or complete. Types include **alopecia areata**, patchy hair loss particularly in the scalp and beard; **alopecia totalis**, complete scalp baldness; and **alopecia universalis**, complete baldness over the entire body related to alopecia areata.

   Diagnosis is made by physical and visual examination and is accompanied by blood and thyroid studies. If an underlying pathology exists, correcting it generally resumes hair growth. Chemotherapeutic agents and hair transplants are proving beneficial.

FACT The average person sheds about 40 pounds of skin in a lifetime!

Key Terms	Definitions
alopecia (al oh PEE shee uh)	hair loss
alopecia areata (al oh PEE shee uh air ee AY tuh)	patchy hair loss of the scalp and beard
alopecia totalis (al oh PEE shee uh toh TAY lis)	complete scalp baldness
alopecia universalis (al oh PEE shee uh yoo ni vur SAY lis)	no body hair at all

Key Term Practice: Alopecia

1. The medical term for hair loss or baldness is _____

2. Complete scalp baldness is called _____.

Autoimmune Disorders

Several **autoimmune disorders** affect the cutaneous membrane. An autoimmune disease is one in which immune cells are directed against the body. In essence, the system that is supposed to protect the body from harm is causing the damage. The common autoimmune disorders with a skin component are dermatomyositis, scleroderma, and systemic lupus erythematosus.

As its name suggests, **dermatomyositis,** is an inflammation of the dermal and muscular layers of tissue; it is often accompanied by muscle weakness and extremely taut skin. **Scleroderma** is characterized by an increase in collagenous connective tissue in the skin, causing the skin to be very tight (Fig. 4-6).

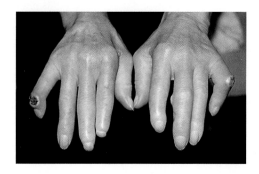

FIGURE 4-6
Scleroderma. An increase in collagenous connective tissue in the skin causes the skin to be very tight. (Reprinted with permission from Goodheart HP. Goodheart's photoguide of common skin disorders. 2nd ed. Philadelphia: Lippincott, Williams & Wilkins, 2003.)

Systemic lupus erythematosus (SLE), frequently shortened to either lupus erythematosus (LE) or lupus, is another autoimmune disease of the connective tissue (Fig. 4-7). Skin redness that occurs in patches is called **erythema,** thus providing the foundation of the term. Skin eruptions are similar to those of **discoid lupus erythematosus** (DLE), in which skin lesions are present. Skin involvement in both SLE and DLE are characterized by an erythematosus malar (pertaining to the cheek) rash. Diagnosis is usually made by blood test, tissue biopsy, patient history, and physical examination. A **biopsy** (bx) involves the excision of living tissue for diagnostic study. General treatment consists of physical exercise, sun avoidance, and immunosuppressive drugs.

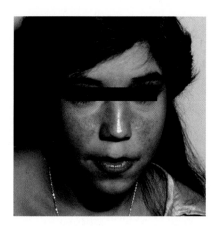

FIGURE 4-7
Systemic lupus erythematosus, or lupus, is an autoimmune disease of connective tissue. A rash on the cheeks characterizes skin involvement. (Reprinted with permission from Goodheart HP. Goodheart's photoguide of common skin disorders. 2nd ed. Philadelphia: Lippincott, Williams & Wilkins, 2003.)

Psoriasis is a chronic, inflammatory autoimmune skin disorder characterized by reddish, cutaneous edema and raised, scaly plaques (hardened patches on skin surface). These plaques sometimes become circumscribed pustules. Signs and symptoms include dry, cracked, and itchy skin spots. The disorder commonly develops on the scalp, elbows, knees, and body trunk. Although psoriasis can occur at any age, disease onset is typically between the ages of 10 and 30 years. It is diagnosed by the presence of white, silvery skin scales. Remissions and exacerbations (flare-ups) commonly occur. Treatment options include UV light therapy to retard cellular division and topical steroid ointments.

Key Terms	Definitions
autoimmune (aw toh i MEWN) **disorders**	conditions in which the immune response is directed toward the self
dermatomyositis (dur muh toh migh oh SIGH tis)	inflammation of skin and muscles
scleroderma (skleer oh DUR muh)	autoimmune disease characterized by increased collagen formation in connective tissues, including skin and organs
systemic lupus erythematosus (LOO pus er ih thee mah TOH sus)	autoimmune disease of connective tissue
erythema (er ih THEE mah)	redness on the skin
discoid lupus erythematosus (dis KOID LOO pus er ih thee mah TOH sus)	autoimmune disease of connective tissue
biopsy (BYE op see)	live tissue excision for diagnostic study
psoriasis (soh RYE uh sis)	autoimmune skin disease characterized by white scaly plaques

Key Term Practice: Autoimmune Disorders

1. Increased collagen formation is seen in this autoimmune disease.

_____

2. _____ is the medical term for the autoimmune disease that is characterized by inflammation of the skin and underlying muscles.

Noncancerous Tumors

Noncancerous skin growths and tumors are classified as either benign or premalignant. **Benign** means that the growth is not **malignant** or does not have a tendency to spread to other body sites to hinder health or cause death. **Premalignant** is a term meaning precancerous, indicating that if the tumor is not treated immediately, it has a chance of developing into **cancer**, malignant tumors that may result in death.

Benign tumors include sebaceous cysts, skin tags (acrochordons or cutaneous papillomas), hemangiomas, keloids, lipomas, and seborrheic keratosis. **Sebaceous cysts** are palpable (capable of being felt), movable, fluid-filled cysts that develop in sebaceous glands. They may take several years to build up, are usually painless, and generally require no treatment, although they may be surgically removed. Frequently occurring in the axillary and cervical regions, **cutaneous papillomas** are flaps of skin held to the body by a thin stalk. They tend to be a nuisance, thus requiring surgical excision because they frequently get caught on clothing.

A benign, reddish purple tumor composed of a mass of blood vessels is termed **hemangioma**, and a **keloid** is an elevated, firm, fibrous hyperplasia that develops at the site of a scar (Fig. 4-8). Keloid borders are typically ill-defined and the condition is observed more commonly in female adults and in dark-skinned people than in others. A benign tumor composed of adipocytes is a **lipoma** or **steatoma**. Laser treatment, corticosteroid injections, and surgery are options to remove or diminish unsightly keloids; liposomes generally do not require treatment.

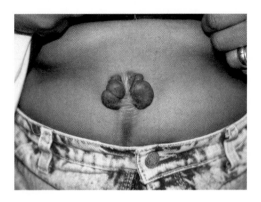

FIGURE 4-8
A keloid is an elevated, firm, fibrous hyperplasia that develops at the edge of a scar. (Reprinted with permission from Goodheart HP. Goodheart's photoguide of common skin disorders. 2nd ed. Philadelphia: Lippincott, Williams & Wilkins, 2003.)

Seborrheic keratosis is a benign tumor composed of squamous and basaloid cells arranged in various patterns that produce a purple-brown papule. Yellow flecks of keratotic material may give the papule a greasy appearance. The cause is unknown; however, their sudden appearance or an increase in their numbers could indicate the presence of an internal malignancy, notably a stomach cancer. Diagnosis is made by visual examination. If treatment is necessary, the options include cryosurgery and curettage. **Cryosurgery** involves the localized freezing of tissue for removal. Once the tissue has been frozen, special instruments aid in the removal of the diseased area. Another surgical method for removing tissue is called **curettage.** With this procedure, a specially designed spoon-shaped instrument, a curet, is used to scrape away tissue.

Two common premalignant skin tumors are actinic keratoses and nevi (moles). Chronic exposure to sunlight may cause areas of rough, vascular skin that eventually form crusts called **actinic keratoses.** The term *actinic* means "pertaining to radiant energy." They can be treated with topical ointments, curettage, and desiccation (drying). **Nevi** refer to any lesions containing melanocytes. They typically appear as round, darkened spots on the skin surface and generally remain benign. When in doubt about a mole, follow the ABCDs of **melanoma** (malignant tumor of melanocytes) to assess the situation. Under this scheme, each letter represents a specific characteristic of the mole's physical appearance (Fig. 4-9):

- A = asymmetry
- B = border

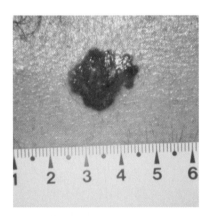

FIGURE 4-9
A melanoma is a malignant tumor of melanocytes. (Reprinted with permission from Goodheart HP. Goodheart's photoguide of common skin disorders. 2nd ed. Philadelphia: Lippincott, Williams & Wilkins, 2003.)

- C = color
- D = diameter

Moles that are symmetrical, have irregular borders, uneven color, and diameters larger than 6 mm (0.24 inch) should be clinically tested.

Key Terms	Definitions
benign (be NINE)	not malignant
malignant (muh LIG nunt)	endangering health or life
premalignant (PREE muh LIG nunt)	precancerous
cancer	malignant tumor that can lead to death
sebaceous cysts (se BAY shus SISTS)	fluid-filled sebaceous glands
cutaneous papillomas (kew TAY nee us pap i LOH muhz)	skin tags
hemangioma (hee man jee OH muh)	benign tumor made up of a blood vessel mass
keloid (KEE loid)	elevated, firm hyperplasia with ill-defined borders at scar site
lipoma (li POH muh)	benign, fatty tumor
steatoma (stee uh TOH muh)	lipoma
seborrheic keratosis (seb oh REE ick kerr uh TOH sis)	benign purple-brown skin tumor
cryosurgery (krye oh SUR juh ree)	localized freezing of diseased tissues for surgical removal
curettage (kewr e TAHZH)	surgical procedure in which tissue is scraped away using a curet
actinic keratoses (ack TIN ick ker uh TOH seez)	premalignant hyperkeratosis
nevus (NEE vus)	lesion containing melanocytes
melanoma (mel uh NOH muh)	malignant tumor of melanocytes

Key Term Practice: Noncancerous Tumors

1. What is the alternate term for skin moles?

_____

2. What are the two terms that refer to a fatty tumor?

_____

Cancerous Tumors

Common skin cancers, **carcinomas**, are malignant tumors of epithelial cells and include basal cell carcinoma, malignant melanoma, and squamous cell carcinoma. **Basal cell carcinoma** is a cancer caused by malignant stem cells in the stratum germinativum, or basal layer. Locally invasive and rarely metastasizing (spreading), it is

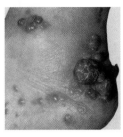

FIGURE 4-10
Kaposi sarcoma is a malignant tumor characterized by multiple bluish-red or brown nodules and plaques, typically in the skin on the extremities. (Reprinted with permission from Roche lexikon medizin. 3rd ed. Munich: Urban & Schwarzenburg, 1993.)

common in individuals with a history of chronic sun exposure. **Malignant melanoma,** the most serious type of skin cancer, is a rapidly spreading cancer of melanocytes. This type of cancer is generally detected by observing mole changes. **Squamous cell carcinoma,** the most common type of skin cancer, develops in the skin's epidermal layer. Both basal cell carcinoma and squamous cell carcinoma form hard coverings resulting from dried skin exudates (fluid) called **crusts** on the skin surface. Squamous cell carcinoma is more serious than basal cell carcinoma as it may metastasize to other body parts. Sun exposure is the primary cause of all skin carcinomas, though malignant melanoma has particular risk factors such as family history, prior case of melanoma, and history of blistering sunburns, that may make an individual more susceptible.

Kaposi sarcoma, occurring often in AIDS (acquired immunodeficiency syndrome) patients, is a tumor characterized by multiple bluish red or brown nodules and plaques (Fig. 4-10). It is typically seen on the extremities. Diagnosis is made by physical and visual examination and biopsy.

Treatment options of the various skin carcinomas are numerous and are case specific. These include, but are not limited to, surgical excision, electrodesiccation, cryosurgery, Mohs surgery, laser surgery, and chemotherapy. **Mohs surgery** is performed under the microscope using zinc oxide paste to remove skin layers. As each cell layer is removed, it is examined under the scope. The procedure ends when all cancerous cells have been removed.

Key Terms	Definitions
carcinomas (kahr si NOH muhs)	malignant tumors composed of anaplastic (abnormally shaped) epithelial cells
basal (BAY sul) **cell carcinoma** (kahr si NOH muh)	cancer of the basal cell layer
malignant melanoma (muh LIG nunt mel uh NOH muh)	cancer of the melanocytes
squamous (SKWAY mus) **cell carcinoma** (kahr si NOH muh)	cancer developing in the epidermis
crusts	hard coverings that result when exudate on the skin dries
Kaposi sarcoma (KAH poh zee sahr KOH muh)	bluish red, brown tumor
Mohs (MOHZ) **surgery**	microscopically controlled cancer surgery

Key Term Practice: Cancerous Tumors

1. _____ is cancer of the melanocytes.

2. Malignant tumors (cancer) are termed _____.

Carbuncles and Furuncles

A **furuncle** (boil) is a localized infection originating in or near a hair follicle that develops into an abscess. An **abscess** is a furuncle involving entire hair follicles and adjoining subcutaneous tissues. A **carbuncle** is a large furuncle or multiple furuncles that form an interconnected mass. Symptoms include erythema, edema, and pain. Both are caused by staphylococcal infection. Treatment consists of the application of warm, moist heat to aid fluid drainage. In several cases, **incision and drainage** (I&D), in which a surgical cut is made to release tissue fluid, and antibiotic therapy may be necessary.

Key Terms	Definitions
furuncle (FEW rung kul)	a boil
abscess (ab SES)	furuncle involving hair follicles and adjacent tissue
carbuncle (KAHR bunk ul)	large furuncle
incision and drainage	surgical cut to drain fluid from tissue

Key Term Practice: Carbuncles and Furuncles

1. I&D is the abbreviation for what procedure?

   _____.

2. What is the medical term for a boil?

   _____.

Clavi and Calluses

A **corn** or **clavus** is a cone-shaped, circumscribed horny layer hyperplasia. Clavi are characterized by epidermal thickening and are found primarily on the toes as a result of pressure or friction. A **callus** is a circumscribed, thickened layer of horny epithelial tissue. Calluses are larger than corns and typically develop on the palms of the hands and the balls of the feet. Pain and tenderness are common symptoms. Repeated trauma, such as from playing stringed musical instruments, engaging in manual labor, and having impaired circulation, may also cause calluses. Treatments include avoiding or removing of the causative agent using creams, and undergoing exfoliation.

Key Terms	Definitions
corn	clavus
clavus (KLAY vus)	corn
callus (KAL us)	thickened layer of horny epithelium

Key Term Practice: Calvi and Calluses

1. Another term for a corn is a _____.

2. _____ typically result from repeated hand trauma, such as playing a guitar.

Decubitus Ulcers

Decubitus ulcers (decub.), also known as pressure sores or bed sores, are caused by a chronic deficiency of blood to tissues subjected to prolonged pressure. **Ulcers** are sores that result from epithelial tissue destruction. Decubitus ulcers are so named because they frequently occur in individuals who have been immobile in the decubitus (recumbent or horizontal) position. Ulcers generally occur over a bony prominence or joint. Thus it is extremely important that bedridden, debilitated, or paralyzed individuals be moved on a regular basis to increase blood flow into tissues. Ulcers can affect all layers of the skin; and the more severe cases penetrate to bone tissue. Signs and symptoms include shiny, red skin in the early stages and blisters, open wounds, and exudates in later stages. Pungent odors are common, because the flesh creates a hospitable environment for microbial activity.

When appropriate, a culture of the tissue may be necessary to choose the appropriate antibiotic therapy. Treatment must be vigorous and rapid to delay further damage to underlying tissue. Options include the use of topical agents, gelatin sponges to absorb excess fluid drainage, karaya gum patches, antibiotics, antiseptic irrigations to flush area, and **débridement**. Débridement involves removal of the necrotized (dead) tissue by sharp dissection, enzymes, or other chemical agents. **Necrosis** (dead tissue) results because there is an interruption in nutrient-rich blood flow to the site. **Gangrene** is the term used to describe necrosis of a body part caused by a lack of blood supply. Ulcers can be prevented or alleviated by changing position frequently, doing range of motion exercises, and using specially designed air mattresses that ease pressure on the tissues.

Key Terms	Definitions
decubitus ulcers (dee KEW bi tus UL surs)	pressure sores
ulcers (UL sur)	interruptions in the integrity of the epithelial tissue
débridement (day breed MAHN)	removal of necrotized tissue from a wound by surgical excision, enzymes, or chemical agents
necrosis (ne KROH sis)	death of living cells or tissue
gangrene (GANG green)	necrosis of a body tissue

Key Term Practice: Decubitus Ulcers

1. What is another term for a pressure sore?

_____.

2. _____ refers to the removal of dead tissue.

Dermatitis

The general term for inflammation of the skin is **dermatitis**. Several types of dermatitis exist, and each has distinguishing skin characteristics. A common form of dermatitis is **contact dermatitis.** Causes of contact dermatitis are varied, ranging from a minor skin irritant resulting from brushing up against a surface to an allergic reaction to food ingested. Symptoms include erythema, edema, and **vesicles**, which are small blisters that leak fluid. **Pruritus** (itching), burning at the site, and stinging sensations are frequent.

Another form of dermatitis is **seborrheic dermatitis.** It is characterized by inflammation of the sebaceous glands. The irritation is greatest in areas of high sebaceous gland concentration, notably the scalp, eyebrows, eyelids, lateral margins of the nose, behind the ears, and on the chest. In infants, it is referred to as **cradle cap.**

Seborrheic dermatitis is not a secondary condition to any other illness, and its cause is not known, thus its onset is **idiopathic**. Individuals with a genetic predisposition may be at an increased risk, and emotional stress may trigger its onset. Diet and food allergies may play a role in its development in infants. Diagnosis is made through patient history and physical assessment. A skin biopsy (tissue excision) may be performed in chronic cases. Seborrheic dermatitis affecting the scalp can be treated using medicated shampoos.

Atopic dermatitis, also known as **eczema,** is another allergic skin disorder (Fig. 4-11). **Atopy** means that the condition is genetically determined. Eczema is the most common inflammatory skin disorder and is characterized by erythema, papules, vesicles, and crusts. A rash with vesicular and **exudative** (leaky) eruptions may also be evident. The condition is intensely pruritic and frequently chronic. Eczema in infants may be linked to milk or orange juice sensitivity.

Treatment of all forms of dermatitis is aimed at controlling inflammation and pruritus and usually involves application of topical steroid creams that contain cortisone or hydrocortisone and possibly administration of an oral steroid. There is no known cure for eczema.

Urticaria, more commonly known as hives, is characterized by pruritus, erythema, and circumscribed, edematous, localized lesions called **wheals.** The condition is generally acute, lasting a few hours; however, chronic cases have been reported. Urticaria is generally caused by allergic reactions to food, drugs, insect bite or stings, or sunlight. Treatment consists of removing the allergen (if known), administering antihistamine medications, or injecting epinephrine in serious cases.

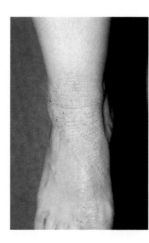

FIGURE 4-11
Eczema, the most common inflammatory skin disorder. (Reprinted with permission from Goodheart HP. Goodheart's photoguide of common skin disorders. 2nd ed. Philadelphia: Lippincott, Williams & Wilkins, 2003.)

Key Terms	Definitions
dermatitis (dur muh TYE tis)	skin inflammation
contact dermatitis (dur muh TYE tis)	skin inflammation caused by an irritant coming in contact with the skin
vesicles (VES i kuls)	blisters that leak fluid
pruritus (proo RYE tus)	itching
seborrheic dermatitis (seb oh REE ick dur muh TYE tis)	inflammation of the skin at the sebaceous glands
cradle cap	seborrheic dermatitis in infants
idiopathic (id ee OH path ick)	of unknown cause
atopic dermatitis (ay TOP ick dur muh TYE tis)	skin inflammation of genetic origin
eczema (ECK zuh muh)	genetic inflammatory skin disorder
atopy (AT uh pee)	genetically determined
exudative (ecks OO duh tiv)	substance that leaks into or out of tissues

urticaria (ur tih KAHR ee ah)	hives marked by redness and swelling
wheals (wheelz)	swellings in specific skin areas

Key Term Practice: Dermatitis

1. Skin inflammation is termed _____.

2. If a disease occurs with no known cause, it is said to be _____.

3. Inflammation of sebaceous glands in infants is commonly called _____.

4. The other medical term for eczema is _____.

5. Another term for hives is _____.

6. The raised bump on the arm after an insect bite could be described as a/an _____.

Dermatophytosis

A fungus called a **dermatophyte** is responsible for skin infections called **dermatophytoses.** The fungi (pl. of fungus) invade the superficial keratinized areas such as the skin, hair, and nails. The lesions of dermatophytoses are called **tinea.** The affected body part gives rise to the medical term describing the infection. For example, **tinea capitis** is a dermatophytosis affecting the scalp (Fig. 4-12), and **tinea corporis** (commonly called ringworm) is found elsewhere on the body (Fig. 4-13). An infection in the groin area is termed **tinea cruris, tinea pedis** (athlete's foot) is on the feet, and **tinea unguium** involves the nails. An exception to the naming rule is **tinea versicolor,** a chronic, superficial fungal infection typically affecting the trunk.

The lesions are generally round, ringed, scaled vesicles that resemble targets. Signs and symptoms can include burning sensations; stinging pruritus; and dry, peeling **fissures** (skin cracks). Characteristics of tinea unguium include thickened, brittle, and dull nails. There usually is no pain or itching.

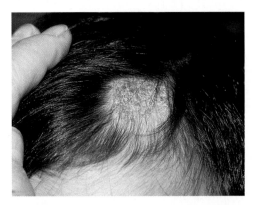

FIGURE 4-12
Tinea capitis, a dermatophytosis affecting the scalp. (Reprinted with permission from Goodheart HP. Goodheart's photoguide of common skin disorders. 2nd ed. Philadelphia: Lippincott, Williams & Wilkins, 2003.)

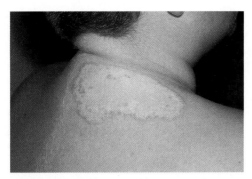

FIGURE 4-13
Tinea corporis, also known as ringworm. (Reprinted with permission from Goodheart HP. Goodheart's photoguide of common skin disorders. 2nd ed. Philadelphia: Lippincott, Williams & Wilkins, 2003.)

Fungal infections invade the skin through cuts, scrapes, or wounds. They are transmitted via direct contact with the fungus or its spores. Identification of specific fungi is made through culturing affected tissue. Treatment options are available, but one must be persistent when attempting to eradicate this type of infection. Along with oral and topical antifungal medications, it is critical that the affected site be kept clean and dry.

Key Terms	Definitions
dermatophyte (der mat oh fite)	type of fungus
dermatophytoses (dur muh toh figh TOH ses)	skin infections caused by fungi
tinea (TIN ee uh)	lesions of dermatophytoses
tinea capitis (TIN ee uh KAP i tis)	fungal infection on the scalp
tinea corporis (TIN ee uh KOR po ris)	fungal infection on the body
tinea cruris (TIN ee uh KROO ris)	fungal infection in the groin region
tinea pedis (TIN ee uh PED is)	fungal infection on the feet
tinea unguium (TIN ee uh UNG gwee um)	fungal infection of the nails
tinea versicolor (TIN ee uh VUR si kul ur)	chronic superficial fungal infection
fissures (FISH urz)	cracks in the skin

Key Term Practice: Dermatophytosis

1. Infections caused by fungi are termed _____.

2. The lesions from a fungal infection are called _____.

Erysipelas

Erysipelas, more commonly known as **cellulitis**, is an acute inflammation of skin and subcutaneous tissue (Fig. 4-14). It results from a diffuse bacterial (*Streptococcus* or *Staphylococcus*) infection. Although it typically occurs on the legs, any part of the body can be affected. Signs and symptoms include erythema, edema, and skin that is hot and tender to touch. Bacteria enter through an excoriation. Definitive diagnosis may include a blood culture to identify the microorganism. Treatment aims include mobilization and elevation of the affected limb, cool magnesium sulfate application, system antibiotics, and **analgesics** (medicines for pain management).

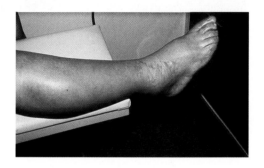

FIGURE 4-14
Cellulitis is an acute inflammation of skin and subcutaneous tissue resulting from diffuse bacterial infection. (Reprinted with permission from Goodheart HP. Goodheart's photoguide of common skin disorders. 2nd ed. Philadelphia: Lippincott, Williams & Wilkins, 2003.)

Key Terms	Definitions
erysipelas (err i SIP e lus)	acute cellulitis of the skin
cellulitis (sell yoo LYE tis)	inflammation of connective tissue, especially of the subcutaneous tissue
analgesics (an al JEE zicks)	drugs that relieve pain

Key Term Practice: Erysipelas

1. Another term for acute cellulitis is _____.

2. Drugs that relieve pain are termed _____.

Hair, Follicle, and Gland Disorders

Folliculitis is an inflammation of hair follicles caused by *Staphylococcus aureus*. Signs and symptoms include erythremic, pustular regions on the thighs, buttocks, beard, and scalp that may be pruritic. A common condition, it affects primarily young adults, and shaving is a precipitating factor. Treatment involves cleansing the affected area daily and applying antiseptics. Untreated folliculitis can lead to carbuncles or furuncles.

Hirsutism is a condition of excessive body hair, particularly in women. In females, the condition causes hair growth in patterns that are typically male. For example, facial hair is very pronounced. It results from a physiological hormone imbalance or steroid use. Excessive growth of normal hair is referred to as **hypertrichosis** and is the condition responsible for the "wolfman" syndrome. When a fungus infects the hair follicle, the resulting hair disease is termed **trichomycosis.**

Rosacea is a chronic, noninfectious disorder characterized by redness on the cheeks, forehead, nose, and chin that results from vascular and follicular dilation (Fig. 4-15). It is often mistaken for a sunburn or acne, hence the older term "acne rosacea." The red mask appearance is referred to as **rosaceiform.** Rosacea has an unknown cause. Treatment consists of avoidance of sunlight, cold weather, and wind; routine use of facial creams is also suggested.

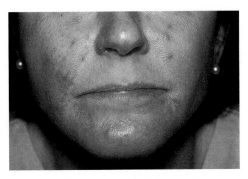

FIGURE 4-15
Rosacea is a chronic, non-infectious disorder characterized by redness on the cheeks, forehead, nose, and chin resulting from vascular and follicular dilation. (Reprinted with permission from Goodheart HP. Goodheart's photoguide of common skin disorders. 2nd ed. Philadelphia: Lippincott, Williams & Wilkins, 2003.)

Rhinophyma is a form of rosacea characterized by expanded blood vessels on the nose and follicular dilation, resulting from hyperplasia of the sebaceous glands and connective tissue. Hence the nose appears red and knobby (Fig. 4-16).

A functional disease of the sebaceous glands characterized by excessive sebum secretion is called **seborrhea**. The oily sebum collects on the skin, forming a greasy coating that eventual transforms to crusts or scales. It occurs in areas where sebaceous glands are most numerous. Signs and symptoms include an oily exudate, slight skin elevation, and perhaps edema, pruritus, and pain on touching. Treatment for rhinophyma and seborrhea includes antiseptic cleansers and medicated facial creams.

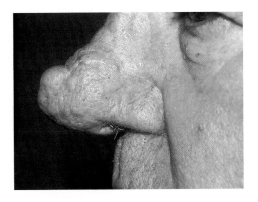

FIGURE 4-16
Rhinophyma. (Reprinted with permission from Goodheart HP. Goodheart's photoguide of common skin disorders. 2nd ed. Philadelphia: Lippincott, Williams & Wilkins, 2003.)

Key Terms	Definitions
folliculitis (fol ick yoo LYE tis)	inflammation of the hair follicles
hirsutism (HER soot izm)	excessive body hair, especially in women
hypertrichosis (high pur tri KOH sis)	excessive growth of normal hair
trichomycosis (trick oh migh KOH sis)	fungal hair disease
rosacea (roh ZAY shee uh)	chronic, noninfectious skin disorder marked by redness on the cheeks, nose, and chin
rosaceiform (roh ZAY shee i form)	the red mask appearance characterizing rosacea
rhinophyma (rye noh FIH muh)	form of rosacea affecting the nose
seborrhea (seb oh REE uh)	disease of the sebaceous glands

Key Term Practice: Hair, Follicle, and Gland Disorders

1. _____ is the term used to describe inflammation of the hair follicles.

2. Another term for wolfman syndrome is _____.

3. Steroid use can result in unusual hairiness in women. This condition is called _____.

Infectious Diseases

Infectious disorders result from bacterial, viral, or other pathogenic invasion. Several forms are described. The causative agent for both herpes zoster (shingles) and varicella (chickenpox) is the varicella-zoster virus (VZV). Affecting children and young adults, **Herpes varicella** is a highly contagious, acute, viral infection. Figure 4-17 illustrates the characteristic cutaneous lesions, macules, vesicles, and crusts of herpes varicella. A small, circumscribed discolored skin spot is termed a **macule.** The macules progress to papules, which eventually form vesicles, which in turn form crusts in the end stage of the disease. Pruritus is intense. The disease is spread directly or indirectly by droplet nuclei from the infected person. People with chickenpox are contagious for 1–2 days before the eruption of the lesions until about day 6, when all lesions are crusty. **Palliative** measures (those that relieve or soothe the symptoms) are the primary treatment options and include anti-itch creams and baths as well as administration of acetaminophen.

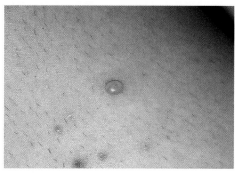

FIGURE 4-17
Chickenpox, or herpes varicella. (Reprinted with permission from Goodheart HP. Goodheart's photoguide of common skin disorders. 2nd ed. Philadelphia: Lippincott, Williams & Wilkins, 2003.)

Herpes zoster is also known as **shingles.** Signs and symptoms include acute inflammation, redness and banding along a dermatome, and pain. A **dermatome** is a specific area of skin innervated by a particular peripheral nerve. The characteristic rash develops along a dermatome, eventually forming vesicles. The vesicles may become pustulant and finally crust (Fig. 4-18). The typical period of duration ranges from 10 days to 5 weeks; however, in some elderly individuals, the disease persists. Although the cause of reactivation of this virus is not clear, stress appears to play a role. Treatment is palliative, and antiviral medication may be administered. There is no cure.

A contagious viral infection in children, **rubella** (German measles) is characterized by fever, pale pink rash, and edema. A similar condition, **rubeola** (measles), is characterized by rose red maculopapular eruptions.

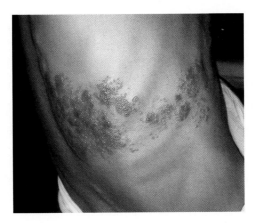

FIGURE 4-18
Shingles, also known as herpes zoster. (Reprinted with permission from Goodheart HP. Goodheart's photoguide of common skin disorders. 2nd ed. Philadelphia: Lippincott, Williams & Wilkins, 2003.)

Impetigo is an acute, contagious inflammatory skin condition caused by streptococci or staphylococci bacteria. Characteristically, vesicles and bullae develop and then burst, forming yellow crusts. The lesions are typically located on the face, arms, legs, and trunk. The causal bacteria are common, and disease occurs as a result of insect bites, anemia, malnutrition, poor hygiene, and nose wiping in children. Diagnosis is made through visual inspection of the characteristic lesions and the Tzanck test. For the **Tzanck test**, a slide smear with Giemsa stain is made from culture taken from the skin blisters. The smear is then examined under the microscope to determine degenerative changes in the epidermal cells. Often, a frozen section (FS), a histologic sample cut from frozen tissues, is used for microscopic study. Impetigo is treated with systemic antibiotic therapy and thorough cleansing. The affected individual must be careful not to spread the disease to other body parts.

Scabies and pediculosis are two common human parasitic insect infections involving the skin and hair. **Scabies,** a contagious skin disorder caused by the *Sarcoptes scabiei* mite, is characterized by intense pruritus and multiform lesions. The itching occurs primarily at night when the female insect burrows beneath the skin to lay eggs.

Pediculosis is a highly contagious skin disease caused by lice infestation. Signs and symptoms include intense pruritus, cutaneous lesions, and nits (eggs) on the hair shafts. Several forms affect humans, each caused by a specific species of louse. *Pediculus humanus capitis* infests the head and scalp, causing **pediculosis capitis. Pediculosis corporis** is caused by *Pediculus humanus corporis,* which infests the skin of the body. *Pthirus pubis,* the crab louse, infests the pubic hair, causing **pediculosis pubis.** When the crab louse spreads over the body to the axillary regions, eyebrows and eyelashes, it causes **pediculosis palpebrarum.**

Mites and lice are transmitted via physical contact with other infected individuals or through contact with their personal belongings, clothes, or bed sheets. Treatment is aimed at removal of the mites, lice, and nits. Lice infestation is treated by using special shampoos, meticulously combing the hair, and cleaning affected personal effects. Scabies treatment involves the use of special shampoos, sulfur creams, and topical steroids.

Verrucae are elevated growths of epidermis, resulting from hyperplasia. **Verruca vulgaris** is a viral disease better known as the common wart. Many warts are caused by papillomaviruses. A verruca is characterized by hard, hyperkeratotic papules commonly occurring on the fingers. The most common type of wart is found on the foot; hence the name **plantar wart**. Plantar warts are small, hard lumps speckled with black dots. The dots are actually clotted blood vessels. Pruritus may be present. Most warts disappear naturally without any treatment. However, treatment in the form of creams, surgical excision, cryosurgery, and electrodesiccation is available.

Key Terms	Definitions
herpes varicella (HUR peez var i SELL uh)	chickenpox
macule (MACK yool)	small, circumscribed discolored skin spot
palliative (PAL ee uh tiv)	relieving or soothing, but not curative, action
herpes zoster (HUR peez ZOS tur)	shingles
shingles	disease caused by VZV
dermatome (DUR muh tome)	area of skin supplied by a sensory nerve
rubella (roo BEL uh)	viral infection; German measles
rubeola (roo BEE oh luh)	measles
impetigo (im pe TYE goh)	contagious skin condition caused by streptococci or staphylococci bacteria
Tzanck (TSANK) test	differential skin test using Giemsa stain and microscopic examination
scabies (SKAY beez)	itch mites
pediculosis (pe dick yoo LOH sis)	skin disease caused by lice
pediculosis capitis (pe dick yoo LOH sis KAP i tis)	lice infestation on the head
pediculosis corporis (pe dick yoo LOH sis KOR puh ris)	lice infestation on the body
pediculosis pubis (pe dick yoo LOH sis PEW bis)	crab lice infestation in the pubic hair
pediculosis palpebrarum (pe dick yoo LOH sis pal pe BRAIR um)	lice infestation in the eyebrows and eyelashes
verruca (ve ROO kuh)	wart
verruca vulgaris (ve ROO kuh vul GAIR us)	common wart
plantar wart	wart on the foot

Key Term Practice: Infectious Diseases

1. An area of skin supplied by a sensory nerve is termed a/an _____.

2. Itch mites are also referred to as _____.

3. Pediculosis _____ is the term used to describe lice infestation on the scalp.

4. The medical term for warts is _____.

Nail Disorders

The fingernails and toenails provide an excellent source for quickly assessing health status as their appearance can often suggest underlying conditions. Many diseases cause nail discoloration, and white patches on the nail beds indicate vitamin and/or mineral deficiency. Diagnosis of nails disorders is usually through physical examination. Correcting underlying pathologies typically corrects nail discoloration.

A basic inflammation of the nail matrix is **onychia.** A suppurative (pus-forming) inflammation occurring around the nail margins caused by infection of the nail bed is called **paronychia.** An ingrown fingernail or toenail is termed **onychocryptosis.** The slow loosening of the nail from the nail bed is called **onycholysis;** the separation begins at the distal free edge and progresses toward the root. **Onychomycosis** is a fungal nail infection.

Edema, erythema, and pain are classic signs and symptoms of nail disorders. Antibiotics and antifungal creams and medications are used to treat these various conditions.

Key Terms	Definitions
onychia (oh NICK ee uh)	inflammation of the nail matrix
paronychia (par oh NICK ee uh)	inflammation with pus at the nail edges
onychocryptosis (on i koh krip TOH sis)	ingrown fingernail or toenail
onycholysis (on i KOL i sis)	loosening of the nail from the nail bed
onychomycosis (on i koh migh KOH sis)	fungal infection of the nail

Key Term Practice: Nail Disorders

1. _____ is the medical term used to describe a fungal infection of the nails.

2. _____ is the medical term for the loosening of the nail from the nail bed.

Pigment Disorders

As discussed previously, skin color variation is a result of genetic, physical, and environmental influences. Alterations in pigmentation are named according to the specific skin abnormality. Diagnosis of pigmentation disorders is made through physical and visual examination.

When skin melanin is lost as a result of a primary disease, the term **leukoderma** is applied. An abnormal thickening, accompanied by abnormal whitening of the epithelium is **leukoplakia.** Skin discoloration as a result of a ruptured blood vessel into the subcutaneous space is known as **ecchymosis.**

Chloasma describes hyperpigmentation occurring on the forehead, temples, cheeks, and nipples during pregnancy, menstruation, or with oral contraceptive use. Childbirth or the discontinuation of oral contraceptives leads to the disappearance of the condition. Depigmenting creams may be applied to lighten the darkened areas.

Although they are not true warts, **seborrheic warts** are characterized by round or oval patches of pigmentation that develop on the skin. The warts generally do not develop until middle age and have a greasy, crusty appearance. **Vitiligo** is a skin disorder characterized by areas of achromia, or regions of no pigmentation (Fig. 4-19). Note that the borders of these achromic regions are hyperpigmented.

Key Terms	Definitions
leukoderma (lew koh DUR muh)	loss of melanin as a result of disease
leukoplakia (lew koh PLAY kee uh)	whitening of the epithelium
ecchymosis (eck i MOH sis)	discoloration because of a ruptured blood vessel

chloasma (kloh AZ muh)	hyperpigmentation caused by hormonal factors
seborrheic (seb oh REE ick) **warts**	pigmented skin with a greasy, crusty appearance
vitiligo (vit i LYE go)	skin disease characterized by patches without pigmentation

Key Term Practice: Pigment Disorders

1. Which skin disease is characterized by regions of no pigmentation?

   _____

2. Whitening of the epithelium is termed _____ .

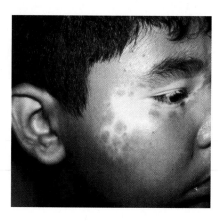

FIGURE 4-19
Vitiligo. This disorder is characterized by regions of no pigmentation with borders that are hyper-pigmented. (Reprinted with permission from Goodheart HP. Goodheart's photoguide of common skin disorders. 2nd ed. Philadelphia: Lippincott, Williams & Wilkins, 2003.)

CLINICAL TERMS

Clinical Dimension	Term	Description
DISORDERS		
	abscess	furuncle involving hair follicles and adjacent tissue
	acne vulgaris	inflammation of the hair follicle and associated sebaceous glands
	actinic keratosis	premalignant hyperkeratosis
	alopecia	hair loss
	alopecia areata	patchy hair loss of the scalp and beard
	alopecia totalis	complete scalp baldness
	alopecia universalis	no body hair at all
	atopic dermatitis	skin inflammation of genetic origin

Clinical Dimension	Term	Definition
	autoimmune disorders	conditions in which the immune response is directed toward the self
	basal cell carcinoma	cancer of the basal cell layer
	burn	tissue reaction as a result of thermal, radioactive, chemical, or electrical insult
	callus	thickened layer of horny epithelium
	cancer	malignant tumor that can lead to death
	carbuncle	large furuncle
	carcinomas	malignant tumor composed of anaplastic (abnormally shaped) epithelial cells
	causalgia	condition characterized by burning sensations
	cellulitis	inflammation of connective tissue, especially of the subcutaneous tissue
	chloasma	hyperpigmentation resulting from hormonal factors
	cicatrix	soft, red fibrous connective tissue
	clavus	corn
	contact dermatitis	skin inflammation caused by an irritant coming in contact with the skin
	corn	clavus
	cradle cap	seborrheic dermatitis in infants
	cutaneous papillomas	skin tags
	decubitus ulcers	pressure sores
	dermatitis	skin inflammation
	dermatomyositis	inflammation of skin and muscles
	dermatophytoses	skin infections caused by fungi
	discoid lupus erythematosus	autoimmune disease of connective tissue
	ecchymosis	discoloration resulting from a ruptured blood vessel
	eczema	genetic inflammatory skin disorder
	elephantiasis	pachyderma
	epidermolysis	dermal–epidermal separation
	erysipelas	acute cellulitis of the skin
	eschar	thick scar that forms over a healed burn
	first-degree burn	damage to the epidermal layer
	fissures	cracks in the skin
	folliculitis	inflammation of the hair follicles
	furuncle	a boil
	gangrene	necrosis of a body tissue
	hemangioma	benign tumor made up of a blood vessel mass

Clinical Dimension	Term	Definition
	herpes varicella	chickenpox
	herpes zoster	shingles
	hirsutism	excessive body hair, especially in women
	hypertrichosis	excessive growth of normal hair
	ichthyosis	hereditary skin condition giving the appearance of scales
	impetigo	contagious skin condition caused by streptococci or staphylococci bacteria
	Kaposi sarcoma	bluish red, brown tumor
	keloid	elevated, firm hyperplasia with ill-defined borders at scar site
	leukoderma	loss of melanin as a result of disease
	lipoma	benign, fatty tumor
	malignant melanoma	cancer of the melanocytes
	melanoma	malignant tumor of melanocytes
	necrosis	death of living cells or tissue
	nevus	lesion containing melanocytes
	onychocryptosis	ingrown fingernail or toenail
	onycholysis	loosening of the nail from the nail bed
	onychomycosis	fungal infection of the nail
	pachydermia	abnormal skin thickening due to filarial infection; elephantiasis
	pediculosis	skin disease caused by lice
	pediculosis capitis	lice infestation on the head
	pediculosis corporis	lice infestation on the body
	pediculosis palpebrarum	lice infestation in the eyebrows and eyelashes
	pediculosis pubis	crab lice infestation in the pubic hair
	pemphigus	skin disorder with groups of bullae
	plantar wart	wart on the foot
	psoriasis	autoimmune skin disease characterized by white scaly plaques
	purpura	condition with purple skin hemorrhages
	rhinophyma	form of rosacea affecting the nose
	rosacea	chronic, noninfectious skin disorder marked by redness on the cheeks, nose, and chin
	rubella	viral infection; German measles
	rubeola	measles
	scabies	itch mites

Clinical Dimension	Term	Definition
	scar	permanent blemish
	scleroderma	autoimmune disease characterized by increased collagen formation in connective tissues, including skin and organs
	sebaceous cysts	fluid-filled sebaceous glands
	seborrhea	disease of the sebaceous glands
	seborrheic dermatitis	inflammation of the skin at the sebaceous glands
	seborrheic keratosis	benign, purple-brown skin tumor
	seborrheic warts	pigmented skin with a greasy, crusty appearance
	second-degree burn	damage to the epidermal and dermal layers
	shingles	disease caused by VZV
	squamous cell carcinoma	cancer developing in the epidermis
	steatoma	lipoma
	systemic lupus erythematosus	autoimmune disease of connective tissue
	third-degree burn	full-thickness burn
	tinea	lesions of dermatophytoses
	tinea capitis	fungal infection on the scalp
	tinea circinata	fungal infection in the skin; ringworm
	tinea corporis	fungal infection on the body
	tinea cruris	fungal infection in the groin region
	tinea pedis	fungal infection on the feet
	tinea unguium	fungal infection of the nails
	tinea versicolor	chronic superficial fungal infection
	trichomycosis	fungal hair disease
	ulcers	interruptions in the integrity of the epithelial tissue
	urticaria	hives marked by redness and swelling
	verruca	warts
	verruca vulgaris	common wart
	vitiligo	skin disease characterized by patches without pigmentation
	xeroderma	extremely dry skin
	xeroderma pigmentosum	genetic skin disease characterized by hypopigmentation and hyperpigmentation

SIGNS AND SYMPTOMS

	abrasion	wearing down of skin by rubbing or scraping
	burrow	channel below the skin caused by a parasite
	bulla	blister or bleb

Clinical Dimension	Term	Definition
	contusion	bruise
	crusts	hard coverings that result when exudate on the skin dries
	edema	swelling
	erythema	redness on the skin
	exanthem	skin eruption
	excoriation	skin abrasion
	exfoliation	peeling and shedding of the epidermis
	lesions	structural or functional alterations
	leukoplakia	whitening of the epithelium
	macule	small, circumscribed discolored skin spot
	nodules	deep, boil-like structures
	onychia	inflammation of the nail matrix
	papule	solid circumscribed skin elevation less than 1 mm in diameter
	paronychia	inflammation with pus at the nail edges
	petechiae	spots of hemorrhaging
	pilonidal cyst	cyst with a clump of hair
	polyp	smooth skin projection
	pruritus	itching
	pustules	skin elevations containing pus
	pyoderma	pus-producing skin lesion
	rosaceiform	the red mask appearance characterizing rosacea
	telangiectasia	dilation of groups of capillaries
	vesicles	blisters that leak fluid
	vibices	linear hemorrhages on the skin surface
	wheals	swellings in specific skin areas
	xanthoma	fat-filled cells in subcutaneous tissue

CLINICAL TESTS AND DIAGNOSTIC PROCEDURES

	Term	Definition
	antinuclear antibody (ANA) test	blood test used in the diagnosis of autoimmune diseases
	biopsy	live tissue excision for diagnostic study
	cauterization	procedure that coagulates or destroys tissue by heat or chemical means
	dermabrasion	procedure that scrapes away skin layers
	electrocautery	procedure that uses a heated wire to destroy tissue
	fluorescent antinuclear antibody (FANA) test	blood test used in the diagnosis of autoimmune diseases

Clinical Dimension	Term	Definition
	galvanocautery	electrocautery
	intradermal test	skin test to identify allergens
	lipectomy	fat excision
	liposuction	fat removal via suction
	Mantoux test	intradermal test to identify tuberculosis
	patch test	skin test to identify allergens
	Schick test	intradermal test to identify diphtheria
	scratch test	skin test to identify allergens
	Tzanck test	differential skin test using Giemsa stain and microscopic examination
	wood lamp examination	placement of hair or skin under UV light to identify the presence of a fungus
TREATMENTS		
	analgesics	drugs that relieve pain
	blepharoplasty	restorative eyelid surgery
	chemabrasion	use of a chemical to peel off skin layers
	cryosurgery	localized freezing of diseased tissues for surgical removal
	curettage	surgical procedure in which tissue is scraped away using a curet
	débridement	excision of necrotized tissue from a wound by surgical excision, enzymes, or chemical agents
	dermatoplasty	skin graft surgery
	diaphoresis	artificially induced perspiration
	electrodesiccation	destruction of growth by a terminal electrode
	incision and drainage	surgical cut to drain fluid from tissue
	Mohs surgery	microscopically controlled cancer surgery
	rhytidectomy	excision of excess wrinkles; facelift
	sclerotherapy	injection of a saline solution into veins to cause their disappearance
	transcutaneous electrical nerve stimulation (TENS)	form of electroanalgesia

Lifespan

During embryologic development, the epidermis is derived from the ectoderm, whereas the dermis and hypodermis are derived from the mesoderm. The ectoderm and mesoderm are two of the three primary germ layers from which all human tissues develop in utero. The skin is nearly developed by the 4th gestational month. Lanugo—soft, downy, peach-fuzz-like hair—covers the fetus beginning around the 5th month.

At birth, the body's skin is covered with vernix caseosa, which literally means "varnish of cheese" and which is produced by the sebaceous glands. Newborn skin is thin, and the presence of milia on the face is common. Milia are small white spots caused by particles clogging the sebaceous glands. These white dots gradually disappear within several weeks.

As children develop, the skin thickens, subcutaneous fat deposition increases, and sweat glands become increasingly functional. During adolescence, there is a marked increase in sebaceous gland activity, often resulting in acne. Skin function and appearance are optimum between the ages of 20 and 40 years. However, many age-associated skin changes are not evident until age 45 years and beyond.

As the integumentary system ages, there are noticeable changes, such as wrinkling, thinner and drier skin, loss of subcutaneous fat, atrophy of sebaceous glands, pigmentation alterations, and a decrease in the number of melanocytes. Owing to the fewer melanocytes, there is less filtering of UV radiation, increasing the risk of skin cancers. Graying hair is a result of the decrease in melanocytes. Moreover, an increase in the size of some melanocytes causes patches of enhanced pigmentation known as age spots.

The decrease in dermal thickness gives aging skin a thin, translucent appearance. Wrinkling occurs as a result of decreased numbers of fibroblasts, which produce collagen and elastic fibers. Thus the skin is less flexible and wrinkling occurs.

Hair and nail growth also diminish with the aging process. It is interesting that beginning around the age of 50 years only about one third of the hair follicles are active. It is also common for hair to become thinner.

Dry skin in the elderly population is attributed to atrophy of sweat and sebaceous glands. Wound healing is delayed in response to decreased blood supply, reduced cell proliferation, and diminished immune response. The immune response is weakened because there are fewer Langerhans cells, which are responsible for resisting disease. Temperature regulation is compromised in aged persons as a result of diminished fat reserves, decreased vascular function, and reduced sweat production.

The skin is the organ that shows the most obvious signs of aging. Proper fluid intake and nutrition, good hygiene, and avoidance of too much UV radiation are essential to maintaining healthy skin throughout the lifespan.

In the News: Necrotizing Fasciitis

Do you remember cases of necrotizing fasciitis, the flesh-eating infection? If not, then here's the news. It sounded like something out of a horror film. Reports from England in 1994, San Francisco in 1996, and Texas in 1998 focused on this disease, when people died as their flesh was literally being eaten away at the rate of several inches per hour. The culprit was the very common bacterium *Streptococcus pyogenes*. The *Streptococcus* killed the infected tissue, thrived in the remaining dead flesh, and produced toxins that diffused into the surrounding healthy tissue to continue the process. The disease was named necrotizing fasciitis because, as the term suggests, it flourished in the fascia (tissue layers under the skin), killing (necrotizing) tissue in its path.

Symptoms of necrotizing fasciitis were described as early as the 5th century B.C.E. by Hippocrates, and more than 2000 cases were reported among soldiers during the Civil War. Signs and symptoms include fever, severe pain and swelling, large fluid-filled purple bullae, and rapid invasive infection of tissue. The release of foul-smelling pus from the vesicles is a telltale sign. Dermal gangrene is often apparent. It often originates from a minor trauma or skin injury that allows the bacteria to gain entry into the body. There are no preventive measures and its onset cannot be predicted. However, for unknown reasons, the flesh-eating strain appears to have a 10-year cycle.

Treatment must be swift to prevent its rampant spread and increase the chances of survival. Urgent tissue excision is usually necessary to remove infected areas and relieve edema. Amputation of limbs is frequently necessary. Antibiotics are useless for the initial infection because they cannot reach the target site owing to inadequate circulatory function in the dead tissue layers. Antibiotic agents also have no effect on the toxins produced by the bacteria. Thus, surgery is the therapy of choice, and broad-spectrum antibiotics are given afterward. Further management involves aggressive antimicrobial therapy, fluid replacement, and the use of a hyperbaric oxygen chamber to promote wound healing.

Flesh-eating bacteria affect between 500 and 1500 people annually in the United States. The mortality rate is 40–60%.

COMMON ABBREVIATIONS

Abbreviation	Term
ABCD	asymmetry, border, color, diameter
AIDS	acquired immunodeficiency syndrome
ANA	antinuclear antibody
ASCP	American Society for Clinical Pathology
bx	biopsy
CAAHEP	Commission on Accreditation of Allied Health Education Programs
CT	cytotechnologist
decub.	decubitus ulcer; bedsore
DLE	discoid lupus erythematosus
FANA	fluorescent antinuclear antibody
FS	frozen section
I&D	incision and drainage
LE	lupus erythematosus
SC	subcutaneous
SLE	systemic lupus erythematosus
subcu.	subcutaneous
subq.	subcutaneous
TENS	transcutaneous electrical nerve stimulation
UV	ultraviolet
VZV	varicella-zoster virus
XDP	xeroderma pigmentosum
XP	xeroderma pigmentosum

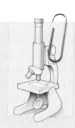

Case Study

Mrs. Walford, a 55-year-old, arrived in her dermatologist's office with a year-long history of a skin lesion on her right temple. History of the present illness indicated that this spot has occasionally bled in response to minor trauma. Surgical, social, and psychosocial histories were unremarkable. Family history was noncontributory.

Mrs. Walford's physical examination revealed that she appeared healthy and was in no acute distress. Because her chief complaint was a neoplasm on the right temple, she was questioned about outdoor activities, sunscreen use, and history of blistering sunburns. It was discovered that in her youth, Mrs. Walford remembered having at least one blistering sunburn. She also stated that she rarely used any type of sunscreen while she gardened, which she engaged in on a regular basis.

Physical examination of the integumentary system revealed the following regarding the lesion:

LOCATION: right temple at temporal hair line
SIZE: 1.7 cm × 1.3 cm
SHAPE: irregular
COLOR: erythematous
ELEVATION: slightly elevated
IRRITATION: slightly irritated

Dr. Byron, her dermatologist, diagnosed probable basal cell carcinoma of right temple and suggested that the most reasonable treatment would be excision of the lesion with pathologic examination of the tissue by a cytotechnologist.

Case Study Questions

Select the best answer to each of the following.

1. **Mrs. Walford made an appointment with her dermatologist for her lesion. Why is this the most appropriate medical specialty for her condition?**

   a. Dermatologists specialize in diseases of the skin and integumentary system; thus Dr. Byron would be a wise choice.

   b. A better choice would have been a family physician because these doctors see a lot of different cases.

   c. She should have gone directly to a pathologist because that specialty area deals with the study of disease.

   d. A dermatologist is okay, but a cytotechnologist is better trained to deal with skin conditions.

2. **What sign or symptom suggested to the doctor that this might be basal cell carcinoma?**

   a. There was nothing in particular to suggest this.

   b. The doctor believed a "better safe than sorry" approach was best.

   c. The lesion had irregular borders, was elevated, and was irritated.

   d. The lesion had been there a long time.

3. **The lesion was described as erythematous. This means the lesion** _____.

   a. has a redness

   b. has a bluish hue

   c. is fluid filled

   d. is hard

4. **What is the significance of the skin being exposed to the sun without using sunscreen?**

   a. There is no significance because sun-exposed skin can hold up to UV radiation.

   b. There is no significance because there is no evidence that sunscreen protects against harmful sun rays.

   c. Continuous sun exposure without sunscreen increases the risk of developing skin cancer.

   d. Sunscreen use has been linked to an increased risk of skin cancer.

5. **Basal cell carcinoma is _____.**

   a. locally invasive, rarely metastasizes, and is common in individuals with a history of chronic sun exposure

   b. the most serious type of skin cancer and is generally associated with changes in a mole

   c. a tumor characterized by multiple bluish red or brown nodules and plaques

   d. a minor lesion that does not require medical treatment

6. **Excision of the lesion with pathologic examination means that the _____.**

   a. growth will be frozen and viewed with the naked eye

   b. lesion will be lanced and the fluid drained

   c. lesion will be removed and grown on a Petri plate

   d. lesion will be removed and evaluated by trained professionals to arrive at a conclusive diagnosis

REAL WORLD REPORT

COMMUNITY HOSPITAL:
DEPARTMENT OF PATHOLOGY

NAME:	Charon Walford
COLLECTION DATE:	05/30/2001
SURGEON:	Richard Kelley
ADMITTER:	Mary Anne Edinburgh
DOB:	02/21/1946
AGE:	55
SEX:	F
CONSULTOR:	Lindsey Limpson
PATH NO.:	F002434
HOSPITAL NO.:	01478
ACCOUNT NO.:	47891s
LOCATION:	Clinic

PATHOLOGIC DIAGNOSIS
Right temple, excisional biopsy: Basal cell carcinoma

COMMENT
- *All* margins of resection are free of neoplasm
- Sources: *Skin,* Rt temple neoplasm

CLINICAL INFORMATION
Excision neoplasm right temple

GROSS DESCRIPTION
In fixative is a solitary elliptical segment of light tan skin measuring 4 × 1.6 × 0.5 cm. A poorly defined gray-tan macular lesion measuring 1.2 × 0.8 cm is present in the center of the specimen, approximately 1 to 2 mm from the short axis margin of resection. All margins are inked in blue. Serial sections across the short axis to include the lesion are submitted in cassette #1. The opposite pointed margins are submitted in cassette #2.

MICROSCOPIC DESCRIPTION
Sections of skin and subcutaneous tissue demonstrate mild hyperkeratosis. The epidermis is focally atrophic. There is mild basophilic degeneration of the reticular collagen. Arising at the dermal–epidermal junction and involving the reticular dermis is a neoplasm consisting of broad-based islands and ribbons of basaloid cells having a hyperchromatic, spindled nucleus with finely stippled chromatin. The peripheral cell layer of these tumor lobules shows prominent palisading. Focal central necrosis is at times identified as well as scattered mitotic figures within the tumor nests. A slightly basophilic fibromyxoid stroma containing chronic inflammation surrounds the tumor nests. All margins of resection are free of neoplasm.

SIGNATURE: Pathologist (signed out 06/01/2001)

REAL WORLD REPORT QUESTIONS

The following exercises review the medical terms used in the preceding medical report. A term that may be unfamiliar is *palisading,* which is used in microbiology to describe cells that are lined up next to each other much like a white picket fence.

1. What is a neoplasm?

   _____

   _____

   _____

2. Hyperkeratosis

   a. Word part *hyper-* = _____

   b. Word part *kerat-* = _____

   c. Word part *-osis* = _____

   d. What does *hyperkeratosis* mean?

      _____

3. What word literally means "a reduction in tissue size"?

   _____

4. The dermal–epidermal junction was mentioned. Refer to the diagram in the text and describe this area.

   _____

   _____

   _____

5. The margins of the section were free of neoplasm, thus _____.

   a. cancerous tissue remains

   b. all the cancerous tissue was removed

REVIEW AND APPLICATION: THREE-LEVEL LEARNING SYSTEM

 LEVEL ONE: REVIEWING FACTS AND TERMS USING RECALL

Match the following terms with the correct definition. Each term is used only once.

    a. burn
    b. keloid
    c. sebaceous
    d. arrector pili
    e. melanocytes
    f. lunula
    g. hypodermis
    h. ceruminous
    i. melanin
    j. hypertrichosis
    k. eponychium
    l. dermis

1. The _____ is the skin layer beneath the epidermis.

2. This layer below the dermis is also called the subcutaneous layer.

_____

3. A dark pigment, _____ is produced by melanocytes.

4. Tissue reaction to heat, radiation, or chemical agents is termed a/an _____.

5. The medical term for excessive hair is _____.

6. Pigment-producing cells are termed _____.

7. An unusually hard, elevated scar is termed a/an _____.

8. The _____ glands produce sebum.

9. The _____ glands produce ear wax.

10. When the _____ muscles contract, goose bumps result.

11. The _____ is the white, moon-shaped growth area of nails.

12. Another term for _____ is cuticle.

Select the best answer to each of the following.

13. This/These type(s) of burn(s) is/are characterized by severe pain; blisters, edema; and slow, complete recovery.

    a. first degree

    b. second degree

    c. fourth degree

    d. a and c

14. Skin functions include _____.

    a. maintaining body temperature and serving as a protective barrier

    b. serving as a protective barrier and synthesizing blood

    c. maintaining body temperature and synthesizing nerve cells

    d. all of the above

15. The correct order of epidermal layers from deep to superficial is _____.

    a. stratum corneum, stratum basale, and stratum granulosum

    b. stratum granulosum, stratum corneum, and stratum basale

    c. stratum basale, stratum corneum, and stratum granulosum

    d. stratum basale, stratum granulosum, and stratum corneum

16. The primary purpose of _____ is to absorb UV radiation to prevent damage to underlying cells.

    a. carotene

    b. melanin

    c. lipocytes

    d. follicles

17. Factors influencing skin color include all of the following *except* _____.

    a. genetics

    b. environment

    c. gender

    d. physiology

18. The correct meaning of the word part *cut-* is _____.
    a. horn
    b. black
    c. skin
    d. carotene

19. The word part _____ means "hair."
    a. trich-
    b. unguo-
    c. onych-
    d. scler-

20. The word part *hidr-* refers to _____.
    a. water
    b. sweat
    c. tissue
    d. a and b

21. The stratum lucidum is _____.
    a. an extra layer found covering the eyes
    b. another skin layer that occurs only in some people
    c. a very thick layer of skin that develops during puberty
    d. a clear layer located on palms and soles of feet

22. Striae occur as a result of _____.
    a. wound healing
    b. clogged sebaceous glands
    c. improper skin formation
    d. weight gain

23. Comedones occur when an enlarged _____ becomes filled with sebum, bacteria, and pigment.
    a. pore
    b. corium
    c. stratum
    d. wart

24. Absence of body hair is termed _____.
    a. hirsutism
    b. seborrhea
    c. alopecia universalis
    d. alopecia areata

25. Fingernails are termed _____.
    a. eponychia
    b. ungues
    c. unguis
    d. phalanges

Define the following word parts.

26. lip- _____

27. dermato- _____

28. xer-, xero- _____

29. melano- _____

30. papulo- _____

LEVEL TWO: REVIEWING CONCEPTS

Select the best answer to each of the following.

31. The skin is an organ because _____.
    a. there are so many different types.
    b. it is composed of two or more kinds of tissue.
    c. it is very large.
    d. it covers the entire body surface.

32. Melanin is important because it _____.
    a. filters UV radiation, thereby preventing damage to underlying tissue
    b. darkens the skin, thereby deterring microbial activity
    c. aids in absorbing nutrients, thus keeping the skin healthy
    d. screens the body of toxins that would otherwise penetrate its surface

33. The skin's outermost membrane is fully keratinized, giving it the name _____.

    a. stratum granulosum

    b. stratum spinosum

    c. stratum corneum

    d. stratum keratin

34. Provide a medical term to complete a meaningful analogy: Stratum is to strata as unguis is to _____.

    a. ungues

    b. uncle

    c. eponychium

    d. fingernail

35. The perionychium can best be described as the _____.

    a. cuticle

    b. nail bed

    c. soft tissue surrounding the nail plate

    d. eponychium

36. The red mask appearance characteristic of rosacea is termed _____.

    a. rosaceiform

    b. epidermolysis

    c. excoriation

    d. exudative

37. Sweat glands are important for _____.

    a. secreting fluids for mating purposes

    b. producing oils to keep the skin soft and pliable

    c. heat regulation

    d. vitamin regulation

38. An epithelial injury that occurs by contact with thermal, radioactive, chemical, or electrical agents is termed a/an _____.

    a. bulla

    b. vesicle

    c. acne

    d. burn

39. Temperature homeostasis suggests that the _____.

    a. body's internal temperature is satisfactory relative to the outside temperature

    b. body cannot keep up with the demands placed on it

    c. skin is capable of producing chemicals

    d. body temperature never fluctuates

40. What word means "under the skin"?

    _____

41. What word means "through the skin"?

    _____

42. *Intradermal* literally means _____.

What is the plural form for each given term?

43. nevus _____

44. bulla _____

45. papule _____

Match the integumentary system disorder with its correct characteristics or definition.

_____ 46. acne vulgaris   a. malignant tumor

_____ 47. alopecia   b. inflammation of a hair follicle associated with a sebaceous gland

_____ 48. clavus

_____ 49. carcinoma   c. corn

_____ 50. decubitus ulcer   d. bed sore

   e. baldness

Match the sign or symptom with its correct definition.

_____ 51. erythema   a. swelling

_____ 52. pruritus   b. patches of redness

_____ 53. edema   c. small, circumscribed discolored skin spot

_____ 54. bulla

   d. itching

_____ 55. macule   e. large, fluid-filled bleb

_____ 56. erysipelas   f. severe skin rash caused by a bacterium

Match the clinical test with its correct definition.

_____ 57. blood test useful for the differential diagnosis of lupus

a. Mantoux test

b. wood lamp examination

c. Schick test

_____ 58. slide smear test done using Giemsa stain

d. Tzank test

e. fluorescent antinuclear antibody (FANA) test

_____ 59. a type of intradermal test for tuberculosis

_____ 60. a type of intradermal test for diphtheria

_____ 61. test done to identify fungal skin infections

Define the following abbreviations.

62. bx. _____

63. decub. _____

64. I&D _____

65. SLE _____

66. UV _____

LEVEL THREE: THINKING CRITICALLY

Select the best answer to each of the following.

67. Mrs. Jones appears weak and is thirsty. After her skin is pinched to test its turgor, it did not respond normally. This indicates that _____.

     a. Mrs. Jones is dehydrated and her skin is quite elastic

     b. Mrs. Jones is not dehydrated and her skin is quite elastic

     c. Mrs. Jones is dehydrated and her skin has lost some elastic properties as a result.

     d. Mrs. Jones is dehydrated but her skin is fine.

68. A family member cannot understand why he is not permitted to visit his brother in the burn unit unless he wears a gown and mask. You explain the reason is because _____.

     a. the skin is the body's first line of defense, and this patient is severely compromised

     b. the immune response of the patient does not operate after a burn

     c. you would not want the family member coming down with a disease from the burned patient

     d. gowns and masks are mandated in the hospital

69. Anna was born with albinism. This places her at increased risk of _____.

     a. autoimmune diseases

     b. infectious skin diseases

     c. vitiligo

     d. sunburn

70. You have just learned that a friend was diagnosed with purpura urticans and another is cyanotic. You know from your medical terminology class that the person with purpura urticans has _____ dots on the skin, and the person with cyanosis has skin appearing _____ in coloration.

     a. purple; bluish

     b. bluish; purple

     c. pink; rosy

     d. yellow; white

71. Noah has just visited Arizona, and he tells you that 90°F in the desert seems cooler than 90°F in the tropical rain forest. Provide a plausible explanation for this statement.

     a. Arizona has a more temperate climate than the tropics, thus he just feels better.

     b. Sweat evaporates more quickly in the tropics than in the desert, thus cooling the body faster.

c. Sweat evaporates more quickly in the dry, arid desert than in the wet, humid tropics, thus cooling the body faster.

d. Sweat radiates more quickly in the desert than in the tropics, thus cooling the body faster.

72. The correct spelling of the word that means "a soft, red, fibrous connective tissue surrounding a wound healing site" is _____.

a. cicatrix

b. cikatrix

c. keloid

d. celoid

73. The correct spelling of the word for the most common inflammatory skin disorder, which is characterized by erythema, papules, vesicles, pruritus, and crusts is _____.

a. petechia

b. petechea

c. eczema

d. egzema

74. The correct word parts meaning "tissue" is _____.

a. histio-, histo-

b. myc-, myco-

c. hidr-, hidro-

d. cry-, cryo-

75. The correct word parts meaning "fungus" is _____.

a. lip-, lipo-

b. myc-, myco-

c. a and b

d. none of these

 # KEY TERMS SPELLING TEST FROM CD-ROM

Use the CD-ROM to test yourself on the spelling of key terms from this chapter. Listen to the terms and write them on a separate sheet of paper. Use a medical dictionary to check your answers.

ANSWERS

WORD GROUPING

Definition	Word Part
beneath	sub-
black	melan-, melano-
blue	cyan-, cyano-
cell	cyt-, -cyte, cyto-
cold	cry-, cryo-
color	chrom-,-chrome, chromat-, chromato-, chromo-
death	necr-, necro-
disease	path-, -pathy-, patho-
dry	xer-, xero-
epidermal scale	squamo-
fat	A. adip-, adipo-
	B. steato-
fatty	lip-, lipo-
fingernail or toenail	onych-, onycho-
fish	ichthy-, ichthyo-
flowing	-rrhea
formation	-plasia
fungus	myc-, myco-
hair	A. pil-, pilo-
	B. trich-, trichi-, tricho-
hardness	sclera-, sclero-
horny tissue or cornea	kerat-, kerato-
pimple, circumscribed solid elevation	papulo-
plants	phyt-, phyto-
pus accumulation	py-, pyo-
red or red blood cell	erythr-, erythro-
sebum (oil)	seb-, sebo-, sebi-
self	aut-, auto-
skin	derm-, derma-, dermat-, dermato-, dermo-
sweat	A. hidr-, hidro
	B. sudor-
tissue	histio-, histo-
tumor	-oma
vesicle, blister	vesic-, vesico-, vesiculo-
wax	cero-
white or white blood cell	leuc-, leuco-, leuk-, leuko-
yellow	xanth-, xantho-

WORD BUILDING

Word Part	Meaning	Common or Known Word	Example Medical Term
adip-, adipo-	fat	adipose	adipocytes
aut-, auto-	self	automobile	autoimmune
cyt-, -cyte, cyto-	cell	cytoplast	erythrocyte
derm-, derma-, dermat-, -dermato-, dermo-	skin	dermis	epidermis
erythr-, erythro-	red or red blood cell	erythrocyte	erythrocyte
histio-, histo-	tissue	histology	histology
lip-, lipo-	fatty	lipid	liposuction
melan-, melano-	black	melanin	melanocyte
path-, patho-, -pathy	disease	pathology	pathophysiology
-rrhea	flowing	diarrhea	seborrhea
scler-, sclero-	hardness	sclera	scleroderma
sub-	beneath	submarine	subcutaneous
vesic-, vesico-, vesiculo-	vesicle, blister	vesicle	vesicle

KEY TERM PRACTICE

Integumentary System Preview

1. a. physical barrier; b. vitamin D synthesis; c. immune function; d. UV radiation filter
2. integument
3. sebaceous
4. dermatology

Skin Layers

1. epidermis
2. subcutaneous
3. dermis
4. A. stratum; B. strata

Skin Color and Birthmarks

1. albinism
2. cyanosis

Hair

1. root; shaft; follicle
2. arrector pili

Glands

1. comedo
2. hidrosis

Nails

1. ungues
2. lunula
3. cuticle

Skin Conditions

1. Causalgia
2. exfoliation

Burns

1. Tissue reaction to thermal, radioactive, chemical, or electrical insult.
2. first-degree; second-degree; third-degree

Alopecia

1. alopecia
2. alopecia totalis

Autoimmune Disorders

1. scleroderma
2. Dermatomyositis

Noncancerous Tumors

1. nevi
2. lipoma; steatoma

Cancerous Tumors

1. Malignant melanoma
2. carcinomas

Carbuncles and Furuncles

1. incision and drainage
2. furuncle

Clavi and Calluses

1. clavus
2. Calluses

Decubitus Ulcers

1. decubitus ulcer
2. Débridement

Dermatitis

1. dermatitis
2. idiopathic
3. cradle cap
4. atopic dermatitis
5. urticaria
6. wheal

Dermatophytosis

1. dermatophytoses
2. tinea

Erysipelas

1. erysipelas
2. analgesics

Hair, Follicle, and Gland Disorders

1. Folliculitis
2. hypertrichosis
3. hirsutism

Infectious Diseases

1. dermatome
2. scabies
3. capitis
4. verrucae

Nail Disorders

1. Onychomycosis
2. Onycholysis

Pigment Disorders

1. vitiligo
2. leukoplakia

CASE STUDY

1. a is the correct answer.
   - b is incorrect because the dermatologist is better trained in skin diseases.
   - c is incorrect because a pathologist's job is studying the actual tissue samples; patient care is reserved for the dermatologist.
   - d is incorrect because cytotechnologists are involved with the laboratory side of patient care and are not trained physicians.
2. c is the correct answer.
   - a, b, and d are incorrect because the shape, color, elevation, and irritation were all abnormal. Time is not necessarily a factor.
3. a is the correct answer.
   - b is incorrect because cyanosis refers to a blue color.
   - c is incorrect because small, fluid-filled raised areas are termed pustules.
   - d is incorrect because erythematous refers to a structure that is red, not hard.
4. c is the correct answer.
   - a, b, and d are all incorrect because sun-exposed skin should be protected. There is an increased risk of nonmalignant and malignant tumors in individuals who regularly engage in outdoor activities without applying skin protection.
5. a is the correct answer.
   - b is incorrect because it describes squamous cell carcinoma.
   - c is incorrect because it describes Kaposi sarcoma.
   - d is incorrect because basal cell carcinoma does require medical treatment for its excision.
6. d is the correct answer.
   - a is incorrect because cultures will be viewed microscopically.
   - b is incorrect because *excision* means it will be removed.
   - c is incorrect. Although cell cultures may be grown on agar in a Petri plate, the "pathologic examination" portion of the question indicates that the cells will be professionally evaluated.

REAL WORLD REPORT

1. A new growth of abnormal cells.
2. A. excessive or above normal; B. horn or hard; C. diseased condition of; D. hypertrophy(excessive cells) of the horny layer of skin
3. atrophic
4. The outer epidermis and the inner dermis are joined together by a polysaccharide gel that "glues" the epidermis to the dermis. This is called the dermal–epidermal junction.
5. B is the correct answer.

REVIEW AND APPLICATION: THREE-LEVEL LEARNING SYSTEM

Level One: Reviewing Facts and Terms Using Recall

1. l
2. g
3. i
4. a
5. j
6. e
7. b
8. c
9. h
10. d
11. f
12. k
13. b
14. a
15. d
16. b
17. c
18. c
19. a
20. b
21. d
22. d
23. a
24. c
25. b
26. fat
27. skin
28. dry
29. black
30. pimple

Level Two: Reviewing Concepts

31. b
32. a
33. c
34. a
35. c
36. a
37. c
38. d
39. a
40. subcutaneous
41. percutaneous
42. within the skin
43. nevi
44. bullae
45. papules
46. b
47. e
48. c
49. a
50. d
51. b
52. d
53. a
54. e
55. c
56. f
57. e
58. d
59. a
60. c
61. b
62. biopsy
63. decubitus
64. incision and drainage
65. systemic lupus erythematosus
66. ultraviolet

Level Three: Thinking Critically

67. c
68. a
69. d
70. a
71. c
72. a
73. c
74. a
75. b

Skeletal System

OBJECTIVES

After completing this chapter, you should be able to:

1. Correctly identify the parts of a typical long bone.
2. Describe the classifications and types of bones.
3. Identify the types of bone cells.
4. Explain bone remodeling and the significance of vitamins, hormones, and exercise in this process.
5. Identify the bones of the human skeleton.
6. Describe various signs, symptoms, clinical tests, diagnostic procedures, and treatments of common skeletal system disorders.
7. Specify anatomical and physiologic alterations throughout the lifespan.
8. Define common abbreviations related to the skeletal system.
9. Correctly define, spell, and pronounce the chapter's medical terms.

INTRODUCTION

Made of bone tissue, the skeletal system plays several important roles in the body. Its functions include maintaining posture, protecting organs, moving the body, storing minerals, and producing blood cells (hemopoiesis). These functions also support other body systems.

Bones create the body's fundamental framework structure. The bones of the feet, legs, pelvis, and backbone carry the weight of the body; and the bones of the arms supplement balance. Bones also provide rigid attachment points for muscles, soft tissues, and organs. The system protects many vital organs, encasing them in tough bone tissue. For example, the skull and vertebrae enclose the central nervous system, the rib cage and shoulder girdle protect the thoracic viscera, and the pelvic girdle shields the reproductive organs and other structures.

Body movement results from the contraction of muscles anchored to bones; joints serve as critical components to mobility. Another key function of the skeletal system is mineral storage; in fact, calcium and phosphorous make up two thirds of bone by weight. Moreover, 95% of calcium and 90% of the body's total phosphorous is found in the bones and teeth. Finally, blood cell production occurs within bone tissue: The red bone marrow produces white blood cells, red blood cells, and platelets.

The interconnectedness of the body's systems is particularly evident when considering the skeletal system. For example, bone is continuously undergoing remodeling, striking a balance between bone breakdown and bone formation. This process works in concert with the endocrine system to regulate the body's hormonal and mineral balance. The dynamic nature of bone is discussed in this chapter.

Professional Profile: Orthopedic Surgeon

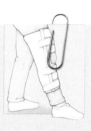

Susan O'Keefe is an orthopedic surgeon who treats a variety of musculoskeletal injuries and disease. She completed an undergraduate degree with a major in biology and then went on to medical school. After graduating with a doctor of medicine (MD) degree, Susan completed a 4-year residency in orthopedic surgery. After her residency, she sat for a national examination and became board certified in orthopedic surgery. Since becoming a surgeon, Susan has had specialized training in pediatric orthopedics and continues with mandated continuing medical education to keep her license current. In the field of orthopedics, women are definitely a minority.

The orthopedic surgeon is responsible for diagnosing and treating skeletal pathology by surgical and conservative means and by the application of mechanical devices. For example, fractures must be identified, reduced and immobilized by open or closed methods, and fixed using corrective appliances. Common corrective devices are braces, casts, and splints.

Orthopedists, as they are commonly called, may work in managed care, private practice, or academic medicine. Although it is one of the most prevalent specialties in medicine, it is not unusual for an orthopedist to work 60 hours a week. Besides performing scheduled surgery and seeing patients with appointments, these specialists often must make emergency visits to hospitals and nursing homes. Thus orthopedists spend time traveling from their office to various facilities to examine patients. They must also be available to field phone calls from patients and consulting professionals.

MEDICAL TERM PARTS

WORD PARTS

Medical term prefixes, suffixes, and combining forms related to the skeletal system are introduced in this section.

Word Parts	Meaning
-blast	immature precursor cell
calc-, calci-, calco-	calcium
calcane-, calcaneo-	calcaneus
carp-, carpo-	carpus (wrist), carpal
chondr-, chondri-, chondrio-, chondro-	cartilage, cartilaginous
-clast	something that breaks; to break
coccy-	coccyx; tailbone
condyl-, condylo-	condyle
cost-, costi-, costo-	rib, costal
crani-, cranio-	cranium, cranial
ethmo-	ethmoid
femoro-	femur, femoral
-genesis	development
hyo-	U-shaped
ili-, ilio-	ilium, iliac
mandibul-, mandibulo-	mandible, mandibular
meat-, meato-	meatus
myel-, myelo-	marrow
orth-, ortho-	straight
osseo-, ossi-	bone
ost-, oste-, osteo-	bone
pelv-, pelvo-	pelvis
peroneo-	peroneal, peroneus
pubo-	pubis, pubic, pubes
scapul-, scapulo-	scapula, scapular
spondyl-, spondylo-	vertebra, vertebral
stern-, sterno-	sternum, sternal, chest
tars-, tarso-	tarsus, tarsal
tibio-	tibia, tibial
vertebr-, vertebro-	vertebrae, vertebral

WORD ETYMOLOGY

Some words have Greek or Latin roots but are not true word parts. This section lists those that are used as medical terms.

Word	Definition
carpus	wrist
cribrum	sieve
dactyl	finger or toe
femur	thigh
malakia	softness
physis	growth
tibia	shinbone

MEDICAL TERM PARTS USED AS PREFIXES

Prefix	Definition
ethmo-	ethmoid
femoro-	femur, femoral
hyo-	U-shaped
peroneo-	peroneal, peroneus
pubo-	pubis, pubic, pubes
tibio-	tibia, tibial

MEDICAL TERM PARTS USED AS SUFFIXES

Suffix	Definition
-blast	immature precursor cell
-clast	something that breaks; to break
-genesis	development

WORD GROUPING

Using the "Medical Term Parts" tables, identify the prefix, suffix, or combining form for each of the following definitions. The first one has been done as an example.

Definition	Word Part
tibia, tibial	tibio-
bone	A.
	B.
calcaneus	

Definition	Word Part
calcium	
carpus (wrist), carpal	
cartilage, cartilaginous	
coccyx; tailbone	
condyle	
cranium, cranial	
development	
ethmoid	
femur, femoral	
ilium, iliac	
immature precursor cell	
mandible, mandibular	
marrow	
meatus	
pelvis	
peroneal, peroneus	
pubis, pubic, pubes	
rib, costal	
scapula, scapular	
something that breaks; to break	
sternum, sternal, chest	
straight	
tarsus, tarsal	
U-shaped	
vertebra, vertebral	A.
	B.

WORD BUILDING

Word parts introduced in the "Medical Term Parts" section are listed in the following table. For this exercise, first supply the meaning of each word part, then use the word part to build a word you already know. The word you list under "Common or Known Word" does not have to be a medical term; a commonly used word is fine. Be sure, however, that the word correctly reflects the meaning. The first one has been done as an example. Check your answers in a dictionary.

Word Part	Meaning	Common or Known Word	Example Medical Term
-genesis	development	histogenesis	osteogenesis
calc-, calci-, calco-			calcium

Word Part	Meaning	Common or Known Word	Example Medical Term
carp-, carpo-			carpal tunnel syndrome
crani-, cranio-			cranial cavity
orth-, ortho-			orthopedics
osseo-, ossi-			ossification
ost-, oste-, osteo-			osteoblast
vertebr-, vertebro-			vertebral column

ANATOMY AND PHYSIOLOGY

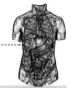

Structures of the Skeletal System

> **FACT** Square inch per square inch, bone is five times stronger than steel!

- Bones of the appendicular skeleton: 126.
- Bones of the axial skeleton: 80.
- Bone cells: osteoblasts, osteoclasts, and osteocytes.
- Cartilage: elastic cartilage, fibrocartilage, and hyaline cartilage.

Skeletal System Preview

The skeletal system is involved with the movement of the body because it provides attachment sites for muscles. It further serves a protective function by enclosing vital organs. Anatomic structures of physiological importance are those associated with bone formation, bone resorption, and blood cell production. In this chapter, the bones of the axial and appendicular skeletons are introduced, and terminology used to describe bone morphology and surface markings is identified. Various types of cartilage important to skeletal tissue are also described.

Numerous structures of the skeletal system are known by eponyms or other common names. Such terms are in regular use in the medical fields.

Bone Anatomy

One way bones can be classified is according to their morphology (shape). **Long bones,** such as those of the arms and legs, have longitudinal axes and expanded ends. The **short bones** of the wrists and ankles are somewhat cube-like, with lengths and widths roughly equal. Ribs, scapulae, and bones of the skull are known as **flat bones,** which are characterized by their plate-like structure and broad surfaces. The **irregular bones** of the vertebrae and face have a variety of shapes and are often connected to several other bones. Round bones, or **sesamoid bones,** such as the patella (kneecap) are small and develop in a joint capsule, where tendons undergo compression. The word *sesamoid* comes from the Greek language and means "shaped like a sesame seed," whereas the term *patella* is a Latin word that means "small, flat dish."

After birth, the skull bones undergo complete closure. During that time, small, irregularly shaped bony sections called **sutural bones,** or **wormian bones,** develop between the cranial bone sutures. A **suture** is the bond formed by fibrous connective tissue between adult skull bones that creates an immovable joint. Wormian bones are generally no larger than the size of a quarter and their edges have the appearance of a jigsaw-puzzle piece. Different types of bones are shown in Figure 5-1.

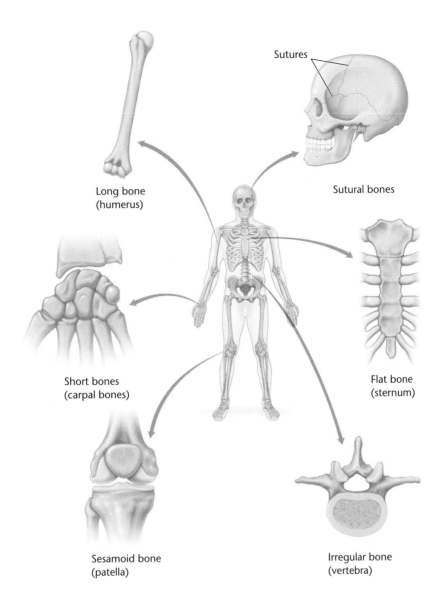

Long bone
(humerus)

Sutures

Sutural bones

Short bones
(carpal bones)

Flat bone
(sternum)

Sesamoid bone
(patella)

Irregular bone
(vertebra)

FIGURE 5-1
Classification of
bones.

The major parts of a typical long bone are proximal epiphysis, diaphysis, distal epiphysis, medullary cavity, periosteum, and articular cartilage (Fig. 5-2). (A medullary cavity and periosteum are also found in other bones.) The proximal **epiphysis** is the expanded end portion of the bone closer to the body's trunk. The shaft of a long bone, providing strong support, is referred to as the **diaphysis.** The distal epiphysis is the expanded end portion of bone farther from the trunk, or the origin (point closest to attachment). The epiphyses cap the ends of long bones, consist of spongy bone surrounded by compact bone, contain red bone marrow, provide attachment for muscles, and serve as the contact point at joints.

The narrow region between the diaphysis and the epiphysis is the **metaphysis.** Bone growth occurs in this region, which is also called the epiphyseal disk, epiphyseal plate, or growth plate. The cavity within the diaphysis of a long bone that is occupied by marrow is called the **medullary (marrow) cavity.** Lining this cavity is a membrane called the **endosteum.** The **periosteum** is the of fibrous connective tissue that encases the surface of a bone. This membrane covers the bone except where tendons and ligaments attach; instead of periosteum, the articular surfaces of bone are protected by articular cartilage.

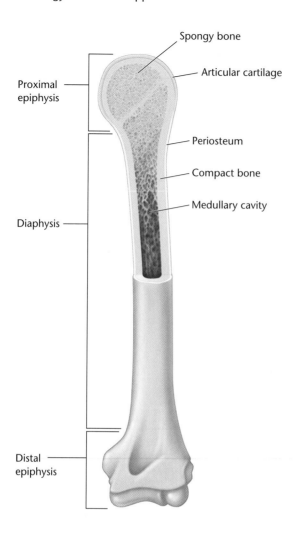

Spongy bone

Articular cartilage

Proximal epiphysis

Periosteum

Compact bone

Medullary cavity

Diaphysis

Distal epiphysis

FIGURE 5-2
Major parts of a long bone.

Articular means pertaining to an articulation, or joint. Articular cartilage covers the ends of bones at synovial joints to facilitate movement and cushion impact. **Synovial joints** are freely movable articulations.

Based on tissue characteristics, two types of bone exist: spongy and compact (Fig. 5-3). **Spongy bone**, also called cancellous or trabecular bone, consists of a network of

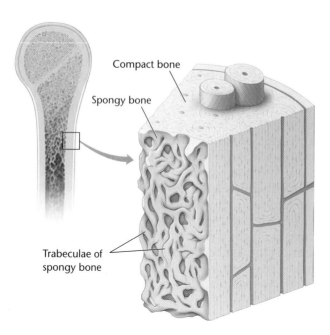

Compact bone

Spongy bone

Trabeculae of spongy bone

FIGURE 5-3
Spongy and compact bone.

struts and plates called **trabeculae.** The branching, lattice-looking trabeculae separate irregular spaces within the spongy portion. These spaces between the plates help reduce the weight of the bone and provide strength. Epiphyses are composed largely of spongy bone with thin layers of compact bone on the surface. Solid, strong **compact** (or dense) **bone** is found on the bone surface. The walls of diaphyses are composed of this tightly packed tissue.

> **FACT** Tooth enamel is the hardest substance in the body; compact bone is the second hardest!

Key Terms	Definitions
long bones	bones found in arms and legs
short bones	bones found in wrists and ankles
flat bones	bones found in ribs, scapulae, and skulls
irregular bones	bones found in vertebrae and faces
sesamoid (SES uh moid) **bones**	small bones that develop in tendons passing over joints that withstand stress
sutural (SUE chur ul) **bones**	irregularly shaped bones between the flat bones of the skull and outlined by sutures
wormian (WUR mee un) **bones**	sutural bones
suture	line of union between two bones
epiphysis (e PIF i sis)	expanded end of a long bone
diaphysis (dye AF i sis)	shaft of a long bone
metaphysis (me TAF i sis)	growing end of a diaphysis
medullary (MED yoo lerr ee) **cavity**	central canal of a long bone
endosteum (en DOS tee um)	membrane lining the medullary cavity in bone
periosteum (perr ee OS tee um)	fibrous membrane covering a bone
articular (ahr TICK yoo lur) **surface**	point where a bone meets another bone; joint surface
synovial (si NOH vee ul) **joints**	freely movable joints
spongy bone	cancellous bone
trabeculae (tra BECK yoo lee)	slender columns of bone in cancellous bone
compact bone	solid bone tissue

Key Term Practice: Bone Anatomy

1. What are the six classes of bone?

   a. _____

   b. _____

   c. _____

   d. _____

   e. _____

   f. _____

2. The term *periosteum* literally means _____.

3. What is the plural form for each given term?

   a. epiphysis = _____

   b. diaphysis = _____

4. What is the alternate term for *spongy bone?*

   _____

5. What is the alternate term for *compact bone?*

   _____

6. What is the singular form of *trabeculae?*

   _____

Bone Marrow, Blood, and Cartilage

Red marrow and yellow marrow are found in bone. **Red bone marrow** is blood cell–forming tissue located in spaces (**interstices**) of spongy bone and within the medullary cavities of long bones. It functions in hemopoiesis, the formation of red blood cells (erythrocytes), certain white blood cells (leukocytes), and blood platelets (thrombocytes). The marrow is called "red" because of the hemoglobin (the oxygen-carrying pigment) contained within red blood cells. Oxygen-saturated blood cells have a reddish hue.

Yellow bone marrow functions as fat-storage tissue, hence its characteristic color. It is found in cavities within certain bones. It is inactive in blood cell production; however, in times of need, it can convert to red bone marrow to manufacture erythrocytes.

Cartilage is nonvascular connective tissue. Its matrix is different from bone tissue. Cells that form cartilage are called **chondrocytes**; they lay down cartilage by dividing and forming more cells and by secreting matrix.

Three types of cartilage are found in humans: fibrocartilage, elastic cartilage, and hyaline cartilage. **Fibrocartilage** is the strongest form and is found in vertebral disks separating vertebrae. The external ear is made of flexible **elastic cartilage**. **Hyaline cartilage** is the most abundant type and serves as the precursor to bone. It is also found covering the ends of long bones and at articular surfaces.

Key Terms	Definitions
red bone marrow	blood-forming tissue in some bone
interstices (in TUR sti siz)	spaces
yellow bone marrow	fat-storage tissue in some bone
cartilage (KAHR ti lij)	nonvascular connective tissue; gristle
chondrocytes (KON droh sites)	cartilage cell

fibrocartilage (figh broh KAHR ti lij)	dense, fibrous connective tissue with masses of cartilage between fibers
elastic cartilage	flexible cartilage containing the protein elastin
hyaline (HIGH uh lin) cartilage	precursor to bone and found on articular surfaces

Key Term Practice: Bone Marrow, Blood, and Cartilage

1. Identify the region in bone where hemopoiesis occurs.

   _____

2. _____ is another term for spaces in cancellous bone.

3. What is the medical term for a cartilage cell?

   _____

4. Identify the three types of cartilage found in the human body.

   a. _____

   b. _____

   c. _____

Bone Development and Remodeling

The process by which bone forms is called **osteogenesis.** Osteogenesis begins during the 6th week of embryonic development, when the germ layers differentiate and mesenchymal cells transform into osteoblasts. Some cells form **intramembranous bone,** which develops from membrane-like layers of primitive connective tissue. Intramembranous bones are the broad, flat skull bones. Other cells form endochondral bone. **Endochondral bones** begin as hyaline cartilage, which is subsequently replaced by bone tissue. Most of the bones of the skeleton are endochondral bones. Osteogenesis occurs through the combined actions of osteoblasts, which build bone, and osteoclasts, which destroy bone. Bone formation is a continuous lifelong process.

A normal physiological process is bone remodeling, in which old bone is destroyed and new bone is formed. The two major types of bone cells responsible for this action are osteoblasts and osteoclasts. **Osteoblasts** are bone-forming cells. They accomplish this task by depositing a bony matrix around themselves. **Osteoclasts** are bone-destroying cells. These cells cause the erosion of bone by breaking it down and resorbing it. Osteoclasts secrete acids, which dissolve the inorganic components of the bone matrix, and lysosomal enzymes, which digest the organic components. Mature bone cells isolated in lacunae, or hollow cavities, are referred to as **osteocytes.** Regulation of bone mass is accomplished by the dual action of osteoclasts and osteoblasts.

The **epiphyseal plate,** a hyaline cartilaginous layer within the epiphysis of a long bone, serves as a growing region. As noted earlier, this structure is also called the epiphyseal disk, metaphysis, and growth plate. The cartilaginous cells of an epiphyseal plate are arranged in four layers, each of which may be several cells thick. The first layer consists of resting cells that anchor the disk to the epiphyseal bony tissue. The second layer consists of cells undergoing mitosis. The third layer is composed of older cells that are enlarging and becoming calcified. Dead cells and calcified intercellular substance make up the fourth layer. This layering process leads to an increase in bone

Mexican Lucia Zarate was the smallest woman in the world at 66 cm (26 inches) and 2.1 kg (4.7 pounds)!

length referred to as **appositional growth.** Long bone growth occurs at the epiphyseal plates. After long bone growth has stopped, a remnant of the plate, the **epiphyseal line,** is evident.

Diametric (thickening or widening) **growth** of bone results from the deposition of compact bone by intramembranous ossification occurring on the outside, just beneath the periosteum. Periosteal osteoblasts add new bone to the region to create a bone-widening effect. As compact bone is forming on the surface, other bone tissue is being eroded away on the inside. This action creates the space for the medullary cavity in the diaphysis, which is filled with marrow. Bone growth is similar to tree growth in that growth is upward, downward, and outward.

Throughout life, osteoclasts are being stimulated to resorb bone tissue at specific sites, and osteoblasts are being activated to replace the bone. This process of resorption and replacement, called **bone remodeling,** is a well-regulated balancing act and is a classic example of a homeostatic mechanism. Remodeling occurs throughout life as a means of maintaining bone tissue.

Vitamins play a pivotal role in bone maintenance. For example, vitamin D is necessary for proper absorption of calcium in the small intestine. The mineral **calcium** is needed to ensure bone strength. In cases of vitamin D deficiency, calcium is poorly absorbed, and thus the inorganic salt portion of bone matrix is deficient in calcium, resulting in deformed bones. Vitamin A is necessary for the bone resorption that occurs during normal development. Vitamin A deficiency may result in retardation of bone development. Vitamin C (ascorbic acid) is necessary for the synthesis of collagen, a substance of bone. Humans and guinea pigs are the only mammals incapable of synthesizing vitamin C; thus it must be obtained from the diet.

Under the direction of hormones, bone mineralization and resorption occur. Hormones are chemical messengers critical to many processes in the body, including bone development. Through hormonal actions, bones will either store calcium or release it into the blood; thus blood calcium concentration is also regulated by bone activity. When blood calcium is low, osteoclasts are stimulated to break down bone tissue, releasing calcium salts from the intercellular matrix into the bloodstream. When circulating blood calcium is high, osteoclast activity is inhibited, and osteoblasts are stimulated to form bone tissue. Excessive calcium is stored in the matrix. This explains why a blood test cannot determine the calcium concentration in bone tissue. Three anomalous substances stored in bone are lead, radium, and strontium. This results when these elements are accidentally ingested.

Thyroid hormone (TH) is important to the **ossification** (bone formation) process. Thyroid hormone causes cartilage in the epiphyseal disks of long bones to be replaced by bone tissue. Excessive TH halts bone growth by causing premature ossification of the disks. On the other hand, TH deficiency may also produce stunted growth; without the normal effect of TH, the pituitary gland fails to secrete enough of another crucial hormone called growth hormone (GH).

Sex hormones, too, play a role in bone development. The hormones promote the formation of bone tissue and stimulate ossification of the epiphyseal plates, thereby causing bones to stop growing. The effect of estrogens is stronger than that of androgens (male sex hormones); hence females typically reach their maximum heights earlier than males.

Physical exercise affects bone structure. When skeletal muscles contract, they pull at their attachments on bones, thus stimulating the bone tissue to thicken and strengthen in what is commonly known as bone **hypertrophy.** Lack of exercise causes bone tissue to waste away; therefore, bones become thinner and weaker or **atrophy.**

FACT *An American, Robert Wadlow, was the tallest man in the world at 8 feet 11 inches (2.72 meters) and 439 pounds (199.13 kg)!*

Key Terms	Definitions
osteogenesis (os tee oh JEN e sis)	development of bony tissue
intramembranous (in truh MEM bruh nus) **bone**	bone formed from connective tissue that is not cartilage

endochondral (en doh KON drul) **bones**	bones formed in which bone tissue replaces cartilage
osteoblasts (OS tee oh blasts)	bone-forming cells
osteoclasts (OS tee oh klasts)	bone-destroying cells
osteocytes (OS tee oh sites)	bone cells
epiphyseal (ep i FIZ ee ul) **plate**	site of bone growth in length
appositional (ap oh ZISH un ul) **growth**	addition of successive layers of bone tissue
epiphyseal (ep i FIZ ee ul) **line**	mark left at the site of the epiphyseal plate after the bone has stopped growing
diametric (dye uh MET rick) **growth**	thickening around the bone's axis
bone remodeling	process of breaking down and building up bone tissue
calcium	mineral essential to bone formation
ossification (os i fi KAY shun)	conversion of cartilage tissue into bone
hypertrophy (high PUR truh fee)	an increase in size
atrophy (AT ruh fee)	a reduction in size

Key Term Practice: Bone Development and Remodeling

1. Identify the two types of bone development.

   _____

2. _____ is the term for bone formation.

3. Mature bone cells are called _____.

4. Bone-forming cells are termed _____, and bone-destroying cells are known as _____.

5. The anatomic term for the growth plate is _____.

6. Bone lengthening is termed _____ growth.

7. Which mineral is necessary for bone formation?

   _____

8. Conversion of cartilage tissue into bone is termed _____.

9. What term means the opposite of *hypertrophy*.

   _____

Axial Skeleton

The two divisions of the skeletal system are the axial and appendicular. The axial skeleton is made up of 80 bones arranged along the longitudinal axis. The **axial** skeleton supports the head, neck, and trunk and their associated organs (Fig. 5-4). The

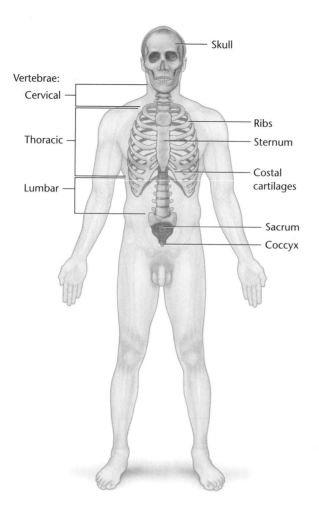

Vertebrae:
Cervical
Thoracic
Lumbar

Skull
Ribs
Sternum
Costal cartilages
Sacrum
Coccyx

FIGURE 5-4
The axial skeleton.

skull, middle ear bones (auditory ossicles), hyoid bone, vertebral column, thoracic cage, sacrum, and coccyx make up the axial portion of the human skeleton.

The 8 bones of the cranium include the **frontal,** two **parietal,** one **occipital,** two **temporal,** the **sphenoid,** and the **ethmoid.** Two bones each of the **maxilla, palatine, zygomatic, lacrimal, nasal, inferior nasal concha (turbinate),** one **vomer,** and one **mandible** bone make up the 14 facial bones. The bones of the skull are shown in Figure 5-5.

Special skull features include fontanelles, sutures, and sinuses. **Fontanelles** (sometimes spelled fontanels) are six membranous regions located between certain cranial bones in the skull of a fetus or infant (Fig. 5-6). They are not ossified at birth. Their purpose is to permit movement between bones so that the developing skull can change size and shape to allow for brain growth and to enable the head to pass easily through the birth canal during parturition (childbirth). The immovable joints that result from fontanelle ossification are termed sutures. The sutures of the adult skull are the coronal, sagittal, lambdoid, and squamous.

Sinuses are mucous membrane–lined spaces within the frontal, sphenoid, ethmoid, and maxilla bones (Fig. 5-7). They lessen the weight of the skull and provide an area of mucous epithelium to the nasal cavity.

The U-shaped **hyoid bone** is unique because it is the only bone in the body that does not articulate with any other bone (Fig. 5-8). It supports the tongue and provides attachment for some muscles. The bone is also known as the "neck bone" in lay terms.

The vertebral column, sternum, and ribs constitute the skeleton of the trunk. Vertebrae serve primarily to support the head and trunk and protect the spinal cord. The typical vertebra has a drum-shaped body, called a **centrum,** which forms the thick

Lateral view

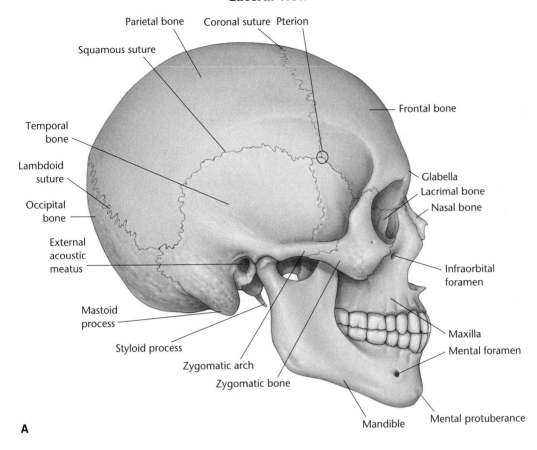

Parietal bone
Squamous suture
Temporal bone
Lambdoid suture
Occipital bone
External acoustic meatus
Mastoid process
Styloid process
Zygomatic arch
Zygomatic bone

Coronal suture Pterion
Frontal bone
Glabella
Lacrimal bone
Nasal bone
Infraorbital foramen
Maxilla
Mental foramen
Mandible Mental protuberance

A

Posterior view

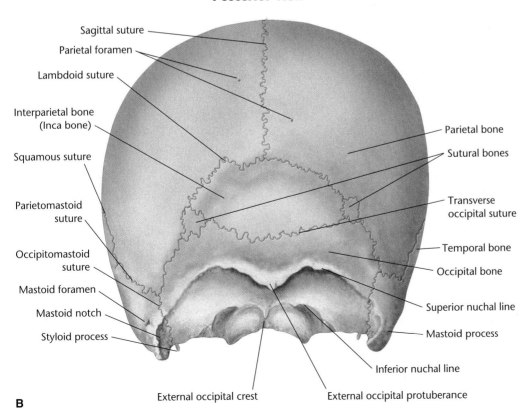

Sagittal suture
Parietal foramen
Lambdoid suture
Interparietal bone (Inca bone)
Squamous suture
Parietomastoid suture
Occipitomastoid suture
Mastoid foramen
Mastoid notch
Styloid process

Parietal bone
Sutural bones
Transverse occipital suture
Temporal bone
Occipital bone
Superior nuchal line
Mastoid process
Inferior nuchal line

External occipital crest External occipital protuberance

B

FIGURE 5-5
The skull bones.
Special skull features
include fontanelles,
sutures, and sinuses.
(Images provided by
Anatomical Chart
Co.)

Superior view

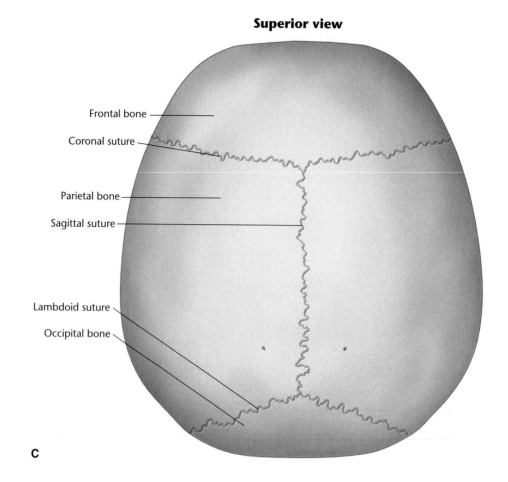

Frontal bone

Coronal suture

Parietal bone

Sagittal suture

Lambdoid suture

Occipital bone

FIGURE 5-5
(Continued)   **C**

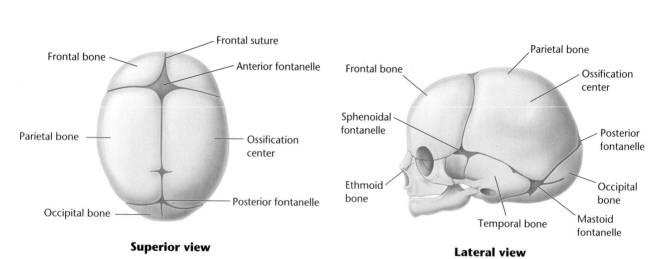

Frontal suture

Frontal bone

Anterior fontanelle

Parietal bone

Ossification center

Occipital bone

Posterior fontanelle

Superior view

Parietal bone

Frontal bone

Ossification center

Sphenoidal fontanelle

Posterior fontanelle

Ethmoid bone

Occipital bone

Temporal bone

Mastoid fontanelle

Lateral view

FIGURE 5-6
Fontanelles are six membranous regions located between certain cranial bones in the skull of a fetus or infant.

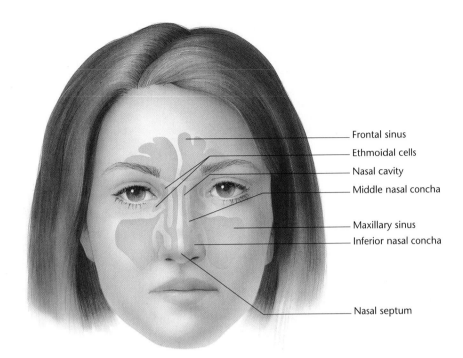

FIGURE 5-7
The paranasal sinuses.
(Image provided by
Anatomical Chart Co.)

- Frontal sinus
- Ethmoidal cells
- Nasal cavity
- Middle nasal concha
- Maxillary sinus
- Inferior nasal concha
- Nasal septum

anterior portion (Fig. 5-9). Projecting posteriorly are two short stalks called **pedicles**, which form sides of the **vertebral foramen.** The spinal cord passes through this hole. Two plates form each **lamina;** the laminae arise from the pedicles and fuse in the back to become the **spinous process.** The **transverse processes** extend laterally from the centrum. Pedicles, laminae, and a spinous process complete the bony vertebral arch around the vertebral foramen, through which the spinal cord passes. Vertebrae have different shapes and sizes along the vertebral column.

Bones of the vertebral column are cervical, thoracic, and lumbar vertebrae, along with the sacrum and coccyx. The 7 vertebrae closest to the head are the cervical

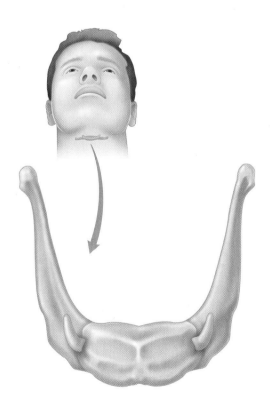

FIGURE 5-8
The U-shaped hyoid
bone.

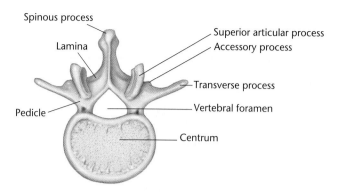

Spinous process

Lamina

Superior articular process

Accessory process

Transverse process

Vertebral foramen

Pedicle

Centrum

Superior view

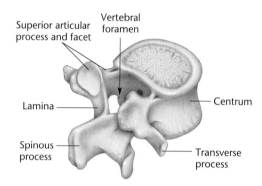

Superior articular process and facet

Vertebral foramen

Lamina

Centrum

Spinous process

Transverse process

Posterolateral oblique view

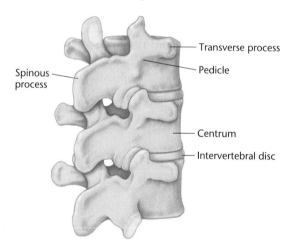

Transverse process

Pedicle

Spinous process

Centrum

Intervertebral disc

Posterolateral view

FIGURE 5-9
Typical vertebra structure. (Top and middle images provided by Anatomical Chart Co.)

vertebrae. They make up the bony axis of the neck, are the smallest vertebrae, yet have the densest bone tissue. They are designated by the letter C and are numbered C1–C7. The first cervical vertebra (C1) is called the atlas and allows the head nod. The second cervical vertebra (C2) is the axis, which enables the head to rotate.

The 12 thoracic (T) vertebrae are larger than the cervical and are adapted to withstand stress. They are designated by the letter *T* and numbered T1–T12. The superior 10 thoracic vertebrae articulate with the ribs; the remaining 2 are attached to the back muscles posteriorly.

The 5 lumbar vertebrae are adapted to support weight. They are designated by the letter *L* and are numbered L1–L5. To help you remember the number of vertebrae in each division from superior to inferior, think about the times of the day when you eat: breakfast at 7, lunch at 12, and dinner at 5.

The sacrum is made up of 5 fused vertebrae that serve as the attachment for the pelvic girdle. The coccyx is made up of 3–5 fused vertebrae. The shape of the sacrum and coccyx forms the pelvic curve. The **sacrum** is wedged between the coxal bones of the pelvis and is united to them at its articular surfaces by fibrocartilage of the sacroiliac joint, the point where the sacrum and ilium join. The **sacral promontory** is the upper anterior margin of the sacrum, which represents the body of the first sacral vertebra. An opening at the inferior tip of the sacral canal is the **sacral hiatus.** The structure of the sacrum and coccyx can be seen in Figure 5-10.

A normal vertebral column has primary and secondary curves that give strength, support, and assistance with balance. Primary curves occur along the thoracic and sacral regions, whereas secondary curves are found in the cervical and lumbar regions. A typical spine is convex through the thoracic region and concave through the cervical and lumbar regions (Fig. 5-11).

The thoracic cage is made up of 24 ribs (12 pairs) and their associated costal cartilages, the thoracic vertebrae, and the sternum (Fig. 5-12). The thoracic skeleton protects the vital chest organs. Superiorly to inferiorly, the sternum is divided into three segments: manubrium, body, and xiphoid process. The 7 pairs of ribs that articulate with the sternum and vertebrae are called true ribs or **vertebrosternal ribs.** The remaining 5 pairs of ribs are called false ribs because they do not directly attach to the sternum. The **vertebrochondral ribs** are pairs 8–10, which articulate with vertebrae and the sternum via the costal cartilage of the last true rib. The floating ribs, pairs 11 and 12, are the **vertebral ribs,** which articulate with the thoracic vertebrae and posterior muscles but not the sternum. The anatomic names aid in identifying the location of each type of rib.

Key Terms	Definitions
axial (ACK see ul)	pertaining to the head, neck, and trunk
frontal (FRUN tul)	forehead bone
parietal (pur RYE e tul) **bones**	superior lateral skull bones
occipital (ock SIP i tul)	back head bone
temporal (TEM puh rul) **bones**	lateral skull bones
sphenoid (SFEE noid)	butterfly-shaped skull bone
ethmoid (ETH moid)	skull bone between sphenoid and nasal bones
maxillae (mack SIL ee)	upper jaw bones
palatine (PAL uh tine) **bones**	L-shaped facial bones
zygomatic (zye goh MAT ick) **bones**	cheek bones
lacrimal (LACK ri mul) **bones**	fingernail-shaped facial bones
nasal (NAY zul)	bones of the nose
inferior nasal conchae (KONG kee)	curved nasal cavity bones
turbinates (TUR bin ates)	conchae
vomer (VOH mur)	thin, vertically positioned bone forming a portion of the septum
mandible (MAN di bul)	lower jawbone
fontanelles (fon tuh NELZ)	membranous space between cranial bones
sinuses	cavity or hollow space in bones
hyoid (HIGH oid) **bone**	bone between the tongue root and larynx (voice box)
centrum (SEN trum)	center of a vertebra

Posterior view

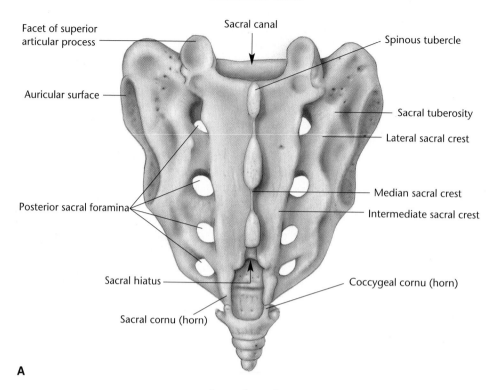

Facet of superior articular process

Auricular surface

Posterior sacral foramina

Sacral hiatus

Sacral cornu (horn)

Sacral canal

Spinous tubercle

Sacral tuberosity

Lateral sacral crest

Median sacral crest

Intermediate sacral crest

Coccygeal cornu (horn)

A

Anterior view

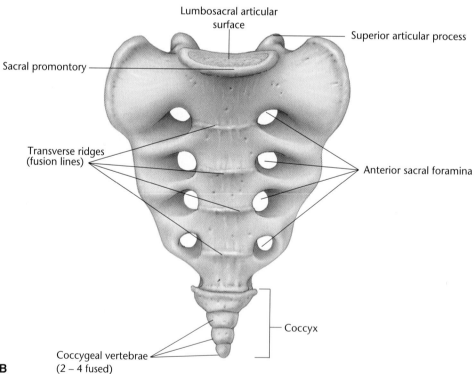

Lumbosacral articular surface

Sacral promontory

Superior articular process

Transverse ridges (fusion lines)

Anterior sacral foramina

Coccyx

Coccygeal vertebrae (2 – 4 fused)

B

FIGURE 5-10
The sacrum. (Images provided by Anatomical Chart Co.)

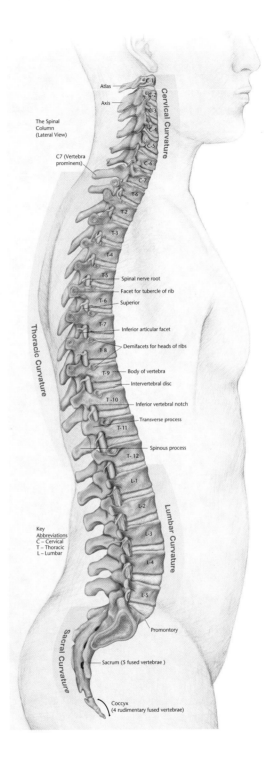

The Spinal Column (Lateral View)

Atlas

Axis

C7 (Vertebra prominens)

Cervical Curvature

C-1
C-2
C-3
C-4
C-5
C-6
C-7

T-6
T-2
T-3
T-4
T-5

Thoracic Curvature

Spinal nerve root
Facet for tubercle of rib
Superior
Inferior articular facet
Demifacets for heads of ribs
Body of vertebra
Intervertebral disc
Inferior vertebral notch
Transverse process
Spinous process

T-6
T-7
T-8
T-9
T-10
T-11
T-12

L-1
L-2
L-3
L-4
L-5

Lumbar Curvature

Key
Abbreviations
C – Cervical
T – Thoracic
L – Lumbar

Promontory

Sacral Curvature

Sacrum (5 fused vertebrae)

Coccyx
(4 rudimentary fused vertebrae)

FIGURE 5-11
The normal spinal column. (Image provided by Anatomical Chart Co.)

Anterior view

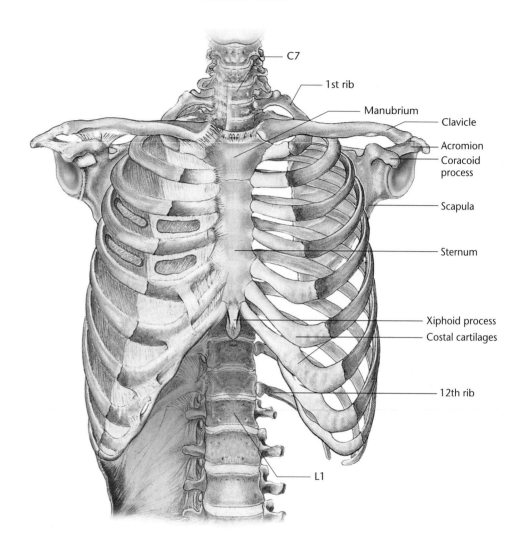

FIGURE 5-12
The thoracic cage.
(Images provided by
Anatomical Chart Co.)

A

pedicles (PED i kuls)	narrow connection between two vertebral structures
vertebral foramen (VUR te brul foh RAY mun)	opening through which spinal cord passes
lamina (LAM i nuh)	thin plate on vertebra
spinous (SPYE nus) **process**	spine-like projection on vertebra
transverse (trans VERCE) **processes**	crosswise projections on vertebra
sacrum (SAY krum)	curved, triangular bone between last lumbar vertebra and coccyx
sacral promontory (SAY krul PROM un to ree)	projection on the sacrum
sacral hiatus (SAY krul high AY tus)	opening in the sacrum
vertebrosternal (VUR te bruh STER nul) **ribs**	rib pairs 1–7; true ribs
vertebrochondral (VUR te bruh KON drul) **ribs**	rib pairs 8–10; false ribs
vertebral (VUR te brul) **ribs**	rib pairs 11 and 12; floating ribs

Posterior view

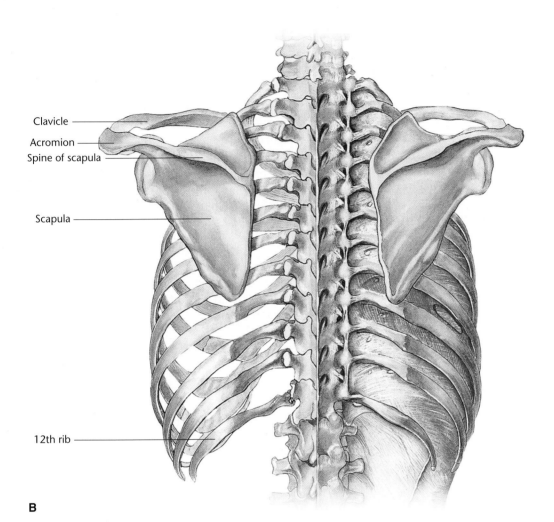

Clavicle

Acromion

Spine of scapula

Scapula

12th rib

FIGURE 5-12
(Continued)

B

Key Term Practice: Axial Skeleton

1. Identify the two divisions of the human skeleton.

   _____

2. Give the medical term for each of the following descriptions.

   a. true ribs _____

   b. rib pairs 8–10 _____

   c. floating ribs _____

3. What is the singular form of each given term?

   a. conchae = _____

   b. maxillae = _____

   c. vertebral foramina = _____

Appendicular Skeleton

Bones that anchor the limbs to the axial skeleton and the bones of the limbs (appendages) make up the **appendicular** skeleton (Fig. 5-13). Appendicular means pertaining to the arms and legs, or appendages. The pectoral girdle, upper limbs, pelvic girdle, and lower limbs are made up of 126 bones. The two primary girdles are the pectoral and pelvic. The two **scapulae** (singular = scapula) and two **clavicles** constitute the pectoral (shoulder) girdle, and the two coxal bones make up the pelvic (hip) girdle.

Each coxal bone of the pelvic girdle consists of three fused components: the **ilium**, **pubis**, and **ischium** (Fig. 5-14). Differences exist between male and female pelves (Fig. 5-15). Female pelvic bones are lighter, thinner, and have less obvious muscular attachment points than their male counterparts. The obturator foramina and the acetabula are smaller and farther apart than those of a male. The **obturator foramen** is a large opening formed by the ischium and pubic bones through which nerves and vessels pass. The **acetabulum** is a cup-like socket where the femur attaches to the hip. The female pelvic cavity is wider in all diameters, and is shorter, roomier, and less funnel shaped than the male pelvic cavity. The distances between the ischial spines and between the ischial tuberosities are greater than in a male. These anatomic differences exist to accommodate childbirth.

The two upper limbs provide muscle attachment points and are adapted for movement. Each upper arm has a **humerus**, and each forearm contains a **radius** and an **ulna**. There are 8 **carpal bones** in each wrist, and 5 **metacarpal bones** and 14 **phalanges** (which make up the fingers) in each hand. The bones of both fingers and

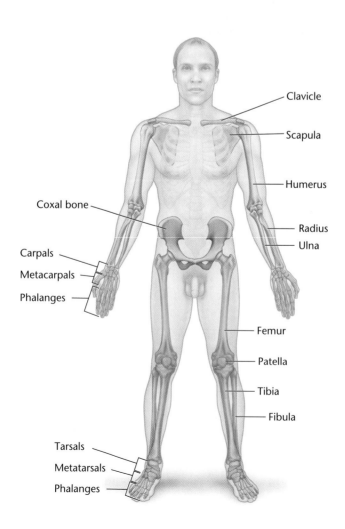

FIGURE 5-13
The appendicular skeleton.

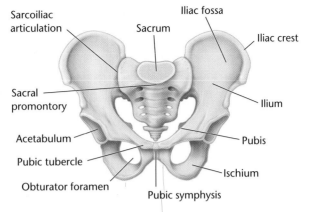

Anterior view

Sarcoiliac articulation
Sacrum
Iliac fossa
Iliac crest
Sacral promontory
Ilium
Acetabulum
Pubis
Pubic tubercle
Obturator foramen
Ischium
Pubic symphysis

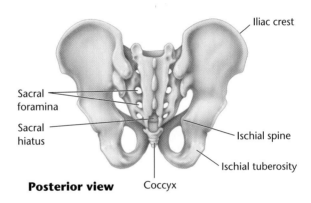

Posterior view

Iliac crest
Sacral foramina
Sacral hiatus
Ischial spine
Ischial tuberosity
Coccyx

FIGURE 5-14
The pelvic girdle consists of three fused components: ilium, pubis, and ischium.

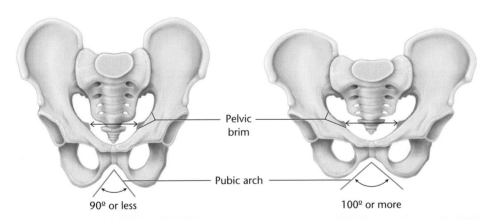

Pelvic brim
Pubic arch
90º or less
100º or more

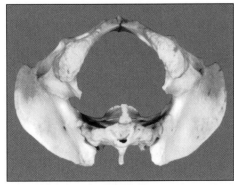

Male

Female

FIGURE 5-15
The male and female pelves. The anatomic differences exist to accommodate childbirth. (Reprinted with permission from Moore KL, Dalley AF II. Clinically oriented anatomy, 4th ed. Baltimore: Lippincott Williams & Wilkins 1999.)

Dorsal view

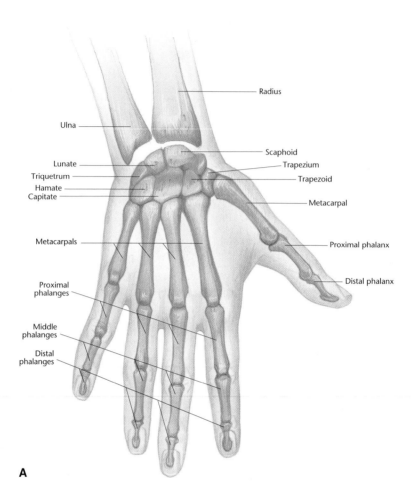

Radius

Ulna

Lunate
Triquetrum
Hamate
Capitate

Scaphoid
Trapezium
Trapezoid

Metacarpal

Metacarpals

Proximal phalanx

Distal phalanx

Proximal
phalanges

Middle
phalanges

Distal
phalanges

FIGURE 5-16
(A–B). Wrist and hand bones. (Images provided by Anatomical Chart Co.)

A

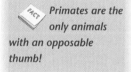

Primates are the only animals with an opposable thumb!

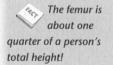

The femur is about one quarter of a person's total height!

toes are referred to as phalanges (singular = phalanx). Phalanx parts are labeled proximal, middle, and distal. The 8 carpal bones are the **scaphoid, lunate, triquetrum, pisiform, trapezium, trapezoid, capitate,** and **hamate** (Fig. 5-16).

The lower extremities function in body support, locomotion, and muscle attachment. The proximal portion of each lower limb has a **femur**, at the knee joint is the **patella**, and the distal portion of the lower limb is made up of the **tibia** and **fibula.** To help you remember the difference between the tibia and the fibula, keep in mind that the *fib*ula is *small*er than the tibia: "to tell a small lie is to fib." The femur is more commonly known as the thigh bone, the patella is the kneecap, and the tibia is the shinbone. Each ankle is made up of 7 **tarsal bones**, and each foot contains 10 **metatarsal bones** and 14 bones that make up the toes (Fig. 5-17). The 7 tarsal bones are the **talus; calcaneus; navicular; cuboid;** and medial, intermediate, and lateral **cuneiform bones.** The toes and fingers are numbered, medially to laterally, I, II, III, IV, and V.

Key Terms	Definitions
appendicular (ap en DICK yoo lur)	pertaining to arms and legs
scapulae (SKAP yoo lee)	triangular bones of the back; shoulder blades
clavicles (KLAV i kuls)	collar bones

Palmar view

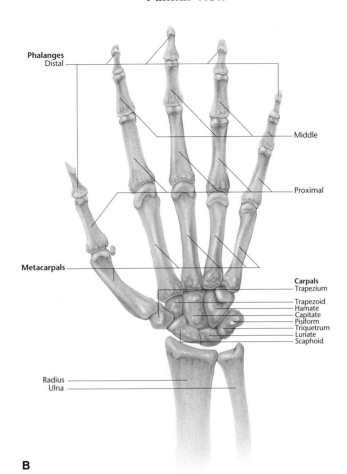

Phalanges
Distal

Middle

Proximal

Metacarpals

Carpals
Trapezium
Trapezoid
Hamate
Capitate
Pisiform
Triquetrum
Lunate
Scaphoid

Radius
Ulna

B

FIGURE 5-16
(Continued)

ilium (IL ee um)	superior broad part of the hip bone
pubis (PEW bis)	front part of the hip bone, forming anterior pelvis
ischium (IS kee um)	inferior part of the hip bone
obturator foramen (OB tew ray tur foh RAY mun)	oval opening between the ischium and pubis
acetabulum (as e TAB yoo lum)	cup-shaped depression on outer hip bone surface for insertion of femur head
humerus (HEW mur us)	upper arm bone
radius (RAY dee us)	outer forearm bone
ulna (UL nuh)	inner forearm bone
carpal (KAHR pul) **bones**	wrist or carpus bones
metacarpal (met uh KAHR pul) **bones**	bones of the hand between the wrist and fingers
phalanges (fa LAN jeez)	bones of the fingers and toes
scaphoid (SKAF oid)	boat-shaped carpal bone
lunate (LEW nate)	a carpal bone

Frontal view

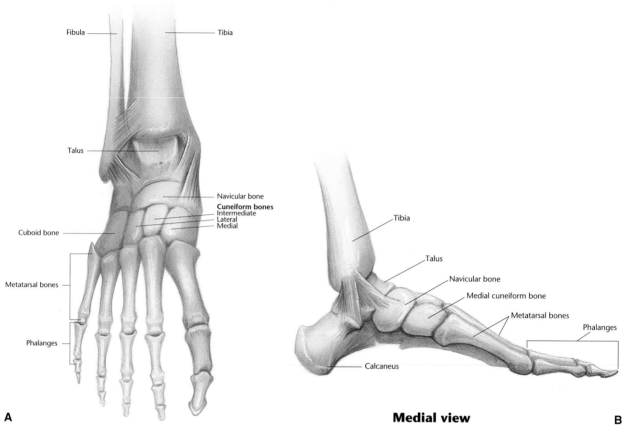

FIGURE 5-17
Ankle and foot bones. (Images provided by Anatomical Chart Co.)

triquetrum (trye KWET rum)	third proximal carpal bone
pisiform (PYE si form)	small, pea-shaped carpal bone
trapezium (tra PEE zee um)	first distal carpal bone
trapezoid (TRAP e zoid)	second distal carpal bone
capitate (KAP i tate)	largest carpal bone
hamate (HAY mate)	hook-shaped carpal bone
femur (FEE mur)	thigh bone
patella (pa TEL uh)	kneecap
tibia (TIB ee uh)	shinbone; larger of two lower leg bones
fibula (FIB yoo luh)	slender lower leg bone
tarsal (TAHR sul) **bones**	ankle or tarsus bones
metatarsal (met uh TAHR sul) **bones**	bones of the foot between the ankle and toes
talus (TAY lus)	ankle bone that connects to lower leg bones
calcaneus (kal KAY nee us)	heel bone

navicular (na VICK yoo lur)	boat-shaped tarsal bone
cuboid (KEW boid)	cube-shaped tarsal bone, between calcaneus and fourth and fifth metatarsals
cuneiform (kew NEE i form) bones	three tarsal bones

Key Term Practice: Appendicular Skeleton

1. What is the singular form for each given term?

   a. phalanges = _____

   b. acetabula = _____

   c. scapulae _____

2. What is the medical term for each of the following descriptions?

   a. shoulder girdle _____

   b. hip girdle _____

Surface Markings

Surface markings are identifiable landmarks on the exterior of bones. Each is designed for a specific purpose, which demonstrates that structure and function are complementary. Figure 5-18 provides examples of surface markings and their associated bones. The markings occur for joint formation, muscle attachment, and passage of nerves and blood vessels. Table 5-1 lists common surface marking terms along with their definitions and an example location. Table 5-2 matches selected surface markings with their associated bones.

THE CLINICAL DIMENSION

Pathology of the Skeletal System

Signs and symptoms of pathologic conditions in bone are often similar to those associated with other body disorders. Those specific to osseous disorders are discussed in this section. Common disorders of the skeletal system are also introduced.

Abnormal Spinal Curvatures

Abnormal curvatures of the spine include kyphosis, lordosis, and scoliosis (Fig. 5-19). **Kyphosis** is an exaggeration of the thoracic curve. Commonly referred to as hunchback or humpback, it is caused by poor posture, tuberculosis, osteochondritis, or ankylosing spondylitis. The person generally has rounded shoulders, and back pain is a regular symptom. Physical examination and x-rays give a definitive diagnosis. Treatment consists of exercises and physical therapy to strengthen the involved muscles.

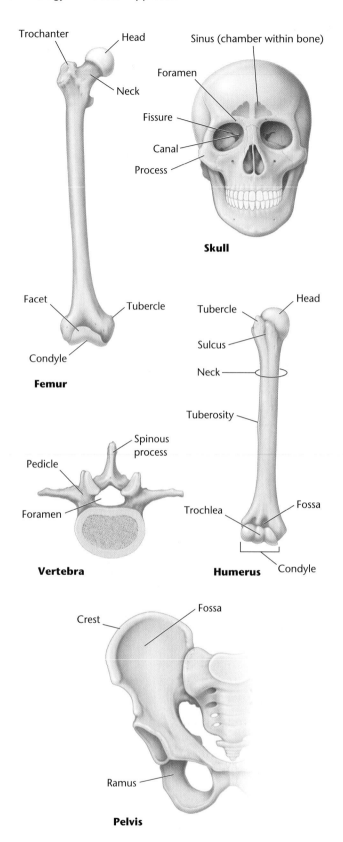

FIGURE 5-18
Surface markings and associated bones.

Labels within figure:
Trochanter, Head, Neck, Sinus (chamber within bone), Foramen, Fissure, Canal, Process, **Skull**

Facet, Tubercle, Condyle, **Femur**

Tubercle, Head, Sulcus, Neck, Tuberosity, Trochlea, Fossa, Condyle, **Humerus**

Pedicle, Spinous process, Foramen, **Vertebra**

Crest, Fossa, Ramus, **Pelvis**

   Lordosis is an abnormal anterior concavity of the lumbar curve. It is frequently called swayback. It is generally caused by excessive abdominal weight from obesity or pregnancy. The person makes a postural adjustment to compensate for the extra girth. Individuals typically have a protruding abdomen and experience back pain as a result of muscle strain. Diagnosis is made by physical examination of the spine

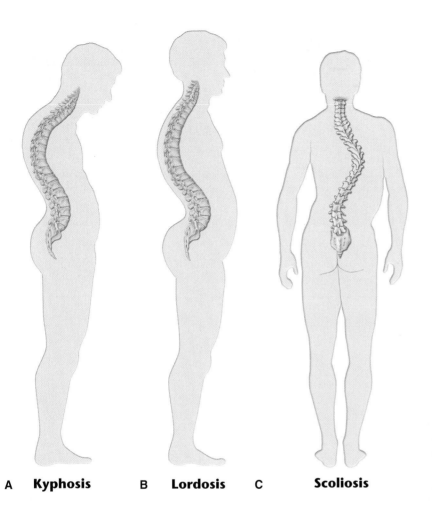

FIGURE 5-19
Abnormal curvatures of the spine. (Images provided by Anatomical Chart Co.)

| A | **Kyphosis** | B | **Lordosis** | C | **Scoliosis** |

in various postures and x-ray evaluation. Treatment is aimed at weight reduction and exercise to strengthen abdominal and back muscles. Untreated lordosis can progress to degenerative lumbar disk disease, which can be treated by a surgical treatment called displacement osteotomy. **Displacement osteotomy** is a surgical intervention in which vertebral bone segments are removed to facilitate spinal realignment.

Scoliosis is an abnormal lateral curvature of the spine that appears S-shaped. A sign of scoliosis is having one shoulder and hip higher than the other. The cause of scoliosis is either genetic or idiopathic (unknown). Physical examination and radiographic studies confirm the diagnosis and determine the degree of curvature. For mild cases, treatment involves exercises to strengthen muscles. Severe scoliosis with a curvature of 40° or more can be treated by surgery or bracing. Attempts should be made to correct kyphosis, lordosis, and scoliosis so that they do not progress to stages that compromise respiratory or cardiac function.

Key Terms	*Definitions*
kyphosis (kigh FOH sis)	angular curve of the thoracic spine
lordosis (lor DOH sis)	forward curve of the lumbar spine
displacement osteotomy (os tee OT uh mee)	surgery to remove vertebral bone segments and change spinal alignment
scoliosis (skoh lee OH sis)	lateral curve of the spine

TABLE 5-1   Bone Surface Markings

Surface Marking	Definition	Example Location
alveolus (al VEE oh lus)	deep pit or socket	alveolus for each tooth in the maxilla
condyle (KON dile)	round knob	occipital condyle
crest	narrow, ridge-like projection	iliac crest
epicondyle (ep i KON dile)	projection superior to a condyle	medial epicondyle of the femur
facet (FAS it)	flattened or shallow articulating surface	costal facet of the thoracic vertebrae
fissure (FISH ur)	narrow, slit-like opening	superior orbital fissure
foramen (foh RAY mun)	rounded opening	obturator foramen
fossa (FOS uh)	flattened or shallow surface	mandibular fossa
fovea (FOH vee uh)	pit or depression	fovea capitis
head	rounded articulating end	head of femur
malleolus (ma LEE oh lus)	process with hammerhead shape	medial malleolus
meatus (mee AY tus)	canal; tube-like passageway	external auditory meatus
plate	flattened process of bone	cribriform plate
process	bony prominence (outgrowth)	mastoid process
sinus	cavity or hollow space	frontal sinus
spinous process (SPYE nus)	sharp, slender spine	spinous process of the scapula
sulcus (SUL kus)	linear groove for a vessel, nerve, or tendon	intertubercular sulcus of the humerus
trochanter (troh KAN tur)	large process found only on the femur	greater trochanter of the femur
tubercle (TEW bur kul)	small, rounded process	greater tubercle of the humerus
tuberosity (tew bur OS i tee)	large, roughened knob-like projection	radial tuberosity

Key Term Practice: Abnormal Spinal Curvatures

1. _____ is abnormal lateral curvature of the spine.

2. Hunchback is another term for this irregular spinal curve.

   _____

Fractures

A **fracture** (Fx) is a break in a bone or tooth. Whenever there is a disruption in bone integrity, the body repairs itself by forming a fracture hematoma and then a callus at the site of injury. Remodeling then completes the task of forming new bone at the fracture area. Fractures in an epiphyseal plate can be serious because this is the area of greatest

TABLE 5-2   Selected Surface Markings Matched with Associated Bones

Marking	Bone
acetabulum (as e TAB yoo lum), greater sciatic (sigh AT ick) notch	coxal bone
acromion (a KROH mee on) process, glenoid (GLEE noid) cavity	scapula
coronoid (KOR o noid) process[a]	mandible
foramen magnum (foh RAY mun MAG num)	occipital bone
greater trochanter (troh KAN tur)	femur
lateral malleolus (ma LEE oh lus)	fibula
linea aspera (LIN ee uh AS per uh)	femur
mastoid (MAS toid) process	temporal bone
medial malleolus (ma LEE oh lus)	tibia
olecranon (oh LECK ruh non) process	ulna
radial tuberosity (RAY dee ul tew bur OS i tee)	radius
sella turcica[b] (SEL uh TUR si kuh)	sphenoid bone
temporal (TEM po rul) process	zygomatic bone
transverse (tans VERCE) process, atlas, pedicle (PED i kul)	vertebra
xiphoid (ZYE foid) process	sternum

[a]*Coronoid* means "curved like a beak."
[b]*Sella* means "saddle."

mitotic activity in a growing bone. Broken bones are frequently accompanied by **crepitus,** the harsh, grating sound heard when broken bone ends rub together. Without proper treatment, the patient risks having one limb shorter than the other. Options for treating fractures include skeletal traction, closed and open reduction, and fixation. **Skeletal traction** is an option for treating some types of bone fractures and involves pulling on a bone structure that is mediated by surgically placed rods, plates, pins, wires, and/or screws in that bone to keep it internally fixed. **Reduction** is the restoration of a part to its normal anatomic relation by surgery or manipulation. **Closed reduction** refers to bone manipulation without skin incision; when skin incision is necessary to restore a dislocated joint or fracture to its anatomic relationships, it is termed an **open reduction.** Two types of **fixation,** the immobilization of a fractured bone, are external and internal. With **external fixation,** splints, dressings, or pins immobilize the fractured bone, whereas **internal fixation** involves the stabilization of fractured bony parts by directly attaching the fragments with surgical wires, screws, pins, rod, or plates.

Table 5.3 identifies and describes several types of fractures, and Figure 5-20 illustrates the more common examples.

Key Terms	Definitions
fracture	break in a bone or tooth
crepitus (KREP i tus)	grating sound heard from broken bone ends rubbing together
skeletal traction	bone pulling mediated by internal fixation with rod, plate, wire, pin, and/or screws

TABLE 5-3 Types of Fractures

Type	Description
Colles (KOL eez) fracture	fracture of the distal end of the radius and ulna with displacement of the hand backward and upward
comminuted (KOM i newt ed) fracture	complete break with bony fragments
complete fracture	break across the entire bone
compound (open) fracture	bone is exposed through injured (open) skin
compression fracture	fracture of vertebra(e) as a result of severe stress; may impinge the spinal cord
greenstick fracture	incomplete break on a convex bone surface (bends like a green tree twig)
impacted fracture	bone fracture in which one bone fragment is driven into the cancellous (spongy) bone of another fragment
Le Fort fracture	bilateral fracture of the maxillae
oblique fracture	bone fracture in which the break occurs at an angle not perpendicular to the bone axis
partial (incomplete) fracture	fracture in which bony fragments remain partially joined
Pott fracture	fracture of the distal end (lateral malleolus) of the fibula
simple (closed) fracture	break is protected by uninjured (closed) skin
spiral fracture	excessive bone twisting
stress fracture	tiny fractures in the subchondral plates caused by excessive mechanical strain
transverse (trans VERCE) fracture	complete break occurring at a right angle to the bone axis

reduction	restoration of a dislocated joint or fractured bone to its anatomic relationships via surgical or manipulative procedures
closed reduction	restoration of a dislocated joint or fractured bone to its anatomic relationships via surgical or manipulative procedures without skin incision
open reduction	restoration of a dislocated joint or fractured bone to its anatomic relationships via surgical or manipulative procedures with skin incision
fixation	immobilizing a fracture
external fixation	immobilizing a fracture by splints, dressings, or pins
internal fixation	immobilizing a fracture by directly attaching the bony fragments together with surgical wires, screws, pins, rods, or plates

Key Term Practice: Fractures

1. A break in a bone is termed a _____.

2. _____ refers to fracture immobilization.

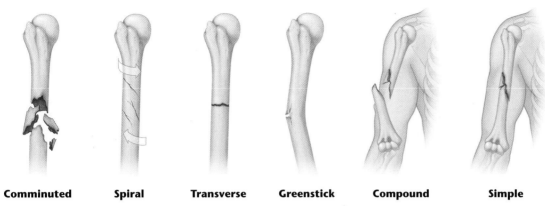

| Comminuted | Spiral | Transverse | Greenstick | Compound | Simple |

FIGURE 5-20
Fractures of the bone.

Genetic Bone Diseases

Marfan syndrome is a heritable disorder of the connective tissue manifested by abnormal skeletal changes. Its signs and symptoms include arched palate, ocular changes, and congenital heart disease (Fig. 5-21). It may go undetected until the occurrence of a life-threatening event such as a ruptured aortic aneurysm. Diagnosis may be made at birth or during early childhood through physical and genetic evaluation. Treatment involves prepubescent hormonal therapy to prevent excessive growth and therapies aimed at preventing glaucoma and hypertension. Cardiac evaluations are continuous.

Another genetic bone disease, characterized by hypoplasia of osteoid tissue and collagen, is **osteogenesis imperfecta** (OI). It is commonly known as "brittle bone disease." This disease is marked by bone fractures resulting from minimal trauma, and individuals with this disease suffer multiple fractures throughout life. Several types exist, and diagnosis is based on clinical manifestations and serologic tests. There is no therapeutic treatment available for type II osteogenesis imperfecta; the remaining types are treated according to individual cases. Research is advancing in this area; however, options are still limited and include surgical placement of rods to encourage bone growth and strengthen tissue and chemical therapies such as bisphosphonate drug compounds that are aimed at stimulating osteoblast activity.

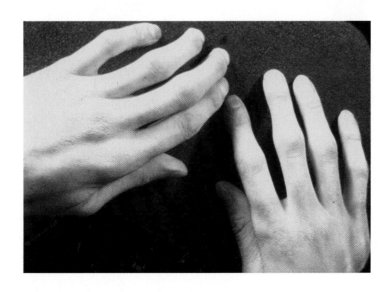

FIGURE 5-21
Skeletal changes as a result of Marfan syndrome. (Reprinted with permission from Rubin E, Farber JL. Pathology, 3rd ed. Philadelphia: Lippincott Williams & Wilkins, 1999.)

Key Terms	Definitions
Marfan (mar FAHN) **syndrome**	genetic disorder of the connective tissue manifested by abnormal skeletal alterations
osteogenesis imperfecta (os tee oh JEN e sis im pur FECK tuh)	brittle bone disease

Key Term Practice: Genetic Bone Diseases

1. What is the medical term for *brittle bone disease?*

_____

Hand and Foot Disorders

The term used to describe adhesion between fingers and toes is **syndactyly.** It refers to digits that have a webbed appearance (Fig. 5-22). This is a feature common to some genetic diseases. **Polydactyly** describes the condition of having an extra digit (Fig. 5-23). Extra fingers or toes are usually surgically removed at birth.

The general medical term used to describe a variety of foot deformities is **talipes.** Most talipes are congenital in origin and are commonly known as clubfoot or equinovarus (Fig. 5-24). Such foot distortions are usually surgically corrected in infancy.

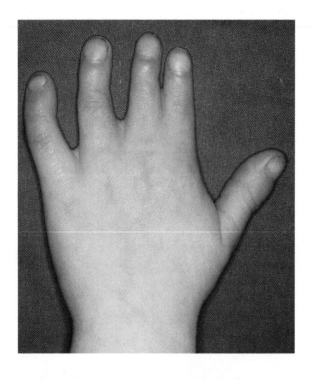

FIGURE 5-22
Syndactyly is an adhesion between fingers or toes common in some genetic disorders. The digits have a webbed appearance. (Photo Courtesy of L Thompson.)

Key Terms	Definitions
syndactyly (sin DACK ti lee)	webbed fingers or toes
polydactyly (pol ee DACK ti lee)	existence of extra fingers or toes
talipes (TAL i peez)	human foot deformity

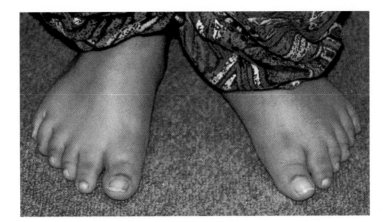

FIGURE 5-23
Polydactyly describes the condition of having an extra digit. (Reprinted with permission from Gold DH, Weingeist TA. Color atlas of the eye in systemic disease. Baltimore: Lippincott Williams & Wilkins, 2001.)

Key Term Practice: Hand and Foot Disorders

1. _____ refers to webbed fingers.

2. The medical term that describes foot deformities such as clubfoot is _____.

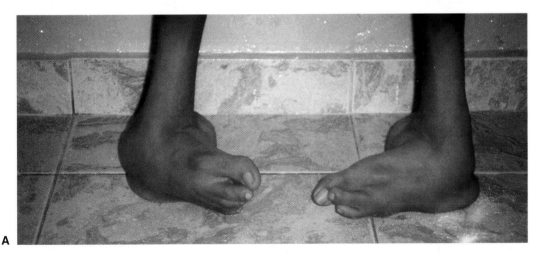

A

Ankle joint (plantarflexed)

Talus (deformed)

Tibionavicular ligament and tendons of extensor digitorum longus, tibialis anterior, and extensor hallucis longus tendons (note tightness)

Calcaneus (inverted)

Bones of forefoot
B (in extreme varus position)

FIGURE 5-24
Talipes. (Photo courtesy of R. A. O'Keefe, M.D.; drawing reprinted with permission from Moore KL, Dalley AF II. Clinically oriented anatomy, 4th ed. Baltimore: Lippincott Williams & Wilkins 1999.)

Hormone and Vitamin Imbalances

Hormone disturbances can lead to overgrowth or undergrowth. **Pituitary dwarfism** results when the hypophysis (pituitary gland) fails to secrete growth hormone (GH), which stimulates cartilage cell reproduction in the epiphyseal plates. In the absence of GH, the long bones of the limbs fail to develop normally. The person is very short, but has normal body proportions. **Pituitary gigantism** results when excessive amounts of GH are released before the epiphyseal plates are ossified. **Acromegaly** is the condition whereby excessive secretion of GH occurs in an adult; hands, feet, and jaw enlargement are hallmark characteristics.

Vitamin intake is essential for normal bone development, and vitamin D is especially critical. If vitamin D intake is inadequate or there is ineffective use of it by the body, calcium absorption is hindered, leading to rickets or osteomalacia. Lack of adequate amounts of sunlight may also cause the condition because sunlight stimulates natural vitamin D synthesis. This condition is referred to as **rickets** when it occurs in children and is called **osteomalacia** if it occurs during adulthood. In both diseases, there is inadequate mineralization of bone. The lack of proper bone formation in children causes the bones to soften and bend under the body's weight. Treatment consists of vitamin D and calcium supplements, calcitonin administration, and/or sunlight exposure. Calcitonin is a viable option in some cases because this hormone decreases the blood concentration of calcium by causing its absorption into bone tissue.

Scurvy is a condition caused by a deficiency of ascorbic acid (vitamin C), which is evidenced by abnormal bone and teeth development. Treatment involves ingesting vitamin C.

Bone inflammation with fibrous nodules and cysts forming in osseous tissue is termed **osteitis fibrosis cystica**. It is characterized by generalized skeletal demineralization and results in decalcification and bone weakening. Loss of bone tissue leads to porous bones and spontaneous fractures are common. The underlying cause is hyperparathyroidism in which excessive parathyroid hormone (PTH) causes undue calcium withdrawal from bones. Treatment is aimed at decreasing the circulating levels of PTH. Surgery is an option if the bones are deformed.

Key Terms	Definitions
pituitary (pi TEW i tayr ee) **dwarfism**	abnormal underdevelopment of bones
pituitary gigantism (pi TEW i terr ee jye GAN tiz um)	excessive bone growth
acromegaly (ack roh MEG uh lee)	condition characterized by overgrowth of bone tissue
rickets	calcium deficiency disease caused by inadequate vitamin D intake in children
osteomalacia (os tee oh muh LAY shee uh)	calcium deficiency disease in adulthood
scurvy (SKUR vee)	nutritional disorder caused by lack of vitamin C
osteitis fibrosis cystica (os tee EYE tis figh BROH sis SIS ti kuh)	bone inflammation with fibrous nodules and cysts

Key Term Practice: Hormone and Vitamin Imbalances

1. Insufficient amounts of vitamin D and calcium in adults is termed _____.

2. _____ results from inadequate amounts of growth hormone during childhood.

Other Bone Disorders

Premature ossification of infant fontanelles is referred to as **craniostenosis.** Cranial sutures form too quickly, before the brain has matured. Its cause is not known, but surgical intervention is necessary to prevent brain damage and mental impairment.

A disease of unknown origin, **osteitis deformans,** also known as Paget disease, is characterized by simultaneous hyperplasia and accelerated deossification, resulting in bone weakness and deformity. Its occurrence can be isolated or widespread within the skeletal system and may be either symptomatic or asymptomatic. Signs and symptoms can include pain, edema, deformity, and hearing loss if the auditory ossicles are involved. Fractures, hypercalcemia, renal calculi (kidney stones), and sarcoma are other possible complications. Diagnosis is made by physical examination, patient history, blood tests, urinalysis (analysis of urine), and radiographic evaluation. No treatment is prescribed for asymptomatic osteitis deformans. Symptomatic disease is treated with analgesics; anti-inflammatory drugs; cytotoxic (cell-killing) agents; and diet therapy consisting of a high-protein, high-calcium, high-vitamin D intake.

Osteomyelitis is an infection of bone characterized by an inflammation of the marrow, periosteum, and hard tissue. It is usually bacterial in origin and the frequent culprit is *Staphylococcus aureus.* Symptoms include pain, tenderness at the site, and malaise. Children with the condition generally are just recovering from a streptococcal infection. Classic signs of advanced infection include subperiosteal abscesses and sequestra. Detached or dead bone fragments within a cavity, abscess, or wound are termed **sequestra** (singular, sequestrum). To determine the extent of infection, erythrocyte sedimentation test (EST), magnetic resonance imaging (MRI), and computerized tomography (CT) scans may be used in diagnosis. Treatment involves long-term antibiotic use, vitamin therapy, analgesics (painkillers), and immobilization to reduce fracture risk. Surgical draining of the abscess may also be required.

Osteoporosis is a decrease in the amount and strength of bone. It is characterized by bone deossification, an enlargement of bone marrow cavities and osteonic spaces, decreased cortical bone (superficial layer of compact bone) and trabeculae, and structural weakness. A photomicrograph of characteristic osteoporosis of the vertebral column is shown in Figure 5-25. It is generally asymptomatic, unless the bone loss

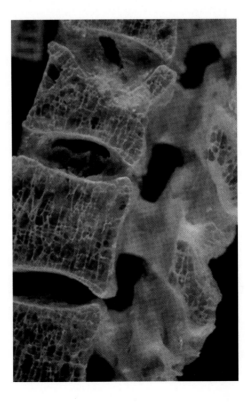

FIGURE 5-25
Osteoporosis of the vertebral column. (Reprinted with permission from Rubin E, Farber JL. Pathology, 3rd ed. Philadelphia: Lippincott Williams & Wilkins, 2000.)

happens in vertebrae or weight-bearing bones. It occurs more frequently in women than in men, and the first indication of dysfunction is often a bone fracture. It is commonly caused by endocrine disorders, dietary factors, or trauma. Blood tests, radiographic films, CT scan, photon absorptiometry, and bone densitometry make the definitive diagnosis. **Photon absorptiometry** measures the uptake of electromagnetic radiation to determine bone density, and a **densitometer** uses x-rays to measure the thickness and mineral density of bone tissue. Through computer analysis, densitometry identifies those at risk of osteoporosis. Treatment options depend on the severity of disease. Increased dietary calcium, vitamin D, and exercise are viable options. Pharmaceutical measures include drugs such as Fosamax and estrogen replacement therapy for postmenopausal women to assist with bone building. Estrogen is an important hormone for osteogenesis. In postmenopausal women, estrogen levels decline; thus replacing the lost estrogen through **estrogen replacement therapy** (ERT) is often beneficial for stimulating bone growth. The term **hormone replacement therapy** (HRT) is frequently used to describe ERT; however, the word *hormone* implies that estrogen is used in combination with another hormone such as progesterone.

The most common skeletal tissue tumor is an **osteochondroma.** It frequently causes **osteophytes,** or bone spurs, at the ends of long bones. Although their cause is unknown, osteochondromas originate in bone or cartilage. An **osteosarcoma** is the most common malignant bone tumor. Treatment options include surgical removal and chemotherapeutic measures, if necessary.

Key Terms	Definitions
craniostenosis (KRAY nee oh stuh NOH sis)	premature ossification of the fontanelles and fusion of the cranial sutures
osteitis deformans (os tee EYE tis de FOR manz)	bone disease characterized by a combination of osseous hyperplasia and accelerated decalcification; Paget disease
osteomyelitis (os tee oh migh e LYE tis)	bacterial infection of bone and associated tissue
sequestra (se KWES truh)	detached bony fragments associated with an abscess or wound
osteoporosis (os tee oh poh ROH sis)	bone deossification
photon absorptiometry (FOH ton ab SOHRP tee OM e tree)	measurement of bone density
densitometer (den si TOM e tur)	instrument used to measure bone density
estrogen (ES troh jen) replacement therapy	administration of the hormone estrogen
hormone replacement therapy	administration of hormones, notably estrogen and progesterone
osteochondroma (os tee oh kon DROH muh)	benign bone tumor
osteophytes (OS tee oh fites)	bony outgrowths
osteosarcoma (os tee oh sahr KOH muh)	osteogenic sarcoma; malignant bone tumor

Key Term Practice: Other Bone Disorders

1. The medical term for a malignant bone tumor is _____.

2. _____ is a bone disease caused by a bacterial infection.

CLINICAL TERMS

Clinical Dimension	Term	Description
DISORDERS		
	acromegaly	condition characterized by overgrowth of bone tissue
	craniostenosis	premature ossification of the fontanelles and fusion of the cranial sutures
	fracture	break in a bone or tooth
	kyphosis	angular curve of the thoracic spine
	lordosis	forward curve of the lumbar spine
	Marfan syndrome	genetic disorder of the connective tissue manifested by abnormal skeletal alterations
	osteitis deformans	bone disease characterized by a combination of osseous hyperplasia and accelerated decalcification; Paget disease
	osteitis fibrosis cystica	bone inflammation with fibrous nodules and cysts
	osteogenesis imperfecta (OI)	brittle bone disease
	osteochondroma	benign bone tumor
	osteomalacia	calcium deficiency disease in adulthood
	osteomyelitis	bacterial infection of bone and associated tissue
	osteoporosis	bone deossification
	osteophytes	bony outgrowths
	osteosarcoma	osteogenic sarcoma; malignant bone tumor
	pituitary dwarfism	abnormal underdevelopment of bones
	pituitary gigantism	excessive bone growth
	polydactyly	existence of extra fingers or toes
	rickets	calcium deficiency disease caused by inadequate vitamin D intake in children
	scoliosis	lateral curve of the spine
	scurvy	nutritional disorder caused by lack of vitamin C
	syndactyly	webbed fingers or toes
	talipes	human foot deformity
SIGNS AND SYMPTOMS		
	crepitus	grating sound heard from broken bone ends rubbing together
	sequestra	detached bony fragments associated with an abscess or wound

Clinical Dimension	Term	Description
CLINICAL TESTS AND DIAGNOSTIC PROCEDURES		
	bone aspiration	withdrawal of fluid from the medullary cavity
	bone scan	radioactive dye administered intravenously
	densitometer	instrument used to measure bone density
	erythrocyte sedimentation est (EST)	measure of the rate of red blood cell sedimentation to determine blood protein status as it pertains to various disorders
	photon absorptiometry	measurement of bone density
TREATMENTS		
	closed reduction	restoration of a dislocated joint or fractured bone to its anatomic relationships via surgical or manipulative procedures without skin incision
	displacement osteotomy	surgery to remove vertebral bone segments and change spinal alignment
	estrogen replacement therapy (ERT)	administration of the hormone estrogen
	external fixation	immobilizing a fracture by splints, dressings, or pins
	fixation	immobilizing a fracture
	hormone replacement therapy (HRT)	administration of hormones, notably estrogen and progesterone
	internal fixation	immobilizing a fracture by directly attaching the bony fragments together with surgical wires, screws, pins, rod, or plates
	open reduction	restoration of a dislocated joint or fractured bone to its anatomic relationships via surgical or manipulative procedures with skin incision
	pulsating electromagnetic fields (PEMFs)	treatment for speeding bone tissue recovery
	reduction	restoration of a part to its normal anatomic relationships via surgical or manipulative procedures
	skeletal traction	bone pulling mediated by internal fixation with rod, plate, wire, pin, and/or screws

Lifespan

Bone formation begins around the 8th week in utero. Ossification continues by both endochondral and intramembranous formation. Because the skeletal system develops in a specific time frame, fetal age can be determined by looking at bone development through x-rays or sonograms. At birth, the head is disproportionately large, and the spine of a newborn appears kyphotic, or concave. At 3 months after birth, the cervical spine becomes lordotic and has an increased ability to hold the head. As the infant matures, normal lordotic curvature of the lumbar region develops. The ability to sit enhances this developmental change.

The bones are essentially ossified at birth; however, the epiphyseal plates will be present until long bone growth ceases, typically around adolescence. At birth, infant legs are bowed as a result of confinement in the womb. As the child ages, the arms and legs undergo rotational and alignment changes. It is not uncommon for children to appear "bowlegged" until 2.5 years of age or "knock kneed" until 6 years. If either condition persists beyond these ages, it is considered pathologic and should be treated. During childhood, the appendicular skeleton grows at a greater rate than the axial skeleton. By age 1, the spine reaches 50% of its total growth.

By age 25, bones are completely ossified. During childhood and adolescence, bone formation exceeds bone resorption. A balance between osteoblastic and osteoclastic activity characterizes adulthood. Osteoclastic activity outpaces osteoblastic activity during late adulthood. Bone mass, except cranial bone mass, begins declining around age 40 years. Calcium loss appears to be the principal effect on the aging process. Furthermore, decreased production of organic matter makes bones more susceptible to fracture. Exercise and proper nutrition can strengthen bones and increase osteoblastic activity at any time during one's life. Thus osteoporosis can be thwarted.

> **FACT** *Newborns have about 300 separated bones, which later ossify into 206!*

In the News: Child Abuse or Osteogenesis Imperfecta?

It is a scenario that is played time and again across the country in America's emergency rooms. A seemingly healthy child is brought to the hospital by loving parents for an unexplained injury. Radiographs reveal that the young person has a recent fracture with evidence of several prior bone breaks. Red flags automatically go up, and the physician alerts social services for suspected child abuse. Despite pleas to the contrary, the parents are prevented from contacting their child and are whisked away and charged with child abuse by the authorities. The child is placed in foster care and the parents enter into a legal battle.

First described in 1840 as a syndrome, osteogenesis imperfecta affects primarily bone tissue. It is characterized by fractures, osteoporosis, and skeletal deformities. In the most severe cases, the child may be born with broken bones, while the less severe forms may not become obvious until the child begins walking.

Although child abuse is a prevalent societal problem, medical and legal authorities should not rush to judge. There may be a perfectly reasonable explanation for the bone fractures. The child may have osteogenesis imperfecta (OI), or brittle bone disease. A genetic disorder, OI affects approximately 1 in 30,000 births. Because of its rareness, physicians and the public alike may be unfamiliar with the disorder, thus confusing it with child abuse. Improved media coverage has increased public awareness.

COMMON ABBREVIATIONS

Abbreviation	Term
C1–C7	cervical vertebrae 1–7
CT	computerized tomography
ERT	estrogen replacement therapy
EST	erythrocyte sedimentation test
Fx	fracture
GH	growth hormone
HRT	hormone replacement therapy
L1–L5	lumbar vertebrae 1–5
MD	doctor of medicine

Abbreviation	Term
MRI	magnetic resonance imaging
OI	osteogenesis imperfecta
PEMF	pulsating electromagnetic field
PTH	parathyroid hormone
T1–T12	thoracic vertebrae 1–12
TH	thyroid hormone

Case Study

Andy Simmons, a 15-year old male, arrived in the emergency room with injuries sustained from a motor vehicle accident. He was conscious and indicated severe pain in his left elbow and right hand. Physical examination revealed that Andy could not flex or extend either his left arm or his right hand. His right hand was missing digits II, III, IV, and V. Blood loss was prevalent. Vital signs were as follows:

HEART RATE	50
RESPIRATIONS	20
TEMPERATURE	35°C
BLOOD PRESSURE	90/50 mm Hg

Intravenous fluid and antibiotic therapy was initiated, and portable x-rays were taken. As the medical team awaited the results from the radiology department, they prepped Andy for orthopedic surgery.

Case Study Questions

Select the best answer to each of the following questions.

1. **Digits II, III, IV, and V have been amputated. That means Andy was missing _____.**
   a. thumb, index finger, middle finger, and ring finger
   b. index finger, middle finger, ring finger, and pinky
   c. pinky, thumb, index finger, and middle finger
   d. all of his fingers plus the thumb

2. **Being unable to flex (decrease the angle between two parts) or extend (increase the angle between two parts) suggests a _____.**
   a. muscle strain
   b. lack of coordination
   c. possible bone fracture at a joint
   d. none of these

3. **What type of fracture was Andy most likely to have sustained?**
   a. compound
   b. Pott
   c. greenstick
   d. Le Fort

4. **What bones may be involved in Andy's injury?**
   a. femur, radius, and tibia
   b. ulna, phalanges, and radius
   c. tibia, fibula, and radius
   d. phalanges, radius, and patella

REAL WORLD REPORT

CENTRAL IMAGING DEPARTMENT

NAME:	Andrew Simmons
DATE ORDERED:	08/27/2003
ORDPHYS:	R. A. O'Keefe, MD
DOB:	07/04/1988
TEST:	Hand, R, Multiple Views;
	Elbow, L, Multiple Views
ATTENDING:	R. A. O'Keefe, MD
REFERRING:	B. A. Saxon, MD
CLINIC:	ER
EXAM DATE:	08/27/03

CLINICAL HISTORY
Injury to right hand, pain. Injury to left elbow, motor vehicle accident.

RIGHT HAND
There has been complete amputation of the second through fifth digits of the hand to the level of the distal shaft of the proximal phalanges. The remainder of the visualized bones are intact. Joint spaces are maintained. Views of the amputated digits demonstrate comminuted fractures involving the mid and distal shafts of the proximal phalanges.

LEFT ELBOW
Multiple views obtained of the left elbow demonstrate the presence of a nondisplaced fracture through the radial head. Metaphyseal cartilage is present. Associated joint effusion is evident.

IMPRESSION
Fracture radial head

DICTATED BY: Jack D. O'Henry, MD

This document has been reviewed and electronically approved by Jack D. O'Henry, MD 08/27/03

REAL WORLD REPORT QUESTIONS

The following exercises review the medical terms in the preceding medical report.

1. The report stated there was complete amputation to the level of the distal shaft of the proximal phalanges.

   a. Distal refers to _____.

   b. Proximal refers to _____.

   c. Thus what section of each phalanx was severed?

   _____

2. Comminuted fractures were observed. Comminuted means that there is a complete break with _____.

3. Metaphyseal cartilage was viewed on the radiograph.

   a. Give an alternate term for metaphyseal cartilage.

   _____

   b. Is this a remarkable finding? Why or why not?

   _____

4. The radial head is fractured.

   a. Identify the bone.

   _____

   b. Is this the proximal or distal portion of the bone?

   _____

REVIEW AND APPLICATION: THREE-LEVEL LEARNING SYSTEM

LEVEL ONE: REVIEWING FACTS AND TERMS USING RECALL

Select the best response to each of the following questions.

1. Functions of the skeletal system include _____.
   a. mineral storage
   b. protection
   c. hemopoiesis
   d. all of these

2. Most of the body's phosphorous and calcium is stored in _____.
   a. bones and teeth
   b. bones and blood
   c. muscle and bone
   d. none of these

3. Which word part means "cartilage"?
   a. osteo-
   b. chondro-
   c. myelo-
   d. peroneo-

4. What does word part *spondylo-* mean?
   a. pelvis
   b. bone
   c. vertebra
   d. straight

5. The _____ is the shaft of a long bone.
   a. diaphysis
   b. epiphysis
   c. metaphysis
   d. head

6. The ends of long bones are called _____.
   a. diaphyses
   b. epiphyses
   c. sutures
   d. metaphyses

7. The medullary cavity can be found _____.
   a. on a bone's exterior
   b. at an articulation
   c. in the bone's interior
   d. in conjunction with hyaline cartilage

8. Another term for *sutural bones* is _____ bones.
   a. cranial
   b. sesamoid
   c. round
   d. wormian

9. Cancellous bone is also known as _____.
   a. cortical bone
   b. compact bone
   c. osteonic bone
   d. spongy bone

10. _____ is the process of bone formation.
    a. Blastogenesis
    b. Osteogenesis
    c. Clastogenesis
    d. Histogenesis

11. _____ are mature bone cells, whereas _____ are bone-forming cells.
    a. Osteocytes; osteoblasts
    b. Osteoblasts; osteocytes
    c. Osteoclasts; osteoblasts
    d. Osteoclasts; osteocytes

12. Long bone growth occurs at the _____.
    a. epiphyseal plate
    b. subchondral plate
    c. appositional line
    d. diaphysis

13. Vitamins essential for bone growth include _____.

   a. vitamin B

   b. vitamin E

   c. vitamin D

   d. vitamin B_{12}

14. _____ marrow functions in fat storage.

   a. Red

   b. Yellow

   c. Blue

   d. Brown

15. Types of cartilage found in the body include _____.

   a. hyaline

   b. elastic

   c. fibrocartilage

   d. all of these

16. The two divisions of the skeleton are axial and _____.

   a. thoracic

   b. appendicular

   c. vertebral

   d. cranial

17. Metatarsal refers to the _____ between the _____ and _____.

   a. hand; wrist; fingers

   b. knee; hip; foot

   c. foot; ankle; toes

   d. elbow; shoulder; wrist

18. Anatomic terminology referring to identifiable landmarks on bone is best described as _____.

   a. surface markings

   b. exterior formations

   c. surface definitions

   d. morphology lines

19. A break in a bone is called a _____.

   a. strain

   b. sprain

   c. fracture

   d. compression

LEVEL TWO: REVIEWING CONCEPTS

Select the best response to each of the following questions.

20. Cervical vertebrae are _____.

   a. numbered T1–T12

   b. identified as C1–C7

   c. inferior to the sacral region

   d. between the thoracic and lumbar vertebrae

21. Epiphyseal plates are present until _____.

   a. birth

   b. adolescence

   c. long bone growth ceases

   d. puberty

22. Endochondral bone formation suggests that _____.

   a. there is medullary involvement

   b. bone cells form from blood

   c. cartilage is involved

   d. membranes will ossify

What is the singular form for each given term?

23. laminae = _____

24. vertebrae = _____

25. sacra = _____

26. humeri = _____

What is the plural form for each given term?

27. ulna = _____

28. phalanx = _____

29. fibula = _____

30. patella = _____

Match the bone with its location.

_____ 31. lacrimal bone   a. upper leg bone

_____ 32. atlas   b. cranium

_____ 33. tibia   c. pectoral girdle

_____ 34. femur   d. lower leg bone

_____ 35. scapula   e. cervical vertebrae

Match the surface marking with its definition.

_____ 36. fovea   a. linear groove

_____ 37. sulcus   b. round projection

_____ 38. condyle   c. pit or depression

_____ 39. tuberosity   d. deep pit or socket

_____ 40. alveolus   e. knob-like protuberance

Match the surface marking with its associated bone.

_____ 41. acetabulum   a. femur

_____ 42. cribriform plate   b. coxal bone

_____ 43. xiphoid process   c. vertebra

_____ 44. greater trochanter   d. ethmoid bone

_____ 45. transverse process   e. sternum

Match the description with the fracture type.

_____ 46. bilateral maxillae fracture   a. simple

_____ 47. broken bone; skin intact   b. Colles

_____ 48. incomplete break; bone bends   c. greenstick

_____ 49. fractured distal radius and ulna   d. compound

_____ 50. broken bone; skin cut   e. Le Fort

Complete the following sentences by inserting the correct word in each sentence. Each word is used only once.

51. _____ is abnormal lateral curvature of the vertebral column.   Scoliosis

52. _____ is an exaggeration of the thoracic curve.   Kyphosis

53. _____ is concavity of the lumbar curve.   Lordosis

Using the following groups of word parts, form a medical term for each definition. Each group of word parts may be used more than once.

54. bone-forming cell = _____   -blast

55. bone softening = _____   chondr-, chondri-, chondrio-, chondro-

56. cartilage cell = _____   -cyte malacia ost-, oste-, osteo-

Provide a medical term to complete a meaningful analogy.

57. Humerus is to appendicular as cranium is to _____.

58. Floating rib is to vertebral as true rib is to _____.

59. Growth hormone (GH) is to pituitary gigantism as parathyroid hormone (PTH) is to _____.

Identify the correctly spelled term in each set.

60. _____

   a. ziphoid

   b. zifoid

   c. xiphoid

   d. xifoid

61. _____

   a. humerous

   b. humerus

   c. humurus

   d. humurous

62. _____

   a. forramen

   b. foramen

   c. foraman

   d. foremon

63. _____

   a. acetabulm

   b. acetabelum

   c. asatabulum

   d. acetabulum

64. _____

   a. ilium bone

   b. illium bone

   c. illeum bone

   d. ileum bone

65. _____

   a. spinus process

   b. spinnus process

   c. spinous process

   d. spineous process

LEVEL THREE: THINKING CRITICALLY

Write a short answer to each of the following questions.

66. Iva is an 80-year-old woman who was hospitalized for a broken hip. This was her first experience with a fracture. Her history and physical (H&P) examination revealed that since the death of her spouse she remained home bound, got very little exercise, and began to experience back pain. Her diet evaluation indicated that she was not eating properly and lacked appropriate dietary intake of calcium, phosphorous, and vitamin D. Without performing any other diagnostic procedure or clinical test, the physician told her she suspected a very common porous bone disorder. What bone disease did the doctor suspect and why?

   _____

   _____

   _____

67. A patient was brought to the emergency room with a compound fracture. After the initial set of x-rays, the radiologist and orthopedic surgeon diagnosed an epiphyseal fracture of the femur and sent the patient to the pediatric ward for surgical treatment. What prompted the pediatric assignment?

   _____

   _____

   _____

KEY TERMS SPELLING TEST FROM CD-ROM

Use the CD-ROM to test yourself on the spelling of the key terms from this chapter. Listen to the terms and write them on a separate sheet of paper. Use a medical dictionary to check your answers.

ANSWERS

WORD GROUPING

Definition	Word Part
tibia, tibial	tibio-
bone	A. osseo-, ossi-
	B. ost-, oste-, osteo-
calcaneus	calcane-, calcaneo-
calcium	calc-, calci-, calco-
carpus (wrist), carpal	carp-, carpo-
cartilage, cartilaginous	chondr-, chondri-, chondrio-, chondro-
coccyx; tailbone	coccy-
condyle	condyl-, condylo-
cranium, cranial	crani-, carnio-
development	-genesis
ethmoid	ethmo-
femur, femoral	femoro-

Definition	Word Part
ilium, iliac	ili-, ilio-
immature precursor cell	-blast
mandible, mandibular	mandibul-, mandibulo-
marrow	myel-, myelo-
meatus	meat-, meato-
pelvis	pelv-, pelvo-
peroneal, peroneus	peroneo-
pubis, pubic, pubes	pubo-
rib, costal	cost-, costi-, costo-
scapula, scapular	scapula, scapulo-
something that breaks; to break	-clast
sternum, sternal, chest	stern-, sterno-
straight	orth-, ortho-
tarsus, tarsal	tars-, tarso-
U-shaped	hyo-
vertebra, vertebral	vertebr-, vertebro-

WORD BUILDING

Word Part	Meaning	Common or Known Word	Example Medical Term
-genesis	development	histogenesis	osteogenesis
calc-, calci-, calco-	calcium	calcium	calcium
carp-, carpo-	carpus (wrist), carpal	carpal	carpal tunnel syndrome
crani-, cranio-	cranium, cranial	cranium	cranial cavity
orth-, ortho-	straight	orthodontist	orthopedics
osseo-, ossi-	bone	ossification	ossification
ost-, oste-, osteo-	bone	osteocytes	osteoblast
vertebr-, vertebro-	vertebrae	vertebrae	vertebral column

KEY TERM PRACTICE

Bone Anatomy

1. a. long; b. short; c. flat; d. irregular; e. sesamoid; f. sutural or wormian
2. around the fibrous membrane
3. a. epiphyses; b. diaphyses
4. cancellous
5. cortical
6. trabecula

Bone Marrow, Blood, and Cartilage

1. red bone marrow
2. Interstices
3. chondrocyte
4. a. fibrocartilage; b. elastic cartilage; c. hyaline cartilage

Bone Development and Remodeling

1. intramembranous; endochondral
2. Osteogenesis
3. osteocytes
4. osteoblasts; osteoclasts
5. epiphyseal plate
6. appositional
7. calcium
8. ossification
9. atrophy

Axial Skeleton

1. axial; appendicular
2. a. vertebrosternal; b. vertebrochondral; c. vertebral
3. a. concha; b. maxilla; c. vertebral foramen

Appendicular Skeleton

1. a. phalanx; b. acetabulum; c. scapula
2. a. pectoral; b. pelvic

Abnormal Spinal Curvatures

1. Scoliosis
2. kyphosis

Fractures

1. fracture
2. Fixation

Genetic Bone Diseases

1. osteogenesis imperfecta

Hand and Foot Disorders

1. Syndactyly
2. talipes

Hormone and Vitamin Imbalances

1. osteomalacia
2. Pituitary dwarfism

Other Bone Disorders

1. osteosarcoma
2. Osteomyelitis

CASE STUDY

1. b is the correct answer.
   - a, c, and d are incorrect; digit counting begins with the pollex (thumb) as number I and continues in order.
2. c is the correct answer.
   - a is incorrect because the person would be able to move the hand or arm, although there may be associated pain.
   - b is incorrect because a lack of coordination would indicate only that moving the hand and arm simultaneously may be difficult.
   - d is incorrect because answer c is correct.
3. a is the correct answer.
   - b is incorrect because this is a fracture of the distal end (lateral malleolus) of the fibula, and Andy's leg was not injured.
   - c is incorrect because this is an incomplete break on a convex bone surface (bends like a green tree twig)
   - d is incorrect because this is a bilateral fracture of the maxillae, and the face was not injured.
4. b is the correct answer.
   - a is incorrect because the femur and tibia are leg bones; but the radius may be involved.
   - c is incorrect because the tibia and fibula are leg bones; but the radius may be involved.
   - d is incorrect because the patella is the knee region; but the phalanges and radius may be involved.

REAL WORLD REPORT

1. a. farther from the point of origin or the midline; b. closer to the point of origin or the midline; c. The sections distal to the first joints were severed. The fingertips plus the next finger section were amputated.
2. bony fragments
3. a. epiphyseal disk, epiphyseal plate, metaphysis, or growth plate; b. This is not a remarkable finding because Andy is only 15 years old; thus his bones have not finished growing. The metaphyseal cartilage indicates that long bone growth is still occurring.
4. a. radius; b. proximal portion of the radius

REVIEW AND APPLICATION: THREE-LEVEL LEARNING SYSTEM

Level One: Reviewing Facts and Terms Using Recall

1. d
2. a
3. b
4. c
5. a
6. b
7. c
8. d
9. d
10. b
11. a
12. a
13. c
14. b
15. d
16. b
17. c
18. a
19. c

Level Two: Reviewing Concepts

20. b
21. c
22. c
23. lamina
24. vertebra
25. sacrum
26. humerus
27. ulnae
28. phalanges
29. fibulae
30. patellae
31. b
32. e
33. d
34. a
35. c
36. c
37. a
38. b
39. e
40. d
41. b
42. d
43. e
44. a
45. c
46. e
47. a
48. c
49. b
50. d
51. Scoliosis
52. Kyphosis
53. Lordosis
54. osteoblast
55. osteomalacia
56. chondrocyte
57. axial
58. vertebrosternal
59. osteitis fibrosis cystica
60. c
61. b
62. b
63. d
64. a
65. c

Level Three: Thinking Critically

66. The doctor suspected osteoporosis because Iva's history fit the classic profile of this degenerative bone disease.
67. The assignment to the pediatric ward was based on the evidence of an epiphyseal fracture. Because children are still growing, they would still have an epiphyseal plate; only a remnant epiphyseal line is present in adults. Thus the patient was a child.

Articulations

OBJECTIVES

After completing this chapter, you should be able to:

1. State the meanings of word parts related to articulations.
2. State the structural and functional classifications of articulations.
3. Identify the various types of joints and associated structures.
4. Identify bones involved with key body articulations.
5. Correctly use terms describing anatomic movement at joints.
6. List the common signs, symptoms, and treatments of various articular diseases.
7. Explain clinical tests and diagnostic procedures related to disorders of articulations.
8. Describe anatomical and physiological alterations of articulations throughout the lifespan.
9. List common abbreviations related to articulations.
10. Define terms used in medical reports involving joint disorders.
11. Correctly define, spell, and pronounce the chapter's medical terms.

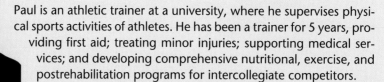

Professional Profile: Athletic Trainer

Paul is an athletic trainer at a university, where he supervises physical sports activities of athletes. He has been a trainer for 5 years, providing first aid; treating minor injuries; supporting medical services; and developing comprehensive nutritional, exercise, and postrehabilitation programs for intercollegiate competitors.

To be an athletic trainer, Paul completed a 4-year undergraduate degree in exercise science. After graduating with a bachelor's degree, he became certified by the National Athletic Trainers Association. His university's internal policy requires certification in cardiopulmonary resuscitation (CPR).

Working with athletes is exciting because the athletic trainer is called into action any time a player sustains an injury. On-the-job training provides valuable experience, and wrapping ankles, wrists, arms, and legs; using gauze and tape; cleaning wounds; applying therapeutic wraps; and operating braces and guards all become second nature.

Physical damage to the body, especially to the joints, is expected for football players during their sport's season. In fact, injuries to the tibiofemoral articulation (knee joint) commonly occur on the field of play and are assessed first by the athletic trainer.

INTRODUCTION

Movement of the body is made possible through the interaction of muscles and bones operating at an articulation. An articulation, or joint, is simply the union of two or more bones. Well-known articulations are the elbow, shoulder, foot, ankle, knee, hip, and vertebral column. Diagnosis of joint disease is made through patient history and physical examination, and laboratory and x-ray data provide supplemental assistance. Joint disorders result from autoimmune diseases, trauma, genetic influences, infection, and the aging process.

Articulations are classified according to the type of tissue that binds the bones together at each joint, the joint's function, or the amount of movement possible at the joint. Joints are designed to withstand stress placed on the body while providing leverage, stability, and balance assistance. Fibrous, cartilaginous, and synovial joints make various movements possible.

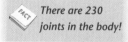

There are 230 joints in the body!

MEDICAL TERM PARTS

WORD PARTS

Medical term prefixes, suffixes, and combining forms related to articulations are introduced in this section.

Word Parts	Meaning
amph-, amphi-	both
ankyl-, ankylo-	bent, crooked
arthr-, arthro-	joint
capsul-, capsulo-	capsule
chondr-, chondri-, chondro-	cartilage
condyl-, condylo-	condyle (rounded part forming a moving joint)
-ectomy	surgical removal
hyal-, hyalo-	glassy, transparent, hyaline

Word Parts	Meaning
menisc-, menisco-	crescent-shaped meniscus (crescent-shaped cartilage disk)
orth-, ortho-	straight
-plasty	plastic surgery; shaping as a result of surgery
spondyl-, spondylo-	vertebra
sym-, syn-	together, with
tendo-, teno-	tendon
troch-, trocho-	round

WORD ETYMOLOGY

Some words have Greek or Latin word roots but are not true word parts. This section lists those that are used as medical terms.

Word	Definition
articulo	to articulate, come together
hallux	great toe
kinetosis	puncture
rheuma	a flux (fluid discharge)
ligamentum	band, ligament

MEDICAL TERM PARTS USED AS PREFIXES

Prefix	Definition
sym-, syn	together, with

MEDICAL TERM PARTS USED AS SUFFIXES

Suffix	Definition
-ectomy	surgical removal
-plasty	plastic surgery; shaping as a result of surgery

WORD GROUPING

Using the "Medical Term Parts" tables, identify the prefix, suffix, or combining form for each of the following definitions. The first one has been done as an example.

Definition	Word Part
round	troch-, trocho-
bent, crooked	

Definition	Word Part
both	
capsule	
cartilage	
condyle (rounded part forming a moving joint)	
crescent-shaped, meniscus (crescent-shaped cartilage disk)	
glassy, transparent, hyaline	
joint	
plastic surgery; shaping as a result of surgery	
straight	
surgical removal	
tendon	
together, with	
vertebra	

WORD BUILDING

Word parts, introduced in the "Medical Term Parts" section, are listed in the following table. For this exercise, first supply the meaning of each word part, then use the word part to build a word you already know. The word you list under "Common or Known Word" does not have to be a medical term; a commonly used word is fine. Be sure, however, that the word correctly reflects the intended meaning. The first one has been done as an example. Check your answers in a dictionary.

Word Part	Meaning	Common or Known Word	Example Medical Term
amph-, amphi-	both	amphibian	amphiarthrosis
arthr-, arthro-			arthroscopy
capsul-, capsulo-			joint capsule
-ectomy			bunionectomy
orth-, ortho-			orthopedics
sym-, syn-			syndesmoses
tendo-, teno-, tenon-			tendonitis

ANATOMY AND PHYSIOLOGY

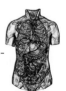

Structures of Articulations

- Articular cartilage
- Bursae
- Joint capsule

- Joints: fibrous, cartilaginous, and synovial
- Ligaments
- Menisci
- Tendons

Articulations Preview

An **articulation**, or joint, is a point of close contact between two or more bones. Articulations operate in concert with the musculoskeletal system. Joints make body movement, such as standing, sitting, and walking, possible. Articulations can be classified according to their function or structure, which determine the type of movement possible. Functional classification is based on the degree of movement and groups the joints as immovable, slightly movable, and freely movable. Structural classification is based on the presence or absence of a synovial cavity and the type of connective tissue found at the joint. Based on structure, articulations may be fibrous, cartilaginous, or synovial.

Ligaments, tendons, and cartilage are key component of joints. Cartilage is tough, white, nonvascular elastic tissue found throughout the body, notably at joints. The sheath of cartilage capping the ends of bones is called **articular cartilage** and serves to reduce friction and absorb shock. For example, between the femur and the tibia, the band of articular cartilage prevents the bone ends from rubbing together and absorbs the shock of walking.

Tendons are nondistensible (nonstretchy), fibrous cords that extend from muscle tissue to insert into bones. These conduits between muscle and bone facilitate motion at joints by attaching to articular structures.

 FACT *Tendons and ligaments have no direct blood supply, so they receive nutrients by diffusion!*

Key Terms	Definitions
articulation (ahr tick yoo LAY shun)	junction of two or more bones or skeletal parts
articular cartilage (ahr TICK yoo lur KAHR ti lij)	cartilage capping the ends of bones at a joint
tendons (TEN dunz)	fibrous bands of tissue at the end of muscles that attach to bone

Key Term Practice: Articulations Preview

1. The tough, fibrous connective tissue capping the ends of bones at joints is termed _____.

2. The term *articulation* means _____ between two bones.

Fibrous Joints

In the structural classification of joints is the type termed fibrous. **Fibrous joints** are found between bones coming into close contact with one another, such as the bones of the skull, between the teeth and jaw, and at the junction of the tibia (shin bone) and fibula (smaller lower leg bone). Structurally, the bones are fastened tightly together with a thin layer of fibrous connective tissue, and functionally, little or no appreciable movement occurs there. A synarthrosis joint is immovable, and an amphiarthrosis joint is slightly movable.

Three categories of fibrous joints exist: gomphoses, sutures, and syndesmoses. A type of joint in which a peg-shaped process fits into a bony socket is called a **gomphosis**

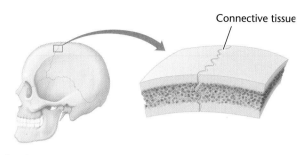

A Suture

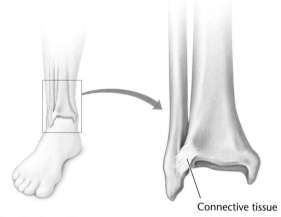

FIGURE 6-1
Fibrous joints. Two
types of fibrous joints
are (**A**) sutures and
(**B**) syndesmoses.

B Syndesmosis

joint. The articulation between the root of a tooth (peg-shaped process) and the jaw
(bony socket) is an example. **Sutures** are immovable joints. Sutures create seams in the
skull when the cranial bones ossify (Fig. 6-1). A **syndesmosis** is a type of joint in which
the bones are united by relatively long fibers of connective tissue. This type is seen at
the distal ends of the tibia and fibula, forming the tibiofibular articulation.

Key Terms	Definitions
fibrous (FIGH brus) **joints**	articulation made of fibrous connective tissue found between bones in close proximity
gomphosis (gom FOH sis)	synarthrosis joint such as a tooth in its socket
sutures (SUE churz)	joint type found in the skull in which the bones are bound together by fibrous connective tissue
syndesmosis (sin dez MOH sis)	articulation in which the bones are held together by fibrous connective tissue

Key Term Practice: Fibrous Joints

1. The medical term for tooth socket is _____.

2. What are the three classes of fibrous joints?

a. _____

b. _____

c. _____

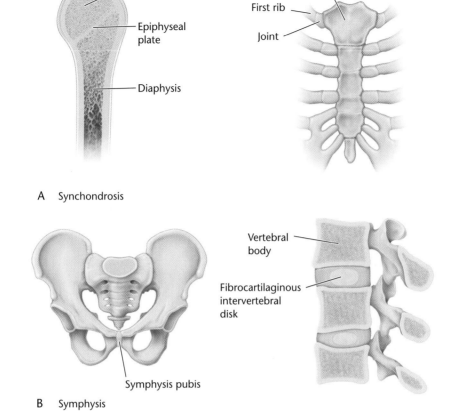

A Synchondrosis

B Symphysis

FIGURE 6-2
Cartilaginous joints. (**A**) Synchondroses and (**B**) symphyses are cartilaginous joints.

Cartilaginous Joints

Structurally, **cartilaginous joints** are composed primarily of nonvascular connective tissue (Fig. 6-2). Cartilaginous joints are either slightly movable (amphiarthroses) or immovable (synarthroses). Symphyses and synchondroses are types of cartilaginous joints. A **symphysis** is a slightly movable joint in which the bones are separated by a pad of fibrocartilage. An example is the **symphysis pubis**, the anterior union of the pubic bones, in the pelvic girdle. Another example is the joint formed by the bodies of two adjacent vertebrae, which are separated by an intervertebral disk. Each **intervertebral disk** is composed of an outer band of fibrous cartilage, called the **annulus fibrosus**, and an inner circle of soft gelatinous material, known as the **nucleus pulposus**. The term *annulus* means "ring-shaped part." The cores of the nucleus pulposus allow the disks to act as shock absorbers. Because each disk is slightly flexible, the combined movement of all of the joints in the vertebral column allows the limited motion that occurs when the back is bent forward or to the side or is twisted. These joints are classified as cartilaginous instead of fibrous because they do allow for some movement, whereas fibrous joints are basically nonmovable.

A type of joint in which the bones are united by bands of hyaline cartilage is called a **synchondrosis**. Hyaline is the transparent material making up the cartilage matrix. An example of this joint is the epiphyseal plate, where the epiphysis (end of a long bone) is joined to the diaphysis (shaft) of an immature long bone.

FACT Humans and giraffes have the same number of cervical vertebrae articulations!

Key Terms	Definitions
cartilaginous (kahr ti LAJ i nus) joints	articulations made of cartilage
symphysis (SIM fi sis)	a slightly movable joint

symphysis pubis (SIM fi sis PEW bis)	the fibrocartilaginous union of the pubic bones
intervertebral (in tur VUR te brul) disk	masses of fibrocartilage between adjacent vertebrae
annulus fibrosus (AN yoo lus figh BROH sus)	layer of fibrocartilage surrounding each intervertebral disk
nucleus pulposus (NEW klee us pul POH sus)	center of the intervertebral disk
synchondrosis (sing kon DROH sis)	joint in which the surfaces are connected by a cartilage plate

Key Term Practice: Cartilaginous Joints

1. The symphysis pubis is an example of a _____ joint.

2. Relative to the degree of movement, cartilaginous joints are _____ movable.

3. The word part *syn-* means _____; the word part _____ means cartilage; thus a *synchondrosis* is a joint whose surfaces are connected by _____.

Synovial Joints

Synovial joints are diarthroses, and most joints in the skeletal system are of this type. They are considered diarthroses because they are freely movable. Figure 6-3 illustrates the structures of synovial joints: articular cartilage, joint capsules, menisci, and a synovial membranes. The fibrous sheet enclosing a synovial joint is called the **joint capsule.** Joint capsules are reinforced by bundles of strong, tough, collagenous fibers

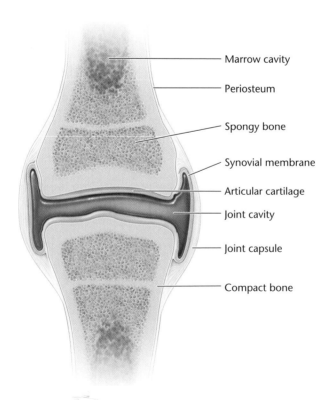

Marrow cavity

Periosteum

Spongy bone

Synovial membrane

Articular cartilage

Joint cavity

Joint capsule

Compact bone

FIGURE 6-3
Structures of a synovial joint.

called **ligaments.** The synovial membrane forms the inner lining of the capsule of a freely movable joint and surrounds a closed sac called the synovial (joint) cavity. The clear viscous fluid secreted by the synovial membrane is called synovial fluid. The functions of the fluid are to moisten and lubricate cartilaginous surfaces within the joint and help supply articular cartilage with nutrients obtained from the blood vessels of the synovial membrane.

Joints have several associated structures that lend support to their form and function. Ligaments help bind the articular ends of the bones together while preventing excess movement at the joint, and tendons attach muscle to bones. **Bursae** are sac-like, fluid-filled structures lined with synovial membrane that occur near a joint. They act as cushions and aid the movement of tendons that glide over bony parts or over other tendons.

Menisci are pieces of fibrocartilage that separate the articulating surfaces of bones in the knee, upper chest where the sternum meets the collar bone (sternoclavicular), and the shoulder (acromioclavicular) joints. They cushion the articulating surfaces and help distribute the body weight onto these surfaces.

Six types of synovial joints are found in the human body. The first type, the **ball-and-socket joint**, is located in the hip and shoulder. **Condyloid joints** are the articulations between the metacarpals (hand) and phalanges (fingers). **Gliding joints** are located at the wrists, ankles, and articular processes of vertebrae. **Hinge joints** are found at the elbows, knees, and phalanges. **Pivot joints** are located at the neck and proximal ends of the radius and ulna. The **saddle joint** is found between the carpal and metacarpal of the thumb.

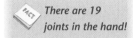 *There are 19 joints in the hand!*

Synovial joints permit several movements. Ball-and-socket joints allow motion and rotational movement in all planes. Condyloid joints allow motion in several planes, but not rotational movement. Back and forth movement is accomplished by gliding joints. The hinge joint has movement in one plane only, much like the hinge on a door. Rotation around a central axis is possible with pivot joints, and the saddle joint where the thumb meets the hand accommodates a variety of movements.

Key Terms	Definitions
synovial (si NOH vee ul) **joints**	freely movable articulations
joint capsule	fibrous sheet enclosing a freely movable joint
ligaments (LIG uh munts)	bands of tough, flexible fibrous connective tissue
bursa (BUR suh)	small sac lined with synovial membrane near a joint
meniscus (me NIS kus)	crescent-shaped wedge of fibrocartilage
ball-and-socket joint	rounded head of one bone fits in the concave surface of another
condyloid (KON di loid) **joints**	joints in which the oval surface of one bone fits into the elliptical surface of another
gliding joints	joints that allow only sliding movements
hinge joints	joins formed by two bones that move in a right angle
pivot joints	joints with rotational movement
saddle joint	thumb joint

Key Term Practice: Synovial Joints

1. Relative to movement, synovial joints are _____ movable.

2. What is the singular form of menisci?

   _____

3. The fibrous sheet enclosing a synovial joint is termed the _____.

4. What is the singular form of bursae?

   _____

Articulations Summary

Table 6-1 summarizes the three types of joint classifications, their functions, and their movements. The functional classification identifies the type of joint according to the degree of movement at that joint. The structural classification indicates the type of connective tissue within the articulation and designates whether a synovial cavity is present.

Selected Articulations

A selection of common body joints are introduced and described in more detail in this section. The medical terms for some of these articulations are provided.

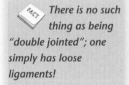

There is no such thing as being "double jointed"; one simply has loose ligaments!

Shoulder

Of all the joints, the **scapulohumeral joint** (shoulder) has the widest range of motion. Owing to the looseness of its attachments and its relatively large articular surface, this joint permits extensive flexibility. The joint itself consists of several stabilizing ligaments that allow movement.

Elbow

The elbow articulation consists of a hinge joint between the humerus and the ulna and a gliding joint between the humerus and the radius. Two ligaments associated with the elbow are the ulnar collateral and radial collateral. Movements possible at the

TABLE 6-1 Joint Classifications

Structural Classification	Functional Classification	Movement
fibrous	suture	synarthrosis (immovable)
	gomphosis	synarthrosis (immovable)
	syndesmosis	amphiarthrosis (slightly movable)
cartilaginous	synchondrosis	synarthrosis (immovable)
	symphysis	amphiarthrosis (slightly movable)
synovial	synovial cavity	diarthrosis (freely movable)

elbow joint are hinge movements, pronation (downward or backward motion), and supination (upward motion).

Hip

The **coxal joint** (hip) is held together by a ring of cartilage in the acetabulum and a joint capsule that is reinforced by ligaments. The articulating parts of the hip are held more closely together than those of the shoulder; thus there is less freedom of movement at the hip joint. Parts of the hip joint are the head of the femur and the cup-shaped acetabulum of the coxal bone, along with several ligaments.

Knee

The **tibiofemoral joint** (knee) is formed by the femur, patella, and tibia. Specifically, the parts of the knee joint are the medial and lateral condyles at the distal end of the femur, the patella, and the medial and lateral condyles at the proximal end of the tibia. The fibula is not involved. The tibia is attached to the femur by two ligaments found inside the joint capsule, the anterior cruciate ligament (ACL) and the posterior cruciate ligament (PCL). The term *cruciate* (KROO shee ayt) means "resembling a cross," and the ACL and PCL intersect in the knee to limit femur movement. Ligamentous injuries to the knee are common in athletes.

Key Terms	*Definitions*
scapulohumeral (skap yoo loh HEW mur ul) **joint**	pertaining to the scapula and humerus; shoulder joint
coxal (KOCK sul) **joint**	hip joint
tibiofemoral (tib ee oh FEM uh rul) **joint**	pertaining to the tibia and femur; knee joint

Key Term Practice: Selected Articulations

1. What is the medical term for each of the following joints?

   a. shoulder _____

   b. hip _____

   c. knee _____

Joint Movements

Articulations enable the body to perform a variety of actions. Specific terms are used to indicate these types of joint movements—for example, abduction, adduction, extension, flexion, and hyperextension (Fig. 6-4). Movement away from the body's midline is termed **abduction**, and movement toward the body's axis is **adduction**. An aid for learning the difference between *ab*duction and *ad*duction is to remember that if somebody is *ab*ducted, he is taken *away*.

Increasing the angle between two bones is referred to as **extension**, and decreasing the angle between two bones is **flexion**. Bringing the lower arm up to "flex" the upper arm muscles is an example of flexion. Moving the arm back to its original

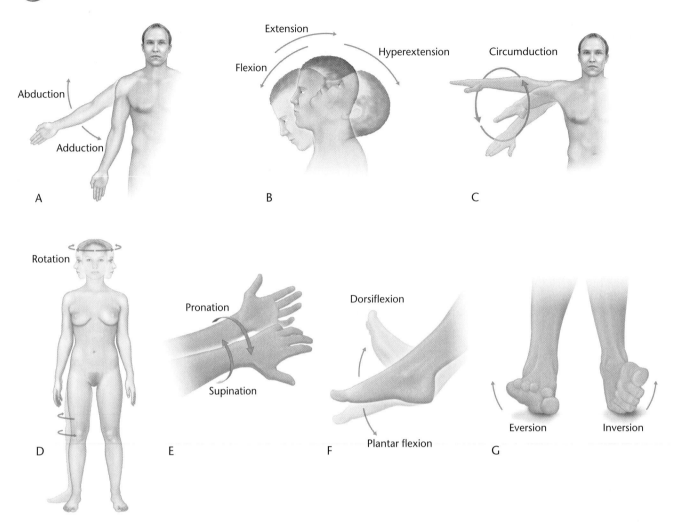

FIGURE 6-4
Movement at joints. Articulations enable the body to perform a variety of actions: (**A**) abduction and adduction; (**B**) hyperextension, extension, and flexion; (**C**) circumduction; (**D**) rotation; (**E**) pronation and supination; (**F**) dorsiflexion and plantar flexion; and (**G**) inversion and eversion.

position is extension. **Hyperextension** is excessive extension of a body part beyond the 180° angle of the anatomic position. Tilting the head back to look up at the sky is an example of hyperextension.

Circular movements are circumduction and rotation and are described as if the person were in the anatomic position. **Circumduction** is movement in a circular motion as when throwing a pitch. **Rotation** involves turning a bone on its own axis. The motion made while turning a key in a lock is a rotational movement.

Turning the palm posteriorly is termed **pronation,** and turning the palm anteriorly is called **supination.** Movement of the forearm into the anatomic position involves pronation. As a tip, associate the *p* in posterior with the *p* in pronation. Another clue is to think about the position of a waiter's hand when she's carrying a bowl of *soup* as the same position as *sup*ination.

Movement terms applied to foot and lower leg include dorsiflexion, plantar flexion, eversion, and inversion. **Dorsiflexion** describes the movement of bending the foot toward the tibia. The opposite of dorsiflexion, bending the foot away from the tibia and pointing the toe, is **plantar flexion.** Movement in which the sole of the foot is turned outward or laterally is **eversion,** and **inversion** is movement of the sole of the foot inward or medially.

Key Terms	Definitions
abduction (ab DUCK shun)	movement away from the body axis
adduction (ad DUCK shun)	movement toward the midline
extension	straightening out; making a flexed part straight
flexion (FLECK shun)	bending movement at a joint
hyperextension	overstraightening; overextending
circumduction (sur kum DUCK shun)	the proximal end is fixed while the distal end moves in a circle
rotation	turning around on an axis or fixed point
pronation (proh NAY shun)	turning the palm posteriorly or downward
supination (sue pi NAY shun)	turning the palm upward
dorsiflexion (dor si FLECK shun)	bending the foot so the toes move upward toward shin
plantar flexion (PLAN tahr FLECK shun)	bending the foot so the toes move downward
eversion (e VUR zhun)	turning outward
inversion (in VUR zhun)	turning inward

Key Term Practice: Joint Movements

1. Turning the head to the side to look out the car window is an example of what type of movement?

   _____

2. The opposite of abduction is _____.

THE CLINICAL DIMENSION

Pathology of Articulations

To treat patients with joint disease requires a complete history and physical examination. Pathological conditions of articulations are associated with musculoskeletal and connective tissue disorders. Articulation disorders may be the result of arthritis, autoimmune diseases, localized trauma, infection, or part of a greater systemic disease that can disturb joint function.

As with other signs and symptoms exhibited by the body, some are common to many dysfunctions, whereas others are specific to articulations. Edema, malaise, and fibrosis are common descriptions of a variety of homeostatic imbalances. Ankylosis, pannus, and synovitis are specific to joints. Clinical tests and diagnostic procedures supplement the history and physical examination of a patient with a joint disorder. Definitive diagnoses often require laboratory data and diagnostic tests.

Arthritis

Arthritis refers to several disorders characterized by inflammation of the joints, often accompanied by stiffness of adjacent structures. Mineral deposits (calcification) may form on bone tissue causing joint inflexibility.

Gouty arthritis, also called **gout**, is a condition in which sodium urate crystals are deposited in the soft tissues of joints, eventually destroying them. Gout affects feet joints, typically the first metatarsal joint of the great toe (hallux). Its cause is thought to be a metabolic or renal disorder. It generally appears in bouts with acute attacks. Signs and symptoms include pain, edema, fever, chills, and headache; however, the person is symptom free between attacks. Figure 6-5 illustrates the **edema** (swelling) associated with gout. The inflammation is the result of excessive fluid accumulation between the tissue cells. Typically, edema is the direct result of a damaged capillary that causes leakage into the surrounding tissue. Damage to a joint can produce localized swelling at the site of injury.

Arthrocentesis and radiographic studies aid in making the diagnosis. For diagnostic and/or therapeutic purposes it may be necessary to extract liquid from the synovial space. Puncturing the joint capsule with a needle to remove the fluid is termed **arthrocentesis**. Arthrocentesis is considered a treatment when the fluid is removed to reduce inflammation and is a diagnostic tool when the fluid is extracted for analysis. The presence of urate crystals in synovial fluid and hyperuricemia typically indicate gout. Treatment involves joint immobilization, ice to reduce edema, anti-inflammatory drugs, low-protein/high-fluid diet, and antihyperuricemic medications.

Lyme arthritis, also known as Lyme disease, is an infectious disease transmitted to humans from the bite of a tick infected with *Borrelia burgdorferi*. Signs and symptoms are overall malaise, flu-like symptoms, joint pain, and a target lesion. **Malaise** is the term for general weakness, fatigue, and discomfort, common symptoms of infection and autoimmune joint disorders. The disease mimics rheumatoid arthritis. Most cases are diagnosed on the basis of the clinical picture, but a definitive diagnosis is made through a positive blood antibody test identifying specific antibodies to the Lyme disease antigen. Treatment begins by removing the tick if still evident, followed by prompt administration of antibiotics. Unfortunately, symptoms may not appear for

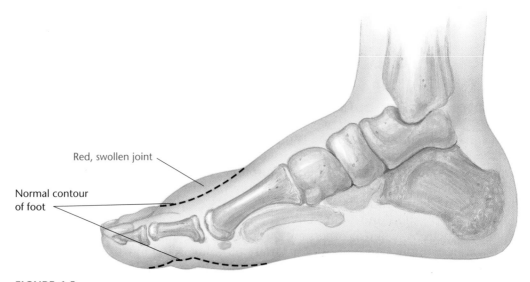

Red, swollen joint

Normal contour of foot

FIGURE 6-5

Gout is a condition in which sodium urate crystals are deposited in the soft tissues of joints, eventually destroying them. (Image provided by Anatomical Chart Co.)

weeks or months after infection. In individuals with a genetic predisposition to the disease, chronic arthritis generally develops. Untreated disease can progress to encephalitis, gastritis, and carditis. Vaccines are available to prevent initial infection, but human vaccines have deleterious side effects.

Osteoarthritis is an age-related degenerative joint disease (DJD) characterized by deterioration of articular cartilage and spur formation, which are bony outgrowths that develop around the joint (Fig. 6-6). Affecting mainly large, weight-bearing joints, this form of arthritis results from normal wear and tear on the articulations. It is characterized by articular cartilage deterioration and osteophyte formation. When the hands are involved, it primarily affects the distal interphalangeal (DIP) joints and

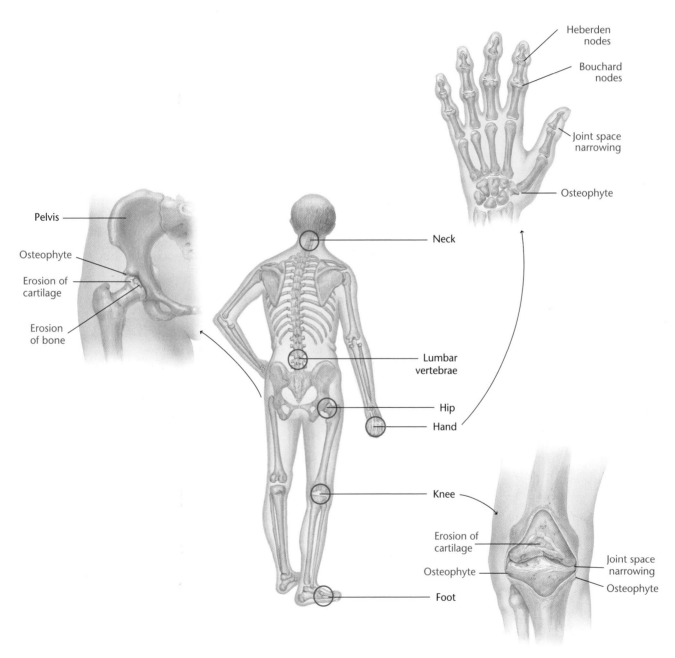

FIGURE 6-6
Joints affected by osteoarthritis. (Images provided by Anatomical Chart Co.)

some proximal interphalangeal (PIP) joints. Characteristic bony overgrowths forming knobby fingers on the DIP joints are termed Heberden nodes, and bony enlargements on the PIP joints are known as Bouchard nodules. Signs and symptoms include achiness and stiffness in the joints, deformity, and crepitus (crackling sound heard when bones rub together). It can be either a primary (main) or secondary (result of another disease) condition. Autoimmune factors may be involved. Diagnosis is made through the history and physical examination, computed tomography (CT) scan, and/or magnetic resonance imaging (MRI) scans. Treatment includes anti-inflammatory medicines, analgesics, and physical therapy (PT) to increase range of motion (ROM) at articulations. Total joint replacement (TJR) and arthrodesis are surgical options for severe cases. **Arthrodesis** is an operation in which the articular surfaces are removed and the articulating bones are surgically fused together.

Key Terms	Definitions
arthritis (ahr THRIGH tis)	joint inflammation
gouty arthritis (GOW tee ahr THRIGH tis)	metabolic disorder causing excessive uric acid production and deposition in joints, often in the great toe; gout
gout (gowt)	metabolic disorder causing excessive uric acid production and deposition in joints, often in the great toe; gouty arthritis
edema (e DEE muh)	swelling; tissue inflammation with fluid accumulation
arthrocentesis (ahr throh sen TEE sis)	incision or puncture into a joint capsule to extract synovial fluid
Lyme arthritis (lime ahr THRIGH tis)	joint inflammation as a result of the bite of a tick infected with *Borrelia burgdorferi*
malaise (mal AIZ)	general weakness, tiredness, and discomfort
osteoarthritis (os tee oh ahr THRIGH tis)	degenerative joint disease characterized by deterioration of articular cartilage and bone hypertrophy
arthrodesis (ahr throh DEE sis)	surgical joint fusion

Key Term Practice: Arthritis

1. What is the alternate term for gout?

   _____

2. What is the plural form for each given term?

   a. arthritis = _____

   b. edema = _____ and _____

   c. arthrocentesis = _____

Autoimmune Diseases

Autoimmune diseases are caused by the reaction of antibodies to naturally occurring substances in the body. Examples of autoimmune diseases affecting articulations are ankylosing spondylitis, rheumatoid arthritis, and systemic lupus erythematosus. **Ankylosing spondylitis** is a chronic, progressive inflammatory disease of the intervertebral spaces that causes abnormal fusion (growing together) of the vertebrae. The vertebral fusion results in a solid, inflexible spinal column. It can also affect the sacroiliac and costovertebral joints. Joint immobility or fixation is referred to as **ankylosis.** Ankylosis is a sign that there is some sort of joint disorder. Edematous joints, fibrosis, kyphosis, and osteoporosis characterize it. Abnormal thickening and scarring of fibrous connective tissue is called **fibrosis.** Fibrosis can also be a consequence of injury, infection, surgery, or lack of oxygen. Symptoms of ankylosing spondylitis include back pain and morning stiffness. It is marked by joint calcification, abnormal hardening caused by calcium salt deposits. Diagnosis is made through the physical examination, x-rays, and MRI evaluations. MRI uses electromagnetic radiation to obtain images of body tissues.

Treatment is supportive and includes physical therapy, acetylsalicylic acid (ASA; commonly known as aspirin), and nonsteroidal anti-inflammatory drugs (NSAIDs; pronounced EN saids). **Nonsteroidal anti-inflammatory drugs** are medicines such as ibuprofen and aspirin that have both analgesic and anti-inflammatory properties.

Rheumatism is the general term used to describe diseases of muscle, tendon, joint, or bone that share characteristics of musculoskeletal pain and stiffness. An example of a rheumatic disease is **rheumatoid arthritis** (RA), a chronic autoimmune disease causing nonspecific joint inflammation. It is a degenerative joint disease characterized by deterioration of articular cartilage and osteophyte formation. Remissions and exacerbations causing progressive damage are common. There is generally symmetrical inflammation of peripheral joints as well as the temporomandibular joint (TMJ). Hallmark signs and symptoms are malaise, synovitis, pannus, fibrosis, cartilage erosion, and ankylosis.

Synovitis means inflammation of the synovium. Synovial inflammation is the body's reaction to injury or infection. **Pannus** is granulation tissue forming from rheumatoid synovium that releases cartilage-destroying enzymes. Pannus is a true phenomenon that makes the inflammatory arthritides different from the post-traumatic or osteoarthritic "wearing away" forms of arthritis. Surgeons often operate to crudely remove pannus in an effort to save the articular cartilage. Be careful with the spelling of this term because the word *panus* describes an inflamed lymph node, something entirely different from the synovial membrane. Diagnosis is made through the history, physical examination, and analysis of synovial fluid. Rheumatoid factor (RF), an indication of the disease found by blood analysis, may or may not be present, making definitive diagnosis difficult. Treatment is supportive and includes rest during periods of flare-ups and physical therapy at other times. Anti-inflammatory analgesics such as ASA also prove beneficial.

A chronic inflammatory connective tissue disorder of unknown origin that affects primarily women, describes **systemic lupus erythematosus** (SLE). This disorder involves several systems because connective tissue is widely dispersed throughout the body. Articular symptoms are observed in 90% of cases of SLE and include arthralgia and polyarthritis. Early-stage SLE is difficult to differentiate from rheumatoid arthritis and other connective tissue disorders. Initial diagnosis is made by the clinical picture and confirmed by SLE antibody tests, which identify markers specific to SLE. Management of SLE depends on its manifestations and severity. Mild SLE is treated with NSAIDs and physical therapy; corticosteroids and immunosuppressive drugs that dampen the immune response are used to treat severe disease. **Corticosteroids** are used in the treatment of joint disorders to relieve swelling. These synthetic drugs are similar to the body's natural steroid hormones produced by the adrenal gland and are generally injected directly into the joint area to reduce inflammation.

Key Terms	Definitions
ankylosing spondylitis (ang i LOH sing spon di LYE tis)	fusion and inflammation of the vertebrae
ankylosis (ang i LOH sis)	joint immobility or fixation
fibrosis (figh BROH sis)	increase in fibrous connective tissue
nonsteroidal (non STEER oid ul) **anti-inflammatory drugs**	medicines that act against tissue inflammation
rheumatism (ROO muh tiz um)	general term for diseases characterized by musculoskeletal pain and stiffness
rheumatoid arthritis (ROO muh toid ahr THRIGH tis)	systemic disease characterized by articular and joint deformity
synovitis (sin oh VYE tis)	inflammation of the synovium
pannus (PAN us)	granulation tissue forming from synovium that releases cartilage-destroying enzymes
systemic lupus erythematosus (LEW pus er ih thee mah TOH sus)	inflammatory disease of the joints and internal organs
corticosteroids (kor ti koh STEER oidz)	synthetic drugs used to reduce inflammation

Key Term Practice: Autoimmune Diseases

1. With ankylosing spondylitis, the back will appear _____.

   a. flexible

   b. inflexible

2. Define the abbreviation *RA*.

   _____

3. What is the plural form of pannus?

   _____

Foot, Ankle, and Knee Disorders

Articular foot disorders are associated with cartilage, whereas extra-articular problems involve tendons, nerves, ligaments, or bones. A **bunion** is a bony protrusion from a metatarsophalangeal (MTP) joint (Fig. 6-7). When the great toe, hallux, is involved, it is termed **hallux valgus**, which literally means bending toward the lateral side of the foot. The condition is associated with flat-footedness and rheumatoid arthritis. Signs and symptoms are pain and joint displacement. Diagnosis is made by physical examination and radiographic studies. Treatment options include analgesics, intra-articular corticosteroid injections, and **bunionectomy.**

Hallux rigidus is a degenerative MTP joint disorder in which articular cartilage at the joint deteriorates, causing bone tissue to rub against other bone tissue. Without the cartilaginous cap to prevent friction, the bone abrasion causes pain, stiffness, and

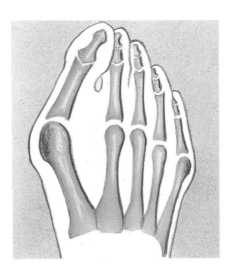

FIGURE 6-7
A bunion is a bony protrusion from a metatarsophalangeal joint. (Image provided by Anatomical Chart Co.)

swelling. Since there is limited range of motion, the toe is rigid, hence the term *rigidus* in its description. The history, physical examination, and radiographic studies confirm the diagnosis. Conservative treatment includes NSAIDs and wearing low-heeled, good-fitting shoes. Depending on severity, cheilectomy, arthrodesis, and arthroplasty are surgical options. The surgical removal of osteophytes and degenerative changes by chiseling away at the bony irregularities is termed **cheilectomy.** Severe trauma, disease, or joint deterioration may necessitate the reconstruction or creation of an artificial joint. This is called **arthroplasty** (Fig. 6-8).

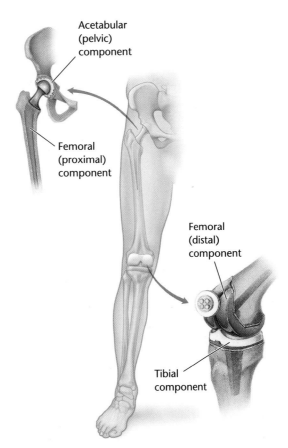

Acetabular (pelvic) component

Femoral (proximal) component

Femoral (distal) component

Tibial component

FIGURE 6-8
Arthroplasty. Arthroplastic surgery includes the reconstruction of a joint and implantation of an artificial joint, such as a hip or knee replacement. (Images provided by Anatomical Chart Co.

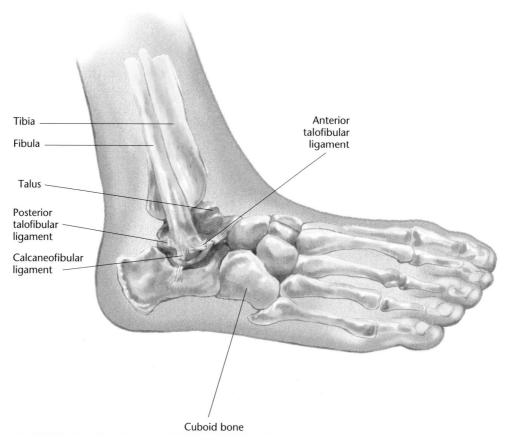

Tibia

Fibula

Talus

Posterior
talofibular
ligament

Calcaneofibular
ligament

Anterior
talofibular
ligament

Cuboid bone

FIGURE 6-9
A sprain is a painful injury to the ligaments of a joint, caused by wrenching or overstretching.
(Image provided by Anatomical Chart Co.)

A **sprain** is a painful injury to the ligaments of a joint caused by wrenching or over-stretching. The ankle is a common site for sprain (Fig. 6-9). Signs and symptoms of mild to moderate sprain include tenderness, swelling, and difficulty moving the joint. Complete ligamentous tears cause swelling and hemorrhage. Treatments for mild to moderate sprains are immobilization and strapping with elastic bandages, followed by light exercise of the affected part. Severe sprains may require cast immobilization or surgery.

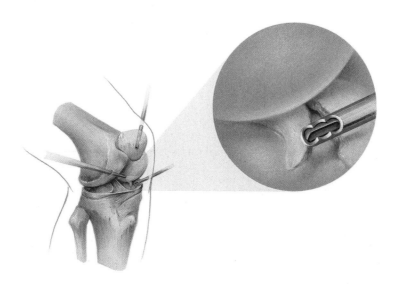

FIGURE 6-10
Arthroscopy. The interior of a joint can be inspected with an arthroscope, or fiberoptic camera. (Image provided by Anatomical Chart Co.)

Tearing of the medial and lateral knee menisci is termed a **torn meniscus.** The ACL of the knee is often involved. It is characterized by acute pain, crepitus, and flexion impairment. The injury is usually sports related and caused by twisting or external rotation while the knee is flexed. Physical examination, x-ray, MRI, or arthrography confirms the diagnosis. Treatment involves arthroscopic surgery and physical therapy. Visual inspection of the joint interior using an **arthroscope** (fiberoptic camera) is termed **arthroscopy** (Fig. 6-10). To obtain an image of the joint interior, **arthrography** may be performed. This involves obtaining a radiograph of the joint space after it has been injected with a contrast medium. Clinicians use these tests to assess the extent of damage, if any, in an articulation.

Key Terms	Definitions
bunion (BUN yun)	swelling of a metatarsophalangeal joint
hallux valgus (HAL ucks VAL gus)	a deformity at the metatarsophalangeal joint that forces the great toe toward the other toes
bunionectomy (bun yun ECK tuh mee)	excision of a bunion
hallux rigidus (HAL ucks RIJ i dus)	limited range of motion at the first metatarsophalangeal joint
cheilectomy (kye LECK toh mee)	chiseling away of bony outgrowths that interfere with joint mobility
arthroplasty (AHR throh plas tee)	joint removal with replacement by artificial joints or prostheses
sprain	stretched ligaments caused by wrenching the joint
torn meniscus (me NIS kus)	meniscus abnormality
arthroscope (ahr THROH skope)	fiberoptic instrument used to view a joint's interior
arthroscopy (ahr THROS kuh pee)	insertion of a fiberoptic lens called an arthroscope directly into the joint for visual examination
arthrography (ahr THROG ruh fee)	x-ray of the joint space after introduction of a contrast medium

Key Term Practice: Foot, Ankle, and Knee Disorders

1. A _____ is a swelling at the metatarsophalangeal joint.

2. Hallux _____ describes the toe deformity resulting in an adducted great toe, whereas hallux _____ refers to a stiff great toe.

3. Ripping of the crescent-shaped cartilage disk as a result of twisting the knee is termed a _____.

4. Arthrography involves the use of _____.

   a. x-rays

   b. sonograms

5. _____ is the medical term to describe joint reconstruction.

Wrist Disorders

Carpal tunnel syndrome is caused by unceasing pressure on the median nerve passing through the tunnel in carpal bones (Fig. 6-11). It results from repetitive movements of the hands and wrists and is characterized by numbness, weakness, and tingling. The physical examination and a positive Tinel's sign are generally enough to diagnose the condition. For the **Tinel's sign test**, the patient's arms are outstretched while the clinician taps the inside affected wrist over the median nerve with a reflex hammer. If the person experiences a "pins and needles" sensation, he or she has tested positive for carpal tunnel syndrome. Treatment involves physical therapy, splinting, or surgery that divides the carpal ligament to relieve median nerve pressure.

A **ganglion** is a benign growth filled with colorless fluid arising from the joint capsule or tendon sheath. Ganglia commonly develop on the wrist. The underlying cause is not known, but fortunately they are painless, creating only an unsightly bump. Diagnosis is made by palpation and needle aspiration. Treatment often is not necessary because they disappear on their own. When treatment is warranted, a needle aspiration to reduce the ganglion's size or a **ganglionectomy** may be performed.

FIGURE 6-11
Carpal tunnel syndrome is caused by constant pressure on the median nerve passing through the tunnel in the carpal bones. (Image provided by Anatomical Chart Co.)

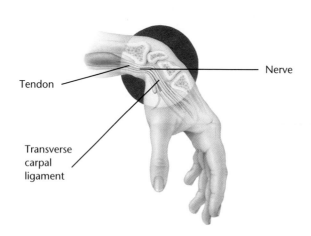

Nerve

Tendon

Transverse carpal ligament

Key Terms	Definitions
carpal (KAHR pul) **tunnel syndrome**	wrist affliction caused by pressure on the median nerve in the carpal bones
Tinel's (tee NELZ) **sign test**	test to assess carpal tunnel syndrome
ganglion (GANG glee un)	cystic localized growth in or around a tendon sheath or joint capsule
ganglionectomy (gang glee un ECK tuh mee)	excision of a ganglion

Key Term Practice: Wrist Disorders

1. Removal of a ganglion is termed _____.

2. What is the plural form of ganglion?

_____

Trauma

Bursitis is an acute or chronic inflammation of the bursae. Signs and symptoms are pain, tenderness, edema, and limited ROM. It results from overuse injuries such as those occurring in tennis players and baseball pitchers whose bursae are subjected to excessive friction. Calcified deposits form in advanced disease. Diagnosis is made through the history and physical examination, ROM as measured by a goniometer, x-rays, and MRI studies.

Articular disorders usually restrict movement. To determine the severity of the joint disease, ROM data are gathered and assessed. To evaluate the flexibility and angle of movement in a joint, the clinician may use an instrument called a **goniometer** (Fig. 6-12). A goniometer is calibrated in degrees to measure the angle of movement at a joint. Treatment of joint diseases involves moist heat, immobilization, NSAIDs, and corticosteroid injections to reduce inflammation. Surgery or aspiration (suction withdrawal) to remove calcified deposits may be necessary.

A **dislocation**, or **luxation**, is a displacement of a bone from its normal joint position. A partial dislocation is called a **subluxation.** It is usually caused by trauma or a sports injury. Typically, the affected joint has an abnormal appearance, is immobile, and shows signs of edema; the patient generally complains of pain. Diagnosis is made through history and physical examination and is confirmed by x-ray. Treatment involves joint reduction (surgical or manipulative procedures) to return the bones to their normal position. Recurring problems may require surgery to tighten the associated joint ligaments.

A **herniated disk** occurs when the center of the intervertebral disk, known as the nucleus pulposus, protrudes through the surrounding fibrocartilage (Fig. 6-13).

Chondromalacia is cartilage softening as a result of strenuous activity or an overuse injury. Athletes generally experience cartilage erosion on the undersurface of the knee joint, which is known as chondromalacia patella. The primary symptom is pain when climbing stairs. Mild forms are treated with rest, isometric exercise, and ice application. Arthroscopic surgery to shave the underside of the patella or to remove excessive tissue may be necessary.

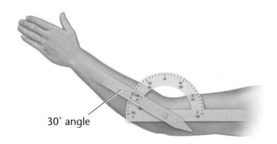

30° angle

FIGURE 6-12
A goniometer is used to measure degree of joint movement.

Key Terms	Definitions
bursitis (bur SIGH tis)	inflammation of a bursa
goniometer (goh nee OM uh tur)	instrument used to measure degree of joint movement
dislocation	displacement of a joint; luxation

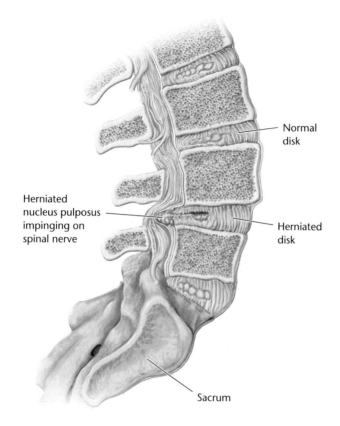

Normal
disk

Herniated
nucleus pulposus
impinging on
spinal nerve

Herniated
disk

FIGURE 6-13
In a herniated disk,
the center of the disk
protrudes through
the surrounding
fibrocartilage and
into the intervertebral
space.

Sacrum

luxation (luck SAY shun)	displacement of a joint; dislocation
subluxation (sub luck SAY shun)	incomplete dislocation
herniated (HUR nee ate ed) disk	condition in which the center of an intravertebral disk protrudes through the fibrocartilage
chondromalacia (kon droh muh LAY shuh)	cartilage softening

 ## Key Term Practice: Trauma

1. Give the medical term for each of the following terms.

    a. dislocation _____

    b. partial dislocation _____

2. _____ is the medical term for bursa inflammation.

3. This instrument is used to measure the degree of movement at a joint.

    _____

CLINICAL TERMS

Clinical Dimension	Term	Description
DISORDERS		
	ankylosing spondylitis	fusion and inflammation of the vertebrae
	ankylosis	joint immobility or fixation
	arthritis	joint inflammation
	bunion	swelling of a metatarsophalangeal joint
	bursitis	inflammation of a bursa
	carpal tunnel syndrome	wrist affliction caused by pressure on the median nerve in the carpal bones
	chondromalacia	cartilage softening
	dislocation	displacement of a joint; luxation
	ganglion	cystic localized growth in or around a tendon sheath or joint capsule
	gout	metabolic disorder causing excessive uric acid production and deposition in joints, often in great toe; gouty arthritis
	gouty arthritis	metabolic disorder causing excessive uric acid production and deposition in joints, often in great toe; gout
	hallux rigidus	limited range of motion at the first metatar sophalangeal joint
	hallux valgus	a deformity at the metatarsophalangeal joint that forces the great toe into adduction
	herniated disk	condition in which the center of an intravertebral disk protrudes through the fibrocartilage
	luxation	displacement of joint; dislocation
	Lyme arthritis	joint inflammation as a result of the bite of a tick infected with *Borrelia burgdorferi*
	osteoarthritis	degenerative joint disease characterized by deterioration of articular cartilage and bone hypertrophy
	rheumatoid arthritis	systemic disease characterized by articular and joint deformity
	rheumatism	general term for diseases characterized by musculoskeletal pain and stiffness
	sprain	stretched ligaments caused by wrenching the joint
	subluxation	incomplete dislocation
	systemic lupus erythematosus (SLE)	autoimmune inflammatory disease of the joints and internal organs
	torn meniscus	meniscus abnormality

Clinical Dimension	Term	Description
SIGNS AND SYMPTOMS		
	ankylosis	joint immobility or fixation
	edema	swelling; tissue inflammation with fluid accumulation
	fibrosis	increase in fibrous connective tissue
	malaise	general weakness, tiredness, and discomfort
	pannus	granulation tissue forming from synovium that releases cartilage-destroying enzymes
	synovitis	inflammation of the synovium
CLINICAL TESTS AND DIAGNOSTIC PROCEDURES		
	arthrography	x-ray of the joint space after introduction of a contrast medium
	arthroscope	fiberoptic instrument used to view a joint's interior
	arthroscopy	insertion of a fiberoptic lens called an arthroscope directly into the joint for visual examination
	goniometer	instrument used to measure degree of joint movement
	Tinel's sign test	test to assess carpal tunnel syndrome
TREATMENTS		
	anti-inflammatory analgesic aspirin	aspirin; acetylsalicylic acid (ASA)
	arthrocentesis	incision or puncture into a joint capsule to extract synovial fluid
	arthrodesis	surgical joint fusion
	arthroplasty	joint removal with replacement by artificial joints or prostheses
	bunionectomy	excision of a bunion
	cheilectomy	chiseling away of bony outgrowths that interfere with joint mobility
	corticosteroids	synthetic drugs used to reduce inflammation
	ganglionectomy	excision of a ganglion
	nonsteroidal anti-inflammatory drugs (NSAIDs)	medicines that act against tissue inflammation

Lifespan

In the fetus, infant, and child, articulations develop along with their corresponding skeletal tissues. Joints and bones are both derived from embryonic mesenchymal tissue.

With the exception of congenital defects, autoimmune diseases, and injuries affecting articulations, joint disorders generally do not appear until advanced age. Congenital articular disorders possibly resulting from intrauterine positioning include hip and knee dislocation. However, joint abuse as a result of overtraining or traumatic exercise can lead to early degenerative diseases or dysfunction. Surgery on articular tissue is also known to hasten the onset of generalized arthritis.

As one ages, fibrous protein strands of collagen form differently, resulting in decreased tissue elasticity and increased joint stiffening. Osteoarthritis appears to be a normal function of aging, and individuals aged 70 years and beyond typically exhibit some degree of degenerative joint disease. Fortunately, with the use of anti-inflammatory drugs coupled with life-long range of motion exercises, arthritis does not have to be totally debilitating.

In the News: Lyme Arthritis

In November 1975, Lyme arthritis, also known as Lyme disease, was first observed in the United States in the towns of Lyme and Old Lyme, Connecticut. The story of its identification is interesting. A woman in the town of Lyme decided to keep a personal journal to track the disease when she realized that neighbors in her community were exhibiting common symptoms of malaise, a bull's-eye-centered rash, and severe joint pain. Between June and September of that same year, 59 cases were observed. Eventually, rheumatologist Dr. Allen Steere and his research group affiliated with Yale University traced the bizarre finding to a tick-borne bacterial infection.

Two years later, the deer tick *Ixodes scapularis* was identified as the vector of disease transmission (Fig. 6-14). It was not until 1982 that Dr. Willy Burgdorfer of the National Institutes of Health discovered that the disease was caused by a bacterium living inside the tick. Today, that microbe is known as *Borrelia burgdorferi*.

Just 10 years later, Lyme arthritis was the most commonly reported tick-borne illness in the continental United States. The disease became a reportable disease (one that must be detailed to public health officials) in 1987. Media coverage in 1988 made the disease more well known; and in 1991, federal funding for research became available.

The cycle of disease transmission to humans involves bacteria, ticks, deer, and tick bites. Ticks normally feed on deer, and the bacteria are often harbored in deer ticks. Deer do not become ill when bitten by affected ticks but spread the ticks to humans in deer habitat areas such as woods and fields. The disease is spread to humans who

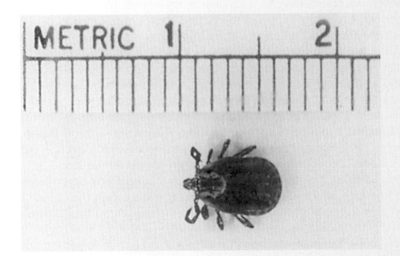

FIGURE 6-14
A deer tick.

are bitten by an infected tick. It is not known for certain whether there has actually been a dramatic spread of the disease or if better diagnosis of the disease has created the impression of increased numbers. The disease has now appeared in nearly every state, and precautions should be taken to avoid contracting it.

COMMON ABBREVIATIONS

Abbreviation	Term
ACL	anterior cruciate ligament
ASA	acetylsalicylic acid (aspirin)
CPR	cardiopulmonary resuscitation
CT	computed tomography
DIP	distal interphalangeal
DJD	degenerative joint disease
MRI	magnetic resonance imaging
MTP	metatarsophalangeal
NSAIDs	nonsteroidal anti-inflammatory drugs
PCL	posterior cruciate ligament
PIP	proximal interphalangeal
PT	physical therapy
RA	rheumatoid arthritis
RF	rheumatoid factor
ROM	range of motion
SLE	systemic lupus erythematosus
TJR	total joint replacement
TMJ	temporomandibular joint

Case Study

Justin Miller is a wide receiver on his college football team. A conscientious athlete, he has strictly adhered to his conditioning plan, which includes weightlifting four times per week, practice six days per week, and nutritious meals. Justin began playing tackle football in grade school. Since that time he has sustained no serious sports-related injuries.

During a Saturday afternoon game, Justin took an unusually hard hit from behind. Justin heard a "crunch" sound and thought something must have "popped." While he lay immobile on the field, Paul, the athletic trainer, rushed to his side. Justin was conscious, able to talk, and had little difficulty moving his extremities. Two other players assisted Justin to his feet. While standing erect, Justin experienced excruciating pain radiating from his cervical and lumbar regions. He also had slight pain while walking.

On the sidelines, the athletic trainer assessed Justin's physical strength, range of motion, and balance, which were unremarkable in all joints except the cervical and lumbar spine and the left tibiofemoral. Joint tenderness was evident in these areas, and edema was noted in the patellar region. Tibiofemoral flexion was slight, and complete extension was not possible. Extension and flexion at the coxal articulation caused considerable pain. Paul administered a therapeutic dosage of an NSAID and recommended that Justin undergo radiographic studies.

Case Study Questions

Select the best answer to each of the following questions.

1. **During his assessment of Justin's injuries, Paul noted edema at the _____.**
   a. knee
   b. shin
   c. hip
   d. neck

2. **The tibiofemoral joint is also known as the _____ joint.**
   a. shoulder
   b. hip
   c. knee
   d. elbow

3. **Normal tibiofemoral joint movements include _____.**
   a. flexion
   b. extension
   c. hyperextension
   d. A and B

4. **NSAIDs were administered to _____.**
   a. reduce swelling
   b. relieve pain
   c. assist with the cartilage growth
   d. A and B

5. **The cervical and lumbar regions refer to the _____.**
   a. head and neck
   b. shoulder and leg
   c. neck and lower back
   d. lower back and knee

6. **Radiographic studies involve the use of _____.**
   a. magnetic fields
   b. sound waves
   c. x-rays
   d. sonograms

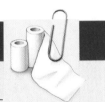

REAL WORLD REPORT

CENTRAL IMAGING DEPARTMENT

NAME:	Justin Miller
DATEORD:	06/06/2003
ORDPHYS:	M. A. Johnson, MD
DOB:	10/13/1983
TEST:	Lumbar, routine, 6 views
ATTENDING:	G. G. Timmons, MD
REFERRING:	D. Brindly, MD
CLINIC:	SM
EXAM DATE:	09/13/2003

CLINICAL INFORMATION: Back pain; injured in football game.

LUMBAR SPINE
Multiple views of the lumbar spine were obtained and show no fracture or subluxation. There is moderate degenerative disk narrowing at L5–S1, which shows degenerative vacuum phenomenon. No spondylolysis or spondylolisthesis is shown.

IMPRESSION
1. No fracture.
2. Moderate degenerative disk narrowing and degenerative vacuum phenomenon at L5–S1.

CERVICAL SPINE
Multiple views of the cervical spine were obtained and show no fracture or subluxation. The intervertebral disk spaces and neuroforamina are maintained. The prevertebral soft tissues are unremarkable.

IMPRESSION
No fracture or subluxation.

TIBIOFEMORAL
Multiple views of the knee were obtained and show no fracture or subluxation. Effusion is evident.

IMPRESSION
No fracture or subluxation.

DICTATED BY: Jack D. O'Henry, MD
This document has been reviewed and electronically approved by Jack D. O'Henry, MD 09/14/03

REAL WORLD REPORT QUESTIONS

The following exercises review the medical terms used in the preceding medical report. Two terms may be unfamiliar: *Vacuum phenomenon* means that there is a stripe on an intervertebral disk that becomes apparent on an x-ray. The word *vacuum* is a misnomer because gas is actually present, and the stripe is a sign of disk degeneration. *Prevertebral tissue* refers to the fascia and muscles on the anterior aspect of the vertebral column.

1. Degenerative disk narrowing was noted. The term *disk* refers to _____.

   a. the vertebral lamina

   b. vertebrae

   c. the intervertebral pad of cartilage

   d. the spinal column

2. *Degenerative disk narrowing* means _____.

   a. the intervertebral disks are showing deterioration

   b. there is bone damage

   c. the vertebrae are normal

   d. a subluxation is present

3. Subluxation refers to a/an _____.

   a. fracture

   b. strain

   c. dislocation

   d. abrasion

4. The report referred to spondylolysis.

   a. The word part *spondylo-* means _____.

   b. The word part *lys-* means _____.

   c. Thus *spondylolysis* means _____.

5. The report referred to spondylolisthesis.

   a. The word part *spondylo-* means _____.

   b. The word part *–esis* means _____.

   c. Thus *spondylolisthesis* means _____.

6. The report referred to neuroforamina. The word part *neuro-* means "nerve or nerve tissue," and the word *foramen* means "opening."

   a. What is the plural form of foramen? _____

   b. Thus *neuroforamina* means _____.

REVIEW AND APPLICATION: THREE-LEVEL LEARNING SYSTEM

LEVEL ONE: REVIEWING FACTS AND TERMS USING RECALL

Select the best response to each of the following questions.

1. The combining form *arthro-* means _____.
   a. anthropology
   b. anthrax
   c. cartilage
   d. joint

2. The combining form *chondro-* means _____.
   a. anthropology
   b. anthrax
   c. cartilage
   d. joint

3. Articulations are classified according to _____.
   a. structure
   b. function
   c. position
   d. A and B

4. Synarthrosis means that the joint bones are _____.
   a. close together
   b. far apart
   c. freely movable
   d. none of these

5. A suture is a type of _____ joint.
   a. fibrous
   b. freely movable
   c. diarthrosis
   d. hematopoietic

6. The symphysis pubis is a type of _____ joint.
   a. gomphotic
   b. cartilaginous
   c. intervertebral
   d. gomphotic and cartilaginous

7. Synovial joints are _____ movable.
   a. not
   b. slightly
   c. freely
   d. somewhat

8. The thumb joint is an example of a _____ joint.
   a. ball-and-socket
   b. saddle
   c. pivot
   d. hinge

9. The alternate name for the knee joint is the _____ joint.
   a. tibiofemoral
   b. tibiopatellar
   c. fibulofemoral
   d. fibulopatellar

10. Fluid-filled sacs in a synovial joint are termed _____.
    a. vursae.
    b. bursae.
    c. menisci.
    d. capsules.

Match the movement with its correct definition.

_____ 11. extension   a. movement away from the midline

_____ 12. abduction   b. increasing the angle between bones

273

_____ 13. pronation   c. turning inward

_____ 14. plantar   d. turning palm
       flexion   downward

_____ 15. inversion   e. pointing toes

Match the sign or symptom with its correct definition.

_____ 16. ankylosis   a. inflammation of
                          synovium

_____ 17. synovitis   b. granulation tissue in
                          synovium

_____ 18. pannus   c. joint fixation

_____ 19. malaise   d. general fatigue

LEVEL TWO: REVIEWING CONCEPTS

Select the best response to the following question.

20. This disease is caused by the bite of a tick infected with _Borrelia burgdorferi_.

    a. Legionnaire's disease

    b. West Nile virus

    c. Lyme arthritis

    d. kennel cough

For each of the following directional terms, what term has the opposite meaning?

21. adduction / _____

22. pronation / _____

23. flexion / _____

24. eversion / _____

25. supination / _____

Fill in the blanks: Use the correct bone terms to complete each of the following statements.

26. The _____ and _____ along with the patella make up the hinge joint at the knee.

27. The _____, _____, and _____ make up the hinge joint at the elbow.

28. The _____ and _____ make up the ball-and-socket joint at the shoulder.

29. The _____ and _____ make up the ball-and-socket joint at the hip.

Match the synovial joint with its type.

_____ 30. ankle   a. hinge

_____ 31. proximal   b. gliding
          radius

_____ 32. fingers   c. pivot

Match the condition with its key characteristics.

_____ 33. hallux   a. autoimmune disease;
          rigidus   deterioration of
                          articular cartilage;
                          degenerative joint
                          disease

_____ 34. ankylosing   b. degenerative joint
          spondylitis   disease affecting the
                          great toe

_____ 35. rheumatoid   c. fusion and
          arthritis   inflammation of
                          vertebrae

Define the following abbreviations.

36. PCL _____

37. DIP _____

38. MTP _____

39. ACL _____

40. NSAIDs _____

Identify the correctly spelled term in each set.

41. _____

    a. pannus

    b. pannis

    c. panis

    d. pannes

42. _____

    a. ankalosis

    b. ankylosis

    c. ankyelosis

    d. anckylosis

43. _____

    a. burcitis

    b. bursitis

    c. bursitus

    d. bersitus

44. _____

    a. lucksation

    b. luxashun

    c. luxtion

    d. luxation

45. _____

    a. rheumatizm

    b. rumatism

    c. rheumatism

    d. rhumatizm

46. _____

    a. abduction

    b. abducsion

    c. abduckshun

    d. abbducshun

Provide a medical term to complete a meaningful analogy.

47. Dislocation is to luxation as joints are to _____.

48. Subluxation is to partial dislocation as great toe is to _____.

LEVEL THREE: THINKING CRITICALLY

Write a short answer to each of the following questions.

49. What types of movement are possible at the scapulohumeral joint?

    _____

    _____

    _____

50. Which articulation is also known as the glenohumeral joint?

    _____

51. Mike is playing in a football game. The pigskin is thrown directly at him, but slightly above his head. He plants his feet firmly to the ground, twists, and extends his arms to make the catch. As he is making this tremendous play, an opposing player hits him on the anterior knee and tackles him. After the down, Mike experiences acute pain and has difficulty walking. Identify a possible knee injury, and cite the bones that make up the tibiofemoral articulation.

    _____

    _____

    _____

KEY TERMS SPELLING TEST FROM CD-ROM

Use the CD-ROM to test yourself on the spelling of key terms from this chapter. Listen to the terms and write them on a separate sheet of paper. Use a medical dictionary to check your answers.

ANSWERS

WORD GROUPING

Definition	Word Part
round	troch-, trocho-
bent, crooked	ankyl-, ankylo-
both	amph-, amphi-
capsule	capsul-, capsulo-
cartilage	chondr-, chondri-, chondro-
condyle (rounded part forming a moving joint)	condyl-, condylo-
crescent-shaped meniscus (crescent-shaped cartilage disk)	menisc-, menisco-
glassy, transparent, hyaline	hyal-, hyalo-
joint	arthr-, arthro-
plastic surgery; shaping as a result of surgery	-plasty
straight	orth-, ortho-
surgical removal	-ectomy
tendon	tendo-, teno-
together, with	sym-, syn-
vertebra	spondyl-, spondylo-

WORD BUILDING

Word Part	Meaning	Common or Known Word	Example Medical Term
amph-, amphi-	both	amphibian	amphiarthrosis
arthr-, arthro-	joint	arthritis	arthroscopy
capsul-, capsulo-	capsule	capsule	joint capsule
-ectomy	surgical removal	appendectomy	bunionectomy
orth-, ortho-	straight	orthodontist	orthopedics
sym-, syn-	together, with	synergy	syndesmoses
tendo-, teno-	tendon	tendon	tendonitis

KEY TERM PRACTICE

Articulations Preview
1. articular cartilage
2. point of contact or junction

Fibrous Joints
1. alveolus
2. a. gomphoses; b. sutures; c. syndesmoses

Cartilaginous Joints
1. cartilaginous
2. slightly
3. together; chondro-; cartilage

Synovial Joints
1. freely
2. meniscus
3. joint capsule
4. bursa

Selected Articulations
1. a. scapulohumeral; b. coxal; c. tibiofemoral

Joint Movements
1. rotation
2. adduction

Arthritis
1. gouty arthritis
2. a. arthritides; b. edemas; edemata; c. arthrocenteses

Autoimmune Diseases
1. b
2. rheumatoid arthritis
3. panni

Foot, Ankle, and Knee Disorders
1. bunion
2. valgus; rigidus
3. torn meniscus
4. a
5. Arthroplasty

Wrist Disorders
1. ganglionectomy
2. ganglia

Trauma
1. a. luxation; b. subluxation
2. Bursitis
3. goniometer

CASE STUDY

1. a is the correct answer.
   - b is incorrect because that region is tibial or crural.
   - c is incorrect because that region is coxal.
   - d is incorrect because that region is cervical.
2. c is the correct answer.
   - a is incorrect because the shoulder joint is known as the scapulohumeral or glenohumeral joint.
   - b is incorrect because the hip joint is also known as the coxal joint.
   - d is incorrect because the elbow joint is also known as the humeroulnar joint.
3. d is the correct answer.
   - c is incorrect because hyperextension is not a normal knee joint movement and would indicate a disorder.
4. d is the correct answer.
   - c is incorrect because NSAIDs do not assist with cartilage growth.
5. c is the correct answer.
   - a is incorrect because the head and neck regions are called cranial and cervical.
   - b is incorrect because the shoulder region is called acromial, femoral describes the upper leg, and tibial refers to the lower leg.
   - d is incorrect because the lumbar region describes the lower back and the patellar region describes the knee.
6. c is the correct answer.
   - a is incorrect because magnetic fields are used in MRI studies.
   - b is incorrect because sound waves are used for ultrasound.
   - d is incorrect because sonograms are the images obtained from ultrasonography.

REAL WORLD REPORT

1. c
2. a
3. c
4. a. vertebra; b. lysis, destruction; c. degeneration or destruction of a vertebra
5. a. vertebra; b. condition or process; c. a condition of the vertebra. Specifically, it refers to forward movement of a lumbar vertebra centrum on the vertebra below it.
6. a. foramina; b. the openings through which the spinal nerves pass

REVIEW AND APPLICATION: THREE-LEVEL LEARNING SYSTEM

Level One: Reviewing Facts and Terms Using Recall

1. d
2. c
3. d
4. a
5. a
6. b
7. c
8. b
9. a
10. b
11. b
12. a
13. d
14. e
15. c
16. c
17. a
18. b
19. d

Level Two: Reviewing Concepts

20. c
21. abduction
22. supination
23. extension
24. inversion
25. pronation
26. femur; tibia
27. radius; ulna; humerus
28. scapula; humerus
29. femur; acetabulum of coxal bone
30. b
31. c
32. a
33. b
34. c
35. a
36. posterior cruciate ligament
37. distal interphalangeal
38. metatarsophalangeal
39. anterior cruciate ligament
40. nonsteroidal anti-inflammatory drugs
41. a
42. b
43. b
44. d
45. c
46. a
47. articulations
48. hallux

Level Three: Thinking Critically

49. abduction, adduction, circumduction, rotation, pronation, and supination
50. scapulohumeral joint
51. Mike may have a torn meniscus or an injury to his ACL or PCL. Bones comprising the tibiofemoral joint include the femur, patella, and tibia.

chapter 7

Muscular System

OBJECTIVES

After completing this chapter, you should be able to:

1. State the meanings of word parts related to the muscular system.
2. State components of muscle tissue and the key characteristics of each muscle type.
3. Describe the underlying premise behind naming muscles.
4. Identify common superficial and deep muscles and their locations.
5. List the common signs, symptoms, and treatments of various muscular system diseases.
6. Explain clinical tests and diagnostic procedures related to the muscular system.
7. Describe anatomical and physiological alterations of muscles throughout the lifespan.
8. List common abbreviations related to the muscular system.
9. Define terms used in medical reports involving muscles
10. Correctly define, spell, and pronounce the chapter's medical terms

Professional Profile: Physical Therapist

Cindy is a licensed physical therapist (PT) who works in private practice. In addition to her master of science (MS) degree in physical therapy, she also holds a doctor of philosophy (PhD) in biomechanics. Physical therapy programs in the United States are now all master's level courses because the bachelor of science (BS) degree has been phased out of existence in these programs. A strong science background is critical to acceptance into a PT program. Once admitted to a program, coursework includes classes in biology, chemistry, physics, biomechanics, neuroanatomy, and gross anatomy.

A physical therapist evaluates and provides treatment to people who have been disabled by injury, pain, disease, physical condition, or medical procedure. PTs restore function, improve mobility, and relieve pain by nonsurgical methods, using physiotherapy. For example, after undergoing a sports injury or fracture repair, a patient often requires physical therapy to regain normal function.

While working in the field for more than 10 years, Cindy has encountered a vast array of musculoskeletal disorders, including those requiring postsurgery rehabilitation. This practice employs a physical therapy assistant (PTA), who works closely under the PT's guidance. The PTA prepares patients for treatment and performs selected therapeutic and evaluative tests.

A major focus of physical therapy is to help patients regain function, develop new physical skills, and enhance their quality of life. A PT undertakes many tasks in the course of his or her practice. The duties of a typical workweek include evaluating patients using appropriate tests and clinical observation, developing individual treatment plans, discussing patient goals, and prescribing therapeutic activities. Therapy programs, which are devised for individual patients, range from exercise and massage to yoga and myofascial release.

A fair amount of client interaction deals with instruction. A PT must also develop the necessary skills to plan and implement a therapy program to match the needs of each patient. In addition, a PT must be able to convey information effectively in both oral and written communication and must maintain accurate, detailed records and documentation.

INTRODUCTION

There are more than 700 muscles in the body, which are responsible for moving the body's framework, maintaining posture, producing heat, and assisting lymph transport. Approximately 40% of a person's weight is attributed to muscle mass, although this percentage can be much higher in trained athletes and body builders. Muscles are arranged in layers; superficial muscles form the surface landmarks easily identified when viewing exposed skin, and deep muscles are visible by dissection or imaging techniques.

Muscles are often considered with the skeletal system; hence the term *musculoskeletal* is used to denote the interaction of bones with muscles. Three types of muscle tissue exist within the body, each with specific locations. All muscular movement is made possible through nervous impulses that act on the tissue, causing contraction, another term for muscle fiber shortening. Muscles, tendon, ligaments, bones, and nerves work in concert to achieve optimal functioning.

Key alterations related to the muscular system are considered in this chapter. Pathological conditions result from infection, trauma, inheritance, or tumors or are secondary to (the result of some other) existing disease. Age-related disorders greatly depend on physical activity level.

MEDICAL TERM PARTS

Medical term prefixes, suffixes, and combining forms related to the muscular system are introduced in this section.

Word Parts	Meaning
brachi-, brachio-	arm, brachial
brachy-	short
bucco-	cheek, mouth
cardi-, cardio-	heart, cardiac
fascio-	fascia
fibr-, fibro-	fiber
kin-, kine-, kino-	movement
kinesi-, kinesio-	movement
kinet-, kineto-	movement
-lemma	sheath, envelope
muscul-, musculo-	muscle
my-, myo-	muscle
peroneo-	pertaining to fibular side of leg
plat-, platy-	flat, broad
pterygo-	wing shaped
rhabd-, rhabdo-	striated
sarc-, sarco-	muscle, flesh
skelet-, skeleto-	skeleton, skeletal
tendo-, teno-	tendon
-troph, troph-, tropho-	nutrition, nourishment

WORD ETYMOLOGY

Some words have Greek or Latin word roots but are not true word parts. This section lists those that are used as medical terms.

Word	Definition
brevis	short
bucca	cheek
femur	thigh
gloutos	buttock
pteron	wing, feather
pteryx	wing
rectur	straight

Word	Definition
teres	round, smooth
vastus	great

MEDICAL TERM PARTS USED AS PREFIXES

Prefix	Definition
brachy-	short
bucco-	cheek, mouth
fascio-	fascia
peroneo-	pertaining to fibular side of leg
pterygo-	wing shaped

MEDICAL TERM PARTS USED AS SUFFIXES

Suffix	Definition
-lemma	sheath, envelope
-troph	nutrition, nourishment

WORD GROUPING

Using the "Medical Term Parts" tables, identify the prefix, suffix, or combining form for each of the following definitions. The first one has been done as an example.

Definition	Word Part
arm, brachial	brachi-, brachio-
cheek, mouth	
fascia	
flat, broad	
fiber	
heart, cardiac	
movement	A. B. C.
muscle	A. B.
muscle, flesh	
nutrition, nourishment	
pertaining to fibular side of leg	
sheath, envelope	

Definition	Word Part
short	
skeleton, skeletal	
striated	
tendon	
wing, wing shaped	

WORD BUILDING

Word parts, introduced in the "Medical Term Parts" section, are listed in the following table. For this exercise, first supply the meaning of each word part, then use the word part to build a word you already know. The word you list under "Common or Known Word" does not have to be a medical term; a commonly used word is fine. Be sure, however, that the word correctly reflects the intended meaning. The first one has been done as an example. Check your answers in a dictionary.

Word Part	Meaning	Common or Known Word	Example Medical Term
muscul-, musculo-	muscle	muscular	musculoskeletal
cardi-, cardio-			cardiomyopathy
skelet-, skeleto-			musculoskeletal
tendo-, teno-			tendonitis

ANATOMY AND PHYSIOLOGY

Structures of the Muscular System

- Muscle cells
- Muscle fibers
- Muscle tissue
- Sarcolemma
- Sarcoplasm

Muscular System Preview

The key characteristic of muscles is their ability to contract when stimulated by nerves to produce movement. When a nerve impulse travels to muscle tissue, it excites the muscle to contract, which is accomplished through the functioning of several structures. **Muscle cells** are called **muscle fibers** because of their thread-like appearance; the terms can be used interchangeably. **Muscle tissue** consists of fibers covered by **sarcolemma**, which is a plasma membrane. **Sarcoplasm** is the name given to the cytoplasm found in a muscle fiber.

Key Terms	*Definitions*
muscle cells	muscle fibers

muscle fibers	muscle cells
muscle tissue	tissue composed of contractile fibers
sarcolemma (sahr koh LEM uh)	sheath surrounding muscle cell
sarcoplasm (SAHR koh plaz um)	intercellular material of a muscle cell

Key Term Practice: Muscular System Preview

1. What is the alternate name for muscle cell?

   _____

2. Which type of tissue is made of contractile fibers?

   _____

3. The word part *sarc-* or *sarco-* means _____ and the word part *-lemma* means _____; thus the word _____ is the sheath or envelope surrounding the muscle cell.

Muscle Fiber

An individual muscle fiber has many parts (Fig. 7-1). As noted earlier, the sarcolemma is the outer cell membrane of a muscle fiber, and the sarcoplasm is the cytosol within a muscle fiber. **Myofibrils** are contractile fibers within muscle; they resemble threads running through muscle tissue. These strands contain contractile proteins that enable the muscle to contract and relax. Sets of myofibrils make up the sarcomere segments of striated muscle. **Sarcomeres** are the structural and functional units of the myofibril that cause the muscle to shorten (contract).

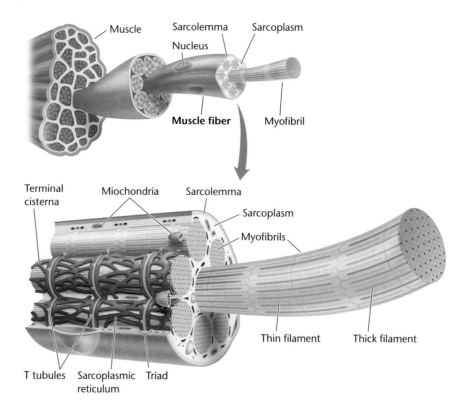

FIGURE 7-1
Muscle fiber structure.

Key Terms	Definitions
myofibrils (migh oh FIGH brilz)	filaments in muscle cytoplasm
sarcomeres (SAHR koh meers)	contractile segment of skeletal muscle tissue

Key Term Practice: Muscle Fiber

1. Contractile segments of muscle tissue are called _____.

2. The word part *my-* or *myo-* refers to _____, and the word part *fibr-* means "fiber"; thus _____ are filaments in muscle cytoplasm.

Muscle Tissue: Skeletal, Smooth, and Cardiac

The three types of muscle tissue are skeletal, smooth, and cardiac. Each has specific characteristics and functions within the body. **Skeletal muscle** is so named because it attaches to the skeletal system (bones) by tendons and provides movement (Fig 7-2). It is also called striated muscle because it has a striped appearance when viewed under the microscope. This muscle type is under voluntary control, giving it its alternate name of voluntary tissue. Skeletal muscle contracts and relaxes rather rapidly, in contrast to smooth muscle.

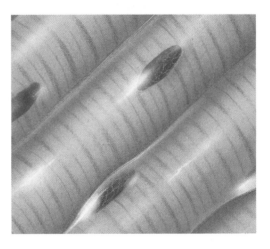

FIGURE 7-2
Skeletal or striated muscle. (Image provided by Anatomical Chart Co.)

Located in the viscera (organs), **smooth muscle** tissue is nonstriated and is involuntarily controlled (Fig. 7-3). Smooth muscle is so named because under a microscope it lacks the stripes of skeletal muscle. Hollow organs and blood vessels are lined with smooth muscle, which contracts and relaxes relatively slowly to permit the rhythmic squeezing action of these structures.

Peristalsis is the term describing rhythmic waves of muscular contractions that occur in the walls of various tubular organs. Through peristaltic actions, contents are moved through the intestines, urine is moved from the kidneys to the urinary bladder, and blood is forced through peripheral vessels outside the heart.

Cardiac muscle tissue is found only in the heart and permits the constant pumping action necessary for circulation (Fig. 7-4). Its appearance is striated, yet it is involuntary muscle. Cardiac fibers are characterized by striated cells, joined end to end, that release large quantities of calcium ions. Cardiac muscle contraction is unique because the fibers contract as a rhythmic unit, are self-stimulated, and remain refractory (unresponsive to neural stimulation) until the contraction is completed.

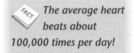

The average heart beats about 100,000 times per day!

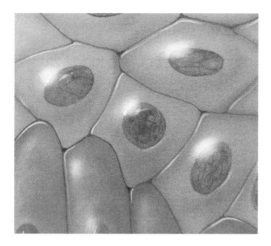

FIGURE 7-3
Smooth muscle lines organs and blood vessels. (Image provided by Anatomical Chart Co.)

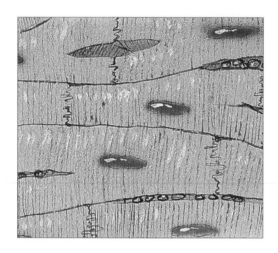

FIGURE 7-4
Cardiac muscle. (Image provided by Anatomical Chart Co.)

Band-like masses of white fibrous connective tissue that attaches muscles to bones are called **tendons**. **Aponeuroses** are sheet-like tendons by which certain muscles are attached to other body parts. An aponeurosis often attaches muscles to other muscles.

Fascia is a sheet of fibrous connective tissue that encloses muscle tissue and separates their layers. Fasciae associated with muscle tissue are deep, subcutaneous, and subserous. Deep fascia surrounds and penetrates the muscles, and subcutaneous fascia lies just beneath the skin. Subserous fascia forms the connective tissue layer of the serous membranes covering organs in various body cavities.

Key Terms	Definitions
skeletal muscle	muscle associated with the skeleton
smooth muscle	muscle in viscera walls and blood vessels
peristalsis (perr i STAHL sis)	progressive waves of contraction
cardiac muscle	heart muscle
tendons (TEN dunz)	fibrous bands or cords attaching muscle to bone or muscle to other body parts
aponeuroses (ap oh new ROH seez)	tendon sheets
fascia (FASH uh)	fibrous tissue between muscles that forms sheaths

Key Term Practice: Muscle Tissue: Skeletal, Smooth, and Cardiac

1. The word part *cardi-* or *cardio-* means _____; thus _____ tissue is found in the heart.

2. What is the singular form of *aponeuroses*. _____

3. What is the plural form of *fascia*._____

4. The term for rhythmic, wave-like contractions that propel food through the digestive tract is _____.

Muscle Movement

Muscles produce movement by pulling on bones. The end of the muscle that is attached to a relatively immovable part is the **origin.** Origins are attached to stationary bone and do not move when contraction occurs. The **insertion** is the end of the muscle that is attached to a movable part. When contraction occurs, the insertion does move. One muscle typically produces movement in one direction, and another muscle produces movement in the opposite direction. An example of the opposing actions of two different muscles on the same body part is seen in the arm: The biceps brachii muscle flexes the arm, whereas the triceps brachii extends the arm. The bones serve as levers, and the joints serve as supporting structures called fulcrums. Levers (bones) pivot about a fulcrum (joint) to move one end (insertion) by applying force to the other (origin). The three types of levers are shown in Figure 7-5.

Contraction is a complicated event; it occurs within the musculature and requires a motor neuron (nerve cell that excites a muscle) and a muscle fiber. **Neuromuscular (NM) junctions** are sites of union between a motor neuron axon (segment carrying an impulse) and a muscle fiber (Fig. 7-6). Motor end plates are the specialized portions of a muscle fiber membrane found at a neuromuscular junction. Neurotransmitters, which play an important role at the junctures, are chemical substances secreted by the terminal end of an axon that stimulate a muscle fiber contraction or an impulse in another neuron. **Acetylcholine** (ACh) is an important neurotransmitter involved in the nerve impulse transmission to muscle tissue.

To elicit a nerve impulse for a muscle contraction, a particular level of stimulation, known as a threshold stimulus, must be exceeded. Contraction of a muscle fiber results from a sliding movement within the myofibrils in which filaments containing the contractile proteins actin and myosin merge. Much of the heat produced in the body is a byproduct of skeletal muscle contraction. Whenever muscles are active, heat is released. This heat is then transported to other tissues via blood.

All the muscle cells controlled by a single motor neuron are referred to as a motor unit. The fewer the muscle fibers in a motor unit, the finer the movements that can be produced by that muscle. For example, human eyes have fewer than 10 muscle fibers per motor unit, whereas back muscles may have 100 or more.

Adenosine triphosphate (ATP) and creatine phosphate (CP) are chemicals necessary for muscle movement. ATP supplies the energy for muscle fiber contraction. CP, which can be used to synthesize ATP as it decomposes, is an energy-storing substance present in muscle tissue. Active muscles depend on the energy-producing process known as cellular respiration because the amount of ATP and CP present in skeletal muscle is not sufficient to support maximal muscle activity for more than a few seconds. For normal muscle functioning, cellular respiration requires an adequate supply of oxygen. Critical oxygen is carried from the lungs to body cells by hemoglobin in erythrocytes (red blood cells). **Myoglobin,** a molecule resembling hemoglobin, takes oxygen from the blood and releases it to muscles.

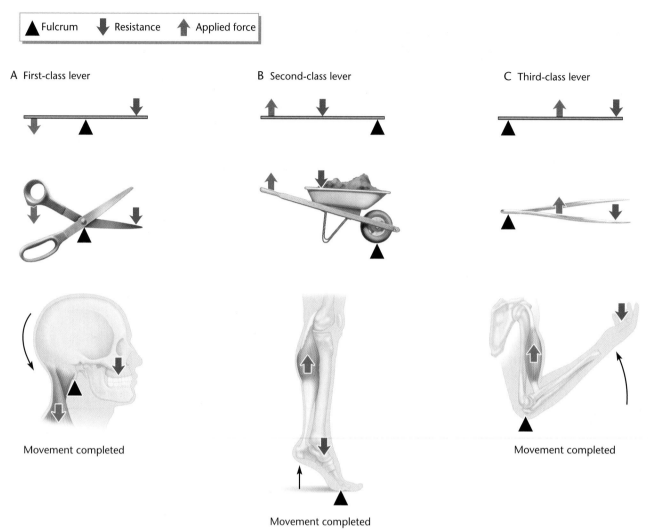

FIGURE 7-5
Three types of levers.

Muscle fatigue occurs when a muscle loses its ability to contract. This results from an interruption of blood supply to the muscle, lack of acetylcholine, or an accumulation of lactic acid as a result of anaerobic respiration. Anaerobic respiration occurs in cells when there is an inadequate oxygen supply. It is interesting to note that trained athletes produce less lactic acid than nonathletes during exercise because the strenuous activity of physical training stimulates new capillary growth within muscles, allowing more oxygen and nutrients to be supplied to the muscle fibers.

Muscle relaxation involves calcium ions (CA^{2+}) and the sarcoplasmic reticulum (SR). The SR is the storage and release site of CA^{2+} in a muscle fiber. After CA^{2+} has been released for muscle contraction, the SR reabsorbs the calcium, thereby halting the contraction process.

 Humans have the same biting force as a shark!

Key Terms	Definitions
origin	muscle end that remains fixed during contraction
insertion	muscle end that moves during contraction
neuromuscular (new roh MUS kew lur) **junctions**	myoneural junctions

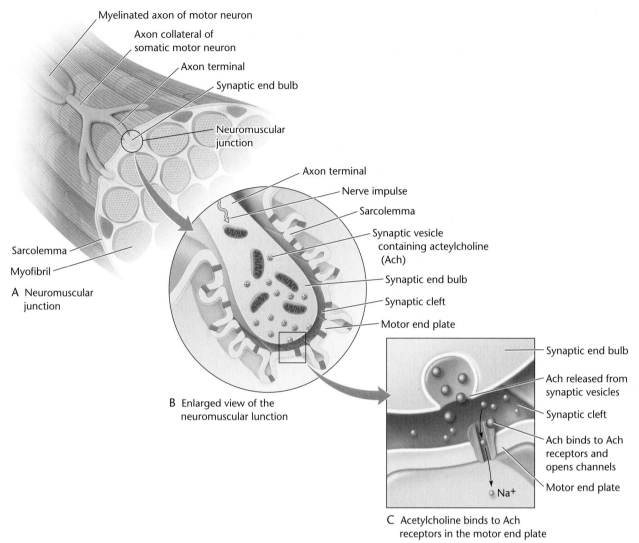

Myelinated axon of motor neuron
Axon collateral of somatic motor neuron
Axon terminal
Synaptic end bulb
Neuromuscular junction

Sarcolemma
Myofibril

A Neuromuscular junction

Axon terminal
Nerve impulse
Sarcolemma
Synaptic vesicle containing acetylcholine (Ach)
Synaptic end bulb
Synaptic cleft
Motor end plate

B Enlarged view of the neuromuscular lunction

Synaptic end bulb
Ach released from synaptic vesicles
Synaptic cleft
Ach binds to Ach receptors and opens channels
Na⁺
Motor end plate

C Acetylcholine binds to Ach receptors in the motor end plate

FIGURE 7-6
Neuromuscular junctions.

acetylcholine (as e til KOH leen)	chemical involved in nerve impulse transmission
adenosine triphosphate (uh DEN oh seen trye FOS fate)	energy source for cells
myoglobin (MIGH oh gloh bin)	muscle hemoglobin; myohemoglobin

Key Term Practice: Muscle Movement

1. The _____ is the immovable muscle attachment, and the _____ moves during a muscle contraction.

2. If *globin* means "protein," *hem-* refers to "blood," and *myo-* means "muscle," then _____ is a blood protein in muscle.

3. Muscle cell energy is supplied in the form of _____.

Muscle Tone

Even when a muscle is not producing movement, enough motor units are stimulated to cause tension. This resting tension is called **muscle tone** and is achieved through sustained contraction of portions of skeletal muscle. Muscle tone is essential for posture and balance.

Atrophy is a term describing muscle tissue wasting as a result of disuse, ischemia (inadequate blood supply to tissue), or nutritional deficiencies. The opposite of atrophy is **hypertrophy**, or enlargement of muscle tissue. Hypertrophic muscles are seen in well-defined body builders. Engaging in repetitive weight-bearing exercises causes muscle tissue to enlarge because more blood and nutrients are delivered to the fibers in response to the greater workload demands.

Key Terms	Definitions
muscle tone	muscle integrity achieved through active contraction of some fibers
atrophy (AT roh fee)	physiological or pathologic reduction in muscle size
hypertrophy (high PUR troh fee)	increase in size

Key Term Practice: Muscle Tone

1. Muscle tension that does not produce movement is termed _____.

2. Exercising with weights will cause muscle _____, or an increase in tissue mass.

Naming Skeletal Muscles

The names of skeletal muscles are based on several factors, such as location, fiber direction, size, number of origins (heads), shape, location of insertion, action, and point of attachment. The names of very small muscles may contain the word *minimi*, and of very large muscles, the word *vastus*. Names indicating a muscle's shape include terms for broad, narrow, long, tapering, short, blunt, triangular, quadrilateral, irregular, flat sheets, or bulky masses. Many muscles have Latin names related to size, function, appearance, or shape.

Action names correspond to directional movements of the muscle. For example, there are abductors, adductors, extensors, and flexors. **Abductors** are muscles that pull a limb away from the midline, and **adductors** pull the limb toward the body's axis. Muscles that straighten or extend an appendage are termed **extensors**, and muscles that bend an appendage at a joint are termed **flexors**. Table 7-1 lists the names and functions of common superficial skeletal muscles. Figure 7-7 locates the muscles in the body.

Key Terms	Definitions
abductors (ab DUCK turz)	muscles that draw a body part away from the axis when contracted
adductors (a DUCK turz)	muscles that draw a body part toward the median when contracted

TABLE 7-1 Selected Superficial Muscles and Functions

Muscle	Functions
adductor longus (a DUCK tur LONG us)	adducts hip; flexes and medially rotates leg
adductor magnus (a DUCK tur MAG nus)	adducts hip; flexes and rotates leg
biceps brachii (BYE seps BRAY kee eye)	supinates forearm; flexes forearm
biceps femoris (BYE seps FEM o ris)	part of hamstring muscle group; moves leg
brachialis (bray kee AY lis)	flexes forearm
brachioradialis (BRAY kee oh ray dee AY lis)	flexes forearm
buccinator[a] (BUK si nay tur)	muscle of smiling; compresses cheeks; involved in mastication (chewing)
corrugator[b] supercilii (kor uh GATE ur sue per SIL ee)	draws eyebrows together to frown
diaphragm[c] (DYE uh fram)	enlarges thoracic cavity
deltoid (DEL toid)	abducts upper arm
epicranius (ep i KRAY nee us)	raises eyebrows, as expression of surprise
external oblique	compresses abdomen; aids in posture
frontalis (frun TAY lis)	raises eyebrows
gastrocnemius (gas trock NEE mee us)	plantar flexion
gluteus maximus (gloo TEE us MACK si mus)	extends thigh
gluteus medius (gloo TEE us MEE dee us)	abducts thigh
gracilis (GRAS i lis)	adducts thigh; flexes and adducts leg
hamstring group	flexes leg; composed of biceps femoris, semimembranosus, and semitendinosus
iliopsoas (il ee oh SOH us)	flexes thigh
infraspinatus (in fruh spye NAY tus)	laterally rotates shoulder
intercostal (in tur KOS tul)	contracts and relaxes rib cage
internal oblique	compresses abdomen
latissimus dorsi (la TIS i mus DOR see)	extends and adducts upper arm
levator ani (le VAY tur AY nigh)	operates with coccygeus muscles
masseter[d] (ma SEE tur)	involved in mastication (chewing)
occipitalis (ock sip i TAL is)	retracts and tenses scalp
opponens pollicis (op OH nenz POL i sis)	pulls thumb across palm to enable finger touching
orbicularis oculi (or bick yoo LAIR is OCK yoo lye)	closes eyelid
orbicularis oris (or bick yoo LAIR is OR is)	compresses lips
pectoralis (peck toh RAH lis) major	pulls arm forward and across chest
pectoralis (peck toh RAH lis) minor	moves scapula against thorax
platysma (pla TIZ muh)	stretches neck from chest to face
pronator teres (proh NAY tur TEER eez)	medial arm rotation
pterygoid[e] (TEER i goid)	involved in opening and closing the jaw; grates teeth during mastication (chewing)

(continues)

TABLE 7-1 **Selected Superficial Muscles and Functions** *(continued)*

Muscle	Functions
quadriceps (KWAH dri seps) group	extends leg; composed of rectus femoris, vastus intermedius, vastus lateralis, and vastus medialis
rectus abdominis (RECK tus ab DOM i nis)	flexes trunk
rectus femoris (RECK tus FEM o ris)	thigh movement
rotator cuff	rotates arm; composed of supraspinatus, infraspinatus, teres minor, subscapularis
rhomboideus (rom BOY dee us) major	raises and adducts scapula
sartorius (sahr TOH ree us)	flexes knee; rotates hip
semimembranosus (sem ee mem bruh NOH sus)	flexes knee; extends and rotates hip
semitendinosus (SEM ee ten di NOH sus)	flexes knee; extends and rotates hip
soleus (SOH lee us)	plantar flexion
splenius capitis (SPLEE nee us KAP i tus)	pulls head into an upright position
sternocleidomastoid[f] (ster noh klye doh MAS toid)	flexes head; prayer muscle
sternohyoid (ster noh IGH oid)	depresses hyoid bone and larynx
subscapularis (sub SKAP yoo lahr ris)	medially rotates shoulder
supinator (SUE pi nay tur)	supinates forearm
supraspinatus (sue pruh spye NAY tus)	abducts shoulder
temporalis (tem poh RAY lis)	closes jaw
teres (TEER eez) major	extends, adducts, and medially rotates shoulder
teres (TEER eez) minor	rotates arm laterally
tibialis (tib ee AY lis) anterior	inverts foot
trapezius (tra PEE zee us)	shrugs shoulders
transversus abdominis (trans VUR sus ab DOM i nis)	compresses abdomen; aids in posture
triceps brachii (TRYE seps BRAY kee eye)	extends forearm
vastus intermedius (VAS tus in tur MEE dee us)	extends knee
vastus lateralis (VAS tus lat ur AL is)	extends knee
vastus medialis (VAS tus mee dee AL is)	extends knee
zygomaticus (zye goh MAT i kus)	draws corner of mouth upward

[a] This muscle is sometimes called the trumpeter muscle because it enables blowing action.

[b] The word *corrugator* is derived from *corrugatus,* meaning "wrinkled," as in a corrugated box.

[c] Watch the spelling of this word; note the silent *g.*

[d] The word *mastication* means "to chew"; hence, this muscle is involved in that action.

[e] The word *pteryx* is Greek for "wing," and the pterygoids are wing-shaped muscles. Think of the winged dinosaur the pterodactyl. Also note that *pt* is pronounced as a "tee."

[f] The origins of this muscle are on the sternum and clavicle, and the insertion is on the mastoid process of the temporal bone; thus, the name sternocleidomastoid.

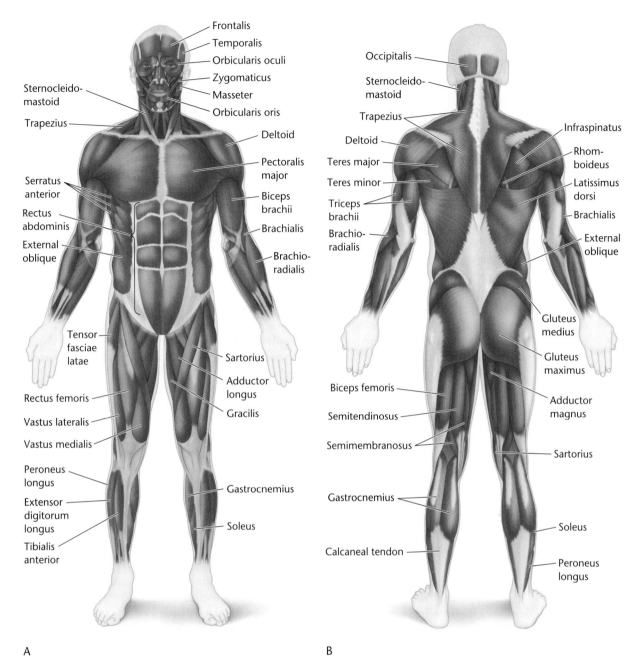

FIGURE 7-7
Anterior (**A**) and posterior (**B**) views of the superficial muscles.

| **extensors** (eck STEN surz) | muscles that extend or stretch a limb or part |
| **flexors** (FLECK surz) | muscles that bend or flex a limb or part |

Key Term Practice: Naming Skeletal Muscles

1. _____ are muscles that would cause the biceps brachii to bulge while "making a muscle."

2. These muscles enable one to lift the legs laterally. _____

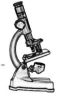

THE CLINICAL DIMENSION

Pathology of the Muscular System

Signs of muscle disorder are often evident during a physical examination and may provide clues to underlying neurologic pathology. Muscle pain and weakness are common symptoms of muscular system disorders. Terms describing signs and symptoms of the muscular system are commonly built from the combining form *my-* or *myo-*. Medical terms pertaining to muscles and tendons often are built from the combining form *fibr-* or *fibro-*, which refers to fiber.

Muscle disorders usually result from trauma, tumor, immune disorder, improper nerve conduction, inheritance, or infection. The following sections discuss a sampling of muscle tissue pathologies.

Myopathies

Myopathy describes any disease of muscles and muscle tissue that is either inherited or acquired. **Botulism** is a serious form of food poisoning caused by eating food contaminated with *Clostridium botulinum* organisms, microbes that thrive in anaerobic conditions. People become infected with the toxin by eating food that has not been canned or cooked appropriately. The toxin produced by *C. botulinum*, botulinus, is the most potent poison known. Botulinus toxin prevents the release of acetylcholine at the neuromuscular junction, thereby causing skeletal muscle paralysis. This is especially critical if the diaphragm and respiratory muscles are involved.

Double vision, light sensitivity, blurred speech, nausea, vomiting, and inability to walk are common signs and symptoms. The potent neurotoxin affects the myoneural junction, preventing the release of ACh and causing muscle weakness and possible respiratory failure. Treatment is supportive. Guanidine hydrochloride, a drug that promotes the release of ACh may be administered. Pulmonary ventilation (artificial breathing machine) may be necessary for severe cases. Recovery is gradual and may take up to one year.

Fibromyalgia is a syndrome of unknown origin characterized by diffuse **myalgia** (muscle pain), stiffness, and tenderness at characteristic joints. Signs include fibrosis and fibrositis. **Fibrosis** is the formation of fibrous tissue where it normally does not exist, and **fibrositis** is inflammation of fibrous tissue. Joint regions typically involved include the antecubital, cervical, sacroiliac, and patellar. Diagnosis is made through patient history and physical examination. Patients usually experience fatigue; sensitivity to noise, light, and odors; and irregular sleep patterns. Treatment includes analgesics, aspirin, and nonsteroidal anti-inflammatory drug (NSAID) administration; stress reduction; and exercise. Chemical therapeutic agents serve to reduce inflammation, alleviate pain, or interfere with the immune response. NSAIDs are commonly prescribed for swelling reduction. Aspirin and analgesics work to lesson pain symptoms.

Muscular dystrophies (MDs) are inherited diseases of muscles characterized by degeneration of individual muscle cells causing progressive muscle weakness. The genetic disorder causes muscle atrophy and muscle to be replaced by fat and connective tissue, both of which cannot contract. Duchenne (pseudohypertrophic) muscular dystrophy (DMD) is the most common type of muscular dystrophy. Pseudohypertrophic MD is an X-linked genetic disorder affecting only females with Turner syndrome and young males. With this disorder, the cytoskeleton protein dystrophin is missing. It is characterized by rapid progression and weakness, and death by approximately age 21 years. The muscles affected by muscular dystrophy are shown in Figure 7-8.

Progression of other dystrophies is usually slow, taking decades unless cardiac tissue is involved. Blood tests used to establish muscle tissue damage include the **alanine aminotransferase test**, the **aspartate aminotransferase test**, and the **creatine phosphokinase** (CPK or CK) **test.** Elevated levels of any of these muscle enzymes indicate

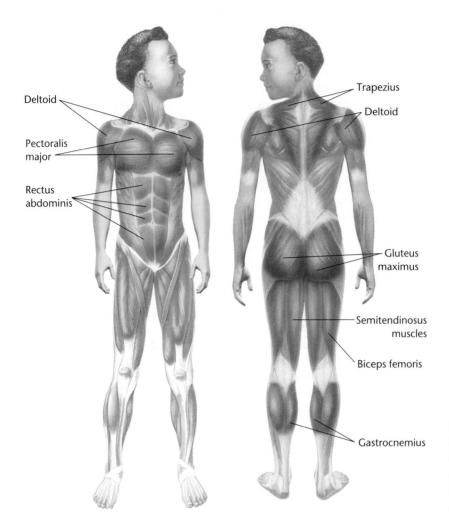

Deltoid

Pectoralis
major

Rectus
abdominis

Trapezius

Deltoid

Gluteus
maximus

Semitendinosus
muscles

Biceps femoris

Gastrocnemius

FIGURE 7-8
Muscles affected by
different types of mus-
cular dystrophy.
(Image provided by
Anatomical Chart Co.)

tissue damage. Urine tests used to assess muscle pathology are the **myoglobin urine test** and the **3-methoxy-4-hydroxymandelic acid test.** Myoglobin in the urine suggests muscle damage. The presence of 3-methoxy-4-hydroxymandelic acid in the urine indicates muscular dystrophy.

Because there is no cure, treatment is limited and involves PT, occupational therapy (OT), and orthopedic procedures. Treatments for many muscle disorders involve PT, OT, rehabilitative exercise, or surgery. The aim of physical therapy is to gain and/or restore function and range of motion in body parts. Occupational therapy helps individuals overcome medical disability and live a quality life with existing disease. A goal of OT is to provide alternative methods, utensils, or skills to assist the activities of daily living (ADLs). Exercise often facilitates physical and emotional well-being.

Immune disorders include myasthenia gravis and polymyositis. **Myasthenia gravis** (MG) is an autoimmune disease marked by the weakness of skeletal muscles, particularly in the face and neck. Like most autoimmune disorders, this condition affects more women than men. All skeletal muscles are involved, and the affected person's face appears expressionless. A lack of the neurotransmitter ACh is probably the culprit of the disease. The resulting difficulty in chewing, swallowing, and talking may be alleviated with rest, allowing muscle strength to be regained. This relaxation period allows time for synthesis and buildup of ACh. Diagnosis is made through the history and physical examination, including electromyography. Treatment options include the administration of drugs, such as cholinesterase inhibitors, to decrease the normal destruction of ACh, thereby making it more available for impulse transmission. These drugs would oppose the effect of the enzyme cholinesterase. Corticosteroid therapy is also administered. Corticosteroids are synthetic drugs used to reduce inflammation and hamper immune function.

Polymyositis (PM) is an autoimmune disease that causes **myositis** (muscle inflammation), myomalacia (muscle tissue softening), and atrophy. Nearly 67% of those afflicted are women. It is called dermatomyositis (DM) when the skin is also involved. The initial signs and symptoms are malaise and fatigue, which progress to an inability to raise arms over the head and difficulty walking. The preliminary diagnosis is made through the history and physical examination, blood tests to rule out other disorders with similar characteristics, and electromyography. **Electromyography** makes use of artificial electrical stimulation of muscles and records the information on an **electromyogram**. The electromyography is a graphed record tracing the electrical activity in a muscle at rest or during contraction. A probe is inserted into the muscle to obtain the results. Electromyography and electromyogram are both abbreviated EMG. Neurologists generally administer EMGs, which can assist in diagnosing disorders such as myasthenia gravis and muscular dystrophy. Elevated CPK levels indicate polymyositis. A muscle biopsy confirms the diagnosis and is the definitive test. In a **muscle biopsy** procedure, tissue specimens are excised for evaluation. This often is the only method for obtaining an accurate diagnosis of some myopathies.

Treatment is aimed at controlling symptoms and impeding the immune response. Steroids such as prednisone are prescribed to minimize inflammation, immunosuppressants are often used to treat the immune component, and physical therapy helps preserve muscle function and prevent further atrophy. There is no known cure, but the disease can be managed fairly successfully.

Key Terms	Definitions
myopathy (migh OP uth ee)	any disease of the muscles
botulism (BOT yoo liz um)	illness acquired by ingesting improperly cooked or canned food containing *Clostridium botulinum*
fibromyalgia (figh broh migh AL juh)	widespread muscle and joint pain of unknown origin
myalgia (migh AL jee uh)	muscle pain
fibrosis (figh BROH sis)	increase in fibrous tissue
fibrositis (figh broh SIGH tis)	inflammation of muscle sheaths and fascial layers
muscular dystrophies (DIS troh feez)	hereditary diseases marked by muscle cell degeneration
alanine aminotransferase (AL uh neen uh mee noh TRANS fur ace) **test**	blood enzyme test to evaluate tissue damage
aspartate aminotransferase (as PAR tate uh mee noh TRANS fur ace) **test**	blood enzyme test to detect tissue damage or muscular dystrophy
creatine phosphokinase (KREE a teen fos foh KIGH nace) **test**	blood enzyme test to detect tissue damage
myoglobin (migh oh GLOH bin) **urine test**	urine test to detect muscle damage
3-methoxy-4-hydroxymandelic (3 muh THOK see 4 high DROCK see man DEL ick) **acid test**	urine test to detect possible muscular dystrophy
myasthenia gravis (migh as THEEN ee uh GRAV is)	autoimmune disease characterized by weakened muscles and chronic fatigue

polymyositis (pol ee migh oh SIGH tis)	autoimmune disease characterized by muscle inflammation and atrophy
myositis (migh oh SIGH tis)	muscle inflammation
electromyography (ee leck troh migh OG ruh fee)	procedure to obtain an electromyogram
electromyogram (ee leck troh MIGH oh gram)	record of muscular activity
muscle biopsy (BYE op see)	tissue sample taken for evaluation

Key Term Practice: Myopathies

1. Identify the autoimmune disease characterized by muscle atrophy and inflammation.

   _____

2. The medical term for muscle pain is _____.

3. Identify three blood enzyme tests useful for detecting muscle tissue damage.

   a. _____

   b. _____

   c. _____

4. EMG is the abbreviation for _____ or _____.

Trauma

A protrusion of an organ through an opening is termed a **hernia.** Hernias can occur when forceful muscle contractions increase abdominopelvic pressure considerably, forcing organ bulging. There are numerous types, but common forms are inguinal, reducible, and strangulated. When an organ extends through the inguinal canal (groin) into the scrotum or labia, it is called an **inguinal hernia** (Fig 7-9). Typically, this type of hernia involves the intestines bulging through the cavity as a result of increased abdominal pressure. Inguinal hernias are more common in males than females.

A **reducible hernia** is one that can be manually manipulated back into the abdominal cavity. A hernia in which the organ cannot be reduced and blood flow is interrupted is termed strangulated. **Strangulated hernias** need to be surgically repaired to prevent obstruction and possible gangrene (death of soft body tissues resulting from interrupted blood supply).

Rotator cuff injuries involve a group of shoulder muscles. Four muscles—supraspinatus, infraspinatus, teres minor, and subscapularis—make up the rotator cuff, and they are easily remembered by the acronym SITS. This type of injury is a consequence of acute trauma, degenerative changes, or overuse as in baseball pitchers. A snapping sound is usually heard when the surrounding tendons tear. There is immediate pain and inability to abduct the arm. Physical evaluation, computed tomography (CT) scan, or magnetic resonance imaging (MRI) studies make the diagnosis. Surgery is required to repair damaged tissue and preserve muscle integrity. Drugs may also be used to manage pain.

Shin splints, a disorder associated with the tibial periosteum and related extensor muscles, occur from tremendous muscle stress caused by running. Inflammation, edema, and pain are common signs and symptoms. Diagnosis is made by physical

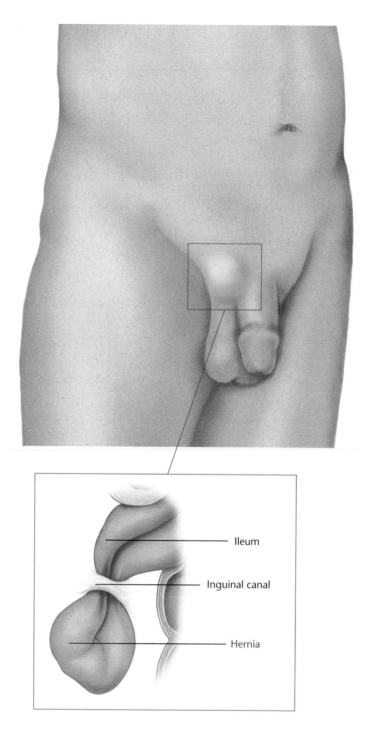

FIGURE 7-9
Hernia. When an organ extends through the inguinal canal (groin) into the scrotum or labia, it is called an inguinal hernia. (Image provided by Anatomical Chart Co.)

Labels in figure:
Ileum
Inguinal canal
Hernia

examination and radiographic studies. The diagnosis is usually confirmed when pain occurs while exercising but disappears during rest. Alternate heat and ice treatments (cold packs) alleviate some symptoms. Analgesics, NSAIDs, rest, good-fitting shoes, and proper exercise techniques are prescribed.

Severed tendon injuries result from trauma or laceration. When severed, the elastic fibrous cord, like a thick rubber band, will snap. The signs and symptoms include pain, inflammation, and immobility of the affected structure. Diagnosis is made through the patient's history, physical examination, and radiographic studies. Treatment involves **tenoplasty**, surgical intervention to repair and attach the cleaved part.

A **strain** is an injury to muscle resulting from overexertion or trauma. Strains involve myotasis (stretching or tearing muscle fibers). Similar to strains, **sprain** injuries are more serious, occur near a joint, and involve breaks in ligaments or tendons. Edema, fibromyositis, and myalgia are signs and symptoms of both. Edema refers to swelling, whereas **fibromyositis** is muscle and tendon inflammation. **Tendonitis**, inflammation of connective tissue surrounding a tendon, especially at the point of its attachment to bone, may occur with sprain injuries (Fig. 7-10). Sprains are caused by acute or accumulative trauma. Diagnosis is made by physical examination and radiographic studies to differentiate between a sprain, strain, and bone fracture. Treatment involves limb elevation, rest, analgesics, and NSAIDs. Because cartilaginous tendons and ligaments have no direct blood supply, these injuries are slow healing and can take up to six weeks for complete recovery.

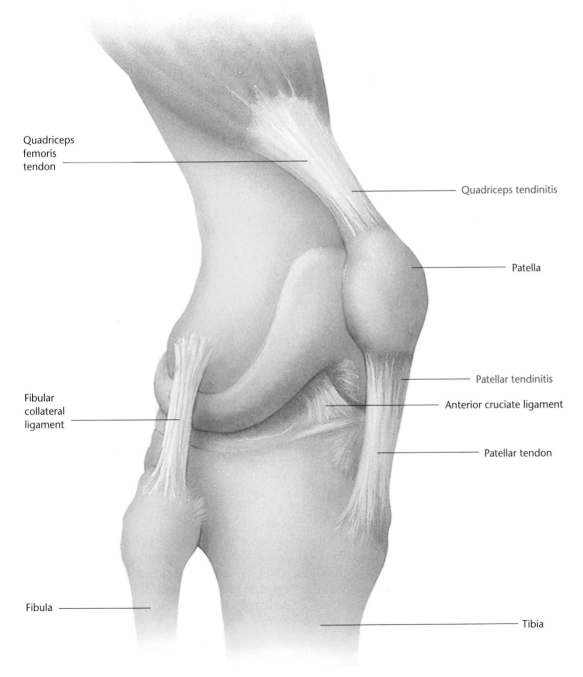

Quadriceps femoris tendon

Quadriceps tendinitis

Patella

Fibular collateral ligament

Patellar tendinitis

Anterior cruciate ligament

Patellar tendon

Fibula

Tibia

FIGURE 7-10
Tendonitis, inflammation of connective tissue surrounding a tendon, may occur with sprain injuries. (Image provided by Anatomical Chart Co.)

Key Terms	Definitions
hernia (HUR nee uh)	protrusion as a result of pressure
inguinal hernia (ING gwi nul HUR nee uh)	organ protrusion in the inguinal region
reducible hernia (HUR nee uh)	organ protrusion that can be manipulated back into the normal position
strangulated hernias (HUR nee uhz)	organ protrusions with interrupted blood flow
shin splints	pain in the anterior tibial region
severed tendon (TEN dun)	lacerated tendon
tenoplasty (TEN oh plas tee)	surgical repair of a tendon
strain	injury from overexertion or trauma; involves the stretching or tearing of muscle fibers
sprain	injury near a joint that involves ligament or tendon damage
fibromyositis (figh broh migh OH sigh tis)	muscle and tendon inflammation
tendonitis (ten dun EYE tis)	tendon inflammation

Key Term Practice: Trauma

1. Identify the three types of hernias.

   a. _____

   b. _____

   c. _____

2. What are the two acceptable plural forms of hernia?

   _____

3. Surgical repair of a tendon is termed _____.

Tumors

Muscle tumors are rare because muscle tissue is not replaced with new growth like bone and many other tissues. However, two skeletal muscle tumors have been identified: rhabdomyosarcoma and rhabdomyoma. A malignant skeletal muscle tumor is called **rhabdomyosarcoma**. A benign tumor is termed **rhabdomyoma**. They are so named because the combining forms *rhabd-* and *rhabdo-* mean "striated," thus indicating their location in skeletal muscle tissue.

Key Terms	Definitions
rhabdomyosarcoma (rab doh migh oh sahr KOH muh)	malignant tumor of skeletal muscle
rhabdomyoma (rab doh migh OH muh)	nonmalignant tumor of skeletal muscle

Key Term Practice: Tumors

1. A malignant tumor of skeletal muscle tissue is termed _____, and a benign skeletal muscle tumor is referred to as a _____.

CLINICAL TERMS

Clinical Dimension	Term	Description
DISORDERS		
	botulism	illness acquired by ingesting improperly cooked or canned food containing *Clostridium botulinum*
	fibromyalgia	widespread muscle and joint pain of unknown origin
	hernia	protrusion as a result of pressure
	inguinal hernia	organ protrusion in the inguinal region
	muscular dystrophies	hereditary diseases marked by muscle cell degeneration
	myasthenia gravis	autoimmune disease characterized by weakened muscles and chronic fatigue
	myopathy	any disease of the muscles
	polymyositis	autoimmune disease characterized by muscle inflammation and atrophy
	reducible hernia	organ protrusion that can be manipulated back into the normal position
	rhabdomyoma	nonmalignant tumor of skeletal muscle
	rhabdomyosarcoma	malignant tumor of skeletal muscle
	severed tendon	lacerated tendon
	shin splints	pain in anterior tibial region
	sprain	injury near a joint that involves ligament or tendon damage
	strain	injury from overexertion or trauma; involves the stretching or tearing of muscle fibers
	strangulated hernias	organ protrusions with interrupted blood flow

Clinical Dimension	Term	Description
SIGNS AND SYMPTOMS		
	atrophy	physiological or pathologic reduction in muscle size
	fibromyositis	muscle and tendon inflammation
	fibrosis	increase in fibrous tissue
	fibrositis	inflammation of muscle sheaths and fascial layers
	myalgia	muscle pain
	myomalacia	muscle tissue softening
	myosclerosis	muscle hardening
	myositis	muscle inflammation
	myotasis	stretched muscle
	tendonitis	tendon inflammation
CLINICAL TESTS AND DIAGNOSTIC PROCEDURES		
	alanine aminotransferase test	blood enzyme test to evaluate tissue damage
	aspartate aminotransferase test	blood enzyme test to detect tissue damage or muscular dystrophy
	creatine phospho-kinase (CPK; CK) test	blood enzyme test to detect tissue damage
	electromyography (EMG)	procedure to obtain an electromyogram
	electromyogram (EMG)	record of muscular activity
	muscle biopsy	tissue sample taken for evaluation
	myoglobin urine test	urine test to detect muscle damage
	3-methoxy-4-hydro-xymandelic acid test	urine test to detect possible muscular dystrophy
	corticosteroids	synthetic drugs used to reduce inflammation
TREATMENTS		
	nonsteroidal anti-inflammatory drugs (NSAIDs)	medicines that act against tissue inflammation
	tenoplasty	surgical repair of a tendon

Lifespan

Muscle tissue is derived from embryonic myoblast cells. Cardiac muscle is operative in 3-week-old embryos. By week 7 in utero, skeletal muscle tissue begins functioning.

Approximately 25% of the body weight of infants is attributed to muscle mass. This proportion increases to approximately 40% in the adult. Most infant muscle mass is contained in the axial musculature; in the adult, 55% of muscle weight is located in lower limbs.

Satellite cells (stem cells that repair damaged tissue) in skeletal muscle allow for limited muscle regeneration. Cardiac satellite cells promote heart tissue regeneration, but damaged tissue is replaced primarily by scar tissue. Smooth muscle tissue remains mitotic (capable of dividing and regenerating) throughout life.

A normal response to aging in skeletal muscle tissue is diminished ATP, CP, glycogen (storage form of glucose), and myoglobin reserves. This leads to a progressive deterioration of tissue. As one ages, skeletal muscles become less elastic, and the reflex response is lessened.

Muscle tissue can grow all through life; exercise exerts its effect by increasing the size of existing muscle fibers. Exercise serves to promote blood flow to muscle tissue, control body weight, and enhance the quality of life. It also augments stability and balance in all life stages.

In the News: Botox

Botulinum toxin is increasing in popularity. It is making its way into mainstream America as a cosmetic treatment for facial wrinkles. Once considered a poison to avoid at all cost, now some people are anxiously awaiting their injections.

Food borne botulism cases in the United States have been linked to peppers, potato salad, sautéed onions, canned tuna, smoked fish, and cold soups. Symptoms appear within 36 hours of eating contaminated cuisine. Antibiotic treatment is of no use because microbial growth does not cause the disease, rather the toxin produced by the bacteria does. Treatment is supportive and may involve pulmonary ventilation. Despite the disease severity, the mortality rate is approximately 10%.

This same toxin is being used to lessen frown and forehead wrinkles. The trade name is Botox, short for botulinum toxin. Botulinum toxin is injected in very low doses into certain facial muscles, causing muscle paralysis and relaxation. This, in turn, eliminates wrinkles because without movement of underlying muscles, the skin does not form the deep creases. The treatment lasts about three months before it must be repeated. The toxin is also used for other neuromuscular conditions such as multiple sclerosis and muscle spasms (involuntary, sudden contractions).

COMMON ABBREVIATIONS

Abbreviation	Term
ACh	acetylcholine
ACL	anterior cruciate ligament
ADLs	activities of daily living
ATP	adenosine triphosphate
BS	bachelor of science
CA^{2+}	calcium ion
CK	creatine kinase
CP	creatine phosphate
CPK	creatine phosphokinase
CT	computed tomography
DM	dermatomyositis
DMD	Duchenne muscular dystrophy
EMG	electromyogram, electromyography
MCL	medial collateral ligament
MDs	muscular dystrophies

Abbreviation	Term
MG	myasthenia gravis
MRI	magnetic resonance imaging
MS	master of science
NM	neuromuscular
NSAID	nonsteroidal anti-inflammatory drug
OT	occupational therapy
PhD	doctor of philosophy
PM	polymyositis
PT	physical therapy
PTA	physical therapy assistant
ROM	range of motion
SITS	supraspinatus, infraspinatus, teres minor, subscapularis muscles
SR	sarcoplasmic reticulum
WFL	within functional limits
WNL	within normal limits

Case Study

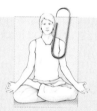

Mrs. Lee, a 45-year-old tax clerk, presented in Cindy's physical therapy office for evaluation and therapy. Her orthopedic surgeon referred her for rehabilitative services after she had been involved in an automobile accident.

Subjective Findings

Mrs. Lee's chief complaints were pain in the right leg and inability to walk. During the casting period, her activity level declined and she engaged in no physical pursuits beyond going to work. Mrs. Lee was able to ambulate using a wheelchair and walker. She noted pain in her right lower extremity of 4 on a 0–10 pain scale. Her goal for physical therapy was to regain mobility.

Objective Findings

Her initial diagnosis was fractured right lateral malleolus, torn right anterior cruciate ligament (ACL), and torn right medial collateral ligament (MCL). Her right fibula was casted inferior to the patella for 7 weeks. There was disruption of the deep fibers of the medial collateral ligament complex. Edema and hemorrhage within the substance of the components of the medial collateral ligament were evident. She supported her weight through her left lower extremity and bilateral upper extremities. Patient's range of motion (ROM) was severely restricted. Several measurements were taken.

Range of Motion

Measure	Right	Left
Knee extension	−40°	0°
Knee flexion	55°	145°
Hip extension	−17°	WFL[a]
Plantar flexion	49°	WNL[a]
Dorsiflexion	−25°	WFL

[a]*WFL,* within functional limits; *WNL,* within normal limits.

Circumference Measurements

Location	Right	Left
Thigh	45 cm	50 cm
Calf	30 cm	35 cm

Case Study Questions

Select the best answer to each of the following questions.

1. **ROM refers to _____.**
   a. range of motion
   b. restriction of motion
   c. range of muscle
   d. reading on measurement

2. **The circumferential measurements revealed that the right leg is smaller than the left. Which of the following is a plausible explanation?**
   a. One leg is usually considerable smaller than the other.
   b. Mrs. Lee is experiencing some atrophy in the muscle tissue owing to disuse.
   c. The physical therapist probably made an error in charting.

3. **The goal of Mrs. Lee's therapy is to _____.**
   a. increase flexion of left knee
   b. decrease flexion of left knee
   c. increase flexion of right knee
   d. decrease flexion of right knee

4. **Other therapy options for Mrs. Lee are _____.**
   a. warm packs to reduce swelling and active exercise to alleviate pain
   b. moist hot packs to reduce swelling and passive exercise to reduce pain
   c. home instruction to increase range of motion and isometric (muscle tension without contraction) exercises to strengthen the shoulder girdle
   d. cold packs to reduce swelling and pain, and range of motion exercises to increase strength

REAL WORLD REPORT

Cindy assessed Mrs. Lee and developed a physical therapy plan. The physical therapy report follows.

PATIENT ASSESSMENT

Patient: Annabelle Lee

Date: August 15, 2003

STRENGTH
Patient demonstrates 5/5 strength for left lower extremity and 2/5 strength throughout right lower extremity, grossly secondary to an inability to move through ROM. Significant atrophy is noted throughout right lower extremity.

GAIT
Patient ambulates only very short distances with the walker and with no weight bearing on the right lower extremity; she uses a "hop-to" gait pattern with the walker.

OTHER
Patient demonstrates significant fear of trying to weight bear on the right lower extremity although minimal to no pain is present when attempting to bear weight.

PROBLEMS
Inability to walk; decreased strength; hip, knee, and ankle contractures; decreased ADLs and mobility; lack of home-exercise program.

EXERCISES

EXERCISE 1: STRETCH GASTROCNEMIUS—SITTING WITH TOWEL
- Perform 1 set of 3 repetitions, twice a day.
- Hold exercise for 30 s.
- Rest 15 s between sets.

EXERCISE 2: STRETCH GASTROCNEMIUS—STANDING
- Perform 1 set of 4 repetitions, twice a day.
- Hold exercise for 30 s.
- Rest 15 s between sets.

EXERCISE 3: STRETCH SOLEUS—STANDING
- Perform 1 set of 4 repetitions, twice a day.
- Hold exercise for 30 s.
- Rest 15 s between sets.

GOALS

SHORT-TERM—AFTER 10 TREATMENTS
- Increase extension of right knee to $-10°$
- Increase flexion of right knee to $75°$
- Patient able to ambulate independently with weight bearing of right lower extremity using walker or appropriate assistive device
- Patient independent with beginning home-exercise program
- Increase hip extension to $10°$
- Increase dorsiflexion of right ankle to $-5°$
- Patient to note 50% improvement in ADLs

LONG-TERM—AFTER 20 TREATMENTS
- Increase right knee ROM to minimum of 3–120°
- Increase dorsiflexion right ankle to minimum of 5°
- Patient able to ambulate independently without use of assistive device with full weight bearing on right lower extremity
- Increase strength of right lower extremity to 5/5
- Independent with advanced home-exercise program

PLAN
Patient to be seen two to three times per week for a total of 10 treatments per prescription and reevaluated at that time. Patient has significant limitations secondary to muscle contracture and expresses fear; additional visits will be required to return the patient to function and normal gait pattern.

Cindy Harst, PT, PhD

REAL WORLD REPORT QUESTIONS

The following exercises review the medical terms in the preceding medical report.

1. Flexion, accomplished by flexor muscles, refers to _____.

   a. increasing the angle between body parts

   b. decreasing the angle between body parts

   c. moving the foot in a circular fashion

   d. standing with the feet facing forward

2. Mrs. Lee has limitations that are secondary to muscle contracture. This means that the muscle contracture _____.

   a. caused her limitations

   b. is the result of her limitations

   c. is going to heal after she can walk

   d. has nothing to do with her range of motion limitations

3. Gastrocnemius stretching exercises were prescribed. These will strengthen muscles in the _____.

   a. hip

   b. thigh

   c. calf

   d. ankle

4. Soleus exercises while standing were given as part of the rehabilitation plan. The action of this muscle is _____.

   a. leg extension

   b. plantar flexion

   c. leg flexion

   d. thigh adduction

REVIEW AND APPLICATION: THREE-LEVEL LEARNING SYSTEM

LEVEL ONE: REVIEWING FACTS AND TERMS USING RECALL

Select the best response to each of the following questions.

1. Functions of the muscular system include _____.

   a. movement

   b. heat production

   c. posture maintenance

   d. all of these

2. The function of the sarcoplasmic reticulum is to _____.

   a. provide structural support

   b. store and release calcium ions

   c. communicate with the sarcolemma

   d. provide cellular energy

3. The functional units of myofibrils are _____.

   a. sarcomeres

   b. myofilaments

   c. actin molecules

   d. myosin molecules

4. Skeletal muscle tissue is also known as _____.

   a. striated

   b. unstriated

   c. involuntary

   d. cardiac

5. Smooth muscle tissue is also known as _____.

   a. striated

   b. unstriated

   c. involuntary

   d. cardiac

6. Heart muscle tissue is also known as_____.

   a. striated

   b. unstriated

   c. involuntary

   d. cardiac

7. This type of muscle tissue is found lining blood vessels.

   a. striated

   b. unstriated

   c. involuntary

   d. cardiac

8. Energy is supplied to muscle fibers in the form of _____.

   a. sucrose

   b. ATP

   c. DNA

   d. RNA

9. Skeletal muscles are named according to _____.

   a. size

   b. location

   c. action

   d. all of these

10. Most muscles have _____ names.

    a. Latin

    b. Spanish

    c. English

    d. German

Match the word part with its meaning.

_____ 11. brachy-   a. skeleton, skeletal

_____ 12. plat-, platy-   b. nutrition, nourishment

_____ 13. -troph, troph-, tropho-   c. muscle

_____ 14. my-, myo-   d. short

_____ 15. skelet-, skeleto-   e. broad, flat

LEVEL TWO: REVIEWING CONCEPTS

Match the disorder with its key characteristics.

_____ 16. strain

_____ 17. sprain

_____ 18. muscular dystrophy

_____ 19. fibromyalgia

_____ 20. rhabdomyosarcoma

a. hereditary muscle disease; muscle atrophy

b. diffuse muscle and joint pain; unknown cause

c. torn muscle

d. muscle, ligament, and/or tendon injury

e. malignant skeletal muscle tumor

Provide a medical term to complete a meaningful analogy.

21. Origin is to immovable as insertion is to _____.

22. Cytoplasm is to sarcoplasm as cell membrane is to _____.

Match the muscle with its location.

_____ 23. rectus abdominis

_____ 24. diaphragm

_____ 25. latissimus dorsi

_____ 26. biceps brachii

_____ 27. masseter

_____ 28. rectus femoris

_____ 29. tibialis anterior

a. upper arm

b. lower leg

c. upper leg

d. thoracic region

e. abdominal region

f. back

g. face

Define the following abbreviations.

30. PM _____

31. ATP _____

32. MD _____

33. CP _____

34. MG _____

For each of the following, indicate whether the test involves urine (U), blood (B), or neither (N).

35. creatine kinase test _____

36. 3-methoxy-4-hydroxymandelic acid _____

37. aspartate aminotransferase _____

38. electromyography _____

Using the following word parts, form a medical term for each definition. Each word part is used only once.

-logy	my-, myo-	kinesi-, kinesio-
-plasty	-pathy	teno-

39. the study of muscles = _____

40. the study of movement = _____

41. repair of a tendon = _____

42. any disease of muscle = _____

Which criterion was used to name each of the following muscles? More than one criterion may be used for each muscle name.

_____ 43. pterygoids

_____ 44. triceps brachii

_____ 45. adductor longus

_____ 46. quadriceps femoris

_____ 47. rectus abdominis

_____ 48. gluteus maximus

a. size

b. location

c. number of heads/origins

d. action

e. appearance

Define the following word parts.

49. fascio- _____

50. sarc-, sarco- _____

51. muscul-, musculo- _____

52. -troph, troph-, tropho- _____

53. pterygo- _____

Identify the correctly spelled term in each set.

54. ____
   a. sarcolemma
   b. sarkolemma
   c. sarcolema
   d. sarrcolemma

55. ____
   a. elecktromyogram
   b. electromiogram
   c. electromyogram
   d. electromighogram

56. ____
   a. insersion
   b. insertion
   c. ensertion
   d. insershun

57. ____
   a. myoglobbin
   b. myoglobin
   c. mioglobin
   d. mygloben

58. ____
   a. atrofee
   b. atrophee
   c. atrophie
   d. atrophy

59. ____
   a. delltoid
   b. deltod
   c. deltoid
   d. deltowd

60. ____
   a. semimembranosus
   b. semimembranosis
   c. sememembranosis
   d. semimembrenosus

LEVEL THREE: THINKING CRITICALLY

Provide the best response to each of the following questions.

61. Jack's physician sent him to the physical therapist for an evaluation. The physical examination revealed that Jack is unable to extend at the knee and cannot flex or laterally rotate his leg. The PT determines which of the following muscles are involved?
   a. biceps brachii and biceps femoris
   b. quadriceps femoris and calcaneal tendon
   c. quadriceps femoris and biceps femoris
   d. rectus abdominis and rectus femoris

62. Which muscle has the following origin and insertion?
   a. Origin: distal lateral end of humerus
   b. Insertion: lateral surface of radius
   c. Muscle: _____

KEY TERMS SPELLING TEST FROM CD-ROM

Use the CD-ROM to test yourself on the spelling of key terms from this chapter. Listen to the terms and write them on a separate sheet of paper. Use a medical dictionary to check your answers.

ANSWERS

WORD GROUPING

Definition	Word Part
arm, brachial	brachi-, brachio-
cheek, mouth	bucco-
fascia	fascio-
fiber	fibr-, fibro-
flat, broad	plat-, platy-
heart, cardiac	cardi-, cardio-
movement	A. kin-, kine-, kino-
	B. kinesi-, kinesio-
	C. kinet-, kineto-
muscle	A. muscul-, musculo-
	B. my-, myo-
muscle, flesh	sarc-, sarco-
nutrition, nourishment	-troph, troph-, tropho-
pertaining to fibular side of leg	peroneo-
sheath, envelope	-lemma
short	brachy-
skeleton, skeletal	skelet-, skeleto-
striated	rhabd-, rhabdo-
tendon	tendo-, teno-
wing, wing shaped	pterygo-

WORD BUILDING

Word Part	Meaning	Common or Known Word	Example Medical Term
muscul-, musculo-	muscle	muscular	musculoskeletal
cardi-, cardio-	heart, cardiac	cardiac	cardiomyopathy
skelet-, skeleto-	skeleton, skeletal	skeleton	musculoskeletal
tendo-, teno-	tendon	tendon	tendonitis

KEY TERM PRACTICE

Muscular System Preview
1. muscle fiber
2. muscle tissue
3. muscle, flesh; envelope, sheath; sarcolemma

Muscle Fiber
1. sarcomeres
2. muscle; myofibrils

Muscle Tissue: Skeletal, Smooth, and Cardiac
1. heart or cardiac; cardiac
2. aponeurosis
3. fasciae
4. peristalsis

Muscle Movement
1. origin; insertion
2. myohemoglobin
3. ATP

Muscle Tone
1. muscle tone
2. hypertrophy

Naming Skeletal Muscles
1. Flexors
2. abductors

Myopathies
1. polymyositis
2. myalgia
3. a. alanine aminotransferase test; b. aspartate aminotransferase test; c. creatine phosphokinase test
4. electromyography; electromyogram

Trauma
1. a. inguinal hernia; b. reducible hernia; c. strangulated hernia
2. hernias and herniae
3. strain
4. tenoplasty

Tumors
1. rhabdomyosarcoma; rhabdomyoma

CASE STUDY

1. a is the correct answer.
   - b, c, and d are incorrect because the abbreviation ROM does not stand for these terms.
2. b is the correct answer.
   - a is incorrect because in the absence of disease, there is little difference in circumference measurements between legs.
   - c is incorrect because the report states that Mrs. Lee injured her right leg, thus the measurements seem to be correct.

3. c is the correct answer.
   - a and b are incorrect because the left leg was not affected.
   - d is incorrect because the goal is to increase the range of motion.
4. d is the correct answer.
   - a and b are incorrect because warm or moist hot packs would not reduce swelling. They would increase circulation to the area and perhaps alleviate pain.
   - c is incorrect because the shoulder girdle was not injured.

REAL WORLD REPORT

1. b
2. a

3. c
4. b

REVIEW AND APPLICATION: THREE-LEVEL LEARNING SYSTEM

Level One: Reviewing Facts and Terms Using Recall

1. d
2. b
3. a
4. a
5. c
6. d
7. c
8. b
9. d
10. a
11. d
12. e
13. b
14. c
15. a

Level Two: Reviewing Concepts

16. c
17. d
18. a
19. b
20. e
21. movable
22. sarcolemma
23. e
24. d
25. f
26. a
27. g
28. c
29. b
30. polymyositis
31. adenosine triphosphate
32. muscular dystrophy
33. creatine phosphate
34. myasthenia gravis
35. b
36. u
37. b
38. n
39. myology
40. kinesiology
41. tenoplasty
42. myopathy
43. e
44. b, c
45. a, d
46. b, c
47. b, e
48. a, b
49. fascia
50. muscle, flesh
51. muscle
52. nutrition, nourishment
53. wing shaped
54. a
55. c
56. b
57. b
58. d
59. c
60. a

Level Three: Thinking Critically

61. c
62. brachioradialis

chapter 8

Nervous System and Special Senses

OBJECTIVES

After completing this chapter, you should be able to:

1. Define the meanings of word parts related to the nervous system.
2. Identify major structures of the brain, ear, and eye.
3. Describe primary functions of brain, ear, and eye parts.
4. Explain different signs, symptoms, and treatments of various nervous system diseases.
5. Explain clinical tests and procedures related to the nervous system.
6. Describe anatomical and physiological alterations throughout the lifespan.
7. List common abbreviations related to the nervous system.
8. Define terms used in medical reports involving the nervous system and special senses.
9. Correctly define, spell, and pronounce the chapter's medical terms.

Professional Profile: Optometric Assistant

Sally is an optometric assistant working in an optometry office. After a patient checks in at the front desk, the optometric assistant is the next person he or she encounters in the office. Sally's job is to collect the patient's history, perform preliminary tests, and orchestrate the flow of services. In addition to preparing and replenishing supplies in the examination and screening rooms, she performs the preliminary tests on patients, including the following: color vision, keratometry, autorefractor, visual fields, pupil distance (PD), visual acuities, and blood pressure. All of this is done before the doctor sees the patient, so accurate charting is crucial. The optometric assistant also files all the charts and previews reports from ophthalmologists and neurologists, checking to be sure that any reports that need immediate attention by the optometrist are placed on his or her desk. Common medical conditions seen in the office include cataracts, macular degeneration, retinopathy, and other sight-related disorders.

Sally's job involves a good deal of interaction with patients because she also teaches contact lens insertion, removal, and care. Optometric assistants are commonly trained on the job by the employer and are frequently cross-trained to perform minor eyeglass repairs. However, Sally recently completed a 1-year optometric assistant program, which included coursework in dispensing, front office skills, lens fabrication, contact lens modification, medical terminology, anatomy, and physiology. She is now certified as an optometric assistant.

INTRODUCTION

The nervous system has one of the most complex body organizations. It plays a role in nearly every function and acts as the primary means of self-protection. Through its actions, distinctly human characteristics such as emotion and thought are achieved and homeostasis is maintained. Nerves and their affiliated structures bring about nearly all of our actions and intellect.

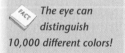

The eye can distinguish 10,000 different colors!

The nervous system and special sense organs receive and interpret stimuli and transmit impulses to effector organs. Because sight, hearing, smell, taste, and equilibrium are specialized functions of the nervous system, they are referred to as special senses. This chapter focuses on specific anatomy, general physiology, and key medical aspects of the nervous system and the special senses.

MEDICAL TERM PARTS

WORD PARTS

Medical term prefixes, suffixes, and combining forms related to the nervous system are introduced in this section.

Word Parts	Meaning
acou-, acouo-	hearing
adren-, adreno-	adrenal
ambly-	dimness
arachn-, arachno-	spider, spider-like

Word Parts	Meaning
astr-, astro-	star-like
audio-	sense of hearing
aur-, auri-, auro-	ear
bleph-, blepharo-	eyelid
caud-, caudo-	tail, caudal
cephal-, cephalo-	head
cerebell-, cerebelli-, cerebello-	cerebellum
cerebr-, cerebri-, cerebro-	cerebrum, cerebral, brain
chem-, chemi-, chemico-, chemio-, chemo-	chemical
choroid-, choroido-	choroid, vascular coat
coccy-	coccyx; tailbone
corne-, corneo-	cornea, corneal
cry-, cryo-	cold, freezing
dendr-, dendro-	tree, tree-like
dextr-, dextro-	right side
dynam-, dynamo-	motion, energy, power
encephal-, encephalo-	brain
equi-	equal, equally
gangli-, ganglio-	ganglion, knot
gli-, glio-	gluey, gelatinous
-glia	neuroglia of a specific kind or size
gloss-, -glossa, glosso-	tongue
hemi-	half
irid-, irido-	iris
isch-, ischo-	stoppage, suppression
-lexia	reading impairment or word recognition impairment
meat-, meato-	meatus, passageway, opening
mening-, meningo-	meninx, meninges, membrane
myel-, myelo-	myelin
neur-, neuro-	nerve, neural, nervous
ocul-, oculo-	eye or ocular
ophthalm-, ophthalmo-	pertaining to the eye
-opia, -opy	defect of the eye
opt-, opto-	optic, vision, eye
ot-, oto-	ear
-phasia, -phasy	speech disorder

Word Parts	Meaning
phot-, photo-	light
presby-, presbyo-	old age
retin-, retino-	retina, retinal
rhod-, rhodo-	red
scler-, sclero-	sclera, scleral
sinistr-, sinistro-	left side
stere-, stereo-	involving three dimensions, involving depth perception
-tome	section, part
-tropia	deviation in the line of vision
-tropic	turning toward
tympan-, tympano-	tympanum, tympanic
vascul-, vasculo-	vascular

WORD ETYMOLOGY

Some words have Greek or Latin word roots but are not true word parts. This section lists those that are used as medical terms.

Word	Definition
afferens	carrying toward
aqua	water
audio	to hear
corpus	body
durus	hard
efferens	to bring out
epilepsia	seizure
glia	glue
lacrima	tear
plexus	braid, network
pons	bridge

MEDICAL TERM PARTS USED AS PREFIXES

Prefix	Definition
ambly-	dimness
coccy-	coccyx; tailbone

MEDICAL TERM PARTS USED AS SUFFIXES

Suffix	Definition
-glia	neuroglia of a specific kind or size
-glossa	tongue
-lexia	reading impairment or word recognition impairment
-opia, -opy	defect of the eye
-phasia, -phasy	speech disorder
-tome	section, part
-tropia	deviation in the line of vision
-tropic	turning toward

WORD GROUPING

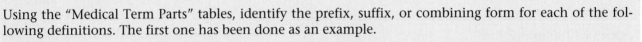

Using the "Medical Term Parts" tables, identify the prefix, suffix, or combining form for each of the following definitions. The first one has been done as an example.

Definition	Word Part
section, part	-tome
adrenal	
brain	
cerebellum	
cerebrum, cerebral, brain	
chemical	
choroid, vascular coat	
coccyx; tailbone	
cold, freezing	
cornea, corneal	
defect of the eye	
deviation in the line of vision	
dimness	
ear	A. B.
equal, equally	
eye or ocular	
eyelid	
ganglion, knot	

Definition	Word Part
gluey, gelatinous	
half	
head	
hearing	
involving three dimensions, involving depth perception	
iris	
left side	
light	
meatus, passageway, opening	
meninx, meninges, membrane	
motion, energy, power	
myelin	
nerve, neural, nervous	
neuroglia of a specific kind or size	
old age	
optic, vision, eye	
pertaining to the eye	
reading impairment or word recognition impairment	
red	
retina, retinal	
right side	
sclera, scleral	
sense of hearing	
speech disorder	
spider, spider-like	
star-like	
stoppage, suppression	
tail, caudal	
tongue	
tree, tree-like	
turning toward	
tympanum, tympanic	
vascular	

WORD BUILDING

Word parts, introduced in the "Medical Term Parts" section, are listed in the following table. For this exercise, first supply the meaning of each word part, then use the word part to build a word you already know. The word you list under "Common or Known Word" does not have to be a medical term; a commonly used word is fine. Be sure, however, that the word correctly reflects the intended meaning. The first one has been done as an example. Check your answers in a dictionary.

Word Part	Meaning	Common or Known Word	Example Medical Term
adren-, adreno-	adrenal	adrenaline	adrenaline
audio-			audiologist
aur-, auri-, auro-			auricle
cerebr-, cerebri-, cerebro-			cerebrum
chem.-, chemi-, chemico-, chemio-, chemo-			chemoreceptor
corne-, corneo-			cornea
dynam-, dynamo-			dynamic equilibrium
irid-, irido-			iridectomy
-lexia			dyslexia
neur-, neuro-			neuron
opt-, opto-			optometry
ot-, oto-			otoscope
phot-, photo-			photoreceptor
retin-, retino-			retina
scler-, sclero-			sclera
stere-, stereo-			stereopsis
vascul-, vasculo-			vascular tunic

ANATOMY AND PHYSIOLOGY

Structures of the Nervous System and Special Senses

- Brain
- Ears
- Eyes
- Nerves
- Nose
- Spinal Cord
- Tongue

Nervous System and Special Senses Preview

The nervous system has two primary divisions, the **central nervous system** (CNS) and the **peripheral nervous system** (PNS). The CNS consists of the brain and spinal cord, and the PNS consists of the auxiliary cranial and spinal nerves that connect the CNS to other body parts (Fig. 8-1).

The complete central nervous system is made up of the brain and spinal cord; but the peripheral nervous system consists of two divisions: the somatic nervous system and the **autonomic nervous system** (ANS), which has two subdivisions. The somatic portion is under voluntary control. The ANS portion is entirely automatic so it cannot be consciously controlled. The subdivisions of the ANS are the sympathetic and parasympathetic nervous systems. The **sympathetic nervous system** prepares the body for stressful and emergency conditions and is frequently called the "fight or flight" response. Another term is the thoracolumbar division because thoracic and lumbar nerve fibers are involved. The **parasympathetic nervous system** is most active under ordinary conditions and is referred to as the "rest and digest" or "rest and repair" response. An alternate term is the craniosacral division.

The nervous system has three general functions: sensory, integrative, and motor. The **sensory** function involves the use of receptors that detect (sense) changes in internal and external body conditions to regulate homeostasis, a condition of balance. The integrative function coordinates the sensory information with internal activity and motor function. Motor function implies skeletal muscle activity in which effectors like muscles respond when they are stimulated by motor impulses.

The **special senses** are olfaction (smelling), gustation (tasting), vision, equilibrium, and hearing. Because the eyes, ears, tongue, and nose are sensory organs of the nervous system involved with the special senses, they are often considered as an integrated whole and are thus discussed within this chapter.

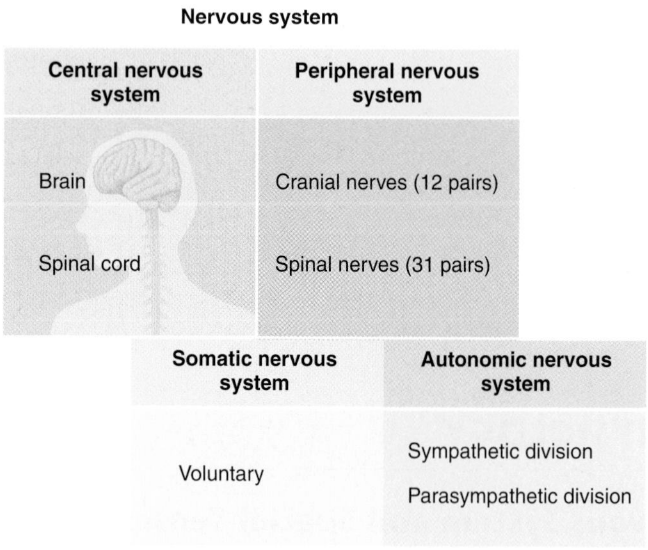

FACT An impulse can travel from the toe to the spinal cord in about 0.01 second!

FIGURE 8-1
Organization of the nervous system.

Key Terms	Definitions
central nervous system	structures supported by the brain and spinal cord
peripheral nervous system	all neural tissue outside the CNS
autonomic (aw tuh NOM ick) **nervous system**	involuntary response by nerve fibers

sympathetic (sim puh THET ick) nervous system	thoracolumbar subdivision of the ANS
parasympathetic (par uh sim puh THET ick) nervous system	craniosacral subdivision of the ANS
sensory (SEN suh ree)	conveying sensation
special senses	the five senses: olfaction, gustation, vision, hearing, and equilibrium

Key Term Practice: Nervous System and Special Senses Preview

1. Identify the two primary divisions of the nervous system. _____

2. What are the two divisions of the autonomic nervous system? _____

Neurons and Neuroglia

Neurons, or nerve cells, are the basic functional units of the nervous system. They are the structural components that react to physical and chemical changes by way of nerve impulse conduction. The basic neuron structure consists of a single cell body, an axon, and multiple dendrites (Fig. 8-2). The cell body, or **soma** (plural = somata), is that portion of a nerve cell that includes a cytoplasmic mass and a nucleus from which the nerve fibers extend. Nerve fibers that conduct electrical impulses, called action potentials, away from the cell body are **axons.** (As a memory aid, associate the *a* in *axon* with the *a* in *away*.) **Dendrites** are sensitive branching nerve fiber extensions that receive information and transmit impulses toward the neuron cell body. The region in which adjacent neurons communicate with one another is termed the **synapse.**

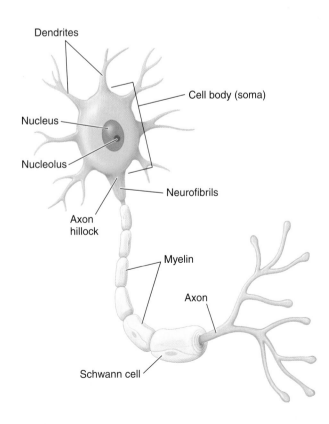

FIGURE 8-2
Neurons are the basic functional units of the nervous system.

The networks of nourishing **neuroglia** (or glial cells) are supporting cells within the CNS and PNS. These accessory cells function in serving as connective tissue by filling spaces and surrounding and supporting parts. Four types of CNS neuroglia are astrocytes, which form the protective blood–brain barrier (BBB); ependymal cells, which line the brain ventricles (spaces) and spinal cord central canals; wandering microglia, which engulf debris; and myelin-forming oligodendrocytes. **Myelin** is an insulating sheath around axons that increases the impulse-transmission rate. Neuroglia of the PNS include satellite cells and Schwann cells. Satellite cells surround neuron cells bodies, and Schwann cells surround peripheral nerve axons forming the **neurilemma.** Schwann cells are like the casings on hot dogs.

> FACT
> There are 100 billion neurons in the body!

Key Terms	Definitions
neurons (NEW ronz)	complete nerve cells
soma (SOH muh)	cell body
axons (ACKS onz)	efferent nerve cells carrying impulses away from the cell body
dendrites (DEN drites)	branched nerve fibers carrying impulses toward the cell body
synapse (SIN aps)	communicating region between neurons
neuroglia (new ROG lee uh)	supporting cells of the CNS
myelin (MIGH e lin)	white, fatty substance forming the nerve sheath
neurilemma (new ri LEM uh)	membrane forming myelin

Key Term Practice: Neurons and Neuroglia

1. What is the plural form of soma? _____

2. What is the medical term for each of the following definitions?

  a. nerve cell _____

  b. cell body _____

Spinal Cord and Spinal Nerves

Attached to the brain, the spinal cord begins at the foramen magnum of the skull and extends to the first lumbar vertebra (Fig. 8-3). Consisting of 31 segments, each of which gives rise to a pair of spinal nerves, the spinal cord is slightly shorter than the vertebral column.

Spinal nerve anatomy consists of a bundle of nerve fibers surrounded by connective tissues. The three layers are the outer **epineurium;** the **perineurium,** which encloses bundles of nerve fibers; and the **endoneurium** surrounding each fiber.

Spinal nerves branch to supply peripheral body regions and are grouped in a numbered sequence according to the level from which they arise (Fig. 8-4). Accordingly, there are 8 pairs of cervical nerves, 12 pairs of thoracic nerves, 5 pairs of lumbar nerves, 5 pairs of sacral nerves, and 1 pair of coccygeal nerves. A group of spinal nerves called the **cauda equina** (horse's tail) extends below the distal end of the spinal cord.

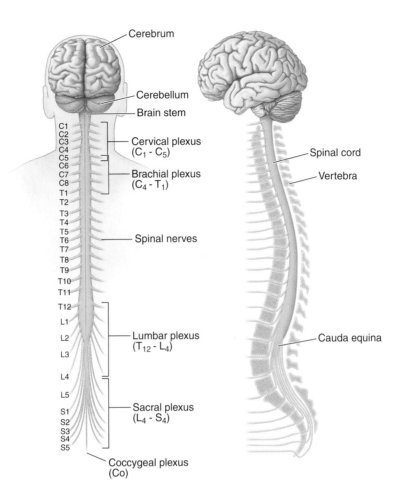

Cerebrum
Cerebellum
Brain stem
C1
C2
C3
C4
C5
C6
C7
C8
T1
T2
T3
T4
T5
T6
T7
T8
T9
T10
T11
T12
L1
L2
L3
L4
L5
S1
S2
S3
S4
S5

Cervical plexus (C$_1$ - C$_5$)
Brachial plexus (C$_4$ - T$_1$)
Spinal nerves
Lumbar plexus (T$_{12}$ - L$_4$)
Sacral plexus (L$_4$ - S$_4$)
Coccygeal plexus (Co)

Spinal cord
Vertebra
Cauda equina

FIGURE 8-3
Spinal nerves branch to supply the peripheral body regions. They are grouped in a numbered sequence.

Associated with the spinal nerves is a structure referred to as a **plexus** (plural = plexuses), or nerve network. Peripheral nerves branching from the spinal cord form plexuses of nerve fibers that are sorted and recombined so all the fibers associated with a particular region reach it together. The **cervical plexus** lies deep in the neck on either side. The **brachial plexus** is made up of the lower four cervical nerves and the first thoracic nerve. Spinal nerves T2–T12 do not form plexuses. The **lumbosacral plexus** consists of some fibers from the last thoracic nerve and the lumbar and sacral nerves. The **coccygeal plexus** innervates the pelvic cavity floor. The interlacing nerve networks of each plexus enable motor functioning in those particular innervated regions.

An area of skin supplied by a single spinal nerve is known as a **dermatome.** All spinal nerves except C1 innervate specific skin segments (Fig. 8-5). When examining and treating patients with spinal nerve damage or disease, clinicians use their knowledge of the dermatomes to determine which segment of the spinal cord is malfunctioning or affected.

The brain is only 2% of a person's total body weight, but it uses 20% of the body's total energy!

Key Terms	Definitions
epineurium (ep i NEW ree um)	connective tissue around a nerve trunk
perineurium (perr i NEW ree um)	connective tissue around a bundle of nerve fibers
endoneurium (en doh NEW ree um)	connective tissue surrounding an individual nerve fiber
cauda equina (KAW duh e KWYE nuh)	roots of the sacral and coccygeal nerves
plexus (PLECK sus)	spinal nerve network

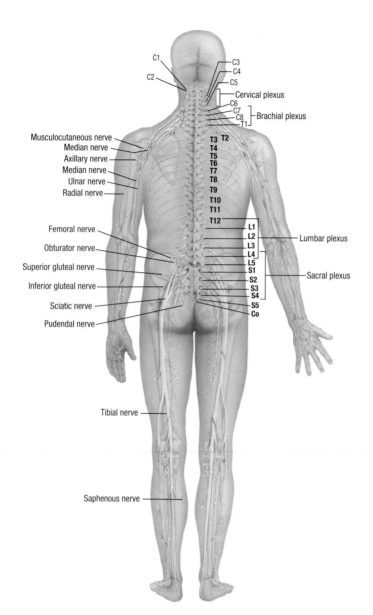

FIGURE 8-4

The nerve plexuses branch from the spinal cord to innervate particular regions of the body. (Images provided by the Anatomical Chart Co.)

cervical plexus (SUR vi kul PLECK sus)	network of interlacing nerves in the cervical region
brachial plexus (BRAY kee ul PLECK sus)	spinal nerve network of the lower four cervical and first thoracic nerves
lumbosacral plexus (lum boh SAY krul PLECK sus)	spinal nerve network of the lumbar and sacral regions
coccygeal plexus (kock SIJ ee ul PLECK sus)	spinal nerve network in the coccyx region
dermatome (DUR muh tome)	area of skin supplied by sensory fibers

Key Term Practice: Spinal Cord and Spinal Nerves

1. From superficial to deep, what are the three layers of connective tissue surrounding a spinal nerve?

   _____

2. A network of nerves is referred to as a/an _____.

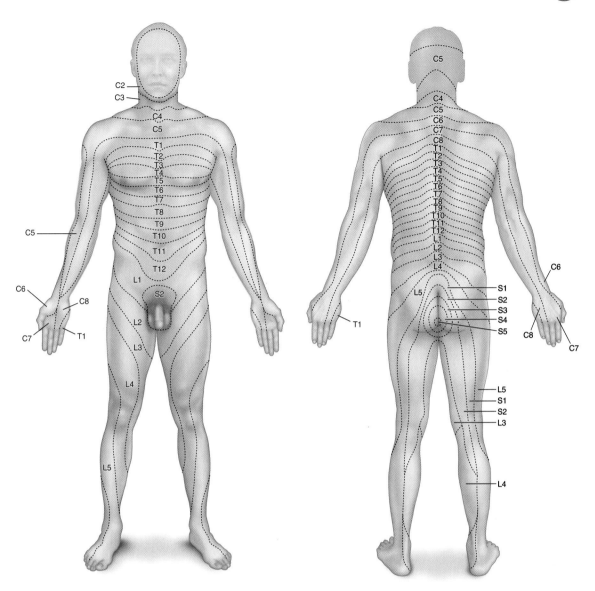

FIGURE 8-5
A dermatome is an area of skin supplied by a single spinal nerve.

Brain and Cranial Nerves

The majority of the body's neural tissue is contained within the brain, which weighs approximately 1.4 kg (3 lb.). Anatomic variations exist among individuals, with men typically having larger brains than females. Despite the difference, intellectual function is equal.

The principal parts of the brain are the cerebrum, cerebellum, and brainstem (Fig. 8-6). Other major landmarks include gyri, sulci, and fissures. Structures contained within the deep portions of the brain are the thalamus, hypothalamus, and pituitary gland.

The **cerebrum** is the largest part of the brain, consisting of two cerebral hemispheres connected by the **corpus callosum**, which is a mass of white matter (myelinated tissue) composed of nerve fibers. The **cerebral cortex**, a superficial layer of gray matter (somata and dendrites of neurons), covers folds of brain tissue called **convolutions**. Raised surface convolutions termed **gyri** (singular = gyrus) increase the surface area of the brain. Shallow depressions called **sulci** (singular = sulcus) and deeper grooves called **fissures** separate gyri. Lobes of the cerebrum correspond to the bone names overlying its surface and are the frontal, parietal, temporal, and occipital.

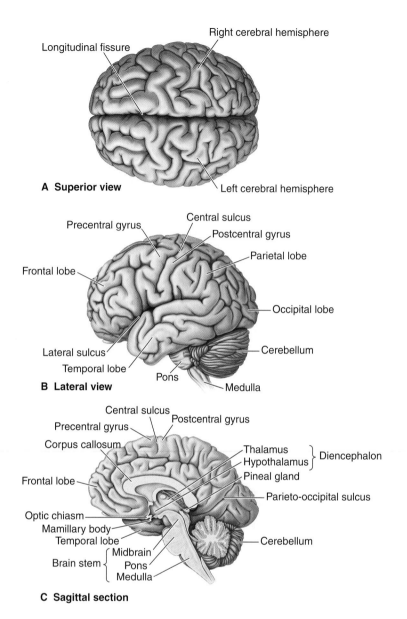

Right cerebral hemisphere

Longitudinal fissure

A Superior view

Left cerebral hemisphere

Central sulcus

Precentral gyrus

Postcentral gyrus

Parietal lobe

Frontal lobe

Occipital lobe

Cerebellum

Lateral sulcus

Temporal lobe

Pons

B Lateral view

Medulla

Central sulcus

Postcentral gyrus

Precentral gyrus

Corpus callosum

Thalamus

Hypothalamus

Diencephalon

Pineal gland

Frontal lobe

Parieto-occipital sulcus

Optic chiasm

Mamillary body

Temporal lobe

Cerebellum

Midbrain

Brain stem

Pons

Medulla

C Sagittal section

FIGURE 8-6

The principle parts of the brain.

The **cerebellum** is the second-largest region of the brain and consists of two hemispheres connected by the **vermis.** The white matter forming a tree-like pattern in the cerebellum is the **arbor vitae.** This portion of the brain functions as a reflex center in the coordination of skeletal muscle movements and in the maintenance of equilibrium. It attaches to the brainstem by three pairs of supporting cerebellar peduncles: the inferior, middle, and superior.

The **brainstem** extends from the base of the cerebrum to the spinal cord. It consists of the diencephalon, midbrain, pons, and medulla oblongata. The **diencephalon** contains the thalamus and hypothalamus. The **thalamus** serves as a central relay station for incoming sensory impulses, and the **hypothalamus** plays a role in homeostatic maintenance. The reflex centers associated with eye and head movements are in the **midbrain** (mesencephalon). The **pons** (metencephalon) separates the midbrain from the medulla oblongata and transmits impulses between the cerebrum and other parts of the nervous system by serving as a relay station for sensory impulses from the peripheral nerves to the brain. It also contains centers that aid in regulating the rate and depth of breathing. The **medulla oblongata** (myelencephalon) is an enlarged continuation of the spinal cord that transmits all ascending and descending impulses. It also contains reflex centers such as the cardiac center for responding to heart function; the

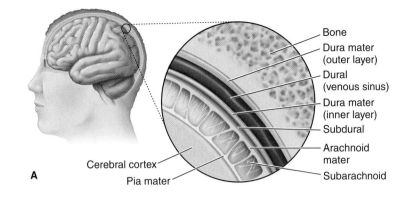

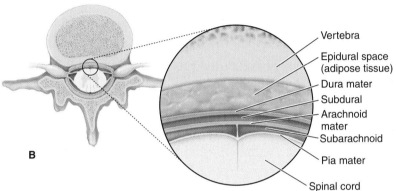

FIGURE 8-7

The meninges are made up of three membranes: the dura mater, arachnoid mater, and pia mater. **(A)** Meninges of the brain. **(B)** Meninges of the spinal cord. (Panel A enlargement: image provided by the Anatomical Chart Co.)

vasomotor center, which is involved with blood vessel constriction and dilation; and the respiratory center, which regulates breathing.

The brain and spinal cord are protected by the surrounding bone tissue, meninges, and cerebrospinal fluid (CSF). Three membranes called **meninges** (singular = meninx) are the dura mater, arachnoid mater, and pia mater (Fig. 8-7). The **dura mater**, whose name literally means "tough mother," is the strong outer layer. In the vertebral column, it forms a tubular sheath around the spinal cord, and it fuses with the internal periosteum (outer bone layer) of the skull bones in the cranial vault. The **arachnoid mater** is the delicate, spiderweb-like middle layer of the meninges that spreads over the brain and spinal cord, but it does not dip into the grooves on their surfaces. The last membrane, **pia mater,** is the inner layer of meninges that encloses the brain and spinal cord. The pia mater contains many nerves as well as blood vessels that aid in nourishing underlying brain and spinal cord cells.

There are three meningeal spaces: epidural, subdural, and subarachnoid (Fig. 8-7). The **epidural** is located between the dura mater and the bony covering of the brain and spinal cord. The **subdural** is found between the dura mater and the arachnoid mater. It secretes lubricating serous fluid. The **subarachnoid** is situated between the arachnoid mater and the pia mater.

The **cerebrospinal fluid** is a liquid that occupies the ventricles of the brain, subarachnoid space, and the central canal of the spinal cord. Normal CSF is clear and sterile. The four interconnected cavities within the cerebral hemispheres and brainstem that are filled with CSF are called **ventricles** (Fig. 8-8). **Choroid plexuses** are vascular complexes in the walls of the third and fourth ventricles that secrete CSF. This fluid circulates through the ventricles to cushion structures, support the brain, and serve as a transport medium for nutrients, hormones, and waste products.

Cranial nerves are components of the PNS that connect directly to the brain but not the spinal cord (Fig. 8-9). There are 12 pairs of cranial nerves, all of which except the first pair, arise from the brainstem. Cranial nerves are designated by the abbreviation CN and are numbered with Roman numerals. The 12 pairs are olfactory (CN I), optic

FIGURE 8-8
The ventricles of the brain consist of four interconnected cavities within the cerebral hemispheres and brainstem and are filled with cerebrospinal fluid. (Image provided by the Anatomical Chart Co.)

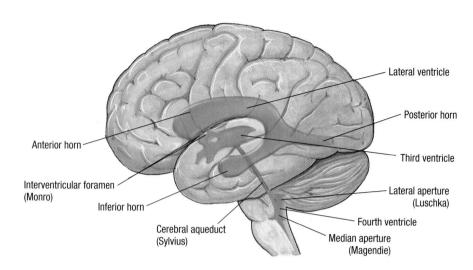

There are about 25 million olfactory receptors!

(CN II), oculomotor (CN III), trochlear (CN IV), trigeminal (CN V), abducens (CN VI), facial (CN VII), vestibulocochlear (CN VIII), glossopharyngeal (CN IX), vagus (CN X), accessory (CN XI), and hypoglossal (CN XII). There are several mnemonic devices, or memory aids, for the cranial nerves. For example, the first letter of each word in the following sentence corresponds to the first letter of each cranial nerve, in order: "*O*h, *o*h, *o*h, *t*o *t*ouch *a*nd *f*eel *v*ery *g*reen *v*egetables, *a*h, *h*eaven."

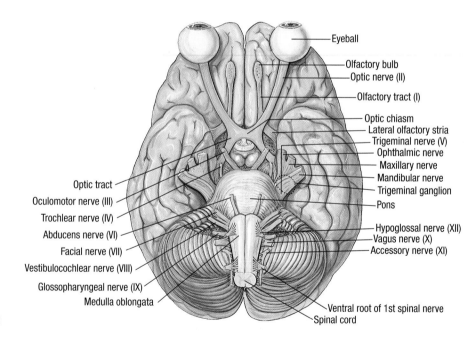

FIGURE 8-9
The cranial nerves connect directly to the brain but not the spinal cord. (Image provided by the Anatomical Chart Co.)

Key Terms	Definitions
cerebrum (se REE brum)	largest portion of the brain; has left and right hemispheres
corpus callosum (KOR pus kuh LOH sum)	broad band of white matter connecting the cerebral hemispheres

cerebral cortex (se REE brul KOR tecks)	outer layer of the cerebrum
convolutions (kon voh LEW shunz)	folds separated by depressions
gyri (JYE rye)	surface convolutions
sulci (SUL sigh)	linear grooves, furrows
fissures (FISH urz)	grooves or clefts
cerebellum (serr e BEL um)	inferior part of the brain between the cerebrum and pons
vermis (VUR mis)	lobe of the cerebellum between the hemispheres
arbor vitae (AHR bur VYE tee)	white section of the cerebellum
brainstem	brain part remaining outside of the cerebrum and cerebellum
diencephalon (dye en CEF uh lon)	brain part containing the thalamus and hypothalamus
thalamus (THAL uh mus)	gray matter on either side of the third ventricle
hypothalamus (high poh THAL uh mus)	region of the diencephalon forming the third ventricle floor
midbrain	middle portion of the brain; mesencephalon
pons (PONZ)	portion of the brain between the medulla and midbrain; metencephalon
medulla oblongata (me DUL uh ob long GAH tuh)	caudal brain part
meninges (me NIN jeez)	three-layered membrane covering the brain and spinal cord
dura mater (DEW ruh MAH tur)	outermost fibrous meninx
arachnoid mater (uh RACK noid MAH tur)	central meninx
pia mater (PEE uh MAH tur)	vascular meninx on the brain and spinal cord surface
epidural (ep i DEW rul)	space between the dura mater and periosteum
subdural (sub DEW rul)	space between the dura mater and arachnoid mater
subarachnoid (sub uh RACK noid)	space between the arachnoid mater and pia mater, filled with CSF
cerebrospinal (serr e broh SPYE nul) fluid	circulating fluid in the ventricles and subarachnoid space
ventricles (VEN tri kulz)	brain cavities
choroid plexuses (KOR oid PLECK sus es)	structures in the ventricles secreting CSF

Key Term Practice: Brain and Cranial Nerves

1. What is the singular form of sulci? _____

2. What are the three primary brain regions? _____

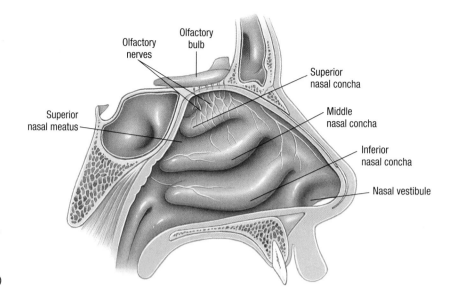

FIGURE 8-10
The olfactory receptors send impulses to the frontal lobe of the cerebrum. (Image provided by the Anatomical Chart Co.)

Olfaction and Gustation

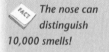

The nose can distinguish 10,000 smells!

The sense of smell is termed **olfaction**. Olfactory receptors are similar to those for taste in that they are chemoreceptors stimulated by chemicals dissolved in liquids. Olfactory and gustatory (taste) receptors function together because food is usually smelled at the same time it is tasted. The nose and olfactory organs contain olfactory receptors that are supported by columnar epithelial cells (Fig 8-10). These specified structures cover the nasal cavity, superior nasal conchae, and septum; their primary function is to allow one to smell. Impulses travel from the olfactory receptors through the olfactory nerves (CN I) to interpreting centers in the frontal lobes of the cerebrum. Seven primary olfactory sensations have been identified: camphoraceous (scent of camphor), musky (scent of musk), floral (scent of flowers), pepperminty (scent of oil of peppermint), ethereal (scent of ether), pungent (scent of spices), and putrid (scent of decaying meat).

Gustation is the term used to describe tasting. Salivary glands aid the function of taste receptors. Before the taste of a particular chemical can be detected, the chemical must first be dissolved in the watery fluid supplied by the salivary glands, surrounding the tongue's taste buds. Figure 8-11 illustrates the structure of the taste buds and papillae. Sensory impulses from taste receptors travel on fibers of the facial (CN VII), glossopharyngeal (CN IX), and vagus nerves (CN X). These impulses are carried to the

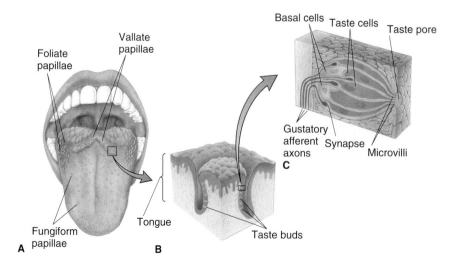

FIGURE 8-11
Taste buds are taste-sensitive structures made up of receptor cells. (Image provided by the Anatomical Chart Co.)

medulla and ascend to the thalamus, from which they are directed to the gustatory cortex in the parietal lobes. Seven primary taste sensations have been isolated: sweet, sour, salty, bitter, metallic, umami, and water. The umami taste is one of chicken broth, beef broth, or Parmesan cheese and is triggered by the presence of amino acids in these foods. Figure 8-12 maps the locations of each of these taste sensations on the tongue. Taste sensation is not likely to diminish with age because taste cells are reproduced continually; in fact, any one of these cells functions for only about 1 week before it is replaced.

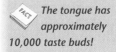 **The tongue has approximately 10,000 taste buds!**

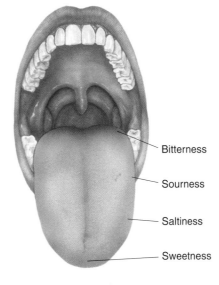

— Bitterness

— Sourness

— Saltiness

— Sweetness

FIGURE 8-12
Regions of the tongue with the lowest thresholds for basic tastes. The center of the tongue has no taste buds. (Image provided by the Anatomical Chart Co.)

Key Terms	Definitions
olfaction (ol FACK shun)	sense of smell
gustation (gus TAY shun)	sense of taste

Key Term Practice: Olfaction and Gustation

1. What is the medical term for the sense of taste? _____

2. _____ is the medical term for the sense of smell.

Ear, Hearing, and Equilibrium

The three anatomic sections making up the ear are the external, middle, and internal (inner). The **external ear** collects sound waves created by vibrating objects (Fig. 8-13). The external ear components are the pinna, ceruminous glands, external auditory meatus, and tympanic membrane (Fig 8-14). The **pinna** or **auricle** is the external cartilaginous structure that directs sound waves. The **ceruminous glands** secrete cerumen, commonly called earwax. Cerumen keeps the tympanic membrane soft and pliable. The **external acoustic meatus** transmits sound waves to the **tympanic membrane,** or eardrum, which in turn transmits pressure waves to the malleus. An alternate term for the tympanic membrane is **myringa.** The external acoustic meatus is that portion of the ear directly exposed to the outside.

The **middle ear** houses the **auditory ossicles,** the three small bones called the **malleus, incus,** and **stapes.** Ossicles conduct and amplify the force of sound waves

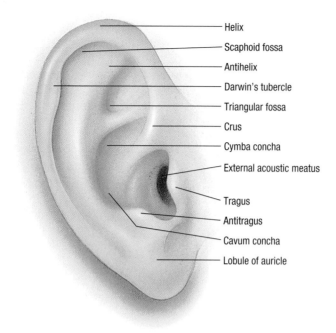

FIGURE 8-13
The external ear collects sound waves created by vibrations. (Image provided by the Anatomical Chart Co.)

Helix
Scaphoid fossa
Antihelix
Darwin's tubercle
Triangular fossa
Crus
Cymba concha
External acoustic meatus
Tragus
Antitragus
Cavum concha
Lobule of auricle

from the tympanic membrane to the oval window of the inner ear. The **internal ear** consists of a complex system of interconnected tubes and chambers along with the **osseous labyrinth** (bony canal in the temporal bone). Structures within the bony (osseous) labyrinth include the semicircular canals, vestibule, and cochlea. The **semicircular canals** are interconnected bony tubes situated in three different planes, and the **vestibule** is the bony chamber between them. The **membranous labyrinth** is a tube that lies within the osseous labyrinth and conforms to its shape. The cochlea houses the **organ of Corti**, which contains the hearing receptors. Fluids associated with the inner ear are endolymph and perilymph.

Skeletal muscles attached to the auditory ossicles act in the tympanic reflex to protect the inner ear from the effects of loud sounds. When the reflex occurs, muscles contract, and the malleus and stapes are moved, resulting in rigidity of the ossicle bridges in the middle ear, thereby reducing its effectiveness in transmitting vibrations to the inner ear.

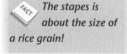

The stapes is about the size of a rice grain!

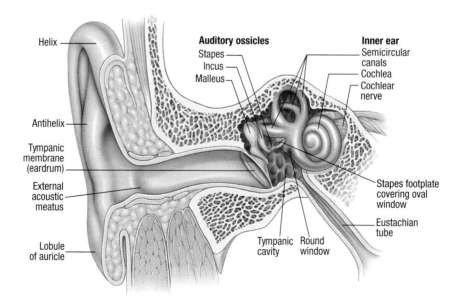

FIGURE 8-14
Structures of the middle and internal ear. (Image provided by the Anatomical Chart Co.)

Helix
Antihelix
Tympanic membrane (eardrum)
External acoustic meatus
Lobule of auricle
Auditory ossicles
Stapes
Incus
Malleus
Tympanic cavity
Round window
Inner ear
Semicircular canals
Cochlea
Cochlear nerve
Stapes footplate covering oval window
Eustachian tube

The **auditory tube** connects the middle ear cavity to the pharynx (throat). Because of the shared connection, it is not uncommon for bacterial and viral infections to migrate between the ear and the throat cavities. The auditory tube also helps maintain equal pressure on both sides of the tympanic membrane. This structure creates the characteristic ear "pop" experienced when changing altitudes.

The **cochlea**, a structure shaped like a coiled snail's shell, is the portion of the inner ear that contains the receptors of hearing. Hearing receptors, also referred to as **hair cells**, are arranged in four parallel rows and possess numerous hair-like processes called **stereocilia** (singular = stereocilium). Different frequencies of vibrations stimulate different sets of receptor cells. Hearing receptors stimulate sensory neurons along a pathway. The pattern of sound wave transmission is as follows:

1. Sound waves enter external auditory meatus.

2. The eardrum reproduces the vibrations.

3. The vibrations move to the auditory ossicles (malleus, incus, and stapes), the oval window, the perilymph in the scala vestibuli, and then to the endolymph of cochlear duct.

4. Neurotransmitters stimulate the ends of nearby sensory neurons.

5. Impulses are triggered on the fibers of the cochlear branch of the vestibulo-cochlear nerve (CN VIII).

6. The auditory cortex of the cerebral temporal lobe interprets the impulses.

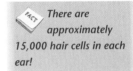

FACT There are approximately 15,000 hair cells in each ear!

Several abbreviations associated with the ear are derived from Latin words. For example, the medical abbreviation for ear is the letter *A,* which stands for the word *auris. Auris dextra* (A.D.) means the "right ear," *auris sinistra* (A.S.) refers to the "left ear." In Latin, *auris uterque* (A.U.) can be translated to mean "each ear" or "both ears."

Ears play an important role in both static and dynamic equilibrium. Static equilibrium is concerned with maintaining the stability of the head and body when they are motionless. Equilibrium sensations enable balance by monitoring head position, acceleration, and rotation. Organs of dynamic and static equilibrium are located in the vestibule (utricle and saccule), and the semicircular ducts maintain dynamic equilibrium.

Key Terms	Definitions
external (ecks TUR nul) **ear**	outer ear
pinna (PIN uh)	projecting ear part; auricle
auricle (AW ri kul)	projecting ear part; pinna
ceruminous (se ROO mi nus) **glands**	cerumen-secreting glands of the external auditory meatus
external acoustic meatus (ecks TUR nul uh KOOS tick mee AY tus)	passageway between the pinna and tympanic membrane
tympanic (tim PAN ick) **membrane**	eardrum; membrane separating the external ear from the middle ear
myringa (mi RING guh)	tympanic membrane
middle ear	tympanic membrane and ossicles
auditory ossicles (AW di tor ee OS i kulz)	small bones of the ear: malleus, incus, stapes
malleus (MAL ee us)	hammer-shaped middle ear bone
incus (ING kus)	anvil-shaped ear bone between the malleus and the stapes

stapes (STAY peez)	stirrup-shaped middle ear bone
internal ear	inner ear
osseous (OS ee us) labyrinth	part of the temporal bone surrounding the inner ear
semicircular canals (sem i SIRR kew lur kuh NALS)	bony tubes situated in three planes
vestibule	chamber between the semicircular canals
membranous (MEM brah nus) labyrinth	canals lining the osseous labyrinth
organ of Corti (KOR tee)	location of the hearing receptors
auditory tube	canal connecting the pharynx with the tympanic cavity
cochlea (KOCK lee uh)	structure that houses the essential organs of hearing
hair cells	epithelial cells with hair-like processes that respond to sound waves and maintain equilibrium
stereocilia (sterr ee oh SIL ee uh)	hair cells involved with balance and equilibrium

Key Term Practice: Ear, Hearing, and Equilibrium

1. What is the plural form of each given term?

   a. pinna = _____

   b. malleus = _____

   c. incus = _____

   d. cochlea = _____

2. What is the singular form of stereocilia? _____

Eye and Vision

In addition to sight, the eyes have a role in maintaining equilibrium. The eyes can detect changes in posture that result from body movements. Such visual information is so important that even if a person suffers damage to the organs of equilibrium in the ear, he or she may be able to maintain normal balance by keeping the eyes open and moving slowly.

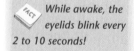

While awake, the eyelids blink every 2 to 10 seconds!

Visual accessory organs have special functions as well. The eyelid serves to protect the eye, and the **conjunctiva** lines the inner surfaces of eyelids. **Lacrimal glands** secrete tears for lubrication and **lysozyme** for antimicrobial actions; extrinsic muscles move the eyes.

Three **tunics** (layers) make up the eyeball: fibrous, vascular, and inner (Fig. 8-15). The **fibrous tunic** is the outer layer and includes the cornea and sclera. The clear **cornea** is the window of the eye that helps focus entering light. The white portion, providing protection and serving as an attachment for extrinsic eye muscles, is the **sclera**.

The **vascular tunic** (uvea) is the middle part, consisting of the choroid, ciliary body, and iris. The nourishing tissue that contains melanocytes, which absorb excess light and keep the inside of the eye dark, is called the **choroid**. The **ciliary body** is the thickest part, forming a ring around the front of the eye. Dividing the space between

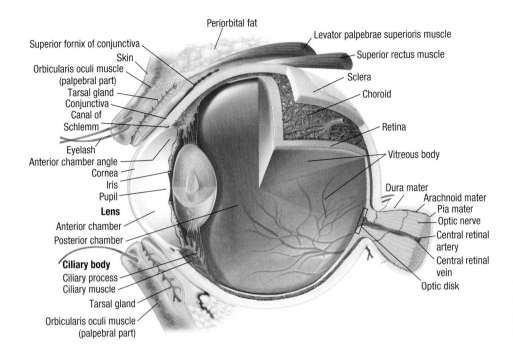

Periorbital fat
Superior fornix of conjunctiva
Skin
Orbicularis oculi muscle
(palpebral part)
Tarsal gland
Conjunctiva
Canal of
Schlemm
Eyelash
Anterior chamber angle
Cornea
Iris
Pupil
Lens
Anterior chamber
Posterior chamber
Ciliary body
Ciliary process
Ciliary muscle
Tarsal gland
Orbicularis oculi muscle
(palpebral part)

Levator palpebrae superioris muscle
Superior rectus muscle
Sclera
Choroid
Retina
Vitreous body
Dura mater
Arachnoid mater
Pia mater
Optic nerve
Central retinal
artery
Central retinal
vein
Optic disk

FIGURE 8-15
The structures of the
eye. (Image provided
by the Anatomical
Chart Co.)

the cornea and the lens is the colored portion of the eye termed the **iris.** The muscular iris controls the amount of light entering the eye through an opening in its center termed the **pupil.** The **lens** is an elastic, transparent structure between the iris and vitreous humor that allows accommodation.

Accommodation is the increase in lens thickness and convexity in response to ciliary muscle contraction to focus an object. It occurs when the lens is focused to view a close object. **Refraction,** the bending of light rays, is necessary for vision. Light rays are focused on the back of the eyeball. When adjusting for a close object, the lens becomes more convex; when focusing on a distant object, the lens becomes more concave. Light rays are refracted primarily by the cornea and lens to focus an image on the retina (Fig. 8-16).

The innermost layer is the **neural tunic,** which includes the retina and the optic nerve. The **retina** contains photoreceptors (visual receptors), and the **optic nerve** (CN II) serves as the connection from the eye to the central nervous system. The **macula** is a region of the retina containing the fovea centralis. The region of greatest visual acuity is found within the **fovea centralis,** an indentation in the central region of the macula. The **optic disk** is the particular location where nerve fibers exit to become part of the optic nerve.

*There are over
1 million
photoreceptors in each
eye!*

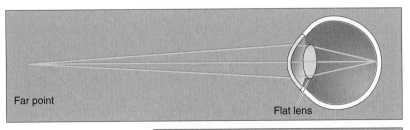
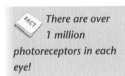

Far point
Flat lens

Near point
Fat lens

FIGURE 8-16
Refraction by the lens
is necessary for vision.
(Image provided by
the Anatomical Chart
Co.)

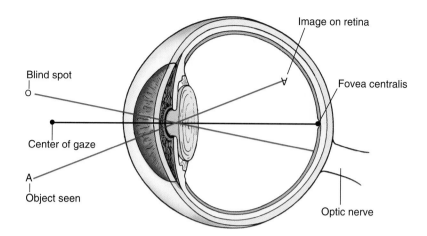

FIGURE 8-17
The visual pathway. (Image provided by the Anatomical Chart Co.)

The chambers of the eyeball are the anterior and posterior, each containing a different fluid, termed a humor. **Aqueous humor** is a watery, nourishing fluid located in the anterior chamber. The **vitreous humor** of the posterior chamber is a transparent, gelatinous fluid, found between the lens and retina; it functions to support internal eye parts while helping the eye maintain its shape.

Rods and cones are important photoreceptors in the retina. **Rods** are responsible for colorless vision in relatively dim light, and **cones** are responsible for color vision. (Think of *cones* for *color*.) Cone vision is more acute than rod vision because impulses originating from the cones are often transmitted to the brain on separate nerve fibers, allowing for sharper vision. Impulses from several rods may be transmitted to the brain on a single sensory nerve fiber; hence images from these cells are not nearly as fine. The visual pathway is as follows (Fig. 8-17):

1. Light stimulates the nerve fibers from the retina that form the optic nerve.
2. From the optic nerve, impulses are transmitted to the optic chiasma, optic tract, and optic radiations.
3. Finally, the impulses reach the visual cortex for interpretation.

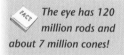

The eye has 120 million rods and about 7 million cones!

The human eye is capable of adapting to both light and dark through the interaction of rods, cones, and pigments. One pigment responsible for this is rhodopsin. **Rhodopsin** (visual purple) is a light-sensitive pigment in rods that decomposes in the presence of light and triggers a complex series of reactions that initiate nerve impulses on the optic nerve.

Common abbreviations for eye terms are O.S., O.D, and O.U. The letter *O* stands for the word *oculus*, referring to the eye. *Oculus sinister* (O.S.) means "left eye." *Oculus dexter* (O.D.) describes the "right eye," and *oculus uterque*, (O.U.) refers to "each eye" or "both eyes." .

Key Terms	Definitions
conjunctiva (kon junk TYE vuh)	mucous membrane covering the anterior eye and eyelids
lacrimal (LACK ri mul) **glands**	tear-secreting glands
lysozyme (LYE soh zime)	antimicrobic enzyme of tears
tunics (TEW nicks)	coats or layers
fibrous tunic	outer eye layer
cornea (KOR nee uh)	transparent anterior part of the eye
sclera (SKLEER uh)	whitish, outer layer of the eyeball
vascular (VAS kew lur) **tunic**	layer containing blood vessels

choroid (KOR oid)	pigmented vascular tunic
ciliary (SIL ee err ee) body	thickening of the vascular tunic
iris (EYE ris)	colored portion of the eyeball
pupil (PEW pil)	opening in the iris
lens (LENZ)	eye portion that refracts light
accommodation	process by which light rays are focused on the retina by changes in the ciliary muscle and lens
refraction (ree FRACK shun)	bending of light rays
neural (NEW rul) tunic	layer of the eye containing the retina
retina (RET i nuh)	light-receptive layer of the optic nerve
optic (OP tick) nerve	CN II
macula (MACK yoo luh)	point of clearest vision; yellow spot on the retina
fovea centralis (FOH vee uh sen TRAY lis)	center of the macula
optic (OP tick) disk	circular area of the retina where fibers converge forming the optic nerve
aqueous (AY kwee us) humor	watery eye secretion
vitreous (VIT ree us) humor	semisolid fluid of eye
rods	rod-shaped photoreceptor concerned with vision in dim light
cones	conical-shaped photoreceptor concerned with color vision
rhodopsin (roh DOP sin)	red pigment of the rods which are bleached by daylight

Key Term Practice: Eye and Vision

1. What is the plural form of each of the following terms?

   a. lens = _____

   b. iris = _____

2. _____ are photoreceptors for color vision.

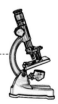

THE CLINICAL DIMENSION

Pathology of the Nervous System and Special Senses

This chapter focuses on the nervous system and includes topics related to the brain, spinal cord, peripheral nerves, ears, eyes, and senses. The following sections outline common signs, symptoms, clinical tests, diagnostic procedures, pathological conditions, and treatments pertinent to the nervous system.

Clinicians working in the neurologic field are varied because the nervous system is so diverse. Health-care workers include audiologists, neurologists, neurosurgeons, optometrists, and ophthalmologists. Neurologists, neurosurgeons, and ophthalmologists are medical doctors (MDs or DOs) with advanced training in neurology, surgery, and ophthalmology. Doctors of optometry, or optometrists, have earned a doctorate degree in the specialized field of optometry. Audiologists are not physicians, but they have specialized degrees and training in the area of audiology.

General Brain Disorders

Pain in the head is termed **cephalalgia**, or headache. There are no pain receptors in the brain, but they do exist in the meninges. Therefore, the pain can be isolated to this region. (This also explains why brain surgery can be performed while the patient is wide awake.) Common types of cephalalgia are tension and vascular. Tension headaches result from strain on facial, neck, and scalp muscles. The vascular form results from edema in arterial vessels. Initial diagnosis is made through history and physical examination.

To rule out underlying pathology, electroencephalography, and computed tomography scans are performed. **Electroencephalography** (EEG) is the recording of the electrical potentials in the brain obtained by an electroencephalograph (EEG). The record itself is termed an electroencephalogram (EEG). A technique for producing images of cross-sections of the body using a computer that processes data from radiographs (x-rays) is termed **computed tomography** (CT).

A **migraine** is a recurrent, severe vascular headache. Migraines are commonly unilateral and associated with vomiting, nausea, visual disturbances, and **photophobia** (sensitivity to light). Sufferers experience auras, flashes appearing as heat waves, jagged lines, flashing lights, and striped vision. Ocular migraines are characterized by the same symptoms but without the headache. Migraines are usually familial and affect women twice as frequently as men. History and physical examination are used for initial diagnosis. Other tests such as magnetic resonance imaging (MRI) and CT scan are given to rule out pathology. Treatment is aimed at making the person comfortable and includes bed rest in a dark, quiet room and prescription medications. Vasoconstrictors to reduce vascular spasms and antiemetics to control vomiting are administered. An agent for preventing or relieving nausea is called an **antiemetic.** The prescription drug Imitrex may also be prescribed. Biofeedback techniques, whereby involuntary processes are perceptible to the senses, are also beneficial to some individuals.

The immediate loss of consciousness resulting from a nonpenetrating head injury that causes a change in skull momentum is called a **concussion.** It is also referred to as being "knocked out" for seconds to a few minutes. Brain electrical activity, but not brain tissue, is altered. The activity generally resolves, yet **amnesia** (loss of memory) may persist for up to 24 hours. Signs and symptoms after regaining consciousness are headache, vomiting, blurred vision, and photophobia. Neurologic examination and history of the injury confirm the diagnosis. Bed rest with waking the person every 4 hours is the only treatment.

Coma is a state of profound unconsciousness from which one cannot be roused. Its causes include ingesting a toxic substance, lack of oxygen, trauma, or disease. Ruling out hypoglycemia (low blood glucose level) is the first step in the diagnosis, followed by a complete neurologic examination that includes an EEG. The **Glasgow coma scale** is used to assess the patient's level of consciousness (LOC) (Fig. 8-18).

Bruising of brain tissue is termed a **contusion.** Headache, hemiparesis, and drowsiness are typical signs and symptoms. **Paresis** means there is a slight paralysis or incomplete loss of muscle power; **hemiparesis** is muscle weakness on one side. Loss of consciousness may be temporary or result in coma. Contusions are more serious than concussions and result from a severe blow to the head. Skull fracture is common. Diagnosis is made by neurologic evaluation and CT scan to identify any bone

Glasgow Coma Score

The GCS is scored between 3 and 15, 3 being the worst, and 15 the best. It is composed of three parameters: Best Eye Response, Best Verbal Response, Best Motor Response, as given below:

Best Eye Response. (4)

1. No eye opening.
2. Eye opening to pain.
3. Eye opening to verbal command.
4. Eyes open spontaneously.

Best Verbal Response. (5)

1. No verbal response
2. Incomprehensible sounds.
3. Inappropriate words.
4. Confused
5. Orientated

Best Motor Response. (6)

1. No motor response.
2. Extension to pain.
3. Flexion to pain.
4. Withdrawal from pain.
5. Localizing pain.
6. Obeys commands.

A Coma Score of 13 or higher correlates with a mild brain injury, 9 to 12 is a moderate injury and 8 or less a severe brain injury.

FIGURE 8-18
The Glasgow Coma Scale is used to assess a patient's level of consciousness.

fractures. Hospitalization is necessary to monitor the patient and provide appropriate treatments as they become necessary.

Epilepsy is a brain disorder characterized by excessive neuronal discharge with accompanying motor, sensory, or psychic dysfunction exhibited as seizures. It results from irregular electrical discharges of brain cells. Cerebral (formerly known as petit mal) and generalized tonic–clonic (also called grand mal) seizures are common types experienced by people with epilepsy. **Cerebral seizures** are recurrent convulsions with blank stares and temporary loss of awareness. A loud cry, falling to the floor, sudden onset of intermittent muscle contractions and relaxations, and loss of consciousness are characteristics of **generalized tonic–clonic seizures**. The cause is either idiopathic or the result of a known brain pathology. An EEG and medical history are used to diagnose epilepsy. Treatment is aimed at patient and family education and the administration of anticonvulsant drugs.

Parkinson disease (PD; parkinsonism) is characterized by progressive degeneration of the dopamine-producing neurons in the substantia nigra of the brain, resulting in insufficient dopamine (DA) in the basal ganglia. Its cause is unknown. Other characteristics include rhythmic muscular tremors, movement rigidity, droopy posture, mask-like appearance, "pill-rolling" tremor of thumb and index finger, and shuffling gait. The disease affects more men than women; the typical age of onset is around 60 years. Physical examination, neurologic evaluation, and history confirm the diagnosis. There is no cure, but drugs such as levodopa, antidepressants, and anticholinergics (drugs that interfere with the neurotransmitter acetylcholine) are used.

Transient refers to something being "present for a short period of time." A **transient ischemic attack** (TIA) is the result of atherosclerotic thrombolytic disease or cerebral embolism. The person experiences blurred vision, hemiparesis, and speech difficulty. A TIA is often a signal of an impending stroke and is frequently caused by a plaque fragment that interrupts vascular flow in the brain. Diagnosis is made through physical examination, MRI, CT scan, and EEG; however, these studies may not always confirm a TIA. Administration of anticoagulants (blood thinners) is the treatment of choice.

Cerebrovascular accidents (CVAs), or strokes, result when brain tissue is destroyed by hemorrhage, thrombosis, or atherosclerosis. *Cerebrovascular* refers to "blood vessels or blood supply to the brain." It often is caused by disruption of blood flow to a particular brain region. Signs and symptoms vary, depending on the area affected by occlusion. Headache, blurred vision, slurred speech, dysphasia, hemiparesis, and facial paralysis are common.

Dysphasia is the loss of or deficiency in ability to use or understand language caused by an acquired brain lesion. Initial diagnosis is made by history and physical examination and confirmed by MRI, CT scan, cerebral angiography, or EEG. With **cerebral angiography**, blood vessel arrangement is mapped by capillaroscopy, fluoroscopy, or radiography after introduction of a dye. Treatment involves the prompt administration of tissue plasminogen activator to thwart blood clotting or anticoagulants. **Tissue plasminogen activator** (TPA or tPA) is a naturally occurring substance that acts as a thrombolytic agent, or a chemical against blood clotting. It is also synthetically manufactured and used for the treatment of stroke, heart attack, and peripheral vascular clotting. Follow-up care in the form of speech therapy and physical rehabilitation is often necessary.

Key Terms	Definitions
cephalalgia (sef uh LAL jee uh)	headache
electroencephalography (ee leck troh en sef uh LOG ruh fee)	method of graphically recording the electrical activity of the brain
computed tomography (toh MOG ruh fee)	imaging method using a computer to reconstruct the anatomic features obtained by x-ray
migraine (MIGH grain)	recurrent, severe vascular headache
photophobia (foh toh FOH bee uh)	eye sensitivity to light
antiemetic (an tee e MET ick)	agent for relieving nausea
concussion (kun KUSH un)	transient, immediate loss of consciousness
amnesia (am NEE zhuh)	loss of memory
coma (KOH muh)	prolonged state of deep unconsciousness
Glasgow (GLAS goh) **coma scale**	scale used to assess the level of consciousness
contusion (kon TEW zhun)	brain tissue bruise
paresis (puh REE sis)	slight paralysis
hemiparesis (hem ee puh REE sis)	muscle weakness on one side

epilepsy (EP i lep see)	brain disorder resulting from an irregular electrical discharge of neurons
cerebral seizures (se REE brul SEE zhurz)	recurrent convulsions with blank stares and temporary loss of awareness
generalized tonic-clonic (TON ick KLO nick) seizure	seizure characterized by collapse, loss of consciousness, and intermittent muscle contractions and relaxations
Parkinson disease	disorder resulting from progressive degeneration of dopamine-producing neurons in the brain
transient ischemic (TRAN zee unt is KEE mick) attack	brain disorder that is not permanent
cerebrovascular (se ree broh VAS kew lur) accidents	strokes
dysphasia (dis FAY zhuh)	difficulty in speaking and understanding written or spoken language as a result of brain injury
cerebral angiography (se REE brul an jee OG ruh fee)	mapping of the cerebral blood vessels using dye and x-rays
tissue plasminogen (plaz MIN oh jen) activator	substance that acts against blood clots

Key Term Practice: General Brain Disorders

1. Which disease is associated with the loss of dopamine-producing neurons on the brain? _____

2. _____ refers to difficulty in speaking and understanding written or spoken language as a result of brain injury.

3. What is the common term for a cerebrovascular accident? _____

Dementia

Dementia is a general term used to describe the progressive loss of intellectual functions while maintaining those of perception, consciousness, and motor control. **Alzheimer disease** (AD) is a disabling dementia of the elderly (primarily) that involves widespread intellectual impairment, personality changes, and sometimes delirium. The disorder is named after Alois Alzheimer, who first described the disease in 1907. It causes characteristic lesions in the cortex (Fig. 8-19). It has an unknown cause, although some research suggests a genetic basis. Diagnosis is made by family history and performance on specific cognitive function tests. Definitive diagnosis is possible only after death, when examination of brain tissue at autopsy reveals β-amyloid senile plaques, neurofibrillary tangles, atrophy, and widened sulci and ventricles. Treatment is palliative; however, newer drug therapies targeting the behavioral aspects are available. Early diagnosis and intervention may delay disease progression.

Huntington chorea is an inherited form of dementia. *Chorea* refers to "widespread involuntary, jerky movements of brief duration." Symptoms appear between 30 and 40 years of age. It is characterized by progressive atrophy of the brain putamen and caudate nucleus. Neurologic examination and family history suggest the disease. Brain scans can demonstrate anatomic brain changes. There is no cure, and drug treatment is provided as a supportive measure.

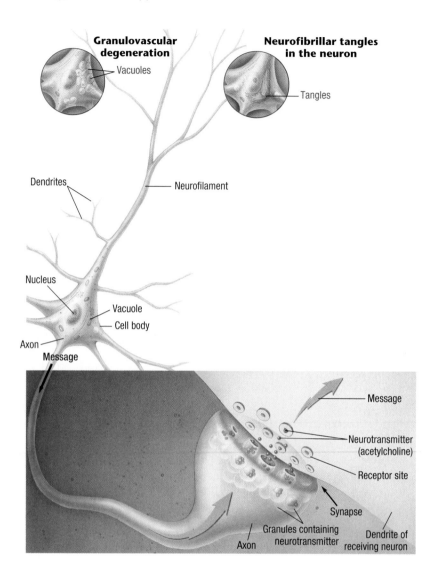

FIGURE 8-19
Tissue changes in Alzheimer disease. (Image provided by the Anatomical Chart Co.)

Key Terms	Definitions
dementia (de MEN shuh)	loss of intellectual and cognitive functions while other brain functions are maintained
Alzheimer (AWLTZ hye mur) disease	degenerative brain disorder that causes dementia; onset is typically late in life
Huntington chorea (koh REE uh)	inherited form of dementia accompanied by atrophy of the cerebral cortex and basal ganglia

Key Term Practice: Dementia

1. The medical term for the progressive deterioration of intellectual functions while other brain functions remain intact is _____.

Brain Neoplasms

A brain neoplasm (abnormal growth) derived from neuroglial cells is termed a **glioma**. A tumor originating from an astrocyte, oligodendrocyte, and ependymal cell is termed an **astrocytoma**, **oligodendroglioma**, and **ependymoma**, respectively. An astrocytoma occurs anywhere in the brain or spinal cord and is typically slow growing. Relatively avascular, an oligodendrocytoma may arise from the brainstem, cerebellum, and spinal cord but most commonly occurs in the frontal lobes. An ependymoma is found in the brain ventricles and is more common in children than in adults. Early signs and symptoms of astrocytomas and oligodendrogliomas are usually headaches or seizures. Signs and symptoms of ependymomas include uncoordinated muscle movement, visual changes, and headache. Gliomas are diagnosed by CT scan and treated by surgery and/or radiation therapy.

Key Terms	*Definitions*
glioma (glye OH muh)	tumor composed of cells derived from neuroglia
astrocytoma (as troh sigh TOH muh)	tumor derived from astrocytes
oligodendroglioma (ol i goh den droh glye OH muh)	tumor derived from oligodendrocytes
ependymoma (ep en digh MOH muh)	tumor derived from ependymal cells

Key Term Practice: Brain Neoplasms

1. Identify the glioma derived from each of the following cell types.

   a. astrocyte _____

   b. ependymal cell _____

   c. oligodendrocyte _____

Pediatric Disorders

A group of motor disorders caused by damage to motor centers of the cerebral cortex, cerebellum, or basal ganglia (four deep masses of gray matter in each hemisphere) during fetal development, childbirth, or early infancy is termed **cerebral palsy** (CP). The word *palsy* means "paralysis or weakness." The disease may result from inadequate oxygen supply while in utero or by an interruption of oxygen-rich blood to the brain during birth. Diagnosis is made by neurologic examination. Treatment options depend on the level of severity. Physical therapy and occupational therapy are often prescribed. Antispasmodic and anticonvulsant drugs are indicated in some cases.

Reye syndrome is an acute illness generally of young children that occurs after a viral infection such as influenza or varicella (chickenpox). Fever, vomiting, brain dysfunction, and liver damage are characteristic signs and symptoms. It can progress from loss of consciousness to coma. There is also fatty invasion of the organs. The cause is unknown, but there is a link between aspirin administration and its onset when a fever is present. The clinician assesses the clinical picture, evaluates the elevated serum ammonia levels, and views the liver biopsy to confirm the diagnosis. Patients are hospitalized so cerebral edema can be monitored.

Key Terms	Definitions
cerebral palsy (se REE brul PAWL zee)	group of motor function diseases
Reye (RYE) **syndrome**	complex of symptoms with liver damage and brain dysfunction that occurs after a viral infection

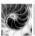

Key Term Practice: Pediatric Disorders

1. A rare and serious childhood disease usually following a respiratory infection and with a known association with aspirin ingestion is termed _____ syndrome.

Cranial Nerve Disorders

Bell palsy is a condition of probable viral infection involving the facial nerve (CN VII). It is characterized by unilateral paralysis of muscles innervated by the facial nerve (Fig. 8-20). Its usual onset occurs while sleeping, so the person wakes up with the condition. Men and women are equally affected, and its onset is between 20 and 60 years. Bell palsy is normally transient, but occasionally it can be permanent. It is diagnosed on the basis of the signs and symptoms, neurologic evaluation, and case history. Analgesics; warm, moist heat; and corticosteroids (immunosuppressive anti-inflammatory drugs) are recommended. Avoidance of extreme temperature variation is also suggested. One can expect complete recovery if it is treated early.

Trigeminal neuralgia, or **tic douloureux**, is a condition of unknown cause marked by sudden, severe pain of one or more branches of the trigeminal nerve (CN V). If the ophthalmic branch is involved, there is pain in the eye and forehead. Nose, upper lip, and cheek pain indicates maxillary branch involvement; and if the mandibular branch is affected the person experiences pain in the lower lip and tongue. It is an occasional **sequela** (plural = sequelae), an aftereffect of a condition that follows infection, with herpes zoster or accompanies multiple sclerosis. The disorder may persist from months to years, but it normally subsides. Patient observation and pain mapping are used to make the diagnosis. For mild episodes, analgesics (pain relievers) are given; severe cases may require surgery.

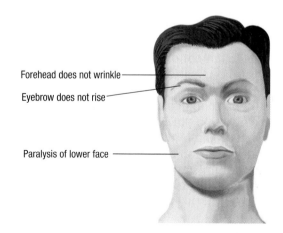

Forehead does not wrinkle

Eyebrow does not rise

Paralysis of lower face

FIGURE 8-20
Bell palsy is characterized by unilateral paralysis of the muscles innervated by the facial nerve. (Image provided by the Anatomical Chart Co.)

Key Terms	Definitions
Bell palsy (PAWL zee)	peripheral paralysis of the muscles innervated by the facial nerve
trigeminal neuralgia (trye JEM i nul new RAL juh)	pain in one or more branches of CN V; tic douloureux
tic douloureux (TIC doo loo RUH)	pain in one or more branches of CN V; trigeminal neuralgia
sequela (se KWEL uh)	aftereffect of a condition, disease, or injury

Key Term Practice: Cranial Nerve Disorders

1. The term _____ refers to the aftereffect of a disease, condition, or injury.

2. Tic douloureux is the alternate term for this disorder, which affects CN V. _____

Spinal Cord and Spinal Nerve Disorders

Amyotrophic lateral sclerosis (ALS) is an idiopathic degenerative disease of upper and lower motor neurons. It is commonly known as Lou Gehrig's disease after the New York Yankees baseball player afflicted with the disorder. *Amyotrophy* means "muscular atrophy." The onset is between the ages of 40 and 70 years, and it affects more men than women. Features of the disease include motor weakness and spastic limbs. The underlying pathology demonstrates neuronal loss in the anterior horns of the spinal cord with degeneration of the tracts. Neurologic evaluation and electromyogram (EMG) studies confirm nerve involvement. Treatment is supportive because there is no cure. Death usually occurs within 10 years of disease onset.

Erb palsy describes upper brachial plexus paralysis. The loss of movement is the result of a lesion of the C5 and C6 nerve roots. It commonly results from a birth injury. The biceps brachii, deltoid, brachialis, and brachioradialis muscles are involved. There is loss of abduction and external rotation of the arm accompanied by weak forearm flexion and supination. The palsy is transient or permanent, depending on the severity of the condition and the individual's response to treatment. Physical therapy and occupation therapy are primary treatment options.

Multiple sclerosis (MS) is an inflammatory disease of the CNS. It is an autoimmune disease in which a previous viral insult manifests as destruction to the myelin sheaths of the CNS neurons, thereby causing an interruption of impulse transmission. There are four major classifications of MS, and general signs and symptoms of its associated syndromes include optic neuritis, weakness, motor difficulty, **vertigo** (the sensation of whirling, tilting, or dizziness that causes balance loss), and faulty speech. Diagnosis is made by physical examination, history, clinical picture, CT scans, and MRI studies. There is no cure. Treatment is supportive and rehabilitative; immunosuppressive drugs may be prescribed.

A **neurilemoma** is the general term used to classify neuromas and schwannomas that are now classified as neurofibromatoses. **Neurofibromatosis** is a genetic disease characterized by neurofibromas (benign tumors arising from the nerve sheath) on the skin along peripheral nerves. Clinical manifestations include headache, **tinnitus** (ringing in one or both ears), vertigo, nausea, and vomiting. CT scan and MRI studies confirm the diagnosis. Treatment involves surgical extraction of the neurilemoma.

Sciatica is neuritis and neuralgia of the sciatic nerve and its branches. It is generally the result of injury to the nerve or its roots from a herniated lower lumbar or upper

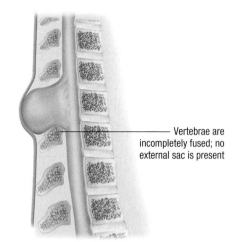

FIGURE 8-21

Spina bifida occulta is caused by the incomplete fusion of the vertebral posterior arch. (Image provided by the Anatomical Chart Co.)

Vertebrae are incompletely fused; no external sac is present

sacral vertebral disk. Typical signs and symptoms are numbness, pain, tingling, and tenderness extending from the hip down to the calf. History and physical examination confirm the diagnosis. Rest, massage therapy, analgesics, muscle relaxants, nonsteroidal anti-inflammatory drugs (NSAIDs), and physical therapy are prescribed. Narcotics are given for severe pain; and in some cases, surgery is an option.

Spina bifida is a congenital defect resulting in improper closure of the vertebral column. It is usually located in the lumbosacral region. Two types exist: spina bifida occulta and spina bifida cystica. **Spina bifida occulta** is caused by the incomplete fusion of the vertebral posterior arch (Fig. 8-21). There is no protrusion of the cord, and the lesion is covered by skin and generally evident only on x-ray evaluation. **Spina bifida cystica** is a severe type characterized by increased intracranial pressure (ICP). Meningocele, hydrocephalus, paraplegia, and the inability to control the urinary bladder and rectum are common. A **meningocele** is a protrusion of the meninges through bone that forms a CSF-filled cyst (Fig. 8-22). **Hydrocephalus** is an accumulation of CSF on the brain (Fig. 8-23); the CSF is not absorbed because some underlying pathology that causes it to pool. Surgery is the only form of treatment.

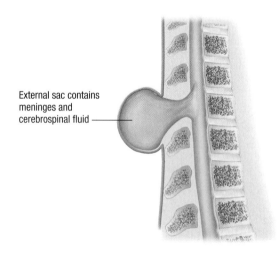

External sac contains meninges and cerebrospinal fluid

FIGURE 8-22

A meningocele is a protrusion of the meninges through bone, causing a cyst filled with cerebrospinal fluid. (Image provided by the Anatomical Chart Co.)

Key Terms	Definitions
amyotrophic (am migh oh TROH fick) **lateral sclerosis** (skle ROH sis)	degenerative disease of the motor neurons
Erb palsy (PAWL zee)	paralysis of the upper brachial plexus

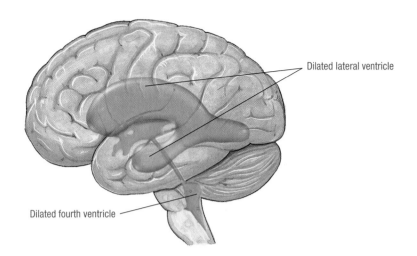

Dilated lateral ventricle

Dilated fourth ventricle

FIGURE 8-23
Hydrocephalus is an accumulation of cerebrospinal fluid on the brain (compare to normal ventricles in Fig. 8-8). (Image provided by the Anatomical Chart Co.)

multiple sclerosis (skle ROH sis)	autoimmune disorder causing destruction of the myelin sheaths
vertigo (VUR ti goh)	dizziness while still
neurofibromatosis (new roh figh broh muh TOH sis)	genetic disease characterized by neurofibromas
tinnitus (ti NIGH tus)	ringing in the ear(s)
sciatica (sigh AT i kuh)	pain and inflammation along the sciatic nerve
spina bifida (SPYE nuh BIF i duh)	congenital defect of incomplete vertebral closure
spina bifida occulta (SPYE nuh BIF i duh ock UL tuh)	incomplete fusion of the posterior arch of vertebra
spina bifida cystica (SPYE nuh BIF i duh SIS ti kuh)	severe type of congenital vertebral defect
meningocele (me NING goh seel)	protrusion of the meninges through bone forming a CSF-filled cyst
hydrocephalus (high droh SEF uh lus)	accumulation of CSF on the brain

Key Term Practice: Spinal Cord and Spinal Nerve Disorders

1. In _____ palsy, the upper brachial plexus is paralyzed.

2. Lou Gehrig's disease is also known as _____.

Infectious Diseases of the Central Nervous System

Brain inflammation is termed **encephalitis.** Viral toxins associated with chickenpox, measles, or mumps may cause the inflammation. Confusion, lethargy, headache, fever, muscle weakness, and visual disturbances are ordinary signs and symptoms. The clinical picture, abnormal EEG, and a **lumbar puncture** (a procedure in which CSF is extracted through a needle inserted into the subarachnoid space) are useful for making the diagnosis. A lumbar puncture is usually performed between the L3 and L4 vertebrae. Evidence of the virus in the blood and CSF indicates encephalitis. Treatment options include antiviral agents, analgesics, and antipyretics to reduce fever.

Guillain-Barré syndrome is an acute, symmetrical, lower motor neuron paralysis of unknown cause. It is thought to be an autoimmune disorder. Advanced cases have trunk and cranial involvement with progression to respiratory failure. It results from demyelinization of the affected nerves. The syndrome follows a respiratory infection, gastroenteritis, or inoculation with the flu vaccine. Diagnosis is made by physical examination, patient history, and elevated protein level in the CSF. Treatment is supportive. If the diaphragm and respiratory muscles are involved, pulmonary ventilation may be necessary. **Plasmapheresis,** a procedure in which whole blood is extracted and the antibodies are removed, lessens the time of duration. Recovery is usually complete.

Meningitis is inflammation of the meninges. It is caused by a bacterial or viral infection. The bacterial form is typically more severe than the viral type. *Haemophilus influenzae, Neisseria meningitides,* and *Streptococcus pneumoniae* are common bacteria associated with its onset. Signs and symptoms include vomiting, headache, and nuchal rigidity. Neck stiffness and resistance to passive movements is termed **nuchal rigidity.** Diagnosis is made through physical and clinical examination. Positive Kernig and Brudzinski signs, increased CSF pressure, and the presence of microbes and white blood cells in the CSF point toward meningitis. A physical finding is the **Kernig sign,** in which the thigh is flexed at a right angle to the trunk, and leg extension at the knee joint is impossible because of pain. Neck flexion that causes hip flexion in the supine position is the **Brudzinski sign.** Aggressive treatment with antibiotics for the bacterial form is essential. Analgesics can be given for pain.

Poliomyelitis is a viral disease characterized by upper respiratory and gastrointestinal symptoms progressing to CNS involvement, causing inflammation of the gray matter (Fig. 8-24). Two forms exist: nonparalytic and paralytic. The disease is preventable through immunization. Malaise, muscle weakness, neck stiffness, vomiting, and flaccid paralysis are common. Isolation of poliovirus from sputum culture, feces, or CSF confirms the diagnosis. Treatment is supportive for mild cases, and pulmonary ventilation may be required for severe cases. Physical therapy may be appropriate after recovery.

Key Terms	Definitions
encephalitis (en sef uh LYE tis)	brain inflammation
lumbar puncture	spinal tap to remove CSF or introduce medications
Guillain-Barré (gee yan-bahr RAY) **syndrome**	acute symmetrical lower motor neuron paralysis
plasmapheresis (plaz muh fuh REE sis)	removal and cleansing of whole blood for reintroduction into the body
meningitis (men in JYE tis)	inflammation of the meninges
nuchal (NEW kul) **rigidity**	stiffness of the neck
Kernig (KER nig) **sign**	leg extension resistance after thigh flexion
Brudzinski (broo JIN skee) **sign**	neck flexion causes hip flexion in the supine position
poliomyelitis (poh lee oh migh e LYE tis)	viral infection resulting in paralysis

Key Term Practice: Infectious Diseases of the Central Nervous System

1. What is the medical term for brain inflammation? _____

2. _____ is the term describing meningeal inflammation.

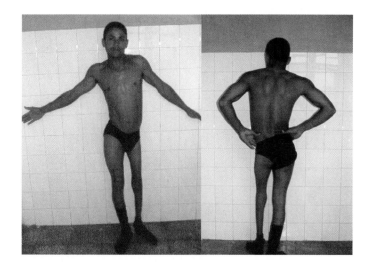

FIGURE 8-24
Poliomyelitis is a viral disease that involves the central nervous system. (Courtesy of Ruth Anne O'Keefe, MD.)

General Eye Disorders

An **ophthalmoscope** is an instrument used to examine the interior of the eye (Fig. 8-25). It consists of a light source and a mirror with a hole in it, through which the observer looks. The eye is illuminated by the light reflected from the mirror into the eye through the pupil. The reflected rays enable visualization of the back of the eyeball.

The loss of transparency of the lens or capsule, **cataract**, leads to cloudy spots on the lens (Fig. 8-26). There is partial or complete opacity of the lens. Cataracts appear to be a normal consequence of aging; however, they may also result from congenital defects, diabetes mellitus, corticosteroid toxicity, lightning flash, or ocular trauma. Signs and symptoms include blurred vision and a milky appearance on the lens. Patients often see haloes around objects. Eye-care professionals diagnose the condition with slit-lamp examination. A **slit-lamp** is an instrument consisting of a microscope combined with

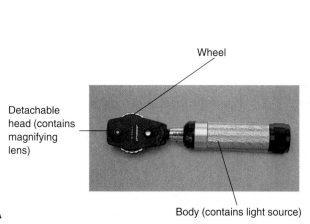

Wheel

Detachable head (contains magnifying lens)

Body (contains light source)

A

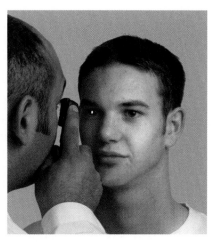

B

FIGURE 8-25
(**A**) An ophthalmoscope is an instrument used to examine the eye. (Reprinted with permission from Weber J, Kelley J. Health assessment in nursing, 2nd ed. Philadelphia: Lippincott Williams & Wilkins, 2003.) (**B**) The interior of the eye. (Reprinted with permission from Bickley LS, Szilagui P. Bates' guide to physical examination and history taking, 8th ed. Philadelphia: Lippincott Williams & Wilkins, 2003.)

FIGURE 8-26
A cataract is characterized by partial or complete opacity of the lens. (Reprinted with permission from Tasman W, Jaeger E. The Willis Eye Hospital atlas of clinical ophthalmology, 2nd ed. Baltimore: Lippincott Williams & Wilkins, 2001.)

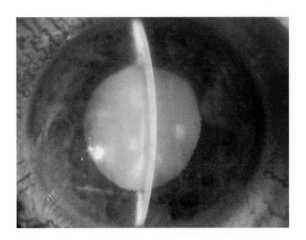

a high-intensity rectangular light source in which the beam can be narrowed into a small stream (slit). Treatment options consist of **extracapsular extraction** (removal of a cataract in one piece), laser surgery, or **phacoemulsification** (use of ultrasonic waves to disintegrate a cataract). *Phakos* is Greek for "lens." The ultrasonic probe pulses the cataract into pieces that are aspirated through a small incision. At the time of treatment, an intraocular lens (IOL) is implanted to replace the faulty one.

Conjunctivitis is inflammation of the conjunctiva caused by viruses, bacteria, or allergy. If pus is present, it is termed "pinkeye." Viral and bacterial forms are highly contagious. Redness, swelling, itching, and tearing commonly occur. Diagnosed by visual examination, it is treated with warm compresses. The eye-care professional may prescribe antibiotics if it is the result of a bacterial infection. The condition usually resolves within two weeks.

Glaucoma is an eye disorder characterized by increased intraocular pressure (IOP), degeneration of the optic nerve head, and visual defects. It may be primary, secondary, or congenital. Glaucoma is a leading cause of blindness in people over 60 years of age. It is caused by an accumulation of aqueous humor. History, eye examination, and **tonometry** (measurement of intraocular pressure using a tonometer) are used to render a diagnosis. Eye drops and laser surgery are viable treatment options.

The medical term for inflammation of the cornea is **keratitis.** It is usually caused by herpes simplex infection or corneal trauma. Visual disturbances, tearing, and photophobia are key characteristics. An eye examination using a slit-lamp confirms the diagnosis. Available treatments include ointments, eye drops, and possibly antibiotics to prevent secondary infection.

An eye abnormality in which both eyes cannot focus on a desired object simultaneously is termed **strabismus.** There are two types: esotropia and erotropia. Esotropia (cross-eyed) is characterized by one eye turning inward, whereas erotropia (walleyed) is characterized by one eye turning outward. Esotropia is usually an **amblyopia**, an abnormal development of visual areas in the brain in response to abnormal visual stimulation during early development. Pathological conditions such as diabetes mellitus, hypertension, and brain trauma may lead to its development in the adult. It is diagnosed by eye examination. Corrective lenses and orthoptic training are treatment options. Visual exercises designed to treat amblyopia and strabismus are termed **orthoptic training.**

Inflammation of the uvea, pigmented vascular layer of the eye, iris, ciliary body, and choroid is termed **uveitis.** It may be idiopathic or caused by infection. It is characterized by pain, blurred vision, and extreme photophobia. Slit-lamp exam provides diagnosis. Treatment consists of managing the underlying cause.

Key Terms	Definitions
ophthalmoscope (off THAL muh skope)	medical instrument used to examine the eye's interior
cataract (KAT uh rakt)	partial or complete opacity of the lens
slit-lamp	instrument used to examine the eye while aiming a light beam directly into it
extracapsular (EKS truh KAP sue lur) **extraction**	cataract removal in one piece
phacoemulsification (fay koh ee mul si fi KAY shun)	ultrasonic technique to disintegrate a cataract
conjunctivitis (kun junk ti VYE tis)	inflammation of the conjunctiva
glaucoma (glaw KOH muh)	eye disease caused by increased intraocular pressure
tonometry (toh NOM e tree)	measurement of eye pressure using a tonometer
keratitis (kehr uh TYE tis)	corneal inflammation
strabismus (stra BIZ mus)	problem related to eye convergence
amblyopia (am blee OH pee uh)	congenital or acquired visual disturbance
orthoptic (or THOP tick) **training**	visual exercises
uveitis (yoo vee EYE tis)	inflammation of the uvea and surrounding tissues

Key Term Practice: General Eye Disorders

1. What is the medical term for partial or complete opacity of the lens? _____

2. A/an _____ is an instrument with a light source and mirror used to examine the interior of the eye through the pupil.

Refractive Errors

In normal eyes, parallel light rays are focused on the retina, forming a sharp image. When the eyes focus the light rays in front of or behind the retina, refractive errors occur. Common refractive errors include astigmatism, myopia, and hyperopia. **Astigmatism** (As) is the medical term for an irregular curvature of the cornea or lens. Its cause is unknown. Focus of light rays does not occur at one retinal point, but rather the rays spread, hampering the focusing ability. Blurred vision is the most common complaint. Examination by an optometrist or ophthalmologist reveals its existence. Treatment involves corrective lenses, contact lenses, or radial keratotomy. **Radial keratotomy** is an invasive surgical procedure in which incisions are made in the cornea. The incisions cause the cornea to flatten to the prescriptive cure for visual acuity (VA). The instrument used to measure the corneal curve is a keratometer.

Common vision disorders are hyperopia, myopia, and presbyopia. A refractive error in which the focus of parallel light rays falls behind the retina is termed **hyperopia**, commonly called farsightedness. It effects near vision; distant vision is not normally affected. In **myopia** (My), or nearsightedness, the focal image is formed in front of the retina. Figure 8-27 illustrates the refractive errors with and corrections for hyperopia and myopia. **Presbyopia** (Pr) is a vision disorder resulting from diminished accommodation owing to impaired lens elasticity. Onset is around the middle 40s. Individuals with presbyopia have difficulty focusing on near objects and reading fine print.

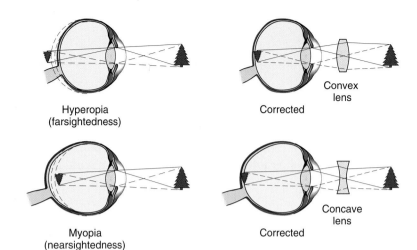

FIGURE 8-27
Two common vision disorders are hyperopia and myopia. (Image provided by the Anatomical Chart Co.)

Blurred vision and squinting are common to all three disorders. Diagnosis is made by physical eye examination. Corrective lenses are used to treat the conditions. Radial keratotomy and LASIK surgery are available for the treatment of myopia. **LASIK surgery** is an acronym for laser-assisted in situ keratomileusis. This treatment for myopia involves a surgical procedure in which a corneal flap is made and the corneal opening is ablated (destroyed). The new flap is then positioned in place.

Key Terms	Definitions
astigmatism (uh STIG muh tiz um)	irregular cornea or lens curvature
radial keratotomy (kerr uh TOM e tree)	surgical procedure for correcting vision
hyperopia (high pur OH pee uh)	farsightedness
myopia (migh OH pee uh)	nearsightedness
presbyopia (prez bee OH pee uh)	accommodation disorder owing to loss of elasticity in the lens
LASIK surgery	laser surgery in which the corneal stoma is ablated and replaced with a new corneal flap

Key Term Practice: Refractive Errors

1. What is the medical term for each of the following eye disorders?

    a. farsightedness _____

    b. nearsightedness _____

2. The word part *presby-* means _____; thus the term _____ refers to age-related vision loss.

Retinal Disorders

Pathological changes of the macula are termed **macular degeneration** or macular dystrophy. These changes occur bilaterally, causing central vision reduction, although peripheral vision remains intact. The cause may be genetic, traumatic, age related, or atherosclerotic. Eye examination and fluorescein angiography provide information for accurate diagnosis. Laser photocoagulation is used to treat the condition. In **laser photocoagulation**, a concentrated light beam is focused on the retina to destroy blood vessels. Recent research suggests zinc supplementation may also be beneficial.

Age-related macular degeneration (AMD) is the leading cause of poor vision in the United States. The two forms are wet and dry, and both are characterized by a decrease in the central vision. The dry form accounts for nearly 90% of AMD cases. Photoreceptors in the macula break down, causing loss of central vision. It usually affects one eye first; the other eye may be affected later. The wet form results from neovascularization from the retina that grows toward the macula. The delicate new vessels leak blood and fluid under the retina, causing the central vision loss. The cause of both forms is unknown. Research suggests the condition may be linked to nutrition, environment, or genes. Blurred and distorted vision is commonly experienced. Angiographic studies confirm the diagnosis. Treatment options consist of laser photocoagulation and photodynamic therapy (PDT) with Visudyne. In **photodynamic therapy with Visudyne**, Visudyne, a light-activated drug, is injected into the bloodstream. After the drug arrives in the retina, the clinician uses a nonthermal laser to activate the drug, closing the vessels without destroying retinal tissue.

A **macular hole** is a full-thickness defect in the retinal center as a result of trauma or aging. Typical onset occurs between the 6th and 8th decade of life. With this condition, the vitreous gel separates from the retinal surface, causing a hole to develop gradually. Infection of the vitreous is termed **endophthalmitis.** Signs and symptoms include the absence of the central field of vision. Other visual disturbances are manifested as wavy lines, and objects with straight profiles, such as trees and telephone poles, also appear wavy. Diagnosis is made by angiography. It is treated by **pars plana vitrectomy**, a procedure in which vitreous gel is removed and replaced with a gas bubble.

Nystagmus is an oscillatory eyeball movement. With this condition, the eyes continually move back and forth involuntarily. Causes of nystagmus can be congenital, acquired, physiologic, or pathological. Blurred vision is the main symptom. Eye examination and visual inspection lead to the diagnosis. Correction of the underlying cause is the best treatment; however, surgery may be an option for some.

Disorders related to the retina are termed retinopathies. **Diabetic retinopathy** is a retinal manifestation secondary to diabetes mellitus. The underlying microvascular disease is the main culprit. Capillary microaneurysms, hemorrhages, and neovascularization (formation of new vessels) result in blindness. **Central serous retinopathy** is caused by leakage of the cellular interconnections under the retina. Fluid accumulates in the macula cause distorted vision. Individuals aged 20–50 years are most affected. Diagnosis of retinopathy is made by complete eye examination, and fluorescein angiography. **Fluorescein angiography** allows the clinician to observe and map the vascular eye patterns, after a yellow dye called fluorescein is injected into a peripheral vein. Central serous retinopathy may be self-limiting or treated by laser surgery. Diabetic retinopathy can be treated, but not cured, by laser photocoagulation or vitrectomy. **Vitrectomy** is the removal of vitreous gel, scar tissue, and accumulated blood. A special vitreous substitute and gas bubble then replace the vitreous humor.

The separation of the retina from the posterior of the eyeball is called a **detached retina.** It usually begins with a retinal tear as the result of eye trauma or vitreous detachment. The retina peels away from the eyeball much like wallpaper comes off a wall. It is characterized by loss of vision, floaters, and flashes. **Floaters**, tiny clumps of gel or cellular debris within the vitreous, are experienced as small specks seen moving across the visual field (VF). The illusion of flashing lights resulting from vitreous gel pulling on the retina is referred to as **flashes.** Retinal evaluation provides confirmation. Treatment is aimed at closing the tear to return the retina to its normal position. Cryotherapy, intraocular gas bubble, laser, scleral buckle, and vitrectomy are other treatment options. **Cryotherapy** involves the freezing of tissue to prevent further damage, and **intraocular gas bubble** treatment involves the injection of a gas bubble into the vitreous cavity. The pressure holds the retina in place until the retinal tear is healed. The body absorbs the gas within several weeks. A **scleral buckle** is a permanent silicone band that attaches to the sclera periphery behind the eye, pulling the retina together.

Key Terms	*Definitions*
macular (MACK yoo lair) **degeneration**	pathological changes of the macula
laser photocoagulation (foh toh koh ag yoo LAY shun)	technique that cauterizes blood vessels with a laser
age-related macular (MACK yoo lair) **degeneration**	disease affecting the macula as a result of aging
photodynamic therapy with Visudyne (VIS yoo dine)	procedure in which the interaction of the drug with a nonthermal laser closes the blood vessels in the retina
macular (MACK yoo lair) **hole**	full-thickness defect of the retinal center
endophthalmitis (en dof thal MIGH tis)	infection in the vitreous
pars plana vitrectomy (PARS PLAY nuh vi TRECK toh mee)	removal of the vitreous and replacement with a gas bubble
nystagmus (nis TAG mus)	oscillatory eyeball movement
diabetic retinopathy (dye uh BET ick ret i NOP uh thee)	retinal disease resulting from diabetes mellitus
central serous retinopathy (ret i NOP uh thee)	retinal disease caused by fluid accumulation in the macula
fluorescein angiography (floo uh RES ee in an jee OG ruh fee)	x-ray mapping of the vascular eye pattern after introduction of a yellow dye
vitrectomy (vi TRECK toh mee)	removal of vitreous humor and replacement with a synthetic vitreous gel
detached retina (RET i nuh)	separation of the retina from its normal position on the posterior eye
floaters	small specks in the field of vision
flashes	illusion of flashing lights in the field of vision
cryotherapy (krye oh THERR uh pee)	tissue freezing
intraocular (in truh OCK yoo lur) **gas bubble**	introduction of a gas bubble into the vitreous cavity
scleral (SKLEER ul) **buckle**	a silicone band is placed to tighten the retina

Key Term Practice: Retinal Disorders

1. Small abnormal flecks seen in the field of vision are termed _____; and the term _____ describes the illusion of flashing lights in the visual field.

2. A surgical operation to remove some or all of the vitreous humor of the eye is called a/an _____.

Eyelid Disorders

Inflammation of the eyelid is termed **blepharitis** (Fig. 8-28). Itching, redness, and crusting around eyelids typify the condition, which is usually caused by allergies or a staphylococcal infection. Diagnosis is based on a visual examination. Saline solution eye washes, ointments, and good eyelid hygiene are recommended. Antibiotics are prescribed in some instances of bacterial infection.

The word for upper eyelid drooping is **blepharoptosis.** It is caused by eyelid muscle weakness that tends to be secondary to diabetes mellitus, muscular dystrophy, myasthenia gravis, tumor, or nerve damage. Diagnosis is made by history, physical examination, and visual inspection. Surgery is the only treatment option to correct a sagging eyelid. Any underlying disease also requires attention.

Hordeolum is an infection of the ciliary glands in the eyelid. It is commonly called a sty. The infectious agent is usually *Staphylococcus.* Signs and symptoms include pain, swelling, and pus formation at the site. Visual examination confirms the diagnosis. Treatment involves applying hot compresses to the area and antibiotics in severe cases.

Inflammation of the eyelid resulting from a blocked tarsal gland is called **chalazion.** Tarsal glands, also known as Meibomian glands, are sebaceous glands found in the eyelids. Redness, pain, swelling, and cyst formation are common. Chalazia are diagnosed by visual examination. Treatment is not usually necessary because they disappear within 2 months. If the condition persists, surgery may be required.

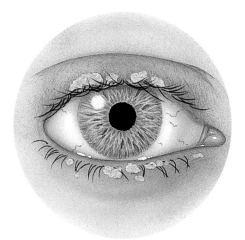

FIGURE 8-28
Blepharitis, or inflammation of the eyelid, is usually caused by allergies or infection. (Image provided by the Anatomical Chart Co.)

Key Terms	Definitions
blepharitis (blef uh RYE tis)	eyelid inflammation
blepharoptosis (blef uh rop TOH sis)	upper eyelid drooping
hordeolum (hor DEE oh lum)	sty
chalazion (kay LAY zee on)	inflammation of the eyelid from a blocked tarsal gland

Key Term Practice: Eyelid Disorders

1. The medical term for a sty is _____.

2. The word part *blephoro-* means _____, the word part *opt-* refers to the _____, and the word part *-ptosis* means "drooping." Therefore, the term _____ means "upper eyelid drooping."

External Ear Disorders and Deafness

Otitis externa is inflammation of external ear. It is also known as swimmer's ear. It is caused by an accumulation of cerumen mixing with water, which creates an environment rich for microbial growth. Signs and symptoms include pain, redness, swelling, hearing loss, and pruritus (itching). Otologic examination and cell culture provide the diagnosis. Treatment consists of washing the ear canal; antibiotics are given if necessary.

Deafness is a lack of hearing or a significant hearing loss. The loss of hearing as a result of improper sound passage through the ossicles is termed **conduction deafness.** **Sensorineural deafness** is hearing loss caused by damage to the cochlea or auditory nerve. Sound waves reach the inner ear, but nerve impulses are not transmitted to the brain. Aging, side effects to some medications, and loud noise are causes. It may be the result of occupational exposure to noise. Patient history, ear examination, and audiometry provide the diagnosis. **Audiometry** is an examination using an audiometer to test the ability of the human ear to detect sounds over a range of frequencies and intensities. The aim of treatment is to reduce environmental noise. Hearing aids may provide some assistance. Sensorineural deafness is irreversible if the cochlea is damaged. **Presbycusis** is sensorineural hearing loss associated with aging. It results from loss of hair cells in the organ of Corti.

Key Terms	Definitions
otitis externa (oh TYE tis ecks TUR nuh)	inflammation of external ear
deafness	partial or complete hearing loss
conduction deafness	hearing loss with ossicle involvement
sensorineural (sen suh ri NEW rul) **deafness**	hearing loss involving a damaged cochlea or auditory nerve
audiometry (aw dee OM e tree)	the quantitative and qualitative evaluation of a person's hearing using an audiometer
presbycusis (prez bee KEW sis)	hearing loss associated with old age

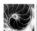

Key Term Practice: External Ear Disorders and Deafness

1. The type of hearing loss associated with a damaged cranial nerve is termed _____.

2. _____ is the medical term for inflammation of the external ear.

Middle Ear and Tympanic Membrane Disorders

Inflammation of middle ear with fluid accumulation behind the tympanic membrane is called **otitis media.** Associated hearing loss and dizziness are common. Infections are the most common cause. Diagnosis is made by otoscopy and tympanogram. **Otoscopy** is the visualization of the auditory tube and tympanic membrane with an otoscope (Fig 8-29). Audiometry reveals hearing loss. Analgesics, decongestants, and antibiotics are conservative treatments. Myringotomy or tympanostomy tubes may be required. An incision through the tympanic membrane to drain fluid or pus buildup is called a **myringotomy.** (Remember that the alternate term for the tympanic membrane is myringa.) **Tympanostomy tubes** are tubes that are inserted through the tympanic membrane to create a passageway for fluid drainage.

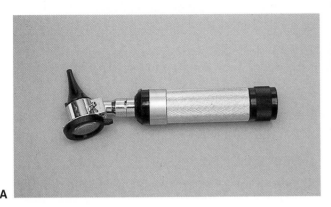

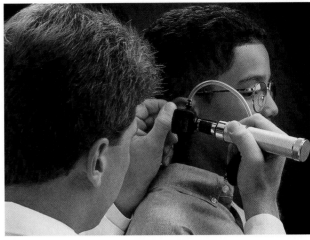

A   B

FIGURE 8-29
(**A**) An otoscope enables visualization of the auditory tube and tympanic membrane. (Reprinted with permission from Taylor C, Lillis C, LeMone P. Fundamentals of nursing: The art and science of nursing care. 4th ed. Philadelphia: Lippincott Williams & Wilkins, 2001). (**B**) The auditory tube and tympanic membrane. (Reprinted with permission from Moore KL, Dalley AF II. Clinical oriented anatomy. 4th ed. Baltimore: Lippincott Williams & Wilkins, 1999.)

An epidermal cyst of the middle ear or mastoid bone is termed a **cholesteatoma** (Fig 8-30). Cholesteatomas may develop in infancy as a result of recurrent otitis media that causes the development of a pocket of skin cells. Vertigo and earache are common. Treatment consists of ear washings and surgical removal of the cyst.

Inflammation of mastoid cells in the mastoid part of the temporal bone is called **mastoiditis.** It is generally the result of untreated otitis media. Pain and edema occur around the mastoid. Diagnosis is made by an ear examination and otoscopy. Antibiotics are usually prescribed; however, severe cases may require mastoidectomy (removal of the mastoid).

An idiopathic middle and inner ear disorder in which new bone is deposited around the oval window and/or cochlea is referred to as **otosclerosis.** The onset is between puberty and age 35 years; the primary sign is conduction deafness. Otoscopic evaluation, history, and audiogram provide a diagnosis. The record of auditory acuity measured by an audiometer is an **audiogram. Stapedectomy,** the surgical removal of the stapes and replacement with a prosthesis, is the available treatment.

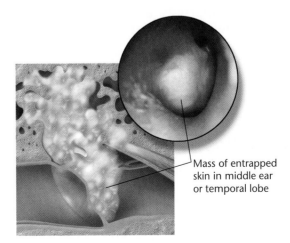

Mass of entrapped skin in middle ear or temporal lobe

FIGURE 8-30
A cholesteatoma is an epidermal cyst of the middle ear or mastoid bone. (Image provided by the Anatomical Chart Co.)

Key Terms	Definitions
otitis media (oh TYE tis MEE dee uh)	acute infection of the middle ear cavity
otoscopy (oh TOS kuh pee)	visualization of the auditory tube and tympanum with an otoscope
myringotomy (mirr in GOT uh mee)	incision through the myringa to drain fluid
tympanostomy (tim puh NOS tuh mee) **tubes**	prosthetic tubes placed as a passageway for fluid drainage
cholesteatoma (koh les tee uh TOH muh)	cyst in the middle ear or mastoid bone
mastoiditis (mas toid EYE tis)	inflammation of the mastoid
otosclerosis (oh toh skle ROH sis)	ear disorder in which new bone is deposited in the inner ear
audiogram (AW dee oh gram)	record of auditory acuity as measured by an audiometer
stapedectomy (stay pe DECK tuh mee)	surgical removal of the stapes

Key Term Practice: Middle Ear and Tympanic Membrane Disorders

1. _____ is the ear disorder in which new bone is deposited in the inner ear.

2. The surgical removal of the stapes is termed _____.

Internal Ear Disorders

Labyrinthitis is an inflammation of the inner ear labyrinth that causes nausea and loss of balance. It is some times called otitis interna. It is caused by a viral or bacterial infection and is marked by fever, nausea, and extreme vertigo. Ear examination and audiometry provide the diagnosis. Treatment involves rest, antibiotics, and an antiemetic, if necessary, for the nausea.

    Ménière disease is an internal ear disorder of unknown origin characterized by deafness, tinnitus, and vertigo. Nausea, vomiting, and nystagmus commonly occur in conjunction with the disease. The onset is usually between the ages of 40 and 50 years. The symptoms and electronystagmography (ENG) confirm the diagnosis. **Electronystagmography** is a method of recording eye movement in response to stimuli. Antinausea and antivomiting medications are prescribed. A nutrition plan that includes the restriction of both salts and fluids is also given. Surgical destruction of the labyrinth may be necessary.

Key Terms	Definitions
labyrinthitis (lab i rin THIGH tis)	infection or inflammation of the inner ear that has a variety of causes
Ménière (mey NYEHR) **disease**	specific disease of the internal ear
electronystagmography (ee leck troh nigh stag MOG ruh fee)	method of recording eye movements in response to stimuli

Key Term Practice: Internal Ear Disorders

1. An illness in which the inner ear becomes inflamed, causing balance loss and nausea, is termed _____.

2. _____ is a method of recording eye movements in response to stimuli.

CLINICAL TERMS

Clinical Dimension	Term	Description
DISORDERS		
	age-related macular degeneration (AMD)	disease affecting the macula of eye as a result of aging
	Alzheimer disease (AD)	degenerative brain disorder that causes dementia; onset is typically late in life
	amblyopia	congenital or acquired visual disturbance
	amnesia	loss of memory
	amyotrophic lateral sclerosis (ALS)	degenerative disease of the motor neurons
	astigmatism (As)	irregular cornea or lens curvature
	astrocytoma	tumor derived from astrocytes
	Bell palsy	peripheral paralysis of the muscles innervated by the facial nerve
	blepharitis	eyelid inflammation
	blepharoptosis	upper eyelid drooping
	cataract	partial or complete opacity of the lens
	central serous retinopathy	retinal disease caused by fluid accumulation in the macula
	cephalalgia	headache
	cerebral palsy (CP)	group of motor function diseases
	cerebral seizures	recurrent convulsions with blank stares and temporary loss of awareness
	cerebrovascular accidents (CVAs)	strokes
	chalazion	inflammation of the eyelid from a blocked tarsal gland
	cholesteatoma	cyst in the middle ear or mastoid bone
	coma	prolonged state of deep unconsciousness
	concussion	transient, immediate loss of consciousness
	conduction deafness	hearing loss with ossicle involvement

Clinical Dimension	Term	Description
	conjunctivitis	inflammation of the conjunctiva
	contusion	brain tissue bruise
	coup–contre coup injury	brain injury occurring at the point of impact and on the opposite side of impact as a result of forward and backward motion within the skull
	cystoid macular edema	accumulation of fluid in the macula of eye, causing swelling
	deafness	partial or complete hearing loss
	dementia	loss of intellectual and cognitive functions while other brain functions are maintained
	detached retina	separation of the retina from its normal position on the posterior eye
	diabetic retinopathy	retinal disease resulting from diabetes mellitus
	ectropion	eyelid eversion
	encephalitis	inflammation of the brain
	endophthalmitis	infection in the vitreous
	entropion	eyelid inversion
	ependymoma	tumor derived from ependymal cells
	epilepsy	brain disorder resulting from an irregular electrical discharge of neurons
	Erb palsy	paralysis of the upper brachial plexus
	generalized tonic–clonic seizure	seizure characterized by collapse, loss of consciousness, and intermittent muscle contractions and relaxations
	glaucoma	eye disease caused by increased intraocular pressure
	glioma	tumor composed of cells derived from neuroglia
	Guillain-Barré syndrome	acute symmetrical lower motor neuron paralysis
	hordeolum	sty
	Huntington chorea	inherited form of dementia accompanied by atrophy of the cerebral cortex and basal ganglia
	hyperopia	farsightedness
	keratitis	corneal inflammation
	labyrinthitis	infection of the inner ear that has a variety of causes
	macular degeneration	pathological changes of the macula
	macular hole	full-thickness defect of the retinal center
	mastoiditis	inflammation of the mastoid

Clinical Dimension	Term	Description
	Ménière disease	specific disease of the inner ear
	meningitis	inflammation of the meninges
	migraine	recurrent, severe vascular headache
	multiple sclerosis	autoimmune disorder causing destruction of the of myelin sheath
	myopia	nearsightedness
	neurofibromatosis	genetic disease characterized by neurofibromas
	nystagmus	oscillatory eyeball movement
	ocular histoplasmosis	fungal disease of the eye
	oligodendroglioma	tumor derived from oligodendrocytes
	otitis externa	inflammation of the external ear
	otitis media	acute infection of the middle ear cavity
	otosclerosis	ear disorder in which new bone is deposited in the inner ear
	Parkinson disease (PD)	disorder resulting from progressive degeneration of dopamine-producing neurons in the brain
	poliomyelitis	viral infection resulting in paralysis
	presbycusis	hearing loss associated with old age
	presbyopia	accommodation disorder owing to loss of elasticity in the lens
	Reye syndrome	complex of symptoms with liver damage and brain dysfunction that occurs after a viral infection
	sciatica	pain and inflammation along the sciatic nerve
	sensorineural deafness	hearing loss involving a damaged cochlea or auditory nerve
	sequela	after effect of a condition, disease, or injury
	spina bifida	congenital defect of incomplete vertebral closure
	spina bifida cystica	severe type of congenital vertebral defect
	spina bifida occulta	incomplete fusion of the posterior arch of vertebra
	strabismus	problem related to eye convergence
	tic douloureux	pain in one or more branches of CN V; trigeminal neuralgia
	transient ischemic attack (TIA)	brain disorder that is not permanent
	trigeminal neuralgia	pain in one or more branches of CN V; tic douloureux
	uveitis	inflammation of the uvea and surrounding tissues

Clinical Dimension	Term	Description
SIGNS AND SYMPTOMS		
	aphasia	partial or total inability to produce and understand speech as a result of brain damage
	aphonia	inability to speak
	apraxia	inability to perform purposeful movements as a result of brain damage
	areflexia	absence of reflexes
	autonomic dysreflexia	several signs evident in quadriplegia
	battle sign	skin discoloration behind the ear that indicates a skull fracture
	Brudzinski sign	neck flexion causes hip flexion in the supine position
	decerebrate posturing	particular body position caused by a lesion of the upper brainstem or bilateral cerebral lesions
	decorticate posturing	particular body position caused by a lesion of the upper brainstem, frontal lobe, or cerebral peduncles
	dysphasia	difficulty in speaking and understanding spoken or written language as a result of brain injury
	flashes	illusion of flashing lights in the field of vision
	floaters	small specks seen in the field of vision
	hemiparesis	muscle weakness on one side
	hydrocephalus	accumulation of CSF on the brain
	Kernig sign	leg extension resistance after thigh flexion
	meningocele	protrusion of the meninges through bone forming a CSF-filled cyst
	nuchal rigidity	stiffness of the neck
	paresis	slight paralysis
	photophobia	eye sensitivity to light
	spastic paralysis	involuntary contractions of affected muscles
	tinnitus	ringing in the ear(s)
	vertigo	dizziness while still
CLINICAL TESTS AND DIAGNOSTIC PROCEDURES		
	amyloid beta-protein precursor test	test that checks CSF levels of amyloid beta-protein
	audiogram	record of auditory acuity as measured by an audiometer
	audiometry	quantitative and qualitative evaluation of a person's hearing using an audiometer
	cerebral angiography	mapping of the cerebral blood vessels using dye and x-rays

Clinical Dimension	Term	Description
	cerebral arteriogram	radiographic mapping of the cerebral arteries
	computed tomography (CT)	imaging method using a computer to reconstruct the anatomic features obtained by x-ray
	electrocochleography	measurement of electrical current in inner ear after sound stimulation
	electroencephalography (EEG)	method of graphically recording the electrical activity of the brain
	electronystagmography (ENG)	method of recording eye movements in response to stimuli
	fluorescein angiography	x-ray mapping of the vascular eye pattern after introduction of a yellow dye
	Glasgow coma scale	scale used to assess the level of consciousness
	indocyanine green angiogram	map of the vascular eye pattern after introduction of a green dye
	lumbar puncture	spinal tap to remove CSF or introduce medications
	ophthalmoscope	medical instrument used to examine the eye's interior
	otoscopy	visualization of the auditory tube and tympanic membrane with an otoscope
	pneumoencephalography (PEG)	image of the brain ventricles after CSF is withdrawn and intermittently replaced with air
	positron emission tomography (PET)	diagnostic medical imaging method capable of displaying metabolic activities of body organs
	slit-lamp	instrument used to examine the eye while aiming a light beam directly into it
	tonometry	measurement of eye pressure using a tonometer
TREATMENTS		
	antiemetic	agent for relieving nausea
	Coumadin	trade name of the anticoagulant drug warfarin
	cranial trephination	excision of a small disk of skull bone using a trephine (also spelled cranial trepanation)
	cryotherapy	tissue freezing
	extracapsular extraction	cataract removal in one piece
	intraocular gas bubble	introduction of a gas bubble into the vitreous cavity
	laser photocoagulation	technique that cauterizes blood vessels with a laser
	LASIK surgery	laser surgery in which the corneal stoma is ablated and replaced with a new corneal flap

Clinical Dimension	Term	Description
	myringotomy	incision through the myringa to drain fluid
	orthoptic training	visual exercises
	pars plana vitrectomy	removal of the vitreous and replacement with a gas bubble
	phacoemulsification	ultrasonic technique to disintegrate a cataract
	photodynamic therapy with Visudyne	procedure in which the interaction of the drug with a nonthermal laser closes the blood vessels in the retina
	plasmapheresis	removal and cleansing of whole blood for reintroduction into the body
	radial keratotomy	surgical procedure for correcting vision
	scleral buckle	a silicone band is placed to tighten the retina
	stapedectomy	surgical removal of the stapes
	tissue plasminogen activator (TPA; tPA)	substance that acts against blood clots
	tympanostomy	prosthetic tubes placed as a passageway for fluid drainage
	vitrectomy	removal of vitreous humor and replacement with a synthetic vitreous gel
	warfarin	anticoagulant drug

Lifespan

Nervous tissue is derived from the embryonic ectoderm germ layer. Cells proliferate and migrate to determined positions before differentiating into the neuroblasts that ultimately transform into the various components of the nervous system.

As neurons mature, most lose their ability to divide, becoming amitotic. In fact, approximately two thirds of nerve cells engage in apoptosis (programmed cell death) between conception and birth. Hippocampus and olfaction cells are the exceptions and retain their mitotic ability throughout life.

During infancy, the nervous system is developing rapidly. Motor control improves with age as myelination occurs. Brain growth continues until approximately age 18.

With respect to the special senses, eye development continues until around age 9, when the eyes reach their adult size. Visual acuity gradually declines in aging persons, and it appears that no one is exempt from corrective lenses in later life. Age-related hearing loss is also prevalent beginning in the 6th or 7th decade of life.

Relative to old age, brain weight and volume decline as a result of neuron death. Mental functioning, however, can remain when there is no neurovascular disease. Moreover, recent research indicates that individuals who maintain intellectual stimulation preserve normal brain function throughout life. Owing to brain plasticity and the ability to learn new information and skills, elderly persons can have high cognitive function; however, the rate at which novel tasks are learned, along with reflex activity, diminishes with age. Other autonomic functions also decline with age.

In the News: Mad Cow Disease

You may want to think twice before eating steak. Remember the news from Great Britain regarding the crisis in its beef supply? The news coverage is justified because mad cow disease has affected nearly 200,000 cattle. The scientific community refers to mad cow disease as bovine spongiform encephalopathy (BSE). Its name is derived from the characteristic sponge-like appearance of infected brains. The cattle disease was first diagnosed in 1986 in Great Britain.

Why the cause for alarm? Mad cow disease belongs to a class of neurologic disorders known as transmissible spongiform encephalopathies (TSEs). Proteinaceous infectious particles that lack nucleic acid, called prions, cause these brain pathologies. Prions cause neurodegenerative disease in both animals and humans. In addition to mad cow disease, other prion diseases are scrapie in sheep, chronic wasting disease in deer and elk, and kuru and Creutzfeldt-Jakob disease (CJD) in humans.

Prions are extremely stable, small, nonliving, particles that elicit no immune response in humans. Thus an individual can be infected for 9 to 21 years without exhibiting any signs of the disease. Variant Creutzfeldt-Jakob disease (vCJD) is a new form transmitted to humans through ingestion of beef infected with BSE. Since 1989, the United States has banned meat from countries with known BSE in the cattle population. Yet, the meat supply can still harbor prions as demonstrated by the fact that one to two cases of prion diseases per million are reported worldwide, and 200 cases per year occur in the United States.

Signs and symptoms of CJD begin rather benignly as forgetfulness and memory impairment. However, they rapidly progress to muscular impairment, personal changes, abnormal gait, dementia, inability to speak, and coma. MRI and EEG are abnormal. Definitive diagnosis is based on pathology evidenced in brain tissue at autopsy. There is no cure, and death usually occurs 1 year after onset of disease symptoms.

COMMON ABBREVIATIONS

Abbreviation	Term
A.D.	right ear
AD	Alzheimer disease
ALS	amyotrophic lateral sclerosis
AMD	age-related macular degeneration
ANS	autonomic nervous system
A.S.	left ear
As	astigmatism
A.U.	each ear; both ears
BBB	blood-brain barrier
BSE	bovine spongiform encephalopathy
CJD	Creutzfeldt-Jacob disease
CN	cranial nerve
CNS	central nervous system
CP	cerebral palsy
CS	cortical sclerosis
CSF	cerebrospinal fluid
CT	computed tomography

Abbreviation	Term
CVA	cerebrovascular accident
DA	dopamine
DO	doctor of ophthalmology
EEG	electroencephalogram; electroencephalograph; electroencephalography
EMG	electromyogram
ENG	electronystagmography
ICP	intracranial pressure
IOL	intraocular lens
IOP	intraocular pressure
J	Jaeger
LASIK	laser-assisted in situ keratomileusis
LOC	level of consciousness
MD	medical doctor
MRI	magnetic resonance imaging
MS	multiple sclerosis
My	myopia
NS	nuclear sclerosis
NSAIDs	nonsteroidal anti-inflammatory drugs
O.D.	right eye
OD	doctor of optometry
O.S.	left eye
O.U.	each eye; both eyes
PD	Parkinson disease; pupil distance
PDT	photodynamic therapy
PEG	pneumoencephalography
PNS	peripheral nervous system
Pr	presbyopia
TIA	transient ischemic attack
TPA or tPA	tissue plasminogen activator
TSE	transmissible spongiform encephalopathy
VA	visual acuity
vCJD	Variant Creutzfeldt-Jacob disease
VF	visual field

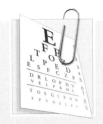

Case Study

Mr. Treeton, a 61-year-old male, visited his optometrist for his annual eye examination. Sally met him and began the initial procedures, including color vision testing, keratometry, autorefraction, visual fields, measuring pupil distance (PD) and visual acuities, and taking his blood pressure. Mr. Treeton's chief complaint was decreased vision in the right eye for approximately 3 weeks. The diminished visual acuity was gradual.

Upon examination by the optometrist, it was discovered that Mr. Treeton had a history of diabetic retinopathy. His medical history indicated that he has had insulin-dependent diabetes mellitus for 13 years, hypertension for 15 years, myocardial infarction, and cardiac arrhythmia. His social history indicated no alcohol or tobacco use. There is a family history of heart disease and hypertension. The following results were obtained.

Visual Acuity

Eye	With Correction	Pinhole	Near
right	20/70	20/40−1	J8
left	20/25−2		J1

Other Measures

Measure	Value
Applanation tensions	18 O.D.; 20 O.S. at 9:20 A.M.
PD	7 cm
Pupils	both pupils are 4 mm in size with brisk response
Blood pressure	170/110
Color vision	7/14 O.D.; 8/14 O.S.

Slit-Lamp Examination

Measure	Right Eye	Left Eye
Conjunctiva	1+ injection	1+ injection
Cornea	clear	clear
Anterior chamber	deep and quiet	deep and quiet
Iris	within normal limits	within normal limits
Lens	2+ NS; 1+ CS	2+ NS

Recommendation

- Fluorescein angiogram to further define.

Case Study Questions

Select the best answer to each of the following questions.

1. Applanation tensions (the force required to flatten a small area of the cornea) are measured by tonometry, which indicates the intraocular pressure. Mr. Treeton's results show _____.

   a. 18 in the left eye and 20 in the right eye
   b. 18 in the right eye and 20 in the left eye
   c. 25 in the left eye and 70 in the right eye
   d. 20 in the left eye and 20 in the right eye

2. The test results for the cornea _____.

   a. are normal
   b. are abnormal
   c. indicate cataracts

3. The PD is 7 cm. This means that the _____ is 7 cm.

   a. average size of each pupil
   b. primary distance between the eyes
   c. distance between the centers of each pupil
   d. photo density

4. Explain the recommended test. Why was this test suggested?

   _____

   _____

   _____

5. The instrument used to view various parts of the eye is called a/an _____.

REAL WORLD REPORT

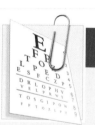

Sally just received Mr. Treeton's fluorescein angiography report.

PATIENT NAME: Randolph Treeton	DATE: July 30, 2003
REFERRED BY: Dr. Vanden	ATTENDING: Dr. Nolen
COLOR VISION: 7/14 O.D.; 8/14 O.S.	CONFRONTATION FIELDS: Full, O.U.

INDIRECT OPHTHALMOSCOPY/BIOMICROSCOPY

RIGHT EYE

The optic nerve head is pink with sharp disc borders. The A/V ratio is 1:2. The mid and far periphery show an occasional intraretinal hemorrhage. There are some fine scattered intravitreal condensations. Views of the macula show scattered microaneurysms with a question of some mild intraretinal thickening adjacent to the fovea. There is no evidence of active neovascularization.

LEFT EYE

The optic nerve head is pink with sharp disc borders. The A/V ratio is 1:2. The mid and far periphery show an occasional intraretinal hemorrhage. Views of the posterior pole show one to two cotton-wool spots nasal to the optic nerve head. There are scattered perimacular microaneurysms but no definite evidence of active neovascularization.

IMPRESSION

- Background diabetic retinopathy.
- Rule out clinically significant macular edema.
- Mild intraretinal ischemia.
- Bilateral vitreous degeneration.
- Nuclear sclerotic and cortical cataractous changes.
- Essential hypertension.

REAL WORLD REPORT QUESTIONS

The following exercises review the medical terms in the preceding medical report.

1. The term *intraretinal hemorrhage* was used for both the right and the left eye.

   a. *Intra-* means

   _____.

   b. *Retinal* refers to the

   _____.

   c. *Hem-* means

   _____.

   d. Thus *intraretinal hemorrhage* means

   _____.

2. The report noted that there was no evidence of neovascularization. *Neovascularization* means

   _____.

3. Perimacular microaneurysms would be located _____ the macula.

   a. around or adjacent to

   b. behind

   c. on

   d. in

4. Macular edema is the medical term for macular_____.

5. Define the following medical terms used in the report.

   a. intraretinal ischemia

   _____

   b. vitreous degeneration

   _____

   c. cortical cataractous changes

   _____

REVIEW AND APPLICATION: THREE-LEVEL LEARNING SYSTEM

LEVEL ONE: REVIEWING FACTS AND TERMS USING RECALL

Select the best response to each of the following questions.

1. The CNS consists of _____.
   a. the brain and spinal cord
   b. the spinal cord and peripheral nerves
   c. CSF and PMS
   d. PNS and motor pathways

2. Supporting cells of the CNS are termed _____.
   a. collaterals
   b. Schwann cells
   c. neuroglia
   d. dendrites

3. Special senses refer to _____.
   a. olfaction
   b. gustation
   c. vision and hearing
   d. all of these

4. A plexus is best described as _____.
   a. tangled auditory tubes
   b. a vision abnormality
   c. a spinal nerve network
   d. a hearing disorder

5. Identify the three meninges of the CNS.
   a. dura mater, pia mater, and subdural mater
   b. dura mater, arachnoid mater, and pia mater
   c. arachnoid mater, pia mater, and subdural mater
   d. epidural mater, subdural mater, and pia mater

6. The largest part of the brain is the _____.
   a. cerebrum
   b. cerebellum
   c. brainstem
   d. pons

7. The white section of the cerebellum is referred to as the _____.
   a. basal ganglia
   b. arbor vitae
   c. pia mater
   d. cerebral peduncles

8. Convolutions are formed by _____.
   a. gyri and fissures
   b. pons and gyri
   c. hemispheres and grooves
   d. cerebri and cerebelli

9. A/an _____ is an area of skin supplied by sensory nerve fibers.
   a. somatotype
   b. fibroderm
   c. epidome
   d. dermatome

10. The myringa is also known as the _____.
    a. pinna
    b. tympanic membrane
    c. auditory tube
    d. cochlea

Match the word part with its correct definition.

_____ 11. equi-   a. dimness

_____ 12. ambly-   b. equal, equally

_____ 13. coccy-   c. left

_____ 14. sinistro-   d. tailbone

_____ 15. dextro-   e. right

Match the ear part with its correct description.

_____ 16. ossicles

_____ 17. pinna

_____ 18. external auditory meatus

_____ 19. semicircular canals

_____ 20. auditory tube

a. connecting canal between pharynx and tympanic cavity

b. malleus, incus, and stapes

c. auricle, outer ear

d. bony tubes positioned in three planes

e. connecting tube between pinna and tympanic membrane

Match the eye part with its correct description.

_____ 21. choroid

_____ 22. pupil

_____ 23. sclera

_____ 24. retina

_____ 25. optic nerve

_____ 26. iris

a. cranial nerve II

b. eyeball outer layer

c. opening

d. pigmented vascular tunic

e. colored portion visible to exterior

f. extension of optic nerve

LEVEL TWO: REVIEWING CONCEPTS

Select the best response to each of the following questions.

27. A patient presents with constant "ringing white noise" in her ears. This is termed _____.

a. reflexia

b. aphonia

c. tinnitus

d. areflexia

28. Jill is standing in her room and experiences dizziness. This describes _____.

a. tinnitus

b. reflexia

c. photophobia

d. vertigo

What is the test or diagnostic procedure described by each of the following definitions?

29. mapping of cerebral blood _____

30. spinal tap to remove CSF _____

31. measurement of intraocular pressure _____

32. measurement of electrical current in the inner ear after sound stimulation _____

33. record of auditory acuity _____

Match the brain disorder with its chief characteristics.

_____ 34. cerebral palsy

_____ 35. Alzheimer disease

_____ 36. Huntington disease

_____ 37. Parkinson disease

_____ 38. transient ischemic attack

a. mini-stroke; nonpermanent brain disorder

b. progressive degeneration of dopamine-producing neurons

c. dementia with neurofibrillary tangles

d. inherited form of dementia; atrophy of cerebral cortex

e. group of motor function diseases

What disorder or disease is described by each of the following key characteristics?

39. peripheral paralysis of facial nerve _____

40. paralysis of upper brachial plexus _____

41. inflammation of meninges _____

Match the eye disorder with its correct definition.

_____ 42. strabismus

_____ 43. macular degeneration

_____ 44. macular hole

_____ 45. nystagmus

_____ 46. blepharitis

_____ 47. chalazion

a. involuntary, oscillatory eyeball movement

b. problem related to eye convergence

c. pathological changes of the macula

d. full-thickness defect of the retinal center

e. inflammation of the eyelid caused by a blocked tarsal gland

f. inflammation of the eyelid caused by allergy or infection

Match the ear disorder with its correct definition.

_____ 48. presbycusis

_____ 49. cholesteatoma

_____ 50. Ménière disease

a. cyst of middle ear or mastoid

b. specific disease of inner ear

c. age-related hearing loss

For each of the following, indicate whether the test involves the eye or the ear.

51. scleral buckle _____

52. vitrectomy _____

53. myringotomy _____

54. stapedectomy _____

55. extracapsular extraction _____

56. tympanostomy _____

Provide a medical term to complete a meaningful analogy.

57. Pinna is to auricle as eardrum is to _____.

58. Rods are to dim vision as _____ are to color vision.

Using the following word parts, form a medical term for each definition. Each word part is used only once.

blephar-	hyper-	-phasia
cerebro-	-itis	retino-
cerebro-	-opia	-spinal
dys-	-pathy	-vascular

59. visual image focused behind the retina; farsightedness _____

60. pertaining to the cerebrum and spinal cord _____

61. pertaining to the blood vessels in the cerebrum _____

62. disease of the retina _____

63. impaired speech _____

64. eyelid inflammation _____

What is the medical term described by each of the following definitions?

65. nerve inflammation _____

66. nerve pain _____

67. disease of the nervous system _____

What is the adjective form for each given term?

68. cornea _____

69. pupil _____

70. dura _____

71. meninges _____

Identify the correctly spelled term in each set.

72. _____

a. astigmatism

b. assitigmatism

c. assigmatizm

d. astimetism

73. _____

   a. cerrebrum

   b. serebrum

   c. cerebrum

   d. cerebrem

74. _____

   a. koroid

   b. choroid

   c. coroid

   d. coroyd

75. _____

   a. demensha

   b. dimentia

   c. dementea

   d. dementia

76. _____

   a. mighgraine

   b. migraine

   c. migrane

   d. meigraine

77. _____

   a. labyrinthitis

   b. labirinthitis

   c. laberinthitis

   d. labarinthitis

78. _____

   a. fakoemulsification

   b. phakoemulsification

   c. phacoemulsification

   d. phackoemulsification

79. _____

   a. polymyelitis

   b. poleomyelitis

   c. poliomyelitis

   d. poleymyelitis

80. _____

   a. vurtigo

   b. vertigo

   c. vertego

   d. vurtego

Define the following abbreviations.

81. ENG _____

82. MS _____

83. CSF _____

84. CVA _____

85. ALS _____

LEVEL THREE: THINKING CRITICALLY

Write a short answer to the following questions.

86. Patient Smith presents with a TIA affecting vision in O.S. Using medical and common terminology, describe what the patient is experiencing.

   _____

   _____

   _____

87. Dr. Xenon orders an EEG on patient Smith to obtain an EEG. Spell out each abbreviation correctly so the sentence makes sense.

   _____

   _____

   _____

KEY TERMS SPELLING TEST FROM CD-ROM

Use the CD-ROM to test yourself on the spelling of key terms from this chapter. Listen to the terms and write them on a separate sheet of paper. Use a medical dictionary to check your answers.

ANSWERS

WORD GROUPING

Definition	Word Part
section, part	-tome
adrenal	adren-, adreno-
brain	encephal-, encephalo-
cerebellum	cerebell-, cerebelli-, cerebello-
cerebrum, cerebral, brain	cerebr-, cerebri-, cerebro-
chemical	chem-, chemi-, chemico-, chemio-, chemo-
choroid, vascular coat	choroid-, choroido-
coccyx; tailbone	coccy-
cold, freezing	cry-, cryo-
cornea, corneal	corne-, corneo-
defect of the eye	-opia, -opy
deviation in the line of vision	-tropia
dimness	ambly-
ear	A. aur-, auri-, auro-
	B. ot-, oto-
equal, equally	equi-
eye or ocular	ocul-, oculo-
eyelid	bleph-, blepharo-
ganglion, knot	gangli-, ganglio-
gluey, gelatinous	gli-, glio-
head	cephal-, cephalo-
hearing	acou-, acouo-
half	hemi-
involving three dimensions, involving depth perception	stere-, stereo-
iris	irid-, irido-
left side	sinistr-, sinistro-
light	phot-, photo-
meatus, passageway, opening	meat-, meato-
meninx, meninges, membrane	mening-, meningo-
motion, energy, power	dynam-, dynamo-
myelin	myel-, myelo-
nerve, neural, nervous	neur-, neuro-
neuroglia of a specific kind or size	-glia
old age	presby-, presbyo-
optic, vision, eye	opt-, opto-
pertaining to the eye	ophthalm-, ophthalmo-
reading impairment or word recognition impairment	-lexia
red	rhod-, rhodo-
retina, retinal	retin-, retino-

Definition	Word Part
right side	dextr-, dextro-
sclera, scleral	scler-, sclero-
sense of hearing	audio-
speech disorder	-phasia, -phasy
spider, spider-like	arachn-, arachno-
star-like	astr-, astro-
stoppage, suppression	isch-, ischo-
tail, caudal	caud-, caudo-
tongue	gloss-, -glossa, glosso-
tree, tree-like	dendr-, dendro-
turning toward	-tropic
tympanum, tympanic	tympan-, tympano-
vascular	vascul-, vasculo-

WORD BUILDING

Word Part	Meaning	Common or Known Word	Example Medical Term
adren-, adreno-	adrenal	adrenaline	adrenaline
audio-	sense of hearing	audio	audiologist
aur-, auri-, auro-	ear	aural	auricle
cerebr-, cerebri-, cerebro-	cerebrum, cerebral, brain	cerebral	cerebrum
chem-, chemi-, chemico-, chemio-, chemo-	chemical	chemotherapy	chemoreceptor
corne-, corneo-	cornea, corneal	cornea	cornea
dynam-, dynamo-	motion, energy, power	dynamite	dynamic equilibrium
irid-, irido-	iris	iridescent	iridectomy
-lexia	reading or word recognition impairment	dyslexia	dyslexia
neur-, neuro-	nerve, neural, nervous	neuron	neuron
opt-, opto-	optic, vision, eye	optical illusion	optometry
ot-, oto-	ear	otitis	otoscope
phot-, photo-	light	photograph	photoreceptor
retin-, retino-	retina, retinal	retina	retina
scler-, sclero-	sclera, scleral	sclera	sclera
stere-, stereo-	involving three dimensions; involving depth perception	stereo	stereopsis
vascul-, vasculo-	vascular	vascular	vascular tunic

KEY TERM PRACTICE

Nervous System and Special Senses Preview

1. central nervous system (CNS); peripheral nervous system (PNS)
2. sympathetic; parasympathetic

Neurons and Neuroglia

1. somata
2. a. neuron; b. soma

Spinal Cord and Spinal Nerves

1. epineurium → perineurium → endoneurium
2. plexus

Brain and Cranial Nerves

1. sulcus
2. cerebrum; cerebellum; brainstem

Olfaction and Gustation

1. gustation
2. Olfaction

Ear, Hearing, and Equilibrium

1. a. pinnae; b. mallei; c. incudes; d. cochleae
2. stereocilium

Eye and Vision

1. lentes; irides
2. Cones

General Brain Disorders

1. Parkinson disease (PD)
2. Dysphasia
3. stroke

Dementia

1. dementia

Brain Neoplasms

1. a. astrocytoma; b. ependymoma; c. oligodendroglioma

Pediatric Disorders

1. Reye

Cranial Nerve Disorders

1. sequela
2. trigeminal neuralgia

Spinal Cord and Spinal Nerve Disorders

1. Erb
2. amyotrophic lateral sclerosis (ALS)

Infectious Diseases of the Central Nervous System

1. encephalitis
2. Meningitis

General Eye Disorders

1. cataract
2. ophthalmoscope

Refractive Errors

1. a. hyperopia; b. myopia
2. old age; presbyopia

Retinal Disorders

1. floaters; flashes
2. vitrectomy

Eyelid Disorders

1. hordeolum
2. eyelid; eye; blepharoptosis

External Ear Disorders and Deafness

1. sensorineural
2. Otitis externa

Middle Ear and Tympanic Membrane Disorders

1. Otosclerosis
2. stapedectomy

Internal Ear Disorders

1. labyrinthitis
2. Electronystagmography

CASE STUDY

1. b is the correct answer.
   - a is incorrect because OD stands for right eye, and OS stands for left eye.
   - c and d are incorrect because these numbers were obtained from the visual acuity test.
2. a is the correct answer.
   - b is incorrect because the cornea should be clear.
   - c is incorrect because the lens appears cloudy with cataracts; this question refers to the cornea.
3. c is the correct answer.
   - a is incorrect because the pupils are not that large, and PD stands for "papillary distance," or distance between the pupils.

   - b is incorrect because the measure *primary distance between the eyes* is a made-up term.
   - d is incorrect because *photo density* is a made-up term.
4. A fluorescein angiogram was suggested because this test can provide a good picture of the retina. Mr. Treeton has diabetes and a history of diabetic retinopathy. The angiogram would give clear visualization of the retinal vessels.
5. slit lamp

REAL WORLD REPORT

1. a. within, in; b. retina; c. blood; d. bleeding within the retina
2. New blood vessel growth where it should not be occurring
3. a

4. swelling
5. a. vascular obstruction within the retina; b. deterioration of the vitreous; c. opacity of the lens cortex (outer portion) is changing; cataract forming on lens cortex

REVIEW AND APPLICATION: THREE-LEVEL LEARNING SYSTEM

Level One: Reviewing Facts and Terms Using Recall

1. a
2. c
3. d
4. c
5. b
6. a
7. b
8. a
9. d
10. b
11. b
12. a
13. d
14. c
15. e
16. b
17. c
18. e
19. d
20. a
21. d
22. c
23. b
24. f
25. a
26. e

Level Two: Reviewing Concepts

27. c
28. d
29. cerebral angiography
30. lumbar puncture
31. tonometry
32. electrocochleography
33. audiogram
34. e
35. c
36. d
37. b
38. a
39. Bell palsy
40. Erb palsy
41. meningitis
42. b
43. c
44. d
45. a
46. f

47. e
48. c
49. a
50. b
51. eye
52. eye
53. ear
54. ear
55. eye
56. ear
57. tympanic membrane or myringa
58. cones
59. hyperopia
60. cerebrospinal
61. cerebrovascular
62. retinopathy
63. dysphasia
64. blepharitis
65. neuritis
66. neuralgia
67. neuropathy
68. corneal
69. pupillary
70. dural
71. meningeal
72. a
73. c
74. b
75. d
76. b
77. a
78. c
79. c
80. b
81. electronystagmography
82. multiple sclerosis
83. cerebrospinal fluid
84. cerebrovascular accident
85. amyotrophic lateral sclerosis

Level Three: Thinking Critically

86. The patient is experiencing a transient ischemic attack or mini-stroke with visual disturbances in the oculus sinister, or left eye.
87. Dr. Xenon orders an electroencephalograph or electroencephalography to obtain an electroencephalogram.

Endocrine System

OBJECTIVES

After completing this chapter, you should be able to:

1. State the meanings of word parts related to the endocrine system.
2. Identify and locate organs and glands of the endocrine system.
3. List key hormones of each gland and name a primary action of the significant hormones.
4. Explain the role of the endocrine system in overall body functioning.
5. Define common signs, symptoms, and treatments of various endocrine system diseases.
6. Explain clinical tests and diagnostic procedures related to the endocrine system.
7. Describe anatomical and physiological alterations of the endocrine system throughout the lifespan.
8. List common abbreviations related to the endocrine system.
9. Define terms used in medical reports involving the endocrine system.
10. Correctly define, spell, and pronounce the chapter's medical terms.

Professional Profile: Licensed Practical Nurse

Justina is a licensed practical nurse (LPN) working in an endocrinology office. She has been a nurse for 20 years, most recently working for an endocrinologist in private practice. The majority of patients seen in this practice have diabetes, but thyroid disorders are also common.

LPN educational programs require less time for completion than do registered nurse (RN) courses of study. Justina's state-approved practical nursing program was offered by a local vocational school and consisted of 1 year of classroom study and supervised clinical practice. Basic nursing concepts and patient care–related subjects are covered during training. She took courses in the following areas: medical terminology, basic anatomy and physiology, medical-surgical nursing, pediatrics, obstetrics, psychiatric nursing, drug administration, nutrition, and first aid.

After successful completion of the educational program, candidates must pass a licensing examination before they can be called an LPN. Although LPNs are not permitted to perform as many procedures as are RNs, their role in the health-care setting is extremely important.

Patients under the care of an endocrinologist, a physician specializing in disorders of glands, must routinely visit the office for follow-up and continuing care. For example, patients with diabetes must chart their daily blood glucose levels, which are reviewed by the staff when determining individual patient protocols. Thyroid disorders often require iodine-uptake tests, which the office interprets to decide on the best treatment options. Keen observational skills are critical to the LPN profession.

INTRODUCTION

After released, hormones exert their effects within minutes or within days!

The endocrine system is involved with complicated mechanisms aimed at maintaining homeostasis, the state of body equilibrium. The word part *endo-* means "inner," and the word part *-crine* refers to "secretion," thus *endocrine* refers to an "internal structure that secretes." The nervous system operates in conjunction with the endocrine system. Hence, the term *neuroendocrine system* is often applied when describing its roles. Two components of the endocrine system are glands and hormones. Glands are organs or clusters of specialized cells, and hormones are chemical messengers. Hormones arrive at their destinations through the systemic circulation and are responsible for starting, stopping, or orchestrating some types of body activity. The endocrine system interacts with every other system to create balance in the body.

Because the endocrine system exerts its effects on so many other body systems, disorders of the endocrine system are often widespread. Signs, symptoms, clinical tests, diagnostic procedures, and treatments of various endocrine diseases are discussed in this chapter.

MEDICAL TERM PARTS

WORD PARTS

Medical term prefixes, suffixes, and combining forms related to the endocrine system are introduced in this section.

Word Parts	Meaning
acr-, acro-	extreme, intense
aden-, adeno-	gland, glandular
adren-, adreno-	adrenal

Word Parts	Meaning
calc-, calci-, calco-	calcium
cortic-, cortico-	cortex, cortical
-crine	secretion, secreting
end-, endo-	within, inner
gluc-, gluco-	glucose
glyc-, glyco-	sweet, sugar, glucose
hypo-	deficient, below normal
lact-, lacti-, lacto-	milk
mel-, meli-, melo-	honey, sugar
myx-, myxo-	mucus, mucous
pancre-, pancreo-	pancreas, pancreatic
para-	alongside
-phage, -phagia, -phagy	eating, eat
thyr-, thyreo-, thyro-	thyroid
toco-	childbirth
-tropic	having an affinity for, attracted to

WORD ETYMOLOGY

Some words have Greek or Latin word roots but are not true word parts. This section lists those that are used as medical terms.

Word	Definition
adenos	a gland
mellitus	honeyed
pancreas	the sweetbread

MEDICAL TERM PARTS USED AS PREFIXES

Prefix	Definition
hypo-	deficient, below normal
para-	alongside
toco-	childbirth

MEDICAL TERM PARTS USED AS SUFFIXES

Suffix	Definition
-crine	secretion, secreting
-phage, -phagia, -phagy	eating, eat
-tropic	having an affinity for, attracted to

WORD GROUPING

Using the "Medical Term Parts" tables, identify the prefix, suffix, or combining form for each of the following definitions. The first one has been done as an example.

Definition	Word Part
glucose	*gluc-, gluco-*
adrenal	
alongside	
calcium	
childbirth	
cortex, cortical	
deficient, below normal	
eating, eat	
extreme, intense	
gland, glandular	
having an affinity for, attracted to	
honey, sugar	
milk	
mucus, mucous	
pancreas, pancreatic	
secretion, secreting	
sweet, sugar, glucose	
thyroid	
within, inner	

WORD BUILDING

Word parts, introduced in the "Medical Term Parts" section, are listed in the following table. For this exercise, first supply the meaning of each word part, then use the word part to build a word you already know. The word you list under "Common or Known Word" does not have to be a medical term; a commonly used word is fine. Be sure, however, that the word correctly reflects the intended meaning. The first one has been done as an example. Check your answers in a dictionary.

Word Part	Meaning	Common or Known Word	Example Medical Term
aden-, adeno-	*gland, glandular*	*adenoid*	adenohypophysis
adren-, adreno-			adrenal gland
end-, endo-			endocrine
gluc-, gluco-			glucose
hypo-			hypoparathyroidism

Word Part	Meaning	Common or Known Word	Example Medical Term
lact-, lacti-, lacto-			prolactin
mel-, meli-, melo-			diabetes mellitus
pancre-, pancreo-			pancreas
para-			parathyroid glands
thyr-, thyreo-, thyro-			thyroid gland

ANATOMY AND PHYSIOLOGY

Structures of the Endocrine System

- Adrenal glands
- Hypothalamus
- Pancreas
- Parathyroid glands
- Pineal gland
- Pituitary gland
- Thymus
- Thyroid gland

Endocrine System Preview

The **endocrine system**, composed of glands and their hormones, ensures internal balance (homeostasis). A **gland** is an organized grouping of cells that function as a secreting or excreting organ. **Secretion** means producing a physiologically active substance, and **excretion** refers to separating matter from blood. Endocrine glands have no ducts, so the blood absorbs their products directly. For this reason, endocrine glands are sometimes referred to as "ductless glands." The **hormones** that they release or secrete are chemical substances formed in one gland and transported in the blood to another site, termed target cells; there they exert their effects. The effects of hormones, such as changing the metabolic or functional activity of other cells, are slower to appear and longer lasting than those of neurotransmitters, supplied by the nervous system.

Target cells play a critical role in the endocrine system. A **target cell** is a cell that responds to a particular hormone. It does so because it has specific receptors to which certain hormone molecules can bind. Think of the hormone and target cell as if they were a lock and key—only one particular hormone can interact with one type of receptor site, much like only one key fitting a specific lock. Two primary types of hormones exist: steroid and nonsteroid. Steroid hormones combine with receptors within the cell nucleus, whereas nonsteroid hormones attach to receptors in the target cell membrane. When the hormone combines with the binding site (receptor attachment), the interaction stimulates activity.

"Tropic," "trophic," and "tropin" hormones are chemical messengers from one gland that stimulate another endocrine gland or organ to secrete its hormones. The word part *-trophic* is derived from the Greek and means "having an affinity for." Thus hormones with *-tropic, -trophic,* or *-tropin* in their names are attracted to, or target, other endocrine structures.

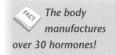

The body manufactures over 30 hormones!

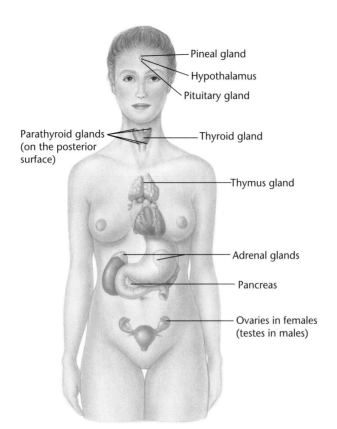

Pineal gland
Hypothalamus
Pituitary gland
Parathyroid glands
(on the posterior surface)
Thyroid gland
Thymus gland
Adrenal glands
Pancreas
Ovaries in females
(testes in males)

FIGURE 9-1
Organs and glands of the endocrine system. (Image provided by the Anatomical Chart Co.)

Figure 9-1 illustrates the major endocrine glands: hypothalamus, pituitary, thyroid, parathyroids, adrenals, pineal, thymus, and pancreas. The pituitary is referred to as the master gland because it controls so many other endocrine structures. Key glands and their particular hormones are discussed in general terms in the following sections.

Key Terms	Definitions
endocrine (EN doh krin) **system**	glands and organs that secrete directly into the bloodstream or lymph; ductless glands
gland	an organized group of cells that function as a secreting or excreting organ
secretion (se KREE shun)	production of a physiologically active substance
excretion (eck SKREE shun)	formation by separating materials from the blood
hormones (HOR mohnz)	chemicals transported by blood or lymph that exerts their effect at a site other than their origin
target cell	cell with a specific receptor for a particular hormone

Key Term Practice: Endocrine System Preview

1. Ductless glands can be found in the _____ system.

2. Chemical messengers called _____ are part of the endocrine system.

3. The formation of a product from materials delivered by the blood is termed _____.

Pituitary Gland (Hypophysis)

The **pituitary gland** is an endocrine gland, about 1 cm (0.4 inch) in diameter, that is attached to the base of the brain in a skull depression called the sella turcica (Fig. 9-2). It is subdivided into two main parts, each of which has two synonymous names. The pituitary gland as a whole is also referred to as the **hypophysis.** Its two lobes are the **adenohypophysis** (anterior pituitary) and **neurohypophysis** (posterior pituitary). Releasing hormones produced by the **hypothalamus**, a region of the diencephalon that forms the floor of the third brain ventricle, control the anterior lobe (Fig. 9-3). Releasing hormones are substances that accelerate the rate of secretion of a given hormone. Hormones secreted by the adenohypophysis are adrenocorticotropic hormone (ACTH), follicle-stimulating hormone (FSH), human growth hormone (hGH), luteinizing hormone (LH), prolactin (PRL), and thyroid-stimulating hormone (TSH).

Only two hormones are associated with the neurohypophysis: antidiuretic hormone (ADH) and oxytocin (OT or OXT). The posterior lobe does not synthesize hormones; it merely stores and releases them. The primary functions and alternate names for each of the pituitary hormones are listed in Table 9-1.

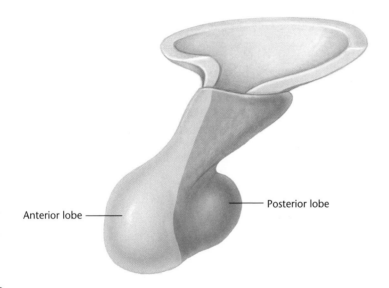

Anterior lobe —————
Posterior lobe

FIGURE 9-2
The anterior lobe of the pituitary gland produces adrenocorticotropic hormone (ACTH), thyroid-stimulating hormone (TSH), human growth hormone (hGH), prolactin (PRL), follicle-stimulating hormone (FSH), luteinizing hormone (LH), and melanocyte-stimulating hormone (MSH). The posterior lobe releases antidiuretic hormone (ADH) and oxytocin (OT). (Image provided by the Anatomical Chart Co.)

Key Terms	Definitions
pituitary (pi TEW i terr ee) **gland**	master gland that orchestrates endocrine function; hypophysis
hypophysis (high POF i sis)	master gland that orchestrates endocrine function; pituitary gland
adenohypophysis (ad e noh high POF i sis)	anterior pituitary, which produces hormones
neurohypophysis (noor oh high POF i sis)	posterior pituitary, which stores and releases hormones
hypothalamus (high poh THAL uh mus)	area at the central underside of the brain that produces releasing hormones

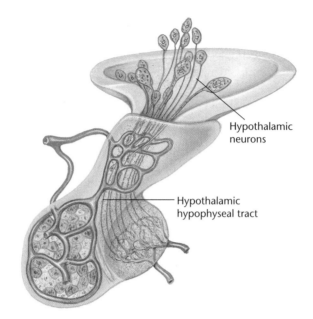

Hypothalamic neurons

Hypothalamic hypophyseal tract

FIGURE 9-3
The hypothalamus produces hormones in the third brain ventricle. (Image provided by the Anatomical Chart Co.)

TABLE 9-1 Pituitary Hormones and Functions

Area of Pituitary	Hormone	Alternate Name(s)	Functions
adenohypophysis (anterior pituitary)	adrenocorticotropic hormone (ACTH)	corticotropin	stimulates the adrenal cortex to produce corticosteroids
	follicle-stimulating hormone (FSH)	follitropin	stimulates the growth of egg follicles (ovary) and sperm production (testicle)
	human growth hormone (hGH)	somatotropin	stimulates protein synthesis and long-bone growth
	luteinizing hormone (LH)	lutropin in females; interstitial cell-stimulating hormone (ICSH) in males	stimulates production of eggs (ovary), secretion of progesterone, and formation of the corpus luteum (tissue mass formed after ovulation)
	prolactin (PRL)	mammotropin	stimulates lactation and secretion of progesterone
	thyroid-stimulating hormone (TSH)	thyrotropin	stimulates release of thyroid gland hormones
neurohypophysis (posterior pituitary)	antidiuretic (ADH) hormone	vasopressin	reduces water excretion by the kidneys
	oxytocin (OT or OXT)	none	stimulates uterine contractions and triggers milk secretion during nursing

Key Term Practice: Pituitary Gland (Hypophysis)

1. What is the alternate term for each of the following structures?

   a. pituitary gland _____

   b. anterior pituitary _____

   c. posterior pituitary _____

2. The hormone that exerts its effects in the adrenal cortex is _____.

3. _____ is the alternate name for prolactin.

Thyroid and Parathyroid Glands

The **thyroid gland** is a bilobed, butterfly-shaped endocrine structure, located just inferior to the larynx (voice box) and anterior to the trachea, that secretes thyroid hormones (Fig. 9-4). The isthmus joins the two lobes. The term *thyroid*, meaning "shield-shaped," is derived from the Greek word for the shields carried by Greek warriors. The gland itself consists of fluid-filled cavities called follicles, which store hormones secreted by follicle cells. Dietary iodine is essential for making thyroid hormones. Iodine can be obtained only by ingesting food containing the mineral.

Hormones associated with this gland are thyroxine, triiodothyronine, and calcitonin. Two thyroid hormones are produced by follicle cells: **tetraiodothyronine** (T_4 or **thyroxine**) and **triiodothyronine** (T_3). Each gets its name from the number of iodine atoms found within its molecule: Thyroxine has four, and triiodothyronine has three. Both increase metabolic rate, enhance protein synthesis, and stimulate the breakdown of lipids. TSH from the hypophysis controls the secretion of hormones from the thyroid gland.

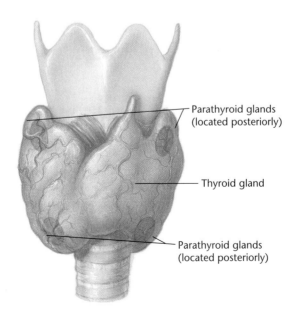

Parathyroid glands (located posteriorly)

Thyroid gland

Parathyroid glands (located posteriorly)

FIGURE 9-4
The thyroid and parathyroid glands. (Image provided by the Anatomical Chart Co.)

Calcitonin (CT), another thyroid hormone, is produced by C (clear) cells, which are endocrinocytes located between the follicle cells and the basement membrane. Calcitonin targets bones and kidneys to regulate blood calcium ion concentrations by lowering the circulating levels.

The **parathyroid glands** are four small endocrine glands that are embedded in the posterior surface of the thyroid gland (Fig. 9-4). The calcium- and phosphorus-regulating hormone produced by chief cells in the glands is **parathyroid hormone** or **parathormone** (PTH). Whereas calcitonin serves to lower blood calcium ion levels, PTH works antagonistically to increase circulating blood calcium ion levels. It does this by stimulating resorption of the mineral from bone tissue. PTH also causes a decrease in blood phosphate (phosphorus ion) concentration by causing the kidneys to conserve calcium and excrete phosphate. This hormone also indirectly stimulates the absorption of calcium from the intestine. A negative-feedback mechanism (a system for adjusting body concentrations of a particular substance) operates to maintain the appropriate levels of circulating calcium and phosphate ions. Through the combined actions of the thyroid and parathyroid hormones, calcium balance in the blood is achieved.

Key Terms	Definitions
thyroid (THIGH roid) **gland**	gland that secretes thyroid hormones
tetraiodothyronine (tet ruh eye oh doh THIGH roh neen)	a thyroid hormone; thyroxine
thyroxine (thigh ROCK seen)	a thyroid hormone; tetraiodothyronine
triiodothyronine (trye eye oh doh THIGH roh neen)	a thyroid hormone
calcitonin (kal si TOH nin)	a thyroid hormone that lowers plasma calcium and phosphate ion levels by inhibiting bone resorption; increases renal excretion of phosphate and calcium
parathyroid (pair uh THIGH roid) **glands**	endocrine glands on the posterior thyroid
parathyroid (pair uh THIGH roid) **hormone**	parathyroid hormone, which regulates blood calcium and phosphorus ion levels; parathormone
parathormone (pair uh THOR mohn)	parathyroid hormone, which regulates blood calcium and phosphorus ion levels; parathyroid hormone

Key Term Practice: Thyroid and Parathyroid Glands

1. The hormone _____ lowers blood calcium levels, whereas the hormone _____ increases their levels.

2. _____ is also known as parathormone.

Pancreas

The **pancreas**, a gland 20–25 cm (8–10 inches) long, is sandwiched between the stomach and the first portion of the small intestine (Fig. 9-5). It has both endocrine and exocrine (digestive enzyme) functions. The exocrine portion secretes pancreatic juice directly into a duct, and the endocrine portion produces hormones. Its endocrine functions are controlled by the pancreatic islets, consisting of four cell types: alpha, beta, delta, and F cells. Each cell type produces a different hormone. These cells were

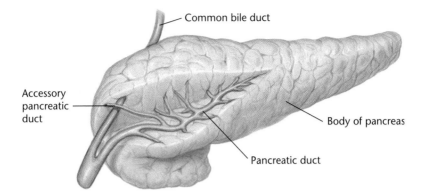

— Common bile duct

Accessory pancreatic duct

Body of pancreas

Pancreatic duct

FIGURE 9-5
The pancreas is nestled between the stomach and the first portion of the small intestine. (Image provided by the Anatomical Chart Co.)

once referred to as the islets of Langerhans, after their discoverer, German pathologist Paul Langerhans. **Pancreatic islets** are responsible for the secretions of glucagon, insulin, somatostatin, and pancreatic polypeptide.

Alpha cells produce **glucagon**, a hormone that removes glucose from storage sites and allows it to be exported to the blood. Glucagon also stimulates the liver to convert glycogen (the stored form of glucose) and carbohydrates to glucose, and it stimulates fat catabolism (break down). The action of **insulin**, produced by beta cells, is opposite that of glucagon; it moves glucose from the blood into the cells. Insulin promotes the formation of glycogen from glucose, inhibits the conversion of noncarbohydrates into glucose, enhances glucose movement, promotes amino acid transport, and enhances protein and fat synthesis. When blood sugar (glucose) levels rise, insulin is released to transport the sugar from the bloodstream into the cells; when blood glucose levels dip, glucagon is secreted to stimulate the liver to release glucose into the blood.

Key Terms	Definitions
pancreas (PAN kree us)	organ with endocrine and exocrine functions
pancreatic (pan kree AT ick) **islets**	the endocrine cells of the pancreas
glucagon (GLOO kuh gon)	pancreatic hormone (from alpha cells) that elevates blood glucose
insulin (IN suh lin)	pancreatic hormone (from beta cells) that lowers blood glucose

Key Term Practice: Pancreas

1. Which hormone elevates blood glucose levels? _____

2. Which hormone lowers blood glucose levels? _____

Adrenal Glands

The **adrenal glands** are pyramid-shaped structures weighing about 7.5 grams (0.15 ounce) positioned above each kidney, forming a cap at its superior border (Fig. 9-6). The word *adrenal* literally means "above the renal" or "above the kidney." The adrenal gland should be thought of as two glands in one because it is composed of medullary and cortical regions that each have different functions. The **adrenal cortex** is the outer portion of the gland and produces aldosterone, cortisol, and some sex hormones. The **adrenal medulla** is the inner portion of the gland and secretes norepinephrine and epinephrine.

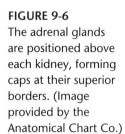

FIGURE 9-6
The adrenal glands are positioned above each kidney, forming caps at their superior borders. (Image provided by the Anatomical Chart Co.)

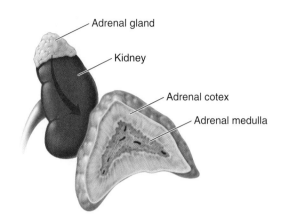

Adrenal gland

Kidney

Adrenal cotex

Adrenal medulla

Aldosterone causes the kidneys to conserve sodium ions (Na^+) and to excrete potassium ions (K^+). This helps maintain blood volume and pressure. The secretion of aldosterone is regulated by a negative-feedback loop: Aldosterone is secreted in response to decreased sodium, increased potassium, or the presence of angiotensin II (another hormone important for blood pressure maintenance). As a memory aid, the letters of the word *salt* are found in *al*dos*te*rone, and sodium is a salt.

Cortisol (hydrocortisone) is secreted in response to tissue damage and causes inflammation at the site. It also regulates blood sugar levels, fat deposition, and protein metabolism. **Androgens**, sex hormones, are produced in the inner zone of the adrenal cortex. This region secretes supplementary sex hormones already produced by the gonads (sex organs). The significance of the androgens produced in the adrenals is not known.

The medullary hormones, epinephrine and norepinephrine, are synthesized from the amino acid tyrosine and are specific in their actions. These hormones take part in nervous system functions such as the fight-or-flight response. Once the hormones are formed, about 10% of medullary cells retain the compound as norepinephrine; the remaining norepinephrine is converted to epinephrine. **Norepinephrine** (NE), also called **noradrenaline**, is unique in that it has the ability to work as either a neurotransmitter or as a hormone. For example, when norepinephrine is released by presynaptic neurons, it diffuses across the cleft and binds to an adrenergic receptor in a postsynaptic neuron, thus it acts as a neurotransmitter. When norepinephrine diffuses into the blood and binds to an adrenergic receptor in a target cell, it is acting as a hormone. Norepinephrine acts to accelerate the heart rate, increase blood flow, increase blood pressure, and increase metabolic rate.

Epinephrine (E; or **adrenaline**) functions to raise heart rate, cause vasodilation, elevate blood pressure, dilate airways, activate the reticular formation of the brain, increase blood glucose levels, and enhance metabolic rate. Epinephrine and norepinephrine are known collectively as catecholamines. The terms noradrenaline and adrenaline may still be used because they describe the source of the hormones as the adrenal glands.

Key Terms	Definitions
adrenal (uh DREE nul) **glands**	endocrine gland on each kidney
adrenal cortex (uh DREE nul KOHR tecks)	outer portion of the adrenal gland
adrenal medulla (uh DREE nul me DEW luh)	inner portion of the adrenal gland
aldosterone (al DOS te rohn)	adrenal hormone of sodium metabolism
cortisol (KOR ti sol)	adrenocortical steroid hormone; hydrocortisone

androgens (AN droh jinz)	hormone promoting male secondary sex characteristics
norepinephrine (nor ep i NEF rin)	adrenal medulla hormone; noradrenaline
noradrenaline (nor uh DREN uh lin)	adrenal medulla hormone; norepinephrine
epinephrine (ep i NEF rin)	adrenal medulla hormone; adrenaline
adrenaline (uh DREN uh lin)	adrenal medulla hormone; epinephrine

Key Term Practice: Adrenal Glands

1. What is the alternate term for each of the following?

   a. epinephrine _____

   b. norepinephrine _____

2. The outer portion of the adrenal gland is termed the _____, and the inner region is known as the _____.

Pineal and Thymus Glands

The **pineal gland (epiphysis cerebri)** is a structure named for its characteristic pine cone shape. It is attached to the thalamus near the roof of the third ventricle in the brain (Fig. 9-7). One function of the gland is **melatonin** secretion, which may influence the onset of sexual maturation. It is also believed to be involved with human biorhythms, or the circadian cycle. The **circadian cycle** repeats approximately every 24 hours (Fig. 9-8).

The **thymus** is situated posterior to the sternum between the lungs (Fig. 9-9). It functions in the secretion of **thymosins**, a group of thymic hormones that affect the maturation and development of lymphocytes (white blood cells), which play a role in immunity.

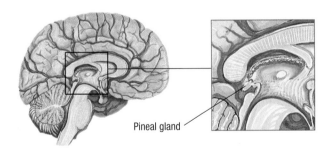

Pineal gland

FIGURE 9-7
The pineal gland is attached to the thalamus near the roof of the third ventricle of the brain. (Image provided by the Anatomical Chart Co.)

Key Terms	Definitions
pineal (PYE nee ul) **gland**	pine cone-shaped organ in the brain that secretes melatonin; epiphysis cerebri
epiphysis cerebri (e PIF i sis SERR e brye)	pine cone-shaped organ in the brain that secretes melatonin; pineal gland

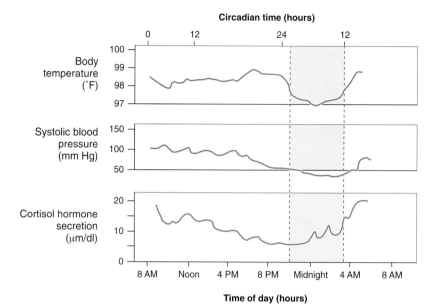

FIGURE 9-8
The circadian cycle repeats at approximately 24-hour intervals, and it may be influenced by melatonin, secreted by the pineal gland.

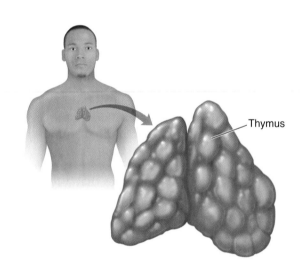

FIGURE 9-9
The thymus is situated just posterior to the sternum between the lungs. (Image of gland provided by the Anatomical Chart Co.)

Thymus

melatonin (mel uh TOH nin)	hormone
circadian (sur KAY dee un) **cycle**	human biorhythm that repeats every 24 hours
thymus (THIGH mus)	organ at the base of the neck associated with lymphocytes and the immune system
thymosins (THIGH moh sins)	thymus gland

Key Term Practice: Pineal and Thymus Glands

1. Hormones from the thymus gland are collectively termed _____.

2. What is the alternative term for the pineal gland? _____

TABLE 9-2 Key Endocrine Glands, Hormones, and Functions

Gland	Hormone	Function
adrenals	aldosterone	causes the kidney to conserve sodium ions (Na^+) and excrete potassium ions (K^+)
	cortisol	causes inflammation in response to tissue damage
	epinephrine (E)	increases the heart rate, blood pressure, and blood glucose levels
	norepinephrine (NE)	increases the heart rate, blood pressure, and metabolic rate
hypothalamus	releasing hormones	affect other glands
pancreas	glucagon	increases blood glucose levels
	insulin	decreases blood glucose levels
parathyroid	parathormone (parathyroid hormone or PTH)	increases blood calcium levels; decreases blood phosphorus levels
pineal	melatonin	influences sexual maturation and the circadian cycle
thymus	thymosins	affect lymphocyte development and immunity
thyroid	calcitonin	lowers blood calcium ion concentration
	triiodothyronine (T_3)	increases metabolic rate
	tetraiodothyronine (T_4 or Thyroxine)	increases metabolic rate; is converted to T_3

Endocrine Overview

Hormones associated with other endocrine glands exert their effects on numerous body tissues, cells, and organs. Hormonal effects are widespread and important for maintaining homeostatic balance. Table 9-2 lists the key endocrine glands, their hormones, and the hormones' functions.

THE CLINICAL DIMENSION

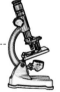

Pathology of the Endocrine System

This section identifies signs and symptoms, pathological conditions, and treatments related to the endocrine system. Endocrine disorders can be assessed through a variety of clinical tests and diagnostic procedures. Laboratory analyses used to evaluate endocrine function include plasma, serum, blood, urine, glucose tolerance, and glycosylated hemoglobin (A_{Ic}) tests. Common disorders and treatments of the endocrine system are described.

Disorders of the endocrine system are generally the result of tumors or the hyperfunction or hypofunction of specific glands. They can also be secondary to some other primary condition. The pathological disorders discussed in this section are commonly associated with endocrine dysfunction.

Adrenal Gland Disorders

Chronic adrenocortical insufficiency is also termed **Addison disease.** In many cases, the cause is unknown, but an autoimmune problem is suspected. In addition to idiopathic Addison disease, adrenal tumors and tuberculosis have been implicated.

Decreased aldosterone levels, weakness, pigmentation blotches on the mucous membranes, skin bronzing, hypotension (low blood pressure), and gastrointestinal distress characterize the disease.

Urine and blood tests show decreased cortisol levels, and adrenal calcification may be evident on **x-ray studies**, radiographic films used to evaluate structures. **Blood tests** are used to evaluate blood components, and **urine ketosteroid tests** to detect androgen metabolites are used. Types of urine ketosteroid tests include the **hydroxycorticosteroid urine test,** which detects the presence of cortisol byproducts, and the **17-ketosteroids** (17-KS) **test,** which detects steroidal metabolites of androgenic and adrenocortical hormones. Treatment involves hormone-replacement therapy, including glucocorticoids and mineralocorticoids. **Hormone-replacement therapy** may be used to restore a normal endocrine function or to alter the secretion of another hormone.

Cushing syndrome is a clinical disorder characterized by adipose deposition in the face and trunk, a "buffalo hump" in the scapular region, hypertension (high blood pressure), fatigue, glycosuria (glucose in the urine), increased susceptibility to infection, muscle weakness, and "moon face" (Fig. 9-10). Its cause is an adrenal cortex tumor, pituitary tumor, overdose reaction to adrenocortical hormone administration, or hypersecretion of cortisol. Physical evaluation and increased cortisol levels in the urine lead to the diagnosis. The treatment depends on the cause. Tumor excision and drugs to suppress ACTH are options.

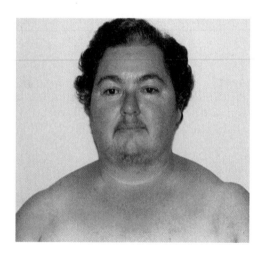

FIGURE 9-10
Cushing syndrome is characterized by adipose deposition in the face and trunk. (Reprinted with permission from Rubin E. Essential Pathology, 3rd ed. Philadelphia: Lippincott Williams & Wilkins, 2000.)

A **pheochromocytoma** is a usually benign neoplasm of the adrenal medulla. It is characterized by irregular heart rate, hypertension, pounding headaches, and excessive catecholamine (epinephrine and norepinephrine) secretion. Increased levels of blood catecholamines (epinephrine and norepinephrine) or radiographic studies confirm the diagnosis. Surgical removal of the tumor is the best treatment.

Excessive output of adrenal androgens leading to the development of masculine traits in females is termed adrenal **virilism.** Its underlying cause is usually adrenal hyperplasia or a tumor. Signs and symptoms include **hirsutism** (excessive hair growth in abnormal locations), baldness, acne, uterine atrophy, clitoris hypertrophy, decreased breast size, and increased masculinity. Diagnostic studies, including a computed tomography (CT) scan or magnetic resonance imaging (MRI), identify tumors. **Computed tomography scans** are cross-sectional body images produced using a computer and x-rays. **Magnetic resonance imaging** is a technique that uses electromagnetic radiation to obtain images. Hydrocortisone, tumor removal, and adrenalectomy are treatment options.

Key Terms	Definitions
Addison disease	primary adrenocortical insufficiency
x-ray studies	radiographic films of structures used for evaluation
blood tests	analyses of blood to evaluate components
urine ketosteroid (kee toh STEER oid) tests	analyses of urine to detect androgen metabolites
hydroxycorticosteroid (high drock see kor ti kos tur oid) urine test	analysis of urine to detect cortisol byproducts
17-ketosteroids (kee toh STEER oidz) test	analysis of urine to detect steroidal metabolites of androgenic and adrenocortical hormones
hormone-replacement therapy	hormone administration to restore normal function
Cushing (KOOSH ing) syndrome	clinical disorder of the adrenal gland characterized by excessive ACTH production
pheochromocytoma (fee oh kroh moh sigh TOH muh)	adrenal medulla tumor
virilism (VIRR i liz um)	development of male secondary sex characteristics in a female
hirsutism (HUR sewt iz um)	abnormal hair growth on a female's face or body
computed tomography scans	computerized x-ray images of internal organs
magnetic resonance imaging	imaging of glands and organs using electromagnetic radiation

Key Term Practice: Adrenal Gland Disorders

1. An alternate medical term for primary adrenocortical insufficiency is _____ disease.

2. A/an _____ is a tumor associated with the adrenal medulla.

Pancreas Disorders

Diabetes mellitus (DM) is a chronic disorder of carbohydrate metabolism. The disease is so named because of the sugary urine that is excreted. The word parts *mel-*, *meli-*, and *melo-* mean "sugar or honey," hence the term *mellitus*. The condition is characterized by inadequate insulin production or decreased cellular sensitivity to insulin. Signs and symptoms include hyperglycemia (elevated blood glucose levels), glycosuria, altered fat and protein metabolism, polyuria (excessive urination), polydipsia (excessive thirst), and polyphagia (excessive appetite or eating). There are three major categories of the disease: type 1, type 2, and type 3.

Type 1 diabetes, a chronic disorder, is known as juvenile-onset diabetes or **insulin-dependent diabetes mellitus** (IDDM), and it begins before age 30 years. The pancreas produces little or no insulin, and individuals with IDDM must take insulin injections. Maturity-onset diabetes (type 2) has a gradual onset and is also called **non-insulin-dependent diabetes mellitus** (NIDDM). The disease generally begins after age 40 years. Type 2 is managed initially with dietary measures. Type 1 is thought to be an autoimmune disorder; research suggests that there may be a genetic predisposition for type 2 diabetes, especially in obese individuals or those with excessive abdominal girth. Diagnosis of diabetes mellitus is made by a positive glucose test, glycosuria, and glucose tolerance test.

The **glucose tolerance test** (GTT) measures serum glucose levels at intervals up to 3 hours. The patient fasts for 12 hours and then ingests a glucose mixture. Blood is drawn before the patient drinks the glucose so clinicians can measure the fasting level; blood is then drawn at half-hour intervals to measure the glucose levels over time. Measuring **glycosylated hemoglobin** assists in evaluating plasma glucose over a 3-month period. The average life span of a red blood cell is 120 days. During the life of a red blood cell, glucose molecules adhere to the cell's hemoglobin, forming glycosylated hemoglobin molecules (A_{Ia}, A_{Ib}, and A_{Ic}). Once formed, the glycosylated hemoglobin remains until red blood cell death. Therefore, evaluating this molecule accesses the effectiveness of the therapy of the patient with diabetes. As yet, there is no standardization for measurement, so glycosylated hemoglobin cannot be used as a definitive diagnostic test for diabetes.

Type 3 diabetes mellitus occurs only during pregnancy and is termed **gestational diabetes mellitus** (GDM). Gestational diabetes has the same signs and symptoms as types 1 and 2. It usually disappears after pregnancy; however, 30–40% of women with GDM develop type 2 diabetes mellitus within 10 years of giving birth. Type 3 may be caused by destruction of insulin by the placenta when there are increased levels of human placental lactogen (hPL). The diagnosis is confirmed by glycosuria and the results of the glucose tolerance test and **postprandial** (after a meal) glucose tests.

The goal of treatment is to control blood glucose levels through exercise, insulin injections, diet, and/or oral drug therapy. Insulin and **oral antidiabetic agents**, hypoglycemic drugs used to decrease blood glucose levels, are used to manage glucose levels in the diabetic patient. Diabetes leads to systemic complications, such as kidney, eye, and nerve damage, so glucose management is life-long and paramount for thwarting future complications.

Hypoglycemia is a decreased blood glucose level, characterized by hunger, nervousness, sweating, and fatigue. If not treated, the signs could progress to convulsions. Hypoglycemia can be caused by fasting, increased insulin secretion, or a pancreatic tumor. A patient with diabetes may become hypoglycemic from an insulin overdose, not eating, or too much exercise. Hypoglycemia is diagnosed by abnormally low blood glucose (< 40 mg/dL in men; < 45 mg/dL in women). Eating food, ingesting glucose tablets, or removing the tumor are the usual treatments.

Key Terms	Definitions
diabetes mellitus (dye uh BEE teez mel EYE tus)	chronic disorder of carbohydrate metabolism
insulin dependent diabetes mellitus (dye uh BEE teez mel EYE tus)	disorder of glucose metabolism occurring before adulthood; type 1 diabetes mellitus
non-insulin-dependent diabetes mellitus (dye uh BEE teez mel EYE tus)	disorder of glucose metabolism occurring in adulthood; type 2 diabetes mellitus
glucose (GLOO koce) **tolerance test**	determination of serum glucose levels at different times after ingestion of a glucose syrup
glycosylated hemoglobin (GLYE koh si lay ted HEE moh gloh bin)	used to test circulating glucose blood levels over the life span of a red blood cell
gestational diabetes mellitus (jes TAY shun ul dye uh BEE teez mel EYE tus)	disorder of glucose metabolism that occurs during pregnancy; type 3 diabetes mellitus
postprandial (pohst PRAN dee ul)	after a meal
oral antidiabetic (AN tee dye uh BET ick) **agents**	drugs used to decrease blood glucose levels
hypoglycemia (high poh glye SEE mee uh)	abnormally low blood glucose level

Key Term Practice: Pancreas Disorders

1. What is the alternative medical term for each of the following?

 a. Type 1 _____

 b. Type 2 _____

 c. Type 3 _____

2. _____ is the term used to describe abnormally low blood glucose levels.

Parathyroid Disorders

Hyperparathyroidism is a condition that results from increased parathyroid gland activity leading to increased PTH levels. The elevated PTH levels cause bone resorption and subsequent elevated calcium ion levels in the blood, a condition called hypercalcemia. The hypercalcemia initiates a cascade of events affecting the functioning of other systems. The cause may be idiopathic or the result of an adenoma (benign tumor). Signs and symptoms are muscle weakness, gastrointestinal upset, nausea, cardiac arrhythmia, renal calculi (kidney stones), and fragile bones that fracture easily.

Elevated PTH levels on radioimmunoassay, blood studies that show increased calcium ion concentration and decreased potassium ion levels, and urinalysis that demonstrates excessive calcium ion levels confirm the diagnosis. **Radioimmunoassay** (RIA) is a method used for detecting antigens, antibodies, enzymes, and hormones using radiolabeled reactants. Treating the underlying cause (tumor removal or parathyroidectomy) alleviates the condition. Surgical removal of one or more of the parathyroid glands is called **parathyroidectomy.**

Parathyroid hormone insufficiency results in **hypoparathyroidism.** The condition is caused by a tumor or by injury to the parathyroid gland. It may also be autoimmune induced or a congenital disorder. Hypoparathyroidism is characterized by hypocalcemia (low blood calcium levels), hyperphosphatemia (elevated blood phosphate levels), and increased neuromuscular excitability (elevated muscle responsiveness to a stimulus). It can progress to seizures and tetany (sustained muscle contractions). Diagnosis is made by the clinical picture, physical examination, and clinical test results. Tests show decreased serum calcium ion levels, increased bone density, and decreased PTH levels on RIA. The **Trousseau sign,** muscle tetany in which carpal spasm is elicited by compressing the brachial region, is also evident (Fig 9-11). Treatment is a high-calcium, low-phosphorus diet supplemented with calcium and vitamin D tablets. (Vitamin D enhances calcium ion absorption.)

Key Terms	Definitions
hyperparathyroidism (high pur pair uh THIGH roid iz um)	increased activity of parathyroid glands causing excessive PTH production
radioimmunoassay (RAY dee oh im yoo noh as say)	test detects antigens, antibodies, enzymes, and hormones using radiolabeled reactants
parathyroidectomy (pair uh thigh roy DECK tuh mee)	parathyroid gland

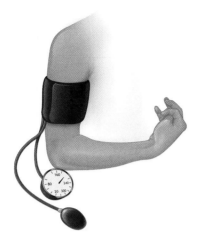

FIGURE 9-11
Trousseau sign is a symptom of hypoparathyroidism in which carpal spasm is elicited by compressing the brachial region.

hypoparathyroidism (high poh pair uh THIGH roid iz um)	inadequate secretion of parathyroid hormones
Trousseau (true SOH) **sign**	carpal spasm elicited when the brachial region is compressed

Key Term Practice: Parathyroid Disorders

1. PTH insufficiency is termed _____.

2. Oversecretion of PTH is called _____.

Pituitary Disorders

Acromegaly is the result of excessive secretion of anterior pituitary hGH in adulthood. It is characterized by overgrowth of bone, connective tissue, and viscera. It is outwardly expressed as enlarged hands, feet, face, and head (Fig. 9-12). The cause is a pituitary tumor or adenoma. Diagnosis is made through visual and physical examination. RIA studies reveal elevated hGH levels. Radiographic and MRI studies show a pituitary lesion. Treatment includes radiation or surgery to remove the tumor.

Like acromegaly, **gigantism** (or giantism) is the result of oversecretion of hGH; but in this case, the excessive production occurs before puberty. The underlying cause is an adenoma. Signs include very long bones and an arched mouth palate. Diagnosis is made by physical examination, elevated hGH on RIA, and evidence of bone thickening. Radiographic studies, CT scans, and MRI scans expose a pituitary lesion. Figure 9-13 shows gigantism and dwarfism, as compared to men of average stature.

Pituitary dwarfism is characterized by abnormal underdevelopment. It is also referred to as hypopituitarism. The disorder is generally a congenital defect or the result of cranial hemorrhage occurring during the birth process. Signs and symptoms include a small body with disproportionate limbs, delayed secondary sexual characteristics, and possible mental retardation (Fig. 9-14). Physical examination demonstrates lipid deposition in the lower trunk. Serum studies show low hGH levels. (Serum is blood plasma without the clotting agent fibrinogen.) Lifelong treatment of the chronic condition is aimed at correcting the imbalance of hormone levels and involves administration of hGH.

In contrast to diabetes mellitus, which is a pancreatic disorder, diabetes insipidus is related to the pituitary. **Diabetes insipidus** results from a deficiency of ADH. It is

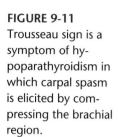

The onset of puberty is between the ages of 9 and 13 years for girls!

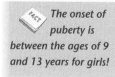

The onset of puberty is between the ages of 10 and 15 years for boys!

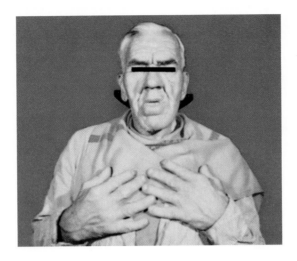

FIGURE 9-12
Acromegaly is the result of excessive secretion of anterior pituitary hGH in adulthood; it is characterized by overgrowth of bone, connective tissue, and viscera. (Reprinted with permission from Willis MC, CMA-AC. Medical terminology: A programmed learning approach to the language of health care. Baltimore: Lippincott Williams & Wilkins, 2002.)

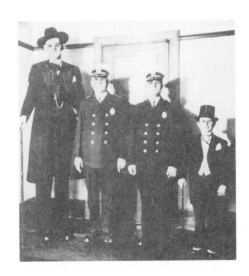

FIGURE 9-13
Gigantism is the result of excessive secretion of anterior pituitary hGH during pre-pubescence. Signs include abnormally long and thick bones. (Reprinted with permission from Tribondeau GA, Patton KT. Anatomy and Physiology, 3rd ed. St. Louis: Mosby, 1996.); p. 16. Tribondeau GA and Patton KT. Yearbook-Yearbook Inc. St. Louis, MO.

characterized by polyuria and compensatory polydipsia. The sequence of urinating and drinking sets up a continuous cycle of attempting to balance the body's water levels. The cause is unknown. Diagnosis is made by patient history of symptoms and a urinalysis that demonstrates a low specific gravity because the urine is extremely dilute. Confirmation of diabetes insipidus is made if the urine output diminishes and the specific gravity increases after administration of ADH. Treatment includes vasopressin injections or nasal spray to increase levels of the hormone.

Developing signs of physical maturity at an unusually early age is termed **precocious puberty.** In girls, it is manifested by pubic and axillary hair, along with breast development before age 8 years. It is marked by pubic and facial hair with increased

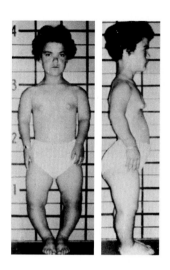

FIGURE 9-14
Pituitary dwarfism is characterized by abnormal underdevelopment. (Reprinted with permission from Saddler T, PhD. Lang man's medical embryology. 9th ed., Ninth Edition Image Bank. Baltimore: Lippincott Williams & Wilkins, 2003.)

gonad size in boys before age 10 years. The cause is pituitary or hypothalamus dysfunction, tumor of the pituitary or hypothalamus, or a testicular tumor in boys. Physical examination and increased hormone levels in the blood and urine provide an accurate diagnosis. Girls also have increased blood FSH and LH levels. Treatment depends on the cause. Tumor removal and hormone therapy to suppress the overactive gland are options.

Key Terms	Definitions
acromegaly (ack roh MEG uh lee)	disorder caused by excessive hGH secretion in adulthood
gigantism (jye GAN tiz um)	disorder from excessive secretion before puberty; giantism
pituitary (pi TEW i terr ee) **dwarfism**	abnormal underdevelopment caused by inadequate hGH levels; hypopituitarism
diabetes insipidus (dye uh BEE teez in SIP i dus)	chronic pituitary disorder causing ADH insufficiency
precocious (pree KOH shus) **puberty**	reaching physical maturity at an unusually early age

Key Term Practice: Pituitary Disorders

1. Excessive growth hormone secretion before puberty can lead to what disorder? _____

2. _____ is characterized by increased bone thickness in the hands and face.

Thyroid Disorders

Hypothyroidism is a condition of diminished thyroid hormone production characterized by low metabolic rate, weight gain, and sluggishness. Congenital, or **infantile hypothyroidism** (formally called cretinism), is caused by a number of factors—for example, failure of the thyroid to position properly, autoimmune disease, and maternal ingestion of medication that interfered with fetal development. In some cases, the thyroid gland may be absent or it fails to produce hormones. Common characteristics are a large, protruding tongue and abdomen, hoarse cry, mental retardation, and depressed muscle tone. It is diagnosed by thyroid gland absence on a CT scan or by a low T_4 level that is accompanied by an increased thyrotropin level. It can be successfully treated with thyroid hormones. If treatment begins early, the individual will have no physiologic manifestations. Thyroid hormone-replacement therapy is necessary throughout life.

A simple **goiter** is an enlargement of the thyroid gland that presents as a large, outwardly obvious swollen mass on the neck (Fig. 9-15). It is also known as nontoxic goiter and results from inadequate iodine ingestion. The lack of iodine causes an increased release of thyrotropin to stimulate the thyroid gland to produce more thyroid hormone. The gland hypertrophies to compensate. Physical examination and blood tests showing an increase in thyrotropin and a decrease in T_3 and T_4 levels confirm the diagnosis. Administration of iodine as potassium iodide or ingestion of iodine-rich foods alleviates the signs. There generally are no symptoms. In some cases, a partial **thyroidectomy** (surgical removal of a portion of the thyroid gland) may be performed.

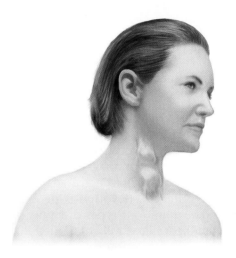

FIGURE 9-15
A simple goiter is an enlargement of the thyroid gland, which presents as a large, swollen mass on the neck. (Image provided by the Anatomical Chart Co.)

Hashimoto disease (Hashimoto thyroiditis) is an autoimmune disease causing chronic thyroiditis. As with most autoimmune diseases, women are more affected than men. The inflammatory response causes diffuse thyroid enlargement. The disease advances to a stage in which the glandular tissue is replaced by fibrous connective tissue. Signs and symptoms include hypothyroidism, cold sensitivity, weight gain, and fatigue. Diagnosis is confirmed by the presence of autoantibodies in the blood and a radioactive iodine uptake (RIU) test.

Thyroid function is evaluated via a **radioactive iodine uptake** (RIU) **test**, which uses radioactive iodine, such as ^{131}I, as a tracer. **Radioiodine**—^{131}I and ^{123}I, radioactive isotopes of iodine—can be delivered intravenously or orally; its dosage is measured in a unit called a microcurie (μCi). ^{131}I is ingested and taken up (absorbed) by the thyroid. A special detector determines the amount taken up over a period of time. This value is then used to assess thyroid function. Lifelong treatment involves the administration (usually orally) of synthetic thyroid hormone.

Overproduction of thyroid hormone is called **hyperthyroidism** or **thyrotoxicosis**. The hypertrophic thyroid may cause a goiter. **Graves disease**, an autoimmune disorder with a familial link, is a form of hyperthyroidism. Signs and symptoms include weight loss and sweating. **Exophthalmos** (abnormal eye protrusion) is characteristic of Graves disease (Fig. 9-16). If not treated, thyrotoxicosis results in **thyroid storm**. Thyroid storm, also termed **thyrotoxic crisis**, is marked by acute hyperthyroidism that can lead to tachycardia (accelerated heart rate), high fever, and muscle weakness. If the crisis does not resolve, coma and possibly death ensue. Diagnosis is based on the clinical manifestations, increased serum T_3 and T_4 levels, and increased uptake of radioiodine as indicated on thyroid function tests. Administering antithyroid drugs to

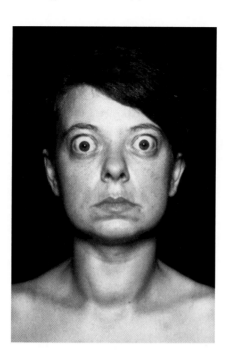

FIGURE 9-16
Overproduction of thyroid hormone may result in Graves disease. Signs and symptoms include weight loss, sweating, and exophthalmos (abnormal eye protrusion). (Reprinted with permission from Rubin E, Farber JL. Pathology, 3rd ed. Philadelphia: Lippincott Williams & Wilkins, 1999.)

decrease thyroid hormone output or radioactive iodine therapy to ablate (remove or destroy unwanted tissue) the thyroid treats hyperthyroidism.

Myxedema occurs in adulthood as an impaired ability of the thyroid gland to produce T_4 hormones. The condition is characterized by water retention (Fig. 9-17). A blood test reveals a decreased T_4 and thyrotropin level. It is treated with administration of synthetic T_4 (levothyroxine sodium or Synthroid).

There are four types of **thyroid cancer** (CA), malignant neoplasm of the thyroid gland: papillary, follicular, medullary, and undifferentiated. Most are medically treatable. A lump in the neck is usually the only sign, although an inflamed lymph node may also be prevalent. Radiographic evidence and needle-aspiration biopsy (tissue excision through a needle for evaluative purposes) are used for diagnosing. Treatments include lobectomy (removal of a thyroid lobe), thyroidectomy (excision of thyroid gland), and radioiodine ablation (destruction of unwanted tissue).

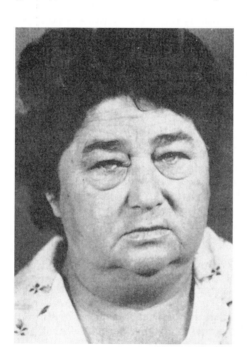

FIGURE 9-17
Myxedema occurs in adulthood as the result of an impaired ability of the thyroid gland to produce T_4 hormones. (Reprinted with permission from Porth CM. Pathophysiology concepts in altered health states, 6th ed. Philadelphia: Lippincott Williams & Wilkins, 2002.)

Key Terms	Definitions
hypothyroidism (high poh THIGH roid izm)	condition of decreased thyroid hormone production
infantile hypothyroidism (high poh THIGH roid izm)	congential form of hypothyroidism
goiter (GOY tur)	enlargement of the thyroid gland
thyroidectomy (thigh roy DECK tuh mee)	partial or complete surgical removal of the thyroid gland
Hashimoto (hah shee MOH toh) **disease**	autoimmune disease causing an inflamed thyroid gland
radioactive iodine uptake test	test to determine the rate of radioiodine absorption in the thyroid
radioiodine (ray dee oh EYE uh dine)	radioactive isotope of iodine
hyperthyroidism (high pur THIGH roid izm)	condition of excessive thyroid hormone production
thyrotoxicosis (thigh roh tock si KOH sis)	condition of excessive thyroid hormone
Graves disease	condition caused by excessive thyroid hormone production; a form of hyperthyroidism
exophthalmos (eck sof THAL mus)	abnormal protrusion of the eyes from their sockets
thyroid (THIGH roid) **storm**	exacerbation of the symptoms of hyperthyroidism; thyrotoxic crisis
thyrotoxic (THIGH roh TOCK sick) **crisis**	exacerbation of the symptoms of hyperthyroidism; thyroid storm
myxedema (mick se DEE muh)	condition caused by decreased thyroid hormone production; a form of hypothyroidism
thyroid (THIGH roid) **cancer**	malignant neoplasm of the thyroid gland

Key Term Practice: Thyroid Disorders

1. The form of hyperthyroidism characterized by exophthalmos is known as _____.

2. Surgical removal of the thyroid gland is termed _____, which is derived from the word part _____, meaning "thyroid," and the word part -*ectomy*, meaning _____.

3. The condition of decreased thyroid hormone production is termed _____.

CLINICAL TERMS

Clinical Dimension	Term	Description
DISORDERS		
	acromegaly	disorder caused by excessive hGH secretion in adulthood
	Addison disease	primary adrenocortical insufficiency
	Cushing syndrome	clinical disorder of the adrenal gland characterized by excessive ACTH production

Clinical Dimension	Term	Description
	diabetes insipidus	chronic pituitary disorder causing ADH insufficiency
	diabetes mellitus (DM)	chronic disorder of carbohydrate metabolism
	gestational diabetes mellitus (GDM)	disorder of glucose metabolism that occurs during pregnancy; type 3 diabetes mellitus
	gigantism	disorder caused by excessive hGH secretion before puberty; giantism
	goiter	enlargement of the thyroid gland
	Graves disease	disorder caused by excessive thyroid hormone production; a form of hyperthyroidism
	Hashimoto disease	autoimmune disease causing an inflamed thyroid gland
	hyperparathyroidism	increased activity of the parathyroid glands causing excessive PTH production
	hyperthyroidism	condition of excessive thyroid hormone production
	hypoparathyroidism	inadequate secretion of parathyroid hormones
	hypothyroidism	condition of decreased thyroid hormone production
	infantile hypothyroidism	congential form of hypothyroidism
	insulin-dependent diabetes mellitus (IDDM)	disorder of glucose metabolism occurring before adulthood; type 1 diabetes mellitus
	myxedema	condition caused by decreased thyroid hormone production; a form of hypothyroidism
	non-insulin-dependent diabetes mellitus (NIDDM)	disorder of glucose metabolism occurring before adulthood; type 2 diabetes mellitus
	pheochromocytoma	adrenal medulla tumor
	pituitary dwarfism	abnormal underdevelopment caused by inadequate hGH levels; hypopituitarism
	precocious puberty	reaching physical maturity at an unusually early age
	thyroid cancer	malignant neoplasm of the thyroid gland
	thyrotoxicosis	condition caused by excessive thyroid hormone production; a form of hyperthyroidism

SIGNS AND SYMPTOMS

	exophthalmos	abnormal protrusion of the eyes from their sockets
	glycosuria	the presence of glucose in the urine, usually indicates diabetes
	gynecomastia	enlarged breasts in males caused by a hormonal imbalance
	hirsutism	abnormal hair growth on a female's face or body
	hyperglycemia	abnormally high blood glucose level
	hypoglycemia	abnormally low blood glucose level

Clinical Dimension	Term	Description
	polydipsia	excessive thirst
	polyphagia	abnormal appetite or excessive hunger
	polyuria	excessive urination
	thyroid storm	exacerbation of the symptoms of hyperthyroidism; thyrotoxic crisis
	thyrotoxic crisis	exacerbation of the symptoms of hyperthyroidism; thyroid storm
	virilism	development of male secondary sex characteristics in a female
	Trousseau sign	carpal spasm elicited when the brachial region is compressed

CLINICAL TESTS AND DIAGNOSTIC PROCEDURES

	Term	Description
	blood tests	analyses of blood to evaluate its components
	computed tomography (CT) scans	computerized x-ray images of internal organs
	glucose tolerance test (GTT)	determination of serum glucose levels at different times after ingestion of a glucose syrup
	glycosylated hemoglobin	used to test circulating glucose blood levels over the life span of a red blood cell
	hydroxycorticosteroid urine test	analysis of urine to detect cortisol byproducts
	^{131}I uptake test	test to determine the rate of radioiodine absorption in the thyroid; radioactive iodide uptake test
	magnetic resonance imaging (MRI)	imaging of glands and organs
	plasma test	analysis of the fluid portion of blood
	17-ketosteroids (17-KS) test	analysis of urine to detect steroidal metabolites of androgenic and adrenocortical hormones
	radioactive iodine uptake (RIU) test	test to determine the rate of radioiodine absorption in the thyroid
	radioimmunoassay (RIA)	test to detect antigens, antibodies, enzymes, and hormones using radioactive reactants
	radioiodine	radioactive isotope of iodine
	radionuclide	radioactive isotope
	serum test	analysis of the plasma without fibrinogen
	thyroid function tests	blood and radionuclide tests to determine thyroid activity
	thyroid scan	image of thyroid produced after ingesting radioiodine
	triiodothyronine (T_3) uptake test	blood test to determine thyroid function
	ultrasound	imaging technique that uses sound waves to examine internal structures

Clinical Dimension	Term	Description
	urine ketosteroid tests	analyses of urine to detect androgen metabolites
	x-ray studies	radiographic films of structures used for evaluation
TREATMENTS		
	adrenalectomy	surgical removal of an adrenal gland
	hormone-replacement therapy (HRT)	hormone administration to restore normal function
	hypophysectomy	surgical removal of the hypophysis (pituitary gland)
	ionizing radiation therapy	use of radioactive isotopes to treat disease
	oral antidiabetic agents	drugs used to decrease blood glucose levels
	pancreatectomy	surgical removal of the pancreas
	parathyroidectomy	removal of the parathyroid gland
	radiation therapy	use of radiation to shrink or destroy a structure
	thyroidectomy	partial or complete surgical removal of the thyroid gland

Lifespan

Endocrine structures develop from all three primary germ layers. Tissue derived from the mesoderm produces steroid hormones; nonsteroid hormone–producing glands are created from endodermal and ectodermal layers.

Endocrine function remains relatively stable throughout life in the absence of overlying disease. Exceptions to this involve the thymus and reproductive glands. The thymus begins to atrophy after puberty, a time when it reaches its greatest mass of about 50 grams; it may be no larger than a walnut during the elderly years. This decrease may be linked to diminished immune response in later years. The decline in female ovary function in the late 40s results in menopause, and testicular testosterone production in males does not decrease until very old age.

Some hormone production declines with age, yet endocrine performance remains intact throughout life. Growth hormone secretion diminishes with age, causing muscle atrophy. Thyroid hormone output decreases, leading to a decline in metabolic rate and fat mobilization.

Epinephrine and norepinephrine levels remain unchanged throughout the aging process. Cortisol and aldosterone levels decrease as the adrenal glands become more fibrous after age 50 years.

Although the pancreas is capable of functioning until death, it becomes slower at insulin release. Furthermore, there is reduced glucose sensitivity, resulting in slower glucose regulation with advancing years.

In the News: DHEA

DHEA may be the snake oil medicine of the early 21st century. You have probably heard of it while watching baseball's home run record breakers or Sunday afternoon football. DHEA is the acronym for dehydroepiandrosterone (dee HEYE droh ep ee an DROS tur ohn), a hormone sold in health food stores to athletes as an alternative to anabolic steroids. The claimed benefits consist of improving energy, boosting strength, and serving as an aging remedy. Since 1994, it has been sold as a dietary supplement; however, it is not a necessary food in the human diet. It is quite popular in the sports culture where athletes tout DHEA's ability to enhance their performance.

Unfortunately, these claims have not been borne out in the scientific research. In fact, what is known about the hormone is quite disturbing. Short-term effects of DHEA use include acne, oily skin, hirsutism, gynecomastia, hepatomegaly, heart arrhythmias, and aggressive behavior. About 20 milligrams of DHEA is secreted naturally by the adrenal cortex in both males and females; DHEA is also secreted in the male testes. The compound is weakly androgenic; but once metabolized, it converts to another hormone—delta-5 androstenediol—that has both androgenic and estrogenic (causing development of female characteristics) effects. This second hormone is the precursor molecule (chemical that leads to) of testosterone.

Efficacy and safety studies are lacking. Because the U.S. Food and Drug Administration (FDA) does not regulate the supplement, labeling can be deceiving. Independent laboratory analyses have shown that the strength of DHEA supplements can range from 0% to 150% of the amount indicated on the bottle. To date, the therapeutic effects have not been realized, and alleged benefits have not been demonstrated in controlled studies. The International Olympic Committee and the National Collegiate Athletic Association (NCAA) have banned its use. The drug can be detected by the 17-ketosteroids urine test.

Research on DHEA is continuing but is still in its infancy. Preliminary results show that it may be beneficial for the treatment of systemic lupus erythematosus and adrenal insufficiency in women because of its androgenic–estrogenic actions. Until more is known, individuals not directly under the care of a physician who can monitor critical physiologic and clinical outcomes should not use DHEA.

COMMON ABBREVIATIONS

Abbreviation	Term
ACTH	adrenocorticotropic hormone; corticotropin
ADH	antidiuretic hormone; vasopressin
A_{Ic}	glycosylated hemoglobin
CA	cancer
CT	calcitonin
CT scan	computed tomography scan
DHEA	dehydroepiandrosterone
DM	diabetes mellitus
E	epinephrine
FDA	Food and Drug Administration
FSH	follicle-stimulating hormone; follitropin
GDM	gestational diabetes mellitus
GTT	glucose tolerance test
hGH	human growth hormone; somatotropin
hPL	human placental lactogen
HRT	hormone-replacement therapy
^{123}I, ^{131}I	radioisotopes of iodine
ICSH	interstitial cell-stimulating hormone
IDDM	insulin-dependent diabetes mellitus

Abbreviation	Term
K^+	potassium ion
17-KS	17-ketosteroids test
LH	luteinizing hormone; lutropin
LPN	licensed practical nurse
μCi	microcurie
MRI	magnetic resonance imaging
MSH	melanocyte-stimulating hormone
NA^+	sodium ion
NCAA	National Collegiate Athletic Association
NE	norepinephrine
NIDDM	non-insulin-dependent diabetes mellitus
OT	oxytocin
OXT	oxytocin
PRL	prolactin; mammotropin
PTH	parathyroid hormone; parathormone
RIU test	radioactive iodine uptake
RIA	radioimmunoassay
RN	registered nurse
T_3	triiodothyronine
T_4	tetraiodothyronine; thyroxine
TSH	thyroid-stimulating hormone; thyrotropin

Case Study

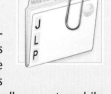

Mr. Cleveland presented in nurse Justina's endocrinology office complaining of weight loss and general malaise. Mr. Cleveland is 50 years old with no medical history of thyroid disease. His vital signs were within normal limits. Over the last 6 months, he had lost 35 pounds without dieting. A routine thyroid palpation—in which the patient swallows water while the clinician applies pressure to the anterior cervical region—indicated a thyroid abnormality. A thyroid ^{131}I uptake and thyroid scan provided the following results:

- Enlarged bilateral lobes. The right thyroid lobe measured $5.6 \times 1.8 \times 3.0$ cm. The left thyroid lobe measured $4.6 \times 2.0 \times 2.0$ cm.
- Abnormal uptake of 78% at 25 h.

Case Study Questions

Select the best answer to each of the following questions.

1. The physician palpated which region of Mr. Cleveland's body?
 a. shoulder
 b. throat
 c. chest
 d. groin

2. A thyroid scan is best described as a _____.
 a. procedure in which x-ray images of the thyroid are produced after the patient ingests a radioactive ion
 b. test in which the patient fasts for 12 h and then ingests a glucose mixture

c. method used for detecting antigens, antibodies, enzymes, and hormones using radiolabeled reactants

d. test that can determine circulating levels of ACTH, CT, LH, and cortisol

3. The ^{131}I test is best described as _____.

a. a urine test to determine cortisol and androgen excretions

b. a measure of serum glucose levels at intervals up to 3 h

c. the test used to determine hyperactivity or hypoactivity of the thyroid gland after the patient ingests radioactive iodine

d. a blood test used to detect iodine

4. Mr. Cleveland's thyroid uptake was measured at 78%. The normal value for thyroid uptake at 24 h is between 9% and 36%. Mr. Cleveland's value suggests _____.

a. hyperthyroidism

b. hypothyroidism

c. hyperparathyroidism

d. hypoparathyroidism

REAL WORLD REPORT

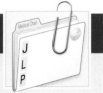

SOUTHWEST IMAGING DEPARTMENT

NAME: Elmer Cleveland

DOB: 02/18/53

DATEORD: 06/06/03

TEST: Localize tumor; whole body

ATTENDING: K. L. Lindau, MD

AGE: 50 years

EXAM DATE: 06/13/03

CLINIC: Nuclear Medical Department

ORDPHYS: K. L. Lindau, MD

CLINICAL DATA
Hyperthyroidism, thyroid carcinoma

---

^{131}I WHOLE-BODY SCAN
A whole-body thyroid scan was obtained 7 days after the patient had been given 105 µCi of iodine-131 orally. This study was compared with previous RIU and scan examination of November 7, 2002.

There is abnormal increased uptake in the region of the thyroid, consistent with the clinical history of thyroid carcinoma. Physiologic uptake is noted in the regions of the pharynx and liver. No abnormal areas of increased uptake seen in the remaining study to suggest metastasis.

IMPRESSION
- Abnormal increased uptake in the region of the thyroid consistent with the clinical history of thyroid carcinoma
- No metastasis seen

Dictated by: J. R. Waterville, MD

REAL WORLD REPORT QUESTIONS

The following exercises review the medical terms in the preceding medical report.

1. Mr. Cleveland was given 105 μCi of iodine-131 orally.

   a. What does 105 μCi mean?

   _____

   b. What is iodine-131 and why is it used?

   _____

   _____

   _____

2. Define the abbreviation RIA. What is an RIA scan?

   _____

   _____

   _____

3. Define hyperthyroidism. _____

4. Identify the targeted organ for the ^{131}I uptake test in this report. _____

REVIEW AND APPLICATION: THREE-LEVEL LEARNING SYSTEM

LEVEL ONE: REVIEWING FACTS AND TERMS USING RECALL

Select the best response to each of the following questions.

1. In the endocrine system, which gland is referred to as the master gland?

   a. hypothalamus

   b. thymus

   c. thyroid

   d. pituitary

2. A _____ cell is one with a specific receptor for a particular hormone.

   a. target

   b. hormone

   c. substrate

   d. precursor

3. Type 3 diabetes mellitus, also known as _____, has an onset during _____.

   a. adult diabetes; puberty

   b. gestational diabetes; pregnancy

   c. gestational diabetes; childbirth

   d. insulin dependent diabetes mellitus; childhood

4. A disorder resulting from excessive human growth hormone secretion before puberty is known as_____.

   a. acromegaly

   b. gigantism

   c. dwarfism

   d. virilism

5. The endocrine system responds faster than the nervous system.

   a. True

   b. False

6. Which hormone is *not* secreted by the adenohypophysis?

   a. ACTH

   b. MSH

   c. ADH

   d. LH

7. The hypophysis is divided into _____ and _____ portions.

   a. primary; secondary

   b. proximal; distal

   c. anterior; posterior

   d. dorsal ; ventral

8. Which area of the hypophysis is merely a storage and releasing site?

   a. neurohypophysis

   b. pars intermedia

   c. epiphysis cerebri

   d. adenohypophysis

9. The anterior pituitary is directed by hormones from the _____.

   a. hypothalamus

   b. neurohypophysis

   c. pineal gland

   d. thyroid gland

10. What is the alternative name for the neurohypophysis.

    a. anterior pituitary

    b. adrenal gland

    c. parathyroids

    d. posterior pituitary

11. Human biorhythms of 24-hour cycles are termed _____ cycles in the medical field.

    a. cyclical

    b. melatonin

    c. circadian

    d. pineal

12. The parathyroid glands are located on the _____

    a. anterior surface of the thyroid gland

    b. posterior surface of the thymus gland

    c. anterior surface of the pituitary gland

    d. posterior surface of the thyroid gland

13. Tetraiodothyronine is also called _____.

    a. T$_3$

    b. T$_4$

    c. thyroxine

    d. b and c

14. The pancreas is situated adjacent to the _____ and _____.

    a. anterior pituitary; posterior pituitary

    b. stomach; small intestine

    c. thyroid; parathyroid

    d. thymus; pineal gland

15. The _____ and _____ are the two portions of the adrenal gland.

    a. outer; cortex

    b. inner; medulla

    c. medulla; cortex

    d. anterior; posterior

16. Polydipsia, polyuria, and polyphagia mean _____, respectively.

    a. excessive thirst, excessive urination, and excessive hunger

    b. excessive urination, excessive thirst, and excessive hunger

    c. excessive hunger, excessive thirst, and excessive urination

    d. excessive appetite, excessive hunger, and excessive thirst

17. The glucose tolerance test is useful for diagnosing _____.

    a. thyroid disorders

    b. pancreatic disorders

    c. parathyroid disorders

    d. pituitary disorders

LEVEL TWO: REVIEWING CONCEPTS

Select the best response to each of the following questions.

18. After eating supper, which hormone is likely to be secreted in greater amounts than while fasting.

    a. insulin

    b. glucagon

    c. ACTH

    d. epinephrine

19. Upon rising in the morning, your body operates this hormone to prevent a hypoglycemic condition.

    a. insulin

    b. glucagon

    c. glucose

    d. glycogen

Provide a medical term to complete a meaningful analogy.

20. The exocrine system is to glands with ducts as the _____ system is to ductless glands.

21. The adenohypophysis is to FSH as the _____ is to OXT.

22. Calcitonin is to PTH as _____ is to glucagon.

23. Adrenocorticotropic hormone is to corticotropin as follicle stimulating hormone is to _____.

What is the alternative term for each of the following?

24. prolactin _____

25. lutropin _____

26. human growth hormone (hGH) _____

27. thyroid stimulating hormone _____

Define the following abbreviations.

28. E _____

29. TSH _____

30. T$_3$ _____

31. OXT _____

32. PRL _____

Match the hormone with its primary target.

_____ 33. hGH   a. kidneys

_____ 34. TSH   b. bones

_____ 35. ADH   c. liver

_____ 36. glucagon   d. thyroid

_____ 37. LH   e. ovaries

Match the hormone with its primary action.

_____ 38. ACTH   a. supplement sex hormones

_____ 39. androgens   b. white blood cell maturation and development

_____ 40. thymosins   c. hypertrophy of body cells

_____ 41. OT   d. uterine contractions

_____ 42. hGH   e. stimulates cortex of adrenal gland to produce corticosteroids

Define the following terms.

43. hyperthyroidism _____

44. hypothyroidism _____

45. hypophysectomy _____

46. hypoglycemia _____

Using the following words and word parts, form a medical term for each definition. Each word or word part is used only once. Build medical terms for each definition using the following word parts.

acro-	-ectomy	epi-
hyper-	-ism	-ine
megal-	nephr-	parathyroid
-sis	thyro-	thyroid
toxico-	-y	

47. removal of thyroid gland _____

48. disorder characterized by oversecretion of growth hormone in adult _____

49. disorder characterized by excessive activity of parathyroids _____

50. toxic disorder of thyroid caused by hyperactivity of gland _____

51. hormone of adrenal medulla _____

Unscramble the letters to form a medical term.

52. rctismien _____

53. xymeedam _____

54. spancrae _____

55. absteeid _____

Match the disorder with its key characteristics.

_____ 56. diabetes mellitus   a. tumor of the adrenal medulla

_____ 57. diabetes insipidus   b. "buffalo hump"; pituitary or adrenal cortex tumor; adipose deposition

_____ 58. Addison disease   c. disorder of carbohydrate metabolism

_____ 59. Cushing syndrome   d. disorder of neurohypophysis

_____ 60. pheochromocytoma   e. primary adrenocortical insufficiency

Identify the correctly spelled term in each set.

61. _____

    a. addrenal medulla   b. adrenal medulla
    c. adrenal medula   d. addrenal meddula

62. _____

    a. adrennocorticotropic

    b. adrenocorticotroppic

    c. adrenocorticotropick

    d. adrenocorticotropic

63. _____

    a. mineralocorticoid

    b. minneralcorticoid

    c. mineralocorrticoid

    d. minerallocorticoid

64. _____

    a. pinneal   b. pineul
    c. pineal   d. peneal

65. _____

    a. gloocagon   b. glucagun
    c. glycagon   d. glucagon

LEVEL THREE: THINKING CRITICALLY

Provide the best answer to each of the following questions.

66. Wendy is highly allergic to bee stings, so when she got stung at a family picnic, her reaction was immediate: She gave herself an injection with an EpiPen. Upon arrival at the emergency room, she presented with increased heart rate, increased blood pressure, airway dilation, and a rise in blood glucose as a result of her EpiPen injection. Given this information, what hormone was probably in her pen? _____

67. Tom went to his physician complaining of polyuria and polydipsia. He said he was constantly thirsty and could not seem to drink enough water. His urine is very pale, and he excretes large volumes. The physician prescribed a short course of vasopressin therapy. What disorder did the physician suspect? _____

 KEY TERMS SPELLING TEST FROM CD-ROM

Use the CD-ROM to test yourself on the spelling of key terms from this chapter. Listen to the terms and write them on a separate sheet of paper. Use a medical dictionary to check your answers.

ANSWERS

WORD GROUPING

Definition	Word Part
glucose	gluc-, gluco-
adrenal	adren-, adreno-
alongside	para-
calcium	calc-, calci-, calco-
childbirth	toco-
cortex, cortical	cortic-, cortico-
deficient, below normal	hypo-
eating, eat	-phage, -phagia, -phagy
extreme, intense	acr-, acro-
gland, glandular	aden-, adeno-
having an affinity for, attracted to	-tropic
honey, sugar	mel-, meli-, melo-
milk	lact-, lacti-, lacto-
mucus, mucous	myx-, myxo-
pancreas, pancreatic	pancre-, pancreo-
secretion, secreting	-crine
sweet, sugar, glucose	glyc-, glyco-
thyroid	thyr-, thyreo-, thyro-
within, inner	end-, endo-

WORD BUILDING

Word Part	Meaning	Common or Known Word	Example Medical Term
aden-, adeno-	gland, glandular	adenoid	adenohypophysis
adren-, adreno-	adrenal	adrenaline	adrenal gland
end-, endo-	within, inner	endoderm	endocrine
gluc-, gluco-	glucose	glucose	glucose
hypo-	deficient, below normal	hypoglycemic	hypoparathyroidism
lact-, lacti-, lacto-	milk	lactose	prolactin
mel-, meli-, melo-	honey, sugar	mellifluous	diabetes mellitus
pancre-, pancreo-	pancreas, pancreatic	pancreas	pancreas
para-	alongside	parasail	parathyroid glands
thyr-, thyreo-, thyro-	thyroid	thyroid	thyroid gland

KEY TERM PRACTICE

Endocrine System Preview
1. endocrine
2. hormones
3. secretion

Pituitary Gland (Hypophysis)
1. a. hypophysis; b. adenohypophysis; c. neurohypophysis
2. adrenocorticotropic hormone (ACTH)
3. Mammotropin

Thyroid and Parathyroid Glands
1. calcitonin (CT); parathyroid hormone or parathormone (PTH)
2. Parathyroid hormone

Pancreas
1. glucagon
2. insulin

Adrenal Glands
1. a. adrenaline; b. noradrenaline
2. adrenal cortex; adrenal medulla

Pineal and Thymus Glands
1. thymosins
2. epiphysis cerebri

Adrenal Gland Disorders
1. Addison
2. pheochromocytoma

Pancreas Disorders
1. a. insulin-dependent diabetes mellitus (IDDM); b. non-insulin-dependent mellitus (NIDDM) or maturity-onset diabetes mellitus; c. gestational diabetes mellitus (GDM)
2. hypoglycemia

Parathyroid Disorders
1. hypoparathyroidism
2. hyperparathyroidism

Pituitary Disorders
1. gigantism
2. acromegaly

Thyroid Disorders
1. Graves disease
2. thyroidectomy; thyro-; removal of an anatomic structure
3. hypothyroidism

CASE STUDY

1. b is the correct answer.
   - a is incorrect because the shoulder is the acromial region.
   - c is incorrect because the chest is the pectoral region.
   - d is incorrect because the groin is the inguinal region.
2. a is the correct answer.
   - b is incorrect because it describes a glucose tolerance test.
   - c is incorrect because it describes a radioimmunoassay.
   - d is incorrect because these levels are determined by a plasma test.

3. c is the correct answer.
   - a is incorrect because urine tests do not require the ingestion of radioactive iodine.
   - b is incorrect because this test describes a glucose tolerance test.
   - d is incorrect because it is not a blood test used to detect iodine.
4. a is the correct answer.
   - b is incorrect because the gland is undergoing hypertrophy and increased thyroid activity, not atrophy and decreased thyroid activity.
   - c and d are incorrect as the thyroid gland was evaluated using this test, not the parathyroid gland, which would require a different testing procedure.

REAL WORLD REPORT

1. a. 105 microcuries.
   b. Also written ^{131}I, it is a radioactive isotope of iodine that is used as a trace in thyroid studies.
2. radioactive iodine uptake; a test that measures the amount of ^{131}I taken up by the thyroid gland

3. a condition in which excessive thyroid hormones are produced.
4. thyroid gland

REVIEW AND APPLICATION: THREE-LEVEL LEARNING SYSTEM

Level One: Reviewing Facts and Terms Using Recall

1. d
2. a
3. b
4. b
5. b
6. c
7. c
8. a
9. a
10. d
11. c
12. d
13. d
14. b
15. c
16. a
17. b

Level Two: Reviewing Concepts

18. a
19. b
20. endocrine
21. neurohypophysis or posterior pituitary
22. insulin
23. follitropin
24. mammotropin
25. luteinizing hormone (LH)
26. somatotropin
27. thyrotropin
28. epinephrine
29. thyroid-stimulating hormone
30. triiodothyronine
31. oxytocin
32. prolactin
33. b
34. d
35. a
36. c

37. e
38. e
39. a
40. b
41. d
42. c
43. disorder caused by excessive secretion of thyroid hormone
44. disorder caused by inadequate secretion of thyroid hormone
45. surgical excision of the hypophysis (pituitary gland)
46. low blood glucose levels
47. thyroidectomy
48. acromegaly
49. hyperparathyroidism
50. thyrotoxicosis
51. epinephrine
52. cretinism
53. myxedema
54. pancreas
55. diabetes
56. c
57. d
58. e
59. b
60. a
61. b
62. d
63. a
64. c
65. d

Level Three: Thinking Critically

66. Hormones of the adrenal medulla—epinephrine and/or norepinephrine—were probably in the injection.
67. The physician suspected diabetes insipidus.

chapter

10

Blood

OBJECTIVES

After completing this chapter, you should be able to:

1. State the meanings of word parts related to blood.
2. Explain the importance of blood to normal physiological functioning.
3. List the various types of blood cells.
4. Identify blood components.
5. Describe the significance of lipoproteins and the role of clotting proteins and enzymes.
6. Summarize the basis for ABO blood groups and Rh factors.
7. Distinguish different signs, symptoms, and treatments of various blood diseases.
8. Explain clinical tests and diagnostic procedures related to blood.
9. Describe anatomical and physiological alterations throughout the lifespan.
10. Define abbreviations related to the blood system.
11. Define terms used in medical reports involving blood.
12. Correctly define, spell, and pronounce the chapter's medical terms.

Professional Profile: Phlebotomist

John is a phlebotomist working in a hospital clinic, which means he collects blood samples from adult and pediatric patients. In addition to performing venipuncture (drawing blood from a vein) and dermal puncture (drawing blood through the skin), the phlebotomist receives and organizes requests for blood collection, prepares the blood for distribution to the laboratory, cleans laboratory glassware and equipment, and records blood collection statistics.

A high school diploma or equivalency is necessary for employment in many settings. In addition, phlebotomy-training programs generally require 40 hours of instruction and 20 hours of hands-on phlebotomy practice. Basic phlebotomy includes knowledge in the areas of infection control, universal precautions and safety, anatomy and physiology of body systems with special emphasis on the blood and circulatory system, appropriate medical terminology, patient and specimen identification, selection of blood collection equipment, skin preparation, and disposal of instruments and materials used in blood collection. Advanced training in infectious disease control and biologic hazards; anticoagulation theory; and specimen collection, transport, processing, and storage is helpful.

After undergoing classroom instruction, phlebotomists may work a short time in the laboratory before taking a licensing examination. The examination consists of both written and practical portions. Some states do not require such licensure. John had to demonstrate successful completion of a phlebotomy-training program from an accredited institution plus have completed at least 100 successful venipunctures and 20 successful dermal punctures.

Attendance at seminars, update sessions, and continuing education workshops is important to honing skills. These programs cover topics such as legal, moral, and ethical issues related to blood collection. Hospitals usually have training on health issues, emphasizing the significance of bloodborne pathogens and the role phlebotomists play in ensuring blood safety.

INTRODUCTION

Blood is vital to life. Homeostasis (internal balance) of the human body depends on the blood because blood serves as the medium by which nutrients and hormones are transported, gas exchange occurs, body temperature is regulated at a constant 37°C (98.6°F), pH levels (7.35–7.45) are maintained, and immunity is provided.

> **FACT** There are about 10 pints of blood in the adult human body!

Blood is pumped through blood vessels for distribution to the body by the cardiovascular system and serves an immune function through interaction with the lymphatic system. Because blood services all body tissues, its disorders often have systemic effects. Blood disorders can be categorized as congenital, infectious, coagulation (clotting), nutritional, and secondary to other diseases. Tumors, toxins (poisons), and trauma can also adversely affect blood delivery.

As a result of its systemic effects, blood can be tested to identify and assess a variety of conditions. This chapter focuses on the significance of blood to human physiology and identifies signs and symptoms, clinical tests and diagnostic procedures, and treatments related to various blood-related problems.

MEDICAL TERM PARTS

WORD PARTS

Medical term prefixes, suffixes, and combining forms related to blood are introduced in this section.

Word Parts	Meaning
alb-, albo-	white, whitish
baso-	basic
bili-	bile, derived from bile
chromat-, chromato-	color
cyan-, cyano-	blue
-cyte	cell
deoxy-	loss of oxygen from a compound
-emia	condition of blood
erythr-, erythro-	red, erythrocyte
fibr-, fibro-	fiber, fibrous
fibrin-, fibrino-	fibrin, fibrinous
granulo-	granular, granules
hem-, hemo-	blood
hemat-, hemato-	blood, pertaining to blood
leuk-, leuko-	white
lymph-, lympho-	lymph, tissue fluid in lymphatic vessel
-lytic	causing destruction
myel-, myelo-	bone marrow
neutr-, neutro-	neutral
nucle-, nucleo-	nucleus
oxy-	presence of oxygen
phag-, phago-	eating, devouring
-phage, -phagia, -phagy	eater
phen-, pheno-	denoting appearance
phleb-, phlebo-	vein, venous
-philia	having an affinity for, craving for
-philic	having an affinity for, craving for
-phoresis	transmission
plasma-	plasma, noncellular blood portion
pluri-	several

Word Parts	Meaning
-poiesis	formation, production
-rrhagia	excessive discharge, hemorrhage
septic-, septico-	sepsis, septic, pathogens or toxins in blood
ser-, seri-, sero-	serum, serous
sidero-	iron
-taxis	movement toward or away from a stimulus
thromb-, thrombo-	blood clot, coagulation, thrombin
verd-, verdo-	green

WORD ETYMOLOGY

Some words have Greek or Latin word roots but are not true word parts. This section lists those that are used as medical terms.

Word	Definition
cytosis	abnormally high number of cells
globin	protein of hemoglobin
immunis	free from service
lympha	clear spring water
philos	fond, loving
purpura	purple
thrombosis	a clotting

MEDICAL TERM PARTS USED AS PREFIXES

Prefix	Definition
baso-	basic
bili-	bile, derived from bile
deoxy-	loss of oxygen from a compound
granulo-	granular, granules
oxy-	presence of oxygen
pluri-	several
sidero-	iron

MEDICAL TERM PARTS USED AS SUFFIXES

Suffix	Definition
-cyte	cell
-emia	condition of blood

Suffix	Definition
-lytic	causing destruction
-penia	deficiency
-phage, -phagia, -phagy	eater
-philia	abnormal tendency toward, affinity for
-philic	having an affinity for, craving for
-phoresis	transmission
-poiesis	formation, production
-rrhagia	excessive discharge, hemorrhage
-taxis	movement toward or away from a stimulus

WORD GROUPING

Using the "Medical Term Parts" tables, identify the prefix, suffix, or combining form for each of the following definitions. The first one has been done as an example.

Definition	Word Part
basic	baso-
bile, derived from bile	
blood	
blood, pertaining to blood	
blood clot, coagulation, thrombin	
blue	
bone marrow	
causing destruction	
cell	
color	
condition of blood	
denoting appearance	
eater	
eating, devouring	
excessive discharge, hemorrhage	
fiber, fibrous	
fibrin, fibrinous	
formation, production	
granular, granules	
green	

Definition	Word Part
having an affinity for, craving for	A.
	B.
iron	
loss of oxygen from a compound	
lymph, tissue fluid in lymphatic vessel	
movement toward or away from a stimulus	
neutral	
nucleus	
plasma, noncellular blood portion	
presence of oxygen	
red, erythrocyte	
sepsis, septic, pathogens or toxins in blood	
serum, serous	
several	
transmission	
vein, venous	
white	
white, whitish	

WORD BUILDING

Word parts, introduced in the "Medical Term Parts" section, are listed in the following table. For this exercise, first supply the meaning of each word part, then use the word part to build a word you already know. The word you list under "Common or Known Word" does not have to be a medical term; a commonly used word is fine. Be sure, however, that the word correctly reflects the intended meaning. The first one has been done as an example.

Word Part	Meaning	Common or Known Word	Example Medical Term
leuk-, leuko-	white	leukemia	leukocyte
alb-, albo-			albumin
cyan-, cyano-			cyanosis
-emia			anemia
fibr-, fibro-			fibrosis
hem-, hemo-			hemostasis
hemat-, hemato-			hematopoiesis
neutr-, neutro-			neutrophil
oxy-			oxygen
phleb-, phlebo-			phlebotomy

Word Part	Meaning	Common or Known Word	Example Medical Term
-philia			hemophilia
pluri-			pluripotent
septic-, septico-			septicemia
ser-, seri-, sero-			serum
thromb-, thrombo-			thrombocyte
verd-, verdo-			biliverdin

ANATOMY AND PHYSIOLOGY

Components of Blood

- Erythrocytes
- Leukocytes
- Lipoproteins
- Thrombocytes
- Plasma

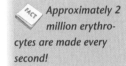

FACT   *Approximately 2 million erythrocytes are made every second!*

Blood Preview

Whole blood is a viscous (thick and sticky) liquid that consists of two major portions: formed elements and plasma. Formed elements are the solid, cellular fractions of blood known as the **packed cell volume** (PCV). The other constituent, **plasma**, is the primary fluid part of whole blood (Fig. 10-1).

Formed elements are composed of three types of blood cells: **erythrocytes** (red blood cells or red corpuscles), **leukocytes** (white blood cells), and **thrombocytes** (platelets). Leukocytes and thrombocytes make up 1% of blood. Plasma lipoproteins are complexes that contain both lipid (fat) and protein (chains of amino acids). Concentrations of specific lipoproteins are correlated with atherosclerosis (hardening of the arteries).

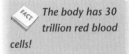

FACT   *The body has 30 trillion red blood cells!*

Each cell type has specific functions and is made by a process termed **hemopoiesis** (**hematopoiesis**), the formation and maturation of blood cells and their derivatives. All blood cells begin as a **pluripotent stem cell**, which differentiates into the various blood cell types. (These cells are commonly referred to as stem cells.) The adjectival term *pluripotent* means that a cell is "capable of producing several other types" of cells.

The percentage of red blood cells (RBCs) within a sample of whole blood is called the **hematocrit** (Hct). The hematocrit of normal blood is approximately 45%; the remaining 55% of whole blood is plasma. Hematocrit values, which are important for assessing human blood disorders, are determined through analysis of a blood sample.

Plasma, the pale yellow, proteinaceous, noncellular part of circulating blood, contains solutes (dissolved substances). Solutes include proteins (albumin, globulin, fibrinogen), enzymes, hormones, electrolytes, lipids, amino acids, glucose, vitamins, antibodies, and nonprotein nitrogenous (NPN) substances (e.g., urea and metabolic wastes). **Albumin** is a protein produced by the liver that provides blood with its

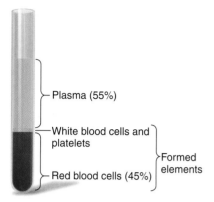

A Major components of whole blood

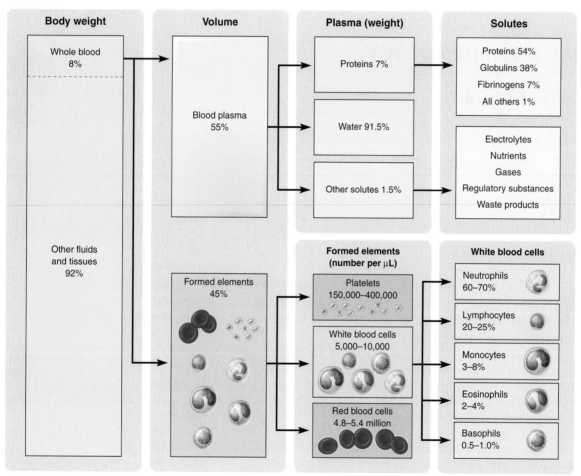

B Components of blood

FIGURE 10-1
The components of blood.

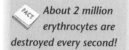
About 2 million erythrocytes are destroyed every second!

viscosity, which is a factor in maintaining blood pressure and blood volume. It makes up about 60% of plasma. **Viscosity** is blood "thickness" or consistency. Approximately 36% of the plasma proteins is **globulin**, a protein group to which the antibodies belong. **Fibrinogen** makes up 4% of plasma proteins and plays an essential role in blood clotting. **Serum** is plasma without the clotting protein fibrinogen. Serum is often considered the fluid portion of coagulated (clotted) blood.

Key Terms	Definitions
packed cell volume	cellular portion of the blood; formed elements
plasma (PLAZ muh)	fluid, noncellular portion of the blood
erythrocytes (e RITH roh sites)	mature red blood cells
leukocytes (LEW koh sites)	white blood cells
thrombocytes (THROM boh sites)	blood platelets
hemopoiesis (hee moh poy EE sis)	blood cell formation and maturation; hematopoiesis
hematopoiesis (hee mat oh poy EE sis)	blood cell formation and maturation; hemopoiesis
pluripotent (ploo RIP oh tent) **stem cell**	blood cell that forms all other blood cells; stem cell
hematocrit (hee MAT oh krit)	percentage of red blood cells in whole blood
albumin (al BEW min)	white-colored protein found in plasma
viscosity (vis KOS i tee)	thickness of a fluid
globulin (GLOB yoo lin)	simple protein found in the plasma
fibrinogen (figh BRIN oh jen)	soluble precursor protein of fibrin
serum (SEER um)	blood plasma minus fibrinogen

Key Term Practice: Blood Preview

1. Identify the two terms that refer to blood formation and maturation. _____

2. What is the medical term for each of the following?

    a. white blood cell _____

    b. red blood cell _____

    c. platelet _____

3. Plasma without clotting proteins is called _____.

Erythrocytes

Erythrocytes are tiny, biconcave, oxygen-carrying disks that are thinner near their centers and thicker around their rims. Erythrocytes do not possess nuclei or mitochondria (energy-producing organelles). Their characteristic red color is caused by the red respiratory protein **hemoglobin** (Hb). A hemoglobin molecule contains two parts: heme and globulin. The heme portion holds an iron atom, and it transports oxygen (O_2), releasing it to tissues. Erythrocyte formation, **erythropoiesis**, is influenced by the endocrine system. The kidneys release the hormone **erythropoietin** (EPO) to promote hemopoiesis. Its secretion is controlled by a negative-feedback mechanism.

Erythrocytes begin their life as a proerythroblast, which is formed from a pluripotent stem cell. They are then changed to an erythroblast and then to a reticulocyte before emerging as a mature red blood cell. A **reticulocyte** is an immature red blood cell that still possesses a nucleus. After the final stage of development, the reticulocyte loses its nucleus and becomes a fully developed red blood cell called an erythrocyte. The loss of the nucleus is important because the space that it previously occupied can be filled with oxygen-rich hemoglobin. Reticulocyte counts increase when there is a significant loss of blood or a decline in blood oxygen levels. This is a compensatory response by the body to enhance the oxygen-carrying capacity of blood.

Erythrocytes are designed to travel easily through blood vessel walls to transport respiratory gases and nutrients. The respiratory system is involved with replenishing the blood's oxygen supply. Within the lungs, carbon dioxide is exchanged for oxygen. Red blood corpuscles carry **oxyhemoglobin** (HbO_2), a compound formed when oxygen combines with hemoglobin. This form of hemoglobin is present in arterial blood.

Erythrocytes have a life span of approximately 120 days. Within this time, old or damaged cells are phagocytized (eaten) by liver and spleen macrophages. In the liver, hemoglobin is decomposed into its heme and globin components, with heme breaking down into iron and a greenish bile pigment, **biliverdin**. Most biliverdin gets converted into a reddish yellow (orange) pigment called **bilirubin**. The bile pigments are excreted in feces, and the iron is recycled for future hemopoiesis.

The red blood cell count is the number of erythrocytes in a cubic millimeter of blood. Typical values are as follows: males have 4,600,000–6,200,000 cells/mm^3, females have 4,200,000–5,400,000 cells/mm^3, and children have 4,500,000–5,100,000 cells/mm^3. A deficiency in the number of erythrocytes is termed **erythropenia**; an excessive amount is called **erythrocytosis**.

Key Terms	Definitions
hemoglobin (HEE muh gloh bin)	iron-containing portion of erythrocyte that reversibly combines with oxygen and transports it
erythropoiesis (e rith roh poy EE sis)	formation of erythrocytes
erythropoietin (e rith roh POY e tin)	hormone released from kidneys necessary for blood cell production
reticulocyte (re TICK yoo loh site)	immature erythrocyte
oxyhemoglobin (ock se HEE muh gloh bin)	oxygen combined with hemoglobin
biliverdin (bil i VER din)	green bile pigment formed from the breakdown of heme
bilirubin (bil i ROO bin)	reddish yellow pigment formed from hemoglobin
erythropenia (e rith roh PEE nee uh)	erythrocyte deficiency
erythrocytosis (e rith roh sigh TOH sis)	elevated erythrocyte count

 ## Key Term Practice: Erythrocytes

1. The formation of red blood cells is called _____.

2. When oxygen combines with hemoglobin, _____ is formed.

3. The reddish yellow bile pigment is termed _____.

Leukocytes

As a group, white blood cells (WBCs) are named leukocytes. The formation of leukocytes is termed **leukopoiesis**. Leukocytes are nucleated cells that lack hemoglobin and contain mitochondria. Five types of leukocytes exist and are classified as granular or agranular (Table 10-1). Granulocytes are leukocytes that contain cytoplasmic granules; agranulocytes are nongranular leukocytes lacking cytoplasmic fragments. Three types of granulocytes are neutrophils, eosinophils, and basophils. The two types of agranulocytes are monocytes and lymphocytes.

Leukocytes aid in the body's defense mechanisms through phagocytosis (the engulfing and ingesting of foreign materials). The granular leukocytes were named according to the dyes that are taken up by their cytoplasmic granules during a specific staining procedure. Neutrophils are stained by neutral dyes, eosinophils by the red acid dye eosin, and basophils by basic (rather than acidic) dyes. Remember that the word part -*phil* means "having an affinity for" something.

Neutrophils are the most numerous and mobile of the leukocyte classes. They contain lysosomes (enzyme-containing organelles) and antibiotic-like proteins called defensins, which increase in number during bacterial infections. Associate the *n* in *nu*merous with the *n* in *n*eutrophils to remember that these "blood hounds" seek out invaders with great force. The lifespan of a neutrophil is about 1 week.

Basophils are similar to eosinophils, have irregularly shaped cytoplasmic granules, and make up less than 1% of the white blood cell count. Basophils release three potent substances: heparin, histamine, and serotonin. During allergic reactions, basophils intensify the response and release **heparin**, an anticoagulant. An **anticoagulant** is a substance that prevents blood clotting. **Histamine**, an inflammation mediator, causes an increase in blood flow to injured tissue. **Serotonin** acts as a vasoconstrictor, causing blood vessels to tighten. The lifespan of a basophil is from a few hours to 3 days.

Eosinophils have a bilobed nucleus and make up 1–3% of the circulating leukocytes. Eosinophils increase during parasitic infections, combat the effect of histamine during allergic reactions, and phagocytize antigen–antibody complexes, which are substances formed during an immune response. They also secrete enzymes that break down blood clots. The lifespan of an eosinophil is 10–12 days.

The largest cells found in blood are the **monocytes.** Some monocytes differentiate into macrophages, which either remain fixed or wander. The wandering macrophages are phagocytic warriors arising from red bone marrow. The term **macrophage** literally means "big eater," and these cells play an important role in infection resistance and the immune response. They are characterized by nuclei that vary in shape and have a life span of several weeks to several months. Normal leukocyte values are 5,000–10,000 cells per/mm^3 of blood.

Lymphocytes have large, round nuclei and have a life span of up to several years. Lymphocytes are derived from lymphoid organs, such as the thymus, bone marrow, spleen, lymph nodes, tonsils, and Peyer patches in the small intestine. Lymphocytes provide specific immune responses by differentiating into T lymphocytes (T cells) or B lymphocytes (B cells). T cells engage in combating viral infections and cancers,

TABLE 10-1 Leukocytes

Type	Subtype
Granular	Neutrophils
	Eosinophils
	Basophils
Agranular	Lymphocytes
	Monocytes

whereas B cells differentiate into antibody-producing plasma cells. Antibodies battle infection and provide **immunity**, or protection against foreign invaders.

White blood cell counts are useful in clinical diagnosing. Determining the percentage of various types of leukocytes is called a **differential** (diff) **white blood cell count** (Fig. 10-2). It is called a differential test because it serves to discriminate (differentiate) the various types of white blood cells and then enumerate (count) them. This value is significant because neutrophils increase during bacterial infections and eosinophils increase during parasitic infections and allergic reactions.

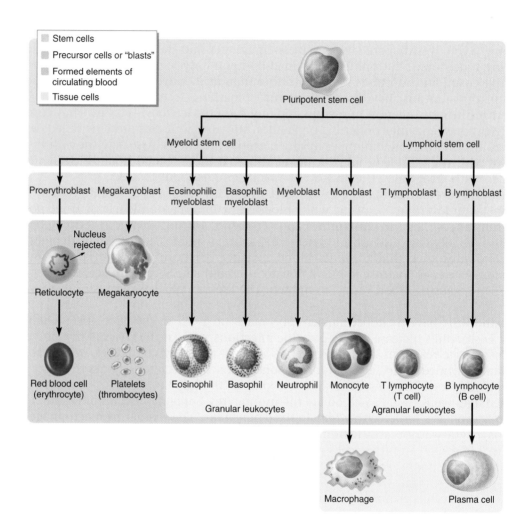

FIGURE 10-2
Blood cell differentiation. A differential white blood count can determine the percentage of various types of leukocytes.

Key Terms	Definitions
leukopoiesis (lew koh poy EE sis)	leukocyte formation
neutrophil (NEW truh fil)	most common type of leukocyte stainable with neutral dye
basophils (BAY soh fils)	type of leukocyte stained by basic dye
heparin (HEP uh rin)	an anticoagulant or antiplatelet factor
anticoagulant (an tee koh AG yoo lunt)	substance that prevents blood clotting
histamine (HIS tuh meen)	chemical that stimulates blood vessel dilation (expansion)

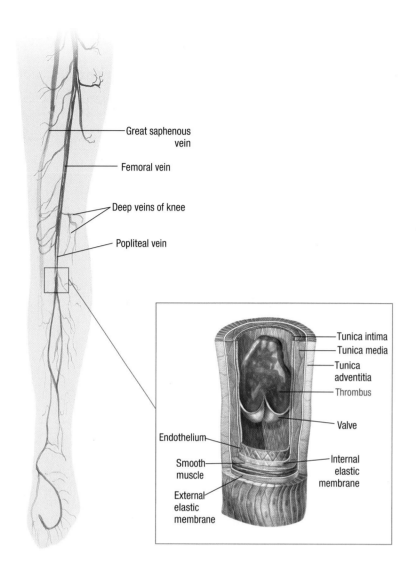

FIGURE 10-3
An embolism is a blood vessel occlusion caused by an embolus. (Image provided by Anatomical Chart Co.)

Key Terms	Definitions
hemorrhage (HEM ur rij)	uncontrolled bleeding
hemostasis (hee moh STAY sis)	stoppage of blood flow through a vessel
coagulation (koh ag yoo LAY shun)	thickening of the blood
prothrombin (proh THROM bin)	precursor molecule to thrombin
thrombin (THROM bin)	enzyme that converts fibrinogen to fibrin to form a clot
fibrin (FIGH brin)	insoluble protein formed from fibrinogen in clotting process
thrombus (THROM bus)	abnormal blood clot that remains at the site of formation
thrombosis (throm BOH sis)	presence of a thrombus; clotting within a blood vessel

serotonin (seer oh TOH nin)	chemical that stimulates blood vessels constriction (narrowing)
eosinophils (ee oh SIN uh fils)	type of leukocyte stained by eosin dye
monocytes (MON oh sites)	leukocytes that are the precursors to macrophages
macrophage (MACK roh faij)	phagocytic cell derived from a monocyte
lymphocytes (LIM foh sites)	leukocyte active in the immune response
immunity (i MEW ni tee)	the resistance to infection
differential (dif ur EN shul) **(diff) white blood cell count**	determines the percentage of each type of leukocyte in a blood sample

Key Term Practice: Leukocytes

1. The most numerous type of leukocyte circulating in blood is a/an _____.

2. What are the two types of agranular leukocytes? _____

Thrombocytes

Thrombocytes are disc-shaped, anucleate, colorless structures. Thrombocytes (**platelets**) are not complete cells but rather are cytoplasmic fragments that represent the smallest of the blood-formed elements. In the presence of cuts, breaks, and interruptions of tissue integrity, platelets release serotonin, which causes contraction of the smooth muscle in vessel walls, thereby reducing blood flow within the vessel. Thrombocytes also prevent entry of pathogens into the body through open wounds by forming scabs; they prevent blood loss by developing clots. They move about in an ameboid manner and have a life span of approximately 10 days. Old thrombocytes are destroyed in the liver and spleen. Thrombocytes number 130,000–360,000 cells/mm^3 of blood.

Key Terms	Definitions
platelet (PLAIT lit)	cytoplasmic fragment that helps control blood loss; thrombocyte

Key Term Practice: Thrombocytes

1. What is the alternate term for platelet?

_____

Plasma

Plasma is the fluid portion of the blood; it transports nutrients and hormones, regulates electrolytes and fluids, and maintains a constant blood pH. Several plasma proteins serve particular functions in the blood: Albumin maintains blood osmotic pressure in the vessels and transports lipids and fat-soluble vitamins; globulins have an immune function; and fibrinogen plays a key role in blood clot formation.

Plasma electrolytes are important for maintaining osmotic pressure and blood pH. **Electrolytes** are minerals such as sodium, chlorine, potassium, bicarbonate, calcium, phosphorous, magnesium, and sulfate whose ions have an electrical charge. Sodium and chloride are the most abundant plasma electrolytes. **Osmotic pressure** is the pressure of fluid in the blood vessels. **Blood pH** is a measure of acidity or alkalinity, and strict parameters must be maintained for organism survival.

Key Terms	Definitions
electrolytes (e LECK troh lites)	circulating plasma ions, such as sodium and chloride
osmotic (oz MOT ick) **pressure**	fluid pressure in the blood vessels
blood pH	a measure of the blood's acidity; the hydrogen ion concentration in the blood

Key Term Practice: Plasma

1. Circulating plasma ions are termed _____.

Lipoproteins

Lipoproteins are a normal constituent of blood. By definition, a **lipoprotein** is a relatively large complex of lipid (fat) and protein. Lipoproteins in the blood are formed by a core of triglycerides surrounded by a surface layer composed of phospholipid, cholesterol (chol), and protein. Cholesterol is a compound important for the synthesis of steroid hormones and cell membranes; however, high levels have been linked to cardiovascular disease and gallstones.

The four primary categories of lipoproteins are very low density lipoprotein (VLDL), intermediate-density lipoprotein (IDL), low-density lipoprotein (LDL), and high density lipoprotein (HDL). **Very low density lipoproteins**, which are produced by liver cells, transport triglycerides (fat molecules containing glycerol and fatty acids) from the intestines and liver to muscles and adipose tissue. **Intermediate-density lipoproteins** are formed from the breakdown of VLDLs. Approximately 50% of IDLs are cleared from the plasma into the liver, and the remaining IDLs are broken down into LDLs. **Low-density lipoproteins** are formed by the conversion of VLDLs. Because most triglycerides have been removed, LDL molecules have a relatively higher cholesterol content than the original VLDL molecules. LDLs transport cholesterol to tissues. **High-density lipoproteins** are formed in the liver and small intestine. HDLs transport cholesterol to the liver for excretion in bile. These molecules have a higher concentration of protein and a lower concentration of lipid, so a high circulating level of HDLs is not linked with cardiovascular disease, as is a high circulating level of LDLs. HDLs are referred to as "good" because they prevent the accumulation of blood cholesterol. LDLs are referred to as "bad" because high levels are correlated with disease.

Key Terms	Definitions
lipoprotein (lip oh PROH teen)	protein combined with a lipid
very low density lipoprotein (lip oh PROH teen)	molecule that transports triglycerides to muscle and adipose tissue
intermediate-density lipoprotein (lip oh PROH teen)	molecule formed from the degradation of a VLDL molecule
low-density lipoprotein	molecule that transports cholesterol to body tissues
high-density lipoprotein (lip oh PROH teen)	molecule that transports cholesterol to the liver

Key Term Practice: Lipoproteins

1. List the four classes of lipoproteins.

   a. _____

   b. _____

   c. _____

   d. _____

Hemostasis

It is critical that the body have a mechanism in place to prevent blood loss after tissue injury. The stoppage of **hemorrhage** (uncontrolled bleeding) is referred to as **hemostasis** and occurs when blood vessels are stimulated to spasm (undergo involuntary contractions) after an injury. **Coagulation** is a hemostatic mechanism in which blood thickens to form clots, which halt bleeding. Clotting factors are agents produced by the body that assist in the hemostatic mechanism. These 12 clotting factors are numbered and identified by Roman numerals (I–XIII; there is no factor VI).

The four plasma components involved with hemostasis are prothrombin, thrombin, fibrinogen, and fibrin. **Prothrombin** is a plasma protein formed in the liver through the action of vitamin K. In the presence of prothrombin activator (PTA), prothrombin is converted to thrombin. **Thrombin** induces clotting by causing the conversion of fibrinogen to fibrin. The basic event for blood clot formation is the conversion of the soluble (easily dissolved) plasma protein fibrinogen into the insoluble (not easily dissolved) plasma protein **fibrin.** The series of events is as follows:

prothrombin → thrombin → fibrinogen → fibrin → clot

Two types of abnormal clots are a thrombus and an embolus. A **thrombus** or **thrombosis** is a blood clot that forms in a vessel and remains at the formation site. An **embolus** is a blood clot that dislodges from its original site and is carried away in the blood, forming an obstruction that blocks blood flow. An **embolism** is a blood vessel occlusion caused by an embolus (Fig. 10-3).

Anticoagulants are substances that prevent blood clotting. Significant anticoagulants are heparin and tissue plasminogen activator. Heparin from basophils and mast cells (cell types present in connective tissue) interferes with the formation of prothrombin activator, thereby providing another method for clot removal. **Tissue plasminogen activator** (TPA) is an enzyme that converts **plasminogen** into **plasmin,** a substance that breaks down blood clots, according to the following schema:

plasminogen + TPA → plasmin → clot dissolution

Figure 10-4 further illustrates hemostasis.

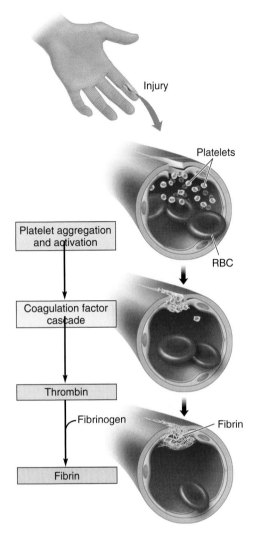

Injury

Platelets

Platelet aggregation and activation

RBC

Coagulation factor cascade

Thrombin

Fibrinogen

Fibrin

Fibrin

FIGURE 10-4
The stoppage of blood flow through a vessel is called hemostasis.

embolus (EM boh lus)	thrombus that migrates and lodges in the bloodstream
embolism (EM boh liz um)	blood vessel occlusion caused by an embolus
tissue plasminogen (plaz MIN oh jen) **activator**	enzyme that converts plasminogen to plasmin
plasminogen (plaz MIN oh jen)	inactive form of plasmin
plasmin (PLAZ min)	enzyme that dissolves clots

Key Term Practice: Hemostasis

1. What is the plural for each given term?

   a. thrombus = _____

   b. embolus = _____

2. A stationary clot is termed a/an _____.

TABLE 10-2 Blood Types

Blood Type	Antigen	Antibody	Preferred Type for Transfusion	Acceptable Type for Transfusion
A	A	B	A	O
B	B	A	B	O
AB	A and B	Neither A nor B	AB	A, B, O
O	Neither A nor B	Both A and B	O	O

Blood Groups

Blood groups (types) are meaningful for blood transfusions, transplants, genetic and anthropological studies, and paternity/maternity legal cases. Typing and cross-matching must be done before a patient receives a blood transfusion because the transfused blood must be compatible with the individual's blood.

Two terms important in the study of blood are agglutinogen and agglutinin. An **agglutinogen** is a substance, usually a protein called an **antigen** (Ag), on the red blood cell membrane. An **agglutinin** is a substance, such as an **antibody** (Ab), dissolved in plasma that causes cells to clump together. Blood types are identified as A, B, AB, and O; the basis of the ABO blood groups involves identifying the antigens present (or absent) on a person's erythrocytes. The terms *antigen* and *antibody* will be used when referring to "agglutinogen" and "agglutinin," respectively. When antibodies detect something foreign (antigen) to the body, they work to get rid of the invader (Table 10-2; Fig. 10-5).

In blood, the resulting antigen–antibody interactions create clumping or agglutination of the blood cells, thereby clogging vessels. To prevent this from happening, cross-matching, or blood typing, must be done before a blood **transfusion** (the transfer of blood from one person to another) occurs.

The two major antigens are A and B. People with type A blood have antigen A and will form antibody B. Type B blood is characterized by antigen B and antibody A. Individuals with blood type AB have both A and B antigens present and will form neither antibody A nor antibody B. Type O blood has no antigens and forms both antibody A and antibody B.

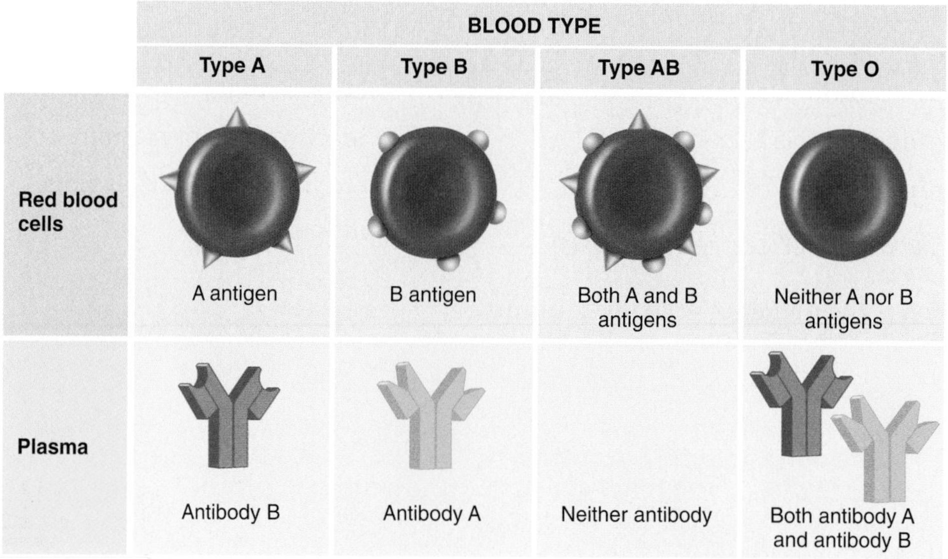

FIGURE 10-5
Blood groups (types) are meaningful for blood transfusions, transplants, genetic and anthropologic studies, and paternity/maternity legal cases.

	BLOOD TYPE			
	Type A	Type B	Type AB	Type O
Red blood cells	A antigen	B antigen	Both A and B antigens	Neither A nor B antigens
Plasma	Antibody B	Antibody A	Neither antibody	Both antibody A and antibody B

A person with type AB blood is called a universal recipient because he or she lacks both antibody A and antibody B; therefore, a person with type AB blood could receive a transfusion of blood of any type. A person with type O blood is referred to as a universal donor because his or her blood lacks antigens A and B; this type can be transfused into people with blood of any type.

In addition to blood types, the Rh factor is also often considered in the medical setting. The Rh factor was discovered when a group of researchers were performing scientific studies on rhesus monkeys. Thus the *Rh* from *rh*esus remains as the medical term. The **Rh factor** is an antigen on the red blood cells. Type Rh positive (Rh+) indicates that Rh antigens are present on the membrane of the erythrocytes. Individuals with type Rh negative (Rh−) blood do not have Rh antigens on the cell membrane. If an Rh− person receives a transfusion of Rh+ blood, the recipient's antibody-producing cells would be stimulated and **agglutination** (clumping) could result. Generally no serious consequences result from an *initial* transfusion of mismatched Rh blood types. As a result, however, the Rh− person is then sensitized to Rh+ blood. Thus if he or she later receives another transfusion of Rh+ blood, the donor's red blood cells will likely agglutinate.

Key Terms	Definitions
agglutinogen (uh GLOO tin oh jen)	protein substance on the red blood cell membrane that reacts to an antibody; antigen
antigen (AN ti jen)	protein substance on the red blood cell membrane that reacts to an antibody; agglutinogen
agglutinin (uh GLOO ti nin)	substance in blood plasma that causes clumping when it interacts with a specific antigen; antibody
antibody (AN tee bod ee)	substance in blood plasma that causes clumping when it interacts with a specific antigen; agglutinin
transfusion (trans FYOO zhun)	transfer of blood from one person to another
Rh factor	a specific antigen found on the red blood cells
agglutination (uh gloo ti NAY shun)	clumping

Key Term Practice: Blood Groups

1. What is the alternative term for each of the following?

    a. antigen _____

    b. antibody _____

THE CLINICAL DIMENSION

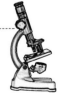

Pathology of the Blood

Signs and symptoms, clinical tests and diagnostic procedures, pathology, and treatments pertaining to the blood are described in this section. Blood pathology may be referred to as dyscrasia, diseases affecting blood cells or platelets.

Anemia

Anemia is a pathologic condition caused by a decreased erythrocyte count, deficient hemoglobin, inadequate erythropoiesis, excessive hemolysis, or a combination of these factors, resulting in overlapping signs and symptoms. Several forms of anemia exist, and most are characterized by erythropenia and deficient hemoglobin caused by blood loss. Defective hemoglobin synthesis, which causes deficient levels, occurs with hereditary anemias. A common characteristic of all forms is the inability of the blood to carry sufficient oxygen to meet the body's demands. Anemia caused by blood loss is **hemorrhagic anemia.** Anemia that results from deficient erythropoiesis, which occurs when the bone marrow is not productive, is **aplastic anemia. Hemolytic anemia** is characterized by hemolysis (bursting red blood cells). The causes of hemolytic anemia include transfusion reaction, autoimmune disease, and mechanical injury. Blood transfusions usually correct the problem.

Transfusions involve the introduction of whole blood or blood components from another person into an individual whose blood volume is diminished or deficient in some way. During an **exchange transfusion,** a person's blood is removed and simultaneously replaced with whole blood from another source. An **autologous transfusion** occurs when an individual has his or her own blood removed and stored for later use. This is also called predonation, and its practice is increasing because of the possibility of unknown and undetected bloodborne pathogens in donated blood.

Two hereditary forms of hemolytic anemia caused by defective hemoglobin synthesis are sickle cell anemia and thalassemia. **Sickle cell anemia,** an inherited chronic disease that occurs almost exclusively in blacks, is characterized by sickle-shaped erythrocytes (Fig. 10-6A). This abnormal morphology inhibits the cells from passing easily through the vasculature. Blood of individuals with the disease contains a form of

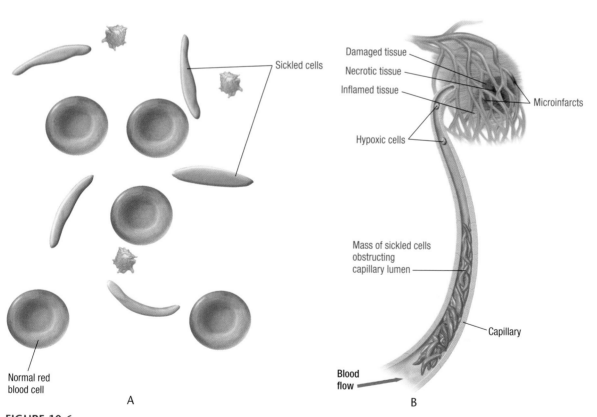

Sickled cells

Normal red blood cell

A

Damaged tissue
Necrotic tissue
Inflamed tissue
Microinfarcts
Hypoxic cells
Mass of sickled cells obstructing capillary lumen
Capillary
Blood flow

B

FIGURE 10-6
Sickle cell anemia is characterized by (**A**) sickle-shaped erythrocytes (**B**) that inhibit cells from passing easily through the vasculature. (Images provided by Anatomical Chart Co.)

hemoglobin called hemoglobin S. Distorted erythrocytes cause plugging of vessels, and these fragile RBCs cannot withstand the mechanical trauma of circulation and eventually lyse (Fig. 10-6B). General signs and symptoms include impaired growth and development, chronic marrow hyperactivity, arthralgia (joint pain), and fever; however, these vary, depending on the severity of the disease. Laboratory findings demonstrate reduced hemoglobin with normal cells. Treatment is primarily symptomatic because no antisickling drugs have been developed. Crises are managed by blood transfusions, oral hydration, and pain medications.

Thalassemia is a chronic, inherited anemia characterized by defective hemoglobin synthesis and ineffective erythropoiesis. It is found in individuals of Mediterranean, African, and Southeast Asian ancestry. Signs and symptoms include **jaundice** (skin yellowness owing to hyperbilirubinemia) and splenomegaly (enlarged spleen). Elevated hemoglobin levels indicate the disease. Blood tests show hypochromic (pale colored) and small erythrocytes (Fig. 10-7). Treatments vary and range from iron-chelation therapy (removal of excessive iron) and blood transfusions to splenectomy (spleen removal).

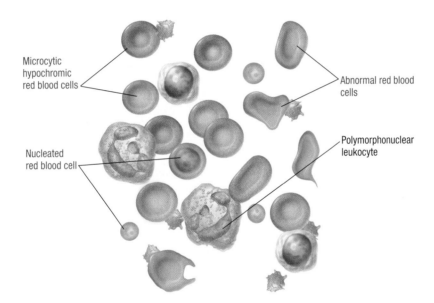

Microcytic hypochromic red blood cells

Nucleated red blood cell

Abnormal red blood cells

Polymorphonuclear leukocyte

FIGURE 10-7
Thalassemia is a chronic, inherited anemia. Signs include jaundice and an enlarged spleen. (Image provided by Anatomical Chart Co.)

Nutritional anemia results from iron, vitamin B_{12}, thiamin, or folate deficiency. These nutrients are required components for normal RBC production. Iron-deficiency anemia is common in premenopausal women. Most nutritional anemias result from inadequate diet, absorption, or use or from increased nutritional requirements. Nutritional anemia can be demonstrated by blood smear (Fig. 10-8). **Pernicious anemia** (PA) results from a vitamin B_{12} deficiency caused by a lack of intrinsic factor. Intrinsic factor, manufactured by parietal cells in the stomach, is required for the absorption of vitamin B_{12}. The term **pernicious** means severe, highly destructive, and potentially fatal. Signs and symptoms include fatigue, impaired pain and temperature sensitivity, and confusion. The Schilling test is used for diagnosis. The **Schilling test** is a diagnostic tool in which radioactive cobalt tagged with vitamin B_{12} is administered orally. Urine samples are then collected and analyzed for the presence of radioactive B_{12} over a 24 hour period. This substance will be decreased in people with pernicious anemia because of their inability to absorb vitamin B_{12}. Treatment for nutritional anemia includes providing the proper nutrient. In cases of PA, vitamin B_{12} injections are given throughout life.

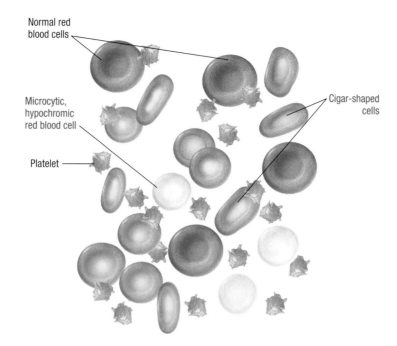

Normal red blood cells

Microcytic, hypochromic red blood cell

Platelet

Cigar-shaped cells

FIGURE 10-8
Nutritional anemia is caused by iron, vitamin B_{12}, thiamin, or folate deficiency. (Image provided by Anatomical Chart Co.)

Key Terms	Definitions
anemia (uh NEE mee uh)	reduced erythrocyte count, hemoglobin, or hematocrit
hemorrhagic anemia (hem uh RAJ ick uh NEE mee uh)	anemia caused by excessive bleeding
aplastic anemia (ay PLAS tick uh NEE mee uh)	anemia caused by production failure in the bone marrow
hemolytic anemia (hee moh LIT ick uh NEE mee uh)	anemia caused by erythrocyte destruction
exchange transfusion	simultaneous blood extraction and replacement
autologous (aw TOL uh gus) **transfusion**	donation of blood for later use by that same person
sickle cell anemia (uh NEE mee uh)	inherited form of anemia in which the erythrocytes are misshaped
thalassemia (thal uh SEE mee uh)	inherited form of hemolytic anemia
jaundice (JAWN dis)	yellowish skin owing to accumulated bilirubin
nutritional anemia (uh NEE mee uh)	anemia caused by nutritional deficiencies
pernicious anemia (pur NISH us uh NEE mee uh)	anemia caused by vitamin B_{12} deficiency secondary to loss of intrinsic factor
pernicious (pur NISH us)	severe, fatal, destructive
Schilling (SHIL ing) **test**	detects pernicious anemia using vitamin B_{12} tagged with radioactive cobalt

Key Term Practice: Anemia

1. Identify two hereditary forms of anemia. _____

2. The form of anemia resulting from direct vitamin B_{12} deficiency is _____.

Bleeding, Coagulation, and Platelet Disorders

Hemophilia is a recessive hereditary bleeding disorder, found almost exclusively in males, caused by a clotting factor deficiency in which one or more specific clotting factors are not naturally formed. Hemarthrosis, hematoma, ecchymosis, and gastrointestinal bleeding characterize it. **Hemarthrosis** is bleeding in the joints. A **hematoma** is an extravascular mass of clotted blood, and **ecchymosis** (bruise) refers to extravasation of blood into soft tissue. **Extravasation** is the term describing the passing of blood outside its proper place into surrounding tissue resulting from a ruptured vessel. The clinical picture, bleeding time, prolonged partial thromboplastin time test, and plasma prothrombin time test lead to the diagnosis.

Bleeding time is the average time it takes for bleeding to stop after the skin has been superficially lanced. **Partial thromboplastin time** (PTT) and **plasma prothrombin time** (PT; protime) are tests used to determine clotting time. Normal PTT is 35–50 seconds. Hemophiliacs and patients on heparin, warfarin, or aspirin may have a prolonged time. This test is usually done every 1–3 months to monitor heparin or other anticoagulant therapies. Normal PT is 9–17 seconds. Prolonged times are seen with hemophilia, infection, heart attack, disseminated intravascular coagulation, and anticoagulant therapy. Treatment involves antihemophilic factor (AHF) transfusions and limiting activities that have the risk of injury. **Antihemophilic factor** is clotting factor VIII, which is administered to individuals with hemophilia to assist with blood coagulation.

Purpura is a condition characterized by hemorrhage into the skin, mucous membranes, and internal organs. Two types are allergic (caused by sensitization to food, drugs, or insect bites) and fibrinolytic (characterized by bleeding and rapid clot fibrinolysis). Typical skin lesions of petechiae (tiny, purplish skin spots), ecchymoses, and vibices (lines of bleeding) vary with the type of purpura. The lesions first appear red, gradually darkening to purple, fading to brown and yellow, and eventually disappearing. The usual duration is 2–3 weeks. No treatment is necessary.

A disorder of the clotting cascade characterized by simultaneous hemorrhage and thrombosis is called **disseminated intravascular coagulation** (DIC). In DIC, fibrin is abnormally generated in the circulating blood. It is usually secondary to another condition such as **septicemia** (blood infection), malignancy (cancer), trauma, or an obstetric complication. Signs and symptoms include venous thrombosis, arterial emboli, and hemorrhage. Laboratory studies, patient history, and the clinical picture confirm the diagnosis. Prolonged PT and PTT are evident. Immediate treatment involves antibiotics (when bacterial infection is present), heparin (unless there is head injury), platelet replacement, and clotting factors. Untreated DIC can be life threatening because hypotension (low blood pressure) develops and the vascular volume is depleted.

A thrombosis is treated with **thrombolytic (thromboclastic)** agents, such as aspirin, streptokinase, and TPA, that break up or dissolve thrombi. Aspirin is considered a thromboclastic substance because it inhibits vasoconstriction and platelet aggregation by blocking the synthesis of thromboxane (a substance formed in platelets). **Streptokinase** and tissue plasminogen activators activate plasminogen to dissolve clots.

A clotting disorder caused by a decreased platelet count is termed **thrombocytopenia**. It is characterized by bleeding from small vessels throughout the body and may be caused by platelet production failure or increased platelet destruction. Signs and symptoms include petechiae and mucosal bleeding. There is generally no bleeding into tissues, as is commonly seen in coagulation disorders. It is diagnosed by history, ruling out any drugs that interfere with platelet formation, blood tests, hemoglobin count, and bone marrow aspiration biopsy. **Complete blood cell** (CBC) **counts** are tests used to evaluate red blood cell levels, hemoglobin levels, and hematocrit. The **RBC count** measures the number of erythrocytes per cubic millimeter of blood. These tests identify types, shapes, and numbers of RBCs, WBCs, and platelets. The **hemoglobin count** measures the grams of hemoglobin per 100 mL of blood. As noted earlier, the measure of the percentage of red blood cells in whole blood is called the hematocrit. The difference between hemoglobin count and hematocrit is that one measures absolute numbers and the other measures percentage volume of RBCs.

A **bone marrow aspiration biopsy** involves the insertion of a needle directly into bone marrow where cells are removed for later examination (Fig. 10-9). This diagnostic procedure is useful for identifying shapes and sizes of erythrocytes and leukocytes. Platelet transfusions are used to treat thrombocytopenia.

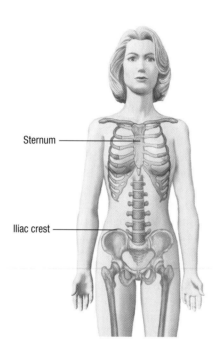

Sternum

Iliac crest

FIGURE 10-9
A bone marrow aspiration biopsy involves placing a needle directly into the bone marrow to remove cells for later examination. The usual sites for biopsy are the sternum and the iliac crest. (Image provided by Anatomical Chart Co.

Key Terms	Definitions
hemophilia (hee moh FIL ee uh)	inherited blood clotting disorder
hemarthrosis (hee mahr THROH sis)	bleeding into a joint
hematoma (hee muh TOH muh)	extravascular mass of clotted blood
ecchymosis (eck i MOH sis)	extravasation of blood into soft tissue; bruise
extravasation (ecks trav uh SAY shun)	passing of blood outside of the vessel into surrounding tissue
bleeding time	average time it takes bleeding to stop after the skin has been superficially lanced
partial thromboplastin (throm boh PLAS tin) **time**	time it takes for blood to clot
plasma prothrombin (proh THROM bin) **time**	test of time it takes for blood to clot
antihemophilic (an tee hee moh FIL ick) **factor**	clotting factor VIII used to treat hemophilia
purpura (PURE pew ruh)	condition characterized by hemorrhage into the skin

disseminated intravascular coagulation (di SEM i nay tid in truh VAS kew lur koh ag yoo LAY shun)	disorder of the clotting cascade characterized by simultaneous bleeding and clotting
septicemia (sep ti SEE mee uh)	bacterial infection of the blood
thrombolytic (throm boh LIT ick)	agent that dissolves a thrombus; thromboclastic
thromboclastic (throm boh KLAS tick)	agent that dissolves a thrombus; thrombolytic
streptokinase (strep toh KIGH nace)	enzyme that destroys blood clots
thrombocytopenia (throm boh sigh toh PEE nee uh)	decreased number of platelets
complete blood cell counts	tests that measure the types of blood cells in a sample of blood
RBC count	erythrocyte count
hemoglobin (HEE muh GLOH bin) **count**	test used to measure hemoglobin content in a blood sample
bone marrow aspiration biopsy (as pi RAY shun BYE op see)	removal of bone marrow for clinical examination

Key Term Practice: Bleeding, Coagulation, and Platelet Disorders

1. Which bleeding disorder is inherited? _____

2. _____ is the clotting disorder caused by a decreased platelet count.

Other Blood Disorders

Because of its very nature, blood is susceptible to an extensive list of disorders. Common blood disorders can be grouped as leukopenia, iron overload, infectious, and myeloproliferative. A total white blood cell count below 5000 cells/mm^3 of blood is referred to as **leukopenia. Neutropenia** is a type of leukopenia characterized by decreased blood neutrophils, which leads to an increased susceptibility to infection. The condition is usually caused by drug toxicity or drug allergy. Weakness, fatigue, fever, and mucous membrane ulcers are common signs and symptoms. The leukopenias are diagnosed via blood studies, and treatment is aimed at controlling infections with antibiotics and removing the allergen.

A chronic iron (Fe) overload disease characterized by iron deposition in the body, hepatomegaly, cirrhosis of the liver, and skin pigmentation is called **hemochromatosis.** The accumulation of hemosiderin, a golden yellow-brown protein, causes skin bronzing and is known as **hemosiderosis.** The origin is either idiopathic or from iron ingestion, iron injection, or a blood transfusion. The condition is diagnosed by the clinical picture, physical examination, and evidence of elevated serum Fe levels. It is treated by phlebotomy until serum Fe levels are restored to normal. **Phlebotomy** is bloodletting for therapeutic purposes to reduce the amount of blood in the body. The term **venesection** is synonymous with phlebotomy.

Commonly referred to as the "kissing disease," **infectious mononucleosis** (IM) is a contagious disease caused by the Epstein-Barr virus (EBV). The virus affects lymphatic tissue and is characterized by leukocytosis accompanied by pharyngitis (inflamed throat), fever, lymphadenopathy (enlarged lymph nodes), and splenomegaly.

Leukocytosis is a condition resulting from a white blood cell count exceeding 10,000 cells/mm^3 of blood. It indicates acute infection but may follow vigorous exercise, emotional disturbance, or excessive loss of body fluids. Blood tests and the clinical picture confirm the diagnosis. Most cases involve children and young adults. Antiviral medications and supportive therapy are the only treatment options. Most patients recover; however, relapses can occur.

Myeloproliferative disorders, such as polycythemia, are characterized by abnormal production of cells from the bone marrow. Erythrocytosis and elevated erythroblast levels typify **polycythemia.** It results from chronic obstructive pulmonary disease, which is caused by decreased oxygen levels (including high altitudes), cardiac disease, and other conditions in which the body compensates for low levels of oxygen in the tissues and blood. **Polycythemia vera** is a form of polycythemia with an unknown origin. It is characterized by bone marrow hyperplasia, leading to erythrocytosis, increased blood volume, and skin redness or cyanosis. **Cyanosis** is bluish skin discoloration owing to poorly oxygenated hemoglobin in the capillaries. An abnormal hematocrit or RBC count diagnoses both conditions. There may also be accompanying splenomegaly. Phlebotomy is used to treat polycythemia.

Multiple myeloma is a condition in which tumors composed of bone marrow–derived cells occur. It is an uncommon disease affecting more men than women. It is characterized by anemia, hemorrhage, recurrent infections, and weakness. Signs include nodular accumulations of abnormal or malignant plasma cells in the bone marrow, especially in the skull, and bone swellings. Radiographs indicating bone lesions, biopsy of the lesions, and evidence of Bence Jones proteins in the serum and urine make the diagnosis (Fig. 10-10). Myeloma cells produce abnormal proteins referred to as Bence Jones proteins. Treatment includes chemotherapy, bone marrow transplant, and plasmapheresis. With **plasmapheresis,** blood is withdrawn from the donor to obtain plasma, followed by the return of the RBCs to the donor. The plasma of the patient is depleted, but the cellular components remain. The median survival of individuals with multiple myeloma is 3 years.

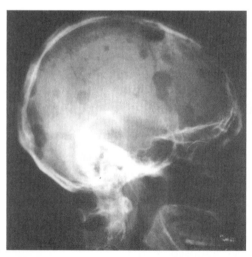
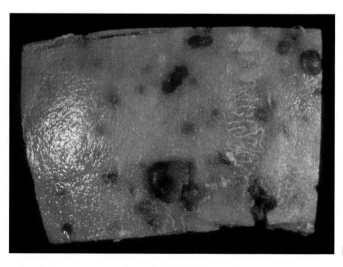

A   B

FIGURE 10-10

Multiple myeloma is characterized by the development of tumors composed of bone marrow–derived cells. (**A**) Numerous punched-out radiolucent areas can be seen. (**B**) Numerous lesions can be seen on the skull from a patient. (Reprinted with permission from Rubin E, Farber JL. Pathology. 3rd ed. Philadelphia: Lippincott Williams & Wilkins, 1999.)

Key Terms	Definitions
leukopenia (lew koh PEE nee uh)	abnormally low leukocyte count
neutropenia (new troh PEE nee uh)	decreased neutrophil levels
hemochromatosis (hee moh kroh muh TOH sis)	chronic disease characterized by iron deposition
hemosiderosis (hee moh sid er OH sis)	accumulation of hemosiderin in tissue
phlebotomy (fle BOT uh mee)	puncture made in a vein to withdraw blood; venesection
venesection (ven i SECK shun)	puncture made in a vein to withdraw blood; phlebotomy
infectious mononucleosis (mon oh new klee OH sis)	viral infection affecting lymphatic tissue
leukocytosis (lew koh sigh TOH sis)	abnormally high leukocyte count
polycythemia (pol ee sigh THEEM ee uh)	abnormally high erythroblast and erythrocyte counts
polycythemia vera (pol ee sigh THEEM ee uh VEER uh)	erythrocytosis of unknown origin
cyanosis (sigh uh NOH sis)	bluish skin discoloration
multiple myeloma (migh eh LOH muh)	tumors composed of cells derived from bone marrow causing nodular accumulations
plasmapheresis (plaz muh fe REE sis)	blood withdrawn to obtain plasma and then reintroduced to the donor without the plasma

Key Term Practice: Other Blood Disorders

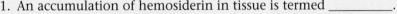

1. An accumulation of hemosiderin in tissue is termed _____.

2. _____ involves withdrawing blood from a donor, removing the plasma, and then reintroducing the blood back into the donor.

Erythroblastosis Fetalis

Erythroblastosis fetalis (hemolytic disease of the newborn; HDN) is a condition involving the Rh blood factor (Fig. 10-11). (*Fetalis* refers to "fetus.") It occurs only in cases in which the mother is Rh− and the fetus is Rh+. During the first pregnancy, this combination is uneventful (causes no problems); however, a subsequent pregnancy is at risk because some Rh+ cells from the first child may have entered the maternal circulation through damaged placental tissues. When this occurs, the mother produces antibodies against the Rh+ blood cells. If a second Rh+ child is conceived, that child is at risk because the anti-Rh antibodies from the maternal circulation can pass through the placenta, enter the fetal blood, and attack the fetal blood cells. The fetus develops erythroblastosis fetalis when the maternal antibodies react with the fetal Rh antigens, causing the fetal RBCs to agglutinate.

A commercial protein preparation, RhoGAM is now administered to Rh− mothers, regardless of the number of pregnancies. This product inhibits the mother's body from forming the anti-Rh antibodies, preventing damage to the fetus.

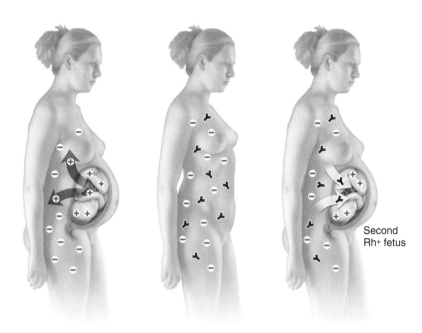

FIGURE 10-11
Erythroblastosis fetalis is a condition involving Rh blood factors, occurring only when the mother is Rh− and the fetus is Rh+. After the first pregnancy, maternal tissues may produce antibodies against fetal Rh+ blood cells.

Second Rh+ fetus

Key Terms	Definitions
erythroblastosis fetalis (e rith roh blas TOH sis fee TAY lis)	condition that occurs when an Rh− mother conceives an Rh+ fetus; hemolytic disease of a newborn
hemolytic (hee moh LIT ick) **disease of the newborn**	condition that occurs when an Rh− mother conceives an Rh+ fetus; erythroblastosis fetalis

Key Term Practice: Erythroblastosis Fetalis

1. The word part *erythro-* means _____; the word part *-blast* means _____; the word part *-osis* refers to _____; and the word *fetalis* means _____. Thus the word _____ describes a condition in which the red blood cells of a fetus are attacked by maternal antibodies.

Leukemia

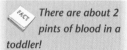
There are about 2 pints of blood in a toddler!

Leukemia is a malignant disease of blood characterized by leukocyte proliferation. The increased WBC production interferes with normal clotting. Leukemias were formally classified as acute or chronic, based on life expectancy, but they are now categorized according to cellular maturity. Because the leukocytes of individuals with leukemia are immature and incapable of fighting infection, a mild infection may be fatal. The disease is further classified on the basis of cell count, cell type, degree of differentiation, and rapidity of onset. Signs and symptoms of all leukemias include joint and bone pain, hepatomegaly, splenomegaly, and enlarged lymph nodes. Leukemia has an unknown cause but may be precipitated by viral infection, chemical exposure, or genetic disposition.

The forms of acute leukemia are acute lymphocytic and acute myelocytic. **Acute lymphocytic leukemia** (ALL) is marked by a rapid onset with severe anemia,

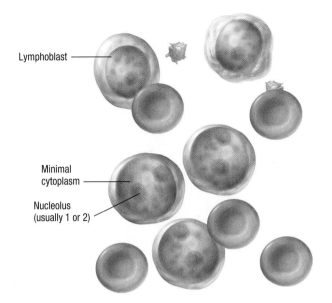

Lymphoblast

Minimal
cytoplasm

Nucleolus
(usually 1 or 2)

FIGURE 10-12
Acute lymphocytic
leukemia is marked by
rapid onset with se-
vere anemia, hemor-
rhage, and increased
susceptibility to infec-
tion. (Image provided
by Anatomical Chart
Co.)

hemorrhage, and increased susceptibility to infection. The affected cells are pre-
dominantly lymphocytes (Fig. 10-12). Although the cause is unknown, the condition can occur after radiation or chemical exposure or viral infection. It is treated by
aggressive chemotherapy, antibiotics, bone marrow transplant, or stem cell transplant.

Chemotherapy, used for disease prevention or treatment, involves the use of
chemical agents (chemotherapeutics) or drugs. Chemotherapeutics that inhibit or
destroy abnormal cells and tumors are termed **antineoplastic drugs. Bone marrow
transplant** (BMTs) and **stem cell transplant** are treatment options for blood diseases. Both procedures require donor tissue. Bone marrow transplants are used as a
last resort when other therapeutic measures fail. It is an extremely dangerous procedure because the recipient's immune response must be suppressed and all malignant
cells destroyed by aggressive treatment before the donor's marrow is intravenously
infused. The new marrow then repopulates the marrow cavity and begins producing
healthy cells. Stem cell transplants involve the transfer of stem cells from one person to another. The aim is to have normal cell proliferation. The survival rate for
ALL is about 50%.

Acute myelocytic leukemia (AML) is a form characterized by uncontrolled
proliferation of bone marrow cells. The cause is unknown but radiation exposure
and viral infections have been implicated. Signs and symptoms include fever,
headache, joint and bone pain, bruising, and enlarged lymphatic organs. The clinical picture, along with blood and bone marrow studies, confirms the diagnosis. It is
treated with chemotherapy and bone marrow or stem cell transplant. The cure rate
is 20–30%.

Increased granulocyte, lymphocyte, and monocyte levels characterize **chronic
lymphocytic leukemia.** The cells appear to be mature and invade lymph nodes and
other lymphoid tissue. Most cases occur in individuals over age 60 years. The onset is
gradual with few early symptoms. Diagnosis is made by blood and marrow studies.
Chemotherapy and radiation are treatment options. The median survival is about 10
years after diagnosis.

Weight loss, fatigue, hepatomegaly, splenomegaly, leukocytosis, thrombocytosis,
bleeding, and bruising characterize **chronic myelocytic leukemia** (Fig. 10-13).
Exposure to ionizing radiation increases the risk of disease. Diagnosis is made by blood
and bone marrow studies. Chronic myelocytic leukemia is treated with antineoplastic
drugs and chemotherapy. Median survival is 5–8 years.

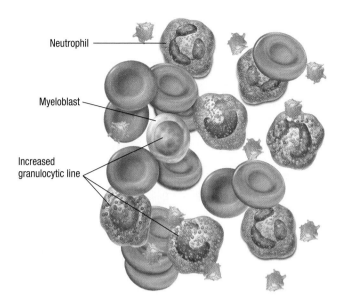

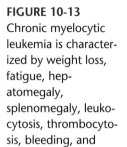

FIGURE 10-13
Chronic myelocytic leukemia is characterized by weight loss, fatigue, hepatomegaly, splenomegaly, leukocytosis, thrombocytosis, bleeding, and bruising. (Image provided by Anatomical Chart Co.)

Key Terms	Definitions
leukemia (lew KEE mee uh)	malignant disease of the blood-forming tissues
acute lymphocytic leukemia (uh KEWT lim foh SIT ick lew KEE mee uh)	leukemia characterized by increased formation of lymphocytes
chemotherapy (kee moh THERR uh pee)	disease prevention or treatment by chemical agents
antineoplastic (an tee nee oh PLAS tick) **drugs**	agents that inhibit or destroy abnormal cells or tumors
bone marrow transplant	transfer of marrow from one person to another
stem cell transplant	transfer of stem cells from one person to another
acute myelocytic leukemia (uh KEWT migh e loh SIT ick lew KEE mee uh)	form of leukemia characterized by the uncontrolled increase of marrow cells
chronic lymphocytic leukemia (KRON ick lim foh SIT ick lew KEE mee uh)	disease characterized by increased granulocyte, lymphocyte, and monocyte levels
chronic myelocytic leukemia (KRON ick migh e loh SIT ick lew KEE mee uh)	disease characterized by increased production of granulocytes by the red bone marrow

Key Term Practice: Leukemia

1. Leukemias with rapid or sudden onset are termed _____.

2. _____ is a malignant blood disease characterized by rapid production of leukocytes.

CLINICAL TERMS

Clinical Dimension	Term	Description
DISORDERS		
	acute lymphocytic leukemia	leukemia characterized by increased formation of lymphocytes
	acute myelocytic leukemia	form of leukemia characterized by the uncontrolled increase of marrow cells
	agranulocytosis	decreased leukocyte levels
	anemia	reduced erythrocyte count, hemoglobin, or hematocrit
	aplastic anemia	anemia caused by production failure in the bone marrow
	chronic lymphocytic leukemia	disease characterized by increased granulocyte, lymphocyte, and monocyte levels
	chronic myelocytic leukemia	disease characterized by increased production of granulocytes by the red bone marrow
	disseminated intravascular coagulation	disorder of the clotting cascade characterized by simultaneous bleeding and clotting
	dyscrasia	any abnormal condition of blood cells
	erythroblastosis fetalis	condition that occurs when an Rh− mother conceives an Rh+ fetus; hemolytic disease of the newborn
	granulocytic leukemia	form of leukemia characterized by uncontrolled proliferation of bone marrow cells
	granulocytosis	increased granulocyte levels
	hemochromatosis	chronic disease characterized by iron deposition
	hemolytic anemia	anemia caused by erythrocyte destruction
	hemolytic disease of the newborn	condition that occurs when an Rh− mother conceives an Rh+ fetus; erythroblastosis fetalis
	hemophilia	inherited blood clotting disorder
	hemorrhagic anemia	anemia caused by excessive bleeding
	hemosiderosis	accumulation of hemosiderin in tissues
	infectious mononucleosis (IM)	viral infection affecting lymphatic tissue
	leukemia	malignant disease of blood-forming tissues
	leukopenia	abnormally low leukocyte count
	microangiopathic hemolytic anemia	anemia caused by bursting blood cells
	multiple myeloma	tumors composed of cells derived from bone marrow causing nodular accumulations
	neutropenia	decreased neutrophil levels
	nutritional anemia	anemia caused by nutritional deficiencies

Clinical Dimension	Term	Description
	pernicious anemia	anemia caused by vitamin B_{12} deficiency secondary to loss of intrinsic factor
	polycythemia	abnormally high erythroblast and erythrocyte counts
	polycythemia vera	erythrocytosis of unknown origin
	purpura	condition characterized by hemorrhage into the skin
	septicemia	bacterial infection of the blood
	sickle cell anemia	inherited form of anemia in which the erythrocytes are misshaped
	thalassemia	inherited form of hemolytic anemia
	thrombocytopenia	decreased number of platelets
SIGNS AND SYMPTOMS		
	cyanosis	bluish skin discoloration
	ecchymosis	extravasation of blood into soft tissue; bruise
	erythrocytosis	elevated erythrocyte count
	erythropenia	erythrocyte deficiency
	extravasation	passing of blood outside of the vessel into surrounding tissue
	hemarthrosis	bleeding into a joint
	hematoma	extravascular mass of clotted blood
	hemorrhage	uncontrolled bleeding
	jaundice	yellowish skin resulting from accumulated bilirubin
	leukocytosis	abnormally high leukocyte count
CLINICAL TESTS AND DIAGNOSTIC PROCEDURES		
	alanine aminotransferase (ALT) test	detects liver dysfunction
	antiglobulin (Coombs) test	detects presence of Rh antibodies
	apheresis	procedure that separates blood into its components
	aspartate aminotransferase (AST) test	detects liver dysfunction or myocardial infarction; SGOT test
	bleeding time	average time it takes for bleeding to stop after the skin has been superficially lanced
	bone marrow aspiration biopsy	removal of bone marrow for clinical examination
	complete blood cell (CBC) counts	measure the types of blood cells in a sample of blood
	differential (diff) white blood cell count	determines the percentage of each type of leukocyte in a blood sample

Clinical Dimension	Term	Description
	erythrocyte sedimentation rate (ESR)	measures the speed at which RBCs settle in a test tube
	hemoglobin count	measures the hemoglobin content in a sample of blood
	hemoglobin electrophoresis	assesses hemoglobin types
	mean corpuscular hemoglobin (MCH)	average amount of hemoglobin in an erythrocyte
	mean corpuscular hemoglobin concentration (MCHC)	average concentration of hemoglobin in a red blood cell
	mean corpuscular volume (MCV)	average volume of a single red blood cell
	partial thromboplastin time (PTT)	time it takes for blood to clot
	phlebotomy	puncture made in a vein to withdraw blood; venesection
	plasma prothrombin time (PT)	time it takes for blood to clot
	platelet count	identifies the number of thrombocytes per cubic millimeter of blood
	prostate-specific antigen (PSA) test	detects prostate cancer
	RBC count	erythrocyte count
	Schilling test	detects pernicious anemia using vitamin B_{12} tagged with radioactive cobalt
	serum glutamic–oxaloacetic transaminase (SGOT) test	detects liver dysfunction or myocardial infarction; AST test
	serum glutamic–pyruvic transaminase (SGPT) test	identifies liver dysfunction
	venesection	puncture made in a vein to withdraw blood; phlebotomy
	white blood cell (WBC) count	identifies the total number of leukocytes in a cubic millimeter of blood

TREATMENTS

	acute normovolemic dilution	treatment used to reduce the blood cell to plasma ratio
	anticoagulant	substance that prevents blood clotting
	antihemophilic factor (AHF)	clotting factor VIII, used to treat hemophilia

Clinical Dimension	Term	Description
	antineoplastic drugs	agents that inhibit or destroy abnormal cells or tumors
	autologous transfusion	donation of blood for later use by that same person
	bone marrow transplant (BMT)	transfer of marrow from one person to another
	chemotherapy	disease prevention or treatment by chemical agents
	exchange transfusion	simultaneous blood extraction and replacement
	packed red blood cells (PRBCs)	stored RBCs given to patients with a low RBC count
	plasmapheresis	blood withdrawn to obtain plasma and then reintroduced to the donor without the plasma
	stem cell transplant	transfer of stem cells from one person to another
	streptokinase	enzyme that dissolves blood clots
	thromboclastic	agent that dissolves a thrombus; thrombolytic
	thrombolytic	agent that dissolves a thrombus; thromboclastic
	transfusion	transfer of blood from one person to another

Lifespan

Blood cells develop from the mesoderm germ layer, one of the primary layers formed early in embryonic life. While in utero, the mesoderm gives rise to other tissues and blood, which then forms from several sites, including the liver and spleen. By the 7th gestational month, the bone marrow takes over the role of hemopoiesis.

Fetal hemoglobin (Hb F) is the form found in the body while still in the womb. It is different from infant and adult hemoglobin; Hb F has a greater affinity for oxygen than does Hb A, the form produced after birth and throughout life. After birth, Hb F is destroyed by the infant's liver and replaced by newly formed Hb A.

Blood disorders that occur early in life, such as hemophilia and von Willebrand disease, a coagulation disorder, are generally genetically determined. Childhood and adolescence is unremarkable relative to blood transformation. Age-related blood changes include decreased hematocrit and blood pooling in the legs that results from ineffective vein valve function. Many disorders are usually secondary to cardiovascular disease. Late-life leukemias may result from declining immune function.

In the News: Blood Doping

Serious athletes go to great lengths to achieve a competitive edge. One such tactic to increase aerobic capacity (the ability of the lungs to exchange respiratory gases) involves autologous transfusion and is termed blood doping. Blood doping is a practice in which one to four units (450–1800 mL) of whole blood are drawn off 3–8 weeks before an athletic event and then reintroduced into the body 1–7 days before the competition. Physiologically, it induces polycythemia. When red blood cell levels decline from the draining process, erythropoietin is released from the kidneys to stimulate RBC production in the marrow. Therefore, red blood cell volume increases on two fronts: as a result of increased production and via reintroduction. Because erythrocytes carry oxygen, the increased numbers of RBCs with their higher oxygen-carrying capacity should enhance performance.

The practice does appear to offer an advantage to endurance athletes. A newer form of blood doping involves the injection of epoetin. Epoetin, also known by the trade names of Procrit and Epogen, is synthetic erythropoietin. The drug has been on the market since 1988 and is beneficial in the treatment of anemia. It is also used in patients with kidney dysfunction. Epoetin injections stimulate RBC formation and have been shown to significantly improve aerobic capacity and endurance exercise performance.

As with any drug whose effects are not monitored by a medical professional, there are inherent risks. Problems associated with the increased hematocrit are related to the higher blood viscosity and include increased blood pressure, decreased cardiac output, and increased risk for heart attack and stroke. Epoetin administration caused the deaths of 18 European bicyclists as a result of heart attack. The International Cycling Union and International Skiing Federation monitor hematocrit and hemoglobin concentrations in competing athletes in an effort to thwart this practice. Moreover, blood doping and/or ancillary epoetin injections are considered a form of cheating and are banned from Olympic games.

COMMON ABBREVIATIONS

Abbreviation	Term
Ab	antibody
Ag	antigen
AHF	antihemophilic factor; factor VIII
ALL	acute lymphocytic leukemia
ALT	alanine aminotransferase
AML	acute myelocytic leukemia
AST	aspartate aminotransferase
B cell	B lymphocyte
BMT	bone marrow transplant
CBC	complete blood (cell) count
chol	cholesterol
DIC	disseminated intravascular coagulation
diff	differential
EBV	Epstein-Barr virus
EPO	erythropoietin
ESR	erythrocyte sedimentation rate
Fe	iron
Hb	hemoglobin
HbO$_2$	oxyhemoglobin
Hct	hematocrit
HDL	high-density lipoprotein
HDN	hemolytic disease of the newborn

Abbreviation	Term
IDL	intermediate-density lipoprotein
IM	infectious mononucleosis
LDL	low-density lipoprotein
MCH	mean corpuscular hemoglobin
MCHC	mean corpuscular hemoglobin concentration
MCV	mean corpuscular volume
NPN	non-protein nitrogenous
O_2	oxygen
PA	pernicious anemia
PCV	packed cell volume
PRBCs	packed red blood cells
protime	plasma prothrombin time
PSA	prostate-specific antigen
PT	plasma prothrombin time
PTA	prothrombin tissue activator
PTT	partial thromboplastin time
RBC	red blood cell
Rh	Rhesus
SGOT	serum glutamic–oxaloacetic transaminase
SGPT	serum glutamic–pyruvic transaminase
T cell	T lymphocyte
TPA	tissue plasminogen activator
VLDL	very low density lipoprotein
WBC	white blood cell

Case Study

Mr. Sanderson, 55 years old, had been sent to the outpatient laboratory where John is the attending phlebotomist. Mr. Sanderson had a history of deep vein thrombosis and neuropathy (nerve disease) secondary to diabetes mellitus. As a monitoring process to evaluate the effectiveness of his medications and assess liver function, Mr. Sanderson was required to have blood studies done on a regular basis.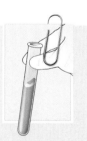

Anthropomorphic data noted that Mr. Sanderson is 6 feet 2 inches tall and weighs 230 lb. The physician ordered complete blood chemistry, immunologic studies, and diagnostic panels. The patient fasted for 12 hr but took his medications the morning of the draw. His medications consisted of a 20-mg tablet of atorvastatin (Lipitor) once per day, a 2-mg tablet of warfarin (Coumadin) once per day, and an 81-mg tablet of aspirin three times per week. Atorvastatin is used in the treatment of hyperlipidemia, and warfarin is an oral anticoagulant.

The blood was drawn and sent for analysis. Immediate results were obtained for PTT, bleeding time, and PT.

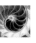

Case Study Questions

Select the best answer to each of the following questions.

1. PTT is the abbreviation for _____.

a. partial thromboplastin time
b. plasma prothrombin time
c. plasma timed test
d. partial thrombocyte test

2. Atorvastatin is used in the treatment of hyperlipidemia. It acts to _____.

a. increase blood lipid levels
b. decrease blood lipid levels
c. keep blood lipid levels constant
d. coagulate blood

3. Warfarin is a drug that _____.

a. promotes clotting
b. inhibits thrombosis
c. promotes lipid formation
d. is used to treat hemophilia

4. Mr. Sanderson's PTT time was 80 sec; the normal range is 35–50 sec. The prolonged time could be caused by _____.

a. warfarin therapy
b. Coumadin therapy
c. aspirin therapy
d. all of these

5. Mr. Sanderson's PT was 18 sec; normal PT time is within 2 sec of the control, which is 11–15 sec. The prolonged time may be the result of _____.

a. fasting
b. vitamin K therapy
c. Coumadin therapy
d. none of these

REAL WORLD REPORT

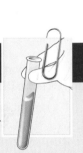

CENTRAL HOSPITAL LABORATORY: LAB ONE

Run Date:	September 29, 2003
Patient Name:	Max Sanderson
Sex:	Male
DOB:	March 3, 1948
Date/Time Last Meal:	09/28/2003 @ 7:30 P.M
Date/Time Collected:	09/29/2003 @ 8:30 A.M.
Date Recd.: 09/29/2003	Date Rptd: 09/29/2003

TEST RESULTS

• Serum: normal

BLOOD CHEMISTRY AND IMMUNOLOGY

Determination	Results	Reference Range	Low	Normal	High
Glucose	85.0 mg/dL	70–125 mg/dL		X	
Fructosamine	1.6 mmol/L	1.2–2.1 mmol/L		X	
BUN	14.0 mg/dL	5–25 mg/dL		X	
Creatinine	1.0 mg/dL	0.5–1.5 mg/dL		X	
Alkaline phosphatase	68.0 U/L	30–115 U/L		X	
Total bilirubin	0.5 mg/dL	0.1–1.2 mg/dL		X	

Determination	Results	Reference Range	Low	Normal	High
AST (SGOT)	22.0 U/L	0–41 U/L		X	
ALT (SGPT)	27.0 U/L	0–45 U/L		X	
Total protein	6.9 g/dL	6.0–8.5 g/dL		X	
Albumin	4.4 g/dL	3.0–5.5 g/dL		X	
Globulin	2.5 g/dL	1.0–4.5 g/dL		X	
Cholesterol	251.0 mg/dL	75–260 mg/dL		X	
Triglycerides	209.0 mg/dL	10–190 mg/dL			X
HDL cholesterol	33.0 mg/dL	31–56 mg/dL		X	
Chol/HDL ratio	7.6	0–4.9			X
LDL cholesterol	176.0 mg/dL	60–160 mg/dL			X
LDL/HDL ratio	5.34	1.82–6.06		X	
PSA	0.2	0.4	X		
HIV	nonreactive	nonreactive			

REAL WORLD REPORT QUESTIONS

The following exercises review the medical terms in the preceding medical report. The central laboratory where John works receives the reports, which are then forwarded to the physician's office. Abnormal values are indicated in some areas.

1. The report indicates that Mr. Sanderson's "Chol/HDL ratio" is high.

   a. Chol is the abbreviation for _____.

   b. HDL is the abbreviation for _____.

2. Mr. Sanderson's LDL cholesterol is also high. LDL is the abbreviation for _____.

3. According to the laboratory report, the patient's AST (SGOT) is within normal limits.

   a. AST is the abbreviation for _____.

   b. SGOT is the abbreviation for _____.

   c. AST and SGOT are synonymous terms. True or False? _____

4. Mr. Sanderson's total bilirubin is within normal limits. Bilirubin is _____.

   a. a bile pigment

   b. a form of PSA

   c. another term for cholesterol

   d. a form of albumin

REVIEW AND APPLICATION: THREE-LEVEL LEARNING SYSTEM

LEVEL ONE: REVIEWING FACTS AND TERMS USING RECALL

Select the best response to each of the following questions.

1. The blood has a role in _____.
   a. nutrient transport
   b. gas exchange
   c. temperature regulation
   d. all of these

2. The word part *-poiesis* means _____.
   a. formation
   b. blood
   c. condition of blood
   d. green colored

3. The word part *leuko-* means _____.
   a. cell
   b. white
   c. red
   d. thrombopenia

4. Thrombosis refers to the presence of _____.
   a. oxygen
   b. hemoglobin
   c. a blood clot in a vessel
   d. biliverdin

5. Hemoglobin without oxygen is called _____.
   a. oxyhemoglobin
   b. deoxyhemoglobin
   c. hemosiderin
   d. a hemocyte

6. A _____ is an immature erythrocyte.
   a. reticulocyte
   b. leukocyte
   c. corpuscle
   d. monocyte

7. Granular leukocytes include _____.
   a. monocytes
   b. lymphocytes
   c. basophils
   d. erythrocytes

8. *Pernicious* means _____.
   a. increased leukocytes levels
   b. decreased leukocyte levels
   c. excessive nutrients
   d. highly destructive and potentially fatal

9. A hematoma is _____.
   a. pain within the blood system
   b. an alternate term for erythrocytes
   c. an extravascular mass of clotted blood
   d. an abnormally low erythrocyte count

10. Cells that assist clot formation are _____.
    a. thrombocytes
    b. eosinophils
    c. agglutinogens
    d. antibodies

11. The fluid portion of blood is called _____.
    a. nonprotein nitrogen substances
    b. plasma
    c. fibrin
    d. thrombin

12. For health reasons, it is better to have a greater circulating level of _____ than _____.

    a. LDL; HDL

    b. VLDL; HDL

    c. fat; cholesterol

    d. HDL; LDL

13. The medical term for stopping blood loss is _____.

    a. thrombostasis

    b. hemostasis

    c. coagustasis

    d. embolism

14. A person with antigens A and B on his or her erythrocytes is said to have type _____ blood.

    a. A

    b. B

    c. AB

    d. O

15. A person with B antibodies has type _____ blood.

    a. A

    b. B

    c. AB

    d. O

16. The universal donor has type _____ blood.

    a. A

    b. B

    c. AB

    d. O

17. Bluish skin coloration is termed _____.

    a. jaundice

    b. cyanosis

    c. bilirubin

    d. biliverdin

18. The average time it takes for bleeding to stop after the skin has been superficially lanced is known as the _____ time.

    a. bleeding

    b. pro

    c. clotting

    c. TPA

19. _____ refers to disease prevention or treatment by chemical agents.

    a. Chemotherapy

    b. Nutritional therapy

    c. Pharmacology

    d. Antineoplasia

LEVEL TWO: REVIEWING CONCEPTS

Select the best response to each of the following questions.

20. Administering synthetic erythropoietin stimulates erythrocyte production. This is known medically as _____.

    a. erythroeisis

    b. cytopenia

    c. proerythroblasts

    d. erythropoiesis

21. Fibrinogen is _____.

    a. soluble and dissolves easily

    b. insoluble and dissolves easily

    c. soluble and does not dissolve

    d. insoluble and does not dissolve

Using the following words and word parts, form a medical term for each definition. Each word or word part is used only once.

    -cyte   erythro-   hemo-
    -philia   phlebo-   -tomy

22. vein incision _____

23. inherited clotting disorder _____

24. red blood cell _____

What is the medical term described by each of following literal meanings?

25. large eater _____

26. affinity for neutral dye _____

27. formation of leukocytes _____

28. blood stoppage _____

29. against clotting _____

30. toxic blood _____

Provide a medical term to complete a meaningful analogy.

31. Leukocytosis is to leukopenia as _____ is to erythropenia.

32. Blue is to cyanosis as _____ is to jaundice.

33. RBC is to erythrocyte as _____ is to leukocyte.

Define the following terms.

34. lipoprotein _____

35. prothrombin _____

36. venesection _____

Define the following abbreviations.

37. Hct _____

38. EPO _____

39. PCV _____

40. CBC _____

Match the disorder with its key characteristics.

_____ 41. disseminated intravascular coagulation   a. viral infection of lymphatic tissue

_____ 42. infectious mononucleosis   b. chronic disease of iron metabolism

_____ 43. chronic lymphocytic leukemia   c. persistent malignant blood disease

_____ 44. hemochromatosis   d. anemia caused by iron or thiamin deficiency

_____ 45. nutritional anemia   e. simultaneous bleeding and clotting

Match the anemia with its chief characteristics.

_____ 46. aplastic anemia   a. anemia with hemoglobin S

_____ 47. hemolytic anemia   b. anemia caused by excessive blood loss

_____ 48. hemorrhagic anemia   c. anemia caused by bone marrow failure

_____ 49. sickle cell anemia   d. anemia caused by RBC destruction

Identify the correctly spelled term in each set.

50. _____
   a. erythrocyte
   b. errythrocyte
   c. erithrocyte
   d. erythracyte

51. _____
   a. aglutinin
   b. egglutinin
   c. agglutinin
   d. agglutinnin

52. _____

   a. hemaglobin

   b. hemeglobin

   c. hemoglobun

   d. hemoglobin

53. _____

   a. pluripotent

   b. pleuripotent

   c. plurepotent

   d. pluripotint

54. _____

   a. albumen

   b. albumin

   c. allbumen

   d. albumine

55. _____

   a. aphoresis

   b. apheresis

   c. aforesis

   d. aphereses

Unscramble the letters to form a medical term.

56. tvineesceno

57. matameho

58. slumboe

59. nistfransuo

60. teauc

LEVEL THREE: THINKING CRITICALLY

Write a short answer to each of the following questions.

61. John Doe has type O blood. What type blood can he successfully receive in a blood transfusion?

   _____

   _____

   _____

62. In what two circumstances might a person simultaneously have a decreased red blood cell count and an increased reticulocyte count?

   _____

   _____

   _____

KEY TERMS SPELLING TEST FROM CD-ROM

Use the CD-ROM to test yourself on the spelling of key terms from this chapter. Listen to the terms and write them on a separate sheet of paper. Use a medical dictionary to check your answers.

ANSWERS

WORD GROUPING

Definition	Word Part
basic	baso-
bile, derived from bile	bili-
blood	hem-, hemo-
blood, pertaining to blood	hemat-, hemato-
blood clot, coagulation, thrombin	thromb-, thrombo-
blue	cyan-, cyano-
bone marrow	myel-, myelo-
causing destruction	-lytic
cell	-cyte
color	chromat-, chromato-
condition of blood	-emia
denoting appearance	phen-, pheno-
eater	-phage, -phagia-, -phagy
eating, devouring	phag-, phago-
excessive discharge, hemorrhage	-rrhagia
fiber, fibrous	fibr-, fibro-
fibrin, fibrinous	fibrin-, fibrino-
formation, production	-poiesis
granular, granules	granulo-
green	verd-, verdo-
having an affinity for, craving for	A. -philia
	B. -philic
iron	sidero-
loss of oxygen from a compound	deoxy-
lymph, tissue fluid in a lymphatic vessel	lymph-, lympho-
movement toward or away from a stimulus	-taxis
neutral	neutr-, neutro-
nucleus	nucle-, nucleo-
plasma, noncellular blood portion	plasma-
presence of oxygen	oxy-
red, erythrocyte	erythr-, erythro-
sepsis, septic, pathogens or toxins in blood	septic-, septico-
serum, serous	ser-, seri-, sero-
several	pluri-
transmission	-phoresis
vein, venous	phleb-, phlebo-
white	leuk-, leuko-
white, whitish	alb-, albo-

WORD BUILDING

Word Part	Meaning	Common or Known Word	Example Medical Term
leuk-, leuko-	white	leukemia	leukocyte
alb-, albo-	white, whitish	albino	albumin
cyan-, cyano-	blue	cyanide	cyanosis
-emia	condition of blood	anemia	anemia
fibr-, fibro-	fiber, fibrous	fiber	fibrosis
hem-, hemo-	blood	hemorrhoids	hemostasis
hemat-, hemato-	blood, pertaining to blood	hematoma	hematopoiesis
neutr-, neutro-	neutral	neutral	neutrophil
oxy-	presence of oxygen	oxygen	oxygen
phleb-, phlebo-	vein, venous	phlebotomist	phlebotomy
-philia	having an affinity for, craving for	pedophilia	hemophilia
pluri-	several	plural	pluripotent
septic-, septico-	sepsis, septic, pathogens or toxins in blood	septic system	septicemia
ser-, seri-, sero-	serum, serous	serum	serum
thromb-, thrombo-	blood clot, coagulation, thrombin	thrombus	thrombocyte
verd-, verdo-	green-	verdant	biliverdin

KEY TERM PRACTICE

Blood Preview
1. hemopoiesis; hematopoiesis
2. a. leukocyte; b. erythrocyte; c. thrombocyte
3. serum

Erythrocytes
1. erythropoiesis
2. oxyhemoglobin (HbO$_2$)
3. bilirubin

Leukocytes
1. neutrophil
2. monocytes; lymphocytes

Thrombocytes
1. thrombocyte

Plasma
1. electrolytes

Lipoproteins
1. a. very low density lipoprotein (VLDL); b. intermediate-density lipoprotein (IDL); c. low-density lipoprotein (LDL); d. high-density lipoprotein (HDL)

Hemostasis
1. a. thrombi; b. emboli
2. thrombus

Blood Groups
1. a. agglutinogen; b. agglutinin

Anemia
1. thalassemia; sickle cell anemia
2. pernicious

Bleeding, Coagulation, and Platelet Disorders
1. hemophilia
2. Thrombocytopenia

Other Blood Disorders
1. hemosiderosis
2. Plasmapheresis

Erythroblastosis Fetalis
1. red; precursor cell; condition of; fetus; erythroblastosis fetalis

Leukemia
1. acute
2. Leukemia

CASE STUDY

1. a is the correct answer.
   - b is incorrect because the abbreviation for plasma prothrombin time is PT.
   - c and d are incorrect because these are made-up tests.
2. b is the correct answer.
   - a and c are incorrect because atorvastatin decreases blood lipid levels.
   - d is incorrect because atorvastatin does not act as a clotting agent.
3. b is the correct answer.
   - a is incorrect because clotting agents enhance clotting.
   - b is incorrect because warfarin is an anticoagulant; drugs typically do not promote fat formation.
   - d is incorrect because hemophilia would be treated with a clotting agent.
4. d is the correct answer.
   - All answers are correct because all these agents act as anticoagulants.
5. c is the correct answer.
   - a is incorrect because fasting does not affect clotting time.
   - b is incorrect because vitamin K therapy acts as a clotting agent and thus would decrease the PT time.
   - d is incorrect because C is the correct answer.

REAL WORLD REPORT

1. a. cholesterol; b. high-density lipoprotein
2. low-density lipoprotein
3. a. aspartate aminotransferase; b. serum glutamic-oxaloacetic transaminase; c. True
4. a

REVIEW AND APPLICATION: THREE-LEVEL LEARNING SYSTEM

Level One: Reviewing Facts and Terms Using Recall

1. d
2. a
3. b
4. c
5. b
6. a
7. c
8. d
9. c
10. a
11. b
12. d
13. b
14. c
15. a
16. d
17. b
18. a
19. a

Level Two: Reviewing Concepts

20. d
21. a
22. phlebotomy
23. hemophilia
24. erythrocyte
25. macrophage
26. neutrophil
27. leukopoiesis
28. hemostasis
29. anticoagulant
30. septicemia
31. erythrocytosis

32. yellow
33. WBC
34. protein combined with lipid (fat)
35. precursor molecule to thrombin
36. phlebotomy; blood removal
37. hematocrit
38. erythropoietin
39. packed cell volume
40. complete blood (cell) count
41. e
42. a
43. c
44. b
45. d
46. c
47. d
48. b
49. a
50. a
51. c
52. d
53. a
54. b
55. b
56. venesection
57. hematoma
58. embolus
59. transfusion
60. acute

Level Three: Thinking Critically

61. John can receive only blood type O.
62. The individual may have severe hemorrhage or low blood oxygen levels.

chapter 11

Cardiovascular System

OBJECTIVES

After completing this chapter, you should be able to:

1. State the meaning of word parts related to the cardiovascular system.
2. Identify common arteries and veins.
3. Identify anatomic features of the heart.
4. Explain how blood pressure is measured.
5. Define common signs, symptoms, and treatments of various cardiovascular system diseases.
6. Explain clinical tests and diagnostic procedures related to the cardiovascular system.
7. Describe anatomical and physiological alterations throughout the lifespan.
8. Define common abbreviations related to the cardiovascular system.
9. Define terms used in medical reports involving the cardiovascular system.
10. Correctly define, spell, and pronounce the chapter's terms.

INTRODUCTION

The cardiovascular (CV) system is composed of the heart, arteries, veins, and capillaries. The heart functions to pump blood that is low in oxygen to the lungs, where it is oxygenated, and then to pump oxygen-rich blood to the entire body. Each day, the heart pumps approximately 7000 L (1855 gallons) of blood throughout the body, ensuring survival.

Arteries, veins, and capillaries make up the body's blood vessels. Capillaries are the smallest of these vessels and the sites of nutrient and gas exchange. Blood courses through blood vessels delivering electrolytes, hormones, nutrients, and oxygen to tissues while simultaneously returning metabolic waste products to proper organs for disposal.

Vital signs—such as blood pressure, pulse, respiratory rate, and temperature—and heart sounds are used to assess the cardiac patient. In addition to normal physiology, common disorders of the cardiovascular system are described in this chapter. Radiography, radionuclide imaging, catheterization, electrocardiography, and echocardiograms provide diagnostic evidence of vascular or cardiac pathology.

FACT *If you strung together all of your blood vessels, they would circle the Earth 2½ times!*

Professional Profile: Registered Nurse in a Cardiovascular Intensive Care Unit

Heidi is a registered nurse (RN) working in the cardiovascular intensive care unit (CVICU) of a public hospital, where she has been employed for 5 years. The CVICU is separate from the intensive care unit (ICU) and receives patients only with cardiovascular or cardiovascular-related disorders. This hospital provides services to patients within a 60-mile radius.

Heidi received her RN diploma and associate of arts (AA) in natural science degree from a hospital-based school of nursing, which has an affiliation with a local college. Her RN program was a "3 + 1" program, which means that after completing the first 3 years of the program, graduates earn a diploma and an AA degree. After the initial 3-year course of study, graduates of the program may continue for 1 year more to earn a bachelor of science in nursing (BSN) degree.

One month after graduating, Heidi passed her National Council Licensure Examination (NCLEX) and began her full-time nursing career, working on the rehabilitation floor. Prospective nurses are required to pass this examination to receive professional licensure in the nursing field. When a position in the CVICU opened up, Heidi applied and was transferred.

Many cardiac patients are in serious condition when they arrive at Heidi's unit. The acuity level ranges from moderate to high. Patients have often undergone major medical procedures, such as coronary artery bypass, valve replacement, and vascular and thoracic surgery. Regardless of the situation, the focus remains on quality care for patients and their families.

As a cardiovascular nurse, one realizes the impact that the cardiovascular system has on every other system in the human body. Therefore, continuing education, attendance at update programs and conferences, and advanced training courses are mandatory. Cardiovascular nurses must also regularly update their advanced cardiac life support (ACLS) certification.

MEDICAL TERM PARTS

WORD PARTS

Medical term prefixes, suffixes, and combining forms related to the nervous system are introduced in this section.

Word Parts	Meaning
angi-, angio-	vessel, vascular
aort-, aorto-	aorta, aortic
apic-, apici-, apico-	apex, apical
arteri-, arterio-	artery, arterial
athero-	fatty, gruel-like, atheroma
atrio-	atrium
automat-, automato-	automatic, spontaneous
brady-	slow
cardi-, cardio-	heart, cardiac
chord-, chordo-	cord
eury-	broad, wide
hepat-, hepato-	liver, hepatic
isch-, ischo-	stoppage, obstruction
parieto-	parietal, forming a wall
phleb-, phlebo-	vein, venous
-pnea	respiratory, respiratory condition
pulmo-	lung, pulmonary
sino-, sinu-	sinus
sphygm-, sphygmo-	pulse
steth-, stetho-	chest or breast
tachy-	rapid, quick, accelerated
vas-, vasi-, vaso-	vessel, vascular
vascul-, vasculo-	small vessel, vascular
veni-, veno-	veins
ventri- ventro-	small cavity, abdomen
ventriculo-	ventricle

WORD ETYMOLOGY

Some words have Greek or Latin word roots but are not true word parts. This section lists those that are used as medical terms.

Word	Definition
bradys	slow
cardia	heart

Word	Definition
cor	heart
corona	crown, garland
kardia	heart
ptysis	a spitting
vena	vein
venter	belly
ventriculus	ventricle

MEDICAL TERM PARTS USED AS PREFIXES

Prefix	Definition
athero-	fatty, gruel-like, atheroma
atrio-	atrium
brady-	slow
eury-	broad, wide
parieto-	parietal, forming a wall
pulmo-	lung, pulmonary
tachy-	rapid, quick, accelerated
ventriculo-	ventricle

MEDICAL TERM PARTS USED AS SUFFIXES

Suffix	Definition
-pnea	respiratory, respiratory condition

WORD GROUPING

Using the "Medical Term Parts" tables, identify the prefix, suffix, or combining form for each of the following definitions. The first one has been done as an example.

Definition	Word Part
heart, cardiac	cardi-, cardio-
aorta, aortic	
apex, apical	
artery, arterial	
atrium	
automatic, spontaneous	
broad, wide	

Definition	Word Part
chest or breast	
cord	
fatty, gruel-like, atheroma	
liver, hepatic	
lung, pulmonary	
parietal, forming a wall	
pulse	
rapid, quick, accelerated	
respiratory, respiratory condition	
sinus	
slow	
small cavity, abdomen	
small vessel, vascular	
stoppage, obstruction	
vein, venous	
veins	
ventricle	
vessel, vascular	A.
	B.

WORD BUILDING

Word parts, introduced in the "Medical Term Parts" section, are listed in the following table. For this exercise, first supply the meaning of each word part, then use the word part to build a word you already know. The word you list under "Common or Known Word" does not have to be a medical term; a commonly used word is fine. Be sure, however, that the word correctly reflects the intended meaning. The first one has been done as an example.

Word Part	Meaning	Common or Known Word	Example Medical Term
hepat-, hepato-	liver, hepatic	hepatitis	hepatic vein
angi-, angio-			angiogram
aort-, aorto-			ascending aorta
arteri-, arterio-			artery
athero-			atherosclerosis
automat-, automato-			automaticity
cardi, cardio-			cardiac
phleb-, phlebo-			thrombophlebitis

Word Part	Meaning	Common or Known Word	Example Medical Term
pulmo-			pulmonary artery
sino-, sinu-			sinoatrial node
steth-, stetho-			stethoscope
tachy-			tachycardia
vascul-, vasculo-			vascular

ANATOMY AND PHYSIOLOGY

Structures of the Cardiovascular System

- Arteries
- Arterioles
- Capillaries
- Heart
- Veins
- Venules

Cardiovascular System Preview

This chapter focuses on the heart and vascular network, otherwise known as the cardiovascular system. The word parts *cardi-* and *cardio-* mean "heart." They are derived from the Latin word for heart, *cardium*, which is based on the Greek term *kardia*. Note the *c* and *k* variation—some terms pertaining to the CV system use the letters interchangeably; for example, both ECG and EKG are acceptable abbreviations for the word *electrocardiogram*. There is a minor difference between the circulatory system and the cardiovascular system. The CV system includes the heart and affiliated blood vessels, and the entire circulatory system includes the cardiovascular system plus the lymphatic vessels, which are outside the CV system.

The **heart** is a four-chambered, pumping organ located in the thoracic cavity. It receives its oxygen and nutrition from the coronary circulation (the heart's blood supply) and delivers oxygen and nutrients to all parts of the body via the blood vessels. The majority of the blood swooshing through the heart's chambers gets distributed to other body regions. The cardiovascular system also includes blood vessels, called arteries, arterioles, veins, venules, and capillaries. **Arteries** carry blood away from the heart, **veins** return blood to the heart, and **capillaries** bridge the smallest arteries (called arterioles) with the smallest veins (venules), thereby providing a closed, continuous circuit of vasculature. As a tip, associate the *a* in *a*rtery with the *a* in *a*way.

Approximately 4000 gallons of blood are pumped through the heart daily!

Most of the body's blood is located in the systemic venous network (64%). Approximately 13% of the blood is distributed in the arterial system, 9% in the pulmonary (lung) circuit, 7% in the heart, and another 7% in systemic capillaries. This chapter discusses significant anatomy and physiology of the heart and identifies important arteries and veins.

Key Terms	Definitions
heart	organ that pumps blood
artery (AHR tur ee)	vessel carrying blood away from the heart
veins	vessels carrying blood toward the heart
capillary (KAP i lair ee)	small blood vessel connecting arteries with veins

Key Term Practice: Cardiovascular System Preview

1. What is the plural form for each given term?

   a. artery = _____

   b. vein = _____

   c. capillary = _____

2. A/an _____ carries blood toward the heart; a/an _____ carries blood away from the heart.

The Heart

Located within the mediastinum of the thorax, the heart is in a tilted position with the inferior **apex** (point) resting on the diaphragm. The **apical heartbeat** can be found by listening between the fifth and sixth ribs, the location of the heart's apex. The bulk of this vital organ lies left of the midsternal line. Its general structure is that of a hollow, funnel-shaped muscular pump; and the average heart is approximately 13 cm (5.2 in.) long and 8 cm (3.2 in.) wide. The heart size, however, depends on the individual and his or her usual level of exercise. Because it is a muscle, aerobic exercise can cause cardiac hypertrophy (increase in size), which in turn enables the heart to thrust more efficiently. The major purpose of cardiac muscle is that of pumping blood, so enhanced function permits improved body tissue perfusion (blood circulation).

Various layers of **pericardium** (*peri-* = "around"; *cardi-* = "heart"), a serous membrane, surround and protect the heart. The **visceral pericardium** is the inner layer that directly covers the heart and is a loose-fitting sac that shields the heart from friction.

The cardiac wall itself is composed of three layers: the outer epicardium, the middle myocardium, and the inner endocardium (Fig. 11-1). The **epicardium** is the protective

> **FACT** *Your heart is about the size of your own clenched fist!*

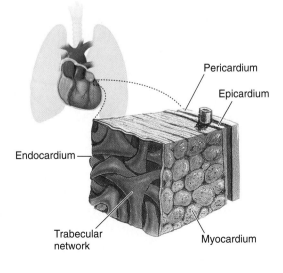

Pericardium

Epicardium

Endocardium

Trabecular network

Myocardium

FIGURE 11-1
The cardiac wall is composed of three layers: epicardium, myocardium, and endocardium.
(Image provided by Anatomical Chart Co.)

serous membrane, and the thick middle **myocardium** (*my-* = "muscle") consists largely of cardiac muscle tissue. Epithelium and connective tissue containing elastic and collagenous fibers make up the inner **endocardium.** This layer is continuous with the endothelium (inner lining) of blood vessels.

Four chambers and four valves are found within the heart (Fig. 11-2). The two upper chambers, called **atria** (sing., **atrium**), have relatively thin walls and receive blood from veins. They are called atria because in early Roman times, the atrium was the room in which guests entered a house. Accordingly, the atrium is the chamber in which blood enters the heart. The two lower chambers, **ventricles,** force blood out of the heart into arteries. The term *ventricle* is derived from Latin and refers to "small

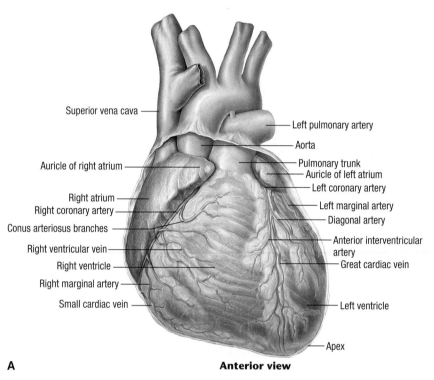

Anterior view

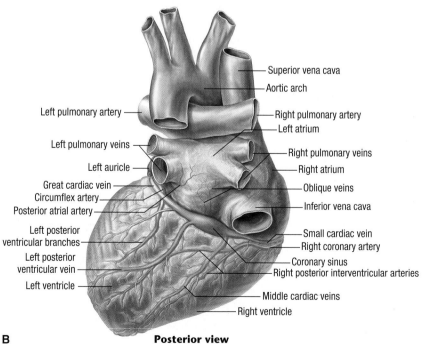

Posterior view

FIGURE 11-2
The heart in (**A**) anterior and (**B**) posterior views. (Images provided by Anatomical Chart Co.)

body cavities," in this case, the two lower heart chambers. The left ventricle has a thicker myocardial wall than the right ventricle because its stronger muscle makes forceful contractions to push blood throughout the whole body system.

The heart has two atrioventricular (AV) valves, called the tricuspid and bicuspid, and two semilunar valves, named the pulmonary and aortic (Fig. 11-3). Valves prevent the backflow of blood during heart contraction or relaxation. The **atrioventricular valves** are so named because they are located between the atria and ventricles and safeguard the openings between the upper and lower chambers, ensuring unidirectional blood flow. The valves are identified according to the number of flaps, called cusps, they contain. The **tricuspid valve**, or **right atrioventricular valve**, is located between the right atrium and right ventricle. (To remember this side, think "*try to be right*" for *tri*cuspid.) Its function is to prevent back flow of blood from the right atrium into the right ventricle during ventricular contraction. Likewise, the **left atrioventricular valve**, also called the **bicuspid valve**, is found between the left atrium and left ventricle. The left AV valve is also called the **mitral valve** because its shape resembles a miter, the hat traditionally worn by bishops.

Chordae tendineae are fibrous cords that look like strings attaching the papillary muscles to the cusps of the AV valves. Chordae tendinea keep the flaps pointing in the correct direction. **Papillary muscles** are bulges in the heart wall from which the chordae tendinea originate. These muscles "tug on the heartstrings."

> FACT The aorta is 2500 times wider than a capillary!

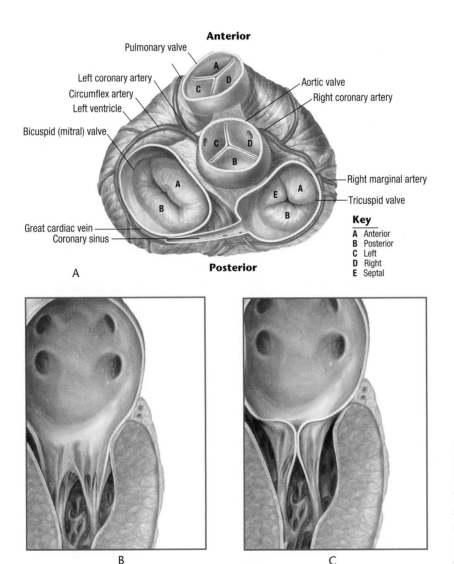

Anterior

Pulmonary valve

Left coronary artery
Circumflex artery
Left ventricle
Bicuspid (mitral) valve

Aortic valve
Right coronary artery

Right marginal artery
Tricuspid valve

Great cardiac vein
Coronary sinus

A

Posterior

Key
A Anterior
B Posterior
C Left
D Right
E Septal

B

C

FIGURE 11-3
(A) The valves of the heart. The atrioventricular valves are shown **(B)** open ar **(C)** closed. (Ima͏͏ provided by Anatomical C'

Two semilunar (SL) valves of the heart are the pulmonary and aortic. These valves are so named because they are shaped like a half moon. The **pulmonary semilunar valve** (PSLV) is located at the entrance to the pulmonary trunk, the vessel that branches into the pulmonary arteries. The function of the PSLV is to prevent blood from moving from the pulmonary trunk into the right ventricle during ventricular relaxation. Located at the entrance to the heart is the **aortic semilunar valve** (ASLV). This valve prevents blood flow from the aorta into the left ventricle during ventricular relaxation. The **aorta** is the largest artery; it branches into several other arteries.

Key Terms	Definitions
apex	lowest, left-most heart point
apical (AY pi kul) **heartbeat**	heartbeat heard at the apex of the heart
pericardium (perr i KAHR dee um)	closed sac encircling the heart
visceral pericardium (VIS ur ul perr i KAHR dee um)	layer directly on the heart
epicardium (ep i KAHR dee um)	outer heart layer
myocardium (migh oh KAHR dee um)	middle layer composed of heart muscle
endocardium (en doh KAHR dee um)	membrane lining the inner heart
atrium (AY tree um)	the two upper heart chamber
ventricle (VEN tri kul)	the two lower heart chamber
atrioventricular (ay tree oh ven TRICK yoo lur) **valve**	valves between the atria and the ventricles; bicuspid and tricuspid valves
tricuspid (trye KUS pid) **valve**	valve between the right ventricle and the right atrium; right atrioventricular valve
right atrioventricular (ay tree oh ven TRICK yoo lur) **valve**	valve between the right ventricle and the right atrium; tricuspid valve
left atrioventricular (ay tree oh ven TRICK yoo lur) **valve**	valve between the left atrium and the left ventricle; bicuspid valve, mitral valve
bicuspid (bye KUS pid) **valve**	valve between the left atrium and the left ventricle; left atrioventricular valve, mitral valve
mitral (MIGH trul) **valve**	valve between the left atrium and the left ventricle; left atrioventricular valve, bicuspid valve
chordae tendineae (KOR dee TEN di nee ee)	tendinous cords in heart
papillary (PAP i lerr ee) **muscle**	muscular eminence from which the chordae tendineae arise
pulmonary semilunar (PUL muh nerr ee sem ee LEW nur) **valve**	valve between the heart and the pulmonary trunk
aortic semilunar (ay OR tick sem ee LEW nur) **valve**	valve between the heart and the aorta
aorta (ay OR tuh)	largest artery, arises from the left ventricle

Key Term Practice: The Heart

1. What is the medical term that means heart muscle? _____

2. What are the terms for the heart valve located between the left atrium and the left ventricle?

    a. _____

    b. _____

    c. _____

Vasculature

Vasculature refers to the arrangement of blood vessels throughout the body. Those vessels (derived from the word part *vas-*, meaning "vessel") include the arteries and arterioles, veins and venules, and the interconnecting capillaries. The vasculature is responsible for delivering nutrients to cells and enabling the important exchange of gases between the blood and tissue fluid.

Arteries are vessels that convey blood away from the heart (Fig. 11-4; Table 11-1). They have three anatomic layers, called tunicae (sing., = **tunica**). The inner layer is named the **tunica intima**, the middle layer is the **tunica media**, and the outer layer is referred to as the **tunica externa** (tunica adventitia). Connections formed between the distal ends of vessels are called **anastomoses**. An anastomosis permits collateral circulation, an alternate blood route in the event of an occluded (obstructed) vessel. These may also be surgically created.

Small arteries that deliver blood from arteries to the capillary network are **arterioles.** By constricting and dilating, arterioles help regulate blood flow from the arteries to the capillaries.

Veins are vessels that return blood to the heart. They are less elastic and have less smooth muscle tissue than arteries (Fig. 11-5). Unlike arteries, veins have valves to prevent backflow of blood. Like arteries, they have three tunicae named the same—intima, media, and externa—but the tunica media is less developed, causing vein walls to be much thinner than arterial walls.

Venules are small vessels that merge with capillaries. In essence, they form a continuous conduit that drains blood from capillaries into veins (Fig. 11-6; Table 11-2). Blood flows through this circuit:

heart → aorta → arteries → arterioles → capillaries → venules → veins → superior and inferior venae cavae → heart

Capillaries are structures that connect arterioles and venules (Fig. 11-7). The capillary network allows for the exchange of microscopic molecules between blood and tissue fluid. They have an extensive branching network so that rapid exchange of materials can occur nearly everywhere throughout the body. Capillaries contain only the tunica intima and are not capable of constricting or dilating. Structures called **precapillary sphincters** regulate blood flow to capillaries.

Key Terms	Definitions
tunica (TEW ni kuh)	layer
tunica intima (TEW ni kuh IN ti muh)	inner layer; tunica interna
tunica media (TEW ni kuh MEE dee uh)	middle layer

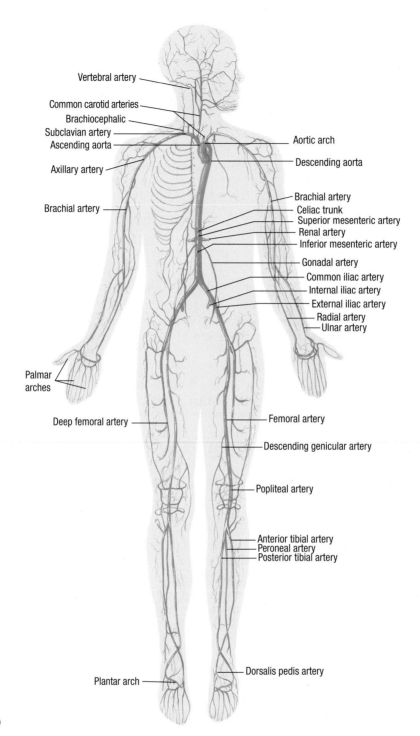

Vertebral artery

Common carotid arteries

Brachiocephalic

Subclavian artery

Ascending aorta

Aortic arch

Descending aorta

Axillary artery

Brachial artery

Brachial artery

Celiac trunk

Superior mesenteric artery

Renal artery

Inferior mesenteric artery

Gonadal artery

Common iliac artery

Internal iliac artery

External iliac artery

Radial artery

Ulnar artery

Palmar arches

Deep femoral artery

Femoral artery

Descending genicular artery

Popliteal artery

Anterior tibial artery

Peroneal artery

Posterior tibial artery

Dorsalis pedis artery

Plantar arch

FIGURE 11-4
The common arteries.
(Image provided by
Anatomical Chart Co.)

TABLE 11-1 Common Systemic Arteries

Common Systemic Arteries	Pronunciations
Cervical Region	
left and right common carotid	ka ROT id
vertebral	VUR te brul
Thoracic and Abdominopelvic Regions	
brachiocephalic trunk	bray kee oh se FAL ick
left and right brachiocephalic	bray kee oh se FAL ick
left and right subclavian	sub KLAY vee un
left and right axillary	ACK si lerr ee
ascending aorta	ay OR tuh
aortic arch	ay OR tick
descending aorta	ay OR tuh
celiac trunk	SEE lee ack
left and right renal	REE nul
superior mesenteric	mez un TERR ick
left and right gonadal	goh NAD ul
inferior mesenteric	mez un TERR ick
left and right common iliac	IL ee ack
left and right internal iliac	IL ee ack
left and right external iliac	IL ee ack
Arms	
left and right radial	RAY dee ul
left and right ulnar	UL nur
left and right palmar arches	PAL mur
Legs	
left and right deep femoral	FEM uh rul
left and right femoral	FEM uh rul
left and right popliteal	pop li TEE ul
left and right peroneal	perr oh NEE ul
left and right posterior tibial	TIB ee ul
left and right anterior tibial	TIB ee ul
left and right dorsalis pedis (top of foot)	dor SAY lis PE dis
left and right plantar arch (bottom of foot)	PLAN tahr

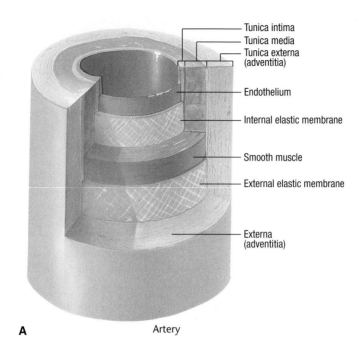

Tunica intima
Tunica media
Tunica externa
(adventitia)

Endothelium

Internal elastic membrane

Smooth muscle

External elastic membrane

Externa
(adventitia)

A Artery

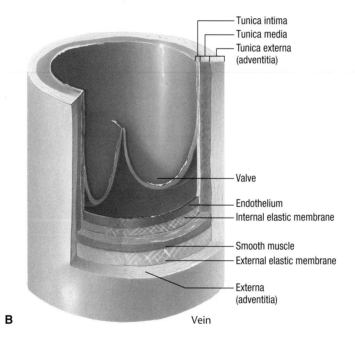

Tunica intima
Tunica media
Tunica externa
(adventitia)

Valve

Endothelium
Internal elastic membrane

Smooth muscle
External elastic membrane

Externa
(adventitia)

B Vein

FIGURE 11-5
(A) The artery wall in cross section. **(B)** The vein wall and valve in cross section. (Images provided by Anatomical Chart Co.)

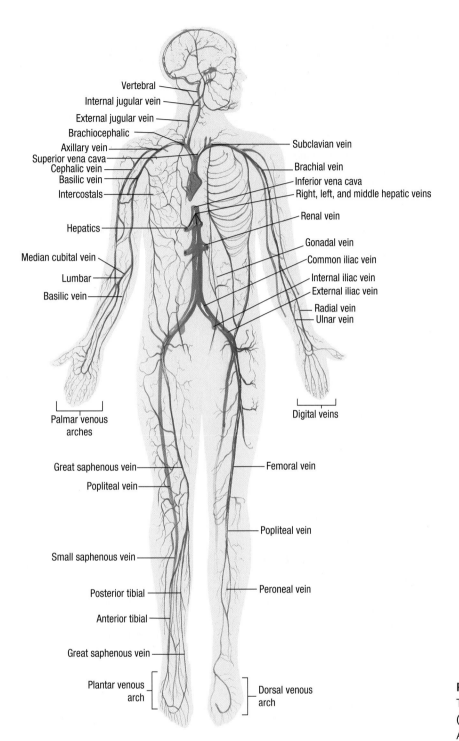

Vertebral
Internal jugular vein
External jugular vein
Brachiocephalic
Axillary vein
Superior vena cava
Cephalic vein
Basilic vein
Intercostals
Hepatics
Median cubital vein
Lumbar
Basilic vein
Palmar venous arches

Subclavian vein
Brachial vein
Inferior vena cava
Right, left, and middle hepatic veins
Renal vein
Gonadal vein
Common iliac vein
Internal iliac vein
External iliac vein
Radial vein
Ulnar vein
Digital veins

Great saphenous vein
Popliteal vein
Small saphenous vein
Posterior tibial
Anterior tibial
Great saphenous vein
Plantar venous arch

Femoral vein
Popliteal vein
Peroneal vein
Dorsal venous arch

FIGURE 11-6
The common veins.
(Image provided by
Anatomical Chart Co.)

TABLE 11-2 Common Systemic Veins

Common Systemic Veins	Pronunciations
Cervical Region	
left and right external jugular	JUG yoo lur
left and right internal jugular	JUG yoo lur
left and right vertebral	VUR te brul
Thoracic and Abdominopelvic Regions	
left and right brachiocephalic	bray kee oh se FAL ick
left and right subclavian	sub KLAY vee un
left and right axillary	ACK si lerr ee
superior vena cava	VEE nuh KAY vuh
intercostals	in tur KOS tulz
hepatics	he PAT icks
inferior vena cava	VEE nuh KAY vuh
left and right renal	REE nul
left and right gonadal	goh NAD ul
left and right lumbar	LUM bahr
left and right common iliac	IL ee ack
left and right internal iliac	IL ee ack
left and right external iliac	IL ee ack
Arms	
left and right cephalic	se FAL ick
left and right basilic	ba SIL ick
left and right median cubital	KEW bi tul
left and right radial	RAY dee ul
left and right median antebrachial	an te BRAY kee ul
left and right ulnar	UL nur
left and right palmar venous arches	PAL mur VEE nus
left and right digital veins	DIJ i tul
Legs	
left and right deep femoral	FEM uh rul
left and right great saphenous	SAF e nus
left and right femoral	FEM uh rul
left and right peroneal	perr oh NEE ul
left and right popliteal	pop li TEE ul
left and right small saphenous	SAF e nus
left and right posterior tibial	TIB ee ul
left and right anterior tibial	TIB ee ul
left and right dorsal venous arch (top of foot)	DOR sul VEE nus
left and right plantar venous arch (bottom of foot)	PLAN tahr VEE nus

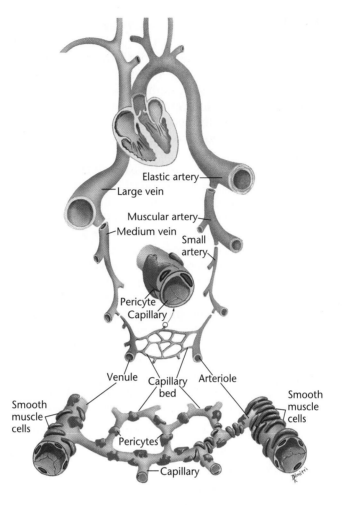

FIGURE 11-7
The capillary network allows for the exchange of molecules between the blood and the tissue fluid. (Reprinted with permission from Rubin E, Farber JL. Pathology. 3rd ed. Philadelphia: Lippincott Williams & Wilkins, 1999.)

tunica externa (TEW ni kuh ecks TUR nuh)	outer layer; tunica adventitia
anastomosis (uh nas toh MOH sis)	intermingling of vessels that grow to bypass an obstruction
arterioles (ahr TEER ee ohlz)	smallest branches of arteries
venules (VEN yoolz)	smallest branches of veins
precapillary sphincters (pree KAP i lerr ee SFINK turz)	structures between capillaries and arterioles that regulate blood flow to capillaries

Key Term Practice: Vasculature

1. What are the three anatomic layers of an artery?

   a. _____

   b. _____

   c. _____

2. The smallest arteries are termed _____.

3. What is the singular form of anastomoses? _____

4. Small veins are termed _____.

Cardiac Blood Flow Pattern

The heart is situated between the lungs to provide ease of access to gas exchange. Blood traveling throughout the systemic circulation releases its oxygen supply along the route. This low-oxygen, high–carbon dioxide blood enters the right side of the heart through the **superior vena cava** and **inferior vena cava** (pl., vena cavae) and **coronary sinus** and is immediately pumped into the **right and left pulmonary arteries,** which transport blood to the right and left lungs. In the lungs, the supply of oxygen is replenished, and the accumulated carbon dioxide is exhaled. The newly oxygenated blood then returns to the left heart via the **right and left pulmonary veins.**

When considering the heart muscle, it is helpful to remember that the left myocardium is thicker because it pumps blood systemically; greater muscle mass is needed to pump oxygenated blood to all parts of the body. The right side of the heart is pumping deoxygenated blood just a short distance to the lungs; therefore, the myocardium on this side is thinner.

Most veins carry deoxygenated blood, and most arteries transport oxygenated blood in the body. However, the pulmonary artery and vein are different: the pulmonary vein carries oxygenated blood, and the pulmonary artery carries deoxygenated blood. If the pathway of blood through the heart is considered, this makes sense because blood enters the lungs through the pulmonary artery to become oxygen rich and exits with oxyhemoglobin through the pulmonary vein. Keep in mind that arteries carry blood away from the heart, while veins carry blood to the heart. Therefore, the pulmonary artery leaves the heart, and the pulmonary vein enters the heart.

The unidirectional passageway of blood through the heart is maintained through the action of the valves (Fig. 11-8). The path is as follows:

1. Inferior vena cava, superior vena cava, and coronary sinus
2. Right atrium
3. Tricuspid valve
4. Right ventricle
5. Pulmonary semilunar valve
6. Right and left pulmonary arteries
7. Right and left lungs
8. Right and left pulmonary veins
9. Left atrium
10. Bicuspid valve
11. Left ventricle

FIGURE 11-8
The unidirectional passage of blood through the heart is maintained by the action of the valves. (Image provided by Anatomical Chart Co.)

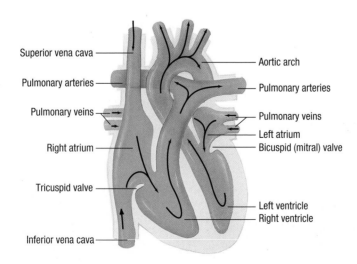

12. Aortic semilunar valve.

13. Aorta.

14. Systemic circulation.

15. Superior vena cava, inferior vena cava, and coronary sinus.

Key Terms	Definitions
superior vena cava (VEE nuh KAY vuh)	vein emptying the blood from the upper (superior) portion of the body into right atrium
inferior vena cava (VEE nuh KAY vuh)	vein emptying the blood from the lower (inferior) portion of the body into right atrium
coronary (KOR uh nerr ee) **sinus**	channel draining the coronary veins into the right atrium
right and left pulmonary (PUL muh nerr ee) **arteries**	vessels that transport blood from the heart to the lungs
right and left pulmonary (PUL muh nerr ee) **veins**	vessels that transport blood from the lungs to the heart

Key Term Practice: Cardiac Blood Flow Pattern

1. What is the plural form of each given term?

   a. vena = _____

   b. cava = _____

Coronary Circulation

The word *corona* means "crown," and the coronary arteries encircle the heart exterior like a crown, supplying the myocardium with blood for nourishment. **Coronary circulation** involves those arteries and veins that supply the heart itself with blood (Fig. 11-9). The deoxygenated blood is returned to the right atrium via the great cardiac vein or the coronary sinus. If blood flow to the heart is chronically interrupted, collateral circulation can develop over time. This formation of new blood vessels is termed **angiogenesis;** new blood vessel development can also occur elsewhere within the body's vascular system.

The right and left coronary arteries, which are the first two branches off the aorta, supply the heart. The **right coronary artery** supplies blood to the right atrium, part of the left atrium, most of the right ventricle, and a portion of the left ventricle. The **left coronary artery** branches into the circumflex artery and the anterior interventricular artery. The **circumflex artery**, which follows the atrioventricular sulcus (superficial groove), supplies blood to the walls of the left atrium and left ventricle.

Key Terms	Definitions
coronary (KOR uh nerr ee) **circulation**	blood supply to the heart tissue
angiogenesis (an jee oh JEN e sis)	formation of new blood vessels
right coronary (KOR uh nerr ee) **artery**	artery supplying blood to the heart tissue

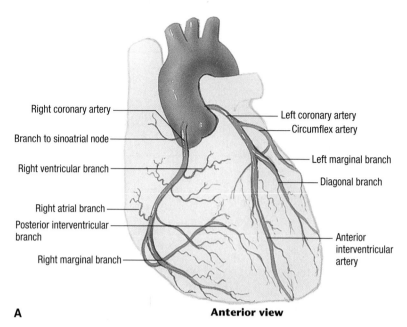

Anterior view

A

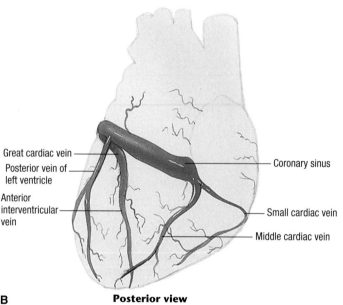

Posterior view

B

FIGURE 11-9
(A) The right and left coronary arteries supply the heart, anterior view. **(B)** The coronary veins, posterior view. (Images provided by Anatomical Chart Co.)

left coronary (KOR uh nerr ee) artery	vessel that branches into the circumflex artery and interventricular artery to supply blood to the heart tissue
circumflex (SUR kum flecks) artery	vessel that supplies blood to the left atrium and left ventricle

 ## Key Term Practice: Coronary Circulation

1. Heart tissue is supplied with oxygen-rich blood via the _____ circulation.

2. The formation of new blood vessels is termed _____.

Cardiac Conduction System

The **cardiac conduction system** involves initiating electrical impulses and conducting them through the entire heart to stimulate contractions (Fig. 11-10). The resulting series of myocardial contractions constitute a complete heartbeat, known as the cardiac cycle. Components of the conduction system include the sinoatrial (SA) node (pacemaker), atrioventricular node, atrioventricular bundle (bundle of His), and conduction myofibers (Purkinje fibers). A node is a circumscribed mass of conduction tissue. Heart impulses originate in the right atrium at the **sinoatrial node;** hence this structure is often referred to as the heart's pacemaker. Impulses then travel to the **atrioventricular node,** a structure in the right atrium near the coronary sinus, where they are delayed for about 0.1 second to allow the atria to contract before the ventricles contract. The stimulus then spreads to the **atrioventricular bundle.** The AV bundle is the only point in the heart where there is an electrical connection between the atria and the ventricles. The AV bundle then divides into two branches, called **right and left bundle branches**, that extend down the sides of the interventricular septum. The septum is the mass of myocardium that separates the ventricles. The **moderator band** is a fibrous right ventricle structure that carries the impulses from the right bundle branch to the papillary muscles of the right ventricle. Last, the **conduction myofibers** are specialized cardiocytes in the heart ventricles that stimulate contraction. These are some times referred to as Purkinje fibers, named after Czech physiologist Jan Purkinje.

During the cardiac cycle, the atrial walls contract while the ventricular walls relax; then as the ventricular walls contract, the atrial walls relax. At the end of each cycle, the atria and ventricles relax for a moment, and then a new cycle begins. The pathway is as follows:

SA node → AV node → right and left bundle branches → conduction myofibers

Cardiac muscle contraction is complicated. To review, think of contraction as depolarization or **systole**, and relaxation as repolarization or **diastole.** Diastole and systole are derived from the Greek language and mean "expansion" and "contraction," respectively. The word part *sy-* means "coming together"; during systole, the ventricular walls come together to contract. The word part *dia-* means "apart"; during diastole, the ventricle walls move apart and relax.

Cardiac tissues contract in much the same manner as other muscle tissue. A membrane at rest is polarized, meaning the interior of the muscle cell is slightly more negative than the cell's exterior. Acids donate protons, creating a negative environment. The amino acid carboxylic acid is the prime amino acid inside the cardiac cell, resulting in its negative charge. The membrane opens up when the neurotransmitter acetylcholine (Ach) is released, and positive sodium ions rush in because opposites

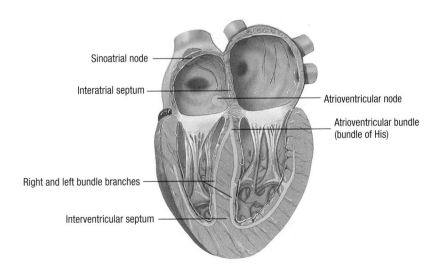

Sinoatrial node

Interatrial septum

Atrioventricular node

Atrioventricular bundle (bundle of His)

Right and left bundle branches

Interventricular septum

FIGURE 11-10

The heart initiates electrical impulses and conducts them through the heart walls to stimulate contractions. (Image provided by Anatomical Chart Co.)

attract. This event causes the sarcoplasmic reticulum to release calcium ions, resulting in muscle contraction, or depolarization. The heart has its own "nervous system" controlled by vagus (cranial nerve X) stimulation and norepinephrine. This cascade of events occurs in less than a half second.

Two ions that influence heart rate are potassium (K^+) and calcium (Ca^{2+}). Hyperkalemia (excessive potassium ions) decreases heart rate and contraction force, and hypokalemia (decreased blood levels of potassium ions) leads to rhythm abnormalities. Hypercalcemia (excessive extracellular calcium ions) increases heart rate and contraction force, and hypocalcemia (decreased levels of calcium ions) results in diminished cardiac function.

The heart exhibits **automaticity**, which is the ability of the cardiac cells to generate electrical impulses to stimulate myocardial contraction in the absence of neural or hormonal input. It is interesting that a heart removed from a living person will continue to beat for nearly 2 minutes as a result of automaticity.

Nervous system involvement in heart rate depends on sympathetic and parasympathetic stimulation. The medulla oblongata, a part of the brainstem, plays a role in increasing or decreasing heart rate and contraction strength. Providing sympathetic stimulation is the **cardioacceleratory center** (CAC), which increases the rate and strength of cardiac contraction; parasympathetic stimulation occurs through the **cardioinhibitory center** (CIC), which decreases heart rate and contraction strength.

> *FACT* *The average heart beats 36 million times per year—more if one exercises!*

Key Terms	Definitions
cardiac (KAHR dee ack) **conduction system**	the system of impulses that guide the heart to contract
sinoatrial (sigh noh AY tree ul) **node**	dense network of conducting fibers at the junction of the superior vena cava and the right atrium, where impulses originate
atrioventricular (ay tree oh ven TRICK yoo lur) **node**	network that divides into two branches
atrioventricular (ay tree oh ven TRICK yoo lur) **bundle**	arises from the atrioventricular node and divides to transmit impulses to the ventricle muscle fibers; bundle of His
right and left bundle branches	conduction fibers that originate at the atrioventricular bundle and separate along the interventricular septum
moderator band	fibrous structure spanning the right ventricle that carries impulses into the papillary muscles
conduction myofibers (migh oh FIGH burz)	heart cells that form the terminal portion of the conducting system that stimulates heart contraction; Purkinje fibers
systole (SIS toh lee)	contraction of the heart
diastole (dye AS toh lee)	relaxation of the heart
automaticity (aw toh muh TISS i tee)	ability to contract without neural stimulation
cardioacceleratory (kahr dee oh ack SEL ur uh tor ee) **center**	sympathetic nervous system area in the brain that quickens the heart rate and strength of contraction
cardioinhibitory (kahr dee oh in HIB i tor ee) **center**	parasympathetic nervous system area in the brain that slows the heart rate and strength of contraction

Key Term Practice: Cardiac Conduction System

1. What is the medical term for each given eponym?

   a. bundle of His _____

   b. Purkinje fibers _____

2. The parasympathetic area that slows heart rate is the _____ center.

Circulatory Routes

Circulatory routes are paths through which blood flows from various organs to the heart. Important circulatory routes of the body are the pulmonary, systemic, and hepatic portal. The **pulmonary circuit** transports deoxygenated blood from the right ventricle to the lungs, where the blood picks up oxygen, and then returns oxygenated blood from the lungs to the left atrium (Fig. 11-11). The **systemic circuit** takes oxygenated blood from the left ventricle to the aorta, which divides into branches that distribute the blood to the rest of the body (Fig 11-12). The **hepatic portal system** collects blood from the pancreas, spleen, stomach, intestines, and gallbladder and transports it to the liver (Fig. 11-13). The word part *hepat-* refers to the "liver," and the Latin word *portare* means "to carry." Consequently, *hepatic portal* refers to "blood being carried to the liver." The liver then uses nutrients and detoxifies the blood before returning it to the heart via the inferior vena cava.

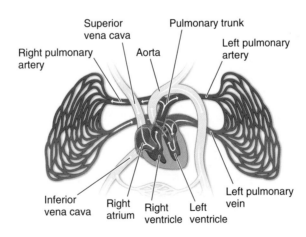

FIGURE 11-11
The pulmonary circuit transports deoxygenated blood from the right ventricle to the lungs (where the blood is oxygenated), and then returns the blood from the lungs to the left atrium.

Key Terms	Definitions
pulmonary (PUL muh nerr ee) **circuit**	circulation of the blood through the lungs via the pulmonary arteries and veins
systemic (sis TEM ick) **circuit**	general circulatory route of the blood throughout the body
hepatic portal (he PAT ick POR tul) **system**	circulation of the blood from the gastrointestinal tract to the liver

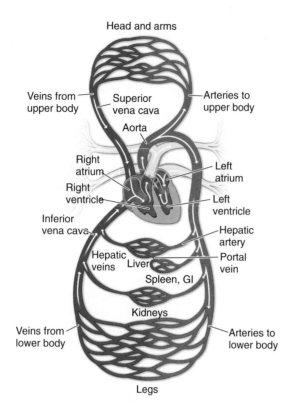

FIGURE 11-12
The systemic circuit takes oxygenated blood from the left ventricle to the aorta, which divides into branches that distribute the blood to the rest of the body.

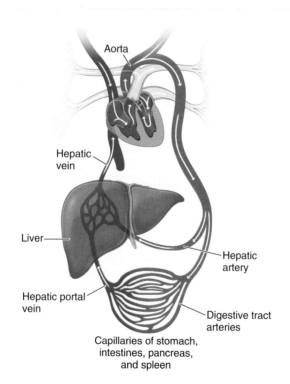

FIGURE 11-13
The hepatic portal system collects blood from the pancreas, spleen, stomach, intestines, and gallbladder and transports it to the liver, where the blood is detoxified before being returned to the heart.

Key Term Practice: Circulatory Routes

1. Circulation of blood through the lungs is termed the _____ circuit.

2. Circulation of blood throughout the body is termed the _____ circuit.

Blood Pressure

Blood pressure (BP) is the force exerted against the arterial walls by the blood. The device used to measure blood pressure is called a **sphygmomanometer.** This instrument has an inflatable cuff, bulb, and gauge that measure pressure in millimeters of mercury, abbreviated mm Hg. The word part *sphygmo-* means "pulse"; thus, this "blood pressure cuff" is an instrument that measures pulsating blood. The measurement indicates the pressure on the arterial wall at the highest and lowest pressures: when the ventricle undergoes systole and diastole. It is written as systolic pressure over diastolic pressure. **Systolic blood pressure** (the top number) represents contraction pressure and **diastolic blood pressure** (the bottom number) represents relaxation or recoil pressure. Associate the *d* in *down* with the *d* in *d*iastolic to remember that diastolic pressure is the number on bottom. A typical blood pressure is 120/80 mm Hg, and optimal blood pressure to reduce the risk of heart disease is lower than 120/80 mm Hg. The 120 represents systolic pressure in millimeters of mercury, and the 80 is the diastolic pressure.

The expansion of an artery with each heartbeat is termed **pulse.** It can be detected by palpating the superficial arteries. Two commonly used pulse points are the common carotid artery in the neck and the radial artery in the wrist. **Pulse pressure** is the difference between systolic and diastolic pressures and provides information about the status of the cardiovascular system. Pulse pressure is increased in conditions such as atherosclerosis. For example, if the blood pressure is 130/80 mm Hg, the pulse pressure is 130 minus 80, which equals 50.

Factors affecting blood pressure are numerous and include chemicals, temperature, emotions, age, sex, and cardiac centers of the autonomic nervous system. Pulse and blood pressure, along with temperature and breathing rate, are **vital signs** directly related to the cardiovascular system. *Vital* refers to "life," and these are objective measures of key parameters in the body.

Listening to sounds made by internal organs, especially the heart and lungs, is called auscultation, and the instrument that enables it is termed a **stethoscope.** The word comes from the Greek *stethos* meaning "chest" and *skopein* meaning "to examine." There are four sounds generated with each cardiac cycle, but in a normal, healthy adult, only the first two, symbolized S1 and S2, are regularly heard. The first typical sound, *lubb,* is produced by the contraction (systole) of ventricles; the second softer sound, *dubb,* is marked by the beginning of ventricular relax (diastole). Both sounds represent the closing of heart valves.

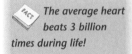

The average heart beats 3 billion times during life!

Key Terms	Definitions
blood pressure	pressure exerted by the circulating blood on the arterial walls
sphygmomanometer (sfig mom muh NOM e tur)	instrument used to measure blood pressure
systolic (sis TOL ick) blood pressure	arterial blood pressure during ventricular contraction

diastolic (dye us TOL ick) **blood pressure**	arterial blood pressure during ventricular relaxation
pulse	palpable thrust of an artery with each heartbeat
pulse pressure	the difference between the systolic and the diastolic blood pressures
vital signs	objective measures of key body parameters, such as temperature, breathing rate, pulse, and blood pressure
stethoscope (STETH uh skope)	instrument used to hear sounds within the body

Key Term Practice: Blood Pressure

1. What is the pulse pressure when the BP is 90/60 mm Hg?

   _____

2. What is the medical term for the instrument that measures blood pressure using a pressure cuff?

   _____

THE CLINICAL DIMENSION

Pathology of the Cardiovascular System

Pathology of the cardiovascular system falls into several broad categories. Many primary diseases have a genetic component or are the result of lifestyle factors. Viral and bacterial infections are implicated in several secondary CV disorders, and congenital diseases are those that are present at birth. Fortunately, a number of treatments are available for the numerous pathologic conditions.

Congenital Heart Defects

Congenital heart defects are conditions present at birth, and congenital vascular disorders are not as common as heart defects. Congenital narrowing of the aorta is termed **aortic coarctation** (Fig. 11-14). It is usually located distal to the subclavian artery and

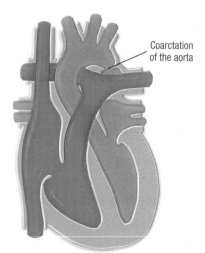

Coarctation
of the aorta

FIGURE 11-14
Aortic coarctation is a congenital narrowing of the aorta. (Image provided by Anatomical Chart Co.)

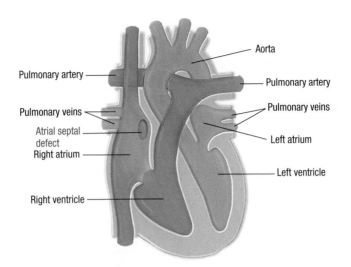

Aorta
Pulmonary artery
Pulmonary artery
Pulmonary veins
Pulmonary veins
Atrial septal defect
Left atrium
Right atrium
Left ventricle
Right ventricle

FIGURE 11-15
An atrial septal defect is an opening in the septum between the atria, causing blood to shunt from the left atrium to the right atrium. (Image provided by Anatomical Chart Co.)

results in upper extremity hypertension (high blood pressure), excessive left ventricular workload, and diminished blood supply to the abdominal organs and lower extremities. The newborn will present with symptoms of congestive heart failure (described later in this chapter) and hypotension (low blood pressure). Older children exhibit upper extremity hypertension. Aortic coarctation is diagnosed by chest x-ray, echocardiogram, and magnetic resonance imaging (MRI) if the previous two are inconclusive.

An **echocardiogram** is a pictorial representation of the heart using ultrasound. Infants younger than 1 year are treated by **aortoplasty** (surgical repair of the aorta); those older than 1 year require aortic resection with anastomosis or enlargement of constricted area using a prosthetic patch.

Atrial septal defect is an opening in the septum between the atria, causing blood to shunt from the left atrium to the right atrium (Fig. 11-15). (The pressure in the left atrium is slightly greater than pressure in the right, so blood flows from high to low.) The right side of the heart becomes overloaded and hypertrophies in response to the greater blood volume.

The condition in which the fetal ductus arteriosus (an opening between the aorta and pulmonary artery) persists after birth is termed **patent ductus arteriosus** (PDA) (Fig. 11-16). *Patent* means "open or exposed." Thus oxygenated blood is pushed back to the lungs. Symptoms include thrill on palpation and signs of congestive heart failure. A **thrill** is a palpable vibration created by turbulent blood flow. The alternate term for thrill is **fremitus.** These vibrations feel like the throat of a purring cat. If the PDA is small, the individual may be asymptomatic. Chest x-ray, abnormal ECG, and echocardiogram are used to make the diagnosis.

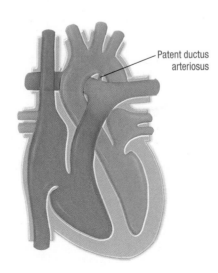

Patent ductus arteriosus

FIGURE 11-16
Patent ductus arteriosus is a condition in which the opening between the aorta and the pulmonary artery persists after birth. (Image provided by Anatomical Chart Co.)

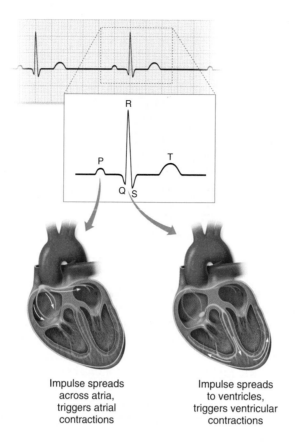

FIGURE 11-17
Correlation of the ECG and the contractions of the heart.

Impulse spreads across atria, triggers atrial contractions

Impulse spreads to ventricles, triggers ventricular contractions

The **electrocardiogram** is an electrical recording of the heart's electrical system on a moving strip of paper. It detects and records electrical potential during contraction. (As noted earlier in this chapter, sometimes electrocardiogram is abbreviated as EKG, which stems from the Greek word *kardia* for "heart.") The letters *P, QRS,* and *T,* are used to represent the record of heart activity. Graphical representation resembles peaks, valleys, dips, and humps (Fig. 11-17). The **P wave** represents atrial contraction and the **QRS complex** demonstrates ventricular contraction. The Q indicates downward deflection, R is upward reflection, and S is downward reflection after the R wave. Atrial relaxation occurs at the same time as ventricular contraction, but it cannot be seen on the ECG because the QRS complex is a bigger event that masks it. The **T wave** shows ventricular relaxation.

As its name suggests, the congenital condition called **tetralogy of Fallot** (*tetra-* = "four") is a complex of four heart defects (Fig. 11-18). These are pulmonary stenosis,

FIGURE 11-18
Tetralogy of Fallot consists of four congenital heart defects: pulmonary stenosis, an opening in the interventricular septum, malposition of the aorta over both ventricles, and right ventricular stenosis. (Image provided by Anatomical Chart Co.)

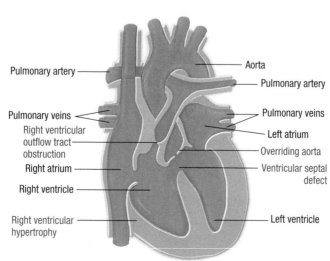

Pulmonary artery

Pulmonary veins

Right ventricular outflow tract obstruction

Right atrium

Right ventricle

Right ventricular hypertrophy

Aorta

Pulmonary artery

Pulmonary veins

Left atrium

Overriding aorta

Ventricular septal defect

Left ventricle

an opening in the interventricular septum, malposition of the aorta over both ventricles, and right ventricular hypertrophy. The abnormally positioned aorta overlaps the ventricular septum, causing it to receive venous as well as arterial blood and leading to cyanosis. Signs and symptoms are **dyspnea** (difficulty breathing or shortness of breath), cyanosis, and restlessness. Chest x-rays reveal the abnormality, and an ECG indicates right ventricular hypertrophy. Treatment involves a patch closure of the septal defect and a resection at the stenosis.

Ventricular septal defect occurs when there is an opening between the two ventricles that allows blood to shuttle back and forth. If the hole does not close, there is risk of right heart failure or left heart failure. A chest x-ray or ECG is used for diagnosis. Treatment includes a patch closure using synthetic material, and cardiopulmonary bypass is necessary during this procedure. Cardiopulmonary bypass involves the use of a **heart–lung machine**, a device in which a pump serves as the heart and a blood oxygenator (artificial lung) provides extracorporal (outside the body) blood circulation during some types of cardiac surgery (Fig. 11-19).

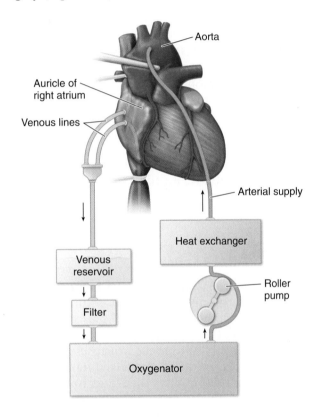

FIGURE 11-19
A heart–lung machine uses a pump that serves both as the heart and as the lungs to provide blood circulation outside the body during cardiac surgery.

Key Terms	Definitions
aortic coarctation (AY or tick koh ark TAY shun)	congenital narrowing of the aorta
echocardiogram (eck oh KAHR dee oh gram)	image of the heart produced by ultrasound
aortoplasty (ay or toh PLAS tee)	surgical repair of the aorta
atrial septal (AY tree ul SEP tul) **defect**	abnormal opening between the atria, allowing blood to shunt back and forth
patent ductus arteriosus (PAT unt DUCK tus ahr teer ee OH sus)	the ductus arteriosus remains open after birth, allowing oxygenated blood back into the lungs
thrill	palpable vibration; fremitus
fremitus (FREM i tus)	palpable vibration; thrill

electrocardiogram (ee leck troh KAHR dee oh gram)	record of the electrical forces producing heart contractions
P wave	section of the ECG showing atria depolarization
QRS complex	section of the ECG showing the duration of ventricular depolarization
T wave	section of the ECG showing ventricular repolarization
tetralogy (te TRAL oh jee) **of Fallot** (fahl OH)	four congenital heart defects appearing together
dyspnea (disp NEE uh)	difficulty breathing or shortness of breath
ventricular septal (ven TRICK yoo lur SEP tul) **defect**	abnormal opening between the ventricles, allowing blood to shunt back and forth
heart–lung machine	device that serves as artificial lungs and heart during some cardiac procedures

Key Term Practice: Congenital Heart Defects

1. Four congenital heart defects—pulmonary stenosis, ventricular septal defect, abnormal aorta positioning, and ventricular hypertrophy—describe this condition.

   _____

2. An opening between the two atria that allows blood to pass back and forth is termed _____; and a similar opening between the ventricles is called _____.

Coronary Artery Disease

Coronary artery disease (CAD) is a condition in which the myocardium receives inadequate blood supply as a result of atherosclerosis, coronary artery spasm, thrombi, or emboli. It is usually caused by **plaque** (accumulation of lipids) on the arterial **lumen**, the space inside the vessel (Fig. 11-20). Hardening of the arteries causing loss of elasticity is termed **arteriosclerosis**, and atherosclerosis represents a major type. Arteriosclerosis characterized by lipid deposition on the tunica intima of large- and medium-size arteries that leads to lumen narrowing, fibrosis, and calcification is

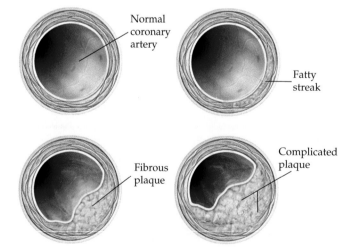

FIGURE 11-20
Coronary artery disease is usually caused by plaque on the arterial lumen. (Image provided by Anatomical Chart Co.)

termed **atherosclerosis.** The word part *athero-* means "fatty or lipid deposit." Treatments of many forms of CAD involve atherectomy or endarterectomy. An **atherectomy** is the surgical removal of an atheroma in an artery, and **endarterectomy** is the surgical excision of atheromatous deposits along with diseased endothelium and significant portions of the arterial lining. The removal results in a smooth lining consisting primarily of tunica externa.

Tests assessing coronary artery function are the exercise stress test and cardiac catheterization. The **exercise stress test** monitors heart rate, blood pressure, and ECG while the patient exercises. Abnormal results indicate coronary artery blockage. During a **cardiac catheterization** procedure, a long, flexible tube is inserted into cardiac vessels via a peripheral artery or vein. Images produced from the procedure can isolate vessel blockage.

CAD has a gradual onset, and early signs and symptoms include ischemia, nausea, and weakness. Advanced signs such as **angina pectoris**—pain in the chest (pectoral region) that radiates to the left shoulder—may not even occur until there is 75% occlusion in a vessel. Angina pectoris is caused by localized **ischemia**, inadequate blood and oxygen supply to heart tissue. Risk factors for CAD are elevated levels of low-density lipoproteins (LDLs), fat and protein molecules that transport cholesterol to cells and tissues; decreased levels of high-density lipoproteins (HDLs), fat and protein molecules that carry cholesterol away from arteries; sedentary lifestyle; and genetic predisposition (hereditary factors that make one more susceptible to disease onset). As a memory tool, think of *H*DLs as *h*ealthy and *h*elpful and *L*DLs are *l*ousy and *l*ethal.

A stress test, thallium scan, cardiac catheterization, ECG, Holter monitor ECG, or angiogram helps make the diagnosis. The **thallium scan** diagnoses coronary artery disease through the use of a radioactive isotope of thallium. Thallium is given via an intravenous drip, and the patient undergoes a physical stress test. The isotope collects in areas of poor circulation and can be seen as an image on the scanner. An **angiogram** is a radiographic visualization of blood vessels after introduction of a radiopaque dye into the bloodstream. The dye enables the vessels to be "mapped."

A **Holter monitor** is a small, portable ECG device that is worn continuously around the neck for 24 hours to record heart activity over an extended time period. During this time, the patient records symptoms and activities in a diary. The resulting graph reflects heart activity under a variety of situations in which the person normally engages.

CAD can be treated with drugs or surgery. Drug therapy includes administration of **vasodilators,** agents that cause blood vessel dilation (expansion) and relaxation. Angioplasty, percutaneous transluminal coronary angioplasty (PTCA), and coronary artery bypass graft (CABG) surgery are invasive options. **Angioplasty** is the reconstructive surgery of diseased vessels. **Percutaneous transluminal coronary angioplasty** is a procedure in which a catheter (cath) is guided into the coronary arteries. Once the catheter is inserted, a balloon catheter is threaded through it and positioned at the occlusion. The balloon is then inflated, expanding the artery and restoring blood flow. **Coronary artery bypass graft surgery** is an operation that creates a detour around obstructions in the coronary vessels. A heart-healthy diet, consisting of low fat and low salt intake, and physical exercise are therapeutic.

> *FACT* *An average blood cell travels about 9 miles per day throughout the body's vasculature!*

Key Terms	Definitions
coronary (KOR uh nerr ee) **artery disease**	condition in which the myocardium receives inadequate blood supply
plaque (PLACK)	lipid deposition on the arterial wall
lumen (LEW min)	space inside the tubular artery
arteriosclerosis (ahr teer ee oh skle ROH sis)	hardening of the arteries

atherosclerosis (ath ur oh skle ROH sis)	plaque formation on the inner arterial wall
atherectomy (ath eh RECK toh mee)	surgical removal of an atheroma in an artery
endoarterectomy (end ahr terr ECK toh mee)	atherectomy that includes removal of diseased endothelium and portions of the arterial linings, leaving a smooth tunica externa
exercise stress test	determines heart rate, blood pressure, and ECG while exercising
cardiac catheterization (KAHR dee ack kath e tur i ZAY shun)	procedure in which a flexible tube is inserted into the coronary vessels via a peripheral artery or vein for imaging purposes
angina pectoris (an JYE nuh PECK to ris)	radiating chest pain
ischemia (is KEE mee uh)	inadequate supply of blood to tissue caused by arterial blockage
thallium (THAL ee um) **scan**	uses radioactive thallium to assess coronary artery disease
angiogram (AN jee oh gram)	radiograph of the blood vessels after injecting a dye into the bloodstream
Holter monitor	ambulatory device for recording ECG over an extended time period
vasodilators (vay zoh dye LAY turz)	drugs that widen blood vessels, decreasing blood flow resistance and blood pressure
angioplasty (AN jee oh plas tee)	reconstructive surgery of diseased vessels
percutaneous transluminal coronary angioplasty (pur kew TAY nee us trans LEW mi nul KOR uh nerr ee AN jee oh plas tee)	procedure in which a balloon catheter is used to restore blood flow in a blocked vessel
coronary (KOR uh nerr ee) **artery bypass graft surgery**	surgically created arterial diversion around an occlusion

Key Term Practice: Coronary Artery Disease

1. Narrowing of the tunica intima, called _____, can lead to arterial wall inelasticity known as _____.

2. The medical term for lipid deposition on the arterial lumen is _____.

Heart Disorders

The cessation of normal, effective heart action is termed **cardiac arrest**. Underlying coronary heart disease that causes ventricular tachycardia and/or ventricular fibrillation usually causes it. **Tachycardia** is a rapid heart rate (more than 100 beats per minute) and **fibrillation** is irregular, uncoordinated, fast contractions. It is usually described as quivering because there are no full contractions. **Palpitation**, fluttering heart, is often associated with irregular rhythm or tachycardia. In some cases, **bradycardia** (heart rate less than 60 beats per minute) leads to cardiac arrest; other situations that can cause bradycardia include respiratory arrest, electrocution, drowning, choking, and trauma. It may also be idiopathic. The diagnosis is based on the absence of a palpable pulse, no respirations, bluish lips and pale skin, and an abnormal ECG.

Cardiopulmonary resuscitation (CPR) combined with cardiac defibrillation must be administered within minutes of the event to prevent death. **Cardiopulmonary resuscitation** is a life-saving procedure that consists of chest compressions that push the heart to stimulate blood flow, alternated with artificial respirations to keep the lungs oxygenated. **Defibrillation** is stopping an asynchronous heart contraction by application of an electrical current via a defibrillator. When defibrillation is provided within 5–7 minutes, the survival rate is approximately 49%. Cardiac drugs are also administered.

The condition called **heart block** occurs when the nerve impulses are abnormal, which results in asynchronous contraction of atria and ventricles. This conduction disturbance may be caused by drugs or by a disturbance of the heart's ability to conduct electrical impulses from the atria to the ventricles via the AV node. An artificial pacemaker may correct this problem. An **artificial pacemaker** is a permanent, battery-operated device that is surgically implanted into the chest wall. The artificial pacemaker assumes the role of the SA node, which is no longer properly regulating heart rate activity.

Cardiac tamponade is heart compression as the result of fluid accumulation in the pericardial sac. Causes include pericardial or myocardial blood vessel breakage. It results in decreased venous return, restricted heart filling, increased systemic pressure, and decreased cardiac output. Signs and symptoms are rapidly falling blood pressure, dyspnea, a weak and thready (lacking fullness) pulse, and decreased consciousness. The clinical picture and normal breath sounds that are accompanied by muffled heart sounds aid in the diagnosis. The sac requires immediate drainage via pericardiocentesis. **Pericardiocentesis** is an invasive procedure in which fluid is aspirated from the pericardial sac (Fig. 11-21). The procedure can also serve as a diagnostic tool because the aspirated fluid can be chemically analyzed for microbes. Surgery may be required to repair the rupture.

Disease of the myocardium is called **cardiomyopathy.** Cardiomyopathy is characterized by ventricular dysfunction and myocardium enlargement. It is diagnosed by the history and physical examination. Cardiomegaly (heart enlargement) is apparent on an echocardiogram, radionuclide scan, or transesophageal echocardiogram; and the ECG is abnormal. A **radionuclide scan** involves the injection of radioactive substances into the bloodstream. Computerized scanning isolates the radioisotope and forms images of the heart. In **transesophageal echocardiography** a combination endoscope/ultrasound

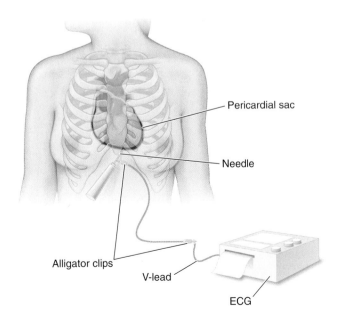

Pericardial sac

Needle

Alligator clips

V-lead

ECG

FIGURE 11-21
Pericardiocentesis is an invasive procedure in which fluid is aspirated from the pericardial sac.

probe is inserted into the esophagus to examine the nearby heart. Pulsating waves from the ultrasound probe create the picture. Three types of cardiomyopathy have been identified: dilated, hypertrophic, and restrictive (Fig. 11-22). Treatment involves the use of drugs to reduce the heart's workload, bedrest, and heart transplant.

Congestive heart failure (CHF) results when the heart cannot supply enough blood to meet the oxygen demands of the body. Blood remains in the heart because the muscle cannot pump it out fast enough, thereby causing an abnormal amount of blood in the veins. Causes include hypertension, CAD, chronic obstructive pulmonary disease (COPD; a progressive lung disease characterized by difficulty breathing), and cardiomyopathy. Common signs and symptoms include increased respiration rate to compensate for the loss of oxygen delivery, distended cervical veins, and edematous extremities, notably the ankles and feet. It is diagnosed by history, physical examination, echocardiogram, and the **aspartate aminotransferase** (AST) test. An alternate term for AST is serum **glutamic-oxaloacetic transaminase** (SGOT), and both terms are used interchangeably. AST (or SGOT) levels rise when congestive heart failure is the result of liver damage. Treatment involves diuretics, vasodilators, and digitalis. **Digitalis** is a drug that increases heart muscle contractility. Pharmacological agents that reduce total blood volume by causing increased urinary output are called **diuretics.**

Known as the "silent killer" because it is frequently asymptomatic, **hypertension** is blood pressure that is higher than normal range for the individual's age and sex. Recent guidelines consider an adult to be hypertensive if the resting blood pressure is consistently 140/90 mm Hg or higher. A resting blood pressure of 120/80 mm Hg is normal.

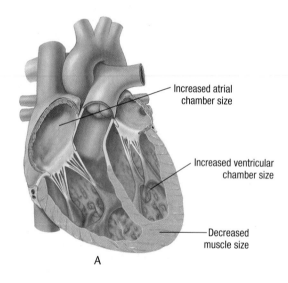

Increased atrial chamber size

Increased ventricular chamber size

Decreased muscle size

A

FIGURE 11-22

The three types of cardiomyopathy are (**A**) dilated, (**B**) hypertrophic, and (**C**) restrictive. (Images provided by Anatomical Chart Co.)

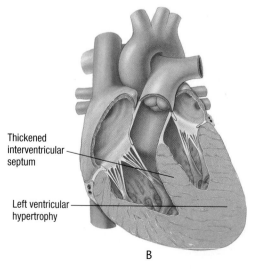

Thickened interventricular septum

Left ventricular hypertrophy

B

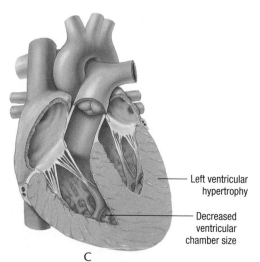

Left ventricular hypertrophy

Decreased ventricular chamber size

C

Key Term Practice: Heart Disorders Associated with the Lungs

1. Fluid filling the air sacs and interstitial tissue of the lung is called _____.

2. The disease characterized by right ventricular hypertrophy resulting from lung disease is termed _____.

Inflammation Disorders

Endocarditis is the inflammation of the endocardium. It is usually secondary to bacterial or fungal infection elsewhere in the body. Individuals with a history of rheumatic disease are at greater risk for endocarditis than the general population. Endocardial inflammation is characterized by growth on the valves that causes improper closure, which can be heard as a murmur. A **murmur** is the blowing or roaring sound heard on cardiac auscultation. Signs and symptoms include fever, chills, fatigue, and generalized weakness. Diagnosis is made through complete blood cell count (CBC); elevated erythrocyte sedimentation rate (ESR); blood cultures to identify the causative microorganism; and detection of **arrhythmia**, an abnormal cardiac rhythm that can result in flutter, fibrillation, or dysrhythmia. **Dysrhythmia** is an abnormality in heart rate, rhythm, or sequence of cardiac activation. Treating the underlying cause with antimicrobics is the first step. After recovery, prophylactic (preventing or helping prevent disease) antibiotics are prescribed to individuals undergoing procedures with risk of bacterial infection. For example, patients with a history of endocarditis take antibiotics before having dental work done.

Inflammation of the myocardium is called **myocarditis**. Its causes are varied and include microbial infection, toxin exposure, and chronic cocaine use. Fatigue, dyspnea, and arrhythmia are common signs and symptoms. Increased cardiac enzyme levels, increased white blood cell count, abnormal ECG, and cardiomegaly confirm the diagnosis. In some cases, a heart tissue biopsy is necessary. Treatment is aimed at managing the underlying cause and providing rest.

Pericarditis is an acute or chronic inflammation of the pericardium. It has varied causes, including bacterial or viral infection, trauma, and neoplastic disease; it may occur secondary to myocardial infarction. Fever, malaise, chest pain, and friction rub (sound resulting from rubbing of two serous surfaces) heard with a stethoscope are common signs and symptoms. Pericarditis is diagnosed through blood studies to determine the causative agent, ECG, and echocardiography. Bacterial cases are treated with antibiotics once the microbe has been identified, analgesics to control pain, and nonsteroidal anti-inflammatory drugs (NSAIDs) for inflammation.

Key Terms	Definitions
endocarditis (en doh kahr DYE tis)	inflammation of the endocardium
murmur	blowing or roaring heart sound
arrhythmia (uh RITH mee uh)	abnormal cardiac rhythm
dysrhythmia (dis RITH mee uh)	an irregularity in the normal heart rhythm
myocarditis (migh oh kahr DYE tis)	inflammation of the myocardium
pericarditis (perr i kahr DYE tis)	inflammation of the pericardium

Key Term Practice: Inflammation Disorders

1. Define the following word parts.

   a. endo- _____

   b. myo- _____

   c. peri- _____

   d. cardi- _____

   e. -itis _____

Shock

Shock results when blood flow to and perfusion of tissues is inadequate. There is reduced venous return to the heart, and the faulty deoxygenated blood return causes collapse (failure) of the cardiovascular system. It may result from inadequate blood volume (hypovolemic shock), inadequate cardiac function (cardiogenic shock), or vasomotor (affecting the blood vessel diameter) tone (neurogenic or septic shock). Signs and symptoms include hypotension, weak pulse, tachycardia, decreased urinary output, coldness, sweating, and irregular respirations. It is diagnosed by the clinical picture and must be treated immediately because it is life-threatening. The form determines the treatment options, but in all cases measures are taken to restore blood pressure and stimulate the heart to contract more forcefully.

Key Terms	Definitions
shock	condition resulting from defective venous return to the heart

Key Term Practice: Shock

1. Sudden collapse of the cardiovascular system is termed _____.

Valvular Heart Disease

Valvular heart diseases are acquired or congenital and cause improper functioning of heart valves. **Rheumatic heart disease** (RHD) is a delayed **sequela** (disorder caused by a preceding disease) of rheumatic fever. That is, RHD is a belated manifestation of rheumatic fever, an acute disease caused by streptococcal A infection. Signs and symptoms of rheumatic fever include fever, sore throat, joint swelling, and heart valve damage. It can be successfully treated with antibiotics. Valvular disturbances and inflammatory lesions in the heart, blood vessels, and joints characterize subsequent rheumatic heart disease. Carditis, arthritis, and skin rash may also be present. Rheumatic heart disease is diagnosed through history of rheumatic fever infection and elevated levels of cardiac enzymes. Surgical repair of damaged heart valves may be necessary.

Mitral insufficiency is also known as mitral incompetence or mitral regurgitation. It is characterized by incomplete closure of the bicuspid (mitral) valve during cardiac systole, thereby allowing blood to re-enter the atrium. A scarred valve that results from rheumatic fever often causes it. Signs and symptoms are fatigue, dyspnea, and heart murmur. Mitral insufficiency is diagnosed through the history, presence of a murmur, ECG, x-ray, or cardiac catheterization. It is treated with bedrest, oxygen therapy, antibiotics, and diuretics.

A benign (mild) condition in which the left atrioventricular flaps do not close properly is termed **mitral valve prolapse** (MVP). Most often it is a congenital disorder in which the chordae tendineae are too long or too short or there is malfunctioning of the papillary muscles. The prolapse (slippage of the valves from their usual position) causes blood regurgitation (backflow). There are usually no signs or symptoms because the volume of blood flowing in the opposite direction through the defective valve is not significant. Mitral valve prolapse is generally discovered during a routine stethoscope auscultation and can be detected at any age. The diagnosis is confirmed by presence of a heart murmur or echocardiogram evidence. Treatment is normally not required but may include avoidance of stimulants such as caffeine, nicotine, and decongestants, and administration of beta-blocker medications.

Mitral stenosis is a condition in which there is an obstruction of blood flow owing to a narrowed valve orifice. The primary cause is rheumatic heart disease. It appears that this is an autoimmune disorder because the antibodies formed after rheumatic fever infection continue to attack the heart tissue. Primary signs and symptoms are cough, dyspnea, and hemoptysis. The diagnosis is confirmed through the presence of a heart murmur and constriction shown by echocardiogram. Treatments include drugs to reduce the heart workload, anticoagulants, **commissurotomy** (surgical division of a stenosed valve), and valve replacement.

Key Terms	Definitions
rheumatic (roo MAT ick) **heart disease**	valvular disease of the heart as a result of rheumatic fever
sequela (se KWEL uh)	disorder caused by a previous disease
mitral (MIGH trul) **insufficiency**	incomplete closure of the bicuspid valve, causing backflow of blood into the atrium from the ventricle
mitral (MIGH trul) **valve prolapse**	improper closure of the bicuspid valve because of abnormal chordae tendineae or papillary muscle failure
mitral stenosis (MIGH trul ste NOH sis)	narrowed mitral valve opening that impedes blood flow
commissurotomy (com i shur OT oh mee)	surgical division of a heart valve

Key Term Practice: Valvular Heart Disease

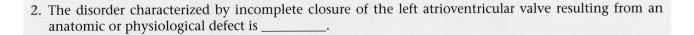

1. Which heart disease results from rheumatic fever infection?

   _____

2. The disorder characterized by incomplete closure of the left atrioventricular valve resulting from an anatomic or physiological defect is _____.

Vein and Artery Disorders

Peripheral vascular disease (PVD) describes progressive occlusions of small arteries and arterioles that supply the extremities. It is a common secondary condition in diabetes mellitus, and atherosclerosis is a primary risk factor. A **vascular murmur** is a finding that originates in blood vessels as a result of turbulent flow. Vascular murmurs create thrills and are common to an **arteriovenous fistula,** a surgically created connection directly between an artery and a vein without the interposition of capillaries. Vascular surgeons perform this procedure on hemodialysis patients to provide circulatory access. Naturally formed AV fistulas do occur, but they are abnormal conditions.

An **aneurysm** is a thin, weakened section of an arterial wall that bulges outward, forming a sac (Fig. 11-26). The localized, abnormal dilation usually progresses in size and causes a **bruit,** which is a swishing sound that results from turbulent blood flow. Medical professionals are taught the phrase "palpate a thrill and auscultate a bruit." The signs and symptoms of aneurysms may include pain, pressure at the site, and hemorrhage. Atherosclerotic plaque buildup causes them. Common sites are the

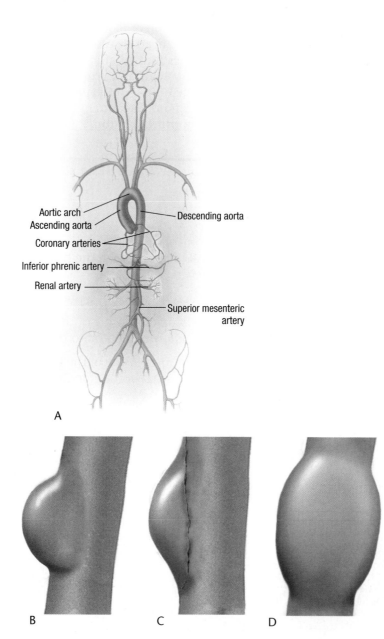

Aortic arch
Ascending aorta
Coronary arteries
Inferior phrenic artery
Renal artery
Descending aorta
Superior mesenteric artery

A

B C D

FIGURE 11-26
An aneurysm is a thin, weakened section of an arterial wall that bulges outward, forming a sac. **(A)** The common sites of aneurysms. The different types of aneurysms are **(B)** saccular, **(C)** dissecting, and **(D)** fusiform. (Images provided by Anatomical Chart Co.)

abdominal aorta between the renal arteries and iliac branches and the thoracic aorta (ascending, arch, or descending).

There are three classifications of aneurysms: saccular, fusiform, and dissecting. As its name suggests, a **saccular aneurysm** is a sac-like bulge on one side of an artery. A **fusiform aneurysm** is an elongated, spindle-shaped dilation of the arterial wall. A **dissecting aneurysm** is a splitting of the arterial wall (usually the intima) layers, creating a bulge between the layers. Dissecting aneurysms are created by blood forcing its way through a tear in the intima between the arterial layers. A **false aneurysm,** or pseudoaneurysm, mimics an aneurysm and is composed of fibrous tissue. A rupture of all arterial layers that causes a swelling in an artery creates a pseudoaneurysm. Hematomas are commonly the underlying cause of aneurysms, which are diagnosed by bruit presence and palpation. Radiographic, CT, and MRI studies reveal their presence. Surgical repair is the primary treatment.

Phlebitis is the term for vein inflammation. Its cause is unknown, and it typically affects lower leg regions. Injury, surgery, and obesity have been implicated as possible causative factors. Other instances include travelers who sit for prolonged periods without changing position, pregnant women, women who have just delivered babies, and smokers who take birth control pills. Pain and edema are frequent signs and symptoms. Phlebitis is diagnosed through the history, physical examination, and visual inspection.

Most cases of phlebitis are acute and resolve, using only analgesics to control pain. Massage is not recommended because this may stimulate either clot formation or emboli release. In elderly, overweight people, who have skin changes from chronic phlebitis, it is as difficult to get the underlying inflamed veins to heal as it is to get the chronically broken down skin (from chronic venous stasis changes) to heal. In some cases, treatment should include elevation of the limbs for improved drainage, antibiotics for underlying skin sepsis, and consideration of blood thinners.

Thrombophlebitis is vein inflammation associated with a thrombus. It is caused by venous stasis or injury affecting the tunica intima. A **deep-venous thrombosis** (DVT) refers to a blood clot in a deep vein. Signs and symptoms include pain, edema, and warmth in the affected area; however, sometimes the phlebitis is silent and the first clinical indication is swelling from the thrombosed veins. It is diagnosed by the clinical picture, physical examination, venography, or Doppler ultrasonography. **Venography** is an x-ray of the veins after injecting a contrast dye that shows up on x-rays; it provides a pictorial venogram or phlebogram. **Doppler ultrasound** is a noninvasive procedure for assessing blood flow velocity, direction, and occlusions. It uses a transducer, which is placed over the blood vessel, and a computer, which analyzes the echoes for aberrations.

The goal of therapy is to dissolve the clot. Anti-clotting agents, such as heparin, are used to dissolve underlying venous clots, and coumarin is used to prevent further clotting in the still-inflamed veins. Because the clot could break loose, migrate, and occlude a major vessel, immobilization of the affected part, along with heparin, is prescribed. Surgical intervention may be necessary.

Abnormal, dilated, **tortuous** (twisted, sinuous, wavy) veins resulting from interference with venous drainage are termed **varicose veins.** Vein wall weakness and defective vein valves, especially in the lower legs, can result in varicose veins. The causes include standing or sitting for prolonged periods allowing blood pooling and pregnancy that creates pressure on veins, thereby compromising blood flow. Leg cramps, pain, and edema are signs and symptoms. Visual inspection and the history lead to the diagnosis.

Treatment options are varied. Exercises, mobility during standing to assist with flow, vein ligation, stripping, and sclerosing solutions are possible medical therapies. The surgical tying off of a vein to close an area's blood supply is termed **vein ligation.** **Vein stripping** refers to removal of a vein after ligation. **Vein sclerosing** involves the introduction of a sclerosing solution that causes the vein to harden and eventually atrophy. After a ligation or sclerosing procedure, collateral circulation develops.

Thromboangiitis obliterans, also called Buerger disease, is thrombosis associated with vessel inflammation in peripheral arteries and veins of the extremities. It is caused by long-term tobacco use. The chief symptom is pain in affected areas and the feet that is aggravated by exercise and relieved by rest. It is diagnosed by the history, physical examination, and arteriography. Treatment involves smoking cessation and surgery in severe cases to create alternate pathways.

Raynaud phenomenon is characterized by intermittent episodes of pallor (pale appearance), cyanosis, or rubor (redness) of fingers and/or toes that is induced by cold or emotions. It is often secondary to or concomitant (existing along) with an autoimmune disease and is more common in women than men. Pain, numbness, and discoloration often occur with this disorder. The effects are the result of artery and arterioles that undergo spasm and constriction. A Raynaud's phenomenon episode resolves after application of warmth. Smoking aggravates the condition. Diagnosis is made by the clinical picture and visual inspection. Treatment involves use of warm compresses, smoking cessation, and avoidance of cold temperatures. Vasodilation therapy may be prescribed.

Key Terms	Definitions
peripheral vascular (pe RIF e rul VAS kew lur) **disease**	progressive disorder caused by occlusions of the small arteries and arterioles that supply the extremities
vascular (VAS kew lur) **murmur**	condition that originates in the blood vessels as a result of turbulent blood flow
arteriovenous fistula (ahr teer ee oh VEE nus FIS tew luh)	direct connection between an artery and a vein with no intervening capillaries
aneurysm (AN yoo riz um)	outward bulge in an artery
bruit (broo EE)	abnormal swishing sound, caused by turbulent blood flow, heard through a stethoscope
saccular aneurysm (SACK yoo lur AN yoo riz um)	sac-shaped outward bulge on an artery
fusiform aneurysm (FEW zi form AN yoo riz um)	spindle-shaped outpouching on an artery
dissecting aneurysm (AN yoo riz um)	bulge between the arterial walls
false aneurysm (AN yoo riz um)	rupture of the arterial walls, causing swelling
phlebitis (fle BYE tis)	vein inflammation
thrombophlebitis (throm boh fle BYE tis)	vein inflammation with thrombus
deep-venous thrombosis (throm BOH sis)	blood clot in a deep vein
venography (vee NOG ruh fee)	x-ray examination of the veins after injecting a dye that absorbs the x-rays
Doppler (DOP lur) **ultrasound**	ultrasound procedure providing images by computer analysis
tortuous (TOR choo us)	turning and bending
varicose (VAR i koce) **veins**	knotted, swollen veins
vein ligation (lye GAY shun)	surgical tying of a vein
vein stripping	surgical removal of a vein
vein sclerosing (skle ROCE ing)	surgical hardening of a vein

thromboangiitis obliterans (throm boh an jee EYE tis uh BLIT ur anz)	combined thrombosis and vessel inflammation
Raynaud (reh NOH) **phenomenon**	artery and arteriole spasms in the fingers and toes causing cold, numb, and painful digits

Key Term Practice: Vein and Artery Disorders

1. _____ is the medical term for vein inflammation.

2. _____ is the word used to describe vein inflammation with clot formation.

CLINICAL TERMS

Clinical Dimension	Term	Description
DISORDERS		
	aneurysm	abnormal, outward bulge on an artery
	aortic coarctation	congenital narrowing of the aorta
	arteriosclerosis	hardening of the arteries
	atherosclerosis	plaque formation on the inner arterial wall
	atrial septal defect	abnormal opening between the atria, allowing blood to shunt back and forth
	cardiac arrest	sudden stoppage of the heartbeat
	cardiac tamponade	heart compression caused by fluid accumulation in pericardial sac
	cardiomyopathy	disease of the heart muscle
	congestive heart failure (CHF)	disease in which the heart muscle cannot keep pace to provide the body with oxygenated blood
	coronary artery disease	condition in which the myocardium receives inadequate blood supply
	cor pulmonale	disease characterized by right ventricular hypertrophy caused by lung disease
	deep-venous thrombosis (DVT)	blood clot in a deep vein
	dissecting aneurysm	bulge between the arterial walls
	endocarditis	inflammation of the endocardium
	false aneurysm	rupture of arterial walls, causing swelling
	fusiform aneurysm	spindle-shaped outpouching on an artery
	heart block	condition caused by an impairment of the conduction system
	hypertension	chronic abnormally high blood pressure

Clinical Dimension	Term	Description
	malignant hypertension	severe high blood pressure of unknown cause
	myocardial infarction (MI)	heart tissue ischemia; heart attack
	mitral insufficiency	incomplete closure of the bicuspid valve, causing backflow of blood into the atrium from the ventricle
	mitral stenosis	narrowed mitral valve opening that impedes blood flow
	mitral valve prolapse (MVP)	improper closure of the bicuspid valve owing to abnormal chordae tendineae or papillary muscle failure
	myocarditis	inflammation of the myocardium
	patent ductus arteriosus	the ductus arteriosis remains open after birth, allowing oxygenated blood back into the lungs
	pericarditis	inflammation of the pericardium
	peripheral vascular disease (PVD)	progressive disorder caused by occlusions of the small arteries and arterioles that supply the extremities
	phlebitis	vein inflammation
	pulmonary edema	fluid leakage into the air sacs and lung tissue caused by left heart failure
	Raynaud phenomenon	artery and arteriole spasms in the fingers and toes, causing cold, numb, and painful digits
	rheumatic heart disease (RHD)	valvular disease of the heart as a result of rheumatic fever
	saccular aneurysm	sac-shaped outward bulge on an artery
	sequela	disorder caused by a previous disease
	shock	condition resulting from defective venous return to the heart
	tetralogy of Fallot	four congenital heart defects appearing together
	thromboangiitis obliterans	combined thrombosis and vessel inflammation
	thrombophlebitis	vein inflammation with thrombus
	varicose veins	knotted, swollen veins
	vascular murmur	condition that originates in the blood vessels as a result of turbulent flow
	ventricular septal defect	abnormal opening between the ventricles, allowing blood to shunt back and forth
SIGNS AND SYMPTOMS		
	angina pectoris	radiating chest pain
	arrhythmia	abnormal cardiac rhythm
	bradycardia	slow heart rate, below 60 beats per minute

Clinical Dimension	Term	Description
	bruit	abnormal swishing sound, caused by turbulent blood flow, heard through a stethoscope
	diaphoresis	profuse sweating
	dyspnea	difficulty breathing or shortness of breath
	dysrhythmia	an irregularity in the normal heart rhythm
	fibrillation	irregular, uncoordinated heart contractions
	fremitus	palpable vibration; thrill
	hemoptysis	bloody sputum
	ischemia	inadequate blood supply to tissue caused by arterial blockage
	murmur	blowing or roaring heart sound
	orthopnea	difficulty breathing except when sitting or standing straight
	palpitation	fluttering heart
	plaque	lipid deposition on the arterial wall
	syncope	loss of consciousness as a result of lack of oxygen to the brain
	tachycardia	rapid heart rate, above 100 beats per minute
	thrill	palpable vibration; fremitus
	tortuous	turning and bending
CLINICAL TESTS AND DIAGNOSTIC PROCEDURES		
	angiogram	radiograph of the blood vessels after injecting a dye into the bloodstream
	aspartate aminotransferase (AST) test	assesses damage to cardiac tissue in CHF; SGOT test
	auscultation	listening to sounds arising from underlying vessels
	cardiac catheterization	procedure in which a flexible tube is inserted into the coronary vessels via a peripheral artery or vein for imaging purposes
	cardiac enzyme test	examines heart muscle enzymes to assess cardiac tissue damage
	CK-BB test	assesses an isoenzyme to diagnose brain infarct or stroke
	CK-MB	assesses an isoenzyme to diagnose cardiac muscle damage
	CK-MM	assesses an isoenzyme to diagnose muscle disease
	creatine kinase (CK) test	assesses creatine kinase, to evaluate cardiac muscle tissue damage

Clinical Dimension	Term	Description
	creatine phosphokinase (CPK) test	assesses phosphocreatine to evaluate cardiac muscle tissue damage
	Doppler ultrasound	ultrasound procedure providing images by computer analysis
	echocardiogram	image of the heart produced by ultrasound
	electrocardiogram (ECG or EKG)	record of the electrical forces producing heart contractions
	exercise stress test	determines heart rate, blood pressure, and ECG while exercising
	Holter monitor	ambulatory device for recording ECG over an extended time period
	lactic dehydrogenase (LDH) test	measures lactic dehydrogenase to assess damage to cardiac tissue
	magnetic resonance imaging (MRI)	imaging technique that uses electromagnetic radiation
	palpation	examination by touch for diagnosing purposes
	pericardiocentesis	drainage of the pericardial sac by a needle or catheter
	positron emission tomography (PET)	imaging method that displays body organs and metabolic activity
	radionuclide scan	computer-generated image made by isolating radionuclides in the bloodstream
	serum glutamic-oxalacetic transaminase (SGOT) test	assesses damage to cardiac tissue in CHF; AST test
	thallium scan	uses radioactive thallium to assess coronary artery disease
	transesophageal echocardiography	ultrasound examination of heart via an endoscope through the esophagus
	venogram	radiograph of a vein via venography
	venography	x-ray examination of the veins after injecting a dye that absorbs the x-rays
TREATMENTS		
	angioplasty	reconstructive surgery of diseased vessels
	angiotensin-converting enzyme (ACE) inhibitors	drugs that act on the kidneys to decrease blood pressure
	aortoplasty	surgical repair of the aorta
	arteriovenous fistula	direct connection between an artery and a vein with no intervening capillaries

Clinical Dimension	Term	Description
	artificial pacemaker	electrical device that restores normal sinoatrial node rhythm
	atherectomy	surgical removal of an atheroma in an artery
	beta-adrenergic blocker	drug that slows the heart rate
	Buerger-Allen exercises	the use of physical forces to prevent pooling of blood in the legs
	bypass surgery	procedure in which blood flow is restored through the creation of a diversionary channel
	calcium channel blocker	drug used to induce muscle relaxation and slow the heart rate
	cardiopulmonary resuscitation (CPR)	emergency technique to restore the heartbeat and breathing by alternating chest compressions with artificial respiration
	cardioversion	converting the heart's electrical pattern, usually from abnormal to normal, with medication or a defibrillator
	commissurotomy	surgical division of a heart valve
	coronary artery bypass graft (CABG) surgery	surgically created arterial diversion around an occlusion
	defibrillation	shocking the heart with a defibrillator to restore the regular heartbeat
	digitalis	drug that increases the strength of heart muscle contraction
	diuretics	drugs that increase urinary excretion
	endarterectomy	atherectomy that includes removal of diseased endothelium and portions of the arterial linings, leaving a smooth tunica externa
	Fowler position	semireclining in bed
	heart–lung machine	device that serves as artificial lungs and heart during some cardiac procedures
	nitroglycerin	fast-acting vasodilator drug
	percutaneous transluminal coronary angioplasty (PTCA)	procedure in which a balloon catheter is used to restore blood flow in a blocked vessel
	vasodilators	drugs that widen blood vessels, decreasing blood flow resistance and blood pressure
	vein ligation	surgical tying of a vein
	vein sclerosing	surgical hardening of a vein
	vein stripping	surgical removal of a vein

Lifespan

Beginning on the 15th day of in utero development, angioblast cells from the mesoderm give rise to blood vessels. The next major feature is the function of the fetal heart, which begins around week 4. Important fetal structures, such as the foramen ovale, ductus arteriosus, and ductus venosus, function until birth. While in utero, the foramen ovale and ductus arteriosus allow blood to bypass the nonfunctioning lungs, and the ductus venosus permits blood to bypass the fetal liver. At birth, the umbilical vein and two umbilical arteries, important structures that enable nutrient and waste exchange between mother and fetus, cease functioning.

As the infant develops, the vasculature increases and the heart tissue grows. Blood pressure is another factor that undergoes considerable change. The average BP for a baby is 90/55 mm Hg. During childhood, there is a gradual increase in both systolic and diastolic measures to the extent that an average BP in adulthood is 120/80. Furthermore, blood pressure gradually increases with aging, and in the elderly it averages 150/90 mm Hg but is not considered hypertensive.

Atherosclerosis is the most common cardiovascular age-related disorder in Western populations; however, little is known of its relationship to aging. It is known that cholesterol deposition is a normal part of aging and begins as fatty streaks (superficial fatty patches on the arterial wall), while still very young. Research has demonstrated that the earliest stage of atherosclerosis is that fatty streak, which lays the foundation for deposition later in life; but the streak appears not to be clinically significant. The only human tissue in which fatty streaks are not evident is fetal. Fatty streaks form fibrous plaques that result in the formation of a connective tissue matrix around age 18 years. At 24 years, about 30% of coronary vessels show evidence of a fatty streak, and at age 40, there is nearly 80% involvement. Fibrous plaques can lead to complicated lesions, which are calcifications of the tunica intima, which may be associated with a clinical event.

The role of cholesterol in aging vessels is still under investigation. To date, there is no strong predictability factor in the elderly population regarding cholesterol levels and heart attack risks. Geriatric research indicates that high cholesterol may serve a protective function in old age because cholesterol in the elderly population may detoxify bacteria.

Cardiac changes with age include an increased incidence of angina, myocardial infarction, and cardiac arrest. There is thickening of the endocardium while myocardial tissue mass may decline. Moreover, cardiac output remains the same, as the resting heart rate decreases, but stroke volume increases. Women lag slightly behind men in incidence of cardiovascular disease until menopause, when the protective effects of estrogen diminish. At age 65 years, the risks of disease are equal for males and females.

Diet modification, aerobic exercise, and cigarette smoking cessation all help lower cardiovascular disease risk and are beneficial for decreasing morbidity. Diet modification can assist in controlling hypertension, and smoking cessation does much for diminishing microvascular (very small blood vessel) disease. In addition, exercise is positively correlated with lowered cardiovascular disease risk and oxygen consumption.

In the News: Aspirin

The phrase is familiar: Aspirin, the wonder drug. Is it really? Or is this marketing hype? The pharmaceutical name for aspirin is acetylsalicylic acid (ASA), and it is a common NSAID. Its properties are numerous, ranging from anti-inflammatory effects to acting as an analgesic, antipyretic (fever reducing), and thrombolytic.

Studies indicate that prophylactic aspirin therapy is beneficial for secondary prevention of vascular events in individuals with a history of CV disease. The U.S. Food and Drug Administration (FDA) has approved aspirin use at 325 mg/day for primary myocardial infarction prevention. Aspirin used clinically at a dosage level of 81 mg/day (baby aspirin) demonstrated antiplatelet effects that last 8–10 days, the lifespan of a thrombocyte (platelet).

Other research has demonstrated that aspirin administration of 325 mg/day decreased the incidence of transient ischemic attacks (TIAs), unstable angina, coronary artery thrombosis with MI, and thrombosis after CABG surgery. Other trials showed that aspirin administration of 325 mg every other day decreased MI incidence 40% in male physicians.

The findings appear promising in terms of disease prevention. Yet, aspirin ingestion of 500 mg/day greatly increases the incidence of gastrointestinal bleeding and may increase the occurrence of peptic ulcer. Therefore, aspirin should be used cautiously as an adjunct therapy and only under the guidance of a health-care professional.

COMMON ABBREVIATIONS

Abbreviation	Term
AA	associate of arts
ACE inhibitors	angiotensin-converting enzyme inhibitors
Ach	acetylcholine
ACLS	advanced cardiac life support
ASA	acetylsalicylic acid
ASLV	aortic semilunar valve
AST	aspartate aminotransferase
AV	atrioventricular; arteriovenous
BP	blood pressure
BSN	bachelor of science in nursing
Ca^{2+}	calcium ion
CABG	coronary artery bypass surgery
CAC	cardioacceleratory center
CAD	coronary artery disease
cath	catheter
CBC	complete blood (cell) count
CHF	congestive heart failure
CIC	cardioinhibitory center
CK	creatine kinase and creatine phosphokinase
CK-BB	creatine phosphokinase brain
CK-MB	creatine phosphokinase muscle and brain
CK-MM	creatine phosphokinase muscle
CO	cardiac output
COPD	chronic obstructive pulmonary disease
CPK	creatine phosphokinase
CPR	cardiopulmonary resuscitation
CV	cardiovascular

Abbreviation	Term
CVA	cerebrovascular accident
CVICU	cardiovascular intensive care unit
DVT	deep venous thrombosis
ECG	electrocardiogram
EKG	electrocardiogram
ESR	erythrocyte sedimentation rate
FDA	U.S. Food and Drug Administration
HDL	high-density lipoprotein
ICU	intensive care unit
K^+	potassium ion
LDH	lactic dehydrogenase
LDL	low-density lipoprotein
MI	myocardial infarction
mm Hg	millimeters of mercury
MRI	magnetic resonance imaging
MVP	mitral valve prolapse
NCLEX	National Council Licensure Examination
NSAIDs	nonsteroidal anti-inflammatory drugs
PDA	patent ductus arteriosus
PET	positron emission tomography
PSLV	pulmonary semilunar valve
PTCA	percutaneous transluminal coronary angioplasty
PVD	peripheral vascular disease
RHD	rheumatic heart disease
RN	registered nurse
SA	sinoatrial
SGOT	serum glutamic-oxalacetic transaminase; AST
SL	semilunar
TIA	transient ischemic attack
2D	two-dimensional

Case Study

Mr. Jay Tigress, age 67 years, was brought to the emergency room by ambulance. Before arrival at the hospital, he had been suffering alternating bouts of diarrhea and vomiting. He had flu-like symptoms and was unable to walk owing to intense weakness. Mr. Tigress stated that he had been unable to keep any food down for several days and last remembered eating some oatmeal and applesauce 2 days earlier. He was extremely confused, but stated he was a diabetic and had not taken his insulin injection in nearly 2 days. Initial examination and blood chemistry profile revealed the following data.

Measure	Value	Measure	Value (Normal Value)
Weight	247 lb	Blood glucose	60 mg/dL (70–110)
BP	90/60 mm Hg	Serum potassium	10 mEq/L (3.8–5.0)
Pulse	50	Serum phosphorus	4.1 mEq/L (1.8–2.6)
Respirations	40	Plasma/serum creatinine	3.2 mEq/L (0.6–1.2)
Temperature	35°C	Serum sodium	100 mEq/L (135–145)
Skin color	pale	CK-MB	65% of total isoenzyme (0–6)

A Foley urinary catheter was inserted; and chest x-rays, ECG, and Doppler ultrasound were ordered. Mr. Tigress was admitted to the CVICU, where Heidi was the charge nurse that night.

Case Study Questions

Select the best answer to each of the following questions.

1. **Mr. Tigress has a BP of 90/60. BP is an abbreviation for _____.**
   a. bicuspid pressure
   b. blood pressure
   c. bradycardia pressure
   d. beating pressure

2. **A BP of 90/60 means _____.**
   a. the systolic pressure is 90 and the diastolic pressure is 60
   b. the diastolic pressure is 90 and the systolic pressure is 60
   c. the pulse pressure is 30
   d. A and C are correct

3. **An ECG was ordered to evaluate _____.**
   a. brain function
   b. cardiac function
   c. liver function
   d. kidney function

4. **An elevated CK-MB is an indication of _____.**
   a. renal failure
   b. liver failure
   c. damaged cardiac tissue
   d. hypertension

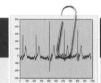

REAL WORLD REPORT

Mr. Tigress was admitted to Heidi's floor, the CVICU, because he was experiencing multiple organ failure secondary to renal failure. His heart was fragile. The following is the cardiologist's report.

CENTRAL HOSPITAL: ECHOCARDIOGRAM REPORT

NAME: Jay Tigress
ATTENDING: J. L. Manjunata, MD
ORDERING: M. M. Isaac, MD

DOB: 01/02/1936
AGE: 67 years
DATE: 04/05/2003

REASON FOR STUDY
• Heart failure

PROCEDURE
The patient underwent M-Mode, 2D, continuous-wave, and pulse-wave Doppler.

RESULTS
- The left ventricle demonstrates mild increase in cavity size with severe systolic dysfunction. Ejection fraction is estimated to be no more than 25%. Hypokinesis is global.
- The right ventricle is normal in size and function.
- Normal size atria and aortic root.
- The mitral valve is mildly thickened. Trivial degree of mitral regurgitation is present.
- The aortic valve was not very well visualized but appears to have normal flow characteristics.
- Tricuspid valve was not very well visualized, but there is no significant (trivial) regurgitation present.
- Pulmonic valve was not visualized.
- Small to moderate size circumferential pericardial effusion that does not seem to be hemodynamically significant.
- No intracardiac mass or thrombi.

CONCLUSION
This is an abnormal study that demonstrates evidence of a mildly dilated left ventricle with severe systolic dysfunction. Ejection fraction is 25%. Mild to moderate circumferential pericardial effusion is present without hemodynamics of significance. No significant valvular abnormalities are seen.

REAL WORLD REPORT QUESTIONS

The following exercises review the medical terms in the preceding medical report. Two terms may be new to you: M-Mode and 2D Doppler. M-Mode Doppler ultrasound is a diagnostic procedure that uses Doppler sound waves so that the echoes displayed correlate to time (T) and motion (M). It is often referred to as TM-Mode Doppler ultrasound. 2D Doppler ultrasound returns a two-dimensional image.

1. The left ventricle demonstrates severe systolic dysfunction. Define *systolic dysfunction* and explain its effects.

   _____

   _____

   _____

2. The report notes that hypokinesis is global.

   a. The word part *hypo-* means _____.

   b. The word part *-kinesis* means _____.

   c. Thus the word *hypokinesis* means _____.

3. The mitral valve is mildly thickened and a trivial degree of regurgitation is present.

   a. Another term for mitral valve is _____.

b. What is another way of stating "trivial degree of mitral valve regurgitation"?

   _____

   _____

   _____

4. Pericardial effusion is present.

   a. The word part *peri-* means _____.

   b. The word part *-cardial* means _____.

   c. Thus the term *pericardial effusion* refers to _____.

5. No significant valvular abnormalities are seen. What valves were evaluated?

   _____

   _____

   _____

REVIEW AND APPLICATION: THREE-LEVEL LEARNING SYSTEM

LEVEL ONE: REVIEWING FACTS AND TERMS USING RECALL

Select the best response to each of the following questions.

1. Components of the cardiovascular system include _____.
   a. the heart
   b. arteries
   c. veins
   d. all of these

2. Which structure is *not* a layer of cardiac tissue?
   a. atrium
   b. endocardium
   c. myocardium
   d. pericardium

3. The two upper chambers of the heart are the _____.
   a. ventricles
   b. atria
   c. semilunar valves
   d. atrioventricular valves

4. The two lower chambers of the heart are the _____.
   a. ventricles
   b. atria
   c. semilunar valves
   d. atrioventricular valves

5. The two semilunar valves are the _____.
   a. aortic and bicuspid
   b. pulmonary and bicuspid
   c. aortic and pulmonary
   d. tricuspid and mitral

6. The term _____ means vein.
   a. arteriole
   b. vena
   c. cava
   d. aorta

7. Pulmonary _____ carry blood to the _____.
   a. veins; lungs
   b. venules; lungs
   c. arteries; lungs
   d. arteries; heart

8. A _____ monitor is a portable _____ machine.
   a. Fowler; sonogram
   b. Holter; sonogram
   c. Fowler; ECG
   d. Holter; ECG

9. The heart's pacemaker is the _____.
   a. sinoatrial node
   b. atrioventricular node
   c. cardiac conduction cycle
   d. atrioventricular bundle

10. The word part *cardio-* refers to _____; the word part *myo-* means _____; and the word part *-pathy* refers to _____.
    a. heart; heart; disease
    b. head; muscle; occupation
    c. heart; muscle; disease
    d. coronary; disease; course of treatment

11. The procedure in which fluid is aspirated from the sac surrounding the heart is termed _____.
    a. myocardiocentesis
    b. pericardiocentesis
    c. endocardiocentesis
    d. cardiac effusion

12. Systolic blood pressure measures arterial blood pressure during ventricular _____.

    a. relaxation

    b. repolarization

    c. fibrillation

    d. contraction

13. The general blood circulatory route through the body is termed the _____ circuit.

    a. pulmonary

    b. systemic

    c. hepatic portal

    d. coronary

LEVEL TWO: REVIEWING CONCEPTS

Select the best response to each of the following questions.

14. Anatomic layers of arteries and veins are termed _____.

Provide a medical term to complete a meaningful analogy.

15. Systole is to diastole as _____ is to repolarization.

16. Tunica interna is to tunica intima as tunica externa is to tunica _____.

17. Veins are to venules as _____ are to arterioles.

Arrange the medical terms so they describe the correct blood flow pattern in the body.

| arteries | aorta | veins |
| venules | capillaries | arterioles |

18. heart → _____ → _____ → _____ → _____ → _____

left ventricle	left atrium
bicuspid valve	lungs
pulmonary arteries	pulmonary veins
right ventricle	tricuspid valve

19. right atrium → _____ → _____ → _____ → _____ → _____ → _____ → _____ → _____

| AV bundle | AV node |
| conduction myofibrils | bundle branches |

20. SA node → _____ → _____ → _____ → _____

Match the term with its definition.

_____ 21. ischemia   a. abnormally slow heart rate

_____ 22. angina   b. pain

_____ 23. bradycardia   c. sound heard in a vessel as a result of turbulent flow

_____ 24. tachycardia   d. interruption of blood flow caused by an obstruction

_____ 25. bruit   e. abnormally rapid heart rate

Match the term with its definition.

_____ 26. venogram   a. radiograph of blood vessels

_____ 27. angiogram   b. phlebogram

_____ 28. pericardio-centesis   c. ultrasound of heart

_____ 29. echocardio-gram   d. monitor of heart rate, BP, and ECG, while on a treadmill

_____ 30. exercise stress test   e. procedure for extracting fluid from pericardial sac

Match the term with its definition.

_____ 31. cardioversion   a. vessel-dilating agent

_____ 32. angioplasty   b. sublingual vasodilator

_____ 33. nitroglycerin   c. surgery of diseased vessels

_____ 34. digitalis

_____ 35. vasodilator

d. shock wave delivered to re-establish normal cardiac rhythm

e. drug that increases heart contractions

Match the term with its definition.

_____ 36. congestive heart failure

_____ 37. congenital heart defect

_____ 38. aneurysm

_____ 39. varicose veins

_____ 40. cardiac arrest

a. stretching of vessel; especially near a valve

b. heart stoppage

c. heart cannot keep up with body's oxygen demands

d. bulging of arterial wall

e. patent ductus arteriosus

Define the following terms.

41. hypertension _____

42. cardiology _____

43. cardiomegaly _____

44. interventricular _____

Using the following word parts, form a medical term for each definition. Each word part is used only once.

cardi-	-itis	phleb-
cardi-	-itis	thrombo-
cardi-	-itis	-um
endo-	myo-	-um
endo-	phleb-	

45. vein inflammation with clot formation _____

46. inner heart lining _____

47. heart muscle _____

48. inflammation of the heart inner lining _____

49. vein inflammation _____

Identify the correctly spelled term in each set.

50. _____

a. infarktion

b. infarction

c. infarckion

d. infarcktion

51. _____

a. cor pulmonale

b. kor pulmonale

c. cor pulmonole

d. kor pulmunale

52. _____

a. cardiac tampanade

b. kardiac tampanade

c. cardiac tamponade

d. cardiack temponade

53. _____

a. anurism

b. aneurizm

c. aneurism

d. aneurysm

54. _____

a. Raynawd

b. Raynoe

c. Raynaud

d. Reynaud

55. _____

a. thromboangitis

b. thromboangiitis

c. thrumboangitis

d. thromboangitiis

Define the following abbreviations.

56. RHD _____

57. CAD _____

58. ASLV _____

59. DVT _____

60. CPR _____

61. PTCA _____

Unscramble the letters to form a medical term.

62. marthahyir

63. rumrum

64. sleup

65. roonyacr

LEVEL THREE: THINKING CRITICALLY

Answer the following questions.

66. List five factors that can influence blood pressure.

   _____

   _____

   _____

67. Explain why there is a difference in muscle wall thickness between the left and the right ventricles.

   _____

   _____

   _____

KEY TERMS SPELLING TEST FROM CD-ROM

Use the CD-ROM to test yourself on the spelling of key terms from this chapter. Listen to the terms and write them on a separate sheet of paper. Use a medical dictionary to check your answers.

ANSWERS

WORD GROUPING

Definition	Word Part
heart, cardiac	cardi-, cardio-
aorta, aortic	aort-, aorto-
apex, apical	apic-, apici-, apico-
artery, arterial	arteri-, arterio-
atrium	atrio-
automatic, spontaneous	automat-, automato-
broad, wide	eury-
chest or breast	steth-, stetho-
cord	chord-, chordo-
fatty, gruel-like, atheroma	athero-
liver, hepatic	hepat-, hepato-
lung, pulmonary	pulmo-
parietal, forming a wall	parieto-
pulse	sphygm-, sphygmo-
rapid, quick, accelerated	tachy-
respiratory, respiratory condition	-pnea
sinus	sino-, sinu-
slow	brady-
small cavity, abdomen	ventri-, ventro-
small vessel, vascular	vascul-, vasculo-
stoppage, obstruction	isch-, ischo-
vein, venous	phleb-, phlebo-
veins	veni-, veno-
ventricle	ventriculo-
vessel, vascular	A. angi-, angio- B. vas-, vasi-, vaso

WORD BUILDING

Word Part	Meaning	Common or Known Word	Example Medical Term
hepat-, hepato-	liver, hepatic	hepatitis	hepatic vein
angi-, angio-	vessel, vascular	angina	angiogram
aort-, aorto-	aorta, aortic	aorta	ascending aorta
arteri-, arterio-	artery, arterial	arteriosclerosis	artery
athero-	fatty, gruel-like, atheroma	atherosclerosis	atherosclerosis
automat-, automato-	automatic, spontaneous	automatic	automaticity
cardi, cardio-	heart, cardiac	cardiac	cardiac
phleb-, phlebo-	vein, venous	phlebotomy	thrombophlebitis
pulmo-	lung, pulmonary	pulmonologist	pulmonary artery
sino-, sinu-	sinus	sinus	sinoatrial node
steth-, stetho-	chest or breast	stethoscope	stethoscope
tachy-	rapid, quick, accelerated	tachymeter	tachycardia
vascul-, vasculo-	small vessel, vascular	vascular	vascular

KEY TERM PRACTICE

Cardiovascular System Preview

1. a. arteries; b. veins; c. capillaries
2. vein; artery

The Heart

1. myocardium
2. a. bicuspid valve; b. mitral valve; c. left atrioventricular valve

Vasculature

1. a. tunica intima; b. tunica media; c. tunica externa
2. arterioles
3. anastomosis
4. venules

Cardiac Blood Flow Pattern

1. a. venae; b. cavae

Coronary Circulation

1. coronary
2. angiogenesis

Cardiac Conduction System

1. a. atrioventricular (AV) bundle; b. conduction myofibers
2. cardioinhibitory

Circulatory Routes

1. pulmonary
2. systemic

Blood Pressure

1. 30
2. sphygmomanometer

Congenital Heart Defects

1. tetralogy of Fallot
2. atrial septal defect; ventricular septal defect

Coronary Artery Disease

1. atherosclerosis; arteriosclerosis
2. plaque

Heart Disorders

1. hypertension
2. Cardiomyopathy

Heart Disorders Associated with the Lungs

1. pulmonary edema
2. cor pulmonale

Inflammation Disorders

1. a. inner; b. muscle; c. around; d. heart; e. inflammation of

Shock

1. shock

Valvular Heart Disease

1. rheumatic heart disease (RHD)
2. mitral valve prolapse

Vein and Artery Disorders

1. Phlebitis
2. Thrombophlebitis

CASE STUDY

1. b is the correct answer.
   - a, c, and d are incorrect because they are fictitious.
2. d is the correct answer.
   - b is incorrect because 90 is the systolic reading and 60 is the diastolic reading.
3. b is the correct answer.
   - a is incorrect because an ECG does not assess brain function.
   - c is incorrect because an ECG does not assess liver function.
   - d is incorrect because an ECG does not assess kidney function.
4. c is the correct answer.
   - a is incorrect because elevated potassium levels do not indicate renal failure.
   - b is incorrect because elevated potassium levels do not indicate liver failure.
   - d is incorrect because Mr. Tigress is experiencing hypotension.

REAL WORLD REPORT

1. Systolic dysfunction means that the contraction of the heart ventricles is not performing optimally. When systolic dysfunction occurs, the force of contraction that enables pumping of the blood through the systemic and pulmonary circuits is diminished.
2. a. diminished, slow, or below; b. motion or movement; c. diminished or slow motion or movement
3. a. bicuspid valve or left atrioventricular valve; b. There is little backflow of blood from the left ventricle into the left atrium, or the mitral valve prolapse is not significant.
4. a. around; b. heart; c. the presence of fluid and/or blood in the area surrounding the heart or in the pericardial space.
5. mitral valve, aortic valve, and tricuspid valve

REVIEW AND APPLICATION: THREE-LEVEL LEARNING SYSTEM

Level One: Reviewing Facts and Terms Using Recall

1. d
2. a
3. b
4. a
5. c
6. b
7. c
8. d
9. a
10. c
11. b
12. d
13. b

Level Two: Reviewing Concepts

14. tunicae
15. depolarization
16. adventitia
17. arteries
18. heart → aorta → arteries → arterioles → capillaries → venules → veins
19. right atrium → tricuspid valve → right ventricle → pulmonary arteries → lungs → pulmonary veins → left atrium → bicuspid valve → left ventricle
20. SA node → AV node → AV bundle → bundle branches → conduction myofibrils
21. d
22. b
23. a
24. e
25. c
26. b
27. a
28. e
29. c
30. d
31. d
32. c
33. b
34. e
35. a
36. c
37. e
38. d
39. a
40. b
41. abnormally high blood pressure
42. study of the heart
43. heart enlargement
44. between the ventricles
45. thrombophlebitis
46. endocardium
47. myocardium
48. endocarditis
49. phlebitis
50. b
51. a
52. c
53. d
54. c
55. b
56. rheumatic heart disease
57. coronary artery disease
58. aortic semilunar valve
59. deep-venous thrombosis
60. cardiopulmonary resuscitation
61. percutaneous transluminal coronary angioplasty
62. arrhythmia
63. murmur
64. pulse
65. coronary

Level Three: Thinking Critically

66. Five factors that can influence blood pressure are blood volume, viscosity, peripheral resistance, chemicals, temperature, and emotions.
67. The left ventricle wall is thicker than the right because this part of the heart is responsible for pumping blood systemically (throughout the body), whereas the right ventricle merely has to push the blood to the nearby lungs.

chapter 12

Lymphatic System and Immunity

OBJECTIVES

- -

After completing this chapter, you should be able to:

1. State the meanings of word parts related to the lymphatic system and immunity.

2. List key functions of the lymphatic system.

3. Describe lymphatic vessels, their locations, and how lymph circulates throughout the body.

4. Identify structures within a typical lymph node.

5. Explain the difference between nonspecific immunity and specific immunity and their function to overall body functioning.

6. Define common signs, symptoms, and treatments of various lymphatic system and immunity diseases.

7. Explain clinical tests and diagnostic procedures related to the lymphatic system and immunity.

8. Describe anatomical and physiological alterations of the lymphatic system and immunity throughout the lifespan.

9. Define common abbreviations related to the lymphatic system and immunity.

10. Define terms used in medical reports involving the lymphatic system and immunity.

11. Correctly define, spell, and pronounce the chapter's medical terms.

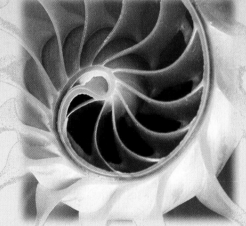

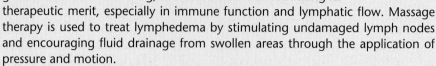

Professional Profile: Massage Therapist

Lee is a massage therapist (MT) who provides treatment by rubbing, kneading, and manipulating the muscles for medical and healing purposes. Massage therapy is a beneficial component to good health and well-being, and research is demonstrating its therapeutic merit, especially in immune function and lymphatic flow. Massage therapy is used to treat lymphedema by stimulating undamaged lymph nodes and encouraging fluid drainage from swollen areas through the application of pressure and motion.

Lee works in a spa environment; however, there is a physician on staff who performs other sorts of treatments, primarily for cancer patients. For each new client, a comprehensive health history is obtained; for established clients, the history is updated before each massage session. As with any allied health profession, the MT must maintain accurate records, document treatments, ensure confidentiality, and be sensitive to age- and gender-related issues.

A typical massage therapy program consists of 720 hours (47 quarter credits) of coursework and clinical internships. The hands-on approach enables students to practice in-class material throughout their educational program. Courses include anatomy, physiology, kinesiology, medical terminology and etymology, first aid, cardiopulmonary resuscitation (CPR), HIV awareness, and herbology along with Swedish massage, sports massage, seated chair massage, prenatal massage, and lymphatic massage. Students also study business and professionalism.

Massage therapy is a discipline in which practice enhances technique. Experience enables the MT to feel for fine nuances in the physical body, observe client reactions, and modify as necessary with greater confidence.

Lee is licensed by the state medical board, the American Massage Therapy Association (AMTA), and the National Certification Examination for Therapeutic Massage and Bodywork (NCETMB). Job satisfaction is high, primarily because the clients almost always feel better after a treatment. The profession is results-oriented, and Lee and the staff physician regularly provide informative community presentations on the benefits of massage.

INTRODUCTION

Protection from disease enables humans to live in a world ripe with microscopic adversity. Discussion about the body's lymphatic system and immune response often sounds like a talk about battles. This is because the body is constantly engaged in a "me versus them" situation with any disease-causing agent. The lymphatic system provides the foundation for immunity and serves as the relentless warrior and constant guard. Through the coordinated actions of the lymphatic system and immunity, millions of infinitesimal organisms are prevented from taking a stronghold.

Distinguishing "self" from "nonself" accomplishes protection. Anything that is nonself, such as a virus, bacterium, or toxin, is eliminated by two specialized mechanisms: nonspecific immunity and specific immunity. Neither type operates in isolation; they are complementary operations that require the coordination of the total immune response.

A common characteristic of all immune disorders is increased susceptibility (likelihood of being affected) to infection, and immunodeficiency diseases result from defective operations of the immune system. Pathology of the lymphatic system and subsequent acute, chronic, or recurrent disease is the topic of "The Clinical Dimension" section of this chapter.

FACT *Microscopic bacteria are about 100 times larger than viruses!*

MEDICAL TERM PARTS

WORD PARTS

Medical term prefixes, suffixes, and combining forms related to the lymphatic system and immunity are introduced in this section.

Word Parts	Meaning
all-, allo-	other, different
aut-, auto-	self, one's own
chyl-, chyli-, chylo-	chyle, fat emulsion in lymph
cellul-, celluli-, cellulo-	cells, cellular
-gen, -gene	substance that produces or generates
heter-, hetero-	other, different
immuno-	safe, protected, immune
iso-	like
lact-, lacti-, lacto-	milk
lymph-, lympho-	lymph
lymphangi-, lymphangio-	lymphatic vessels
lymphaden-, lymphadeno-	lymph nodes
path-, patho-	disease, pathologic
phag-, phago-	eating, feeding
rhin-, rhino-	nose, nasal
splen-, spleno-	spleen
thym-, thymo-, thymi-	thymus
tonsill-, tonsillo-	tonsil
tox-, toxi-, toxo-	toxic, poisonous
xeno-	strange, foreign

WORD ETYMOLOGY

Some words have Greek or Latin word roots but are not true word parts. This section lists those that are used as medical terms.

Word	Definition
globulus	globule
gramma	something written
immunitas	immune
lympha	spring water
masso	to knead
scintilla	spark

MEDICAL TERM PARTS USED AS PREFIXES

Prefix	Definition
immuno-	safe, protected, immune
iso-	like
xeno-	strange, foreign

MEDICAL TERM PARTS USED AS SUFFIXES

Suffix	Definition
-gen, -gene	substance that produces or generates

WORD GROUPING

Using the "Medical Term Parts" tables, identify the prefix, suffix, or combining form for each of the following definitions. The first one has been done as an example.

Definition	Word Part
chyle, fat emulsion in lymph	chyl-, chyli-, chylo-
cells, cellular	
disease, pathologic	
eating, feeding	
like	
lymph	
lymphatic vessels	
lymph nodes	
milk	
nose, nasal	
other, different	A. B.
safe, protected, immune	
self, one's own	
spleen	
strange, foreign	
substance that produces or generates	
tonsil	
toxic, poisonous	
thymus	

WORD BUILDING

Word parts, introduced in the "Medical Term Parts" section, are listed in the following table. For this exercise, first supply the meaning of each word part, then use the word part to build a word you already know. The word you list under "Common or Known Word" does not have to be a medical term; a commonly used word is fine. Be sure, however, that the word correctly reflects the intended meaning. The first one has been done as an example.

Word Part	Meaning	Common or Known Word	Example Medical Term
xeno-	strange, foreign	xenolith	xenograft
all-, allo-			allogeneic
aut-, auto-			autoimmune
cellul-, celluli-, cellulo-			cellular immunity
-gen, -gene			antigen
heter-, hetero-			heterograft
immuno-			immunologic response
iso-			isograft
lact-, lacti-, lacto-			lacteal
lymph-, lympho-			lymph node
path-, patho-			pathogen
phag-, phago-			phagocyte
rhin-, rhino-			rhinitis
thym-, thymo-, thymi-			thymus gland
tonsill-, tonsillo-			tonsillitis
tox-, toxi-, toxo-			lymphotoxin

ANATOMY AND PHYSIOLOGY

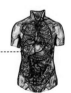

Structures and Components of the Lymphatic System and Immunity

- Lymphatics (lymphatic vessels)
- Lymph nodes
- Lymphocytes
- Nonspecific immunity
- Specific immunity
- Spleen
- Thymus
- Tonsils

Lymphatic System and Immunity Preview

The lymphatic system and immunity are considered together because each supports the other, and both are important for a healthy immune response. Structures of the lymphatic system are lymph nodes, lymphocytes, and lymphatic vessels; lymphatic organs are the spleen, thymus, and tonsils (Fig. 12-1). Lymphatic vessels, or **lymphatics,** transport lymph in a system separate from the blood vasculature. The lymphatic vessels serve as the conduit between the lymphatic system and the vascular (blood vessel) system. The lymphatic system returns tissue fluid to the bloodstream,

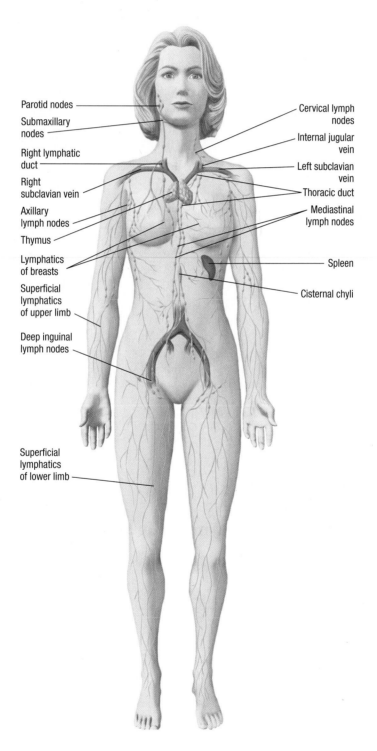

FIGURE 12-1

Structures and components of the lymphatic system. (Image provided by Anatomical Chart Co.)

provides defense against **pathogens** (disease-causing agents), and removes proteins from interstitial (between cells or tissues) spaces. The exchange occurs at lymphatic capillaries, which are more porous than blood capillaries. Their permeable structure enables the vessels to collect products such as interstitial fluid formed from blood plasma that has escaped the vasculature and surrounding tissues.

Furthermore, the lymphatic system also plays an integral part in maintaining the body's fluid balance. Upon entry into the lymphatic vessel, the fluid is termed **lymph.** So that lymph may eventually re-enter the blood, it is transported to collecting ducts that empty into the bloodstream through the right and left subclavian veins.

The lymph is filtered through **lymph nodes**, bean-shaped structures distributed along lymphatics much like beads on a necklace. **Lymphocytes** are white blood cells (cells that protect the body against infection in the immune response) formed in lymphatic tissue throughout the body. Based on surface molecules and function, lymphocytes are grouped into two categories: T and B cells.

The **thymus**, or thymus gland, is a pyramid-shaped organ consisting of two lobes located in the mediastinum, directly posterior to the sternum. It functions in immunity by promoting the maturation of T cells. The **spleen**, a large mass of lymphatic tissue located in the left hypochondriac region, is a nonvital organ involved with lymphocyte production, and **tonsils** are masses of partially encapsulated lymphatic tissue.

Another function of the lymphatic system is the transport of lipids from the intestinal tract to the circulatory system. A special structure called a lacteal; it is located at the terminal end of a lymphatic vessel in an intestinal villus, a finger-shaped vascular extension that increases the absorptive surface area of the intestinal lumen. **Lacteals** carry recently absorbed fats from the small intestine to the thoracic duct, which empties into the blood. These fats are milky white globules called **chyle.** The word part *lact-* refers to "milk," and the fluid from lacteals is milky in color.

The ability of the body to resist disease, **immunity**, is provided by nonspecific and specific defenses. **Nonspecific immunity** is imprecise and defends the body through the action of T cells, whereas **specific immunity** is aimed directly at particular agents through the action of B cells. Both work simultaneously on a continuous basis.

Basic terms associated with the immune response are antibody (Ab), antigen (Ag), and immunoglobulin (Ig). **Antigens** are foreign proteins or nonself substances that trigger immune responses by causing the formation of **antibodies**, proteins that respond to the presence of an antigen to eliminate it. Likewise, immunoglobulins are native glycoproteins that act like antibodies. For example, bacteria and viruses contain antigens that stimulate antibody or immunoglobulin formation.

FACT There are 100 million trillion antibodies circulating in the blood!

Key Terms	Definitions
lymphatics (lim FAT icks)	collecting vessels formed from merging lymphatic capillaries that convey lymph
pathogens (PATH oh jenz)	disease-causing agents
lymph (LIMF)	fluid in the lymphatic vessels
lymph (LIMF) **nodes**	bean-shaped masses of lymphatic tissue
lymphocytes (LIM foh sites)	leukocytes (white blood cells) found in lymphatic tissue
thymus (THY mus)	lymph organ, located in the anteriosuperior mediastinum
spleen	largest lymphatic organ, located on left side, inferior to the diaphragm

tonsils	groups of lymphatic tissue in the oral cavity
lacteals (LACK tee ulz)	lymphatics in small intestine that transport chyle
chyle (KILE)	emulsion of fat droplets in the lymph
immunity	ability to resist and overcome disease
nonspecific immunity	generalized resistance to disease, accomplished by T cells
specific immunity	resistance against specific agents, carried out by B cells
antigens (AN ti jenz)	substances that provoke an immune response
antibodies (AN tee bod eez)	substances produced in the body that react to an antigen

Key Term Practice: Lymphatic System and Immunity Preview

1. The word part _____ refers to "lymph," and the word part _____ means "cell." So a _____ is a "white blood cell in lymphatic tissue."

2. Identify two types of immunity. _____

Lymph Nodes, Lymphocytes, and Lymphatics

The volume of a typical cell is 1000 times the volume of a virus!

Bean-shaped structures located along lymphatics are called lymph nodes. Lymph nodes contain phagocytic cells, which digest foreign substances, and germinal centers, which produce lymphocytes. Their size varies, ranging from 1 to 20 mm. Lymph is filtered through lymph nodes to sift out pathogens, such as viruses and bacteria.

Lymph nodes have several distinct regions (Fig. 12-2). The capsule is the outer layer of dense connective tissue encircling the entire node, and the cortex is the outer region of the node. **Lymph nodules** are the functional units of a lymph node located within the cortical portion. These are areas of dense masses of lymphocytes and macrophages (large phagocytic cells derived from monocytes present in blood and

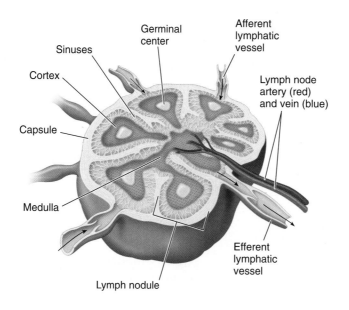

Germinal center

Afferent lymphatic vessel

Sinuses

Cortex

Lymph node artery (red) and vein (blue)

Capsule

Medulla

Efferent lymphatic vessel

Lymph nodule

FIGURE 12-2
Lymph nodes have several distinct regions.

lymph). The inner region, medulla, contains T cells. Lymph enters the node through the afferent vessel and exits through the efferent vessel toward the venous circulation. (Associate the *e* in *e*xit with the *e* in *e*fferent.) Areas of rapidly dividing lymphocytes within the lymph nodules are termed **germinal centers.** When an infection is present, the germinal centers form and release lymphocytes for combat.

Lymph nodes occur in groups throughout the body, except in structures that lack lymphatics, such as avascular tissue, the brain and spinal cord, bone marrow, and teeth. Lymph node clusters are found in the axillary, cervical, thoracic, inguinal, intestinal, mammary, and tonsil regions. Lymph nodes in the axillary regions receive lymph primarily from the arms and mammary glands.

Lymphatics begin as capillaries where lymph capillaries interlace with the capillary beds of the cardiovascular system, forming vast networks (Fig. 12-3). Lymphatic vessels run along side blood vessels. Subcutaneous lymphatic vessels are next to veins, and visceral lymphatics are adjacent to arteries.

Lymphatics merge to form greater vessels called trunks, which eventually become ducts. Two large collecting ducts—called the thoracic (left thoracic) duct and right lymphatic (right thoracic) duct—drain the lymphatic trunks (Fig. 12-4). These ducts are the largest lymphatic vessels and drain into the left and right subclavian veins. Valves prevent blood from entering the lymphatic ducts. The **thoracic duct** drains all but the upper right body quadrant into the left subclavian vein. The smaller **right lymphatic duct** collects lymph from the upper right body quadrant superior to the diaphragm, including the right arm and right regions of the thorax, cervix, and cranium, and drains into the right subclavian vein. The pathway of lymph is as follows:

interstitial fluid → lymph capillaries → lymphatics → lymph trunks → thoracic duct
   or right lymphatic duct → right or left subclavian vein

Because lymphatic vessels are not connected to a pumping organ such as the heart, lymph circulation results from other body movements, collectively called lymphokinetic factors. These **lymphokinetic factors** include actions such as arterial pulses, passive compression of soft body tissues, postural changes, skeletal muscle contractions, and respiratory movements that result in lymph flow.

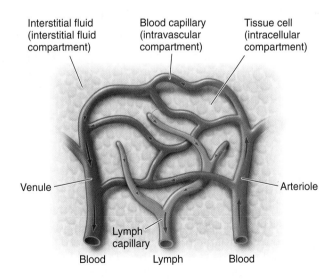

Interstitial fluid (interstitial fluid compartment)

Blood capillary (intravascular compartment)

Tissue cell (intracellular compartment)

Venule

Arteriole

Lymph capillary

Blood   Lymph   Blood

FIGURE 12-3
The structural relationship between a capillary bed of the blood vascular system and the lymphatic capillaries.

Key Terms	Definitions
lymph nodules (LIMF NOD yoolz)	areas of lymphocyte formation within the lymph nodes
germinal (JUR mi nul) **centers**	areas of rapidly dividing lymphocytes within the lymph nodules

thoracic (thoh RAS ick) duct	main lymphatic duct, draining lymph from the trunk and returning it to the bloodstream via the left subclavian vein
right lymphatic (lim FAT ick) duct	main lymphatic duct, draining lymph from the upper right body quadrant and returning it to the bloodstream via the right subclavian vein
lymphokinetic (lim foh ki NET ick) factors	body actions that contribute to lymph circulation

Key Term Practice: Lymph Nodes, Lymphocytes, and Lymphatics

1. The _____ drains the upper right body quadrant superior to the diaphragm.

2. _____ factors encourage lymph flow.

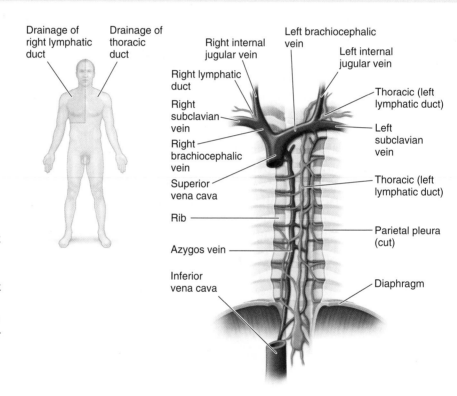

FIGURE 12-4
The thoracic (left thoracic) duct drains all but the upper right body quadrant into the left subclavian vein. The smaller right lymphatic (right thoracic) duct collects lymph from the upper right body quadrant and drains into the right subclavian vein.

Tonsils, Thymus, and Spleen

Tonsils are oval masses of lymphatic tissue, and five are found in the oral region: left and right lingual, left and right palatine, and a single pharyngeal tonsil (Fig. 12-5). The left and right lingual tonsils are located under the tongue base, the palatines are found at the sides of the posterior throat opening, and the pharyngeal tonsil is located near the opening of the nasal cavity at the posterior superior wall of the nasopharynx. The pharyngeal tonsil is also called the **adenoid.**

As noted earlier, the thymus is a lymphatic gland located in the mediastinum and is important to promoting T cell maturation. Immature T cells travel from red bone marrow to the thymus, where a hormone secreted by the gland, **thymosin,** enables lymphocytes to develop into mature T cells. In a child, the thymus is an important site of immunity. This organ hypertrophies from birth to puberty, when it reaches its maximum size of about 40 g. Thereafter, it begins to atrophy, and much of its tissue is replaced by fat so that only a remnant remains in an elderly person (see Fig. 9-9).

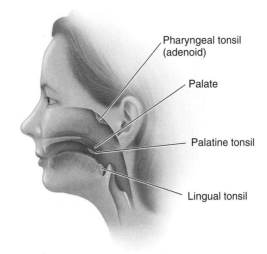

FIGURE 12-5
The tonsils are oval masses of lymphatic tissue found in the oral region.

The spleen is about 12 cm (5 in.) in length with two distinct regions: white pulp and red pulp (Fig. 12-6). The white pulp is active in the immune response, and the red pulp serves as a blood reservoir. In addition to its roles related to hematopoiesis (blood formation), blood storage, blood filtration, and antibody production, it is involved with the **phagocytosis** (the engulfing and ingesting) of bacteria and old cells. The spleen hypertrophies during infection and atrophies in old age.

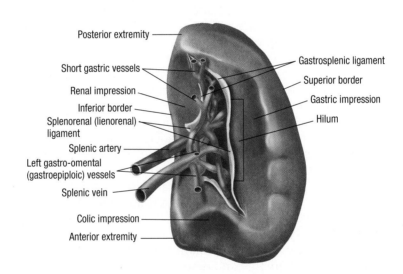

FIGURE 12-6
The spleen is involved with phagocytosis of bacteria and old cells. (Image provided by Anatomical Chart Co.)

Key Terms	Definitions
adenoid (AD e noid)	the pharyngeal tonsil
thymosin (THIGH moh sin)	hormone that aids in T cell maturation
phagocytosis (fag oh sigh TOH sis)	ingestion of particles

Key Term Practice: Tonsils, Thymus, and Spleen

1. What is the alternate term for the pharyngeal tonsil? _____

2. _____ is a hormone produced by the thymus that aids in T cell maturation.

Nonspecific Defenses: T Cells and Cellular Immunity

The body uses several lines of defense to prevent illness. **Cellular immunity** is the direct attack on a pathogen by T cells. The ability to ward off or not to succumb to disease is termed **resistance.** Lack of resistance and disposition to disease development is called **susceptibility.**

The likelihood of being sick varies among individuals; however, stress is a major risk factor for disease. Stress is known to affect the entire body, and may diminish the immune response. Current research demonstrates a link between the mind and the body's resistance or susceptibility to disease and physiological decline. **Psychoneuroimmunology** (PNI) is an emerging field that studies this association between the psyche and the body.

Nonspecific defenses and barriers work in concert with the immune system to prevent **infection,** the condition caused by the presence of a pathogen. Phagocytes and the population of T cells carry out nonspecific immunity. **Phagocytes** are white blood cells (neutrophils and monocytes) that ingest and destroy microbes by phagocytosis. The term literally means "eating cells." Abnormal cells are detected through **immunologic surveillance,** the unceasing monitoring that occurs in the body, because they have chemicals (antigens) on their surfaces that are foreign to the body. **Alveolar macrophages,** or phagocytic dust cells, found within the lungs, engulf debris and foreign compounds. Phagocytic cells in the liver, lungs, lymph nodes, and spleen make up the **reticuloendothelial system** (RES), which is also called the **monocyte–macrophage system.**

Once the trespasser has made its way inside the body, additional nonspecific defenses, such as complement and interferons, take charge. **Complement** is so named because it works together with (or complements) the other nonspecific defenses. In actuality, it is a group of approximately 34 proteins, found in the bloodstream, which destroy pathogen cell walls, stimulate inflammation, and help attract phagocytes to foreign cells. **Interferons** (IFNs) are antimicrobial glycoproteins produced in response to viral invasion. Their presence stimulates cytotoxic T cell activity and amplifies macrophage action.

Numerous classes of **T cells,** a lymphocyte type essential for various aspects of immunity, play roles in combating invaders. T cells originate in the red bone marrow but mature in the thymus gland, hence the *T* indicates it is from the *t*hymus. T lymphocytes proliferate into various T cell populations: cytotoxic T cells, helper T cells, amplifier T cells, suppressor T cells, and memory cytoxic T cells.

Cytotoxic T (T_c) **cells,** also called natural killer (NK) T cells or CD8$^+$ T cells, attack cells that have specific antigens on their surfaces. T_c cells produce poisonous substances called **lymphotoxins** that lyse (break down) antigens on self cells that have been invaded by a foreign substance. T_c cells engage in cell-to-cell combat by secreting toxins that puncture and destroy other cells

Helper T (T_H) **cells** (also known as CD4$^+$ T cells) cooperate with B cells, which are important in specific immunity, to amplify antibody production. They also secrete the cytokine interleukin 2, a protein that stimulates the proliferation of cytotoxic T cells and B cells. Helper T cells are aptly named for they assist in recruiting other T cell populations.

Cells that produce lymphokines, immune substances released by lymphocytes that influence the behavior of other immune cells, are termed **amplifier T cells.** They stimulate T cells, suppressor T cells, and plasma cells to increase their functions.

Suppressor T (T_S) **cells** depress the responses of other T cells and B cells. It is believed that they secrete suppression factors that prevent the destruction of uninfected self cells and act to wind down the immune reaction after the initial response. **Memory T_C cells** are long-lived T lymphocytes that respond to subsequent invasion by the same antigen. These cells lay in wait for the reappearance of a specific antigen.

Key Terms	Definitions
cellular immunity	immune response propagated by macrophages and T cells
resistance	ability to ward off infection
susceptibility	ability to develop disease
psychoneuroimmunology (sigh koh new roh im yoo NOL uh jee)	field of science that deals with the interaction of the mind and the immune system on overall health
infection	invasion of the host by pathogens
phagocyte (FAG oh site)	white blood cell that engulfs and digests foreign debris or particles
immunologic (im yoo noh LOJ ick) **surveillance**	the body's monitoring of tissues
alveolar macrophage (al VEE uh lur MACK roh faij)	phagocytic cell in lung tissue
reticuloendothelial (re tick yoo loh en doh THEE lee ul) **system**	fixed phagocytes in the liver, lungs, lymph nodes, and spleen; monocyte–macrophage system
monocyte–macrophage (MON oh site–MACK roh faij) **system**	fixed phagocytes in the liver, lungs, lymph nodes, and spleen; reticuloendothelial system
complement	proteins involved in destroying foreign cells
interferons (in tur FEER onz)	set of proteins that increase cellular resistance
T cells	lymphocytes derived from the thymus
cytotoxic (sigh toh TOCK sick) **T cells**	cells that attack cells displaying abnormal surface antigens; NK T cells, $CD8^+$ T cells
lymphotoxins (lim foh TOCK sinz)	poisonous substances that break apart cells with foreign antigens
helper T cells	cells that stimulate the activation of B cells and T cells; $CD4^+$ T cells
amplifier T cells	cells that stimulate the function of T cells, T_S cells, and plasma cells
suppressor T cells	cells that modulate T cell and B cell activity
memory T_C cells	cells that can respond to subsequent encounters with a specific antigen

Key Term Practice: Nonspecific Defenses: T Cells and Cellular Immunity

1. What is the alternative term for the reticuloendothelial system or stationary phagocytes in the liver, spleen, lymph nodes, and lungs? _____

2. Poisonous substances circulating in lymph that destroy cells with foreign antigens are called _____.

Specific Defenses: B Cells and Humoral Immunity

Specific body defense mechanisms involve the production of a specific lymphocyte or antibody against a specific antigen to confer resistance to disease. B cells and humoral immunity provide specific defenses. **B cells**, also called B lymphocytes, are another type of white blood cell formed in bone marrow and the fetal liver and spleen. *B* cells are derived from *b*one marrow. B cells circulate freely, searching for antigens. They are capable of producing two kinds of cells: plasma cells and memory cells (memory B cells). Plasma cells are **clones**, daughter cell lymphocytes that are genetically alike and capable of responding to the same specific antigen. These antibodies circulate and bind to the antigens that stimulated their proliferation. These cells, found in circulating blood and lymph, form **plasma cells** that eventually create antibodies in response to an antigen. There are two possible scenarios for the creation of antibodies:

B cell → plasma cell → antibody

B cell → memory cell → antibody

From a molecular perspective, antibodies are Y-shaped proteins with a variable region and a constant region (Fig. 12-7). The variable region, which differs among antibodies, provides antigen specificity and combines with antigens. The constant region consists of amino acids and remains unchanged.

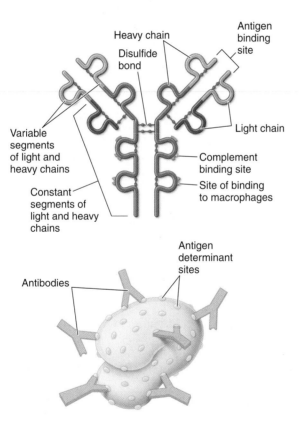

FIGURE 12-7
Antibodies are Y-shaped proteins with a variable region and a constant region.

Humoral immunity is the direct attack by antibodies circulating in body fluids, especially blood serum. (The word *humor* is a medieval term for any of the body's four main fluids: blood, yellow bile, black bile, and lymph.) Antigens stimulate the production of an antibody. Examples of antigens are insect toxins, microbial structures, viral coats, incompatible blood cells, and molecules on pollen or other foreign bodies. The antibody is a specific protein produced by B cell–derived plasma cells in response to the presence of a particular antigen. Antibodies are made only if an abnormal antigen is detected.

Gammaglobulin (γ-globulin) is a general term designating the various immunoglobulins making up a part of humoral immunity. A globulin is a family of proteins precipitated from serum or plasma. **Immunoglobulins** are native glycoprotein molecules produced by white blood cells during an immune response that function like antibodies. There are five classes of immunoglobulins: IgA, IgD, IgE, IgG, and IgM. If placed in another order, they spell *MADGE*. These antibodies circulate in blood plasma, lymph, and extracellular fluids and bind to specific antigens. IgA is found in exocrine secretions and is effective against bacterial and viral infections. IgD is found on the surfaces of B cells and is known to play a role in the activation of the B cell to which it binds; but not much else is known about IgD. IgE is found in exocrine gland secretions and promotes allergic reactions. Approximately 80% of the immunoglobulins are type IgG, found in plasma and breast milk. IgM is an antibody found in plasma that responds to certain antigens in food, bacteria, and cross-matched blood.

Key Terms	Definitions
B cells	lymphocytes that differentiate into plasma cells when stimulated by an antigen
clones	identical cells derived from a single cell (parent cell)
plasma (PLAZ muh) **cells**	antibody-producing cells derived from B cells
humoral (HUGH mor ul) **immunity**	immune response maintained by antibodies
immunoglobulins (im yoo noh GLOB yoo linz)	glycoproteins produced by white blood cells that function as antibodies

Key Term Practice: Specific Defenses: B Cells and Humoral Immunity

1. Antibody-producing cells are termed _____.

2. Humoral immunity is mediated by _____.

Immune Activation

Specific and nonspecific defenses work in concert to ward off invading disease-causing agents. Once a pathogen enters the body, a series of steps activates the immune response. First, macrophages present the strange antigens to T cells and B cells, and the body recognizes the antigen as foreign, or nonself. The body is able to differentiate between cells that belong (self) from cells that do not belong (nonself) via a mechanism called the **major histocompatibility complex** (MHC), also known as **human leukocyte antigens** (HLAs). The MHC is a cluster of genes that determine the recognizable pattern on cell membrane surfaces. If an unfamiliar protein is found, it signals the immune system that an invader is present. No two people, except identical twins, possess the same set of MHC molecules.

Next, lymphocytes proliferate (reproduce) and produce millions of other identical lymphocytes (clones or daughter cells) against the nonself antigen. B cells also develop into antibody-producing plasma cells. Antibodies are extremely selective, and they are synthesized for a particular antigen. Therefore, if several different antigens are present, the antibodies produced must be different. For example, when antigen X is present, only antibody X can act on it, much like there is only one key for each lock. Several keys may be available, but only one will work. When the antibody encounters the precise antigen, it binds to it, forming an **antigen–antibody complex**, a clumping of material. The complex is then phagocytosed by macrophages or lysed by complement proteins. Through the combined actions of nonspecific defense mechanisms, lymphocytes, and antibodies, the foreign substance is destroyed or rendered harmless in most cases.

The initial response to antigen exposure is called the **primary response.** It occurs when the antigen is first encountered. After this primary response, long-lived B cells give rise to **memory cells,** antibody-secreting cells. Memory cells respond only to a later invasion of the same antigen. The subsequent reaction from memory cells is termed the **secondary response** because it is a repeat encounter with a particular antigen. If the body encounters that particular antigen again, the memory cells "remember" the first exposure, recognize the antigen, and take action by releasing the specific antibody. This immunologic reaction to a previously encountered antigen is also referred to as the **anamnestic response.** (*Amnesia* means "loss of memory" and the word part *-an* means "against," so the term literally means "against memory loss"—remembering.) Essentially, it is memory recall. Memory cells provide the foundation for immunity to diseases after their first occurrence. That is why individuals generally have each childhood disease, such as chickenpox, only once in their lifetime. Immunologic surveillance is a never-ending practice.

Key Terms	Definitions
major histocompatibility (his toh kom pat i BIL i tee) **complex**	segment of a chromosome that determines a person's leukocyte antigens and lymphocyte characteristics; human leukocyte antigen
human leukocyte antigens (LEW koh site AN ti jenz)	segment of a chromosome that determines a person's leukocyte antigens and lymphocyte characteristics; major histocompatibility complex
antigen–antibody (AN ti jen–AN tee bod ee) **complex**	specific agglutination of a known antigen with its antibody
primary response	systemic immune reaction to the first encounter with a foreign antigen
memory cells	cells that remember specific antigens
secondary response	immune reaction to a second (or later) encounter with a known antigen
anamnestic (an am NES tick) **response**	immune response initiated by memory recall

Key Term Practice: Immune Activation

1. The alternate term for _____ is human leukocyte antigens (HLAs).

2. The structure formed from the clumping of an antibody with an antigen is termed a/an _____.

Pharmaceutics and Acquired Immunity

Human immunity can be acquired. Two pharmaceutical agents that assist in the immune response are antibiotics and vaccines. As its name suggests, an **antibiotic** is a substance "against life." Antibiotics are chemical agents that are synthetically produced or derived from bacteria or fungi. They function by either killing or inactivating bacteria in the body. The significant word is *bacteria;* antibiotics are effective only against bacteria. **Vaccines**—chemical preparations containing weakened or dead microbes that cause a particular disease—are administered to stimulate antibody and subsequent memory cell production.

TABLE 12-1 Acquired Immunity

Type	Active	Passive
natural	exposure to antigen	transfer of antibodies across the placenta or from breast milk
artificial	immunization	immunoglobulin injection

Vaccines are administered for immunization purposes. **Immunization** provides immunity because the antigen stimulates antibody production. Types of vaccines include attenuated and inactivated. With an **attenuated vaccine**, the disease-producing ability of the antigen has been lessened or eliminated by heat or chemical measures. After inoculation, mild symptoms may result in some people owing to variations in individual immune systems. **Inactivated vaccines** contain only bacterial cell walls or viral coats. Inactivated vaccines may not stimulate as strong an immune response as do attenuated vaccines, and the immunity conferred may not be long lasting. Booster shots are frequently required after inactivated vaccine administration.

Vaccines are basically harmless when given as an injection, oral preparation, or inhalent. The body recognizes the antigen as foreign, mounts an immune response, and produces memory cells, so that any future encounter with the pathogen will be swiftly eliminated.

Acquired immunity is obtained through natural or artificial means (Table 12-1). Natural implies that no pharmaceutical agents or outside therapy was used; artificial immunity, however, is acquired through medical intervention. Genetically determined, **natural immunity** is innate (inborn) immunity present at birth and requires no previous antigen exposure. **Artificial immunity** is not present at birth and is obtained after antigen exposure. Furthermore, acquired immunity is either active or passive, each with two subtypes. Antibodies that develop in response to the presence of antigens produce **active immunity**. Active immunity is called on when a pathogen initiates an immune response. The transfer of antibodies or immunoglobulins from one person to another produces **passive immunity**. These antibodies provide short-term immunity without stimulating an immune response.

The two types of active immunity are natural and artificial. **Natural active immunity** develops after exposure to an antigen. For example, a person is infected with virus X. An immune response occurs and memory cells are made. Later, the previously made antibodies will combat any subsequent exposure to viral infection X. **Artificial active immunity** develops after the individual receives a dosage of an antigen to prevent disease. Vaccination is an example of artificial active immunity.

Natural passive immunity and artificial passive immunity are two types of passive immunity. The transfer of maternal IgG antibodies across the placenta or through breast milk to an infant provides **natural passive immunity. Artificial passive immunity** develops through immunoglobulin injection. For example, intravenous immunoglobulins are given for a particular infection.

> As a result of worldwide vaccination efforts, smallpox was declared eradicated in 1980; however, bioterrorism threatens this achievement.

Key Terms	Definitions
antibiotic (an tee bye OT ick)	drug used against a bacterial infection
vaccines (vack SEENZ)	drugs administered to induce an immune response
immunization (im yoo ni ZAY shun)	providing immunity through antibody stimulation via a vaccine
attenuated vaccine (vack SEEN)	vaccine in which the antigen's ability to produce disease has been lessened or eliminated

inactivated vaccines (vack SEENZ)	vaccines in which only the viral coat or bacterial cell wall are present
natural immunity	innate immunity
artificial immunity	immunity developed after reaction to an antigen
active immunity	immunity as a result of a disease or antigen exposure
passive immunity	immunity acquired through antibody transfer from another person
natural active immunity	immunity resulting from environmental antigen exposure
artificial active immunity	artificially acquired active immunity
natural passive immunity	naturally acquired passive immunity
artificial passive immunity	artificially acquired passive immunity

Key Term Practice: Acquired Immunity

1. Innate immunity, with which humans are born, is termed _____ immunity.

2. Antibiotics should be administered to combat viral infections. True or False? _____

THE CLINICAL DIMENSION

Pathology of the Lymphatic System and Immunity

Pathology related to the lymphatic system and immunity can be grouped into five basic categories: autoimmune diseases, hypersensitivity responses, immunodeficiency disorders, infections, and tumors. Many of these disorders seem to have a genetic component.

Autoimmune Diseases

Autoimmune diseases are caused by the body's inability to distinguish its own cells from foreign material, causing the body to direct antibodies against naturally occurring substances. Because most autoimmune diseases have effects that are manifested in a particular body system, these conditions are discussed in each relevant chapter. Some common autoimmune diseases are Addison disease, chronic hepatitis, glomerulonephritis, Graves disease, hemolytic anemia, hypoparathyroidism, insulin-dependent diabetes mellitus, multiple sclerosis, myasthenia gravis, pernicious anemia, polymyositis, psoriasis, rheumatic fever, rheumatoid arthritis (RA), scleroderma, Sjögren syndrome, system lupus erythematosus (SLE), thrombocytopenia, thyroiditis, ulcerative colitis, and vitiligo.

Sjögren syndrome is an autoimmune disease characterized by keratoconjunctivitis (inflammation of the eye's conjunctiva and cornea) sicca, rhinitis sicca, and polyarthritis. **Sicca** is the medical term for dryness. It is seen in menopausal women and is often associated with rheumatoid arthritis.

Key Terms	Definitions
autoimmune (aw toh i MEWN) **diseases**	disorders that result from the immune response directed against the host
Sjögren (SHOE greyn) **syndrome**	autoimmune disease marked by dry skin, dry nasal membranes, and multiple areas of arthritis
sicca (SICK uh)	dryness

Key Term Practice: Autoimmune Diseases

1. A disease in which antibodies attack the self is termed a/an _____.

2. What is the medical term for dryness? _____

Hypersensitivity Disorders

Hypersensitivity refers to an abnormal, overreaction to an allergen (antigen). Hypersensitivity disorders are characterized by an exaggerated reaction to a stimulus. Examples of disproportionate responses include allergies, asthma, and anaphylaxis. Foods such as shellfish and peanuts trigger hypersensitivity reactions in susceptible persons. Effects of hypersensitivity disorders are generally mild. One treatment for hypersensitivity is desensitization; however, it is not effective for the majority of the population. **Desensitization** is a treatment for allergies that makes the individual insensitive to an antigen through antigen administration. Small amounts of the protein are injected over a period of time, initiating antibody production so that eventually the person will no longer mount a hypersensitivity reaction. This treatment is also called **antianaphylaxis.**

An extreme sensitivity reaction to a normally harmless substance that is touched, breathed in, or ingested is termed **allergy.** Common examples are allergic rhinitis and latex allergy. **Allergic rhinitis** is an allergic reaction to an inhaled particle. Runny nose, itchy eyes, and congestion characterize it. If it occurs seasonally in response to trees, grasses, weeds, or flowers, it is called **hay fever;** year-round occurrence is termed **perennial allergic rhinitis.** Both are treated with decongestants and antihistamines. **Decongestants** are pharmaceutical agents that reduce or relieve nasal congestion, which often accompanies allergies. Drugs that prevent or diminish histamine effects are **antihistamines.** Histamine is a potent capillary dilator, which is evident in the face during an allergic reaction by nasal swelling, itchy eyes, and swollen cheeks. As the name suggests, antihistamines counter the effects of histamine to reduce the signs and symptoms.

An emerging allergy, particularly in the health-care field, is the hypersensitivity to latex, called **latex allergy.** Latex is a sap derived from the rubber tree that can cause localized irritation on the skin or systemic effects that are life threatening.

Various skin tests are diagnostic tools for determining sensitivity or immunity to specific antigens that are applied to or injected into the skin. Common skin tests include the exposure test, intradermal test, patch test, and prick test. The **exposure test** is used to identify previous exposure to fungi or parasites. The **intradermal test** involves the injection of a small amount of antigen into the skin. Positive exposure and intradermal tests are indicated by a **wheal** (raised reddened area) that appears on the skin surface. A test for allergens in which a patch is saturated with allergens and then applied to the skin for a period of time is the **patch test.** The **prick test** is one in which a small amount of antigen is poked into the skin. Positive tests are indicated by erythema, a round hard swelling, or itching.

A chronic, reactive airway disorder characterized by bronchospasm and mucus secretion is called **asthma.** Asthma is often caused by allergies. Other signs and symptoms include coughing, difficulty breathing, and a feeling of tightness in the chest. Several types exist. **Acute asthma** has a sudden onset. **Extrinsic asthma** is caused by sensitivity to inhalants, drugs, foods, pollen, mold, animal dander, or environmental allergen. When the cause cannot be determined, and extrinsic asthma has been ruled out, the condition is called **intrinsic asthma. Status asthmaticus** is persistent asthma that can lead to respiratory distress and failure. Treatment for all forms involves bronchodilator use. **Bronchodilators** are drugs that widen and relax pulmonary passages, thereby making breathing easier. In some cases, preventive maintenance drugs are used.

An immediate hypersensitivity reaction resulting from **sensitization** (reactive to pollen, serum, or antigen) to a foreign body or drug is called **anaphylaxis.** IgE is responsible for the systemic manifestations. **Acute anaphylaxis** is an immediate, severe hypersensitivity reaction to an allergen with systemic effects. Localized anaphylactic reactions include hay fever, asthma, eczema, and hives. It is characterized by pruritic urticaria (itchy hives), edema, bronchial constriction causing respiratory distress, and shock. The effects of acute anaphylaxis range from mild to fatal. If not treated, it can lead to anaphylactic shock, which is marked by an extreme drop in blood pressure, itching, swelling, and difficulty breathing.

Key Terms	*Definitions*
hypersensitivity (high pur sen si TIV i tee)	abnormal sensitivity to an allergen
desensitization (dee sen si ti ZAY shun)	procedure for making a person insensitive to an antigen; antianaphylaxis
antianaphylaxis (an tee an uh fi LACK sis)	procedure for making a person insensitive to an antigen; desensitization
allergy	abnormal reactivity to a subsequent antigen exposure
allergic rhinitis (rye NIGH tis)	nasal mucous membrane inflammation caused by allergen inhalation
hay fever	allergy to seasonal plant allergens
perennial allergic rhinitis (rye NIGH tis)	year-round allergy to environmental allergens
decongestants	drugs that relieve nasal congestion
antihistamines	drugs that work against histamine
latex (LAY tecks) **allergy**	hypersensitivity to products made from the sap of the rubber plant
exposure test	identifies previous contact with fungal or parasitic organisms
intradermal (in truh DUR mul) **test**	detects sensitivity to an antigen injected into the skin
wheal	raised, reddened area caused by a sensitivity reaction
patch test	determines sensitivity to an antigen
prick test	detects a reaction to an antigen
asthma (AZ muh)	respiratory disease often caused by allergies
acute asthma (AZ muh)	sudden, severe asthma that causes coughing and difficulty breathing

extrinsic asthma (ecks TRIN sick AZ muh)	asthma caused by an environmental allergen
intrinsic asthma (in TRIN sick AZ muh)	asthma of unknown cause
status asthmaticus (STAT us az MAT i kus)	long-lasting, persistent asthma
bronchodilators (bronk oh dye LAY turz)	drugs that expand the air passageways to the lungs
sensitization (sen si ti ZAY shun)	becoming reactive to pollen, serum, or antigen
anaphylaxis (an uh fi LACK sis)	extreme reaction to an antigen, protein, or drug
acute anaphylaxis (an uh fi LACK sis)	immediate hypersensitivity

Key Term Practice: Hypersensitivity Disorders

1. Seasonal allergies are called _____, and allergies that last throughout the entire year are referred to as _____.

2. Inflammation of the nasal mucosal resulting from allergies is known as _____.

Immunodeficiency Disorders

Immunodeficiency disorders are characterized by the inability to mount an adequate immune response to disease. These disorders are either innate or acquired.

Acquired immunodeficiency syndrome (AIDS) is the disease caused by infection with the retrovirus **human immunodeficiency virus** (HIV). A retrovirus is a type of virus whose genetic information is found in its RNA rather than its DNA. The HIV binds to T_H cell receptors. This virus cannot survive outside living cells and is transmitted via body fluids, blood, and contaminated needles. HIV attacks T_H cells and renders them incapable of mounting an immune response; thus it hinders the very system meant to protect the body. AIDS lowers the body's immunity by decreasing the number of helper T cells, reversing the ratio of helper T cells to suppressor T cells, and allowing malignancy of lymphoid tissue to develop.

Manifestations of the disease may not appear for several years after infection, as the virus remains latent. Despite its latency, disease transmission is possible throughout the course of disease development, beginning with the initial infection when it may not be apparent.

As impairment of the immune system progresses, signs and symptoms, collectively referred to as **AIDS-related complex**, such as **lymphadenopathy** (lymph node enlargement), weight loss, **fever** (abnormally high body temperature), fatigue, diarrhea, night sweats, and increased disease susceptibility, become obvious (Fig. 12-8). AIDS is advanced HIV infection characterized by diminished immune response, high fevers, *Pneumocystis carinii* pneumonia, Kaposi sarcoma, and an increase in opportunistic infections.

An **opportunistic infection** occurs when a microbe that naturally inhabits the body causes disease or when a relatively minor disease becomes life threatening as a result of impaired immune function. Common infections in the AIDS patient are tuberculosis, herpes simplex, herpes zoster, *Candida albicans*, and toxoplasmosis. End stages are marked by neurologic involvement. Diagnosis is made by enzyme-linked immunosorbent assay and confirmed by western blot test. An **enzyme-linked immunosorbent assay** (ELISA; pronounced ee LYE suh) is a technique that determines the presence of foreign proteins by using an enzyme that bonds to its antigen or antibody, forming a complex that is then used to identify antibodies to bacteria, viruses, DNA allergens, and immunoglobulins. The **western blot test** is a specific electrophoresis procedure used to detect the presence of antibodies to viral proteins in a

FIGURE 12-8
Lymphadenopathy is the enlargement of lymph nodes, as demonstrated by these cervical nodes. (Image provided by Stedman's.)

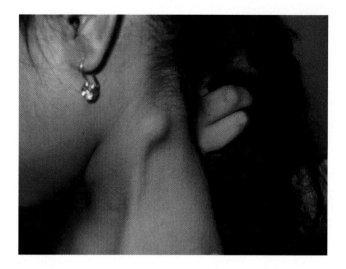

blood sample. The western blot test serves as a follow-up test to a positive ELISA test because it is more sensitive.

There is no cure for AIDS, and treatment is aimed at improving the patient's immune status and preventing infections. Pharmacological therapy consists of antiviral, reverse transcriptase (RT), and protease inhibitor drugs given in combinations often called "cocktails." **Immunotherapy** (serotherapy), therapy that boosts the immune system function—for example, with monoclonal antibodies—is used to treat AIDS when other treatments fail. In **monoclonal antibody** (MAB or MoAb) treatment, an immunoglobulin molecule (antibody) is cloned to establish cell lines of specific antibodies against a particular antigen.

Severe combined immunodeficiency (SCID) syndrome is an inherited disorder characterized by the impairment of cell-mediated and humoral immunity. The first sign is chronic infections early in infancy once maternal-transferred immunity has waned. Initial diagnosis is made by clinical history of low-grade fever and recurring infections. It is confirmed by lymph node biopsy that demonstrates absent lymph follicles and blood tests that indicate low B cell and T cell counts. Individuals with SCID are placed in a completely sterile environment to prevent infections. Currently, the only other treatment option remains a bone marrow transplant to restore immune function. The much-publicized case of David, the boy who lived in a plastic bubble, illustrated this often-fatal infirmity.

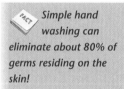 *Simple hand washing can eliminate about 80% of germs residing on the skin!*

Key Terms	Definitions
acquired immunodeficiency (im yoo noh de FISH un see) **syndrome**	disease caused by HIV
human immunodeficiency virus (im yoo noh de FISH un see)	retrovirus that causes AIDS
AIDS-related complex	signs and symptoms related to AIDS
lymphadenopathy (lim fad e NOP uh thee)	lymph node enlargement owing to an underlying pathology
fever	abnormally high body temperature
opportunistic infection	harmless microbes that cause pathology when the host's immune response is impaired
enzyme-linked immunosorbent (im yoo noh SOR bent) **assay**	technique that determines the presence of foreign proteins using an enzyme that bonds to its antigen or antibody, forming a complex

western blot test	type of electrophoresis that separates protein precipitates formed by immunologic reactions
immunotherapy (im yoo noh THERR uh pee)	therapy that boosts immune system function
monoclonal antibody (mon oh KLOH nul AN tee bod ee)	specific antibody produced in large quantities by clones of a cell
severe combined immunodeficiency (im yoo noh de FISH un see) syndrome	disorder in which both humoral and cell-mediated immunity are impaired

Key Term Practice: Immunodeficiency Disorders

1. What does SCID stand for? _____

2. Identify the virus that causes AIDS. _____

Infections

Infections and **lymphangitis** (inflammation of lymph tissue) are common to lymphatic organs because these structures are involved with pathogen eradication. **Elephantiasis**, also termed **filariasis**, is a chronic disease characterized by enlargement of subcutaneous and cutaneous tissue due to lymphatic obstruction and lymphedema (Fig. 12-9). **Lymphedema** is the swelling of extremity lymph vessels caused by the accumulation of tissue fluid and lymph in the interstitial spaces (Fig. 12-10). The legs and male scrotum are primarily affected in elephantiasis. It is caused by the filaria (parasitic roundworm) *Wuchereria bancrofti*, which infects lymphatic tissues. The disease is common in tropical and subtropical regions and is diagnosed by the presence of microfilariae in blood smears. It is treated with diethylcarbamazine and metronidazole drugs.

An acute disorder caused by the Epstein-Barr virus (EBV) is **infectious mononucleosis**, known as mono or the "kissing disease." Signs and symptoms are fever, fatigue, generalized malaise, lymph node enlargement, and sore throat. The virus infects B cells, and latent infections are common. Once afflicted, the individual carries the virus for life. The clinical and physical pictures provide the initial diagnosis, and blood tests indicating elevated lymphocytes confirm the findings. Treatment options are antiviral medication administration and rest.

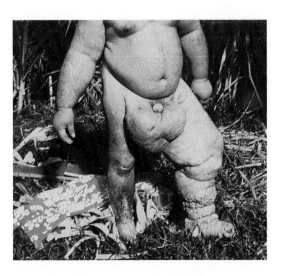

FIGURE 12-9
Elephantiasis is a condition caused by a roundworm that results in lymphedema caused by lymphatic obstruction. (Reprinted with permission from Rubin E, Farber JL. Pathology. 3rd ed. Philadelphia: Lippincott Williams & Wilkins, 1999.)

Tonsillitis is inflammation of the tonsils, usually affecting the pharyngeal tonsils, generally caused by a bacterial or viral infection. It is characterized by swelling and pain, sore throat, and fever. When the pharynx (region between mouth and esophagus) is involved, it is termed **tonsillopharyngitis**, and mouth breathing may become difficult. It is diagnosed by the clinical picture and identification of the culprit organism by a throat swab. When tonsillitis is bacterial in origin, antibiotics are prescribed. **Tonsillectomy** (removal of the tonsils) is performed only as a last resort because the tonsils play a key role in fighting infection.

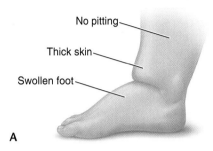

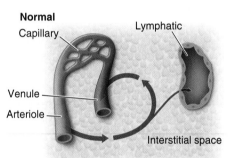

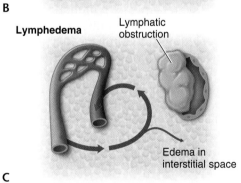

FIGURE 12-10
Lymphedema is the swelling of extremity lymph vessels caused by the accumulation of tissue fluid and lymph in the interstitial spaces. **(A)** Swollen leg. Mechanism of lymphedema **(B)** and **(C)**.

Key Terms	Definitions
lymphangitis (lim fan JYE tis)	inflammation of the lymph vessels
elephantiasis (el e fan TYE uh sis)	disease caused by *Wuchereria bancrofti;* filariasis
filariasis (fil uh RYE uh sis)	disease caused by *Wuchereria bancrofti;* elephantiasis
lymphedema (lim fe DEE muh)	lymph tissue swelling in the extremities
infectious mononucleosis (mon oh new klee OH sis)	disease caused by EBV characterized by an increased number of monocytes
tonsillitis (ton si LYE tis)	inflammation of the tonsils
tonsillopharyngitis (ton si loh fair in JYE tis)	inflammation of the tonsils and pharynx
tonsillectomy (ton sil LECK toh mee)	surgical removal of the tonsils

Key Term Practice: Infections

1. _____ refers to tonsil inflammation.

2. Inflammation of the tonsils and pharynx is called _____.

3. Surgical removal of the tonsils is termed _____.

Tumors

Tumors are abnormal, uncontrolled growths that may occur in lymphatic vessels, tissues, and organs. These structures have no physiological function and are classified as benign (having a mild or harmless effect) or malignant (capable of spreading and causing harm). Malignant lymph cells, or cancerous neoplasms of lymphatic structures, are termed **lymphomas.** Monoclonal antibody treatments are effective for treating cancer when they are tagged with a radionuclide to deliver radiation to cancerous tissue.

The medical term for cancer originating in lymphatic tissue is **malignant lymphoma. Hodgkin disease** (HD) is a malignant lymphoma affecting lymph nodes and lymph organs. It is characterized by lymphadenopathy and sometimes **splenomegaly** (enlarged spleen) and hepatomegaly, but there is no pain. Reed-Sternberg (or Sternberg-Reed) cells, large transformed lymphocytes with one or two large nuclei, are typical of HD. Approximately 40% of lymphomas are Hodgkin type with bipolar distribution; they generally affect individuals who are between 15 and 35 years old or over age 50. It may be precipitated by a viral infection. The clinical picture and scintigraphy or lymphangiography makes the diagnosis.

Scintigraphy is a diagnostic procedure allowing for the examination of lymphatics after injection of a radionuclide. After lymphatic absorption of the radioactive substance, the scanner detects the radioactive tracer and makes a photographic recording, or **scintigram,** of radionuclide distribution using a gamma camera. An alternate term for scintigram is **scintiscan.** Scintigraphic studies are useful for measuring lymphatic metastases. **Lymphangiography** involves the injection of dye into lymphatic vessels for localization. The nodes absorb the dye and x-ray images reveal nodal conditions. It is used to stage (determine the level of disease progression) the disease, locate the source of the lymphedema, and evaluate the treatment.

Total nodal radiation, immunosuppressive drugs (such as azathioprine), corticosteroids, and chemotherapy are used in treating the disease. **Radiation therapy,** or **radiotherapy,** applies radiation to the lymph nodes to treat neoplastic disease. X-rays are aimed at the tumor to kill cancerous cells. **Azathioprine** (AZT) is a synthetic drug that suppresses the body's immune response. **Corticosteroids** are drugs with identical molecular formulas as naturally occurring steroid hormones from the cortical adrenal gland. Corticosteroids have both anti-inflammatory and immunosuppressive actions.

Toxic immunosuppressive drugs for the treatment of Hodgkin disease and tumors of the lymphatic system are cyclosporine and cyclophosphamide. **Cyclosporine** is an immunosuppressant drug derived from soil fungi that selectively depresses T_H cells, and **cyclophosphamide** suppresses B cell activity and antibody formation. **Cytotoxic drugs** are nonselective immunosuppressive drugs. Although the target is immune cells, these pharmacological agents kill all replicating cells. A common four-drug chemotherapy regimen for the treatment of Hodgkin disease is **mechlorethamine, oncovin, prednisone, and procarbazine** (MOPP). (Mechlorethamine is also called nitrogen mustard, and Oncovin is known as vincristine.)

Non-Hodgkin lymphoma (NHL) is the general term used to describe the diverse group of other lymphomas. Some evidence suggests that these lymphomas have a genetic predisposition. **Burkitt lymphoma,** a rare malignant tumor affecting white blood cells, is an example of an NHL (Fig. 12-11). This cancer, occurring primarily in children, usually affects the retroperitoneal area and mandible but not the lymph nodes and bone marrow. Viral infections, including EBV, have been implicated in the disease. A clinical history of fever and night sweats provides the initial diagnosis. Advanced disease is marked by hepatomegaly and splenomegaly, and tissue biopsy is used to confirm the diagnosis. Treatment of NHL may be unnecessary until later stages, in which radiation, chemotherapy, and bone marrow transplants (discussed later in this chapter) may be used.

Kaposi sarcoma is cancer of the lymphatic cell membranes and connective tissues. It is marked by purplish red skin patches and occurs more often in AIDS patients than in other individuals. Treatment measures are primarily supportive.

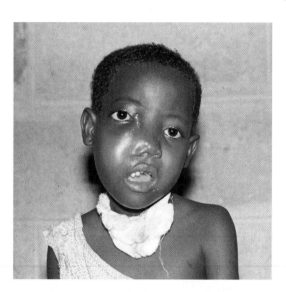

FIGURE 12-11
Burkitt lymphoma is a rare malignant tumor affecting the white blood cells. (Reprinted with permission from Rubin E, Farber JL. Pathology. 3rd ed. Philadelphia: Lippincott Williams & Wilkins, 1999.)

Key Terms	*Definitions*
lymphomas (lim FOH muz)	neoplasms of lymphatic tissue
malignant lymphoma (lim FOH muh)	cancer of the lymphatic tissues
Hodgkin (HOJ kin) **disease**	type of malignant lymphoma characterized by progressive enlargement of the lymph nodes and spleen and sometimes the liver
splenomegaly (splee noh MEG uh lee)	enlarged spleen
scintigraphy (sin TIG ruh fee)	procedure in which lymphatic absorption of a radioactive substance leads to a computer-created image using a scintillation (gamma) camera
scintigram (SIN ti gram)	photographic recording of radionuclide uptake; scintiscan
scintiscan (SIN ti skan)	photographic recording of radionuclide uptake; scintigram
lymphangiography (lim fan jee OG ruh fee)	image of the lymphatic vessels using an injected dye
radiation therapy	treating a disease by using targeted x-rays; another term for radiotherapy
radiotherapy	treating a disease by using targeted x-rays; radiation therapy
azathioprine (ay zuh THIGH oh preen)	immunosuppressive drug
corticosteroids (kor ti koh STEER oidz)	anti-inflammatory, immunosuppressant drugs

cyclosporine (sigh kloh SPOR een)	immunosuppressive drug
cyclophosphamide (sigh kloh FOS fuh mide)	immunosuppressive drug
cytotoxic (sigh toh TOCK sick) **drugs**	chemical agents that kill cells
mechlorethamine, oncovin, prednisone, (meck lor ETH uh meen, on KOH vin, PRED ni sohn) **and procarbazine** (proh KAR buh zeen)	combination of chemotherapeutic drugs used in the treatment of Hodgkin disease
non-Hodgkin (HOJ kin) **lymphoma**	malignant lymphoma that is not Hodgkin disease
Burkitt (BUR kit) **lymphoma**	malignant lymphoma involving the retroperitoneal area and mandible, but not the lymph nodes, bone marrow, and spleen
Kaposi sarcoma (KA poh zee sahr KOH muh)	cancer of the lymphatic connective tissue

Key Term Practice: Tumors

1. Neoplasm of the lymphatic tissue is termed _____.

2. Cancer of the lymphatic tissues characterized by reddish blue or purplish skin nodules is _____.

Transplants

Transplants involve the removal of tissue from one site or person and the placement of it in another site or person. The immune system is of great concern when dealing with tissue or organ transplants because the body recognizes the imported tissue as foreign. Medical transplants are performed out of necessity, and compatibility—the congruity that exists between the donor and recipient tissue—is a major factor. To reduce the risk of tissue rejection in transplant surgery, the MHC must be considered before organ transplant procedures can occur so that the tissue that is transplanted is as close to the recipient's as possible. Cyclosporine drugs that dampen the immune response are used primarily to prevent organ and tissue rejection in transplant surgery. If the immune response is impeded, the body will not mount a full-blown attack on the implanted tissue. As a result, however, the generalized risk of infection also increases.

Grafts are any living tissues or organs used for transplantation. Typically, portions are transplanted to another body part to replace nonfunctional or absent tissue. **Bone marrow transplants** involve extracting cells from functioning red bone marrow and transferring them to an immunosuppressed patient.

Several types of transplants exist. Allogeneic transplants or **allografts** (*allo-* = "other, different") occur between genetically nonidentical members of the same species. For example, allografts take place between compatible donor (usually a sibling or close family member) and recipient. An **autograft** (*auto-* = "self") or autologous transplant uses the patient's own tissue, which is collected and used immediately or frozen for later use. Stem cell (undifferentiated cell from which other cells are derived) transplants are a common type of autologous graft. An **isograft** (*iso-* = "like"), or syngraft or isogeneic transplant, is tissue taken from a genetically identical twin for transference to the recipient. Tissue transplant from a different species, such as using valves from a pig for human valve replacement, is termed **xenograft** (*xeno-* = "strange, foreign") or heterograft.

Graft versus host (GVH) **disease** is an immune reaction in transplant recipients. It occurs most frequently with bone marrow transplants in which the donor's marrow immune cells attack the recipient's tissues. The situation is complicated by the fact that the bone marrow recipient is already immunosuppressed to receive the transplant. The newly transplanted donor's cells react against the recipient's (host's) antigens, creating systemic effects. Signs and symptoms include rash, diarrhea, gastrointestinal distress, and hepatosplenomegaly. Treatment depends on the individual patient. If the condition is not resolved, it could lead to death.

Immunosuppressive drugs are used to overcome tissue rejection. Some are selective in their actions, and others target the entire immune response. **Tissue rejection** involves antibody production against the proteins (antigens) in a transplanted organ. Drugs that affect T cell activity by depleting their numbers include **antilymphocyte serum** or **antilymphocyte globulin.** These drugs are used to hamper T cell–mediated immunity and are beneficial in the prevention of tissue and organ rejection.

Key Terms	Definitions
transplants	tissue transfers between compatible donor and recipient
grafts	tissues used for transplant
bone marrow transplants	bone marrow cells collected and transferred from one individual to another
allografts (AL oh grafts)	transplants between compatible donor and recipient of the same species; allogeneic transplant
autograft (AW toh graft)	transplant tissue sample taken from the same person; autologous transplant
isograft (EYE soh graft)	transplant between identical twins; syngraft
xenograft (ZEE noh graft)	transplant between two different species
graft versus host disease	immunologic reaction involving the attack of host cells by donor immune cells
tissue rejection	destruction of transplanted tissue by the immune response
antilymphocyte serum (an tee LIM foh site SEER um)	agent that depletes T cell numbers
antilymphocyte globulin (an tee LIM foh site GLOB yoo lin)	agent that interferes with cellular immunity by depleting T cell numbers

Key Term Practice: Transplants

1. Graft versus host disease results when _____.

   A. host cells attack the transplanted tissue

   B. donor tissue immune cells attack the host tissue

2. What is the term described by each of the following definitions?

   A. transplant tissue between identical twins _____

   B. transplant tissue sample taken from same person _____

   C. transplant tissue between two different species _____

   D. transplant between compatible donor and recipient _____

CLINICAL TERMS

Clinical Dimension	Term	Description
DISORDERS		
	acquired hypogammaglobulinemia	disease caused by decreased plasma gammaglobulin; common variable immunodeficiency (CVID)
	acquired immunodeficiency syndrome (AIDS)	disease caused by HIV
	acute anaphylaxis	immediate hypersensitivity
	acute asthma	sudden, severe asthma that causes coughing and difficulty breathing
	agammaglobulinemia	antibody deficiency
	allergic rhinitis	nasal mucous membrane inflammation caused by allergen inhalation
	allergy	abnormal reactivity to a subsequent antigen exposure
	anaphylaxis	extreme reaction to an antigen, protein, or drug
	asthma	respiratory disease often caused by allergies
	autoimmune diseases	disorders that result from the immune response directed against the host
	Burkitt lymphoma	malignant lymphoma involving the retroperitoneal area and mandible, but not the lymph nodes, bone marrow, and spleen
	chronic mucocutaneous candidiasis (CMC)	mucous membrane and skin infections as a result of impaired antibody response to fungi
	common variable immunodeficiency (CVID) syndrome	disease caused by decreased plasma gammaglobulin; acquired hypogammaglobulinemia
	congenital thymic hypoplasia	underdevelopment or absence of the thymus; DiGeorge syndrome
	DiGeorge syndrome	underdevelopment or absence of the thymus; congenital thymic hypoplasia
	elephantiasis	disease caused by *Wuchereria bancrofti*; filariasis
	extrinsic asthma	asthma caused by an environmental allergen
	filariasis	disease caused by *Wuchereria bancrofti*; elephantiasis
	graft versus host disease	immunologic reaction involving the attack of host cells by donor immune cells

Clinical Dimension	Term	Description
	hay fever	allergy to seasonal plant allergens
	Hodgkin disease (HD)	type of malignant lymphoma characterized by progressive enlargement of the lymph nodes and spleen and sometimes the liver
	human immunodeficiency virus (HIV)	retrovirus that causes AIDS
	hypersensitivity	abnormal sensitivity to an allergen
	hypersplenism	group of conditions in which the cellular components of the blood are removed by the spleen
	infectious mononucleosis	disease caused by EBV characterized by an increased number of monocytes
	intrinsic asthma	asthma of unknown cause
	Kaposi sarcoma	cancer of the lymphatic connective tissue
	latex allergy	hypersensitivity to products made from the sap of the rubber plant
	lymphomas	neoplasms of the lymphatic tissue
	malignant lymphoma	cancer of the lymphatic tissues
	multiple myeloma	uncommon disorder affecting more men than women characterized by uncontrolled plasma cell proliferation, tumor formation, skeletal and renal disease, abnormal immunoglobulin synthesis, and bone marrow dysfunction
	non-Hodgkin lymphoma (NHL)	malignant lymphoma that is not Hodgkin disease
	opportunistic infection	harmless microbes that causes pathology when the host's immune response is impaired
	perennial allergic rhinitis	year-round allergy to environmental allergens
	selective immunoglobulin A deficiency	disorder caused by iga deficiency
	sensitization	becoming reactive to pollen, serum, or an antigen
	severe combined immunodeficiency (SCID) syndrome	disorder in which both humoral and cell-mediated immunity are impaired
	Sjögren syndrome	autoimmune disease marked by dry skin and nasal membranes, and multiple areas of arthritis

Clinical Dimension	Term	Description
	status asthmaticus	long-lasting, persistent asthma
	thymoma	usually benign tumor of the thymus; some forms are associated with myasthenia gravis
	tissue rejection	destruction of transplanted tissue by the immune response
	Wiskott-Aldrich syndrome	X-linked disorder characterized by decreased B cell and T cell function
	X-linked agammaglobulinemia	condition marked by decreased serum immunoglobulin concentration and antibody deficiency
SIGNS AND SYMPTOMS		
	AIDS-related complex	signs and symptoms related to AIDS
	fever	abnormally high body temperature
	lymphadenopathy	lymph enlargement owing to an erlying pathology
	lymphangitis	inflammation of the lymph vessels
	lymphedema	lymph tissue swelling in the extremities
	sicca	dryness
	splenomegaly	enlarged spleen
	tonsillitis	inflammation of the tonsils
	tonsillopharyngitis	inflammation of the tonsils and pharynx
	wheal	raised, reddened area caused by a sensitivity reaction
CLINICAL TESTS AND DIAGNOSTIC PROCEDURES		
	antibody titer	blood test that determines the antibody level against a particular antigen; used to determine the body's previous exposure to a particular antigen
	antiglobulin test	detects antibodies or complement in the blood; Coombs test
	biopsy	surgical extraction of a tissue sample for laboratory examination
	Coombs test	detects antibodies or complement in the blood; antiglobulin test
	enzyme-linked immunosorbent assay (ELISA)	technique that determines the presence of foreign proteins using an enzyme that bonds to its antigen or antibody, forming a complex
	exposure test	identifies previous contact with fungal or parasitic organisms

Clinical Dimension	Term	Description
	human leukocyte antigen (HLA) test	determines degrees of compatibility for tissue transplant
	immunoelectrophoresis	technique used for the identification of proteins through immunologic reactions
	intradermal test	detects sensitivity to an antigen injected into the skin
	lymphangiography	image of the lymphatic vessels using an injected dye
	nuclear scan	image formed after introduction of radionuclides
	patch test	determines sensitivity to an antigen
	prick test	detects a reaction to an antigen
	scintigram	photographic recording of radionuclide uptake; scintiscan
	scintigraphy	procedure in which lymphatic absorption of a radioactive substance leads to a computer-created image using a scintillation (gamma) camera
	scintiscan	photographic recording of radionuclide uptake; scintigram
	tuberculin skin test	detects past or present tuberculosis infection
	western blot	type of electrophoresis that separates protein precipitates formed by immunologic reactions
TREATMENTS		
	allogeneic transplant	transplant between compatible donor and recipient of the same species; allograft
	allografts	transplants between compatible donor and recipient of the same species; allogeneic transplant
	antianaphylaxis	procedure for making a person insensitive to an antigen; desensitization
	antihistamines	drugs that work against histamine
	antilymphocyte serum	agent that depletes T cell numbers
	antilymphocyte globulin	agent that interferes with cellular immunity by depleting T cell numbers
	autograft	transplant tissue sample taken from the same person; autologous transplant

Clinical Dimension	Term	Description
	autologous transplant	transplant tissue sample taken from the same person; autograft
	azathioprine (AZT)	immunosuppressive drug
	bone marrow transplants	bone marrow cells collected and transferred from one individual to another
	bronchodilators	drugs that expand the air passageways to the lungs
	corticosteroids	anti-inflammatory, immunosuppressant drugs
	cyclophosphamide	immunosuppressive drug
	cyclosporine	immunosuppressive drug
	cytotoxic drugs	chemical agents that kill cells
	decongestants	drugs that relieve nasal congestion
	desensitization	procedure for making a person insensitive to an antigen; antianaphylaxis
	grafts	tissues used for transplant
	heterograft	transplant between two different species; xenograft
	immunotherapy	therapy that boosts immune system function
	isogeneic transplant	transplant between identical twins; syngraft or isograft
	isograft	transplant between identical twins; syngraft
	mechlorethamine, Oncovin, prednisone, and procarbazine (MOPP)	combination of chemotherapeutic drugs used in the treatment of Hodgkin disease
	monoclonal antibody	specific antibody produced in large quantities by clones of a cell
	radiation therapy	treating a disease by using targeted x-rays; radiotherapy
	radiotherapy	treating a disease by using targeted x-rays; radiation therapy
	syngraft	transplant between identical twins; isograft or isogeneic transplant
	tonsillectomy	surgical removal of the tonsils
	transplants	tissue transfers between compatible donor and recipient
	xenograft	transplant between two different species

Lifespan

Lymphatic system development begins early in embryonic life. By the 5th gestational week, lymphatic vessels and nodes are apparent. Except for the thymus gland, which is derived from the endoderm, lymphatic vessels and organs are derived from the mesodermic layer. The vessels originate from lymph sacs that developed from veins. Lymphocytes are derived from hematopoietic (blood) tissue.

The thymus gland is of particular importance regarding immune function. At birth, the thymus is relatively large and continues to grow until puberty and early adolescence, when it reaches its maximum size. Thereafter, it gradually diminishes in size and function. As the thymus gland continues to atrophy, T cells decline in number, and the remaining T cells fail to function as well as their predecessors. In this sense, the thymus loses a portion of its ability to protect against the invasion of bacteria and viruses. It may also fail to protect against abnormal cell growth, as in cancers.

The human immune system becomes less efficient throughout the aging process, but the relationship between decreased immune response and aging is not well understood. Decreased function may be the result of diminished organ reserve. Along with the functional decline, autoantibodies within the blood tend to rise, thereby increasing the risk of developing autoimmune diseases. The B cells also function less well; thus their capacity to form clones and release specific antibodies is diminished in elderly immune systems. Moreover, the antibodies that are produced are directed at the body's own tissue, increasing the risk of developing autoimmune diseases.

Other age-related changes in immunity are delayed hypersensitivity, decreased lymphocyte response to antigens, decreased antibody titer (blood test used to determine the concentration of an antibody) after vaccination, slower antibody response, increased susceptibility to infections, and prolonged infectious episodes. Conversely, some elderly persons have no immunologic changes and have immune systems that are as vigorous as when they were young.

In the News: Antibiotic Resistance

Have you heard of a "superinfection?" This is one that is extremely difficult to treat with available antibiotics because of resistant strains of bacteria. An increasing public health problem currently in the news is antibiotic resistance. The overuse of antibiotics through a variety of means has created disease-causing microbes that are remarkably resilient to drugs meant to kill them.

According to the Centers for Disease Control and Prevention (CDC), bacterial infections worldwide are becoming resistant to drugs that once were effective. Bacteria develop resistance to drugs via a few mechanisms. Bacteria destroy the effect of the chemotherapeutic drug or antibiotic, they mutate to avoid the sensitive step that the drug is designed to affect, or they evolve in way that does not allow the drug to enter.

The problem stems from several causes—namely, unneeded, intensive overuse of antibiotics. Each year, nearly 50 million of the 150 million prescriptions for antibiotics are unnecessary in the United States. For example, too many antibiotics are prescribed for viral infections, for which they offer no benefit; and taking an antibiotic for a virus-based infection increases the risk of a future drug-resistant infection. Compounding the problem is the fact that antibiotics are not always taken as prescribed. Patients cut short the course of treatment because symptoms have disappeared. Failing to adhere to prescription instructions may not kill all the bacteria, allowing the remaining microbes to become drug resilient. Antimicrobial agents are cropping up in soaps, detergents, lotions, and countless other household items; and there is no proven benefit of these products to public health. This adds to the predicament. Simple soap with good hand washing will suffice. Antibacterial products should be reserved for the health-care setting and for individuals with compromised immune systems.

New drug development cannot keep pace with the rate of microbial resistance. Unless drastic measures are taken now, these superbugs may be the rule instead of the exception.

COMMON ABBREVIATIONS

Abbreviation	Term
Ab	antibody
Ag	antigen
AIDS	acquired immunodeficiency syndrome
AMTA	American Massage Therapy Association
AZT	azathioprine
CDC	Centers for Disease Control and Prevention
CMC	chronic mucocutaneous candidiasis
CPR	cardiopulmonary resuscitation
CVID	common variable immunodeficiency
EBV	Epstein-Barr virus
ELISA	enzyme-linked immunosorbent assay
γ-globulin	gammaglobulin
GVH	graft versus host
HIV	human immunovirus
HLA	human leukocyte antigen; MHC
HD	Hodgkin disease
IFN	interferon
Ig	immunoglobulin
KS	Kaposi sarcoma
MAB	monoclonal antibody
MoAb	monoclonal antibody
MHC	major histocompatibility complex; HLA
MOPP	mechlorethamine, Oncovin, prednisone, procarbazine
MT	massage therapist
NCETMB	National Certification Examination for Therapeutic Massage and Bodywork
NHL	non-Hodgkin lymphoma
NK cells	natural killer cells
NSAID	nonsteroidal anti-inflammatory drug
PNI	psychoneuroimmunology
RA	rheumatoid arthritis
RES	reticuloendothelial system
RT	reverse transcriptase
SCID	severe combined immunodeficiency

Abbreviation	Term
SLE	systemic lupus erythematosus
T_C cells	cytotoxic T cell
T_H cells	helper T cell
T_S cells	suppressor T cell

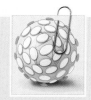

Case Study

Mrs. Eleanor Chime is 67 years old and has a history of melanoma (malignant neoplasm derived from skin melanocytes) on her back. The melanoma metastasized to regional lymph nodes with concomitant splenomegaly and hepatomegaly. Her lungs and brain are not affected.

She is not very ambulatory because of arthritis and suffers from lymphedema, notably in her legs. Analgesics and nonsteroidal anti-inflammatory drugs (NSAIDs) provide some relief. Mrs. Chime's oncologist recommended massage therapy for lymphedema relief.

Case Study Questions

Select the best answer to each of the following questions.

1. **Splenomegaly is best described as** _____.

   a. enlargement of the spleen
   b. papule on the epidermis
   c. cancer of the spleen
   d. non-Hodgkin lymphoma

2. **Lymphedema is best described as** _____.

   a. enlargement of the lymph nodes
   b. swelling of lymphatic tissue
   c. an autoimmune disease
   d. all of these

3. **Lymphedema could result from** _____.

   a. obstructed lymphatics
   b. immobility
   c. decreased fluid intake
   d. a and b

4. **Why might Mrs. Chime experience relief after having massage therapy?**

   a. The oils used increase lymph flow.
   b. Manual manipulation and compression serve as lymphokinetic factors that enhance lymph flow.
   c. Reclining while receiving a massage increases lymph flow.
   d. Massage therapy is counterintuitive, and the benefit she proclaims is merely perceived and not actual.

REAL WORLD REPORT

Mrs. Chime brought her medical report to the spa so that the physician on staff and Lee could review it. Her oncologist believes that massage therapy will assist with her persistent lymphedema.

CENTRAL NUCLEAR MEDICINE IMAGING

NAME: Eleanor Chime	DOB: January 23, 1936
AGE: 67	EXAM DATE: May 3, 2003
DATEORD: May 2, 2003	ORDPHYS: R. J. Meter, DO

CLINICAL INFORMATION: Melanoma in the back; persistent lymphedema

LYMPHOSCINTIGRAPHY

After four separate intradermal injections of technetium-99m sulfur colloid (each injection contains approximately 90 mCi) surrounding the previous excisional biopsy at the dorsal aspect of the upper lumbar region, scintigraphic evaluation was obtained.

The lymphatic drainage was noted toward the right axilla soon after the injection was completed. There are two separate areas of prominent radionuclide concentration within the right-side axillary lymph nodes. The lateral projection show also two additional areas of mildly to moderately increased lymph nodal uptake adjacent to the above-described prominent lymph nodal uptake. There was no lymphatic drainage noted in the groin region.

At the end of the scintigraphic study, the two prominent uptakes in the right axillary lymph nodes were localized using a small amount of radioisotopic marker and the corresponding areas were marked on the skin. The patient tolerated the procedure well and left the department for sentinel node sampling.

DICTATED BY: E. Matters, MD

This document has been reviewed and electronically approved.

REAL WORLD REPORT QUESTIONS

The following exercises review the medical terms in the preceding medical report. Two terms may be new to you. Technetium-99m is used as a radiopharmaceutical for scanning purposes. The abbreviation mCi stands for millicurie, which is a unit of radioactivity equal to 3.7×10^7 disintegrations per second.

1. Mrs. Chime was sent for sentinel node sampling. A sentinel node is the most important node that draws from the area of the tumor. Nodes adjacent to the tumor that receive drainage from the tumor site are sentinel nodes. If the sentinel node does not show cancerous cells during microscopic examination, it may not be necessary to remove any more lymph nodes. Define the following medical terms or phrases.

a. scintigraphic study _____

b. biopsy _____

c. dorsal aspect _____

d. upper lumbar region _____

e. right-side axillary lymph nodes _____

f. increased nodal uptake refers to _____

g. lymphedema _____

REVIEW AND APPLICATION: THREE-LEVEL LEARNING SYSTEM

LEVEL ONE: REVIEWING FACTS AND TERMS USING RECALL

Select the best response to each of the following questions.

1. Interstitial fluid that has entered a lymphatic vessel is termed _____.

    a. plasma

    b. blood

    c. lymph

    d. serum

2. The lymphatic organ located in the mediastinum deep to the sternum is the _____.

    a. thymus

    b. thyroid

    c. parathyroid

    d. spleen

3. _____ is the medical term describing fat globules transported by lacteals.

    a. Lacteal

    b. Chyle

    c. Lymph

    d. Antibody

4. The _____ duct(s) drain(s) the entire body except the upper right quadrant.

    a. right lymphatic

    b. left lymphatic

    c. thoracic

    d. b and c

5. The _____ vessel carries lymph into a node, and the _____ vessel conveys filtered lymph out of the node.

    a. afferent; efferent

    b. efferent; afferent

    c. arterial; venous

    d. capillary; lymphatic

6. A tumor of the lymphatic system is termed a _____.

    a. capsule

    b. lymphocyte

    c. lymphoma

    d. lymph node

7. Disease resistance as a result of antibodies is called _____ defense.

    a. nonspecific

    b. specific

    c. physical

    d. symbiotic

8. Inflammation of the tonsils is termed _____.

    a. tonsillopharyngitis

    b. tonsillectomy

    c. pharyngitis

    d. tonsillitis

9. Proteins that increase cellular resistance are termed _____.

    a. interferons

    b. antigens

    c. macrophages

    d. phagocytes

10. Alveolar macrophages are found in the _____.

    a. spleen

    b. lymph nodes

    c. lungs

    d. intestines

11. _____ is the ability to ward off infection.

    a. Susceptibility

    b. Resistance

    c. Fever

    d. Complement

12. Cellular immunity involves _____.

   a. T cells

   b. antibodies

   c. memory cells

   d. plasma cells

13. Memory recall and action to a previously encountered antigen is known as the _____ response.

   a. primary

   b. tertiary

   c. anamnestic

   d. clone

14. Immune reaction to a first encounter is called the _____ response.

   a. plasma

   b. primary

   c. secondary

   d. HLA

15. T cells mature in the _____.

   a. thyroid

   b. tonsils

   c. T lymphocytes

   d. thymus

16. An alternative term for immunoglobulin is _____.

   a. antigen

   b. complex

   c. CD4$^+$ cell

   d. antibody

17. The type of immunity present after recovering from an infection is _____ immunity.

   a. natural active

   b. natural passive

   c. artificial

   d. innate

18. The immunity conferred to an infant through breast milk is called _____ immunity.

   a. natural active

   b. natural passive

   c. innate

   d. artificial

LEVEL TWO: REVIEWING CONCEPTS

Select the best response to each of the following questions.

19. _____ are chemical agents given to induce an immune response.

   a. Cytotoxic drugs

   b. Antibiotics

   c. Vaccines

   d. Immunosuppressants

20. Which of the following are lymphokinetic factors?

   a. skeletal muscle contractions

   b. arterial pulses

   c. postural changes

   d. all of the above

21. Which pathway correctly identifies lymph flow through the body?

   a. interstitial fluid → lymph trunks → lymph capillaries → thoracic duct or right lymphatic duct

   b. thoracic duct or right lymphatic duct → lymph trunks → lymphatic capillaries → interstitial fluid

   c. lymph capillaries → lymphatics → lymphatic trunks → thoracic duct or right lymphatic duct

   d. lymphatics → lymph capillaries → lymphatic trunks → interstitial fluid

Match the T cell type with its description.

_____ 22. helper T cell

_____ 23. suppressor T cell

_____ 24. cytotoxic T cell

_____ 25. memory T cell

a. halts the immune response of killer T cells

b. long-lived cell that responds to future encounters with a known antigen

c. assists other T cells in their actions

d. directly attacks foreign antigens

Match the drug with its classification or mode of action.

_____ 26. antilymphocyte serum

_____ 27. corticosteroid

_____ 28. cyclosporine

_____ 29. cytotoxic drugs

a. anti-inflammatory, immunosuppressant

b. nonselective, replicating cell killer

c. T cell depleter

d. immunosuppressant, selective T_H depressor

Match the graft type with its definition.

_____ 30. allograft

_____ 31. autograft

_____ 32. isograft

_____ 33. xenograft

a. tissue from same species

b. tissue from different species

c. tissue from self

d. tissue from identical twin

Match the test with its description.

_____ 34. HLA test

_____ 35. biopsy

_____ 36. western blot test

a. confirmation test for HIV; detects antibodies

b. radionuclides used to provide images of organs

_____ 37. nuclear scan

_____ 38. lymphangiography

c. test used to determine compatibility in transplant procedures between donor and patients through antigen detection

d. dye injected into lymphatic vessels for x-ray revelation

e. extraction of tissue sample for examination

Match the pathologic condition with its key characteristics.

_____ 39. severe combined immunodeficiency (SCID) syndrome

_____ 40. anaphylaxis

_____ 41. acquired immunodeficiency syndrome (AIDS)

_____ 42. asthma

_____ 43. perennial allergic rhinitis

a. disease caused by HIV

b. extreme sensitivity to antigen, protein, or drug

c. inherited disorder; absence of immune system

d. year-round allergy to environmental allergens

e. respiratory disease often caused by llergies

Select the best response to each of the following questions.

44. Lymph vessels are most similar to _____.

a. arteries with valves

b. veins with valves

c. arterioles with capillaries

d. venules with capillaries

45. Lymph flow would be the greatest _____.

    a. during sleep

    b. during flight in an aircraft

    c. while bathing

    d. while exercising

46. Lymphatic obstruction resulting from infection in the thumb might cause enlarged lymph nodes in the _____ region.

    a. cervical

    b. axillary

    c. pelvic

    d. inguinal

47. HIV is transmitted to people by _____.

    a. body fluids and blood

    b. skin touching

    c. contaminated needle sharing

    d. a and c

Fill in the blank; use the correct lymphatic system or immunity term to complete the statement.

48. A two-dimensional image of an organ obtained using a scintiscanner is termed a/an _____.

Provide the best response to each of the following questions.

49. Autoimmune diseases occur when the tolerance to self antigens is lost. True or false? _____

50. Do individuals on immunosuppressive drugs have a greater or a lesser risk of succumbing to infection? _____

Provide a medical term to complete a meaningful analogy.

51. Hepatomegaly is to enlarged liver as _____ is to enlarged spleen.

52. Allogeneic transplant is to allograft as _____ is to syngraft or isogeneic transplant.

53. Cytotoxic T cells are to CD8$^+$ cells as _____ are to CD4$^+$ cells.

Define the following abbreviations.

54. AZT _____

55. HD _____

56. Ag _____

57. AIDS _____

58. Ab _____

59. GVH _____

60. Ig _____

Using the following word parts, form a medical term for each definition. Each word part is used only once.

| -angiogram | -ectomy | lymph- |
| lymphadeno- | -pathy | splen- |

61. removal of the spleen _____

62. enlarged lymph nodes _____

63. x-ray of lymphatic tissue after dye injection _____

Define each of the following terms.

64. splenomegaly _____

65. lymphoma _____

66. lymphadenectomy _____

Identify the correctly spelled term in each set.

67. ____

    a. lymphangitis

    b. lymphoangitis

    c. limfangitis

    d. lymphengitis

68. ____

    a. anephylaxis

    b. enaphylaxis

    c. anaphylaxes

    d. anaphylaxis

69. _____

   a. imunodeficiency

   b. immunodeficiency

   c. imunnodeficiency

   d. imminudeficiency

70. _____

   a. humoral

   b. hummoral

   c. humorel

   d. humorol

71. _____

   a. elefantiasis

   b. elephantiasis

   c. elefanntiasis

   d. elephantasis

Unscramble the letters to form a medical term.

72. fragtonex _____

73. mylph _____

74. mathas _____

75. shinriit _____

76. minutyim _____

LEVEL THREE: THINKING CRITICALLY

Write a short answer to each of the following questions.

77. Heinz has been feeling a bit under the weather, but he does not have the flu. Upon physical examination, it was discovered that his lymph nodes in the cervical region were slightly enlarged and palpable. Provide a plausible explanation.

   _____

   _____

   _____

78. Carla is a 3rd-year nursing student. A blood test showed she had antibodies to EBV but she denies being sick with EBV. Explain why she has antibodies to EBV.

   _____

   _____

   _____

KEY TERMS SPELLING TEST FROM CD-ROM

Use the CD-ROM to test yourself on the spelling of key terms from this chapter. Listen to the terms and write them on a separate sheet of paper. Use a medical dictionary to check your answers.

ANSWERS

WORD GROUPING

Definition	Word Part
chyle, fat emulsion in lymph	chyl-, chyli-, chylo-
cells, cellular	cellul-, celluli-, cellulo-
disease, pathologic	patho, patho-
eating, feeding	phag-, phago-
like	iso-
lymph	lymph-, lympho-
lymphatic vessels	lymphangi-, lymphangio-
lymph nodes	lymphaden-, lynphadeno-
milk	lact-, lacti-, lacto-
nose, nasal	rhin-, rhino-
other, different	A. all-, allo-
	B. heter-, hetero-
safe, protected, immune	immuno-
self, one's own	aut-, auto-
spleen	splen-, spleno-
strange, foreign	xeno-
substance that produces or generates	-gen, -gene
tonsil	tonsil-, tonsillo-
toxic, poisonous	tox-, toxi-, toxo-
thymus	thym-, thymo-, thymi-

WORD BUILDING

Word Part	Meaning	Common or Known Word	Example Medical Term
xeno-	strange, foreign	xenolith	xenograft
all-, allo-	other, different	allograft	allogeneic
aut-, auto-	self, one's own	autonomous	autoimmune
cellul-, celluli-, cellulo-	cells, cellular	cellular	cellular immunity
-gen, -gene	substance that produces or generates	antigen	antigen
heter-, hetero-	other, different	heterosexual	heterograft
immuno-	safe, protected, immune	immunology	immunologic response
iso-	like	isolate	isograft
lact-, lacti-, lacto-	milk	lactate	lacteal
lymph-, lympho-	lymph	lymphoma	lymph node
path-, patho-	disease, pathologic	pathophysiology	pathogen
phag-, phago-	eating, feeding	phagocytosis	phagocyte
rhin-, rhino-	nose, nasal	rhinoceros	rhinitis
thym-, thymo-, thymi-	thymus	thyme	thymus gland
tonsill-, tonsillo-	tonsil	tonsillectomy	tonsillitis
tox-, toxi-, toxo-	toxic, poisonous	toxic	lymphotoxin

KEY TERM PRACTICE

Lymphatic System and Immunity Preview
1. lympho-; -cyte; lymphocyte
2. nonspecific immunity; specific immunity

Lymph Nodes, Lymphocytes, and Lymphatics
1. right lymphatic duct
2. Lymphokinetic

Tonsils, Thymus, and Spleen
1. adenoid
2. Thymosin

Nonspecific Defenses: T Cells and Cellular Immunity
1. monocyte–macrophage system
2. lymphotoxins

Specific Defenses: B Cells and Humoral Immunity
1. plasma cells
2. antibodies

Immune Activation
1. major histocompatibility complex (MHC)
2. antigen–antibody complex

Acquired Immunity
1. innate
2. false

Autoimmune Diseases
1. autoimmune disease
2. sicca

Hypersensitivity Disorders
1. hay fever; perennial allergic rhinitis
2. allergic rhinitis

Immunodeficiency Disorders
1. severe combined immunodeficiency disease
2. human immunodeficiency virus (HIV)

Infections
1. Tonsillitis
2. tonsillopharyngitis
3. tonsillectomy

Tumors
1. lymphoma
2. Kaposi sarcoma

Transplants
1. b
2. a. isograft, syngraft, or isogeneic transplant; b. autograft or autologous transplant; c. xenograft or heterograft; d. allogeneic transplant or allograft

CASE STUDY

1. a is the correct answer.
   - b is incorrect because a papule is a small hard bump on the skin.
   - c is incorrect because the word part *-megaly* refers to "enlarged."
   - d is incorrect because splenomegaly refers to an enlargement of the spleen.
2. b is the correct answer.
   - a is incorrect because the word part *-edema* refers to "swelling" not "enlargement."
   - c is incorrect because an autoimmune disease is characterized by the body attacking itself because it can no longer recognize self from nonself tissue.
   - d is incorrect because answers a and c are incorrect.
3. d is the correct answer.
   - c is incorrect because a decreased fluid intake does not cause lymphedema; in fact, fluid restriction often lessens the severity of the swelling.
4. b is the correct answer.
   - a is incorrect because the oils have nothing to do with moving lymphatic fluid.
   - c is incorrect because movement, not reclining, contributes to lymph movement; in fact, elevating a body part will move lymph as a result of gravity.
   - d is incorrect because massage therapy is beneficial for enhancing fluid movement, especially when the body part does not get much exercise. Furthermore, perceived benefits are also beneficial because there is a strong link between psychological and physiological well-being.

REAL WORLD REPORT

1. a. an evaluation of lymph nodes via a two-dimensional image produced by radioactive tracer distribution;
   b. surgical extraction of tissue for examination purposes;
   c. the back side of the body;
   d. the small of the back;
   e. those located in the armpit region on the anatomic right side of the body;
   f. an area in which the radioactive material (technetium-99m) was dense;
   g. swelling in the extremities as a result of lymph accumulation

REVIEW AND APPLICATION: THREE-LEVEL LEARNING SYSTEM

Level One: Reviewing Facts and Terms Using Recall

1. c
2. a
3. b
4. d
5. a
6. c
7. b
8. d
9. a
10. c
11. b
12. a
13. c
14. b
15. d
16. d
17. a
18. b

Level Two: Reviewing Concepts

19. c
20. d
21. c
22. c
23. a
24. d
25. b
26. c
27. a
28. d
29. b
30. a
31. c
32. d
33. b
34. c
35. e
36. a
37. b
38. d
39. c
40. b
41. a
42. e
43. d
44. b
45. d
46. b
47. d
48. scintigram
49. true
50. greater
51. splenomegaly
52. isograft
53. helper T cells (T_H cells)
54. azathioprine
55. Hodgkin disease
56. antigen
57. acquired immunodeficiency syndrome
58. antibody
59. graft verus host
60. immunoglobulin
61. splenectomy
62. lymphadenopathy
63. lymphangiogram
64. enlarged spleen
65. tumor of lymph tissue
66. removal of lymph node
67. a
68. d
69. b
70. a
71. b
72. xenograft
73. lymph
74. asthma
75. rhinitis
76. immunity

Level Three: Thinking Critically

77. Heinz probably has an infection because enlarged lymph nodes are an indication that the body is mounting an immune response.
78. The Epstein-Barr virus causes infectious mononucleosis. Once infected with the virus, the virus will always remain in the body, although there may be no outward signs or symptoms after recovery. However, circulating antibodies indicate either previous infection or exposure.

13

Respiratory System

OBJECTIVES

After completing this chapter, you should be able to:

1. State the meaning of word parts related to the respiratory system.
2. Identify and locate key structures of the respiratory system.
3. Explain functions of the respiratory system.
4. Describe how inhalation and exhalation occur.
5. Define various pulmonary volumes and capacities.
6. Define common signs, symptoms, and treatments of various respiratory system diseases.
7. Explain clinical tests and diagnostic procedures related to this system.
8. Describe anatomical and physiological alterations of the respiratory system throughout the lifespan.
9. Define common abbreviations related to the respiratory system.
10. Define terms used in medical reports involving the respiratory system.
11. Correctly define, spell, and pronounce the chapter's medical terms.

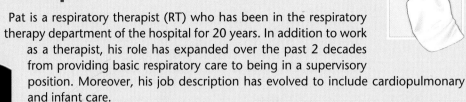

Professional Profile: Respiratory Therapist

Pat is a respiratory therapist (RT) who has been in the respiratory therapy department of the hospital for 20 years. In addition to work as a therapist, his role has expanded over the past 2 decades from providing basic respiratory care to being in a supervisory position. Moreover, his job description has evolved to include cardiopulmonary and infant care.

Daily activities of work in a hospital include pulmonary function testing and patient breathing treatments. Spirometry and blood gas concentration analyses are also routinely performed. Math skills are used daily for computing medication dosages and gas concentrations.

Pat treats patients of all ages with various types of disorders, along with those requiring emergency care. Patients who need respiratory care are treated with oxygen, oxygen mixtures, chest physiotherapy ("poundings" or percussion to dislodge mucus), and aerosol medications. RTs place Venturi masks and nasal cannulas on patients and monitor patients who are on ventilators that deliver pressurized oxygen. When making treatment decisions, physicians rely on the records kept by RTs.

Typical respiratory therapy programs take 2 years to complete. Along with focal respiratory therapy courses, other areas of study within the curriculum include medical terminology, human anatomy and physiology, chemistry, physics, microbiology, and mathematics. Respiratory therapy courses cover procedures, equipment, and clinical tests.

After completing the formalized education, the prospective RT must pass at least one of two examinations offered by the National Board for Respiratory Care (NBRC): certified respiratory therapist (CRT) and registered respiratory therapist (RRT). Either one is the standard for licensure in many states, but the RRT is needed if the therapist is to become a supervisor.

INTRODUCTION

Every cell in the body requires oxygen. The general purposes of the respiratory system are filtering incoming air, transporting air from the environment to the lungs, and exchanging gases to meet the cells' oxygen requirement. The respiratory system engages in trading carbon dioxide (CO_2) for oxygen (O_2) on a continuous basis (Fig. 13-1). The capillary network in close proximity to these alveoli takes up the oxygen. The red blood cells then distribute the oxygen to all body parts. Oxygen delivery is a critical component for normal functioning of every system.

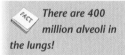
There are 400 million alveoli in the lungs!

Common signs and symptoms of pulmonary disorders are coughing, shortness of breath, and cyanosis (bluish coloration in the mucous membranes resulting from low blood oxygen levels). Pulmonary function tests and diagnostic procedures related to respiratory disorders are highlighted in this chapter.

MEDICAL TERM PARTS

WORD PARTS

Medical term prefixes, suffixes, and combining forms related to the respiratory system are introduced in this section.

Word Parts	Meaning
alveoli-, alveolo-	alveolus (air cell), alveolar
anthrac-, anthraco-	coal, charcoal, carbon, anthrax

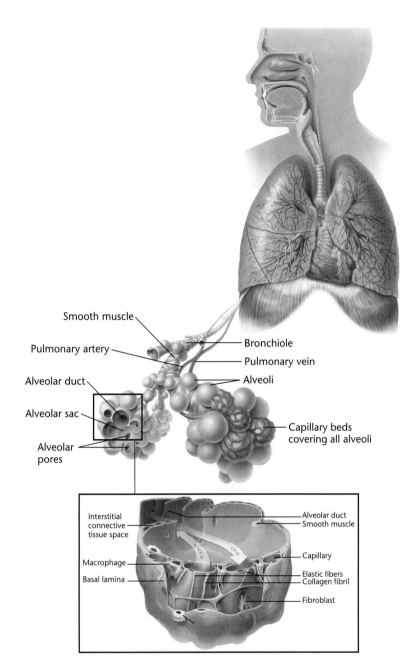

FIGURE 13-1
The respiratory system engages in trading carbon dioxide (CO_2) for oxygen (O_2) on a continuous basis. (Images provided by Anatomical Chart Co.)

Word Parts	Meaning
atel-, atelo-	imperfect, incomplete
brady-	slow
bronch-, bronchi-, broncho-	bronchus, bronchial, windpipe
-capnia	presence of carbon dioxide
chron-, chrono-	time
eu-	normal, true
laryng-, laryngo-	larynx, laryngeal
muc-, muci-, muco-	mucus
nas-, naso-	nose, nasal

Word Parts	Meaning
oro-	mouth, oral
orth-, ortho-	straight
oxy-	presence of oxygen
pharyng-, pharyngo-	pharynx, pharyngeal, throat
phon-, phono-	sound, speech, voice sounds
phren-, phreno-	diaphragm
pleur-, pleuro-	pleura, pleural, lung membrane
-pnea	respiration, respiratory condition
pneum-, pneumo-, pneumon-, pneumono-	air, gas, lung
pulmo-, pulmon-, pulmono-	lung, pulmonary
rhin-, rhino-	nose, nasal, nose-like
spir-, spiro-	breathing
tachy-	rapid, accelerated
thorac-, thoraci-, thoraco-	thorax, thoracic
trache-, tracheo-	trachea, tracheal

WORD ETYMOLOGY

Some words have Greek or Latin word roots but are not true word parts. This section lists those that are used as medical terms.

Word	Definition
bronchus	windpipe
ectasis	a stretching
lobos	lobe
ptysis	act of spitting
sinus	cavity
thorax	breastplate

MEDICAL TERM PARTS USED AS PREFIXES

Prefix	Definition
brady-	slow
eu-	normal, true
oro-	mouth, oral
oxy-	presence of oxygen
tachy-	rapid, accelerated

MEDICAL TERM PARTS USED AS SUFFIXES

Suffix	Definition
-capnia	presence of carbon dioxide
-pnea	respiration, respiratory condition

WORD GROUPING

Using the "Medical Term Parts" tables, identify the prefix, suffix, or combining form for each of the following definitions. The first one has been done as an example.

Definition	Word Part
imperfect, incomplete	atel-, atelo-
air, gas, lung	
alveolus (air cell), alveolar	
breathing	
bronchus, bronchial, windpipe	
coal, charcoal, carbon, anthrax	
diaphragm	
larynx, laryngeal	
lung, pulmonary	
mouth, oral	
mucus	
normal, true	
nose, nasal	
nose, nasal, nose-like	
pharynx, pharyngeal, throat	
pleura, pleural, lung membrane	
presence of carbon dioxide	
presence of oxygen	
rapid, accelerated	
respiration, respiratory condition	
slow	
sound, speech, voice sounds	
straight	
thorax, thoracic	
time	
trachea, tracheal	

WORD BUILDING

Word parts, introduced in the "Medical Term Parts" section, are listed in the following table. For this exercise, first supply the meaning of each word part, then use the word part to build a word you already know. The word you list under "Common or Known Word" does not have to be a medical term; a commonly used word is fine. Be sure, however, that the word correctly reflects the intended meaning. The first one has been done as an example.

Word Part	Meaning	Common or Known Word	Example Medical Term
orth-, ortho-	straight	orthodontics	orthopnea
anthrac-, anthraco-			anthracosis
bronch-, bronchi, broncho			bronchoscopy
chron-, chrono-			chronic
laryng-, laryngo-			laryngospasm
muc-, muci-, muco-			mucus
nas-, naso-			nasal cavity
oro-			oral cavity
phon-, phono-			aphonia
-pnea			apnea
pneum-, pneumo-, pneumon-, pneumono-			pneumonia
pulmo-, pulmon-, pulmono-			pulmonary
tachy-			tachypnea
thorac-, thoraci-, thoraco-			thoracentesis
trache-, tracheo-			tracheostomy

ANATOMY AND PHYSIOLOGY

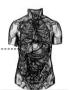

Structures of the Respiratory System

- Bronchial tree: bronchi, bronchioles, and alveoli
- Larynx
- Lungs
- Nasal cavity
- Nose
- Pharynx
- Sinuses
- Trachea

Respiratory System Preview

The respiratory system has two portions: the upper respiratory tract and the lower respiratory tract (Fig. 13-2). The upper structures are the nose, nasal cavity, sinuses, and pharynx. Lower respiratory structures include the larynx (voice box), trachea (windpipe), bronchial tree, and lungs. Consider the *L* as a memory aid: *l*ower structures include the *l*arynx through the *l*ungs. The mouth and nose are structures through which air is breathed, and in the **nasal cavity** are other formations, such as nares and conchae. Four pairs of **sinuses**, air-filled cavities in the face and skull bones that open into the nasal passages, lessen the weight of the skull. The region between the mouth and the esophagus is the **pharynx**, commonly called the throat. *Pharynx* and *larynx* have tricky pronunciations. They are pronounced FAIR inks and LAIR inks, respectively.

The **larynx**, located between the tongue root and the top of the trachea, is the most superior structure of the lower respiratory system. The tube that conducts air from the larynx to the bronchial tree is the **trachea**. The **bronchial tree** begins with the left bronchus and right bronchus, which branch into bronchioles that ultimately terminate as alveoli in each lung. These structures are air-passage tubes leading from the trachea to the lungs. The right and left **lungs** are the respiratory organs, located in the rib cage, in which inhaled oxygen is transferred to the blood and carbon dioxide is removed from the blood.

> **FACT** It is physically impossible to swallow and inhale simultaneously!

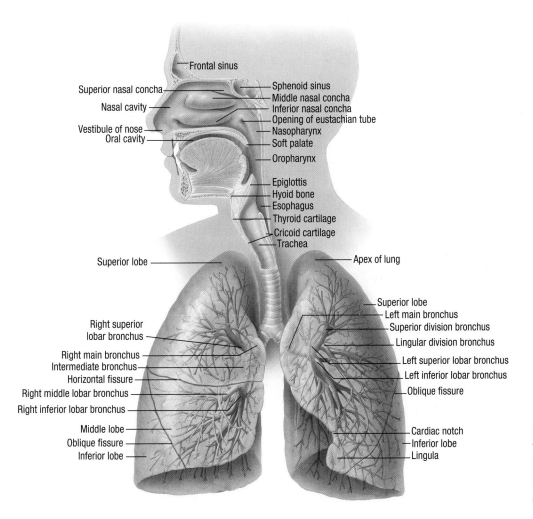

FIGURE 13-2
The structures of the respiratory system. (Image provided by Anatomical Chart Co.)

Key Terms	Definitions
nasal cavity (KAV i tee)	region between the nostrils
sinuses	cavities within the skull bones
pharynx (FAIR inks)	musculomembranous tube extending from the back of the tongue to the esophagus; throat
larynx (LAIR inks)	voice box
trachea (TRAY kee uh)	cartilaginous membranous tube extending from the larynx to the bronchi; windpipe
bronchial (BRONK ee ul) **tree**	branches of the bronchi
lungs	organs of pulmonary ventilation (breathing)

Key Term Practice: Respiratory System Preview

1. What is the plural form for each given term?

   a. pharynx = _____

   b. larynx = _____

2. The word part *bronch-* means _____.

Nose and Nasal Cavity

Skull and facial bone formations provide many of the structures associated with the nose and nasal cavity, including nares, conchae, vestibule, septum and cribriform plate (Fig. 13-3). The **nares** (sing., naris) are nostrils opening out of the nose. The **conchae** (sing., concha), or turbinates, are scroll-shaped projections on the lateral walls of the nasal passages that deflect air; they are divided into the superior, middle, and inferior nasal conchae. The **vestibule** is the space between the flexible tissues of the nose containing vibrissae, fine hairs that filter and screen particulate matter. The cartilaginous membrane that separates the nasal cavity and nostrils into right and left sides is the **septum.**

Separating the roof of the nose from the cranial cavity is the **cribriform plate.** *Cribriform* means "with small holes like a sieve," and these tiny openings within the plate permit branches of the olfactory nerve (cranial nerve I) to enter the cranial cavity, permitting the sense of smell.

Key Terms	Definitions
nares (NAY res)	nostrils
conchae (KONG kee)	projections on the lateral walls of the nasal passages; turbinates
vestibule	nose chamber
septum (SEP tum)	cartilaginous partition dividing the nasal cavity into right and left portions
cribriform (KRIB ri form) **plate**	perforated bone in the skull

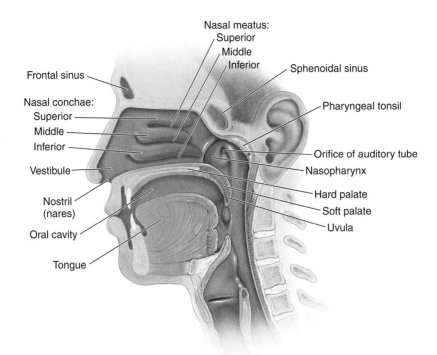

Nasal meatus:
Superior
Middle
Inferior

Frontal sinus

Sphenoidal sinus

Nasal conchae:
Superior
Middle
Inferior

Pharyngeal tonsil

Vestibule

Orifice of auditory tube

Nostril
(nares)

Nasopharynx

Hard palate

Oral cavity

Soft palate

Tongue

Uvula

FIGURE 13-3
The nasal cavity,
sagittal section.

Key Term Practice: Nose and Nasal Cavity

1. What is the singular form for each given term?

   a. nares = _____

   b. conchae = _____

2. Structures within the nasal passages that deflect air are termed _____.

Paranasal Sinuses

Paranasal sinuses are hollow, air-filled spaces in the bones of the face that are lined with mucous membrane. Four major pairs of sinuses, whose names correspond to the bones in which they are located, exist in the cranium (Fig. 13-4). These are the maxillary, frontal, ethmoidal, and sphenoidal sinuses. The **maxillary sinuses** are the largest and are situated within the maxillary bones. The frontal bone, located above the eyes near the midline, contains the **frontal sinuses.** Two groups of small air cells make up the **ethmoidal sinuses,** located in the ethmoid bone found on either side of the upper portion of the nasal cavity. The sphenoid bone is located above the posterior portion of the nasal cavity and contains the **sphenoidal sinuses.**

The paranasal sinuses not only lessen the weight of the skull but also serve as resonance chambers for sound. This is readily understood by anyone experiencing a common head cold: When the sinuses are "plugged," one's voice sounds different because the sound waves are not being conducted across clear air space but rather through the fluid-filled cavities, creating a muffled sound.

The sinuses also drain mucous secretions into the nose. If drainage from the sinuses to the nasal cavity is blocked because of an infection or allergic reaction, the membranes become inflamed and swollen. The accumulation of fluids increases pressure in the sinuses, resulting in a headache.

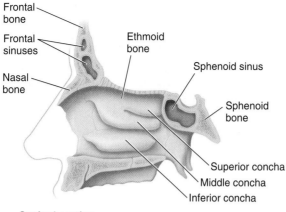

Sagittal section

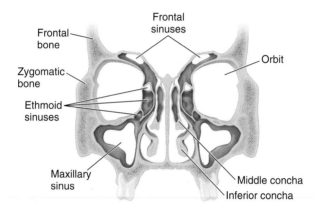

FIGURE 13-4
The paranasal sinuses reduce the weight of the skull, serve as resonance chambers for sound, and drain mucous secretions into the nose.

Anterior section

Key Terms	Definitions
maxillary (MACK si lerr ee) **sinuses**	paranasal sinuses in the maxillae
frontal sinuses	paranasal sinuses in the frontal bone
ethmoidal (eth MOY dul) **sinuses**	paranasal sinuses in the ethmoid bone
sphenoidal (sfe NOY dul) **sinuses**	paranasal sinuses in the sphenoid bone

 Key Term Practice: Paranasal Sinuses

1. Identify the four pairs of paranasal sinuses.

   a. _____

   b. _____

   c. _____

   d. _____

Pharynx

The pharynx, commonly called the throat, connects the oral and nasal cavities to the esophagus and trachea. It is located behind the oral cavity between the nasal cavity and the larynx and serves as a passageway for air to reach the larynx. Also part of the digestive system, it is a pathway for food from the oral cavity to the esophagus. The pharynx also aids in speech by forming vowel sounds.

From superior to inferior, there are three anatomic regions of the pharynx: nasopharynx, oropharynx, and laryngopharynx (Fig. 13-5). The **nasopharynx** is the upper portion situated behind and above the soft palate and is continuous with the nasal passages. The auditory tubes open into this part, and the pharyngeal tonsils are located on its posterior wall. This explains why ear infections commonly spread to the throat and vice versa. The next segment, located below the soft palate and above the larynx and extending from the oral cavity to the hyoid bone, is the **oropharynx**. It contains the palatine tonsils and functions in both digestion and respiration. Located immediately posterior to the larynx is the most inferior section of the pharynx, the **laryngopharynx**. It connects the oropharynx to the esophagus and functions in both digestion and respiration.

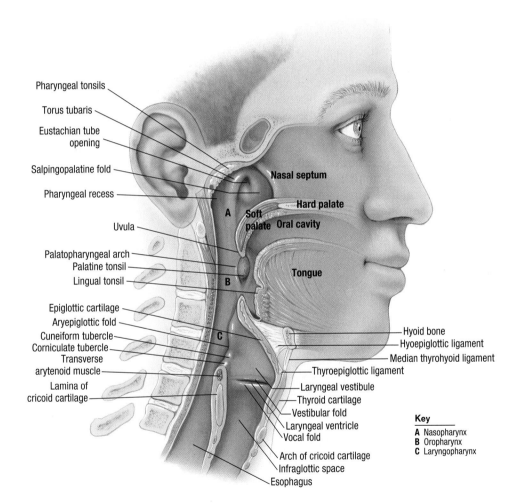

Labels (top to bottom, left side):
Pharyngeal tonsils
Torus tubaris
Eustachian tube opening
Salpingopalatine fold
Pharyngeal recess
Uvula
Palatopharyngeal arch
Palatine tonsil
Lingual tonsil
Epiglottic cartilage
Aryepiglottic fold
Cuneiform tubercle
Corniculate tubercle
Transverse arytenoid muscle
Lamina of cricoid cartilage

Labels (right side):
Nasal septum
Hard palate
Soft palate
Oral cavity
Tongue
Hyoid bone
Hyoepiglottic ligament
Median thyrohyoid ligament
Thyroepiglottic ligament
Laryngeal vestibule
Thyroid cartilage
Vestibular fold
Laryngeal ventricle
Vocal fold
Arch of cricoid cartilage
Infraglottic space
Esophagus

A Nasopharynx
B Oropharynx
C Laryngopharynx

Key
A Nasopharynx
B Oropharynx
C Laryngopharynx

FIGURE 13-5
The pharynx, commonly called the throat, connects the oral and nasal cavities to the esophagus and trachea. (Image provided by Anatomical Chart Co.)

Key Terms	Definitions
nasopharynx (nay zoh FAIR inks)	region of the pharynx behind the nasal cavity
oropharynx (or oh FAIR inks)	region of the pharynx situated near the back of the mouth
laryngopharynx (la ring oh FAIR inks)	lower-most region of the pharynx situated near the larynx

Key Term Practice: Pharynx

1. The word part *naso-* refers to _____; so the region of the pharynx near the nasal passage is termed the _____.

2. _____ refers to "the mouth;" so the region of the pharynx extending from the oral cavity is the _____.

3. The word part _____ means "larynx;" therefore, the _____ is the region of the pharynx posterior to the larynx.

Larynx

The larynx is a musculocartilaginous enlargement in the airway between the pharynx and the top of the trachea (Fig. 13-6). Associate the *L* in *lower* with the *L* in *larynx* to remember that the larynx is lower than (inferior to) the pharynx. It is often called the voice box because it contains the vocal cords. Air enters the larynx through a slit-like opening called the **glottis**. A shoehorn-shaped flap of cartilage known as the **epiglottis** protects the glottis. The epiglottis covers the glottis during swallowing to prevent solid food or liquids from entering the respiratory tract.

There are two types of vocal cords: false and true (Fig. 13-7). **False vocal cords**, also known as **upper vestibular folds**, do not function in sound production. Muscle fibers within these folds help close the larynx during swallowing. The **true vocal cords** are the lower vocal folds that contain elastic fibers that vibrate to produce sound. The two vocal folds surround the glottis.

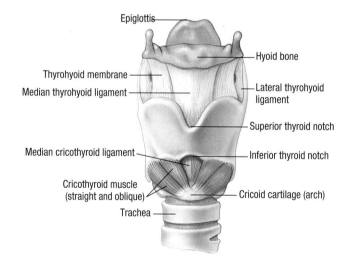

FIGURE 13-6
The larynx, often called the voice box, anterior view. (Image provided by Anatomical Chart Co.)

Key Terms	Definitions
glottis (GLOT is)	the space between the vocal folds
epiglottis (ep i GLOT is)	elastic cartilage that guards the glottis during swallowing
false vocal cords	folds in the larynx that do not produce sound; upper vestibular folds

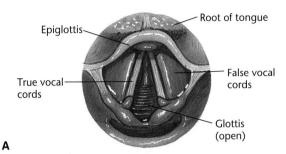
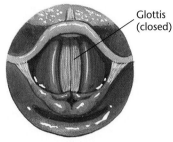

Epiglottis

Root of tongue

True vocal cords

False vocal cords

Glottis (open)

A

Glottis (closed)

B

FIGURE 13-7
The vocal cords (**A**) with glottis open and (**B**) glottis closed. (Images provided by Anatomical Chart Co.)

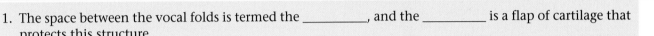

upper vestibular (ves TIB yoo lur) **folds**	folds in the larynx that do not produce sound; false vocal cords
true vocal cords	vocal folds that produce sound

Key Term Practice: Larynx

1. The space between the vocal folds is termed the _____, and the _____ is a flap of cartilage that protects this structure.

2. The vocal folds capable of producing sound are termed _____.

Trachea and Bronchial Tree

The trachea (windpipe) is a flexible, cylindrical tube extending from the larynx into the thorax, where it bifurcates (divides) into the right and left bronchi. The tracheal wall itself has approximately 20 C-shaped open rings of hyaline cartilage arranged one above the other that wrap around the anterior side to prevent collapse. The cartilage does not form a complete circle because the smooth esophagus (food tube) is nestled against its posterior. Functions of the trachea include transporting air between the larynx and the primary bronchi and protecting the bronchial tree from inhaled particles.

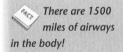

There are 1500 miles of airways in the body!

The bronchial tree is the branched airway segment leading from the trachea to the air sacs (alveoli) in the lungs. The **carina** of the trachea is the V-shaped cartilage ridge at the trachea's base that separates, forming the openings of the primary bronchi. Right and left branches of the bronchial tree in descending order are the primary bronchi, secondary (lobar) bronchi, tertiary (segmental) bronchi, bronchioles, terminal bronchioles, respiratory bronchioles, alveolar ducts, alveolar sacs, and alveoli.

The **primary bronchi,** consisting of right and left bronchi, are the main segments that branch into the lobar bronchi or secondary bronchi. The right primary bronchus is larger in diameter and slightly more vertical than the left; thus an accidentally inhaled object is more likely to become lodged in the right lung than in the left. There are two lobar bronchi on the left and three on the right, which branch into segmental bronchi. The left lung contains 8 segmental bronchi and the right lung contains 10. Segmental bronchi divide into tertiary bronchi, which branch to form bronchioles. **Bronchioles** further subdivide to form **terminal bronchioles;** there are between 50 and 80 per lobule.

The nasal cavity, pharynx, larynx, trachea, bronchi, and terminal bronchioles make up the **conducting airway**, or the parts of the respiratory tract that are involved with air distribution.

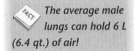

The average male lungs can hold 6 L (6.4 qt.) of air!

As the branch tubes become finer and finer, the amount of cartilage decreases and finally disappears in the small bronchioles to permit diffusion of respiratory gases across their surfaces. There are two or more **respiratory bronchioles** at each terminal bronchiole; a few air sacs capable of gas exchange bud from the sides of the terminal

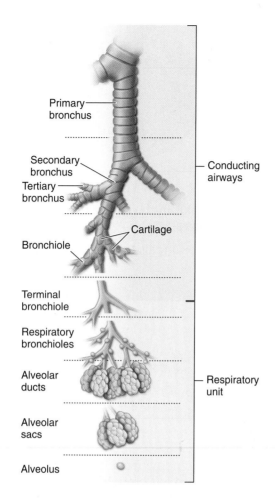

Primary bronchus

Secondary bronchus

Tertiary bronchus

Cartilage

Bronchiole

Conducting airways

Terminal bronchiole

Respiratory bronchioles

Alveolar ducts

Alveolar sacs

Respiratory unit

Alveolus

FIGURE 13-8
The conducting airways are the primary bronchi, bronchioles, and terminal bronchioles. The respiratory airways are the respiratory bronchioles, alveolar ducts, alveolar sacs, and alveoli.

bronchioles. Between 2 and 10 **alveolar ducts** are formed from each respiratory bronchiole. **Alveolar sacs** are outpouches of the alveolar ducts. The minute **alveoli**, which permit gas diffusion, are the ends of the lungs' bronchial trees. There are approximately 150 million alveoli in each lung, representing 30% of the body's entire surface area. Each alveolus is only about 0.02 cm (0.008 in.) in diameter.

The respiratory bronchioles and alveoli are structures of gas exchange and are considered the **respiratory airway**. The pathway of air is as follows (Fig. 13-8):

primary bronchi → secondary bronchi → tertiary bronchi → bronchioles → terminal bronchioles → respiratory bronchioles → alveolar ducts → alveolar sacs → alveoli

Primary gas diffusion occurs between the alveoli and pulmonary capillaries. The **diffusion capacity** of the lungs is the amount of gas (oxygen) taken up by the pulmonary capillaries per minute. Diffusion capacity is abbreviated with the letter D; a subscript letter indicates the location, and the gas being measured is also noted. For example, $D_L O_2$ stands for the diffusion capacity of oxygen (O_2) in the lungs (L). The tracheobronchial tree is shown in Figure 13-9.

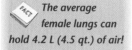

The average female lungs can hold 4.2 L (4.5 qt.) of air!

Key Terms	Definitions
carina (kuh RYE nuh)	cartilaginous ridge that separates the openings of the two primary bronchi
primary bronchi (BRONK eye)	the two branches off the trachea
bronchioles (BRONK ee ohlz)	subdivision of the tertiary bronchi

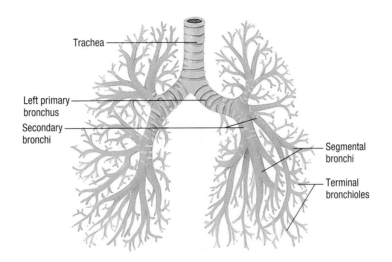

terminal bronchioles (BRONK ee ohlz)	subdivision of the bronchioles
conducting airway	respiratory structures involved with air distribution
respiratory bronchioles (RES pi ruh tor ee BRONK ee ohlz)	last bronchiolar subdivision and the first portion of the lungs capable of gas exchange
alveolar (al VEE oh lur) **ducts**	air passages branching from the respiratory bronchioles to the alveolar sacs
alveolar (al VEE oh lur) **sacs**	branches off the alveolar ducts
alveoli (al VEE oh lye)	lung section where gases pass between air and blood
respiratory (RES pi ruh tor ee) **airway**	respiratory structures involved with gas exchange
diffusion capacity	amount of gas taken up by the pulmonary capillaries per minute

Key Term Practice: Trachea and Bronchial Tree

1. The first branches of the respiratory tree off the trachea are the _____.

2. The last two structures of the bronchial tree are the _____ and _____.

Lungs

The lungs are paired, spongy-like organs of breathing located in the thoracic cavity, which are separated by the mediastinum (Fig. 13-10). Two separate membranes, the visceral and parietal pleura, enclose the lungs. The **visceral pleura** is an inner layer of serous membrane attached to the outside surface of each lung, and the outer **parietal pleura** lines the inner wall of the thoracic cavity. The pleural surfaces are lubricated by serous fluid to reduce friction, and the interaction between these membranes is significant to physical lung action. Water molecules in serous fluid have a great attraction to one another, creating a force called **surface tension.** The liquid on the membranes creates surface tension, which enables the parietal pleura and visceral pleura to expand the entire lung in all directions within the chest cavity during breathing.

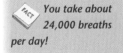

You take about 24,000 breaths per day!

Surface tension is what makes it difficult to separate two wet microscope slides or two pieces of damp plastic wrap. If two wet slides are held close to each other, they are drawn together by surface tension. This same thing happens between the two pleural membranes of the lungs.

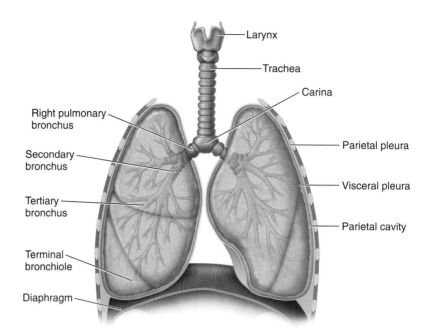

The right and left lung lobes are anatomically different because the heart occupies a portion of the left side of the body. The right lung has three lobes—the superior, middle, and inferior—which are separated by two fissures. It also has 10 bronchiole segments. The left lung is composed of only the superior and inferior lobes, which are separated by one fissure; it also contains the cardiac notch, a divot occupied by the heart. The left lung contains 8 bronchiole segments. Each lung lobe is further subdivided by connective tissue into lobules.

Alveoli, located at the terminal ends of respiratory sacs, are the basic functional units of the lungs because they are the sites of gas exchange. Alveoli are lined with simple squamous epithelium that allows for the oxygen–carbon dioxide swap. In these tiny, thin-walled structures, oxygen leaves the lungs and enters the bloodstream while carbon dioxide leaves the blood to be blown off during exhalation.

Two types of **pneumocytes**, or lung cells, are found within the alveolar walls. Type 1 pneumocytes are thin, delicate cells made of squamous epithelium that permit diffusion. Type 2 cells, also called **septal cells**, secrete surfactant. **Surfactant** is a normal lipoprotein that reduces the surface tension within the alveoli, thus preventing the alveolar walls from sticking together. Surfactant also reduces the surface tension so that the pleural membranes can be separated and the lungs can expand and contract. This is important because the surface tension between the adjacent moist membranes would otherwise cause alveolar collapse.

Key Terms	Definitions
visceral pleura (VIS ur ul PLOOR uh)	serous membrane on the lung surface
parietal pleura (puh RYE e tul PLOOR uh)	serous membrane lining the thoracic cavity
surface tension	contractile force at the surface of a liquid
pneumocytes (NEW moh sites)	lung cells
septal (SEP tul) **cell**	surfactant-secreting cell on the alveoli
surfactant (sur FACK tunt)	substance that reduces the surface tension of the alveolar mucosa

Key Term Practice: Lungs

1. The _____ pleura is the membrane directly on the lung surface, and the _____ pleura lines the thoracic cavity around the lung.

2. The word part *pneumo-* means _____, and the word part *-cyte* refers to "cell," so lung cells are termed _____.

Functions of the Respiratory System

The respiratory system functions to deliver oxygen to cells via the bloodstream while simultaneously removing the metabolic waste product carbon dioxide. Blood pH and acid–base balance are also maintained by the respiratory system. The pH is a measure of blood acidity or alkalinity, a critical factor for blood.

Another function is warming and moistening incoming air. The nasal epithelium is a mucous membrane containing an extensive network of blood vessels. As air passes across the surface, heat radiates from the underlying vessels and warms it. Cilia (hair-like cellular projections) trap particles, which are either expelled through coughing or sneezing, or swallowed, thereby filtering the air.

Inhalation and exhalation are required for normal functioning. Air intake through the mouth or nose for delivery to the lungs is termed **inhalation**, and breathing out is termed **exhalation.** Exhaled air contains the waste products of cellular metabolism, primarily carbon dioxide. The entire procedure of gas exchange between the external atmosphere and body cells is termed **respiration**. This process depends on **pulmonary ventilation**, the act of breathing using the lungs (*pulmon-*, "lung"), which provides the necessary oxygen for respiration to occur. From a strict biologic perspective, respiration occurs at the cellular level and depends on ventilation; however, the term *respiration* is often used synonymously with *breathing* (inspiration and expiration).

Inspiration and expiration result from changes in the size of the thoracic cavity. Muscles involved with breathing include the internal and external intercostals (between the ribs), abdominal muscles, scalenes, sternocleidomastoids, and the diaphragm. The **diaphragm** is a musculotendinous partition separating the thorax and abdomen that serves as the main muscle of breathing. (When pronouncing the word, notice the silent *g*.) The nerve responsible for transmitting important signals to this breathing muscle is the **phrenic nerve** (*phren-*, "diaphragm").

During inspiration (breathing in or inhalation), pressure inside the lungs and alveoli is reduced as the diaphragm moves downward, expanding the thoracic cage upward and outward. Because the outside air has a greater pressure, the result is lung expansion. **Compliance**, also called distensibility, is the ease with which the lungs can be expanded as a result of pressure changes occurring during breathing. Compliance decreases as lung volume increases.

During expiration (breathing out or exhalation), the diaphragm and external intercostal muscles relax, making the chest cavity smaller and causing a decrease in lung volume. A relaxed diaphragm appears dome shaped, thus aiding with air compression. Internal intercostal muscles simultaneously contract, causing air to be pushed up, and expiration occurs.

Breathing is controlled by a group of neurons in the brainstem (midbrain, pons, and medulla oblongata) called the respiratory center, which is composed of three regulatory areas: medullary rhythmicity, pneumotaxic, and the apneustic. Located within the medulla oblongata, the **medullary rhythmicity area** establishes the basic rhythm of breathing. The **pneumotaxic area**, located in the pons, regulates

FACT A sneeze can spew a fine mist of spray 10 feet (3.05 meters)!

FACT Approximately 1.63 gallons (6.17 liters) of air are breathed in every minute!

the rate of breathing by limiting the duration of each inspiration. Also located in the pons, the **apneustic area** coordinates the transition between an inspiration and expiration.

Modified respiratory movements, also called nonrespiratory air movements, are actions that involve the respiratory system, but are not directly involved with breathing. Modified respiratory movements include coughing, crying, hiccupping, laughing, sighing, sneezing, talking, and yawning. A cough (**tussis**) is a rapid rush of air to remove the substance that triggered the reflex. Sneezing clears the upper respiratory passages rather than the lower ones. Hiccupping is the result of a laryngospasm that occurs from an abrupt, involuntary contraction of the diaphragm, which causes an intake of breath and closes the vocal folds. Yawning is thought to aid respiration by providing an occasional deep breath. During **eupnea** (*eu-*, "normal"; *-pnea*, "respiration"), normal quiet breathing, not all alveoli are ventilated and some blood may pass through without being well oxygenated. This low blood oxygen concentration somehow triggers the yawn reflex.

Particles from a sneeze fly at a rate of 103 miles per hour!

Key Terms

Key Terms	Definitions
inhalation (in huh LAY shun)	process of inspiring or inhaling
exhalation (ecks huh LAY shun)	process of expiring or exhaling
respiration (res pi RAY shun)	chemical processes occurring in tissues for gas exchange; breathing
pulmonary (PUL moh nerr ee) **ventilation**	breathing, respiration
diaphragm (DYE uh fram)	curved muscular membrane separating the abdomen from the thoracic region
phrenic (FREN ick) **nerve**	nerve supplying the diaphragm
compliance	the ease with which the lungs can expand and contract
medullary rhythmicity (MED yoo lerr ee rith MIS i tee) **area**	brain region that sets the breathing pattern
pneumotaxic (new moh TACK sick) **area**	brain region that controls the respiration rate
apneustic (ap NEW stick) **area**	brain region that coordinates the transition between inhalation and exhalation
modified respiratory (RES pi ruh tor ee) **movements**	actions of the respiratory system not directly involved with breathing
tussis (TUS is)	cough
eupnea (yoop NEE uh)	normal breathing

Key Term Practice: Functions of the Respiratory System

1. _____ is breathing in, and _____ is breathing out.

2. The medical term for breathing is _____, which is derived from the word part _____, which means "lungs."

3. Coughing, sneezing, and laughing are examples of _____.

TABLE 13-1 Pulmonary Volumes and Capacities

Volume	Description	Average Value
tidal volume (TV)	volume of air entering or exiting the lungs during normal breathing	500 cc
inspiratory reserve volume (IRV)	volume of air entering the lungs plus the tidal volume during forced inhalation	3000 cc
expiratory reserve volume (ERV)	volume of air exiting the lungs plus the tidal volume during forced exhalation	1000 cc
vital capacity (VC)	maximum volume of air that can be exhaled after taking the deepest possible breath (VC = TV + IRV + ERV)	4500 cc
residual volume (RV)	volume of air in the lungs at all times	1500 cc
total lung capacity (TLC)	volume of air that the lungs can hold (TLC = VC + RV)	6000 cc

Pulmonary Volumes and Capacities

Pulmonary volumes and capacities are useful for assessing respiratory function (Table 13-1). The instrument used to measure them is a **spirometer**, and this device is used for pulmonary function tests. The **pulmonary function test** (PFT) is a series of tests using diagnostic spirometry that determines lung volumes and capacities. These tests, involving the person directly and requiring active breathing, are useful in the differential diagnosis of and the determination of the extent of pulmonary disease. They are also called ventilation tests. Important physiological values are identified.

Tidal volume (TV) is the volume of air that can be moved into or out of the lungs during eupnea. The average tidal volume is approximately 500 cc. Think of it as ebbing and flowing like the ocean tide. The volume that can be inhaled with forced breathing in addition to tidal volume is termed the **inspiratory reserve volume** (IRV). The **expiratory reserve volume** (ERV) is the volume of air that can be exhaled during forced breathing in addition to tidal volume. The average IRV is about 3000 cc and the average ERV is roughly 1000 cc.

Vital capacity (VC) is the maximum amount of air a person can exhale after taking the deepest breath possible. The average vital capacity is approximately 4500 cc. **Residual volume** (RV) is the volume that remains in the lungs at all times and averages 1500 cc. **Total lung capacity** (TLC) is the total volume of air that the lungs can hold, about 6000 cc.

Anatomic dead space is the amount of air entering the respiratory tract during breathing that fails to reach the alveoli. This volume, about 1500 cc, remains in the trachea, bronchi, and terminal bronchioles. Because gas exchanges do not occur through walls of these passages, that air is said to occupy anatomic dead space.

Key Terms	Definitions
spirometer (spye ROM e tur)	device that measures inhaled and exhaled air volumes
pulmonary (PUL moh nerr ee) **function test**	measures lung volumes and capacities
tidal volume	amount of air moved in a single breath; tidal air
inspiratory (in SPYE ruh tor ee) **reserve volume**	amount of air that can be forcefully breathed in after involuntary inhalation

expiratory (eck SPYE ruh tor ee) **reserve volume**	amount of air that can be forcefully expired after involuntary exhalation
vital capacity	amount of air that can be expired from the lungs after the deepest possible inspiration
residual volume	amount of air remaining in the lungs after complete expiration; residual air
total lung capacity	total amount of air the lungs can hold
anatomic dead space	space that contains air not reaching the alveoli

Key Term Practice: Pulmonary Volumes and Capacities

1. The instrument used to measure pulmonary volumes and capacities is termed a/an _____.

2. _____ describes normal, nonforced breathing.

THE CLINICAL DIMENSION

Pathology of the Respiratory System

Signs and symptoms of respiratory disorders are generally marked by abnormal breathing patterns, sounds, and mucus production; visible physical manifestations; and physiological alterations. Common indications, tests, and treatments of respiratory system disorders are reviewed in this section. Treatment of respiratory disorders is aimed at increasing lung function and enhancing oxygen delivery or use.

Altered Breathing

The normal resting breathing rate for an adult is 12–20 respirations per minute. **Apnea** refers to the temporary absence of respiration, and several forms exist. For example, **reflex apnea** is the temporary loss of breath owing to a sudden painful or cold stimulation to the skin. Hence an infant gasps after receiving an injection or a person gasps in response to the chill of a cold shower. **Sleep apnea** occurs during sleep and is associated with frequent awakening and daytime sleepiness. **Bradypnea** is an abnormally slow breath rate, usually less than 12 breaths per minute. **Hyperpnea** is an involuntary, compensatory increased breathing rate to meet an increased oxygen demand. This deep, fast breathing is common after physical exercise. An abnormally rapid breathing rate is **tachypnea.** It is usually greater than 20 breaths per minute.

Other terms associated with altered breathing resulting from abnormal gas levels are asphyxia, hyperventilation, and hypoventilation. **Asphyxia** is impaired or absent exchange of oxygen and carbon dioxide during ventilation that results in suffocation. **Hyperventilation** is excessive inhalation and exhalation that leads to decreased alveolar CO_2 levels. **Hypoventilation** is decreased breathing rate that often results in increased levels of CO_2.

Biot respirations are an irregular breathing pattern represented by alternating periods of apnea with four or five breaths having the same depth. Biot respirations result from lesions in the respiratory centers in the brainstem. An alternating pattern of apnea and deep, rapid breathing is termed **Cheyne-Stokes respiration,** after

Scottish doctor John Cheyne and Irish doctor William Stokes. Cheyne-Stokes breathing is characterized as rhythmic waxing and waning of respirations. It is commonly observed in comatose patients and often indicates impending death. **Kussmaul respirations** are described as "air hunger" because the respirations are rapid and deep without pauses. They are characteristic of diabetic or other causes of acidosis.

Key Terms	Definitions
apnea (AP nee uh)	cessation of breathing
reflex apnea (AP nee uh)	sudden, temporary loss of breath; gasp
sleep apnea (AP nee uh)	cessation of breathing during sleep that causes one to awaken and is associated with daytime sleepiness
bradypnea (brad ip NEE uh)	abnormally slow breathing rate
hyperpnea (high pur NEE uh)	increased rate and depth of breathing
tachypnea (tack ip NEE uh)	rapid breathing rate
asphyxia (as FICK see uh)	impaired or absent oxygen exchange that results in suffocation
hyperventilation (high pur ven ti LAY shun)	abnormal rapid, deep breathing leading to low alveolar carbon dioxide levels
hypoventilation (high poh ven ti LAY shun)	reduced respiratory rate resulting in high alveolar carbon dioxide levels
Biot respirations (bee OH res pi RAY shunz)	alternating periods of apnea with breaths of the same depth
Cheyne- (CHAIN) **Stokes respiration** (res pi RAY shun)	hyperpnea alternating with apnea
Kussmaul respirations (KOOS mawl res pi RAY shunz)	air hunger

Key Term Practice: Altered Breathing

1. The word part _____ refers to "slow," and the word part _____ refers to "respiration;" so, the term _____ describes a slow breathing rate.

2. The word part *tachy-* means _____, and the word part *-pnea* means _____; so, the term _____ describes a rapid breathing rate.

Cardiovascular Disorders Affecting Lungs

A **pulmonary embolism** is a blood clot or mass that lodges in a pulmonary artery, obstructing blood flow. An embolism often originates in a deep vein and travels to the lungs (Fig.13-11). A common pathway is as follows:

leg vein → inferior vena cava → right atrium → right ventricle → pulmonary artery

Signs and symptoms include **dyspnea** (shortness of breath or difficulty breathing), tachypnea, and chest pain. If the embolism is large, **cyanosis** (bluish coloration of skin and mucous membranes because of diminished oxygen levels), shock, or sudden death is likely. The clinical picture, rale presence, magnetic resonance imaging (MRI) studies, x-ray, or pulmonary angiogram diagnoses an embolism.

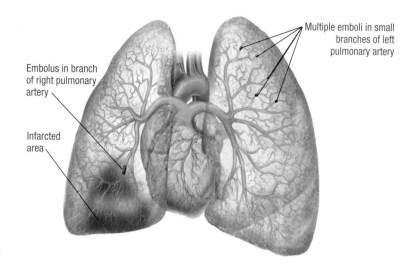

Multiple emboli in small
branches of left
pulmonary artery

Embolus in branch
of right pulmonary
artery

Infarcted
area

FIGURE 13-11
Common sites of
pulmonary emboli.
(Image provided by
Anatomical Chart Co.)

Rales are abnormal hissing, whistling, or rattling lung or airway sounds heard on auscultation. **Auscultation** (listening to sounds made by the respiratory structures with a stethoscope) and **percussion** (thumping on the chest during auscultation) are commonly the first steps in diagnosing lung conditions. Although rales are subjectively characterized, they fall into categories such as coarse, medium, fine moist (gurgling), and dry. Rales are the result of turbulent airflow. Oxygen therapy, mucolytics (mucus-thinning agents), anticoagulants, and thrombolytics are prescribed.

Oxygen therapy involves oxygen being delivered by nasal cannula, Venturi mask, or an oxygen tent. A flexible tube inserted into the nostrils to deliver oxygen through the nasal passages is called a **nasal cannula; Venturi mask** is a facial mask worn by the patient that delivers a precise, continuous high-flow oxygen mixture. A **resuscitation bag** is an inflatable, balloon-like device that can be attached to an oxygen face mask, endotracheal tube, or tracheostomy tube to pump oxygen or air into lungs. The bag allows for manual ventilation. A **nebulizer** is a device that delivers a fine mist or spray for inhalation drug delivery. It is also known as an **atomizer. Oxygen tents** are transparent, plastic tent-like structures that enclose a patient in bed while pumping oxygen into the enclosure to assist with breathing. Emboli prevention is key in susceptible patients, such as those with thrombophlebitis or individuals who are immobile for long periods of time.

An **endotracheal tube** is a flexible tube inserted into the mouth or nose and passed through the glottis to deliver positive-pressure oxygen to lungs. Trache tubes, as they are commonly called, are used to facilitate breathing during surgery or when respiratory assistance is needed. A flexible tube inserted into the tracheal opening to deliver oxygen to the lungs is termed a **tracheostomy tube.** The tube is inserted inferior to an obstruction to effectively provide oxygen (Fig. 13-12).

Key Terms	Definitions
pulmonary embolism (PUL moh nerr ee EM boh liz um)	blood clot in a pulmonary artery
dyspnea (disp NEE uh)	labored breathing
cyanosis (sigh uh NOH sis)	bluish colored tissue owing to a lack of oxygen in the blood
rales (RAHLZ)	abnormal hissing or whistling respiratory sounds
auscultation (aws kul TAY shun)	listening to body sounds using a stethoscope

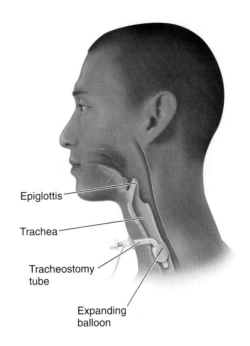

Epiglottis

Trachea

Tracheostomy
tube

Expanding
balloon

FIGURE 13-12
A tracheostomy tube
is a flexible tube
inserted into the
trachea to deliver
oxygen to the lungs.

percussion	technique of hitting the back and chest during auscultation or to loosen mucus so that it can be coughed out
oxygen therapy	supplying oxygen via a nasal cannula, Venturi mask, or oxygen tent
nasal cannula (KAN yoo luh)	flexible tube placed in the nostrils to deliver oxygen
Venturi (ven TUE ree) **mask**	face mask that delivers oxygen
resuscitation (ree sus i TAY shun) **bag**	bag that is manually pumped to deliver air or oxygen
nebulizer (NEB yoo lye zur)	device for administering medicinal liquid in the form of a spray to be breathed through the mouth or nose; atomizer
atomizer (AT uh migh zur)	device for administering medicinal liquid in the form of a spray to be breathed through the mouth or nose; nebulizer
oxygen tent	structure that surrounds a patient in bed to supply oxygen
endotracheal (en doh TRAY kee ul) **tube**	tube passed through the mouth or nose to the trachea
tracheostomy (tray kee OS toh mee) **tube**	tube placed through a hole in the trachea

Key Term Practice: Cardiovascular Disorders Affecting Lungs

1. A/An _____ is a blood clot in the pulmonary artery.

2. The prefix *dys-* means "impaired or abnormal" and the word part _____ means "respiration;" so the term _____ means impaired breathing.

Cystic Fibrosis

Cystic fibrosis (CF), also referred to as mucoviscidosis, is an inherited disorder of the exocrine glands resulting in the production of excessive, thick mucus, which ultimately obstructs the gastrointestinal tract and lungs. Pulmonary failure is the primary cause of death. The disease manifests in infancy and childhood. Because the onset of symptoms begins early in life, children are taught to pronounce this difficult term by calling it "65 roses."

Characteristics of the disease include pancreatic enzyme deficiency, progressive infectious pulmonary disease, malabsorption of nutrients, and elevated sodium chloride concentrations in the sweat. Chronic tussis with purulent sputum production is symptomatic of lung involvement. **Sputum** is material discharged from the air passages, throat, and mouth. Containing a mixture of saliva, mucus, pus, microbes, and/or inhaled particulate matter, it is **expectorated** (coughed up), and then spit out or swallowed. Sputum is commonly called **phlegm**, although technically phlegm is viscid, stringy mucus secreted by the walls of the respiratory passages. Labored breathing as a result of airway obstruction results in **hypoxia** (extreme deficiency or absence of oxygen in the tissues), finger clubbing, and cyanosis. Overly rounded fingertips resulting from long-term decreased oxygen supply to the extremities is termed **clubbing of fingers** (Fig. 13-13).

Diagnosis is confirmed by physical examination, family history, pulmonary function tests, tests measuring oxygen levels, chest x-rays, and sweat tests. The **peak expiratory flow** (PEF) test uses a peak expiratory flow meter to measure the volume of air after forced expiration. It is also used to monitor asthma and drug therapy in lung diseases. **Pulse oximetry** measures the degree of oxygen saturation in the blood using a photoelectric instrument called a **pulse oximeter.** The pulse oximeter is clipped to a fingertip or ear lobe and is usually left in place on hospital patients so that oxygen levels can be continuously monitored.

Although a fatal disease, advances in research and an intense effort by the scientific community in developing new therapies have greatly increased the life expectancy of CF patients (Fig. 13-14). The management plan includes careful use of antibiotics to

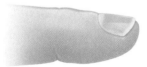
Normal

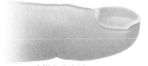
Mild clubbing

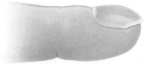
Increased curvature of nail

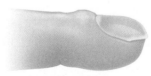
Severe clubbing

FIGURE 13-13
Clubbing of fingers results from a long-term decreased oxygen supply to the extremities.

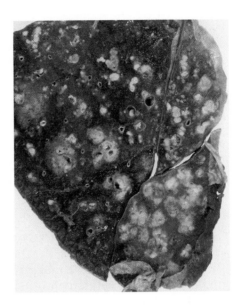

FIGURE 13-14
A lung affected by end-stage cystic fibrosis. (Reprinted with permission from Cagle PT. Color atlas and text of pulmonary pathology. Philadelphia: Lippincott Williams & Wilkins, 2005.)

control pulmonary infection, aggressive chemotherapeutic pulmonary measures to thin mucus secretions, postural drainage to evacuate excess mucus, a flutter device to loosen mucus secretions in the lungs, oxygen infusion to inflate the lungs, and—as a last resort—lung transplantation.

Noninvasive measures can assist with breathing. Positioning the body in various poses to allow gravity to move secretions out of the lungs and bronchial tree to be coughed out is termed **postural drainage** (PD). Percussion often accompanies postural drainage poses, especially in CF patients. This form of percussion involves cupping the hands and striking chest and back over the lung fields to loosen mucus secretions so they can be coughed out and expectorated. Percussions are commonly called "poundings." A recent innovation, the therapy vest, increases the efficacy of displacing the mucus from more areas of the lung fields.

Key Terms	Definitions
cystic fibrosis (SIS tick figh BROH sis)	inherited disorder characterized by thick mucus secretions that block the internal passages, including the lungs
sputum (SPEW tum)	fluid or semifluid mucus mixture
expectorated (eck speck toh RATE ed)	coughed up from the airway
phlegm (FLEM)	thick mucus
hypoxia (high POCK see uh)	oxygen deprivation in the tissues; stage before anoxia
clubbing of fingers	fingertips that are rounded like a club
peak expiratory (eck SPYE ruh tor ee) **flow**	uses a PEF meter to measure the volume of air after forced expiration
pulse oximetry (ock SIM e tree)	measurement of oxygen in the blood
pulse oximeter (ock SIM e tur)	small instrument that measures the amount of oxygen in blood
postural (POS chur ul) **drainage**	positioning the body to allow gravity to drain mucus from areas of the lungs

Key Term Practice: Cystic Fibrosis

1. The word part _____ means "below normal;" an abnormally low oxygen level in tissues is termed _____.

2. An inherited disorder characterized by abnormal mucus production that clogs airways is termed _____.

Chronic Obstructive Pulmonary Disease

Chronic obstructive pulmonary disease (COPD) is a general term describing various lung diseases with permanent or temporary narrowing of the small bronchi, including asthma, bronchiectasis, bronchitis, emphysema, and pneumoconiosis. In all cases, there is inadequate gas exchange owing to the inability to freely ventilate the lungs. COPDs tend to be progressive and irreversible.

Bronchiectasis is chronic dilation of the respiratory passages, causing tussis and excessive mucus production. It is characterized by saccular (sac-shaped) or tubular dilation of the bronchus or bronchi resulting from obstruction and infection. It takes several years to develop and is caused by smoking, obstruction, or corrosive gas inhalation. Other signs include **mucopurulent** (pertaining to mucus with pus) sputum, **hemoptysis** (blood-stained sputum), and recurrent pneumonia. The history and physical examination, x-rays, computerized tomography (CT) scans, bronchoscopy, sputum culture, and pulmonary function tests diagnose bronchiectasis.

Bronchoscopy uses a thin, lighted instrument called a **bronchoscope**, which is inserted into the mouth and down the trachea to the bronchi, enabling the clinician to visually inspect the structures. If necessary, lung tissue can be removed (**lung biopsy**) or other foreign matter can be extracted for evaluation. Lung biopsies are used to test for pathology. Bronchodilators, postural drainage, and avoidance of irritants are treatment options. **Bronchodilators** are drugs that ease breathing by relaxing the air passages.

Bronchitis is inflammation of the bronchial mucous membranes, causing breathing problems and coughing episodes. Two forms exist: acute and chronic. **Acute bronchitis** is characterized by a sharp, rapid onset with a short duration. It is caused by infectious agents in the lower respiratory tract; signs and symptoms include cough, variable sputum production, fever, substernal soreness, and rales. The symptoms subside within 1 week, but the cough persists for 2–3 weeks. **Chronic bronchitis** is long lasting and is typified by excessive mucus secretion with chronic, productive (sputum-producing) cough (Fig. 13-15). It can lead to asthma and often occurs with emphysema, tuberculosis, and heart failure. Signs and symptoms of all forms include dyspnea, wheezing, fever, and cough. Bronchitis is diagnosed by the clinical picture, x-ray studies of the lungs, pulmonary function tests, and blood/sputum analyses. Treatment options include increasing fluid intake, humidifying rooms, using bronchodilators, and smoking cessation.

Emphysema involves an anatomic alteration of the lungs characterized by air space enlargement distal to the terminal bronchioles and destructive changes to the alveolar walls (Fig. 13-16). The deterioration of the alveoli leads to loss of elasticity. Breathing and gas exchange are hindered. Signs and symptoms include gradual breathing difficulty, dyspnea, tachypnea, wheezing, persistent cough, reduced expiratory volume, rhonchi, and inflated lungs at the end of expiration. Progression of the disease is marked by **barrel chest** (increased anteroposterior diameter of the chest, resembling a barrel shape), circumoral (surrounding mouth) cyanosis, and right

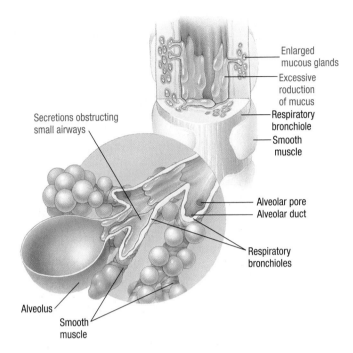

FIGURE 13-15
Bronchitis is an inflammation of the bronchial mucous membranes that results in breathing problems and coughing episodes. (Image provided by Anatomical Chart Co.)

ventricular heart failure. Long-term cigarette smoking, repeated respiratory infections, exposure to environmental hazards, or α_1-antitrypsin (α_1-antiprotease) deficiency are causes. Diagnosis is made by clinical history and physical examination, PFT, and x-rays. Pulmonary function tests reveal increased TV and RV and decreased VC. Radiographic studies show translucent-appearing lungs, flattened diaphragm, and cardiomegaly. Treatments include smoking cessation, increased protein intake, vitamin supplements, oxygen therapy, bronchodilators, and possible prophylactic (preventive) antibiotics. Emphysema is a frequent cause of death in smokers.

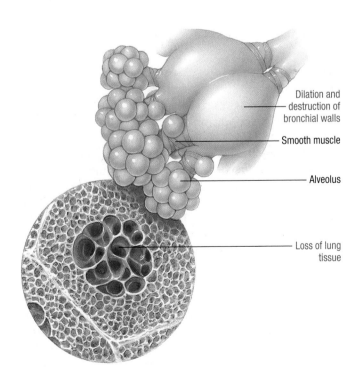

FIGURE 13-16
Emphysema results in an anatomic alteration of the lungs, characterized by air space enlargement and destructive changes to the alveolar walls, leading to loss of elasticity. (Image provided by Anatomical Chart Co.)

Key Terms	Definitions
chronic obstructive pulmonary (PUL moh nerr ee) **disease**	general term describing permanent or temporary lung disease affecting the bronchial tree
bronchiectasis (bronk ee ECK tuh sis)	chronic dilation of the airways
mucopurulent (mew koh PEW roo lunt)	pertaining to mucus with pus
hemoptysis (hee MOP ti sis)	coughing up blood or bloody mucus
bronchoscopy (brong KOS kuh pee)	procedure for viewing the inside of the respiratory structures using a bronchoscope
bronchoscope (BRONK oh skope)	thin, lighted instrument used in bronchoscopy
lung biopsy (BYE op see)	removal of lung tissue for diagnostic evaluation
bronchodilators (bronk oh DYE lay turz)	drugs that ease breathing by relaxing the air passages
bronchitis (bron KIGH tis)	inflammation of the bronchial tubes
acute bronchitis (bron KIGH tis)	sudden and short-lasting inflammation of the bronchial tubes
chronic bronchitis (bron KIGH tis)	long-lasting inflammation of the bronchial tubes
emphysema (em fi SEE muh)	chronic lung disorder characterized by enlarged air sacs
barrel chest	rounded chest cavity

Key Term Practice: Chronic Obstructive Pulmonary Disease

1. The word part _____ refers to "the bronchus," and _____ is the suffix for "inflammation;" therefore, the term _____ describes inflammation of the bronchial passages.

2. Short-term bronchial inflammation is termed _____, and long-term bronchial inflammation is known as _____.

Asthma

Asthma is a disease of the respiratory system caused by increased airway responsiveness to stimuli. The condition is characterized by the narrowing and constriction of the air passages (Fig. 13-17). Signs and symptoms include coughing, chest tightness, dyspnea, shallow respirations, rhonchi, wheezing, bronchospasms, and mucus production. A coarse rale produced by air passage through a partially obstructed bronchus is referred to as a **rhonchus**. A **wheeze** is a whistling or sighing noise that indicates mucus buildup. Some wheezes can be heard without a stethoscope. A **bronchospasm** is the temporary narrowing of a bronchial tube resulting from involuntary contraction of the smooth muscle. Individuals with asthma have greater difficulty exhaling than inhaling.

Two forms of asthma exist: extrinsic (allergic) and intrinsic (nonallergic). Each may have a hereditary component. Asthma is diagnosed by pulmonary function tests, peak airflow measurements, history, and physical examination. **Bronchial asthma** is characterized by attacks of dyspnea and bronchial tube spasms. It is frequently caused by an allergic reaction and results in partial closure of the air passages, inflammation, inflated alveoli, and excess mucus production. Treatments include allergen avoidance, bronchodilators (drugs that increase the diameter of the pulmonary air passages), and anti-inflammatories.

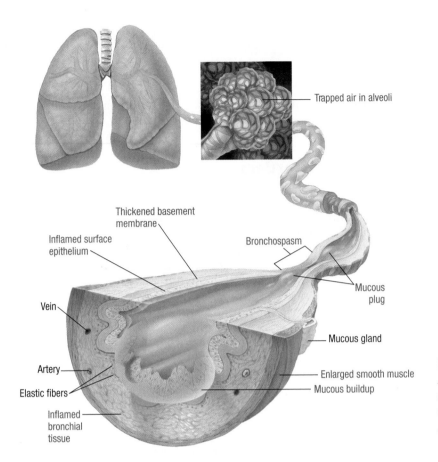

FIGURE 13-17
Asthma results in restricted airways. (Image provided by Anatomical Chart Co.)

Exercise-induced asthma, or exercise-induced bronchospasm, is bronchoconstriction caused by exercise. Exercise normally results in relaxation of the bronchial tree smooth muscle; however, in people with asthma, bronchospasm and mucus secretion follow the initial bronchodilation. The episode normally occurs within 5–15 minutes after exercise. It is diagnosed by the clinical picture and spirometric evaluation. Treatment is usually not necessary because recovery is spontaneous, occurring 30–90 minutes after exercise.

Key Terms	Definitions
asthma (AZ muh)	breathing disorder characterized by chest tightness and airway constriction
rhonchus (RONK us)	harsh, rattling, whistling sound
wheeze	audible whistling breath sound
bronchospasm (BRONK oh spaz um)	involuntary contraction of the bronchial smooth muscle
bronchial asthma (BRONK ee ul AZ muh)	form of asthma with attacks of dyspnea and bronchial spasms
exercise-induced asthma (AZ muh)	form of asthma with bronchoconstriction caused by exercise

Key Term Practice: Asthma

1. The medical term for a harsh rattling sound is _____.

2. A/An _____ describes the involuntary contraction of the bronchial smooth muscle.

Inhalation Disorders

Any lung disease caused by dust inhalation, especially mineral dusts that produce fibrosis of pulmonary tissue, is termed **pneumoconiosis.** The term *coniosis* means "disease or morbid condition caused by dust inhalation." Pneumoconiosis is frequently occupational and may develop after 2–30 years of daily exposure. The average time for disease development appears to be 10 years. It is characterized by progressive, chronic lung inflammation. Dyspnea, dry cough that becomes productive, tachypnea, malaise (generalized tiredness), and recurrent infections are hallmarks of advanced disease. Numerous forms exist, including anthracosis, asbestosis, berylliosis, and silicosis.

Anthracosis, also called black lung disease, results from inhalation of smoke or coal dust and is common in coal miners. **Asbestosis** is caused by prolonged exposure to asbestos dust, **berylliosis** is caused by exposure to beryllium salts, and **silicosis** occurs in quarry workers and stone masons who inhale silica dust. Treatment is symptomatic and supportive because there is no cure. Bronchodilators, oxygen therapy, physical therapy, and corticosteroids may be helpful.

Key Terms	Definitions
pneumoconiosis (new moh koh nee OH sis)	disease caused by inhaling mineral or metallic dust over a long period of time
anthracosis (an thruh KOH sis)	pneumoconiosis caused by inhalation of coal dust
asbestosis (as bes TOH sis)	pneumoconiosis caused by inhalation of asbestos fibers
berylliosis (be ril ee OH sis)	pneumoconiosis caused by inhalation of beryllium
silicosis (sil i KOH sis)	pneumoconiosis caused by inhalation of silica dust

Key Term Practice: Inhalation Disorders

1. The general term used to describe lung diseases caused by mineral dust inhalation is _____, which is derived from the word part _____, meaning "lung" and the word *coniosis*, which refers to a "condition caused by dust inhalation."

2. The word part _____ means "coal," and *-osis* is a suffix meaning _____; so _____ is a lung condition caused by inhaling coal dust.

Upper Respiratory Disorders

An **upper respiratory infection** (URI) is an acute infection causing inflammation that affects the upper respiratory structures. Signs and symptoms vary with the particular strain of microbe and can include nasal congestion, sneezing, watery eyes, sore throat, voice hoarseness, and coughing. Headache, fever, chills, and malaise may also occur. Roughly half of all adult cases of URI are caused by **rhinoviruses**, RNA viruses that infect the upper respiratory system. The diagnosis is made by assessing the common signs and symptoms and, if necessary, sputum or nasal cultures. There is no cure; treatment consists of rest, drinking plenty of fluids, nutrition therapy, and decongestants. **Decongestants** reduce or relieve congestion.

Nasal polyps are spherical or oval masses projecting from the nasal mucosa into the nasal cavity. They usually are not harmful, but large ones may interfere with nose breathing. Polyps are caused by overproduction of mucus, usually resulting from **allergic rhinitis**, nasal mucosa inflammation as a result of allergen reaction. They are identified using a **nasal speculum**, an instrument that enables viewing of the nasal cavity interior. Polyps can be surgically removed or treated with a steroid injection directly into the mass.

Acute rhinitis, also called **nasal catarrh** is an inflammation of the nasal mucous membranes and is characterized by sneezing, **lacrimation** (production of tears), and **coryza** (secretion of watery mucus discharged from the nose). More commonly known as the common head cold, this viral infection differs from other viral-based illness such as influenza in that it is not accompanied by fever. Rhinitis is treated symptomatically.

Inflammation of mucous membranes of any of the paranasal sinuses is **sinusitis**. It is characterized by pain, headache, and pressure. Nasal discharge is usually yellow-green, indicating the infection is bacterial in origin. The patient history is generally enough to confirm the diagnosis. X-ray scans, if necessary, may reveal fluid-filled cavities that appear white; air-filled cavities appear dark on x-ray films. Sinusitis is treated with antibiotics if the causative agent is bacterial. Decongestants, antihistamines, and analgesics may also provide relief.

Pharyngitis, commonly known as a sore throat, is an inflammation of the pharynx. Dry, painful throat; chills; fever; **dysphonia** (voice impairment or hoarseness); **dysphagia** (difficulty swallowing); and a red, swollen pharynx typify the condition. It is caused by a viral or bacterial infection or by chemical or smoke inhalation. Physical examination and patient history confirm the diagnosis. Antibiotics are prescribed for a bacterial infection; otherwise, the treatment involves soothing throat lozenges, getting plenty of rest and fluids, and using over-the-counter medications to treat symptoms.

Key Terms	Definitions
upper respiratory (RES pi ruh tor ee) **infection**	viral or bacterial infection of the nose, nasal cavity, sinuses, and/or pharynx
rhinoviruses (rye noh VYE rus ez)	any of many RNA viruses that cause upper respiratory tract infections
decongestant	drug that reduces congestion
nasal polyp (POL ip)	benign growth on the nasal mucosa
allergic rhinitis (rye NIGH tis)	nasal inflammation resulting from an allergy
nasal speculum (SPECK yoo lum)	instrument for viewing the nasal cavity
acute rhinitis (rye NIGH tis)	inflammation of the nasal cavity caused by infection; nasal catarrh, coryza
nasal catarrh (kuh TAHR)	inflammation of the nasal cavity caused by infection; acute rhinitis, coryza
lacrimation (lack ri MAY shun)	tear production
coryza (koh RYE zuh)	runny nose
sinusitis (sigh nuh SIGH tis)	inflammation of the paranasal sinuses
pharyngitis (fair in JYE tis)	inflammation of the pharynx; sore throat

| **dysphonia** (dis FOH nee uh) | impaired voice |
| **dysphagia** (dis FAY jee uh) | swallowing difficulty |

Key Term Practice: Upper Respiratory Disorders

1. What is the plural form of pharyngitis? _____

2. The word part *rhin-* means _____, and the word part _____ means "inflammation;" therefore, an inflammation of the nasal cavity is termed _____.

Lower Respiratory Disorders

Inflammation of the larynx is termed **laryngitis**, which is usually accompanied by hoarseness, **aphonia** (loss of voice), and coughing. Depending on the causative agent, sore throat, fever, and malaise may also occur. It can be viral or bacterial in origin and frequently is a concomitant (occurs along with) condition with other conditions such as syphilis and tuberculosis. Tonsillitis, sinusitis, smoke or chemical inhalation, and excessive voice use are also common causes of laryngitis. The diagnosis is made by the patient history and physical examination, although laryngoscopy may be performed for confirmation purposes.

Examination of the larynx with a **laryngoscope**, a tubular instrument with a light and telescope for viewing purposes, is termed **laryngoscopy**. In addition to diagnostic purposes, laryngoscopy may also be used to facilitate the passage of a breathing tube through the larynx. Treatment involves voice rest, humidity therapy to thin the mucus secretions, increased fluid intake, and throat lozenges.

Histoplasmosis is a mild respiratory infection caused by the fungus *Histoplasma capsulatum,* which can progress to systemic involvement. It is initially asymptomatic; then dyspnea, malaise, fever, splenomegaly (enlarged spleen), and hepatomegaly (enlarged liver) occur. Infection results from inhaling contaminated dust or bird feces particles. Histoplasmosis is diagnosed by skin test, blood studies, and sputum or tissue samples confirming the presence of the fungus. Antifungal drugs are used to treat the condition.

Lung inflammation with exudate is termed **pneumonia** (Fig. 13-18). The condition is caused by viral or bacterial infection or, less commonly, a chemical or physical irritant. Common pneumonia-causing microorganisms are *Klebsiella pneumoniae, Streptococcus pneumoniae,* and *Mycoplasma pneumoniae.* In addition to viral and bacterial types, **aspiration pneumonia** is a form that results from the inhalation of foreign material, such as food or vomit, into the bronchi. It can also develop secondary to the presence of fluid, blood, saliva, or gastric contents in the airways. When the pneumonia affects one or more lobes, or part of a lobe, it is termed **lobar pneumonia.**

Cough, fever, and dyspnea are major signs and symptoms. Chest pain depends on the area of lung field affected. Pneumonia is diagnosed by the history and physical examination, x-ray evaluations, sputum studies, and blood culture. The type of cytology studies used in the diagnosis of pneumonia are termed **sputum studies;** these tests look for the presence of abnormal cells. Sputum is also often obtained for **culture and sensitivity** (C&S) **studies,** whereby the sample is grown on nutritive media, and infectious microbes (causative agents) are identified and tested for antibiotic sensitivity. Once the organism is known, appropriate antimicrobial therapy can be initiated. Management involves treating the underlying cause, bedrest, fluids, and postural drainage. Fluid aspiration from the lung may also be required.

An infection and inflammation of lungs relatively common in young children and the elderly is **respiratory syncytial virus** (RSV) **pneumonia.** It produces cold-like symptoms, nasal congestion, otitis media (middle ear infection), coughing, fever, malaise, and lethargy. The greatest number of cases occurs between December and

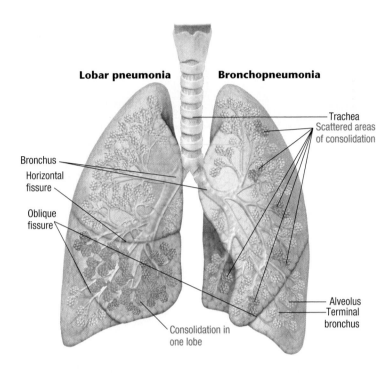

FIGURE 13-18
Lobar and broncho-
pneumonia. (Image
provided by
Anatomical Chart Co.)

March. It is a viral infection spread by contact with secretions of infected individuals. RSV pneumonia is diagnosed by the patient's history, physical examination, and sputum culture. It is treated with antiviral medications, rest, and fluid intake.

Influenza, commonly called the flu, is an acute respiratory infection caused by a specific virus. Because there is usually an epidemic every 1–4 years, annual preventive vaccination programs are initiated during early fall. Sudden onset, cough, headache, runny nose, fever, chills, and myalgia characterize influenza. Complications include bronchitis, sinusitis, and otitis media. Three general types—designated A, B, and C— have been identified, but mutant strains are prevalent. Influenza is rapidly transmitted among people because of the short incubation period of 1–3 days, and it tends to be more serious in the young, elderly, and immunocompromised. It is spread through inhalation of the virus, and the signs and symptoms are often indistinguishable from the common cold. Definitive diagnosis is made by isolation of the virus from throat culture. There is no cure, so the condition is treated symptomatically. Rest and increased fluid intake are generally prescribed. Vaccines are administered before an outbreak, and individuals typically require 2–4 weeks to develop active immunity.

Legionellosis, or **Legionnaires disease**, is a form of pneumonia caused by the *Legionella pneumophila* bacterium. The microbe causes acute lobar pneumonia and affects other body systems. Renal, intestinal, neurologic, and hepatic symptoms are common. It was first recognized in an outbreak in July 1976, at an American Legion conference in Philadelphia. It is spread mainly by water droplets in air-conditioning systems; warm, moist environments such as spas and hot tubs; and grocery store vegetable misting systems. The incubation period for legionellosis is about 7 days, but ranges from 2 to 10 days. *L. pneumophila* infection is not contagious. Signs and symptoms include malaise, headache, cough, chills, fever, chest pain, dyspnea, and myalgia. The diagnosis is based on the history and physical examination, x-rays, and blood sputum studies. Presence of the bacterium in the sputum or urine confirms the diagnosis. Antibiotic therapy is necessary, and prevention measures are used to avoid outbreaks.

Tuberculosis (TB) is an infectious disease caused by *Mycobacterium tuberculosis* in which rounded swellings, called tubercles, form on the mucous membranes, especially in the lungs (Fig. 13-19). Although it infects lung tissue primarily, it can attack most body organs. It is characterized by fever, weight loss, tussis, chest pain, and hemoptysis. It is transmitted when one inhales droplets containing the microbe after an

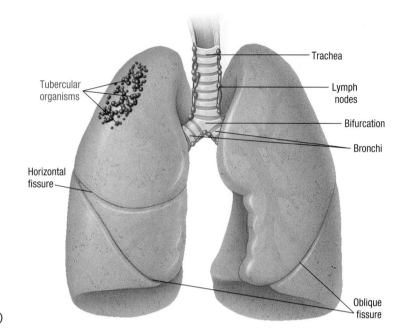

Trachea

Lymph nodes

Bifurcation

Bronchi

Tubercular organisms

Horizontal fissure

Oblique fissure

FIGURE 13-19 Tuberculosis is an infectious disease in which rounded swellings called tubercles form on mucous membranes. (Image provided by Anatomical Chart Co.)

infected person coughs or sneezes. It is diagnosed by a positive Mantoux test followed by chest x-rays that reveal walled-off tubercles in the lungs. The acid-fast bacilli (AFB) staining procedure is useful for detecting **acid-fast bacilli**, such as *M. tuberculosis*. Sputum cultures identifying the AFB also provide confirmation. Tuberculosis is treated aggressively with isoniazid (INH) and rifampin.

Key Terms	Definitions
laryngitis (lair in JYE tis)	larynx inflammation
aphonia (ay FOH nee uh)	loss of the voice
laryngoscope (la RING goh skope)	lighted instrument with a short metal or plastic tube used for examining the larynx
laryngoscopy (lair ing GOS kuh pee)	visual examination of the larynx using a laryngoscope
histoplasmosis (his toh plaz MOH sis)	fungal infection of the lungs
pneumonia (new MOH nee uh)	inflammation of the lungs
aspiration pneumonia (as pi RAY shun new MOH nee uh)	inflammation of the lungs that results from inhaling a substance into the lung field
lobar pneumonia (LOH bar new MOH nee uh)	inflammation of the lungs affecting one or more lobes or parts of a lobe
sputum (SPEW tum) **studies**	evaluation of substances found in sputum
culture and sensitivity studies	identify microbes and the effectiveness of various antibiotics
respiratory syncytial (RES pi ruh tor ee sin SISH ul) **virus pneumonia** (new MOH nee uh)	lung inflammation caused by RSV
influenza (in floo EN zuh)	viral infection producing fever, sore throat, cough, and muscle pain; flu

legionellosis (lee juh nell OH sis)	pneumonia caused by *Legionella pneumophila;* Legionnaires disease
Legionnaires (lee juh NAIRZ) **disease**	pneumonia caused by *Legionella pneumophila;* legionellosis
tuberculosis (tew bur kew LOH sis)	infectious disease affecting the lungs caused by *Mycobacterium tuberculosis*
acid-fast bacilli (buh SIL eye)	microbes that can be identified using the acid-fast staining procedure for the identification of the tuberculosis organism

Key Term Practice: Lower Respiratory Disorders

1. Inflammation of the lung field is termed _____.

2. An infectious disease affecting the lungs that is caused by *Mycobacterium tuberculosis* is called _____.

Lung Cancer

Tumors of the lung tissue are termed **lung cancer** (Fig. 13-20). It is the leading cause of cancer deaths in the United States. Early stages are asymptomatic, but later the affected individual experiences cough, wheezing, and hemoptysis. Common sites of metastasis (tumor spread) are the brain, liver, bone, and skin. Cigarette smoking or passive exposure to cigarette smoke causes 85–90% of all lung carcinomas. Lung cancer is initially diagnosed by chest x-rays and sputum studies. Tissue biopsy indicating the presence of cancerous cells confirms the diagnosis. It is treated aggressively by surgery, radiation, and chemotherapy.

Mesothelioma is a rare malignant or benign neoplasm derived from the pleura and peritoneum. Most cases of mesothelioma are malignant. It is composed of fibrous tissue that grows in sheets over the viscera. Macrophages released to the site lead to a chronic inflammatory state that is thought to contribute to the disease. An association between asbestos exposure and disease development has been established. The cancer

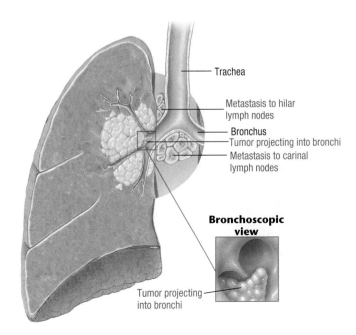

FIGURE 13-20 Cancer of the right lung, anterior view. (Image provided by Anatomical Chart Co.)

is usually asymptomatic in the early stages but progresses to include signs and symptoms of dyspnea and pleuritic pain. Chest x-rays identify the cancer. Treatment includes radiation, chemotherapy, and partial or complete **lobectomy** (surgical removal of all or part of a lung).

Key Terms	Definitions
lung cancer	carcinoma of the lung tissue
mesothelioma (mez oh thee lee OH muh)	cancer derived from the pleura and peritoneum, associated with asbestos exposure
lobectomy (loh BECK toh mee)	surgical removal of all or part of a lung

Key Term Practice: Lung Cancer

1. Carcinoma of the lung tissue is termed _____.

2. Surgical removal of all or part of a lung is termed _____.

Pneumothorax and Hemothorax

The abnormal presence of air or gas in the pleural cavity, which causes pain and difficulty breathing, is a **pneumothorax** (Fig. 13-21). Pneumothoraces result in collapse or partial collapse of the lung. They are characterized by severe dyspnea; sudden chest pain; and rapid, weak pulse. Causes of a pneumothorax include alveoli erosion from tumor or disease, spontaneous tear, improper artificial ventilation, or traumatic injury.

Types of pneumothorax are closed, open, and tension. In a **closed pneumothorax**, air enters the pleural cavity from the lung itself. In an **open pneumothorax**, atmospheric air enters the space surrounding the lungs directly from the environment. A **tension pneumothorax** is characterized by air in the pleural cavity that causes compression of the thoracic organs, resulting in a mediastinal shift. Consequently, the

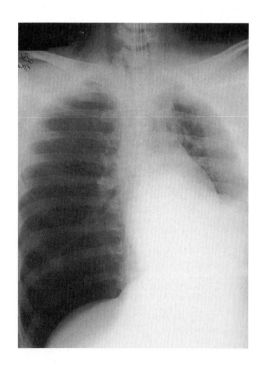

FIGURE 13-21
A pneumothorax is the result of the abnormal presence of air or gas in the pleural cavity. It causes pain and difficulty breathing. (From Fleisher GR, MD, Ludwig S, MD, Baskin MN, MD. Atlas of Pediatric Emergency Medicine. Philadelphia: Lippincott Williams & Wilkins, 2004.)

organs are displaced and normal blood flow to and from the heart is impeded. Diagnosis is made by the history and physical examination and confirmed through chest x-rays and the presence of diminished breath sounds. Abnormal breath sounds are termed **adventitious.** Treatment involves placing the person in the Fowler or semi-Fowler position (sitting position or semireclining position in bed), oxygen therapy, and thoracentesis. **Thoracentesis** is a needle aspiration of intrapleural space for fluid or air withdrawal. Removed fluid can then be analyzed for infection or pathology.

Blood accumulation in the thoracic or pleural cavity is termed **hemothorax.** It is caused by trauma or pulmonary vessel tear. Signs and symptoms are similar to those of pneumothorax. Hemothorax is diagnosed by diminished or absent breath sounds, chest x-rays indicating blood in pleural cavity, and patient distress. Medical intervention involves treating the underlying cause, thoracentesis, and blood replacement if necessary.

Key Terms	*Definitions*
pneumothorax (new moh THOR acks)	air or gas in the pleural cavity surrounding the lungs
closed pneumothorax (new moh THOR acks)	air in the pleural cavity that comes from the lungs
open pneumothorax (new moh THOR acks)	air in the pleural cavity that comes directly from the atmosphere
tension pneumothorax (new moh THOR acks)	air in the pleural cavity that compresses the organs, hindering blood flow
adventitious (ad ven TISH us)	abnormal breath sounds
thoracentesis (thoh ruh sen TEE sis)	surgical procedure in which a needle is inserted through the chest wall to extract air, fluid, or blood
hemothorax (hee moh THOR acks)	blood in the pleural cavity

Key Term Practice: Pneumothorax and Hemothorax

1. _____ is the general term for air in the pleural cavity; _____ is the medical term for blood in the pleural cavity.

2. List three types of pneumothoraces.

   a. _____

   b. _____

   c. _____

Respiratory Acidosis and Respiratory Alkalosis

Both respiratory acidosis and respiratory alkalosis are related to respiratory function. **Respiratory acidosis** is low blood pH resulting from the retention of carbon dioxide, causing an increased partial pressure of carbon dioxide (Pco_2). Partial pressure (P, or p) is the pressure exerted by one gas within a mixture of gases. A sign of respiratory acidosis is decreased respiratory rate. Underlying causes may be COPD, pulmonary embolus, or neuromuscular disease. **Respiratory alkalosis** is caused by accelerated pulmonary elimination of carbon dioxide, causing a decreased Pco_2. Underlying causes contributing to the disorder include exercise, anxiety, and Gram-negative (G−) bacterial blood poisoning. Treatment involves restoring normal breathing patterns.

Key Terms	Definitions
respiratory acidosis (RES pi ruh tor ee as i DOH sis)	low blood pH caused by carbon dioxide retention
respiratory alkalosis (RES pi ruh tor ee al kuh LOH sis)	increased blood pH owing to elimination of too much carbon dioxide

Key Term Practice: Respiratory Acidosis and Respiratory Alkalosis

1. Respiratory _____ results in elevated blood pH levels, and respiratory _____ results in below normal blood pH levels.

Respiratory Syndromes

As a group, respiratory syndromes can be life-threatening. **Adult respiratory distress syndrome** (ARDS) is caused by the inability of the lungs to take in oxygen and is characterized by **hypercapnia** (excessive amount of carbon dioxide in the blood), **acidemia** (acidic blood from decreased pH levels), and severe **hypoxemia** (inadequate amount of oxygen in the blood). ARDS is typified by severe dyspnea, rapid and shallow respirations, cyanosis, rales, rhonchi, and wheezing. The cause is pulmonary edema and respiratory failure when the alveoli fill with exudate.

Pulmonary edema occurs when extravascular fluid accumulates in the lung field and alveoli, producing severe dyspnea (Fig. 13-22). Pulmonary edema is commonly

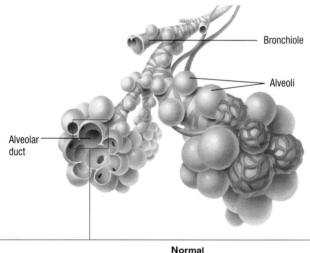
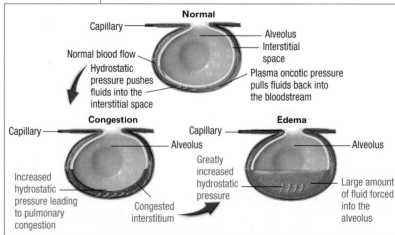

FIGURE 13-22
Pulmonary edema occurs when extravascular fluid accumulates in the lung and alveoli. (Image provided by Anatomical Chart Co.)

caused by left heart failure. The syndrome results in pulmonary hypertension, decreased compliance, decreased functional residual capacity, and hypoxemia. Radiologic studies confirm the clinical picture. Treatment entails oxygen therapy and positive end-expiratory pressure (PEEP). Air administered under positive pressure during expiration to keep the alveoli expanded is termed **positive end-expiratory pressure**.

Infant respiratory distress syndrome (IRDS) is a disease of unknown cause that affects newborns and premature infants during the first few days after birth. It is also known as **neonatal respiratory distress syndrome** (NRDS) and **hyaline membrane disease** (HMD). Respiratory distress, nasal flaring, cyanosis, alveolar collapse, and loss of surfactant are characteristics. Abnormal hyaline membrane lines the alveoli and alveolar ducts when disease persists over a few hours. The disorder is diagnosed by arterial blood gases that show inadequate gas exchange and chest x-rays that reveal the presence of the hyaline membrane. **Arterial blood gas** (ABG) studies measure pH and the pressures of carbon dioxide, oxygen, and bicarbonate ion (HCO_3^-) concentration.

Treatments include mechanical ventilation, PEEP, and aerosol surfactant administration. A **mechanical ventilator**, often referred to as a respirator, supplies negative or positive pressure to the lungs to support breathing. **Continuous positive-airway pressure** (CPAP) supplies positive pressure throughout the entire respiratory cycle.

Sudden infant death syndrome (SIDS) is the sudden, unexpected, unexplained death of an apparently healthy infant. It occurs most commonly in infants between 1 and 4 months old during sleep. Autopsies reveal no conclusive evidence to support a cause of this syndrome. Leading hypotheses suggest an immature ventilatory and arousal response to hypoxemia or hypercapnia, abnormal surfactant, or pulmonary edema in response to viral respiratory tract infections. It is known that the incidence is greater in homes in which the infant is exposed to cigarette smoking while in utero and after birth. Other risk factors include inadequate prenatal care, low birth weight, young maternal age, and maternal hard drug use. Since 1992, the American Academy of Pediatrics has recommended that infants be placed on their backs while sleeping. Although back sleeping is no guarantee against SIDS, research has shown this is a safer sleeping position for infants. Alternative names include cot death, crib death, and sleep apnea syndrome.

Respiratory failure occurs when the respiratory system cannot keep pace with the body's demand for oxygen. Insufficient carbon dioxide is eliminated. The buildup of carbon dioxide results in hypercapnia. If the situation does not resolve, coma ensues. Treatment of respiratory failure entails mechanical ventilation.

Key Terms	Definitions
adult respiratory (RES pi ruh tor ee) **distress syndrome**	disorder marked by hypercapnia, acidemia, and severe hypoxemia resulting in cyanosis
hypercapnia (high pur KAP nee uh)	too much carbon dioxide in the blood
acidemia (as i DEE mee uh)	abnormally low blood pH
hypoxemia (high pock SEE mee uh)	inadequate oxygen in the blood
pulmonary edema (PUL moh nerr ee e DEE muh)	fluid accumulation in the lungs causing breathing difficulty
positive end-expiratory (eck SPYE ruh tor ee) **pressure**	positive-pressure air delivered during expiration
infant respiratory (RES pi ruh tor ee) **distress syndrome**	disorder marked by breathing difficulty and cyanosis in the infant or newborn; NRDS, HMD
neonatal respiratory (RES pi ruh tor ee) **distress syndrome**	disorder marked by breathing difficulty and cyanosis in the infant or newborn; IRDS, HMD

hyaline (HIGH uh lin) **membrane disease**	disorder marked by breathing difficulty and cyanosis in the infant or newborn; IRDS, NRDS
arterial (ahr TEER ee ul) **blood gas**	evaluation of blood pH, CO_2, O_2, and HCO_3^-
mechanical ventilator	machine for moving air into and out of a person's lungs
continuous positive-airway pressure	positive-pressure air delivered throughout the respiratory cycle
sudden infant death syndrome	sudden, unexpected, unexplained death of a sleeping infant
respiratory (RES pi ruh tor ee) **failure**	respiratory system is unable to meet the oxygen demands of the body, and carbon dioxide levels increase

Key Term Practice: Respiratory Syndromes

1. What condition results when the body cannot keep pace with oxygen demands and the carbon dioxide levels rise? _____

2. The unexplained death of an otherwise healthy infant that occurs during sleep is known as _____.

Trauma and Poisoning

Flail chest is a condition with multiple rib fractures occurring with or without sternal fracture. Flail chest results in **paradoxical** (contrary to usual) chest wall movement, resulting from trauma to the rib cage and muscles, hindering their function in breathing (Fig. 13-23). The physical examination, clinical picture, and chest x-ray confirm the diagnosis. Treatment consists of healing the rib fracture(s) and possible mechanical ventilation or oxygen administration.

Carbon monoxide (CO) is a colorless, odorless gas that forms from the burning of carbon-containing fuels with insufficient air turnover. **Carbon monoxide poisoning** occurs when CO instead of oxygen combines with hemoglobin (Hb) molecules. This results in hypoxia. When CO combines with Hb, the hemoglobin does not readily release its oxygen, and hence the skin appears a cherry red color because the hemoglobin is saturated. Tissues are really anoxic, or deprived of oxygen. Symptoms and signs of CO poisoning are shallow breathing and ruddy complexion. Carbon monoxide does not easily dissociate from hemoglobin, so individuals suffering from CO poisoning must be treated in hyperbaric oxygen chambers that are pressurized to force oxygen into the blood.

Key Terms	Definitions
flail chest	fracture of the rib cage that causes paradoxical chest wall movement
paradoxical (pair uh DOCK si kul)	contrary to usual movement
carbon monoxide poisoning	disorder resulting from hemoglobin combining with CO instead of oxygen

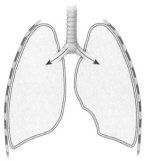

A Normal respiration, inspiration

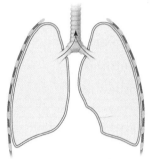

B Normal respiration, expiration

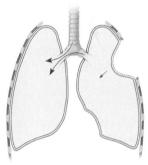

C Flail chest; unstable chest wall sucks in on inspiration

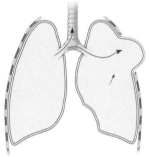

D Flail chest; expiration causes unstable area to balloon out

FIGURE 13-23
Flail chest is a condition of paradoxical chest wall movement, resulting from trauma to the rib cage and muscles.

Key Term Practice: Trauma and Poisoning

1. A rib cage fracture causing paradoxical breathing describes _____.

2. _____ occurs when carbon monoxide instead of oxygen is attached to hemoglobin.

CLINICAL TERMS

Clinical Dimension	Term	Description
DISORDERS		
	acidemia	abnormally low blood pH
	acute bronchitis	sudden and short-lasting inflammation of the bronchial tubes
	acute rhinitis	inflammation of the nasal cavity caused by infection; nasal catarrh, coryza
	adult respiratory distress syndrome (ARDS)	disorder marked by hypercapnia, acidemia, and severe hypoxemia resulting in cyanosis
	allergic rhinitis	nasal inflammation resulting from an allergy
	altitude sickness	disorder characterized by respiratory distress and joint pain caused by the rapid ascent to high altitude; mountain sickness

Clinical Dimension	Term	Description
	anoxia	total lack of oxygen in tissues
	anthracosis	pneumoconiosis caused by inhalation of coal dust
	asbestosis	pneumoconiosis caused by inhalation of asbestos fibers
	asphyxia	impaired or absent oxygen exchange that results in suffocation
	aspiration pneumonia	inflammation of the lungs that results from inhaling a substance into the lung field
	asthma	breathing disorder characterized by chest tightness and airway constriction
	atelectasis	partial or complete collapse of the lung usually caused by an obstructed bronchus
	bends, the	disorder characterized by respiratory distress and joint pain caused by deep-water diving when there is swift reduction in air pressure; decompression sickness, caisson disease
	berylliosis	pneumoconiosis caused by inhalation of beryllium
	bronchiectasis	chronic dilation of the airways
	bronchitis	inflammation of the bronchial tubes
	bronchial asthma	form of asthma with attacks of dyspnea and bronchial spasms
	caisson disease	disorder characterized by respiratory distress and joint pain caused by deep-water diving when there is swift reduction in air pressure; decompression sickness, the bends
	carbon monoxide poisoning	disorder resulting from hemoglobin combining with CO instead of oxygen
	catarrh	inflammation of the mucous membranes of the air passages in the head and throat with discharge
	catarrhal laryngitis	inflammation of the laryngeal mucous membranes with mucoid exudate
	chronic bronchitis	long-lasting inflammation of the bronchial tubes
	chronic obstructive pulmonary disease (COPD)	general term describing permanent or temporary lung disease affecting the bronchial tree
	closed pneumothorax	air in the pleural cavity that comes from the lungs
	croup	laryngotracheobronchitis in infants and children caused by parainfluenza viruses and characterized by a barking cough
	cystic fibrosis (CF)	inherited disorder characterized by thick mucus secretions that block the internal passages, including the lungs

Clinical Dimension	Term	Description
	decompression sickness	disorder characterized by respiratory distress and joint pain caused by deep-water diving when there is swift reduction in air pressure; caisson disease, the bends
	diphtheria	infectious disease caused by *Corynebacterium diphtheriae* that results in severe inflammation of the pharynx, nose, and sometimes the tracheobronchial tree
	emphysema	chronic lung condition characterized by enlarged air sacs
	exercise-induced asthma	form of asthma with bronchoconstriction caused by exercise
	flail chest	fracture of the rib cage that causes paradoxical chest wall movement
	hemothorax	blood in the pleural cavity
	histoplasmosis	fungal infection of the lungs
	hyaline membrane disease (HMD)	disorder marked by breathing difficulty and cyanosis in the infant or newborn; IRDS, NRDS,
	hypercapnia	too much carbon dioxide in the blood
	hyperventilation	abnormal rapid, deep breathing that leads to low alveolar carbon dioxide levels
	hypoventilation	reduced respiratory rate that results in high alveolar carbon dioxide levels
	hypoxemia	inadequate oxygen in the blood
	hypoxia	oxygen deprivation in the tissues; stage before anoxia
	influenza	viral infection producing fever, sore throat, cough, and muscle pain; flu
	infant respiratory distress syndrome (IRDS)	disorder marked by breathing difficulty and cyanosis in the infant or newborn; NRDS, HMD
	laryngitis	larynx inflammation
	Legionnaires disease	pneumonia caused by *Legionella pneumophila*; legionellosis
	legionellosis	pneumonia caused by *Legionella pneumophila*; Legionnaires disease
	lobar pneumonia	inflammation of the lungs affecting one or more lobes or parts of a lobe
	lung cancer	carcinoma of the lung tissue
	mesothelioma	cancer derived from the pleura and peritoneum, associated with asbestos exposure
	mountain sickness	disorder characterized by respiratory distress and joint pain caused by the rapid ascent to high altitude; altitude sickness

Clinical Dimension	Term	Description
	mucoviscidosis	inherited disorder characterized by widespread exocrine dysfunction and pulmonary disease caused by excess mucus production in the respiratory tract; cystic fibrosis
	nasal catarrh	inflammation of the nasal cavity caused by infection; acute rhinitis, coryza
	nasal polyps	benign growths on the nasal mucosa
	neonatal respiratory distress syndrome (NRDS)	disorder marked by breathing difficulty and cyanosis in the infant or newborn; IRDS, HMD
	open pneumothorax	air in the pleural cavity that comes directly from the atmosphere
	pertussis	acute, infectious inflammation of the larynx, trachea, and bronchi caused by *Bordetella pertussis* characterized by spasmodic coughing that ends in a noisy inspiratory stridor, giving rise to the term *whooping cough*
	pharyngitis	inflammation of the pharynx; sore throat
	pleurisy	inflammation of the pleural membrane with exudation; pleuritis
	pleuritis	inflammation of pleural membrane with exudation; pleurisy
	pneumoconiosis	disease caused by inhaling mineral or metallic dust over a long period of time
	pneumonia	inflammation of the lungs
	pneumothorax	air or gas in the pleural cavity surrounding the lungs
	Pontiac fever	mild form of legionellosis without the accompanying pneumonia
	pulmonary edema	fluid accumulation in the lungs causing breathing difficulty
	pulmonary abscess	necrosis within the lung tissue
	pulmonary embolism	blood clot lodged in a pulmonary artery
	respiratory acidosis	low blood pH owing to carbon dioxide retention
	respiratory alkalosis	increased blood pH owing to elimination of too much carbon dioxide
	respiratory failure	respiratory system is unable to meet the oxygen demands of the body, and carbon dioxide levels increase
	respiratory syncytial virus (RSV) pneumonia	lung inflammation caused by RSV
	sarcoidosis	systemic granulomatous disease of unknown cause that specifically involves the lungs and results in interstitial fibrosis

Clinical Dimension	Term	Description
	silicosis	pneumoconiosis caused by inhalation of silica dust
	sinusitis	inflammation of the paranasal sinuses
	sleep apnea	cessation of breathing during sleep that causes one to awaken and is associated with daytime sleepiness
	sudden infant death syndrome (SIDS)	sudden, unexpected, unexplained death of a sleeping infant
	tension pneumothorax	air in the pleural cavity that compresses the organs, hindering blood flow
	tuberculosis	infectious disease affecting the lungs caused by *Mycobacterium tuberculosis*
	upper respiratory infection (URI)	viral or bacterial infection of the nose, nasal cavity, sinuses, and/or pharynx
SIGNS AND SYMPTOMS		
	aphonia	loss of the voice
	apnea	cessation of breathing
	anosmia	loss of the sense of smell, common in frontal lobe tumors
	barrel chest	rounded chest cavity
	Biot respirations	alternating periods of apnea with breaths of the same depth
	bradypnea	abnormally slow breathing rate
	bronchospasm	involuntary contraction of the bronchial smooth muscle
	chest retraction	visible chest depression in the area surrounding the costals (ribs)
	Cheyne-Stokes respirations	hyperpnea alternating with apnea
	clubbing of fingers	fingertips that are rounded like a club
	coryza	runny nose
	cyanosis	bluish colored tissues resulting from a lack of oxygen in the blood
	dry cough	nonproductive tussis; cough without mucus production
	dysphagia	swallowing difficulty
	dysphonia	impaired voice
	dyspnea	labored breathing
	epistaxis	nosebleed
	exudate	mucous material composed of tissue fluid and cellular debris that is deposited on tissue surfaces as a result of inflammation
	friction rub	lung sound heard during auscultation produced by the rubbing of two serous surfaces

Clinical Dimension	Term	Description
	hemoptysis	coughing up blood or bloody mucus
	hyperpnea	increased rate and depth of breathing
	Kussmaul respirations	air hunger
	lacrimation	tear production
	mucopurulent	pertaining to mucus with pus
	nonproductive cough	dry tussis; cough without mucus production
	orthopnea	breathing difficulty except when in an upright position
	phlegm	thick mucus
	productive cough	tussis with mucus production
	rales	abnormal hissing or respiratory sounds
	reflex apnea	sudden, temporary loss of breath; gasp
	rhonchus	harsh, rattling, whistling sound
	sputum	fluid or semifluid mucus mixture
	stridor	harsh sound heard on inhalation that is caused by air passing through a constricted passage
	subcutaneous crepitus	popping sound heard under the skin resulting from gas accumulation that occurs with pneumothorax
	suppurative	forming pus
	tachypnea	rapid breathing rate
	tactile fremitus	vibration felt by the hand on chest while a person talks
	tussis	cough
	wheeze	audible whistling breath sound

CLINICAL TESTS AND DIAGNOSTIC PROCEDURES

Clinical Dimension	Term	Description
	acid-fast stain	procedure that identifies acid-fast bacilli (AFB), such as *Mycobacterium tuberculosis*, the causative agent of tuberculosis
	α_1-antiprotease test	blood test to determine the levels of the glycoprotein α_1-antitrypsin
	α_1-antitrypsin test	blood test to determine the levels of the glycoprotein α_1-antitrypsin
	arterial blood gases (ABGs)	evaluation of blood pH, CO_2, O_2, and HCO_2^-
	auscultation	listening to body sounds using a stethoscope
	bronchoscope	thin, lighted instrument used in bronchoscopy
	bronchoscopy	procedure for viewing the inside of the respiratory structures using a bronchoscope
	chest x-ray	radiographic study of the internal chest organs
	computerized tomography (CT) scan	radiologic imaging method using axial tomography and a computer screen

Clinical Dimension	Term	Description
	culture and sensitivity (C&S) studies	identify microbes and the effectiveness of various antibiotics
	diffusion capacity	measure of gas exchange between alveoli and pulmonary capillary blood
	laryngoscope	lighted instrument with a short metal or plastic tube used for examining the larynx
	laryngoscopy	visual examination of the larynx using a laryngoscope
	lung biopsy	removal of lung tissue for diagnostic evaluation
	lung scan	lung image obtained by using radioisotopes
	magnetic resonance imaging (MRI)	use of electromagnetic radiation to obtain images of body tissue and organs
	Mantoux test	intradermal test used to establish past or present tuberculosis infection
	mediastinoscope	lighted instrument used in mediastinoscopy
	mediastinoscopy	procedure of viewing the mediastinum using a mediastinoscope
	nasal speculum	instrument for viewing the nasal cavity
	palpation	examining the body by touch
	peak expiratory flow (PEF)	uses a PEF meter to measure the volume of air after forced expiration
	pulmonary angiography	x-ray examination of the lungs' blood vessels after injection of a contrast medium
	pulmonary function test (PFT)	measures lung volumes and capacities
	pulse oximeter	instrument that measures the amount of oxygen in the blood
	pulse oximetry	measurement of oxygen in the blood
	sputum studies	evaluation of substances found in the sputum
	thoracentesis	surgical procedure in which a needle is inserted through the chest wall to extract air, fluid, or blood
	transillumination	shining a bright light through a cavity to detect abnormality
	tuberculin skin test	intradermal test, such as the Mantoux test, used to establish past or present tuberculosis infection
	ventilation perfusion scan	combination of radioactive gas inhalation and radioactive dye vessel uptake to provide an image of the lung tissue
TREATMENTS		
	antitussive	drug that prevents or improves coughing
	atomizer	device for administering medicinal liquid in the form of a spray to be breathed through the mouth or nose; nebulizer

Clinical Dimension	Term	Description
	bronchodilators	drugs that ease breathing by relaxing the air passages
	chest tube	tube inserted into the pleural cavity to remove fluid or air
	continuous positive-airway pressure (CPAP)	positive-pressure air delivered throughout the respiratory cycle
	decongestants	drugs that reduce congestion
	endotracheal tube	tube passed through the mouth or nose to the trachea
	expectorant	drug that stimulates phlegm secretion to be coughed out
	isoniazid	drug used to treat tuberculosis
	lobectomy	surgical removal of all or part of a lung lobe
	lung reduction	excision of diseased lung tissue to enhance the function of the remaining healthy lung tissue
	mechanical ventilator	machine for moving air into and out of a person's lungs
	mucolytic	drug that breaks down mucus
	nasal cannula	flexible tube placed in the nostrils to deliver oxygen
	nebulizer	device for administering medicinal liquid in the form of a spray to be breathed through the mouth or nose; atomizer
	oxygen tents	structures that surround a patient in bed to supply oxygen
	oxygen therapy	supplying oxygen via a nasal cannula, Venturi mask, or oxygen tent
	percussion	technique of hitting the back and chest auscultation or to loosen mucus so that it can be coughed out
	pneumonectomy	surgical removal of a lung
	positive end-expiratory pressure (PEEP)	positive-pressure air delivered during expiration
	postural drainage (PD)	positioning the body to allow gravity to drain mucus from areas of the lungs
	resuscitation bag	bag that is manually pumped to deliver air or oxygen
	therapy vest	inflatable vest that vibrates and percusses to dislodge mucus in the lung fields so that it can be coughed out; used in the treatment of cystic fibrosis
	thoracostomy	surgical opening made in the chest wall
	tracheostomy	surgical opening into the trachea
	tracheostomy tube	tube placed through a hole in the trachea
	tuberculostatic	drug that inhibits tubercle growth of tuberculosis bacteria
	Venturi mask	face mask that delivers oxygen

Lifespan

The development of the respiratory system begins early in the gestational period. During the 4th week of embryonic growth, the upper respiratory structures begin forming, and lower respiratory structures are evident at the 5th embryonic week. The remaining respiratory passages and lungs develop from the mesoderm by the 8th week. Bronchial tree structures are completely formed by the 16th week of fetal life, and by the 6th gestational month, alveoli are formed. Surfactant production begins by 20–24 weeks of gestation and is secreted into fetal airways around week 30.

Respiratory structures are nonfunctional while in utero, and the lungs are even fluid filled. The necessary oxygen is delivered to the fetus via the placenta. At birth, the lungs do function, but will not totally inflate for nearly 3 weeks. Premature infants born at 28–30 weeks can breathe on their own provided there is adequate surfactant production.

Although their respiratory systems are complete, newborn infants are fragile in terms of respiratory function. Newborns are quite susceptible to upper respiratory infections owing to immunologic immaturity. In addition, their tonsils and epiglottis are rather large, so infants are obligatory nose breathers up to 3 months. Mouth breathing would not supply enough oxygen for adequate lung inflation; therefore, nasal congestion in young infants can be a serious problem.

Neonates and children have fewer alveoli than adults, but alveolar numbers increase until approximately age 8 years. The metabolic rate in children is greater than in adults; accordingly, oxygen consumption per body weight is higher. If children grow up in a home where cigarette smoke is prevalent, they may never attain optimal respiratory capacity and their organ reserve will be diminished.

With aging, lung tissue becomes less elastic and more rigid. Arthritic changes in the rib cage alter pulmonary function, and there is a decline in blood oxygen levels and lung capacity. The vital capacity can diminish up to 35% by age 70 years. Respiratory muscle strength and endurance decrease up to 20%, but these values can be enhanced with physical exercise. Blood pH and P_{CO_2} remain relatively constant with advancing age.

COPD is not a normal change of aging. Older adults are more susceptible to respiratory infections and pulmonary disorders such as pneumonia, influenza, and bronchitis partially because of decreased alveolar macrophage activity and diminished ciliary action. As of 2001, pneumonia and influenza were the fifth leading cause of death in people older than 65 years, thus it is critical to administer pneumococcal and flu vaccines to this group.

In the News: Hypothermia and the Diving Reflex

It's a miracle! A young boy has an underwater accident while sledding on a cold winter day. After being submerged in icy, frigid lake water for over a half hour, he is rushed to the hospital, where he later recovers with no long-lasting damage. His is not an isolated incident; such cases have been reported over the past 30 years. What is preventing death in these near-drowning victims?

A person can survive immersion in cold water because of two factors: hypothermia and the diving reflex. Hypothermia sets in when the body loses heat faster than it can generate it. Hypothermia occurs in water 25 times faster than in air of the same temperature.

The diving reflex is the physiologic mechanism that enables air-breathing, water-dwelling mammals—such as whales—to remain submerged for extended periods without surfacing for oxygen. In humans, the diving reflex is initiated when the body suddenly comes in contact with cold water. Immediately, blood flow is shunted to the vital areas of the heart, lungs, and brain and is shut off from the extremities and gut. Peripheral arteries constrict, the heart rate becomes bradycardic, and the oxygen supply to heart and brain is enhanced. Laryngospasm protects against water inhalation. The cold water reduces the need for oxygen in body tissues. In warm water, hypoxia would lead to irreversible brain damage within 5 minutes; but in cold water, victims have survived hypoxia lasting 2 hours.

Investigations of near-drowning survival are based on documentation from available case studies, so data are limited. Although the relationship between hypothermia and the diving reflex remains unclear, it is known that an accident victim should not be considered dead until he or she is "warm and dead" because this phenomenon demonstrates that a cold body could be very much alive.

COMMON ABBREVIATIONS

Abbreviation	Term
ABG	arterial blood gas
AFB	acid fast bacilli
ARDS	adult respiratory distress syndrome
CF	cystic fibrosis
CO	carbon monoxide
CO_2	carbon dioxide
COPD	chronic obstructive pulmonary disease
CPAP	continuous positive-airway pressure
CRT	certified respiratory therapist
C&S	culture and sensitivity
CT	computerized tomography
D_LO_2	lung diffusion capacity for oxygen
ERV	expiratory reserve volume
FEV1	forced expiratory volume at 1 second
FVC	forced vital capacity
G−	Gram negative
HCO_3^-	bicarbonate ion
HMD	hyaline membrane disease
INH	isoniazid; isonicotinic acid hydrazide
IRDS	infant respiratory distress syndrome
IRV	inspiratory reserve volume
MRI	magnetic resonance imaging
NBRC	National Board for Respiratory Care
NRDS	neonatal respiratory distress syndrome
O_2	oxygen
P	partial pressure
P_{CO_2}	partial pressure of carbon dioxide
PD	postural drainage
PEEP	positive end-expiratory pressure
PEF	peak expiratory flow

Abbreviation	Term
PFT	pulmonary function test
RRT	registered respiratory therapist
RSV	respiratory syncytial virus
RT	respiratory therapist
RV	residual volume
SIDS	sudden infant death syndrome
TB	tuberculosis
TLC	total lung capacity
TV	tidal volume
URI	upper respiratory infection
VC	vital capacity

Case Study

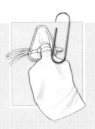

Mrs. June Sawyer, age 55 years, has a history of COPD with severe pulmonary fibrosis. She presented in her physician's office with dyspnea, vomiting, headache, and dizziness as her chief complaints. The physical examination revealed nothing remarkable. Partial CT scans of the sinuses were ordered. Soft tissue and bone windows were used for the examination. The following results were obtained:

- Clear sinuses
- Clear nasal airway
- Normal nasal conchae
- No soft tissue masses
- No bone destructive changes
- No nasal cavity soft tissue displacement
- Normal orbital contents

The physician ordered pulmonary function tests.

Case Study Questions

Select the best answer to each of the following questions.

1. **Mrs. Sawyer presented with dyspnea. Dyspnea means _____.**
   a. being off balance
   b. thirsty
   c. difficulty swallowing
   d. breathing difficulty

2. **Her nasal conchae are normal. These structures _____.**
   a. deflect inhaled air
   b. filter inhaled air
   c. lessen the skull weight
   d. should appear abnormal on a CT scan

3. **The nasal cavity soft tissue refers to the _____.**
   a. external nares
   b. septum
   c. lungs
   d. sinuses

4. **Given the clinical picture and the results of this CT study, Mrs. Sawyer _____.**
   a. probably has a sinus infection
   b. is suffering from TB
   c. does not have a sinus infection
   d. is healthy and requires no further treatment

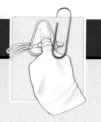

REAL WORLD REPORT

Mrs. June Sawyer's family physician sent her to the respiratory therapy department for a complete pulmonary function test. The examination revealed the following results.

CENTRAL HOSPITAL: PULMONARY CARE UNIT

NAME: June Sawyer

SEX: Female

ORDERPHYS: R. L. Keefer, MD

DOB: February 9, 1948

AGE: 55

EXAM DATE: November 1, 2003

INDICATION FOR STUDY
Pulmonary function studies were done on this patient, who has a history of chronic obstructive pulmonary disease and severe pulmonary fibrosis.

SPIROMETRY
Spirometry showed severe reduction in forced vital capacity, profound reduction in forced expiratory volume at 1 s (FEV1), with severe reduction in the FEV1 to forced vital capacity (FVC) ratio (FEV1/FVC). Midexpiratory flow rates were profoundly reduced. Borderline improvement was noted in forced vital capacity after bronchodilator treatment. Maximum voluntary ventilation was severely reduced.

LUNG VOLUMES
Lung volumes measured by body plethysmography showed increased total lung capacity with marked increase in residual volume.

AIRWAY MECHANICS
Airway resistance was markedly increased and airway conductance was reduced.

DIFFUSION
Diffusion capacity was severely reduced.

OVERALL IMPRESSION
Overall, this study shows evidence of profound obstructive ventilatory impairment associated with severe overinflation and severe diffusion abnormalities consistent with severe chronic obstructive pulmonary disease and emphysema.

Dictated by: M. E. Chabath, MD

REAL WORLD REPORT QUESTIONS

The following exercises review the medical terms in the preceding medical report. A term with which you may not be familiar is *plethysmography.* (pleth iz MOG ruh fee). *Plethysmos* is the Greek term for "increase"; thus plethysmography is a technique to measure increased lung volume or other changes.

1. The pulmonary function tests are done to
   _____.

2. The tests involved spirometry.

   a. Spirometry measures _____.

   b. Vital capacity is _____.

   c. Bronchodilator treatment is used to _____.

3. Lung volumes were measured. Define the following terms.

   a. TLC = _____

   b. residual volume = _____

4. The report indicated that there was reduced conductance. What structures are involved in the conducting airway?

   _____

   _____

   _____

5. What is diffusion capacity and how is the term abbreviated?

   _____

   _____

   _____

6. What type of COPD does Mrs. Sawyer have?

   _____

REVIEW AND APPLICATION: THREE-LEVEL LEARNING SYSTEM

LEVEL ONE: REVIEWING FACTS AND TERMS USING RECALL

Select the best response to each of the following questions.

1. Cavities within skull bones that lighten the weight of the cranium are called _____.

   a. conchae

   b. sinuses

   c. polyps

   d. passages

2. _____ is oxygen use occurring at the cellular level.

   a. Respiration

   b. Pulmonation

   c. Ventilation

   d. Inhalation

3. The _____ is a cartilaginous partition separating the nasal cavity into left and right sections.

   a. cribriform plate

   b. choanae

   c. septum

   d. vestibule

4. The medical term for a cough is _____.

   a. tussis

   b. expectorate

   c. phlegm

   d. sputum

5. The anatomic structure that covers the trachea during swallowing is the _____.

   a. glottis

   b. epiglottis

   c. cricoid cartilage

   d. upper vestibular fold

6. Vocal folds and the space between them is the _____.

   a. epiglottis

   b. false vocal cords

   c. epiglottic cartilage

   d. glottis

7. Identify the form of lung cancer in which fibrous tissue derived from the pleura forms and grows in sheets over the viscera.

   a. tussis

   b. pertussis

   c. mesothelioma

   d. emphysema

8. Structures of the conducting airway of the respiratory system include _____.

   a. larynx, pharynx, and alveoli

   b. trachea, bronchi, and alveoli

   c. respiratory bronchioles, alveoli, and terminal bronchioles

   d. larynx, bronchi, and terminal bronchioles

9. Structures of the respiratory airway include _____.

   a. respiratory bronchioles and alveoli

   b. trachea and alveoli

   c. terminal bronchioles and respiratory bronchioles

   d. bronchi and trachea

10. Type 2 pneumocytes are also called _____ cells.

    a. surfactant

    b. septal

    c. pleural

    d. visceral

11. The substance secreted by pneumocytes that decreases alveolar surface tension is _____.

    a. antitrypsin

    b. antiprotease

    c. $alpha_1$

    d. surfactant

12. The ease with which the lungs can expand with respect to pressure changes is known as _____.

    a. pulmonary ventilation

    b. compliance

    c. expiration

    d. apneusis

13. Cessation of breathing is known as _____.

    a. eupnea

    b. dyspnea

    c. bradypnea

    d. apnea

14. Pulmonary function tests use a device called a _____.

    a. ventilator

    b. respirator

    c. spirometer

    d. nasal cannula

15. Chronic dilation of the respiratory passages causing tussis is termed _____.

    a. bradypnea

    b. hyperventilation

    c. bronchiectasis

    d. hyperpnea

16. An abnormally rapid breathing rate is _____.

    a. tachypnea

    b. Biot respirations

    c. hypoventilation

    d. bradypnea

17. _____ is an abnormal hissing or whistling lung sound.

    a. Sputum

    b. Rale

    c. Phlegm

    d. Dysphonia

18. A flexible tube inserted into the mouth or nose to deliver oxygen to the lungs is a/an _____.

    a. bronchoscopy

    b. thoracotomy

    c. endotracheal tube

    d. auscultation

19. Identify the instrument that measures the amount of oxygen in blood.

    a. lung scan

    b. MRI machine

    c. spirometer

    d. pulse oximeter

20. Normal breathing is controlled by respiratory centers in the _____.

    a. brainstem

    b. lungs

    c. spinal cord

    d. arteries

LEVEL TWO: REVIEWING CONCEPTS

Select the best response to the following question.

21. As the bronchial tree branches into smaller structures, the amount of cartilage _____.

    a. increases

    b. decreases

Provide a medical term to complete a meaningful analogy.

22. Inspiration is to expiration as hypoventilation is to _____

23. Inhalation is to exhalation as _____ is to alkalosis.

24. _____ is to slow respiration rate as tachypnea is to abnormally high respiration rate.

Match the breathing type with its correct definition.

_____ 25. Kussmaul respirations

a. alternating apnea with breathing of same depth

_____ 26. hyperpnea

b. hyperpnea alternating with apnea

_____ 27. Biot respirations

c. air hunger

_____ 28. bradypnea

d. increased rate and depth of breathing

_____ 29. Cheyne-Stokes respirations

e. abnormally slow breathing rate

Match each term with its correct definition.

_____ 30. aphonia

a. thick mucus that is abnormally produced

_____ 31. dysphonia

b. loss of voice

_____ 32. tussis

c. impaired voice

_____ 33. phlegm

d. coarse rale produced by air passage through a partially obstructed

_____ 34. rhonchus

e. cough

Define the following terms.

35. coughing up blood or bloody sputum _____

36. audible whistling breath sound that can be heard without using a stethoscope _____

37. loss of sense of smell _____

38. difficulty swallowing _____

39. too much carbon dioxide in the blood _____

40. inadequate oxygen in the blood _____

Match the medical term with its definition

_____ 41. spirometer

a. amount of air moved in a single breath

_____ 42. expiratory reserve volume (ERV)

b. amount of air forcefully expired after normal expiration

_____ 43. tidal volume (TV)

c. device that measures inhaled and exhaled air volumes

_____ 44. eupnea

d. amount of air in the lungs at all times

_____ 45. residual volume (RV)

e. normal breathing

Match the medical term with its definition.

_____ 46. total lung capacity

a. space containing air that does not reach alveoli

_____ 47. asphyxia

b. amount of air forcefully breathed in

_____ 48. inspiratory reserve volume (IRV)

c. amount of air expired after deepest possible breath

_____ 49. vital capacity (VC)

d. amount of air the lungs can hold

_____ 50. anatomic dead space

e. impaired oxygen exchange resulting in suffocation

Match the disorder with its description.

_____ 51. cystic fibrosis (CF)

a. COPD with enlarged air sacs

_____ 52. emphysema

b. genetic disorder with abnormally thick mucus secretion

_____ 53. bronchiectasis   c. pneumoconiosis caused by silica inhalation

_____ 54. anthracosis   d. chronic dilation of airways

_____ 55. silicosis   e. pneumoconiosis caused by asbestos

Match the drug therapy with its description.

_____ 56. isoniazid   a. drug that reduces congestion

_____ 57. bronchodilator   b. drug used to treat TB

_____ 58. expectorant   c. drug that relaxes bronchial smooth muscles

_____ 59. decongestant   d. drug that stimulates phlegm secretion to be coughed out

Define the following terms.

60. pulmonology _____

61. pneumonitis _____

62. hypercapnia _____

63. tracheotomy _____

Using the following word parts, form a medical term for each definition. Each word part is used only once.

broncho-

bronchiole

centesis

-ectomy

-itis

laryngo-

spasm

thorac-

64. surgical puncture of thorax to remove fluid _____

65. surgical removal of larynx _____

66. involuntary contraction of bronchus _____

67. inflammation of bronchiole _____

Define the following abbreviations.

68. AFB _____

69. SIDS _____

70. COPD _____

71. PEEP _____

72. C&S _____

73. URI _____

Unscramble the letters to form a medical term.

74. yegnxo _____

75. nalnacu _____

76. tyorrerispa _____

77. finezanlu _____

78. mustpu _____

Identify the correctly spelled term in each set.

_____ 79.   a. resusitation   b. resuscitation
             c. resusutation   d. rescuscitation

_____ 80.   a. paradoxical   b. paridoxical
             c. pearadoxical   d. paradocsical

_____ 81.   a. legionelosis   b. legionellosis
             c. legunellosis   d. legunullosis

_____ 82.   a. neumonia   b. pnumonia
             c. pneumonia   d. pneumonuh

_____ 83.   a. tuburculosis   b. tubercolosis
             c. terberculosis d. tuberculosis

_____ 84.   a. rinitis   b. rhinitis
             c. rhynitis   d. rhinitus

LEVEL THREE: THINKING CRITICALLY

Provide a short answer to each of the following questions.

85. Joey was sucking on a throat lozenge when he accidentally choked. The lozenge became wedged in his right bronchus. Provide a plausible explanation for it to be in the right bronchus instead of the left.

_____

_____

_____

86. If an individual loses the gag reflex, a protective mechanism to prevent choking, food particles can be accidentally inhaled. What type of lung disorder is likely to develop? _____

KEY TERMS SPELLING TEST FROM CD-ROM

Use the CD-ROM to test yourself on the spelling of key terms from this chapter. Listen to the terms and write them on a separate sheet of paper. Use a medical dictionary to check your answers.

ANSWERS

WORD GROUPING

Definition	Word Part
imperfect, incomplete	atel-, atelo-
air, gas, lung	pneum-, pneumo-, pneumon-, pneumono-
alveolus (air cell), alveolar	alveoli-, alveolo-
breathing	spir-, spiro-
bronchus, bronchial, windpipe	bronch-, bronchi-, broncho-
coal, charcoal, carbon, anthrax	anthrac-, anthraco-
diaphragm	phren-, phreno-
larynx, laryngeal	laryng-, laryngo-
lung, pulmonary	pulmo-, pulmon-, pulmono-
mouth, oral	oro-
mucus	muc-, muci-, muco-
normal, true	eu-
nose, nasal	nas-, naso-
nose, nasal, nose-like	rhin-, rhino-
pharynx, pharyngeal, throat	pharyng-, pharyngo-
pleura, pleural, lung membrane	pleur-, pleuro-
presence of carbon dioxide	-capnia
presence of oxygen	oxy-
rapid, accelerated	tachy-
respiration, respiratory condition	-pnea
slow	brady-
sound, speech, voice sounds	phon-, phono-
straight	orth-, ortho-
thorax, thoracic	thorac-, thoraci-, thoraco-
time	chron-, chrono-
trachea, tracheal	trache-, tracheo-

WORD BUILDING

Word Part	Meaning	Common or Known Word	Example Medical Term
orth-, ortho-	straight	orthodontics	orthopnea
anthrac-, anthraco-	coal, charcoal, carbon, anthrax	anthrax	anthracosis
bronch-, bronchi, broncho	bronchus, bronchial, windpipe	bronchitis	bronchoscopy
chron-, chrono-	time	chronometer	chronic
laryng-, laryngo-	larynx, laryngeal	laryngitis	laryngospasm
muc-, muci-, muco-	mucus	mucous membrane	mucus
nas-, naso-	nose, nasal	nasogastric	nasal cavity
oro-	mouth, oral	orator	oral cavity
phon-, phono-	sound, speech, voice sounds	phonetics	aphonia
-pnea	respiration, respiratory condition	sleep apnea	apnea
pneum-, pneumo-, pneumon-, pneumono-	air, gas, lung	pneumonia	pneumonia
pulmo-, pulmon-, pulmono-	lung, pulmonary	pulmonologist	pulmonary
tachy-	rapid, accelerated	tachymeter	tachypnea
thorac-, thoraci-, thoraco-	thorax, thoracic	thoracic	thoracentesis
trache-, tracheo-	trachea, tracheal	tracheitis	tracheostomy

KEY TERM PRACTICE

Respiratory System Preview
1. a. pharynges; b. larynges
2. bronchus, bronchial, windpipe

Nose and Nasal Cavity
1. a. naris; b. concha
2. conchae

Paranasal Sinuses
1. a. maxillary; b. frontal; c. ethmoidal; d. sphenoidal

Pharynx
1. nose, nasal; nasopharynx
2. Oro-; oropharynx
3. laryng-, laryngo-; laryngopharynx

Larynx
1. glottis; epiglottis
2. true vocal cords

Trachea and Bronchial Tree
1. primary bronchi
2. alveolar sacs; alveoli

Lungs
1. visceral; parietal
2. lung; pneumocytes

Functions of the Respiratory System
1. Inhalation; exhalation
2. pulmonary ventilation; pulmo-, pulmon-, pulmono-
3. modified or nonrespiratory movements

Pulmonary Volumes and Capacities
1. spirometer
2. Eupnea

Altered Breathing
1. brady-; -pnea; bradypnea
2. rapid, accelerated; respiration; tachypnea

Cardiovascular Disorders Affecting Lungs
1. pulmonary embolism
2. -pnea; dyspnea

Cystic Fibrosis
1. hypo-; hypoxia
2. cystic fibrosis

Chronic Obstructive Pulmonary Disease
1. bronch-, bronchi-, broncho-; -itis; bronchitis
2. acute bronchitis; chronic bronchitis

Asthma
1. rhonchus
2. bronchospasm

Inhalation Disorders
1. pneumoconiosis; pneumo-
2. anthrac-; condition of; anthracosis

Upper Respiratory Disorders
1. pharyngitides
2. nose, nasal; -itis; rhinitis

Lower Respiratory Disorders
1. pneumonia
2. tuberculosis

Lung Cancer
1. lung cancer
2. lobectomy

Pneumothorax and Hemothorax
1. Pneumothorax; hemothorax
2. a. open; b. closed; c. tension

Respiratory Acidosis and Respiratory Alkalosis
1. alkalosis; acidosis

Respiratory Syndromes
1. respiratory failure
2. sudden infant death syndrome (SIDS)

Trauma and Poisoning
1. flail chest
2. Carbon monoxide poisoning

CASE STUDY

1. The correct answer is d.
   - a is incorrect because being off balance describes vertigo.
   - b is incorrect because thirsty describes dipsia.
   - c is incorrect because difficulty swallowing describes dysphagia.
2. The correct answer is a.
   - b is incorrect because nose hairs filter inhaled air.
   - c is incorrect because sinuses lessen the weight of the skull.
   - d is incorrect because an abnormal appearance on a CT scan indicates pathology.
3. b is the correct answer.
   - a is incorrect because the external nares are nostrils.
   - c is incorrect because the lungs are not found in the nasal cavity.
   - d is incorrect because the sinuses are not soft tissue but rather are spaces located within the skull bones.
4. c is the correct answer.
   - a is incorrect because the report indicated clear sinuses; thus she does not have an infection.
   - b is incorrect because a CT scan of the skull would not indicate TB infection; a lung x-ray would be needed.
   - d is incorrect because she is experiencing dyspnea, vomiting, and dizziness, which are all abnormal signs and symptoms; thus further study is warranted.

REAL WORLD REPORT

1. evaluate and assess lung function and performance
2. a. lung capacities and volumes; b. the amount of air that can be exhaled from the lungs after the deepest possible breath; c. expand and relax the breathing passages, especially those of the bronchial tree.
3. a. total lung capacity; b. the amount of air that is constantly present in the lungs
4. nasal cavity, pharynx, larynx, trachea, bronchi, and terminal bronchioles
5. a. Diffusion capacity is the amount of a gas taken up by pulmonary capillaries per minute. It is abbreviated with the letter D followed by a subscript letter indicating location (L for lung), followed by the gas (O_2 for oxygen) that is measured across the membrane: D_LO_2.
6. emphysema.

REVIEW AND APPLICATION: THREE-LEVEL LEARNING SYSTEM

Level One: Reviewing Facts and Terms Using Recall

1. b
2. a
3. c
4. a
5. b
6. d
7. c
8. d
9. a
10. b
11. d
12. b
13. d
14. c
15. c
16. a
17. b
18. c
19. d
20. a

Level Two: Reviewing Concepts

21. b. decreases
22. hyperventilation
23. acidosis
24. Bradypnea
25. c
26. d
27. a
28. e
29. b
30. b
31. c
32. e
33. a
34. d
35. hemoptysis
36. wheeze
37. anosmia
38. dysphagia
39. hypercapnia
40. hypoxemia
41. c
42. b
43. a
44. e
45. d
46. d
47. e
48. b
49. c
50. a
51. b
52. a
53. d
54. e
55. c
56. b
57. c
58. d
59. a
60. study of the lungs
61. inflammation of lung
62. excessive carbon dioxide in blood
63. surgical opening in trachea
64. thoracentesis
65. laryngectomy
66. bronchospasm
67. bronchiolitis
68. acid-fast bacilli
69. sudden infant death syndrome
70. chronic obstructive pulmonary disease
71. positive end-expiratory pressure
72. culture and sensitivity
73. upper respiratory infection
74. oxygen
75. cannula
76. respiratory
77. influenza
78. sputum
79. b
80. a
81. b
82. c
83. d
84. b

Level Three: Thinking Critically

85. Inhaled particles are more likely to be lodged in the right bronchus than the left because the right bronchus is slightly larger in diameter and positioned in a more vertical direction than the left bronchus.
86. Aspiration pneumonia is the type of pneumonia likely to result from inhaled food particles into the lower airways.

Digestive System

OBJECTIVES

After completing this chapter, you should be able to:

1. State the meanings of word parts related to the digestive system.
2. Identify and locate organs of the digestive system.
3. Outline the pathway of food through the gastrointestinal tract.
4. Describe the role of enzymes in the digestive process.
5. List the nutrients necessary for life.
6. Define common signs, symptoms, and treatments of various digestive system diseases.
7. Explain clinical tests and diagnostic procedures related to the digestive system.
8. Describe anatomical and physiological alterations throughout the lifespan.
9. Define abbreviations related to the digestive system.
10. Define terms used in medical reports involving the digestive system.
11. Define word parts related to the digestive system.
12. Correctly define, spell, and pronounce the chapter's medical terms.

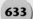

Professional Profile: Registered Dietitian

Jane is a registered dietitian (RD) who works in a clinical setting and who has specialized in renal and diabetic care. (Note that *dietician* is an accepted spelling variation of *dietitian*.) She plans nutrition programs and provides nutritional services to diabetic patients, many of whom already have renal failure and require hemodialysis (artificial blood filtering).

As a registered dietitian, Jane assesses the nutritional needs of patients on an individual basis. She focuses on the development and implementation of dietary programs while educating people on their specific food requirements and restrictions. In the dialysis unit, nutritional reports are generated monthly for evaluation. Much of Jane's time is spent in conference with physicians and other members of the patient's health-care team so that the medical and nutritional needs can be coordinated.

Jane completed a bachelor of science degree in dietetics from a program accredited by the American Dietetic Association (ADA). There are two parts to the curriculum: theory and practice. The academic component (theory) is referred to as the didactic program in dietetics. Students take a variety of courses, including biology, anatomy, physiology, medical terminology, food and nutrition science, chemistry, biochemistry, accounting, management, statistics, sociology, microbiology, business, and communication. After finishing their coursework, students must complete a dietetic internship (practice); Jane's was a 900-hour supervised practicum. Finally, the prospective RD must pass the national registration examination administered by the Commission on Dietetic Registration (CDR) to obtain the credentials to practice.

Jane is both a licensed dietitian (LD), and an RD with the ADA. She took advanced training to obtain certification in both renal nutrition and diabetes education. To maintain her registrations, Jane must participate in continuing professional education.

INTRODUCTION

The digestive system is also referred to as the gastrointestinal (GI) system because it involves the stomach (gastro-) and intestines (intestinal). The primary functions of the system are digestion and elimination. Digestion involves the breakdown of food into smaller, usable forms to keep the body healthy, and elimination is the expulsion of digestive waste products through feces.

The purpose of digestion is to alter the physical and chemical composition of foodstuffs so that they can be absorbed for cellular use. One digestive system action is to supply the blood with vital nutrients to be delivered to the body's cells. Digestion begins in the mouth as soon as food mixes with saliva. When food particles progress through the intestinal tracts, movements of organs and secretions supplied by accessory structures continue the process. The body's cells use the end products of digestion, and waste substances become excrement. Other functions and activities of this system and its parts, along with congenital and structural abnormalities, are described in this chapter.

Nutrition is a key aspect of total body health and must be considered with digestive processes. The field is expanding as the connection between nutrition and health becomes further defined. Nutrition is one area in which intervention strategies can be immediately implemented and positive outcomes easily achieved.

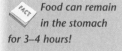

Food can remain in the stomach for 3–4 hours!

MEDICAL TERM PARTS

WORD PARTS

Medical term prefixes, suffixes, and combining forms related to the digestive system are introduced in this section.

Word Parts	Meaning
alveol-, alveolo-	alveolus (tooth socket), alveolar
amino-	chemical compound containing $-NH_2$
amyl-, amylo-	starch
appendico-	an appendix
-ase	enzyme
bili-	bile
bucco-	cheek
calori-	heat
cec-, ceco-	blind (closed), cecum
celi-, celio-	abdomen, belly
cephal-, cephalo-	head
cheil-, cheilo-	lip
chol-, chole-, cholo-	bile
cholangi-, cholangio-	bile duct, biliary passage
chyl-, chyli-, chylo-	chyle (milky fluid taken up by intestines)
col-, coli-, colo-	colon
dent-, denti-, dento-	tooth, dental
duoden-, duodeno-	duodenum, duodenal
emet-, emeto-	vomiting, emesis
enter-, entero-	intestine
epiplo-	omentum (apron), epiploon (omentum)
esoph-, esopho-	esophagus, esophageal
galact-, galacto-	milk
gastr-, gastro-	stomach, gastric
gloss-, -glossa, glosso-	tongue
gluco-, glyc-, glyco-	glucose, sugar
hepat-, hepato-	liver
hernio-	hernia
ile-, ileo-	ileum, ileal
jejun-, jejuno-	pertaining to the jejunum
lingu-, lingua-, lungui-, linguo-	tongue
lip-, lipo-	lipid, fat

Word Parts	Meaning
lith-, litho-	stone, calculus
oro-	mouth, oral
palato-	palate
pancre-, pancreo-	pancreas, pancreatic
peritoneo-	peritoneum
-phagia	eating or swallowing
pharyng-, pharyngo-	pharynx, pharyngeal
proct-, procto-	anus and rectum
pylor-, pyloro-	muscular opening, pylorus
rect-, recto-	rectum, rectal
sacchar-, sacchari-, saccharo-	sugar
sial-, sialo-	saliva, salivary
sigmoid-, sigmoido-	sigmoid, S-shaped
stomat-, stomato-	mouth
uvul-, uvulo-	uvula
vermi-	worm, worm-like

WORD ETYMOLOGY

Some words have Greek or Latin word roots but are not true word parts. This section lists those that are used as medical terms.

Word	Definition
bilis	bile
cholecyst	gallbladder
diverticulum	a by-road
gingiva	gum
kolon	colon
pepsis	digestion
polypus	mass of tissue bulging from the normal surface level
vitalis	life

MEDICAL TERM PARTS USED AS PREFIXES

Prefix	Definition
amino-	chemical compound containing -NH_2
appendico-	an appendix

Prefix	Definition
bili-	bile
bucco-	cheek
calori-	heat
epiplo-	omentum (apron), epiploon (omentum)
hernio-	hernia
oro-	mouth, oral
palato-	palate
peritoneo-	peritoneum
vermi-	worm, worm-like

MEDICAL TERM PARTS USED AS SUFFIXES

Suffix	Definition
-ase	enzyme
-glossa	tongue
-phagia	eating or swallowing

WORD GROUPING

Using the "Medical Term Parts" tables, identify the prefix, suffix, or combining form for each of the following definitions. The first one has been done as an example.

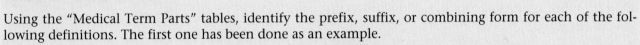

Definition	Word Part
an appendix	appendico-
abdomen, belly	
alveolus (tooth socket), alveolar	
anus and rectum	
bile	A.
	B.
bile duct, biliary passage	
blind (closed), cecum	
cheek	
chemical compound containing -NH_2	
chyle (milky fluid taken up by intestines)	
colon	
duodenum, duodenal	
eating or swallowing	

Definition	Word Part
esophagus, esophageal	
enzyme	
glucose, sugar	
head	
heat	
hernia	
ileum, ileal	
intestine	
lip	
lipid, fat	
liver	
milk	
mouth	
mouth, oral	
muscular opening, pylorus	
omentum (apron), epiploon (omentum)	
palate	
pancreas, pancreatic	
peritoneum	
pertaining to the jejunum	
pharynx, pharyngeal	
rectum, rectal	
saliva, salivary	
sigmoid, S-shaped	
starch	
stomach, gastric	
stone, calculus	
sugar	
tongue	A. B.
tooth, dental	
uvula	
vomiting, emesis	
worm, worm-like	

WORD BUILDING

Word parts, introduced in the "Medical Term Parts" section, are listed in the following table. For this exercise, first supply the meaning of each word part, then use the word part to build a word you already know. The word you list under "Common or Known Word" does not have to be a medical term; a commonly used word is fine. Be sure, however, that the word correctly reflects the intended meaning. The first one has been done as an example.

Word Part	Meaning	Common or Known Word	Example Medical Term
amino-	chemical compound containing -NH$_2$	amino acid	amino acid
-ase			maltase
bucco-			buccal phase
calori-			kilocalorie
cephal-, cephalo-			cephalic phase
chol-, chole-, cholo-			cholecystokinin
col-, coli-, colo-			colon
dent-, denti-, dento-			dentition
duoden-, duodeno-			duodenum
galact-, galacto-			galactose
gastr-, gastro-			gastric juice
gluco-, glyc-, glyco-			gluconeogenesis
hepat-, hepato-			hepatocytes
hernio-			herniorrhaphy
lip-, lipo-			lipase
pancre-, pancreo-			pancreas
pharyng-, pharyngo-			pharyngeal phase
proct-, procto-			proctologist
sacchar-, sacchari-, saccharo-			monosaccharide

ANATOMY AND PHYSIOLOGY

Structures of the Digestive System

- Esophagus
- Gallbladder
- Large intestine
- Liver
- Oral cavity (salivary glands, teeth, and tongue)
- Pancreas
- Small intestine
- Stomach

Digestive System Preview

The digestive tract, or **alimentary canal**, is the passageway between the mouth and anus, the openings to the exterior. The term *aliment* refers to "food." The digestive system transforms food into usable body substances and eliminates nonusable waste products. The organs responsible for these actions are the oral cavity structures (salivary glands, teeth, and tongue), esophagus, stomach, small and large intestines, gallbladder, liver, and pancreas (Fig. 14-1). Through the actions of the various digestive structures, the primary functions of digestion, ingestion, peristalsis, mechanical and chemical catabolism, secretion, absorption, and elimination are performed.

Digestion, the breaking down of food particles into practical forms, begins in the mouth with salivary gland enzymes, the teeth, and the tongue. From the oral cavity, food is swallowed into the esophagus, a muscular transport tube to the stomach. After mechanical (muscular mixing) and chemical (enzymatic) digestion in the stomach, the changed food particles enter the small intestine, where they undergo further alterations, ultimately emptying into the large intestine and then to the outside.

Chemical and mechanical digestion are crucial to food breakdown. **Chemical digestion** is enzymatically controlled and refers to the catabolic reactions in which large carbohydrates (sugars), lipids (fats), and protein molecules (amino acid groups) are broken down into smaller, usable forms. **Mechanical digestion**, chewing and stomach churning, involves movements that aid chemical digestion. The GI tract has both mixing and propelling movements. Smooth muscles in relatively small segments of the alimentary canal undergo contractions to accomplish mixing movements. These rhythmic, wave-like motions, called **peristalsis**, are responsible for the propelling movements that squeeze the contents through the length of the digestive tract. A ring of successive contractions in the tube wall creates these peristaltic waves. As the wave moves along, it pushes the contents ahead of it through the tube, and the substances in the alimentary tract are mixed with digestive secretions. This chapter provides greater explanation for the vital tasks accomplished by the digestive system.

FACT *It takes approximately 10 seconds for food to reach the stomach after swallowing!*

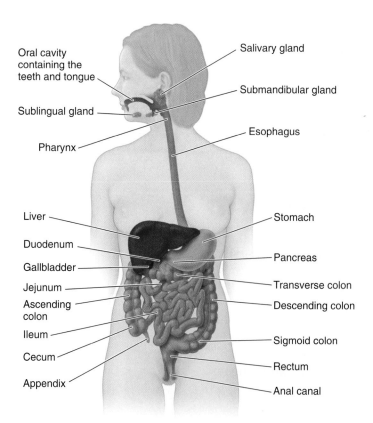

FIGURE 14-1
The digestive tract is the passageway between the mouth and the anus, the two openings to the exterior.

Oral cavity containing the teeth and tongue

Sublingual gland

Pharynx

Salivary gland

Submandibular gland

Esophagus

Liver

Duodenum

Gallbladder

Jejunum

Ascending colon

Ileum

Cecum

Appendix

Stomach

Pancreas

Transverse colon

Descending colon

Sigmoid colon

Rectum

Anal canal

Key Terms	Definitions
alimentary (al i MEN tuh ree) **canal**	digestive tube from the mouth to the anus
digestion	the conversion of food into usable substances through the actions of enzymes and movements
chemical digestion	the breaking down of food by enzymes
mechanical digestion	the breaking down of food by forces of movement
peristalsis (perr i STAL sis)	progressive waves of contractions in GI tract

Key Term Practice: Digestive System Preview

1. What are the two types of digestion that occur in the gastrointestinal tract? _____

2. What is the term for the digestive tract that is derived from the word *aliment*, which means "food"? _____

Oral Cavity

The oral cavity (mouth), the region including cheeks, lips, tongue, palate, teeth, and gums has several functions. The mouth prepares food for digestion. Once food enters the mouth, salivation begins to lubricate food. **Salivary glands** are exocrine structures that secrete 1–1.5 L (1.06–1.59 qt.) of saliva per day into the oral cavity through ducts.

Three major salivary glands are the parotid, submandibular (submaxillary), and sublingual (Fig. 14-2). Serous cells within the glands secrete digestive enzymes, and mucous cells secrete mucus. The largest salivary glands are the **parotid glands**, located in front of the ear between the skin and the masseter muscle, which secrete the enzyme salivary amylase. The **submandibular glands** are located midway along the inner side of the jaw on the floor of the mouth and produce viscid saliva. **Sublingual glands** are found below the tongue under the mouth floor mucosa and secrete mucus.

Digestive functions of saliva include moistening food, binding food particles together, and beginning carbohydrate digestion through the action of salivary amylase. Salivary amylase splits starch and glycogen (the storage form of glucose) into

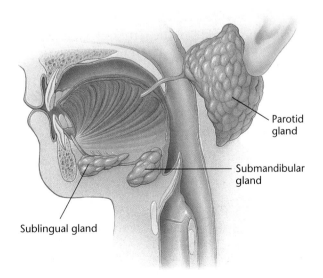

Parotid gland

Submandibular gland

Sublingual gland

FIGURE 14-2
The salivary glands secrete digestive enzymes and mucus. (Image provided by Anatomical Chart Co.)

disaccharides (sugars formed from two single sugar molecules, such as common table sugar, sucrose). Saliva contains bicarbonate ions, which buffer acids, so that the average pH in the mouth is between 6.5 and 7.5. Saliva also cleanses the **dentes** (teeth; sing., dens), which aid in mechanical digestion.

Through **mastication** (chewing), food is mechanically reduced in size to form a round food mass called a **bolus**. Composed of skeletal muscle tissue, the tongue is a mucous membrane–covered structure containing papillae. **Papillae** are small, conical projections on the tongue surface, some of which contain taste buds. The act of swallowing is called **deglutition**, and the entire process of taking in food and swallowing it is termed **ingestion**.

The pharynx receives the bolus and autonomically (automatically under nervous influence) continues deglutition to the esophagus. When the bolus contacts the pharyngeal wall, the **uvula**, a fleshy V-shaped extension hanging from the soft palate above the tongue, closes and seals the nasopharynx. The bolus is then transported through the esophagus to the stomach via peristaltic waves.

Key Terms	Definitions
salivary (SAL i verr ee) **glands**	exocrine structures that secrete saliva
parotid (puh ROT id) **glands**	salivary glands in front of and below the external ears
submandibular (sub man DIB yoo lur) **glands**	salivary glands below mandible
sublingual (sub LING gwul) **glands**	salivary glands beneath tongue
dentes (DEN teez)	teeth; calcified organs used for chewing
mastication (mas ti KAY shun)	chewing
bolus (BOH lus)	rounded food mass made by the mouth
papillae (pa PIL ee)	small projections
deglutition (dee gloo TISH un)	swallowing
ingestion (in JES chun)	taking food into the body
uvula (YOO vew luh)	appendage hanging from the soft palate

Key Term Practice: Oral Cavity

1. Provide the singular and plural forms of the term meaning small projections on the tongue surface.

   singular = _____

   plural = _____

2. Provide the singular and plural forms of the term describing the structure hanging from the soft palate.

   singular = _____

   plural = _____

3. The word part *sub-* means _____, and the word part *lingua-* means _____, so the salivary gland beneath the tongue is the _____ gland.

Teeth

Teeth are important structures for the digestive system as a whole. Dental succession, or **dentition,** refers to the type, number, arrangement, and process of teeth development. The 20 **deciduous** (primary) **teeth** are shed and replaced by the permanent teeth (Fig. 14-3). *Deciduous* means "shed at a particular stage," as in deciduous trees, whose leaves fall off during the autumn. The 32 **permanent** (secondary) **teeth** are the final adult teeth.

Different kinds of teeth are adapted to handle foods in various ways, such as biting, grasping, and grinding. The eight **incisors** are adapted for biting, the four **cuspids** (canines) grasp and tear food, and the eight **bicuspids** (premolars) and 12 **molars** do the job of grinding. One can remember the types of teeth from anterior to posterior by using the mnemonic device I C B M.

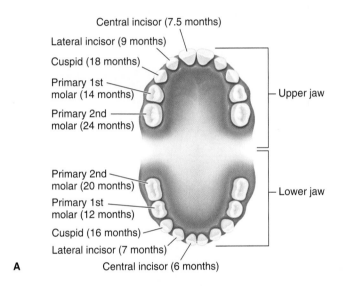

Central incisor (7.5 months)
Lateral incisor (9 months)
Cuspid (18 months)
Primary 1st molar (14 months)
Primary 2nd molar (24 months)
Upper jaw

Primary 2nd molar (20 months)
Primary 1st molar (12 months)
Cuspid (16 months)
Lateral incisor (7 months)
Central incisor (6 months)
Lower jaw

A

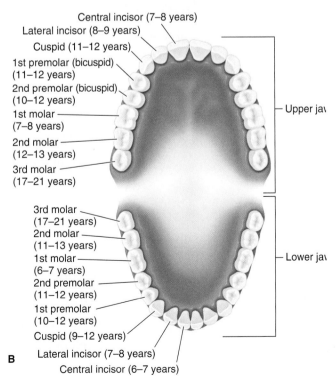

Central incisor (7–8 years)
Lateral incisor (8–9 years)
Cuspid (11–12 years)
1st premolar (bicuspid) (11–12 years)
2nd premolar (bicuspid) (10–12 years)
1st molar (7–8 years)
2nd molar (12–13 years)
3rd molar (17–21 years)
Upper jaw

3rd molar (17–21 years)
2nd molar (11–13 years)
1st molar (6–7 years)
2nd premolar (11–12 years)
1st premolar (10–12 years)
Cuspid (9–12 years)
Lateral incisor (7–8 years)
Central incisor (6–7 years)
Lower jaw

B

FIGURE 14-3 **(A)** Deciduous teeth and **(B)** permanent teeth are adapted to handle foods in various ways.

The typical tooth structure consists of a crown, neck, and root; and teeth are composed of cementum, enamel, dentin, pulp, nerves, and blood vessels (Fig. 14-4). The **gingiva** is the mucous membrane surrounding the teeth and is more commonly known as the gum. The **crown** extends beyond the gingiva (gum) line; the **neck** is the portion at the gingiva between the root and the crown. The ridge of bone in each maxilla and mandible that surrounds and supports the teeth is referred to as the **alveolar process** or **alveolar bone**, which are synonymous terms.

Roots anchor teeth to the alveolar bone by collagenous fibers of the **periodontal ligament**, which passes between the cementum and the alveolar bone. The **root canal** is the tooth cavity containing pulp, nerves, and vessels. **Enamel**, the hardest substance in the human body, covers the dentin of the crown and consists of calcium salts in a crystalline form. **Dentin** forms the bulk of a tooth below the enamel. It is similar to bone, but harder. The pulp cavity is surrounded by dentin and contains blood vessels, nerves, and connective tissue called pulp. **Pulp** is the soft, internal portion of the tooth. **Cementum** is the bone-like material enclosing the roots that "cements" the teeth to the periodontal ligament.

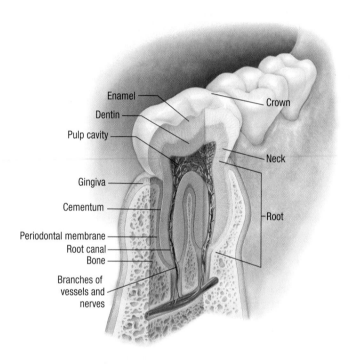

FIGURE 14-4
The typical tooth structure. (Image provided by Anatomical Chart Co.)

Key Terms	Definitions
dentition (den TISH un)	collective term for the teeth collectively
deciduous (de SID yoo us) **teeth**	the 20 primary teeth
permanent teeth	the 32 adult teeth
incisors (in SIGH zurz)	front cutting teeth (four in upper jaw, four in lower jaw)
cuspids (KUS pidz)	teeth with only one point; canines
bicuspids (bye KUS pidz)	teeth with two points; premolars
molars (MOH lurz)	teeth that grind and pulverize
gingiva (JIN ji vuh)	mucous membrane covering the alveolar process; gum

crown	top part of a tooth
neck	area between the crown and the root of a tooth
alveolar (al VEE oh lur) **process**	bony ridge of the maxilla and mandible for teeth; alveolar bone
alveolar (al VEE oh lur) **bone**	bony ridge of the maxilla and mandible for teeth; alveolar process
roots	parts of teeth embedded in tissue
periodontal ligament (perr ee oh DON tul LIG uh munt)	connective tissue surrounding the tooth's root attaching it to the alveolar bone
root canal	tooth cavity in the root containing pulp, nerves, and blood vessels
enamel	calcified substance covering the tooth's crown
dentin (DEN tin)	calcified tooth tissue over the roots, surrounding the pulp, and covered by cementum
pulp	soft interior of the tooth
cementum (se MEN tum)	bony tissue covering the tooth's root

Key Term Practice: Teeth

1. What are the four types of adult teeth?

   a. _____

   b. _____

   c. _____

   d. _____

2. What is the plural form of cementum? _____

Esophagus

The upper gastrointestinal (UGI) tract includes the esophagus, stomach, and duodenum (first segment of the small intestine). The collapsible, muscular tube extending from the pharynx to the stomach that connects the oral cavity to the stomach is the **esophagus**. It is about 25 cm (10 in.) in length and is sometimes called the gullet.

The four layers of the alimentary canal wall from inside (deep) to outside (superficial) are the mucosa (mucous membrane), submucosa, muscularis (muscular layer), and serosa (serous layer) (Fig. 14-5). These strata enable movement and absorption. The **mucosa** absorbs nutrients and secretes mucus, and the **submucosa** nourishes the digestive tract through its rich vascular network. The submucosa also contains nerves and lymphatic vessels. The **muscularis** is composed of circular and longitudinal muscle fibers that are adapted for movement. The **serosa** secretes serous fluid to lubricate the tract.

The mucosa of the esophagus is composed of stratified squamous epithelium so it resists abrasion. The opening where the esophagus passes through the diaphragm is termed the **esophageal hiatus**. *Hiatus* means "an opening in an organ." The diaphragmatic constriction, or **lower esophageal sphincter** (LES), at this point helps prevent the regurgitation of food from the stomach into the esophagus.

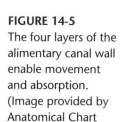

FIGURE 14-5
The four layers of the alimentary canal wall enable movement and absorption. (Image provided by Anatomical Chart Co.)

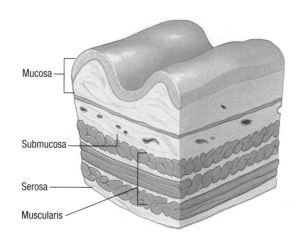

Key Terms	Definitions
esophagus (ee SOF uh gus)	musculomembranous tube extending from the pharynx to the stomach
mucosa (mew KOH suh)	mucous membrane that secretes mucus
submucosa (sub mew KOH suh)	layer of fibrous connective tissue attached to the mucosa
muscularis (mus kew LAIR is)	muscular layer of a tubular organ
serosa (se ROH suh)	serous membrane that secretes serous fluid
esophageal hiatus (ee sof uh JEE ul high AY tus)	opening in the diaphragm for the esophagus
lower esophageal sphincter (ee sof uh JEE ul SFINK tur)	circular band of muscle between the stomach and the esophagus that prevents backflow of stomach contents into the esophagus

 Key Term Practice: Esophagus

1. What are the singular and plural forms of the term describing the muscular tube connecting the throat with the stomach?

   singular = _____

   plural = _____

2. The opening in the diaphragm through which the esophagus passes is termed the _____.

Stomach

The **stomach** begins at the inferior portion of the esophagus and ends at the pyloric sphincter, the valve between the stomach and the small intestine. The stomach is a J-shaped organ that lies mostly left of the midline, inferior to the diaphragm. It receives the bolus from the esophagus and aids in mechanical and chemical digestion. The three-layered muscularis is composed of multidirectional muscle fibers that assist mechanical stomach movement.

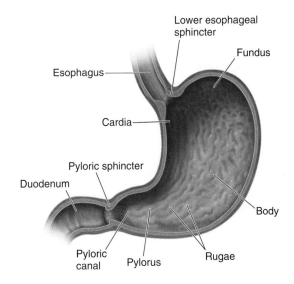

FIGURE 14-6
The stomach has four main anatomic regions.

The stomach has four main anatomic regions: cardia, fundus, body, and pylorus (Fig. 14-6). The **cardia** is nearest the esophageal opening and is the smallest part. Located above the cardia is a dome-shaped temporary storage area called the **fundus**. Swallowed air often fills this area. **Eructation** refers to the belching or burping of stomach air. The main centrally located part of the stomach is referred to as the body. Gastric glands in the body secrete acids and enzymes. Last, the **pylorus** narrows and becomes the pyloric canal, which connects to the duodenum at the pyloric sphincter, a muscular band that prevents backflow.

The stomach has rugae, specialized secreting cells, and a muscularis. **Rugae** are natural folds that allow the stomach to **distend** (stretch). Specialized cells include mucous, chief, and parietal. As their name suggests, **mucous cells** produce mucus, which protects the stomach and prevents it from digesting itself. **Chief cells** or **zymogenic cells** secrete **pepsinogen**, a protein-digesting enzyme that is ultimately converted to pepsin in the presence of hydrochloric acid (HCl). Hydrochloric acid provides the necessary acidic environment for the conversion of pepsinogen to pepsin.

Pepsin is an enzyme that digests protein and is most active in acidic environments. **Parietal cells** secrete intrinsic factor and hydrochloric acid. **Intrinsic factor** is a glycoprotein that facilitates the absorption of vitamin B_{12} in the small intestine. Without intrinsic factor, the body cannot absorb this vital nutrient.

Key Terms	Definitions
stomach	organ in which food is stored after swallowing and that secretes gastric juice to aid digestion
cardia (KAHR dee uh)	stomach area adjacent to the esophagus
fundus (FUN dus)	dome-shaped stomach region
eructation (ee ruck TAY shun)	belching, burping
pylorus (pye LOR us)	region of the stomach opening into the small intestine
rugae (ROO gee)	stomach folds or wrinkles
distend	stretch
mucous (MEW kus) **cells**	cells that secrete mucus

chief cells	stomach cells that secrete pepsinogen; zymogenic cells
zymogenic (zye moh JEN ick) **cells**	stomach cells that secrete pepsinogen; chief cells
pepsinogen (pep SIN oh jen)	pepsin antecedent
pepsin (PEP sin)	proteinase of gastric juice
parietal (puh RYE e tul) **cells**	gastric cells that secrete HCl and intrinsic factor
intrinsic factor	substance produced by gastric cells that enables the absorption of vitamin B_{12}

Key Term Practice: Stomach

1. List three of the four regions of the stomach.

    a. _____

    b. _____

    c. _____

2. _____ is a substance necessary for the absorption of vitamin B_{12} in the intestinal mucosa.

FACT *It may take up to 3 hours for food to move through the intestinal tract!*

Pancreas

The **pancreas**, about 15 cm (6 in.) in length, is an elongated, somewhat flattened organ located posterior to the stomach within the fold of the duodenum (Fig. 14-7). It is conveniently located so that it may secrete digestive pancreatic juices directly into the small intestine. The pancreas is an endocrine gland when secreting insulin (from beta cells) and glucagon (from alpha cells) and an exocrine gland when secreting alkaline digestive juices (from acinar cells). (The term *acinus* refers to sacs in exocrine

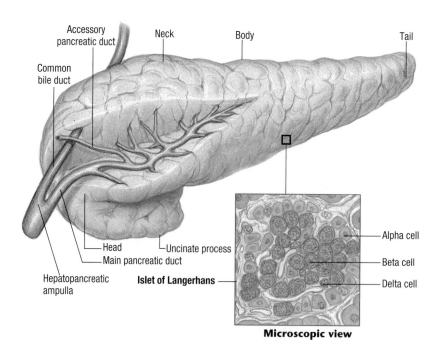

FIGURE 14-7
The pancreas plays an important role in the digestive process, secreting alkaline digestive juices from acinar cells. (Image provided by Anatomical Chart Co.)

Accessory pancreatic duct
Common bile duct
Neck
Body
Tail
Head
Uncinate process
Main pancreatic duct
Hepatopancreatic ampulla
Islet of Langerhans
Alpha cell
Beta cell
Delta cell
Microscopic view

structures.) It plays an important role in the digestion process when acting as an exocrine gland.

Regions of the pancreas are the head, body, and tail. The head is situated near the duodenum; the body is the central portion; and the tail is the short, bluntly rounded part. Extending the length of the pancreas is a tube called the **pancreatic duct.** This duct connects to the duodenum at the common bile duct, the same place where the bile duct from the liver and gallbladder joins the duodenum. **Acinar cells** secrete **pancreatic juice**, an alkaline mixture of digestive enzymes, water, and ions. Alkaline pancreatic juice enzymes catabolize different types of nutrients.

Key Terms	Definitions
pancreas (PAN kree us)	gland with endocrine and exocrine functions located next to the duodenum
pancreatic (pan kree AT ick) **duct**	pancreas excretory canal emptying into the duodenum
acinar (AS i nur) **cells**	pancreatic cells that secrete pancreatic juice and enzymes
pancreatic (pan kree AT ick) **juice**	alkaline secretion containing proteolytic, lipolytic, and amylolytic enzymes

Key Term Practice: Pancreas

1. What is the plural form of pancreas? _____

2. The term *acinum* refers to "exocrine cells"; cells within the pancreas that secrete digestive juices are termed _____ cells.

Peritoneal Membranes

The **peritoneum** is a smooth, transparent membrane lining the abdominal cavity. This membrane doubles back over the surfaces of abdominal organs, surrounding them and forming a continuous sac. Extensions of the peritoneum include the mesentery, mesocolon, falciform ligament, lesser omentum, and greater omentum (Fig. 14-8). The membrane supporting the intestines to keep them in place is the **mesentery**, and the **mesocolon** holds the colon to the posterior abdominal wall. A suspensory ligament extending from the liver to the duodenum and diaphragm is termed the **falciform ligament.** (*Falciform* means "sickle shaped.") The **lesser omentum** is a peritoneal fold that extends from the stomach to the liver, and the **greater omentum** is an apron-like structure that extends over the small intestines. (The term *omentum* means "apron.") Both omenta store fat and hold the viscera in place.

Key Terms	Definitions
peritoneum (perr i toh NEE um)	serous membrane that lines the abdominal cavity and surrounds the abdominal organs
mesentery (MEZ en terr ee)	membrane that attaches the small intestines to the posterior abdominal wall
mesocolon (mez oh KOH lun)	membrane connecting the colon with the posterior abdominal wall

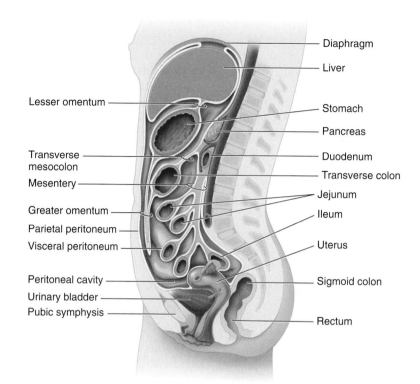

FIGURE 14-8
The peritoneum is a membrane that doubles back over the surfaces of abdominal organs, surrounding them and forming a continuous sac.

falciform ligament (FAL si form LIG uh munt)	mesentery of the liver extending from the diaphragm to the umbilicus
lesser omentum (oh MEN tum)	peritoneal fold extending from the lesser curvature of the stomach to transverse fissure of the liver
greater omentum (oh MEN tum)	peritoneal fold extending from the greater curvature of the stomach, covering intestines, and fusing with the transverse mesocolon

Key Term Practice: Peritoneal Membranes

1. The membrane lining the abdominal cavity is termed the _____.

2. The omenta within the abdominal cavity are the _____ and _____.

Liver and Gallbladder

The **liver** is a vascular, glandular organ that secretes bile, stores and filters blood, and plays a role in many metabolic functions (Fig. 14-9). It is the largest organ in the body, weighing about 1.5 kg (3.3 lb.), and is located in the upper right and central portions of the abdominal cavity, just inferior to the diaphragm. A fibrous capsule encloses this extensively vascular organ. Structurally, it is divided into lobes with smaller subdivisions called lobules. The falciform ligament separates the right and left lobes and attaches the liver to the anterior abdominal wall. The four lobes of the liver are the left, right, caudate, and quadrate lobes. Caudate refers to the tail-like appendage of that lobe, and quadrate indicates the square shape of that lobe. Both the caudate and the quadrate lobes are located on the right side.

Lobules are the functional units of the liver that contain hepatocytes, sinusoids, stellate reticuloendothelial cells, and central veins. Liver cells, or **hepatocytes**, secrete

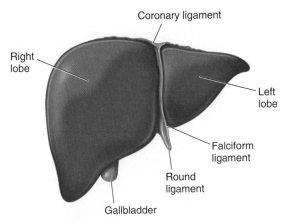

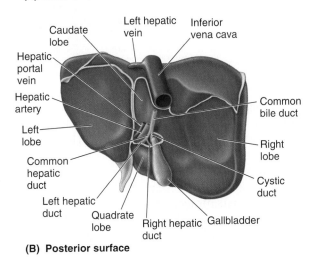

FIGURE 14-9
The liver secretes bile, stores and filters blood, and plays a role in many metabolic functions.

bile that is transported to the gallbladder for storage. Because hepatocytes can regenerate, liver tissue can regrow.

Bile is a yellowish green fluid that emulsifies (disperses and suspends) fats in water-soluble salts to make them more water soluble. Bile is composed of bile salts, bile pigments, cholesterol, and electrolytes. **Electrolytes** are minerals such as sodium, potassium, phosphorus, and calcium that are dissolved in the body's fluids. Bile salts have digestive functions; and the bile pigments bilirubin and biliverdin are the products of red blood cell breakdown. Hepatic cells use cholesterol to produce bile salts, but cholesterol has no special function in bile or the alimentary canal. In addition to emulsification, the bile salts aid in the absorption of fatty acids, cholesterol, and certain vitamins. Bile salts are reabsorbed in the small intestine.

Bile follows a pathway from the bile canal to the small intestine. Bile from the lobules is carried to hepatic ducts by the bile canals. The left hepatic duct drains the left and caudate lobes, and the right hepatic duct drains the right and quadrate liver lobes. The hepatic ducts unite to form the **common hepatic duct.** Bile from the common hepatic duct takes one of two courses: It may flow into the common bile duct, which empties into the duodenum, or it may enter the **cystic duct,** which enters the gallbladder. The cystic duct from the gallbladder and the common hepatic ducts from the liver each carry bile and merge to form the **common bile duct** (CBD). Thus the three ducts common to the liver are the common hepatic duct, cystic duct, and common bile duct (Fig. 14-10).

The **hepatic portal vein** transports blood from the intestinal capillaries to the liver sinusoids. **Sinusoids** are the spaces through which venous blood trickles. Sinusoids within the liver filter blood by removing damaged red blood cells and foreign

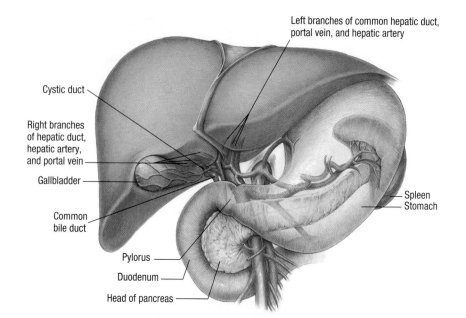

Left branches of common hepatic duct, portal vein, and hepatic artery

Cystic duct

Right branches of hepatic duct, hepatic artery, and portal vein

Gallbladder

Common bile duct

Pylorus

Duodenum

Head of pancreas

Spleen
Stomach

FIGURE 14-10
The three ducts common to the liver are the common hepatic duct, cystic duct, and common bile duct. (Image provided by Anatomical Chart Co.)

substances by phagocytosis. Phagocytic cells lining the sinusoids are termed **Kupffer cells,** or **stellate cells.** Sinusoids ultimately empty into **central veins** that drain into hepatic veins, which drain the liver. Hepatic veins terminate in three large veins that open into the inferior vena cava.

Metabolism refers to the sum of the chemical and physical changes occurring in the body and consists of anabolism and catabolism. Anabolism is the body's ability to convert small molecules into larger ones, and catabolism refers to converting large molecules into smaller particles. The liver functions in carbohydrate metabolism by making glycogen, converting glycogen to glucose, or producing glucose from sources other than sugar. **Glycogenesis** is the conversion of glucose to glycogen, **glycogenolysis** is changing of glycogen to glucose, and **gluconeogenesis** involves converting noncarbohydrates to glucose. Remember that the word part *glyco-* refers to "glucose" (sugar), the word part *-genesis* means "formation of something," and the word *lysis* describes "breaking apart."

Another complementary digestive gland that appears as a small, muscular sac located in a hollow fossa (pit) on the right underside of the liver is the greenish colored **gallbladder.** The word *gall"* means "bile," and this organ concentrates and stores bile until it is needed for digestive processes in the small intestine. The gallbladder releases between 600 and 1000 mL (20 and 33.8 oz.) of bile per day, and 40–70 mL (1.4–2.4 oz.) of bile is stored per day. Bile is ejected into the common bile duct under the influence of the intestinal hormone, cholecystokinin (CCK; or pancreozymin). The word part *chole-* refers to "bile," and this hormone is released after fat ingestion. The fat-soluble vitamins (A, D, E, and K) depend on bile for their absorption. The liver reabsorbs much of the bile secreted.

> **FACT** *If 90% of a healthy liver were to be removed, the remaining portion could regrow an entire organ—if the person survives the trauma!*

Key Terms	Definitions
liver	largest body organ; located beneath the diaphragm and primarily on the right side of the abdominal region; and has a role in metabolism, digestion, and detoxification of body substances
lobules (LOB yoolz)	small lobe or lobe subdivision
hepatocyte (HEP a toh site)	liver cell

bile	alkaline fluid secreted by the liver and passed into the duodenum
electrolytes (ee LECK troh lites)	minerals (ions) dissolved in solution and circulating in body fluids
common hepatic (he PAT ick) **duct**	duct formed by the union of the left hepatic duct and right hepatic duct
cystic duct	duct of the gallbladder
common bile duct	duct formed by the union of the cystic duct and hepatic ducts
hepatic (he PAT ick) **portal vein**	vessel formed at the junction of the superior mesenteric and splenic veins that delivers blood from the digestive system to the liver
sinusoids (SIGH nuh soidz)	spaces within the liver
Kupffer (KUP fur) **cells**	fixed macrophages lining the hepatic sinusoids; stellate cells
stellate (STEL ate) **cells**	fixed macrophages lining the hepatic sinusoids; Kupffer cells
central veins	veins that drain the sinusoids
metabolism (muh TAB oh liz um)	chemical and physical activity consisting of anabolism and catabolism
glycogenesis (glye koh JEN e sis)	glycogen formation
glycogenolysis (glye koh jen OL i sis)	glucose liberation from glycogen
gluconeogenesis (gloo koh nee oh JEN e sis)	glucose formation
gallbladder	musculomembranous organ found on the undersurface of the liver's right lobe that stores and concentrates bile

Key Term Practice: Liver and Gallbladder

1. What is the term described by each of the following definitions?

   a. glucose formation _____

   b. glycogen formation _____

   c. glycogen break down _____

2. Identify the duct formed by the union of the cystic and hepatic ducts. _____

3. The word part *chole-* means _____.

Small Intestine

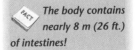

FACT *The body contains nearly 8 m (26 ft.) of intestines!*

The term *small* used to describe the small intestine is deceptive. *Small* is used to indicate the narrow diameter of this portion of the intestine. However, the small intestine is quite lengthy, considerably longer than the large intestine. The **small intestine** is the segment of the GI tract between the stomach and the large intestine.

It is approximately 6.4 m (21 ft.) long and extends from the **pyloric sphincter** (end part of stomach, called the pylorus) to the ileocecal valve (beginning of the large intestine, called the cecum). Most food digestion and nutrient absorption occurs in the small intestine.

The three major parts of the small intestine are the duodenum, jejunum, and ileum (Fig. 14-11). The **duodenum**, which lies behind the parietal peritoneum and is about 30 cm (12 in.) long, is the first portion of the small intestine and leads from the stomach to the jejunum. The duodenal segment receives acidic chyme from the stomach, bile from the gallbladder, and pancreatic juice from the pancreas. The **jejunum**, located between the duodenum and ileum, makes up the next section of the intestine. Approximately 2.4 m (8 ft.) long, this section is where most chemical digestion and nutrient absorption occurs. The **ileum** is the remaining portion between the jejunum and the beginning of the large intestine called the cecum. The ileum is about 3.7 m (12 ft.) long. Note the spelling of this term so you do not to confuse it with the large coxal bone, the il*i*um.

Villi and **microvilli**, hair-like extensions on the intestinal wall, function to increase the absorptive surface area of the lining within its limited space. The villi and microvilli resemble a fine carpet of velvet on the intestinal lumen. These structures absorb monosaccharides, amino acids, fatty acids, glycerol, water, and electrolytes. Other structures known as the **plicae** are circular folds in the intestinal lining, which also increase the absorptive surface area.

Movement of intestinal contents is under nervous control. Major mixing movements are called **segmentation**, and other movements are a result of peristalsis. The growling stomach and intestinal sounds often heard are called **borborygmi** and result from **flatus** (gas in the GI tract) gurgling through fluid.

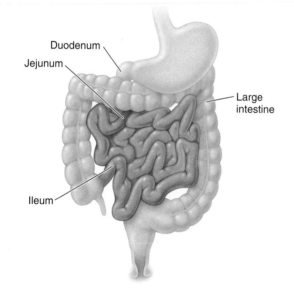

FIGURE 14-11
Most food digestion and nutrient absorption occurs in the small intestine. (Image provided by Anatomical Chart Co.)

Key Terms	Definitions
small intestine (in TES tin)	proximal portion of intestine between stomach and large intestine involved with nutrient absorption
pyloric sphincter (pye LOH rick SFINK tur)	circular muscle enclosing pylorus between the stomach and the small intestine
duodenum (dew oh DEE num)	first part of small intestine beginning at pylorus
jejunum (je JOO num)	part of small intestine between duodenum and ileum

ileum (IL ee um)	last part of small intestine between jejunum and large intestine
villi (VIL eye)	elongated finger-like projections from the intestinal mucosa
microvilli (migh kroh VIL eye)	hair-like projections that increase absorptive surface area of intestines
plicae (PLYE see)	circular folds of small intestine
segmentation	intestinal churning and mixing movements
borborygmi (bor boh RIG migh)	GI sounds caused by flatus
flatus (FLAY tus)	gas or air in the GI tract

Key Term Practice: Small Intestine

1. Provide the singular and plural forms of the medical terms for the segments of the small intestine.

    a. _____

    b. _____

    c. _____

2. Provide the singular and plural forms for the medical term described by each of the following definitions.

    a. hair-like projections in the intestine that increase the absorptive surface area _____

    b. circular folds in the small intestine _____

Large Intestine

The **large intestine**, or large bowel, extends from the **ileocecal valve** (the circular muscle between the ileum and the cecum) to the anus, an opening leading to the outside. It is approximately 1.5 m (5 ft.) long. The last stage of chemical digestion in the large intestine occurs through the actions of bacteria rather than by intestinal enzymes. Its general functions include receiving undigested wastes from the small intestine; secreting mucus; reabsorbing water and electrolytes; absorbing vitamins K, B_{12}, thiamin, and riboflavin synthesized by intestinal bacteria; and storing fecal material before defecation. Most water is reabsorbed in the large intestine, and diarrhea results when excess fluid and electrolytes are not absorbed back into the body through the intestinal wall. This is usually the result of a bacterial infection.

The large intestine is anatomically divided into the cecum, colon, rectum, and anal canal (Fig. 14-12). The **cecum** is the beginning, pouch-like portion of the large intestine to which the small intestine is connected. Attached to the cecum is a worm-like lymphatic structure known as the **vermiform appendix** or appendix. Although its size and shape varies considerably among individuals, it averages 9 cm (3.5 in.) in length. There is no known function for the appendix in humans. The **colon**, with four subdivisions—ascending, transverse, descending, and sigmoid—is commonly referred to as the large intestine.

The **ascending colon** is the region from the cecum to the hepatic flexure, the bend at the liver border that creates a right angle between the transverse colon and the

FACT Partially digested food may remain in the large intestine anywhere from 18 hours to 2 days!

FACT Approximately 2 cm (0.8 in) of bacteria line the large intestine!

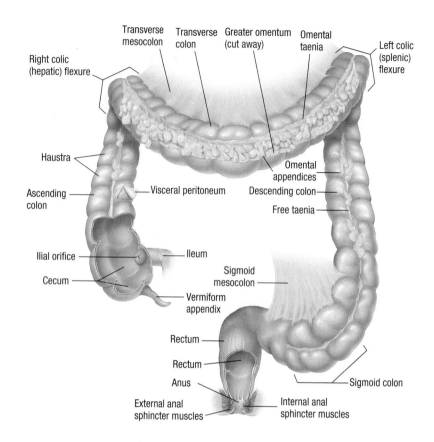

FIGURE 14-12
The large intestine is anatomically divided into the cecum, colon, rectum, and anal canal. (Image provided by Anatomical Chart Co.)

ascending colon. The **transverse colon** is the horizontal section between the hepatic **flexure** (bend) and the splenic flexure, the region closest to the spleen. The transverse colon then turns inferiorly to become the **descending colon**, which ends at the sigmoid colon. The **sigmoid colon** continues to the rectum. It is so named because it is derived from the Greek letter sigma (ς) which looks like a truncated *S*.

The terminal part of the digestive tube between the sigmoid colon and the anus is the **rectum**. The rectum follows the sacral curve. The **anal canal** is the inferior outlet of the digestive tube ending at the **anus**, the opening to the exterior. Anal sphincters control the passage of materials to the outside. The **internal anal sphincter** is a circular band of involuntary smooth muscle in the muscularis, and the **external anal sphincter** is made of voluntary skeletal muscle. The external anal sphincter controls the passage of formed stool.

Defecation is the medical term for the elimination of feces from the large intestine. It is more commonly known as a bowel movement (BM). The composition of **feces**, or body stool, includes undigested food, bacteria, water, and bile pigments. During defecation, internal abdominal pressure increases and forces the feces into the rectum. Peristaltic waves are triggered, and the internal and external anal sphincters relax. Feces are then forced to the outside.

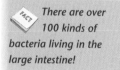

There are over 100 kinds of bacteria living in the large intestine!

Key Terms	Definitions
large intestine (in TES tin)	distal portion of the intestine between the ileum and the anus that forms, stores, and expels waste matter
ileocecal (il ee oh SEE kul) **valve**	sphincter between the ileum and the cecum
cecum (SEE kum)	pouch where the large intestine begins

vermiform (VUR mi form) **appendix**	small structure projecting from the cecum
colon (KOH lun)	large intestine, beginning at the cecum and ending at the sigmoid colon
ascending colon (KOH lun)	section of the large intestine from the cecum to the hepatic flexure
transverse colon (KOH lun)	section of the large intestine between the hepatic flexure and the splenic flexure
flexure (FLECK shur)	bend
descending colon (KOH lun)	section of the large intestine between the splenic flexure and the sigmoid colon
sigmoid colon (SIG moid KOH lun)	section of the large intestine between the descending colon and the rectum
rectum (RECK tum)	section of the large intestine between the sigmoid colon and the anal canal
anal canal	terminal portion of the large intestine between the rectum and the anus
anus (AY nus)	termination of the large intestine
internal anal sphincter (SFINK tur)	ring of involuntary muscle at the anal orifice
external anal sphincter (SFINK tur)	ring of voluntary muscle at the anal opening
defecation (def e KAY shun)	bowel evacuation
feces (FEE seez)	solid body waste material excreted from the bowels

Key Term Practice: Large Intestine

1. What are the four divisions of the colon?

   a. _____

   b. _____

   c. _____

   d. _____

Gastrointestinal Activity

Once food has entered the body, digestion begins. *Gastric* means "pertaining to the stomach," and gastric secretions are regulated by nervous responses. The secretions are enhanced by parasympathetic impulses and the hormone gastrin. The presence of food in the small intestine inhibits gastric secretions. When partially digested food mixed with gastric secretions leaves the stomach and enters the small intestine, it appears thick and pasty and is termed **chyme.** (*Chymos* is the Greek term for "juice.")

Parasympathetic and sympathetic impulses affect this alimentary canal movement. Parasympathetic impulses cause an increase in the activities of the digestive system. Sympathetic impulses have the opposite effect and inhibit various digestive actions by contracting certain sphincter muscles that control movement through the canal. Remember that the parasympathetic division is the "rest and digest" portion, so it is highly active during the digestive process.

As the stomach fills, the muscular wall stretches and the internal pressure remains constant. Chyme is moved by peristalsis to the pyloric region of the stomach. The pyloric region then pumps chyme into the small intestine. The actual rate of emptying depends on fluidity of the chyme and the type of food present. For example, fatty foods take longer to reach the small intestine. The upper part of the small intestine then fills, and **enterogastric reflexes** inhibit peristalsis in the stomach. The enterogastric reflex begins in the small intestine (entero-) and ends in the stomach (-gastro). As a result of this reflex, fewer parasympathetic impulses travel to the stomach, and peristaltic waves are inhibited; thus the intestine is filled less rapidly.

Chemical digestion involves a series of enzymatically controlled catabolic (breaking down) reactions. **Enzymes** are proteins synthesized by the body to promote biochemical reactions by acting as catalysts. **Catalysts** accelerate the rate of chemical reactions without being changed or used up in the process. Enzymes have specific pH levels for optimal functioning and can be activated or inactivated by agents that physically or chemically alter their molecular structures. Enzymes generally end in the suffix -ase and their word parts are useful in identifying the types of food they metabolize. For example, **lipase** (*lip-*, "lipid") breaks down lipids, and **amylase** (*amyl-*, "starch") breaks down starches.

After digestion, absorption occurs. **Absorption** is the passage of digestion end products such as amino acids, fats, and sugars from the alimentary canal into the blood or lymph for distribution to body cells. Absorption of nutrients does not occur in the stomach because the gastric wall is impermeable to most matter.

Emesis (expulsion of stomach contents or vomiting) is the result of a complex nervous reflex triggered by irritation. Sensory impulses travel from the site of gastric stimulation to the vomiting center in the medulla oblongata. The diaphragm moves downward over the stomach and squeezes it on all sides. Motor responses then cause the contents to be dispelled. These involuntary muscle spasms cause the discharge of gastric substances through the mouth. Three types of vomiting are cyclic (recurring attacks), dry (attempts are made to vomit but nothing is expelled), and projectile (ejection of vomit with great force).

> Because men produce more alcohol dehydrogenase (an enzyme that metabolizes ethyl alcohol) than women, pound for pound, women who imbibe alcoholic drinks tend to become intoxicated faster than men!

Key Terms	Definitions
chyme (KIME)	viscid fluid stomach contents, consisting of food mixed with gastric secretions, that enters the duodenum
enterogastric (en tur oh GAS trick) **reflexes**	nervous system actions that inhibit stomach peristalsis
enzyme (EN zyme)	proteinaceous, catalytic substance
catalyst (KAT uh list)	substance that alters the speed of chemical reactions
lipase (LIP ase)	fat-splitting enzyme
amylase (AM il ace)	starch- and glycogen-splitting enzyme
absorption	to take up or assimilate digestive products through the gastrointestinal mucosa
emesis (EM e sis)	vomiting

Key Term Practice: Gastrointestinal Activity

1. Physiological catalysts involved with digestion are termed _____.

2. _____ is the passage of digested products into the blood.

3. What is the medical term that means the ejection of stomach contents through the mouth?_____

Nutrition

Nutrients, the chemical substances in food necessary for normal body functioning, are carbohydrates, proteins, lipids, vitamins, minerals, and water. Carbohydrates, lipids, and proteins provide energy to the body in the form of a **kilocalorie** (kcal), commonly referred to as a calorie: 1 g of carbohydrate equals 4 kcal, 1 g of protein equals 4 kcal, and 1 g of fat equals 9 kcal. The **basal metabolic rate** (BMR) is the average caloric expenditure of a person under basal (basic, fundamental) conditions. Water (H_2O) is considered a nutrient because it is essential for life.

Carbohydrates (CHOs) are organic compounds that contain carbon (C), hydrogen (H), and oxygen (O). **Saccharides** (sugars), starches, and celluloses are all carbohydrates. Carbohydrates can be classified as **monosaccharides** (simple sugars), **disaccharides** (two monosaccharides), and **polysaccharides** (complex sugars) (Table 14-1). Examples of monosaccharides are **glucose** (simple sugar; $C_6H_{12}O_6$), **galactose** (simple sugar that constitutes milk sugar), and **fructose** (fruit sugar). **Lactose** (milk sugar), **maltose** (malt sugar), and **sucrose** (table sugar) are disaccharides. Polysaccharides are **starch** (plant polysaccharide digestible by humans), **glycogen** (animal storage form of glucose), and **cellulose** (plant fiber not digestible by humans).

Proteins are compounds of carbon, hydrogen, oxygen, and nitrogen made into amino acid chains. **Amino acids** contain the compound $-NH_2$ and are the building blocks of proteins. Two types, essential and nonessential, exist. Essential amino acids must be derived from food because the body either does not make them at all or does not make them in sufficient supply to meet its demands. The body manufactures nonessential amino acids; therefore, they are not essential in the diet. Fat and fat-like substances that are insoluble in water but soluble in fat solvents are termed **lipids**. Lipids are composed mostly of triglycerides, the primary storage form of fat in the body.

Vitamins are organic (carbon-containing) compounds naturally occurring in foodstuffs required for normal growth and maintenance. (The word *vitamin* is derived from the Latin word *vitalis*, meaning "life.") Vitamins must be obtained through food because the body does not manufacture them. However, intestinal bacteria do synthesize vitamin K and some B vitamins. Because vitamins are calorie free, they provide no energy source, yet they are essential for metabolic pathways and energy transformation. Vitamins are classified as fat soluble or water soluble. The fat-soluble vitamins are A, D, E, and K; all others are water soluble. Fat-soluble vitamins are absorbed with fats and can be stored in the body; bile salts promote their absorption.

Minerals are inorganic elements that play important roles in physiological systems, such as muscle contraction, nerve impulse transmission, and electrolyte balance. Minerals in the body are identified as bulk or trace, depending on the amount necessary. Common bulk body minerals are calcium, potassium, chlorine, sodium, phosphorus, and magnesium. These elements serve as electrolytes. Trace minerals are chromium, cobalt, copper, iodine, iron, manganese, selenium, sulfur, and zinc.

TABLE 14-1 Common Sugars

Saccharide	Composition
lactose	glucose + galactose
maltose	glucose + glucose
sucrose	glucose + fructose
polysaccharide	long chains of glucose

Key Terms	Definitions
kilocalorie (KIL oh kal oh ree)	unit of energy-producing potential in food
basal metabolic (met uh BOL ick) **rate**	quantity of energy the body expends performing basic physiological tasks
carbohydrate	organic compound containing carbon, hydrogen, and oxygen
saccharide (SACK uh ride)	compound with a sugar base
monosaccharide (mon oh SACK uh ride)	simple carbohydrate
disaccharide (dye SACK uh ride)	carbohydrate made up of two monosaccharides
polysaccharide (pol ee SACK uh ride)	carbohydrate made up of many monosaccharides
glucose (GLOO koce)	a monosaccharide ($C_6H_{12}O_6$)
galactose (guh LACK toce)	a monosaccharide component of lactose
fructose (FROOK toce)	the monosaccharide in fruits and honey
lactose (LACK toce)	the disaccharide in milk
maltose (MAWL toce)	a disaccharide, $C_{12}H_{22}O_{11}$
sucrose (SUE kroce)	a disaccharide found in sugarcane and sugar beets
starch	a plant carbohydrate, $C_6H_{10}O_5$
glycogen (GLYE koh jin)	a polysaccharide formed of glucose and stored in the liver and muscle tissue
cellulose (SEL yoo loce)	a nonstarch plant polysaccharide
protein	a compound made of amino acids
amino (uh MEE noh) **acid**	the building block of proteins
lipid (LIP id)	fat
vitamin	organic substance necessary for normal metabolism
mineral	inorganic substance ingested for normal health and maintenance

Key Term Practice: Nutrition

1. The word part *di-* means _____, and the word part *sacchar-* means _____; so a compound with two simple sugars is called a _____.

2. The building blocks of protein are called _____.

THE CLINICAL DIMENSION

Pathology of the Digestive System

Diagnosing and treating digestive system disorders require a comprehensive, balanced approach. Evaluation tools are numerous and must be used in conjunction with the detailed history and physical examination. This section describes the medical management of common gastrointestinal pathologies.

Oral Cavity Disorders

Missing teeth may result from decay, accident, or congenital disorders. Impacted teeth occur because of the lack of jaw space to accommodate the teeth. This is a common occurrence with third molars (wisdom teeth) when adjacent teeth block their eruption. A dentist diagnoses teeth abnormalities with x-rays. Implants and bridges may be used to replace absent teeth. Treatment of **malocclusion**, or misaligned teeth, involves extraction or orthodontics. **Orthodontics** is the branch of dentistry that uses devices to move the teeth or adjust the underlying bone.

Periodontal disease refers to pathology of the mouth, including the alveolar bone, periodontal membrane, and cementum, and is marked by **gingivitis** (inflammation and degeneration of gingivae). **Dental caries,** commonly called cavities or tooth decay, results when bacteria in plaque destroy tooth tissue. In dentistry, **plaque** refers to an abnormal buildup of saliva, mucus, bacteria, and food residues on the tooth surface that causes tooth or gingival disease. In the process of breaking down sugars, the bacteria form enamel-eroding acids. Periodontal disease and dental caries often have overlapping signs and symptoms. Signs and symptoms of caries include temperature and sweet sensitivity, **halitosis** (offensive breath odor), pain, or an **abscess** (pus-filled sac around root). Radiographic studies confirm the diagnosis. Treatment involves removal of the diseased portion, filling in the space or performing a root canal (removal of the infected pulp, filling the canal with an impervious material, and sealing the canal in the roots to prevent subsequent infection), and sometimes extraction. Good oral hygiene, which includes brushing, flossing, and regular professional cleaning is a preventive measure.

Discolored teeth that are not characteristically white have several underlying causes. With age, teeth become darker, and smoking and food stains can result in tooth discoloration. Tetracycline drugs taken during pregnancy can affect the tooth color of the developing child; and when taken by children, the drug can effect the color of the permanent dentition. Oral examination provides the diagnosis. Treatment options include teeth cleaning with a rotary polisher, bleaches, synthetic veneers, caps, and crowns. Veneers, caps, and crowns create artificial tooth surfaces.

Temporomandibular joint (TMJ) **syndrome** is an inflammation or disease of the mandible and temporal bone articulation characterized by limited jaw movement and pain. Clicking sounds while chewing are common. It can be caused by malocclusion, arthritis, or degenerative joint disease. The oral examination and x-rays diagnose it. The treatment depends on the underlying cause. Options include cortisone injection, grinding the teeth surfaces, or wearing specially created mouth appliances to correct the bite.

A white painful oral ulcer of unknown cause is known as an **aphtha.** Its appearance is correlated with stress or illness. It is diagnosed by oral examination and usually heals spontaneously within 1–2 weeks. Antiseptic or steroid mouthwashes may be used to treat it. The term *aphthae stomatitis* refers specifically to several ulcers occurring on oral mucous membranes.

Herpes simplex virus 1 (HSV-1) causes **cold sores** (fever blisters), small painful blisters on or near the lips or inside the mouth. They often recur at irregular intervals. The virus enters the body through interruptions in the mucous membranes or skin. Tingling and numbness in the area may precede their onset. Visual examination is enough for a clear diagnosis. Topical creams and ice application are treatments.

White spots on the tongue and buccal mucous membrane characterize **thrush,** caused by *Candida albicans.* It occurs most commonly in infants and young children. The organism is part of the normal mouth flora; however, antibiotic use, impaired immunity, or lowered resistance disrupts the natural balance, thereby creating the condition. Oral examination or lesion analysis confirms the diagnosis. It is treated with antifungal medications. Eating yogurt containing active yeast cultures while taking antibiotics is a preventive measure for thwarting thrush onset. (The microbes in yogurt assist in maintaining stability by restoring microbial life that is killed by the antibiotics.)

A noncontagious infection of the oral membranes and gingivae is termed **necrotizing ulcerative gingivitis.** Microorganisms that are normally present in the mouth, which overpopulate as a result of poor hygiene, vitamin B deficiency, or immune disorder, cause the condition. Painful, swollen gums, metallic taste, and halitosis are characteristic signs and symptoms. Contributing factors include stress, cigarette smoking, and infection. It is diagnosed by dental examination. Treatments are antibiotics, hydrogen peroxide mouthwash, and professional teeth cleaning.

Oral leukoplakia is an abnormal thickening and whitening of mucous membranes. It may be a precancerous condition. The tongue and mouth are rough, and the hardened surface is sensitive to heat. It is diagnosed by oral examination. A tissue biopsy is warranted if the condition does not resolve within 2–3 weeks. Treatment involves identifying the source of irritation (such as ill-fitting dentures) and eliminating it.

Key Terms	Definitions
malocclusion (mal oh KLOO zhun)	abnormal positioning of the teeth upon jaw closure
orthodontics (or thoh DON ticks)	dentistry concerned with the prevention and correction of teeth irregularity
periodontal (perr ee oh DON tul) **disease**	term describing pathology of gums, teeth, and underlying bone
gingivitis (jin ji VYE tis)	inflammation of the gums around the roots of the teeth
dental caries (KAIR eez)	progressive tooth decay
plaque (PLACK)	hardened film of saliva, mucus, bacteria, and food on the tooth surface
halitosis (hal i TOH sis)	bad breath
abscess (AB ses)	pus-filled cavity created by bacterial infection and inflammation
temporomandibular (tem puh roh man DIB yoo lur) **joint syndrome**	inflammation of the mandible and temporal bone articulation characterized by limited jaw movement and pain
aphtha (AF thuh)	white oral ulcer of unknown cause
herpes simplex (HUR peez SIM plecks) **virus 1**	virus that causes cold sores
cold sore	small painful blister in the mouth or on the surrounding lips; fever blister
thrush	fungal infection of the mouth characterized by white patches
necrotizing ulcerative gingivitis (NECK roh tize ing UL sur uh tiv jin ji VYE tis)	painful ulcerative condition of the mouth caused by normal mouth microbes
oral leukoplakia (lew koh PLAY kee uh)	thickened white patches inside the mouth

Key Term Practice: Oral Cavity Disorders

1. *Candida albicans* is the causative agent for which oral cavity disorder? _____

2. Which virus causes cold sores? _____

Ulcers

An **ulcer** is a slow-healing sore on the surface of an organ or tissue produced from the shedding of necrotic (dead) tissue (Fig. 14-13). **Peptic ulcers** are tissue interruptions in the mucosa, submucosa, and muscularis in the GI tract area exposed to acidic pepsin gastric juice, such as the esophagus, stomach, and duodenum. The type depends on its location. A **gastric ulcer** is an interruption of the epithelial surface in the stomach with inflammation. A **duodenal ulcer** is a peptic ulcer in the first section of the small intestine. Signs and symptoms of ulcers affecting the GI tract include epigastric pain, heartburn, pain that occurs 2 hours after eating, occult blood, and bloody stools. Heartburn is named for its burning or warm sensation felt beneath the sternum. Its cause is esophageal **regurgitation**, backflow of the stomach contents into the esophagus and possibly the mouth with no ensuing vomiting. An alternate term for heartburn is **pyrosis**, derived from the word part *pyr-*, which means "burning sensation." Associated causes are *Helicobacter pylori* infection, nonsteroidal anti-inflammatory drug (NSAID) use, alcohol and aspirin overuse, smoking, and psychogenic stress.

Diagnosis is made by the history and physical examination, serum gastrin test, barium studies, endoscopy, diagnostic studies indicating the presence of *H. pylori* infection, stool samples, and biopsy to rule out (R/O) or confirm cancer. Normally, the acidity of the stomach creates an inhospitable environment for microbial growth. However, *H.*

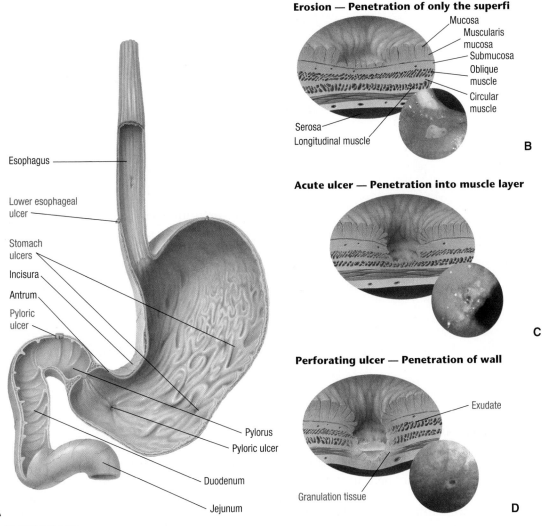

FIGURE 14-13
Common ulcer sites and types. (Image provided by Anatomical Chart Co.)

pylori is an acidophile (acid lover) that thrives well in the low pH of gastric secretions. It is so named because it was originally identified in the pyloric region of the stomach. The **serum gastrin test** evaluates adult gastrin levels in blood serum. Elevated gastrin levels may be a sign of pernicious anemia, gastric ulcers, or pancreatic tumor. Treatment choices consist of diet and lifestyle modifications, increased exercise, antacids, antibiotics, histamine 2 (H_2) receptor–blocking agents, and proton pump inhibitors.

Drugs that prevent, counteract, or neutralize acidity, especially in the stomach are termed **antacids**. **Antibiotics** are synthetic chemical agents, derived from microorganisms, that kill or inhibit bacterial growth. They are used to treat ulcers caused by bacteria, primarily *H. pylori*. Drugs that block gastric secretions are **H_2 receptor antagonists**. Agonists attach to specific receptor molecules as if they were the substances that would normally bind there. **Proton pump inhibitors** are drugs that suppress gastric acid secretion. Inhibitors slow or halt physiological processes by interfering with the exchange of hydrogen ions (H^+) and potassium ions (K^+) in the stomach.

Key Terms	Definitions
ulcer (UL sur)	slow-healing sore on the surface of an organ or tissue resulting from tissue necrosis
peptic ulcer (PEP tick UL sur)	mucous membrane erosion of the upper GI tract caused by excessive secretion of acid
gastric ulcer (GAS trick UL sur)	sore on the stomach membrane lining
duodenal ulcer (dew oh DEE nul UL sur)	sore on the duodenum membrane lining
regurgitation (ree gur ji TAY shun)	bringing undigested food up from the stomach to the esophagus or mouth
pyrosis (pye ROH sis)	uncomfortable burning sensation in the lower chest; heartburn
serum gastrin (SEER um GAS trin) **test**	gastric and intestinal hormone found in blood serum
antacid	substance that neutralizes acid
antibiotic	chemical agent that inhibits bacterial growth
H_2 receptor antagonist (ant AG uh nist)	drug that blocks gastric secretions
proton pump inhibitor	drug that suppresses gastric acid secretions

Key Term Practice: Ulcers

1. A/an _____ is a slow-healing sore on the surface of an organ or tissue.

2. A sore on the membrane lining the stomach is termed a/an _____ ulcer, from the word part _____, which refers to stomach.

Appendicitis

Inflammation of the vermiform appendix is called **appendicitis**. Signs and symptoms of appendicitis are pain in the right lower quadrant, nausea, vomiting, constipation, or diarrhea. The medical term for stomach discomfort with food aversion and a tendency to vomit is **nausea**. Bowel evacuation occurring at long intervals, usually with great difficulty, is **constipation**. Feces are generally hard and dry with constipation. The opposite of constipation is increased frequency of watery stools, termed **diarrhea**.

Diarrhea, constipation, and **fecal incontinence** (involuntary bowel evacuation) may have accompanying excessive gas or air in the GI tract known as **flatulence.**

The cause of appendicitis is poorly understood, but the condition results in an obstructed structure in which bacteria multiply, compromise circulation, and create infection (Fig. 14-14). It most commonly occurs between the ages of 20 and 40.

The history and physical examination, McBurney point tenderness, and rebound pain are used for diagnosis. The **McBurney point** is a 5.08-cm (2-in.) spot located over the appendix base where extreme sensitivity indicates appendicitis. The **Aaron sign** refers to pain when pressure is applied over the McBurney point. **Rebound pain,** also called the **Blumberg sign,** is soreness that is greater at a sensitive site after releasing palpating pressure. It assists in distinguishing between appendicitis pain (great rebound pain) and gas pain. Another test for appendicitis is the **Rovsing sign,** pain in the right lower quadrant when pressure is applied to the left lower quadrant. Appendicitis is treated by appendectomy and broad-spectrum antibiotic therapy.

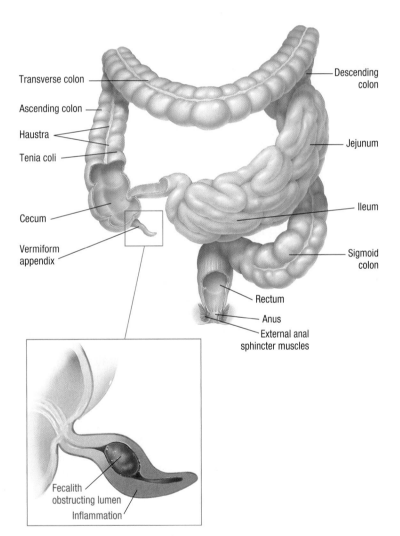

Transverse colon

Ascending colon

Haustra

Tenia coli

Cecum

Vermiform appendix

Descending colon

Jejunum

Ileum

Sigmoid colon

Rectum

Anus

External anal sphincter muscles

Fecalith obstructing lumen

Inflammation

FIGURE 14-14
Inflammation of the vermiform appendix is called appendicitis. (Image provided by Anatomical Chart Co.)

Key Terms	Definitions
appendicitis (a pen di SIGH tis)	inflammation of the appendix with severe pain
nausea (NAW zee uh)	unsettling feeling in the stomach with the urge to vomit
constipation	difficulty eliminating feces

diarrhea (dye uh REE uh)	increased water content in the stools
fecal incontinence (FEE kul in KON ti nence)	inability to control defecation
flatulence (FLAT yoo lens)	excessive gas in the GI tract
McBurney point	site of extreme tenderness indicating appendicitis
Aaron sign	pain in the abdominal region over the McBurney point that is elicited when pressure is applied and indicates appendicitis
rebound pain	after applying pressure to a spot, the pain is greater when the pressure is removed; Blumberg sign
Blumberg sign	after applying pressure to a spot, the pain is greater when the pressure is removed; rebound pain
Rovsing sign	pressure on the left lower quadrant causes pain in the right lower quadrant in acute appendicitis

Key Term Practice: Appendicitis

1. Increased water content in the stools is termed _____.

2. _____ is the term describing inflammation of the appendix.

Gallbladder Disorders

Inflammation of the gallbladder is termed **cholecystitis**. This condition is so called because the prefix *chole-* refers to "gall," a term that means "bile." Adding the suffix *-itis* for "inflammation" creates the term *cholecystitis*. **Cholelithiasis** refers to the formation or presence of calculi (stones) in the gallbladder or bile duct (Fig. 14-15). (The word part *litho-* means "stone or calculus.") Gallstones develop by several processes. For example, if the bile is too concentrated, hepatic cells create too much cholesterol, which comes out of solution and forms crystals, or if the gallbladder is inflamed, gallstones may form. Although the stones are formed from cholesterol, their course of development is not known. The person may be asymptomatic unless there is an obstruction present. Signs and symptoms may include colicky pain, epigastric or right upper quadrant pain radiating to the scapular region, and jaundice.

Colic is acute abdominal pain that increases in severity, reaches a peak, and then slowly subsides. It is usually the result of colonic smooth muscle contractions. Cholelithiasis is often associated with a high calorie/high cholesterol diet and obesity. **Obesity** is an excessive accumulation of fat beyond physical requirements. It is characterized by body weight that is > 20% greater than the recommended weight for a person's height. Cholelithiasis is diagnosed through the history and physical examination, ultrasonography, radioisotope scan, oral cholecystogram, and intravenous cholangiogram.

A **cholecystogram** is a radiograph of the gallbladder taken after the patient has swallowed a contrast medium that shows up in an x-ray image. The **cholangiogram** is an x-ray image of the bile ducts after dye introduction. Cholangiography can be performed using an intravenous or percutaneous method. With intravenous cholangiography, intravenously administered dye is concentrated in the liver and then released into the bile duct, at which point x-rays are taken. The percutaneous method involves guiding a catheter, using ultrasonography, directly into the bile duct. Dye is then injected into the catheter and an x-ray is taken. Elevated bilirubin levels indicate obstruction of the common bile duct. Conservative treatment options include diet

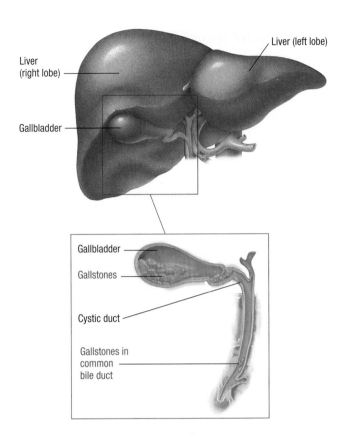

Liver (left lobe)

Liver (right lobe)

Gallbladder

Gallbladder

Gallstones

Cystic duct

Gallstones in common bile duct

FIGURE 14-15
Cholelithiasis of the gallbladder. (Image provided by Anatomical Chart Co.)

therapy to decrease fat intake and exercise to lose weight. Laparoscopic cholecystectomy or extracorporeal shock wave lithotripsy (ESWL) may also be used. The excision of the gallbladder and cystic duct is termed **cholecystectomy**. The surgical procedure can be performed using a **laparoscope** (peritoneoscope), a tube-shaped instrument that is inserted through the abdominal wall for viewing the internal organs. **Extracorporeal shock wave lithotripsy** involves directing high-energy sound waves to the site of the gallstone or other stone concentration to destroy it. The pieces are then small enough to pass normally through the structure.

> FACT Approximately 700 million pounds (318 kg) of peanut butter is consumed in the United States yearly!

Key Terms	Definitions
cholecystitis (koh lee sis TIGH tis)	inflammation of the gallbladder
cholelithiasis (koh lee li THIGH uh sis)	gallstones in the gallbladder or bile ducts
colic (KOL ick)	attack of abdominal pain caused by colonic spasms
obesity	body weight > 20% greater than the recommended weight for sex and height
cholecystogram (kohl ee SIS toh gram)	radiograph of the gallbladder
cholangiogram (kohl AN jee oh gram)	x-ray of the bile ducts after introduction of a contrast dye
cholecystectomy (koh lee sis TECK toh mee)	surgical removal of the gallbladder
laparoscope (LAP uh roh skope)	instrument used to view the inside of the body through a small incision
extracorporeal (ecks truh kor POH ree ul) **shock wave lithotripsy** (lith oh TRIP see)	fragmentation of stones using ultrasound shock waves so that the pulverized pieces can pass naturally

Key Term Practice: Gallbladder Disorders

1. The formation or presence of gallbladder calculi is termed _____.

2. The word part *cholangio-* means _____, and the word part *-gram* refers to a picture; so _____ is an x-ray image of the bile ducts after dye injection.

Pancreas Disorders

Chronic or acute inflammation of the pancreas is known as **pancreatitis.** Signs and symptoms are edema, inflammation, pain radiating to the back, nausea, vomiting, diaphoresis (profuse sweating), tachycardia (rapid heart rate), and tender abdomen. Advanced cases lead to malabsorption and diabetes mellitus. Causes of pancreatitis are varied and include autodigestion from digestive juices secreted, alcoholism, biliary tract disease, infection, trauma, drugs, hyperlipidemia, and gallstones. The history and physical examination, x-rays, sonograms, computerized tomography (CT) scan, hyperglycemia (increased blood glucose), and increased serum amylase and lipase levels within the first 3 days of the attack, confirm the diagnosis. Elevated **serum amylase** occurs with pancreatic disease and pancreatic duct obstruction. Increased **serum lipase** levels result from acute pancreatitis. **Urine amylase** amounts increase 7–10 days after the onset of pancreatic disease. Treatment includes intravenous electrolyte replacement, nothing ingested by mouth, feeding by a nasogastric tube, antibiotics if an infection is present, and pain medications. At times it is necessary to bypass the oral cavity to deliver nutrients, dyes, or medications directly into the stomach. This is accomplished by means of a **nasogastric (NG) tube,** a flexible structure inserted through the nose that ends in the stomach.

A genetic disease starting in infancy that affects various exocrine glands in addition to respiratory structures is **cystic fibrosis** (CF). Secretion of thick mucus that blocks internal passages, absence of pancreatic enzymes, and inadequate absorption of fat-soluble vitamins characterize the disease. Signs and symptoms include frequent respiratory infections, **anorexia** (appetite loss), and failure to gain weight. It is diagnosed by the history and physical examination and a sweat test revealing elevated sodium and chloride levels. Treatment aimed at the digestive malfunction includes vitamin and mineral supplementation, diet therapy, and ingestion of pancreatic enzymes to assist with food metabolism.

Key Terms	Definitions
pancreatitis (pan kree uh TYE tis)	pancreas inflammation
serum amylase (SEER um AM il ace)	test measuring pancreatic enzyme levels of amylase
serum lipase (SEER um LIP ace)	test measuring pancreatic enzyme levels of lipase
urine amylase (YOOR in AM il ace)	test measuring pancreatic enzyme levels of urine amylase
nasogastric (nay zoh GAS trick) **tube**	small hose from the nose to the stomach for feeding purposes
cystic fibrosis (SIS tick figh BROH sis)	hereditary disease associated with dysfunction of the exocrine glands
anorexia (an oh RECK see uh)	loss of appetite

Key Term Practice: Pancreas Disorders

1. The word part _____ means "pancreas" and the word part *-itis* means _____; thus inflammation of the pancreas is termed _____.

2. The medical term for loss of appetite is _____.

Eating, Nutritional, and Metabolic Disorders

Malnutrition results from a lack of healthy foods or an excessive intake of unhealthy foods in the diet leading to physical illness. **Primary malnutrition** is a condition resulting from an inadequate diet. **Secondary malnutrition** results when an individual's pathology makes a normally adequate diet insufficient. For example, a person with cystic fibrosis may eat a balanced, nutrient-rich diet, but many fat-soluble vitamins will not be adequately absorbed as a result of the disease.

Anorexia nervosa is a psychological eating disorder marked by profound food aversion and fear of becoming overweight that leads to emaciation and malnutrition. **Emaciation** describes an extremely lean somatotype caused by starvation that leads to muscle atrophy and depletion of fat reserves. The person denies hunger pains and self-imposes starvation. It occurs more commonly in females who hold a distorted body image, are excessive exercisers, strive for high achievement, and have a compulsive personality. In addition to severe weight and appetite loss, other signs are hypotension (low blood pressure), bradycardia (slow heart rate), and hypothermia (abnormally low body temperature). Serious ill health and death can result without intervention. Treatment includes psychiatric counseling, hospitalization to monitor food intake and electrolytes, and diet therapy.

Bulimia is a condition characterized by bouts of overeating followed by undereating, laxative use, or self-induced vomiting. The individual engages in binge eating to overcome an insatiable appetite but then attempts to purge the body of the recently eaten food. Thus it is commonly called the binge–purge syndrome. Bulimia is associated with depression and anxiety about weight gain and obesity. Common signs are laxative and diuretic abuse, along with tooth decay owing to erosion caused by vomited acidic gastric secretions. Other signs and symptoms mimic those of anorexia nervosa. The person often vomits in secret and denies it when questioned. The cause is unknown. The history and physical examination provide the diagnosis. Treatment for this life-threatening disease requires a multidimensional approach that includes diet therapy and counseling.

Two types of protein-energy malnutrition (PEM) are kwashiorkor and marasmus. **Kwashiorkor** is a type of malnutrition in children characterized by deficiency of calories in general and of protein in particular. A Ghanaian term, *kwashiorkor* means "the evil spirit that infects the first child when the second child is born." It is a common disorder in African children weaned from protein-rich breast milk to a traditional cornmeal diet that is deficient in quality and quantity of protein. Signs and symptoms include edema, ascitic (fluid-filled) abdomen, lethargy, failure to grow, skin and hair changes, fatty liver, and weakness. Sometimes mental retardation results owing to the lack of constituent proteins for neuron development.

Occurring in children, **marasmus** is chronic, severe wasting of body tissues caused by malnutrition. It is referred to as the disease of starvation. Marasmus is characterized by loss of subcutaneous fat, inelastic, wrinkled skin, loss of muscle tissue and strength, failure to grow, lethargy, and hypoproteinemia. It is difficult to distinguish between these two PEM diseases, and recent research suggests that they are stages of the same disease, because marasmus (deficiency of all nutrients) can progress to kwashiorkor. Diagnosis is made by the history and physical examination. Treatment involves nutrition therapy that includes a diet adequate in necessary nutrients.

FACT Americans eat nearly 2 billion pounds (900 million kg) of chocolate annually!

Phenylketonuria (PKU) is an inborn (genetic) error of metabolism characterized by an inability to metabolize the essential amino acid phenylalanine to the nonessential amino acid tyrosine. The genetic mutation causes the body to lack phenylalanine hydroxylase, the enzyme necessary for the conversion. Signs and symptoms include excessive amounts of phenylalanine in the blood and phenylpyruvic acid in the urine, eczema, fair hair, seizures, and neuronal function impairment. If not treated, it can result in mental retardation. It is diagnosed shortly after birth by elevated plasma concentration of phenylalanine after milk or formula ingestion. Treatment involves controlling the amount of phenylalanine in the diet, especially during childhood when the nervous system is developing. Adults with PKU can relax their dietary restrictions; pregnant women, however, must adhere to the strict phenylalanine-restricted diet to protect the fetus. Diet sodas carry a warning label for people with PKU that states the drink contains phenylalanine.

Key Terms	Definitions
primary malnutrition	ill health resulting from an inadequate diet
secondary malnutrition	ill health resulting from a disease process that makes a normally healthy diet inadequate
anorexia nervosa (an oh RECK see uh nur VOH suh)	disorder characterized by not eating because of a morbid fear of weight gain
emaciation (ee may see AY shun)	excessive leanness caused by muscle wasting
bulimia (bew LIM ee uh)	disorder characterized by binge eating and self-induced purging
kwashiorkor (kwah shee OR kor)	malnutrition in children caused by inadequate intake of protein
marasmus (muh RAZ mus)	severe malnutrition in children
phenylketonuria (fen il kee toh NEW ree uh)	hereditary metabolic disorder characterized by a deficiency of phenylalanine hydroxylase

Key Term Practice: Eating, Nutritional, and Metabolic Disorders

1. _____ is the eating disorder marked by self-induced vomiting after eating.

2. Which type of malnutrition results from an inadequate diet? _____

Gastroesophageal Disorders

Gastroesophageal reflux disease (GERD) is characterized by regurgitation from the stomach into the esophagus often resulting in belching with vomitus in the mouth (Fig. 14-16). Coughing and wheezing resulting from oropharynx irritation are common. GERD leads to dysphagia, esophageal ulcers, and esophageal hemorrhage. **Dysphagia**—from the word part *-phagia,* which designates a "condition involving eating or swallowing"—means difficulty swallowing. Be sure not to confuse this term with *dysphasia,* whose word part *-phasia* means "speech disorder or difficulty speaking." Think *g* for *g*astric, as in dysphagia and *s* for *s*peech, as in dysphasia. Tooth enamel erosion occurs from the acidic chyme in the mouth. Causes include overeating and pregnancy, which increase abdominal pressure; hiatal hernia (protrusion of the stomach through the diaphragm hiatus); some medications; coffee; and alcohol.

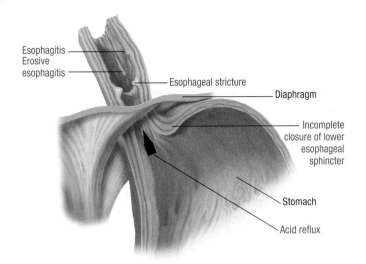

Esophagitis
Erosive esophagitis
Esophageal stricture
Diaphragm
Incomplete closure of lower esophageal sphincter
Stomach
Acid reflux

FIGURE 14-16
Gastroesophageal reflux disease is characterized by regurgitation from the stomach into the esophagus. (Image provided by Anatomical Chart Co.)

The clinical picture and history, barium swallow, endoscopy, or biopsy confirms the diagnosis. Barium is a radiographic contrast medium used for GI studies. Barium sulfate ($BaSO_4$) is a whitish yellowish, odorless powder that is used in medical tests because x-rays cannot penetrate it, so it serves as a contrast medium that is easily viewed. The **barium swallow** examination is a series of x-rays taken after the ingestion of barium sulfate. This test determines pharyngeal and esophageal abnormalities, identifies tumors, and demonstrates the presence of a hiatal hernia. A series of x-rays taken of the stomach and duodenum after swallowing barium sulfate is termed an **upper GI series**.

Esophagogastroduodenoscopy, esophagoscopy, and gastroscopy are performed with a fiber optic instrument called an **endoscope** that allows for visual examination of the organ interior. The endoscope is inserted into the oral cavity and thread through the esophagus for **esophagoscopy**, farther to the stomach for **gastroscopy**, and ending in the duodenum for the **esophagogastroduodenoscopy** (EGD). The endoscope is also used for biopsy, which is tissue removal for diagnostic study.

Mild cases of GERD are treated by elevating the head and chest after eating, ingesting small meals to prevent overstretching the stomach, eating the last meal at least 4 hours before sleeping, losing weight if overweight, limiting alcohol consumption, and eliminating smoking. Severe cases can be treated pharmacologically with H_2-receptor antagonists and proton pump inhibitors.

Dilated, varicose esophageal veins are termed **esophageal varices.** The swollen, twisted veins could rupture. Esophageal varices, common complications with liver cirrhosis (fibrous liver), are caused by the pressure that develops from poor venous return to the liver. Diagnosis is made by physical examination, clinical picture, history of cirrhosis, and endoscopy. Treatment is aimed at controlling bleeding. Ice water lavage and epigastric tamponade are also used. A **lavage** is a washing out or flushing of a body organ. The plugging of the epigastric region with a cylindrical stopper of soft material to halt bleeding or provide hemostasis is termed **epigastric tamponade.**

Key Terms	Definitions
gastroesophageal (gas troh ee sof uh JEE ul) **reflex disease**	disorder of regurgitation into esophagus
dysphagia (dis FAY jee uh)	difficulty swallowing
barium (BAIR ee um) **swallow**	radiographic study of the pharynx and esophagus after ingestion of barium sulfate
upper GI series	x-rays of the GI tract after swallowing barium sulfate

endoscope (EN doh skope)	fiberoptic scope for viewing inside the body
esophagoscopy (ee sof uh GOS kuh pee)	endoscopic examination for viewing the esophagus
gastroscopy (gas TROS kuh pee)	endoscopic examination for viewing the stomach
esophagogastroduodenoscopy (ee sof uh goh gas troh DEW oh den os koh pee)	endoscopic examination for viewing the esophagus, stomach, and duodenum
esophageal varices (ee sof uh JEE ul VAIR i seez)	twisted, swollen veins in the esophagus
lavage (lah VAHJ)	washing out of a hollow organ using a flow of water
epigastric tamponade (ep i GAS trick tam puh NADE)	insertion of a tampon (plug) in the epigastric region to control bleeding

Key Term Practice: Gastroesophageal Disorders

1. GERD is the abbreviation for _____.

2. Dilated varicose veins in the esophagus are termed _____

Hernias

A **hernia** is an abnormal protrusion of an organ through the wall of its cavity. Hernias usually occur in the abdominal cavity. An **abdominal hernia** results when a weak area of muscle allows an abdominal organ to protrude through the abdominal wall; the umbilicus is a common site. An **inguinal hernia** is one in which an organ extends through the inguinal canal into the scrotum (in males) or the labia (in females); this type occurs most often in males (see Fig. 7-9). If the organ can be manipulated back into the abdominal cavity, it is said to be a **reducible hernia.** A **strangulated hernia** results when the intestinal organ is not reducible and the blood flow is interrupted. Fecal obstruction and intestinal gangrene are complications of a strangulated hernia. These types of hernia are characterized by pain radiating from the site. Causes include trauma, excessive abdominal pressure caused by heavy lifting, or increased pressure resulting from pregnancy.

Palpation, radiographic studies, and the Valsalva maneuver are used for diagnosis. The **Valsalva maneuver** is elicited when the patient forcefully exhales while closing the mouth and nose. This movement increases intrathoracic pressure and impedes venous return to the heart, causing a hernia to become more pronounced. Treatment depends on the type. Some may be reducible by manual manipulation, whereas others may require a herniorrhaphy or truss. Surgical repair of a hernia is called **herniorrhaphy.** Hernias may be treated using a **truss,** a mechanical apparatus that applies pressure to a herniated area to prevent recurrence.

Protrusion of the stomach through the esophageal hiatus is termed **hiatal hernia** (Fig. 14-17). It is associated with esophageal regurgitation and GERD. It can have an unknown cause; be a congenital defect; or result from obesity, old age, or trauma. The initial diagnosis is made by x-ray evaluation and confirmed through barium radiographic studies and/or endoscopy. Conservative treatments, such as eating smaller portions and remaining upright after meals to allow gravity to assist in keeping the food down, are applied first. **Cholinergics,** pharmacological agents that mimic acetylcholine may be used to strengthen the sphincter muscles. Surgical repair is used as a last resort.

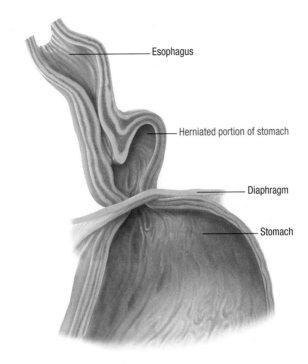

Esophagus

Herniated portion of stomach

Diaphragm

Stomach

FIGURE 14-17
Hiatal hernia. (Image
provided by
Anatomical Chart
Co.)

Key Terms	Definitions
hernia (HUR nee uh)	abnormal protrusion of an organ through a wall or cavity
abdominal hernia (ab DOM i nul HUR nee uh)	abnormal protrusion of an organ through a wall or cavity in the abdominal region
inguinal hernia (ING gwi nul HUR nee uh)	abnormal protrusion of an organ through a wall or cavity in the groin area
reducible hernia (re DEW si bul HUR nee uh)	abnormal protrusion of an organ through a wall or cavity that can be physically manipulated back into normal position
strangulated hernia (HUR nee uh)	abnormal protrusion of the intestine obstructing blood and fecal current
Valsalva (vahl SAHL vuh) **maneuver**	action of exhaling when the mouth and nostrils are closed, forcing air into the middle ears via the eustachian tubes
herniorrhaphy (hur nee OR uh fee)	surgical repair of an opening in the wall of a body or cavity
truss	device that applies pressure to a hernia to stop it from enlarging or protruding
hiatal hernia (high AY tul HUR nee uh)	protrusion of the stomach through the opening in the diaphragm for the esophagus
cholinergics (koh lin UR jicks)	drugs that mimic acetylcholine activity to strengthen the esophageal sphincter

Key Term Practice: Hernias

1. Which type of hernia results from a protrusion of the stomach through the diaphragm? _____

2. The word part *hernio-* refers to a/an _____.

Small Intestine Disorders

Commonly known as "traveler's diarrhea," **gastroenteritis** is inflammation of stomach and intestinal mucosa. The acidity of the stomach generally protects the GI tract from bacterial invasion; however, in some instances the microbes are able to survive and cause infection. Bacteria, toxins produced by bacteria, and parasites cause gastroenteritis. One contracts the illness by ingesting contaminated food or water. Stress is also a culprit. Signs and symptoms are diarrhea, cramps, and mucus and blood in the stool. The history and physical examination, along with a stool sample to identify the causative agent, are used for diagnosis. Treatment depends on the cause, but the condition is usually self-limiting and resolves with simple hydration therapy.

Celiac means "involving the abdomen." **Celiac disease** is a disorder caused by gluten sensitivity or intolerance that hinders the digestive system's ability to metabolize fat. Gluten is a protein in wheat. Alternate names include **gluten enteropathy**, a disease of the intestine, and **celiac sprue**, which is a malabsorption syndrome. Malnutrition, abnormal stools, anemia, edema, skeletal disorders, and peripheral neuropathy characterize this malabsorption syndrome. Signs and symptoms include weight loss, anorexia, diarrhea, flatulence, steatorrhea, and abdominal distension. Greasy, fatty stool is termed **steatorrhea**. Fatty stools float in water owing to their high fat content. It is diagnosed by tests indicating abnormal-appearing villi and a positive response to a gluten-free diet. The disease may have a genetic component and is thought to be an immune reaction to gluten.

Celiac disease is treated by strict adherence to a gluten-free diet and corticosteroid drugs aimed at diminishing the immune response. This disease is associated with the development of abdominal lymphoma.

Short bowel syndrome is a condition characterized by insufficient length of functioning small intestine. The lessened length leads to inadequate nutrient absorption. Its causes include surgical removal of bowel or disease that has altered the length of functioning tissue. Signs and symptoms are steatorrhea, weight loss, and manifestations of malnutrition such as brittle hair and nails. The history and physical examination provide the diagnosis. The underlying cause is treated, and vitamin and mineral supplements are administered.

Key Terms	Definitions
gastroenteritis (gas troh en tur EYE tis)	stomach and intestine inflammation resulting from infection
celiac (SEE lee ack) **disease**	malabsorption disorder caused by gluten sensitivity; celiac sprue, gluten enteropathy
gluten enteropathy (GLOO tin en tur OP uh thee)	malabsorption disorder caused by gluten sensitivity; celiac sprue, celiac disease
celiac sprue (SEE lee ack SPROO)	malabsorption disorder caused by gluten sensitivity; celiac disease, gluten enteropathy
steatorrhea (stee uh toh REE uh)	fatty stools

short bowel syndrome	less than normal small intestine length leading to inadequate nutrient absorption

Key Term Practice: Small Intestine Disorders

1. Inflammation of the stomach and intestines is termed _____, which is derived from the word part _____, meaning "stomach"; the word part _____, meaning "intestines"; and the suffix _____, meaning "inflammation."

2. The medical term for fatty stool is _____.

Large Intestine Disorders

The inability of contents to pass through the intestine is termed **ileus.** Obstruction or muscular inadequacy prohibits peristalsis. Adhesions, calculi, surgical or traumatic injury, infection, or tumors may be the cause of the obstruction. Signs and symptoms include extreme pain and vomiting. Treatment involves removing the source of obstruction or restoring muscle activity.

Inflammatory bowel disease (IBD) is a general term used to describe bowel disorders that cause irritation, swelling, and tenderness. Crohn disease and ulcerative colitis are two types of inflammatory bowel diseases. **Crohn disease**, also known as **regional enteritis**, is a chronic inflammatory disorder of the intestines, usually affecting the terminal ileum but possibly affecting the colon or proximal small intestine (Fig. 14-18). It is characterized by cramps, abdominal pain, diarrhea, fever, anorexia, and weight loss. The cause is unknown; it may have a genetic component, and autoimmunity has been implicated.

Regional enteritis is diagnosed by barium enema radiographic studies revealing diseased strictures (constricted segments) that are separated by normal bowel. Colonoscopy may also have diagnostic value. There is no cure, so the disease is treated symptomatically using anticholinergics and immunosuppressive drugs. **Anticholinergics** block or neutralize the effects of acetylcholine (Ach) activity. Agents that inhibit the immune response are termed **immunosuppressants.**

Similar sounding conditions are diverticulosis and diverticulitis. An outpouching or sac arising from the intestine is termed a **diverticulum.** Presence of diverticula (the plural form of diverticulum) is called **diverticulosis.** The disorder is usually asymptomatic with no inflammation. If signs and symptoms are present, they tend to be occasional pain, flatulence, and constipation. The cause of diverticulosis is inadequate fiber intake that prevents the bowel lumen from fully expanding thereby creating diverticula pouches. It is more common after age 35 years. Treatment consists of increasing fluids and fiber in the diet, decreasing stress, and exercising. Anticholinergic drugs may be prescribed.

Diverticulitis results when fecal matter is trapped in diverticula (Fig. 14-19). (One has to have diverticulosis to be afflicted with diverticulitis.) Signs and symptoms of diverticulitis include severe abdominal pain, fever, and bloody stools. If the wall is perforated, **peritonitis** (inflammation of the peritoneum with abdominal distension) can result. Chronic forms of diverticulitis create adhesions (intestinal fibrous unions), abscesses (localized pus collections), and fistulas (abnormal passages between two hollow structures). The cause is a low fiber diet that is often accompanied by inadequate fluid intake. The clinical picture, sigmoidoscopy, colonoscopy, and barium enema study (if the intestine is not perforated) provide the diagnosis. Treatments are increased fluid and fiber intake and a regimen of exercise. Surgery may be necessary to remove any diseased intestinal portions.

Dilated, tortuous veins in the lower rectal or anal wall are called **hemorrhoids** (piles). Internal (toward the interior) hemorrhoids are located within the rectal wall;

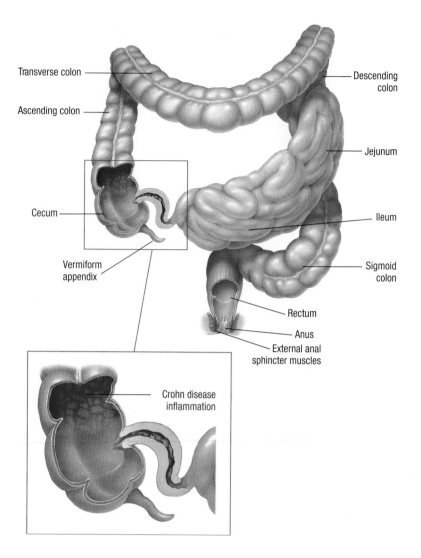

Transverse colon

Descending colon

Ascending colon

Jejunum

Cecum

Ileum

Vermiform appendix

Sigmoid colon

Rectum

Anus

External anal sphincter muscles

Crohn disease inflammation

FIGURE 14-18
Crohn disease is a chronic inflammatory disorder of the intestines. (Image provided by Anatomical Chart Co.)

external (toward the outside) hemorrhoids are found in the anal wall. Pain, pruritus (itching), protrusion through the anus, hematochezia, and bleeding, especially after defecation, are common signs and symptoms. **Hematochezia**, or **hemochezia**, refers to bright red blood discharged from the rectum. The term is used to distinguish this type of blood from the passage of dark bloody stools altered by intestinal juices called **melena.** Causes include constipation, straining while defecating, and pregnancy. Visual examination is generally all that is necessary to confirm the diagnosis.

Treatments include relieving constipation, increasing dietary fiber, anti-inflammatory drugs, and topical anti-itch creams. Ligation, cryosurgery, or hemorrhoidectomy may be necessary. An operation that ties a bleeding vessel with a knotted ligature is called **ligation. Cryosurgery** involves a localized freezing of the bleeding hemorrhoid site, and surgical removal of hemorrhoids is termed **hemorrhoidectomy.**

Key Terms	Definitions
ileus (IL ee us)	peristalsis failure causing intestinal obstruction
inflammatory bowel disease	disorder that causes inflammation of the bowel
Crohn (KROHN) **disease**	chronic lower intestinal tract disease marked by scarring and obstruction; regional enteritis

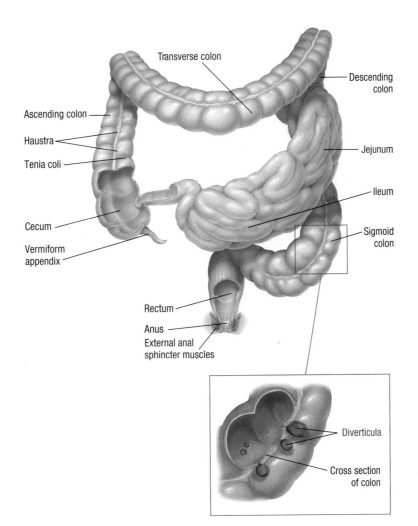

FIGURE 14-19
Diverticulosis is caused by inadequate fiber intake. (Image provided by Anatomical Chart Co.)

regional enteritis (en tur EYE tis)	chronic lower intestinal tract disease marked by scarring and obstruction; Crohn disease
anticholinergic (an tee koh lin UR jicks)	cholinergic- (Ach-) blocking agent
immunosuppressant (im yoo noh suh PRES unt)	drug that hampers the immune response
diverticulum (dye vur TICK yoo lum)	abnormal pouch in the lining of the mucous membrane of the bowel
diverticulosis (dye vur tick yoo LOH sis)	presence of abnormal protrusions (diverticula) in the bowel wall
diverticulitis (dye vur tick yoo LYE tis)	inflammation of the diverticula
peritonitis (perr i toh NIGH tis)	inflammation of the peritoneum, the membrane lining the abdomen
hemorrhoid (HEM uh roidz)	painful varicose vein in the rectum and anal canal
hematochezia (hee muh toh KEE zee uh)	passage of blood in the feces; hemochezia
hemochezia (hee moh KEE zee uh)	passage of blood in the feces; hematochezia
melena (me LEE nuh)	dark-colored stools caused by bowel bleeding
ligation (lye GAY shun)	tying around a structure during surgery with a ligature

cryosurgery (krye oh SUR juh ree)	surgery in which extremely cold temperatures are applied to destroy tissue or stop bleeding
hemorrhoidectomy (hem oh roid ECK tuh mee)	surgical removal of hemorrhoids

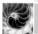

Key Term Practice: Large Intestine Disorders

1. The word part _____ refers to "the peritoneum" and the word part _____ means "inflammation;" so inflammation of the peritoneum is termed _____.

2. What is the surgical procedure in which extremely cold temperatures are used to destroy tissue or stop bleeding? _____

3. What are the singular and plural forms for the medical term describing abnormal pouches of the bowel mucosa?

   singular = _____

   plural = _____

Colon Disorders

Colitis is a general term used to describe inflammation of the colon. Signs and symptoms include diarrhea, abdominal cramps, or constipation. **Pseudomembranous enterocolitis** is a condition of a membranous-appearing bowel mucosa. The primary sign is diarrhea. Its cause is antibiotic use that destroys the normal intestinal flora. It is diagnosed by the history and physical examination and scanning studies if necessary. Treatment options include changing to another antibiotic or eating yogurt containing active cultures while taking antibiotics to maintain the intestinal microflora balance.

   Irritable bowel syndrome (IBS) is a condition characterized by recurrent pain with constipation or diarrhea or alternating attacks of these (Fig. 14-20). If the primary problem is constipation, it is called **spastic colon** or **spastic colitis**. Its cause may be

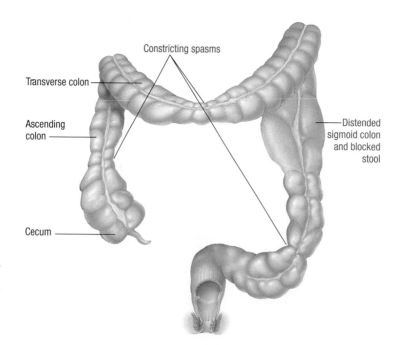

Constricting spasms

Transverse colon

Ascending colon

Cecum

Distended sigmoid colon and blocked stool

FIGURE 14-20
Irritable bowel syndrome is a condition characterized by recurrent pain with constipation or diarrhea or alternating attacks of both. (Image provided by Anatomical Chart Co.)

psychological, with emotions affecting intestinal motility. It is diagnosed by the history and physical examination. Treatment involves ingesting bulking agents or fiber and possibly taking anticholinergic drugs.

Ulcerative colitis is an inflammatory disease of unknown cause affecting the colon's mucosa and submucosa. The **fulminant** form is sudden, severe, intense, and of short duration. Signs and symptoms include abdominal pain, diarrhea, rectal bleeding, and mucoid stool. Its cause is unknown, but it may have a genetic component. The history and physical examination, barium enema studies, colonoscopy, and biopsy are used for diagnosis. Treatment involves eating a well-balanced diet. Anticholinergic drugs and corticosteroids may be prescribed. Surgical removal of a severely diseased portion may be necessary because ulcerative colitis is associated with the development of colon cancer.

Colorectal cancer is the term used to describe several forms of cancer within the colon and/or rectum. Signs and symptoms are anemia, occult blood, diarrhea, constipation, **dyspepsia** (indigestion), and pain or it may be totally asymptomatic. The term **occult** means frank (hidden condition), not obvious, or not readily determined. The **fecal occult blood test** is the analysis of feces to determine the abnormal presence of blood in the stool. The cause is unknown, but there are several predisposing factors, including diets high in red meat, fat, and refined foods and low in fiber. Crohn disease and polyps (growths on the intestinal wall) are also associated with the development of cancer (Fig. 14-21).

After the initial history and physical examination, guaiac test, barium enema, sigmoidoscopy, colonoscopy, CT scan, or magnetic resonance imaging (MRI) studies confirm the diagnosis. The **guaiac test** is used to test for occult blood. With this test, an acetic acid or alcohol solution of guaiac resin (found in some wood) and hydrogen peroxide is mixed with the fecal sample. Blue color formation indicates a positive test for occult blood. The lower GI studies generally evaluate the status of the colon. The infusion of barium sulfate into the rectum and colon for diagnostic x-ray evaluation is termed **barium enema** (BE).

Colonoscopy and sigmoidoscopy are performed with an endoscope that is inserted into the anus and through the rectum for viewing the interior of the large intestine. **Colonoscopy** is visual examination of the entire large intestine to the cecum, while **sigmoidoscopy** examines the interior of the rectum and sigmoid colon. Biopsies can

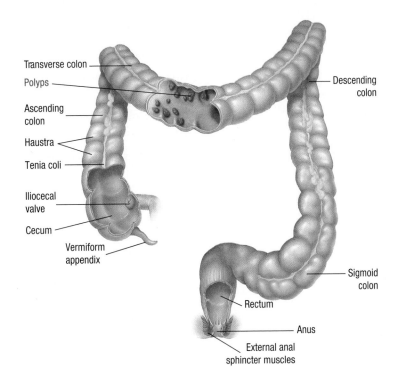

Transverse colon
Polyps
Descending colon
Ascending colon
Haustra
Tenia coli
Iliocecal valve
Cecum
Vermiform appendix
Sigmoid colon
Rectum
Anus
External anal sphincter muscles

FIGURE 14-21
Polyps are associated with the development of cancer. (Image provided by Anatomical Chart Co.)

be obtained through the endoscope. These tests are performed to detect tumors, ulcers, or polyps.

Treatments include surgery, colostomy, chemotherapy, and radiation therapy. A **colostomy** is the surgical formation of an artificial anus in the anterior abdominal wall or loin from the colon; a **cecostomy** is the surgical formation of an artificial anus in the abdominal wall from the cecum; **sigmoidostomy** is an artificial anus made from the sigmoid colon. Colon cancer is shown in Figure 14-22.

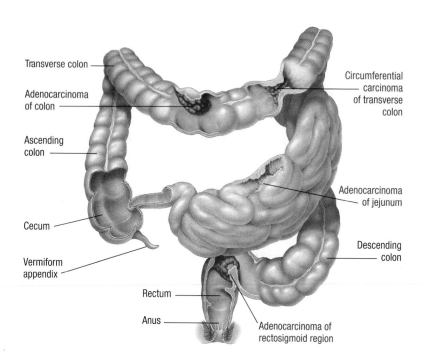

Transverse colon

Adenocarcinoma of colon

Ascending colon

Cecum

Vermiform appendix

Circumferential carcinoma of transverse colon

Adenocarcinoma of jejunum

Descending colon

Rectum

Anus

Adenocarcinoma of rectosigmoid region

FIGURE 14-22
Types of colorectal cancer. (Image provided by Anatomical Chart Co.)

Key Terms	Definitions
colitis (koh LYE tis)	inflammation of the colon
pseudomembranous enterocolitis (sue doh MEM bruh nus en tur oh koh LYE tis)	inflammation in which the bowel mucosa has a membranous appearance
irritable bowel syndrome	disease causing alternating attacks of diarrhea and constipation
spastic colon (SPAS tick KOH lun)	irritable bowel syndrome with constipation; spastic colitis
spastic colitis (SPAS tick koh LYE tis)	irritable bowel syndrome with constipation; spastic colon
ulcerative colitis (UL sur uh tiv koh LYE tis)	inflammation of the colon accompanied by sores on the bowel wall
fulminant (FUL mi nunt)	sudden onset with severe symptoms of short duration
colorectal cancer	umbrella term for various cancers within the colon and/or rectum
dyspepsia (dis PEP see uh)	indigestion, difficulty digesting food

occult	hidden or difficult to detect
fecal (FEE kul) **occult blood test**	determines the presence of hidden blood in the stool
guaiac (GWYE ack) **test**	tool for detecting hidden blood in the feces
barium enema (BAIR ee um EN e muh)	introduction of barium sulfate into the large intestine through the anus for diagnostic purposes
colonoscopy (KOH lun OS kuh pee)	visual examination of the colon
sigmoidoscopy (sig moi DOS koh pee)	visual examination of the sigmoid colon
colostomy (koh LOS tuh mee)	surgical construction of an artificial opening between the colon and the exterior
cecostomy (see KOS toh mee)	surgical construction of an artificial opening made to the exterior from the cecum
sigmoidostomy (sig moi DOS toh mee)	surgical construction of an artificial opening to the exterior from the sigmoid colon

Key Term Practice: Colon Disorders

1. Inflammation of the colon is termed _____, which is derived from the word part _____, meaning "colon," and the suffix _____, meaning "inflammation."

2. A/an _____ describes a visual examination of the colon.

Liver Disorders

Cirrhosis of the liver is chronic, progressive, irreversible diffuse liver fibrosis (widespread fibrous tissue). It is a degenerative disease characterized by the replacement of healthy hepatocytes with scar tissue, creating a nodular condition known as hobnail liver (Fig. 14-23). The resultant scar tissue interferes with normal trickling of

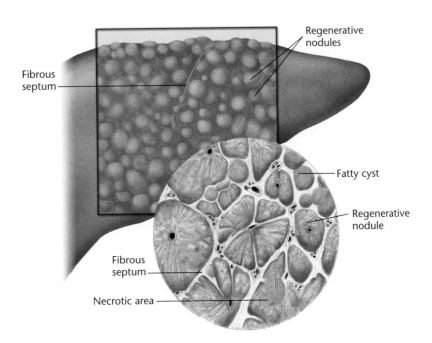

Fibrous septum

Regenerative nodules

Fatty cyst

Regenerative nodule

Fibrous septum

Necrotic area

FIGURE 14-23
Cirrhosis of the liver is chronic, progressive, irreversible diffuse liver fibrosis. (Image provided by Anatomical Chart Co.)

venous blood through the liver for cleansing. The causes range from idiopathic (no known origin) and toxic chemicals to chronic alcoholism, hepatitis, and parasites. Individuals suffering a cirrhotic liver may be symptom free. Signs and symptoms include weight loss, decreased appetite, nausea, vomiting, indigestion, abnormal abdominal distention, and jaundice. It is diagnosed by the history and physical examination, radiographic studies, blood studies demonstrating elevated liver enzymes and bilirubin, liver scan, and biopsy to determine extent of damage. Treatment includes prohibiting alcohol intake, nutrition therapy, and diuretics to reduce fluid volumes are prescribed. Liver transplant is the only cure.

Liver inflammation causing fever, jaundice, abdominal pain, and weakness is termed **hepatitis**. Hepatitis is either viral or nonviral. Nonviral forms result from environmental toxins or drugs that adversely affect the liver causing hepatitis. Viral forms have been categorized according to the six types that have been identified: A, B, C, D, E, and G. Each is abbreviated accordingly: hepatitis A virus (HAV), hepatitis B virus (HBV), hepatitis C virus (HCV), hepatitis D virus (HDV), hepatitis E (HEV), and hepatitis G virus (HGV). Hepatitis A, also known as infectious hepatitis, is transmitted through a fecal–oral route because it results from the ingestion of water, milk, shellfish, or food contaminated with virus-infected feces. Hepatitis B is called serum hepatitis because the virus is transmitted through contact with infected blood, blood products, or bodily fluids. Hepatitis C, formerly referred to as non-A, non-B hepatitis, is transmitted through contaminated blood transfusion before 1990 (when testing began) or by sharing of contaminated needles among intravenous drug users. Hepatitis D occurs in individuals already infected with hepatitis B, and its transmission is the same as hepatitis B. Hepatitis E is also transmitted via the fecal–oral route and is the most common form of hepatitis worldwide, except in the United States. The most recently described hepatitis form is hepatitis G, which occurs in the same populations as hepatitis C. Little is known about this variant strain. Hepatitis is diagnosed through a hepatitis profile that identities hepatitis antibodies.

Hepatitis virus studies are blood tests performed to detect the presence of antibodies to the various hepatitis viruses. Other blood tests indicate elevated alanine transaminase (ALT) and aspartate transaminase (AST), prolonged prothrombin time (PT), and increased total serum bilirubin. **Total serum bilirubin tests** evaluate serum bilirubin levels for adults and newborns. Excessive levels are signs of hepatitis, erythroblastosis fetalis (in newborns), obstruction, hemolysis, cirrhosis, infection, or cancer. The **urine bilirubin test** detects for the abnormal presence of bilirubin in urine. Detectable bilirubin is an indication of bile duct obstruction, hepatitis, liver cirrhosis, or liver cancer.

Common enzyme tests are **aspartate aminotransferase** or **serum glutamic oxaloacetic transaminase** (SGOT), **alanine aminotransferase** or **serum glutamic pyruvic transaminase** (SGPT), **alkaline phosphatase** (ALP) or **isoenzyme ALP$_1$, 5'**-nucleotidase, and **gamma-glutamyl transferase** (GGT) or **gamma-glutamyl transpeptidase** (GGTP). Elevated levels of all these enzymes are observed in liver disease.

The **plasma ammonia test** measures adult levels of blood plasma ammonia, which are elevated in liver disease. **Serum protein tests** measure the levels of albumin and globulin in blood serum; decreased levels of albumin and increased levels of globulin are seen in chronic liver disease. Another blood test, **prothrombin time test**, measures the amount of time it takes blood to clot. Prolonged times occur with liver disease, vitamin K deficiency, and anticlotting medications such as warfarin.

Urinalysis reveals proteinuria (protein in urine) and bilirubinuria (bilirubin in urine). Hepatitis is treated symptomatically with plenty of bed rest. Immunoglobulin may be administered to lessen the severity of the disease. Vaccination with Havrix at least 2 weeks before virus exposure confers immunity to hepatitis A. Boosters are necessary every 6–12 months. The duration of immunity has not been established.

Key Terms	Definitions
cirrhosis (si ROH sis)	chronic, progressive liver disease characterized by the replacement of hepatocytes with scar tissue
hepatitis (hep uh TYE tis)	liver inflammation
hepatitis (hep uh TYE tis) **virus studies**	tests for antibodies to various hepatitis viruses
total serum bilirubin (SEER um bil i ROO bin) **tests**	measures the bile pigment bilirubin in the blood
urine bilirubin (YOOR in bil i ROO bin) **test**	measures the bile pigment bilirubin in the urine
aspartate aminotransferase (as PAHR tate uh mee noh TRANS fur ace)	enzyme test used to assess damage to liver tissue; SGOT test
serum glutamic oxaloacetic transaminase (SEER um gloo TAM ick ock sul oh uh SEE tick trans AM i nace)	enzyme test used to assess damage to liver tissue; AST test
alanine aminotransferase (AL uh neen uh mee noh TRANS fur ace)	enzyme test used to assess damage to liver tissue; SGPT test
serum glutamic pyruvic transaminase (SEER um gloo TAM ick PYE roo vick trans AM i nace)	enzyme test used to assess damage to liver tissue; ALT test
alkaline phosphatase (AL kuh line FOS fuh tace)	enzyme test used to assess damage to liver tissue; isoenzyme ALP_1 test
isoenzyme (eye soh EN zime) ALP_1	enzyme test used to assess damage to liver tissue; alkaline phosphatase test
5′-nucleotidase (new klee oh TIGH dace)	enzyme test used to assess damage to liver tissue
gamma-glutamyl transferase (GAM uh–GLOO tuh mil TRANS fur ace)	enzyme test used to assess damage to liver tissue
gamma-glutamyl transpeptidase (GAM uh–GLOO tuh mil TRANS pep ti dace)	enzyme test used to assess damage to liver tissue
plasma ammonia test	diagnostic tool to evaluate blood plasma levels of ammonia
serum (SEER um) **protein tests**	diagnostic tools to evaluate blood serum levels of albumin and globulin
prothrombin (proh THROM bin) **time test**	measures blood clotting time

Key Term Practice: Liver Disorders

1. List the six forms of hepatitis.

a. _____

b. _____

c. _____

d. _____

e. _____

f. _____

CLINICAL TERMS

Clinical Dimension	Term	Description
DISORDERS		
	abdominal hernia	abnormal protrusion of an organ through a wall or cavity in the abdominal region
	abscess	pus-filled cavity created by bacterial infection and inflammation
	achalasia	a condition that occurs in newborns in which the esophageal sphincter does not open because the smooth muscle fails to relax
	anorexia nervosa	disorder characterized by not eating because of a morbid fear of weight gain
	aphtha	white ulcer of unknown cause
	appendicitis	inflammation of the appendix with severe pain
	bulimia	disorder characterized by binge eating and self-induced purging
	cachexia	condition of extreme weight loss and muscle atrophy resulting from chronic disease
	celiac disease	malabsorption disorder caused by gluten sensitivity; celiac sprue, gluten enteropathy
	celiac sprue	malabsorption disorder caused by gluten sensitivity; celiac disease, gluten enteropathy
	chalasia	relaxation of the lower esophageal sphincter in newborns resulting in projectile vomiting
	cholecystitis	inflammation of the gallbladder
	cholelithiasis	gallstones in the gallbladder or bile ducts
	cirrhosis	chronic, progressive liver disease characterized by the replacement of hepatocytes with scar tissue
	cold sores	small, painful blisters in the mouth or on the surrounding lips; fever blister
	colitis	inflammation of the colon
	colorectal cancer	umbrella term for various cancers within the colon and/or rectum
	Crohn disease	chronic lower intestinal tract disease marked by scarring and obstruction; regional enteritis
	cystic fibrosis (CF)	hereditary disease associated with dysfunction of the exocrine glands
	dental caries	progressive tooth decay
	diverticulitis	inflammation of the diverticula
	diverticulosis	presence of abnormal protrusions (diverticula) in the bowel wall
	diverticulum	abnormal pouch in the lining of the mucous membrane of the bowel

Clinical Dimension	Term	Description
	duodenal ulcer	sore on the duodenum membrane lining
	dysentery	inflammation of the intestines, particularly the colon, accompanied by pain that is caused by chemical irritants, bacteria, protozoa, or parasites
	esophageal varices	twisted, swollen veins in the esophagus
	fecal incontinence	inability to control defecation
	gastric ulcer	sore on the stomach membrane lining
	gastroenteritis	stomach and intestine inflammation resulting from infection
	gastroesophageal reflex disease (GERD)	disorder of regurgitation into the esophagus
	gluten enteropathy	malabsorption disorder caused by gluten sensitivity; celiac disease, celiac sprue
	hemorrhoids	painful varicose veins in the rectum and anal canal
	hepatitis	liver inflammation
	hernia	abnormal protrusion of an organ through a wall or cavity
	hiatal hernia	protrusion of the stomach through the opening in the diaphragm for the esophagus
	hyperbilirubinemia	excessive bilirubin in the blood
	ileus	peristalsis failure causing intestinal obstruction
	inflammatory bowel disease (IBD)	disorder that causes inflammation of the bowel
	inguinal hernia	abnormal protrusion of an organ through a wall or cavity in the groin area
	intussusception	sliding of a segment of a tubular organ into another portion, especially in bowel, creating an obstruction or swelling
	irritable bowel syndrome (IBS)	disorder causing alternating attacks of diarrhea and constipation
	kwashiorkor	malnutrition in children caused by inadequate intake of protein
	malocclusion	abnormal positioning of the teeth upon jaw closure
	marasmus	severe malnutrition in children
	necrotizing ulcerative gingivitis	painful ulcerative condition of the mouth caused by normal mouth microbes
	obesity	body weight > 20% greater than the recommended weight for sex and height
	oral leukoplakia	thickened white patches inside the mouth
	pancreatitis	pancreas inflammation
	peptic ulcers	mucous membrane erosions of the upper GI tract caused by excessive secretion of acid

Clinical Dimension	Term	Description
	periodontal disease	term describing pathology of gums, teeth, and underlying bone
	peritonitis	inflammation of the peritoneum, the membrane lining the abdomen
	phenylketonuria (PKU)	hereditary metabolic disorder characterized by a deficiency of phenylalanine hydroxylase
	plaque	hardened film of saliva, mucus, bacteria, and food on the tooth surface
	primary malnutrition	ill health resulting from an inadequate diet
	pseudomembranous enterocolitis	inflammation in which the bowel mucosa has a membranous appearance
	reducible hernia	abnormal protrusion of an organ through a wall or cavity that can be physically manipulated back into normal position
	regional enteritis	chronic lower intestinal tract disease marked by scarring and obstruction; Crohn disease
	secondary malnutrition	ill health resulting from a disease process that makes a normal healthy diet inadequate
	short bowel syndrome	less than normal small intestine length leading to inadequate nutrient absorption
	spastic colon	irritable bowel syndrome with constipation; spastic colitis
	spastic colitis	irritable bowel syndrome with constipation; spastic colon
	stomatitis	inflammation of the soft tissues of the mouth
	strangulated hernia	abnormal protrusion of the intestine obstructing blood and fecal current
	temporomandibular joint (TMJ) syndrome	inflammation of the mandible and temporal bone articulation characterized by limited jaw movement and pain
	thrush	fungal infection of the mouth characterized by white patches
	ulcer	slow-healing sore on the surface of an organ or tissue resulting from tissue necrosis
	ulcerative colitis	inflammation of the colon accompanied by sores on the bowel wall
	volvulus	abnormal twisting of the intestines
SIGNS AND SYMPTOMS		
	anorexia	loss of appetite
	ascites	accumulation of serous fluid in the peritoneal cavity
	bruxism	unconscious habit of grinding or gritting teeth
	colic	attack of abdominal pain caused by colonic spasms

Clinical Dimension	Term	Description
	constipation	difficulty eliminating feces
	Cullen sign	hemorrhagic patches around the umbilicus that indicate internal bleeding
	diarrhea	increased water content in the stools
	dyspepsia	indigestion, difficulty digesting food
	dysphagia	difficulty swallowing
	emaciation	excessive leanness caused by muscle wasting
	flatulence	excessive gas in the GI tract
	fulminant	sudden onset with severe symptoms of short duration
	gingivitis	inflammation of the gums around the roots of the teeth
	Grey Turner sign	bruise-like discoloration on flank, which indicates pancreatitis
	halitosis	bad breath
	hematochezia	passage of blood in the feces; hemochezia
	hemochezia	passage of blood in the feces; hematochezia
	hypervitaminosis	excessive vitamin intake
	McBurney point	site of extreme tenderness indicating appendicitis
	melena	dark-colored stools caused by bowel bleeding
	nausea	unsettling feeling in the stomach with the urge to vomit
	occult blood	blood in vomit or feces that requires diagnostic screening for detection
	pica	the desire for strange food that is caused by emotional distress, pregnancy, and malnutrition
	pyrosis	uncomfortable burning sensation in the lower chest; heartburn
	regurgitation	bringing undigested food up from the stomach to the esophagus or mouth
	steatorrhea	fatty stools

CLINICAL TESTS AND DIAGNOSTIC PROCEDURES

	Aaron sign	pain in the abdominal region over McBurney point that is elicited when pressure is applied, indicates appendicitis
	abdominocentesis	paracentesis of abdomen
	acid reflux test	measure of pH at the esophageal sphincter after HCl introduction
	alanine aminotransferase (ALT)	enzyme test used to assess damage to liver tissue; SGPT test

Clinical Dimension	Term	Description
	alkaline phosphatase (ALP)	enzyme test used to assess damage to liver tissue; isoenzyme ALP_1 test
	arteriography	radiographic examination of the arteries after injection with a contrast dye
	aspartate aminotransferase (AST)	enzyme test used to assess damage to liver tissue; SGOT test
	barium enema	introduction of barium sulfate into the large intestine through the anus for radiographic diagnostic purposes
	barium swallow	radiographic study of pharynx and esophagus following ingestion of barium sulfate
	basal gastric secretion test	test to monitor the pH level while the patient is fasting
	bitewing dental x-rays	x-ray film with flapped edges used for radiographic examination of the teeth
	Blumberg sign	after applying pressure to a spot, the pain is greater when the pressure is removed; rebound pain
	carcinoembryonic antigen	antigen seen in carcinomas of the digestive system
	cholangiogram	x-ray of the bile ducts after introduction of a contrast dye
	cholecystogram	radiograph of the gallbladder
	colonoscopy	visual examination of the colon
	computerized tomography (CT) scan	ionizing x-rays passed through a patient at specific angles to produce images of internal body organs and structures
	culture and sensitivity (C&S) test	identification and examination of microbes and their responsiveness to specific antibiotics
	endoscopic retrograde cholangiopancreatogram (ERCP)	image of the bile duct system using a duodenoscope
	endoscopy	endoscopic examination of the body interior
	esophagogastroduodenoscopy (EGD)	endoscopic examination for viewing the esophagus, stomach, and duodenum
	esophagoscopy	endoscopic examination for viewing the esophagus
	fecal fat content test	measures the amount of lipid present in the stool
	fecal occult blood test	determines the presence of hidden blood in the stool
	5'-nucleotidase	enzyme test used to assess damage to liver tissue
	gamma-glutamyl transferase (GGT)	enzyme test used to assess damage to liver tissue

Clinical Dimension	Term	Description
	gamma-glutamyl transpeptidase (GGTP)	enzyme test used to assess damage to liver tissue
	gastric acid stimulation test	test to monitor the pH level after stimulating gastric secretion
	gastroscopy	endoscopic examination for viewing stomach
	guaiac test	tool for detecting hidden blood in the feces
	hepatitis virus studies	tests for antibodies to various hepatitis viruses
	isoenzyme ALP_1	enzyme test used to assess damage to liver tissue; alkaline phosphatase test
	lactose tolerance test	hydrogen analysis of the breath and glucose monitoring to detect the inability to digest lactose
	magnetic resonance imaging (MRI)	electromagnetic radiation is used to obtain computer images of soft body tissues
	paracentesis	needle puncture of a fluid-filled space to withdraw fluid
	periapical x-rays	radiographic study of the teeth
	plasma ammonia test	diagnostic tool to evaluate blood plasma levels of ammonia
	prothrombin time test	measures blood clotting time
	ptyalography	x-ray study of the salivary glands; sialography
	radioisotope scan	visualization of radioisotope deposition in the patient
	rebound pain	after applying pressure to a spot, the pain is greater when the pressure is removed; Blumberg sign
	Rovsing sign	pressure on left lower quadrant causes pain in right lower quadrant in acute appendicitis
	serum amylase	test measuring pancreatic enzyme levels of amylase
	serum electrolytes	evaluation of the ions in the blood
	serum gastrin test	gastric and intestinal hormone found in blood serum
	serum glutamic oxaloacetic transaminase (SGOT)	enzyme test used to assess damage to liver tissue; AST test
	serum glutamic pyruvic transaminase (SGPT)	enzyme test used to assess damage to liver tissue; ALT test
	serum lipase	test measuring pancreatic enzyme levels of lipase
	serum protein tests	diagnostic tools to evaluate blood serum levels of albumin and globulin
	sialography	x-ray study of the salivary glands; ptyalography
	sigmoidoscopy	visual examination of the sigmoid colon
	sweat electrolytes	evaluation of ions in the exocrine secretions

Clinical Dimension	Term	Description
	total serum bilirubin tests	measures the bile pigment bilirubin in the serum
	ultrasonography	pulse echo diagnosis in which sound waves are reflected from body organs to produce images
	upper GI series	x-rays of the GI tract after swallowing barium sulfate
	urine amylase	test measuring pancreatic enzyme levels of urine amylase
	urine bilirubin test	measures the bile pigment bilirubin in the urine
	Valsalva maneuver	action of exhaling when the mouth and nostrils are closed, forcing air into middle ear via the eustachian tubes
	x-rays	high-energy electromagnetic radiation used to produce images of internal body structures
TREATMENTS		
	antacids	substances that neutralizes acids
	antibiotics	chemical agents that inhibit bacterial growth
	anticholinergics	cholinergic- (Ach-) blocking agents
	cecostomy	surgical creation of an artificial opening to the exterior from the cecum
	cholecystectomy	surgical removal of the gallbladder
	cholinergics	drugs that mimic acetylcholine activity to strengthen the esophageal sphincter
	colostomy	surgical creation of an artificial opening between the colon and the exterior
	cryosurgery	surgery in which extremely cold temperatures are applied to destroy tissue or stop bleeding
	epigastric tamponade	insertion of a tampon (plug) in the epigastric region during surgery to control bleeding
	extracorporeal shock wave lithotripsy (ESWL)	fragmentation of stones using ultrasound shock waves so that the pulverized pieces can pass naturally
	H_2 receptor antagonists	drugs that block gastric secretions
	hemorrhoidectomy	surgical removal of hemorrhoids
	herniorrhaphy	surgical repair of an opening in the wall of a body or cavity
	immunosuppressant	drug that hampers the immune response
	laparoscope	instrument used to view the inside of the body
	lavage	washing out of a hollow organ using a flow of water
	ligation	tying around a structure during surgery with a ligature

Clinical Dimension	Term	Description
	nasogastric tube	small hose from the nose to the stomach for feeding purposes
	proton pump inhibitors	drugs that suppress gastric acid secretions
	sigmoidostomy	surgical creation of an artificial opening to the exterior from the sigmoid colon
	transplant	placing an organ or tissue from one person into another
	truss	device that applies pressure to a hernia to stop it from enlarging or protruding

A to Z *Lifespan*

The digestive system changes throughout life, beginning with its formation during embryonic development. By the 8th gestational week, the continuous mouth to anus tube is formed. Glandular organs develop as outpouchings of this tube.

Oral cavity changes are evident with age. During the first few years of life, primary teeth appear and are later replaced by permanent teeth, starting around age 7 years. Dentition development is extremely variable, however, and some infants may be born with an erupted tooth whereas some children may not develop their secondary teeth until they are in their teens. Childhood dentition is shown in Figure 14-24.

Common age-associated alterations include the wearing down of enamel and dentin, a decline in the number of taste buds, and decreased saliva production. Tooth loss and poor-fitting dentures are familiar complaints in the elderly and can lead to loss of appetite and subsequent malnutrition. Esophageal, gastric, and intestinal motility also lessen with age. Diminished intrinsic factor and HCl production are commonplace. Nutrient absorption is decreased because of impaired blood flow and motility. Although constipation is associated with old age, this is a myth. Age-related constipation is not caused by an aging GI tract but rather by lifestyle factors such as a low-fiber diet, decreased fluid intake, dehydration, and/or physical immobility.

Hepatocyte regeneration in the liver decreases, resulting in diminished liver size and weight. Liver function remains intact and underlying pathology generally

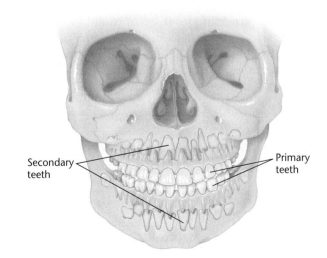

Secondary teeth

Primary teeth

FIGURE 14-24
Dental succession. (Image provided by Anatomical Chart Co.)

A person will process 50 tons of food in the GI system in a lifetime!

causes alterations. Liver blood flow decreases with age, thereby affecting drug metabolism.

Other glandular organs may or may not demonstrate age-associated transformation. Anatomic pancreas changes consist of fatty acid deposits, fibrosis, and atrophy, but dysfunction is abnormal. No observable gallbladder changes accompany aging.

In the News: Obesity in America

Government agencies and scientific health organizations now use data collected by the National Center for Health Statistics (NCHS) and the Centers for Disease Control and Prevention (CDC) from cross-sectional surveys to establish statistically significant information relative to obesity. These continuous surveys have been the standard since 1999; and since 1991, obesity has increased by nearly 60% in American adults.

According to the most recent National Health and Nutrition Examination Survey (NHANES), nearly two-thirds of adults in the United States are overweight; of these two-thirds, 30.5% are obese. Overweight and obesity are known risk factors for several disorders, including diabetes mellitus; cardiovascular disease; gallbladder disease; respiratory disorders; and cancers of the breast, colon, gallbladder, kidney, rectum, and uterus.

Findings from the studies indicate that in the United States, approximately 300,000 deaths annually can be attributed to unhealthy dietary habits, lack of physical activity, and sedentary behavior. Nearly 64.5% of Americans older than 20 years are considered overweight, and nearly one third of them are obese. Despite the known and publicized risks associated with being overweight, the prevalence has steadily increased between both genders and across all ages, ethnic groups, and educational levels. Although there is no accepted definition distinguishing overweight from obesity in the 6- to 19-year-old age group, 15.3% of children aged 6–11 years and 15.5% of adolescents age 12–19 years are overweight.

Another striking discovery is that among individuals with non–insulin dependent diabetes, 67% have a body mass index (BMI) > 27 and 46% have a BMI > 30. The BMI is an indicator of the appropriateness of a person's weight for his or her height and provides a fairly accurate estimate of body fat content. Underweight is a BMI < 18.5, normal is between 18.5 and 25, overweight is between 25 and 30, and obese is 30 or higher.

The figures are nearly as staggering for the prevalence of high blood cholesterol, cancer, and mortality. Diabetes increased by 33% during the 1990s. In 2002, medical spending related to overweight and obesity was estimated to be as much as $92.6 billion, accounting for 9.1% of total U.S. health expenditures.

Americans appear to be quite concerned about their weight problem. In fact, nearly $33 billion is spent annually on weight-loss products and services. However, less than one third (31.8%) of the adult population engages in physical activity, a known factor for reducing obesity and disease risk.

COMMON ABBREVIATIONS

Abbreviation	Term
Ach	acetylcholine
ADA	American Dietetic Association
ALP	alkaline phosphatase
ALT	alanine aminotransferase

Abbreviation	Term
AST	aspartate aminotransferase
$BaSO_4$	barium sulfate
BE	barium enema
BM	bowel movement
BMI	body mass index
BMR	basal metabolic rate
BUN	blood, urea, nitrogen
C	carbon
CCK	cholecystokinin
CBD	common bile duct
CDC	Centers for Disease Control and Prevention
CDR	Commission on Dietetic Registration
CF	cystic fibrosis
CHO	carbohydrate
$C_6H_{12}O_6$	glucose
$C_6H_{10}O_5$	starch
$C_{12}H_{22}O_{11}$	maltose
CRF	chronic renal failure
C&S	culture and sensitivity
CT	computerized tomography
EGD	esophagogastroduodenoscopy
ERCP	endoscopic retrograde cholangiopancreatography
ESRD	end-stage renal disease
ESWL	extracorporeal shock wave lithotripsy
GERD	gastroesophageal reflux disease
GGT	gamma-glutamyl transferase
GGTP	gamma-glutamyl transpeptidase
GI	gastrointestinal
H	hydrogen
H^+	hydrogen ion
H_2	histamine 2
HAV	hepatitis A virus
HBV	hepatitis B virus
HCl	hydrochloric acid
HCV	hepatitis C virus
HDV	hepatitis D virus
HEV	hepatitis E virus
HGV	hepatitis G virus
H_2O	water
HSV-1	herpes simplex virus 1
IBD	inflammatory bowel disease

Abbreviation	Term
IBS	irritable bowel syndrome
K^+	potassium ion
kcal	kilocalorie
LD	licensed dietitian
LES	lower esophageal sphincter
MRI	magnetic resonance imaging
NHANES	National Health and Nutrition Examination Survey
NCHS	National Center for Health Statistics
NG	nasogastric
NSAID	nonsteroidal anti-inflammatory drug
O	oxygen
PEM	protein-energy malnutrition
PKU	phenylketonuria
PT	prothrombin time
RD	registered dietitian
R/O	rule out
SGOT	serum glutamic oxalacetic transaminase
SGPT	serum glutamic pyruvic transaminase
TMJ	temporomandibular joint
UGI	upper gastrointestinal

Case Study

Mr. Tom Lynn is a 67-year-old with diabetes and end-stage renal disease (ESRD) who has just started hemodialysis. ESRD is characterized by scarred, atrophied kidneys with little to no function resulting from chronic renal failure (CRF). Unfortunately, it is a common manifestation of diabetes mellitus. Hemodialysis (pronounced hee moh dye AL i sis) involves cleansing the blood through a semipermeable membrane. *Dialysis* refers to "the separation of substances in fluid." When the kidneys can no longer filter the blood, an artificial means in the form of hemodialysis is necessary to exchange the patient's "dirty" electrolyte-laden blood with clean, electrolyte-balanced blood.

As a newcomer to dialysis, Mr. Lynn must meet with Jane, the RD, to determine his nutrient needs while suffering from CRF. Actual nutrient amounts are highly individualized, and renal diets are challenging. The following table identifies the dietary nutrient parameters for a hemodialysis patient such as Mr. Lynn.

Nutrient	Amount
energy (kcal/kg)	30–35
protein (g/kg)	1.2–1.4
fluid (mL)	500–750 plus daily urine output; 1000 if anuric
sodium (g)	2–3
potassium (g/kg)	3–4
phosphorus (mg/g protein)	12–15
calcium (mg)	1000–1500

Mr. Lynn weighs 236 lb. His medication list includes a specially formulated renal vitamin supplement and a phosphate binder to help maintain serum phosphorus between 4.5 and 6.0 mg/dL.

Case Study Questions

Select the best answer to each of the following questions.

1. **Hemodialysis refers to _____.**
   a. urine cleansing
   b. blood cleansing
   c. blood transfusion
   d. electrolyte equilibrium

2. **Sodium, potassium, phosphorus, and calcium are known collectively as _____.**
   a. organic compounds
   b. minerals
   c. electrolytes
   d. B and C are correct

Calculate the answer for each of the following questions.

3. **To maintain a constant weight of 236 lb., Mr. Lynn's energy requirements are determined by using the guidelines identified for a renal diet. If there are 2.2 kg per pound, what is his weight in kilograms?**

   _____

4. **What are Mr. Lynn's energy requirements in kilocalories per kilogram?**

   _____

REAL WORLD REPORT

After Mr. Lynn had received dialysis for 5 months, Jane discussed the results of the latest report with him. The goals of nutrition therapy are to delay renal failure progression, prevent the toxic buildup of metabolic wastes, maintain the best possible nutrition status, and improve the patient's well-being.

MONTHLY HEMODIALYSIS—NUTRITIONAL STATUS LABORATORY REPORT

Patient Name: Tom Lynn
Age: 67 years
Date: August 30–September 30, 2004
Dry Weight: 95.70 kg
Dialysis Regimen: M, W, F 12:30–17:30

Test(acceptable range)	Patient Results		Low	Normal	High
BUN (8–20 mg/dL)	10			X	
albumin (3.5–5.0 g/kg)	3.9			X	
potassium (3.5–6.0 g/kg)		6.6			X
phosphorus (4.5–6.0 mg/g protein)		7.4			X
calcium (9.5–11.5 mg)	9.5			X	
glucose (80–120 mg/dL)	102			X	
average fluid gain (2–4 lb)		6.4			X

REAL WORLD REPORT QUESTIONS

The following exercises review the medical terms in the preceding medical report. Three terms may not be familiar to you: BUN (blood, urea, nitrogen) is a waste product of protein metabolism. Albumin is a blood protein used in clotting and warding off infection. Average fluid gain is the amount of fluid gained between dialysis treatments.

1. In which categories are Mr. Lynn's laboratory values abnormal? _____

2. On the day of the laboratory studies, what did Mr. Lynn weigh in kilograms?

3. According to the report, what was Mr. Lynn's average fluid gain between visits? _____

4. Potassium, phosphorus, and calcium are classified as _____.

5. Define glucose. _____

REVIEW AND APPLICATION: THREE-LEVEL LEARNING SYSTEM

LEVEL ONE: REVIEWING FACTS AND TERMS USING RECALL

Select the best response to each of the following questions.

1. The conversion of food into usable forms by the body is termed _____.

   a. digestion

   b. deglutition

   c. mastication

   d. defecation

2. The peritoneal fold covering the stomach and intestines is the _____.

   a. mesocolon

   b. greater omentum

   c. peritoneum

   d. lesser omentum

3. The propelling movements by which food and digestive products move through the intestines is termed _____.

   a. segmentation

   b. chyme

   c. propulsion

   d. peristalsis

4. _____ are the units of energy in food.

   a. Basal metabolic rates

   b. Kilocalories

   c. Saccharides

   d. Catalysts

5. Organic compounds containing C, H, and O are called _____.

   a. vitamins

   b. minerals

   c. amino acids

   d. carbohydrates

6. Inorganic elements ingested for health and physiologic functions are _____.

   a. fats

   b. fatty acids

   c. minerals

   d. vitamins

7. _____ is the storage form of glucose in muscle tissue.

   a. Sucrose

   b. Glycerol

   c. Glycogen

   d. Protein

8. A _____ is a rounded food mass formed in the mouth.

   a. bolus

   b. pulp

   c. chyme

   d. dentin

9. Salivary glands located beneath the tongue are the _____.

   a. parotid glands

   b. submandibular glands

   c. sublingual glands

   d. masseter glands

10. The calcified substance covering a tooth crown is _____.

    a. cementum

    b. pulp

    c. dentin

    d. enamel

11. The three primary parts of a tooth are _____.

    a. crown, alveolar bone, and pulp

    b. root, neck, and crown

c. root canal, periodontal ligament, and gingivae

d. pulp cavity, cementum, and enamel

12. Excessive leanness owing to muscle wasting is termed _____.

    a. emaciation

    b. bulimia

    c. anorexia

    d. marasmus

13. _____ is the medical term for peristalsis failure that causes intestinal obstruction.

    a. Colitis

    b. Phenylketonuria

    c. Ileus

    d. Hernia

14. Folds in the stomach are termed _____.

    a. plicae

    b. rugae

    c. sphincters

    d. villi

15. The enzyme that breaks down fat is _____.

    a. lipase

    b. salivary amylase

    c. alcohol dehydrogenase

    d. nuclease

16. The _____ cells are pancreatic cells that secrete pancreatic juice and enzymes.

    a. alpha

    b. acinar

    c. beta

    d. delta

17. The duct formed by the union of the left hepatic duct and the right hepatic duct is the _____ duct.

    a. cystic

    b. common hepatic

c. common bile

d. central

18. The _____ duct exits the gallbladder.

    a. common hepatic

    b. common bile

    c. cystic

    d. pancreatic

19. Kupffer cells are also called _____.

    a. stellate cells

    b. sinusoids

    c. hepatocytes

    d. lobules

20. Inflammation of the gallbladder is known as _____.

    a. cholelithiasis

    b. chylomicrons

    c. cholecystokinin

    d. cholecystitis

21. Microscopic, hair-like intestinal structures that increase the absorptive surface area are termed _____.

    a. lacteals

    b. brush border

    c. microvilli

    d. micelles

22. _____ is the medical term for belching.

    a. Eructation

    b. Bruxism

    c. Flatus

    d. Borborygmi

23. Gas or air in the gastrointestinal tract is called _____.

    a. borborygmi

    b. lactate

    c. enterocrinin

    d. flatus

24. The section of the large intestine beginning at the cecum is the _____.

   a. anus

   b. colon

   c. rectum

   d. anal canal

25. The hardened film on a tooth surface is called _____.

   a. gingiva

   b. plaque

   c. periodontal disease

   d. oral leukoplakia

26. The _____ is the large intestine section between the sigmoid colon and the anal canal.

   a. rectum

   b. anus

   c. transverse colon

   d. ascending colon

LEVEL TWO: REVIEWING CONCEPTS

Select the best response to each of the following questions.

27. Identify the correct order of structures through which food travels in the GI tract.

   a. pharynx → esophagus → small intestine → stomach → large intestine

   b. esophagus → pharynx → small intestine → stomach → large intestine

   c. pharynx → esophagus → stomach → small intestine → large intestine

   d. esophagus → pharynx → stomach → small intestine → large intestine

28. Identify the correct tissue layers of the alimentary canal from superficial to deep.

   a. serosa → muscularis → submucosa → mucosa

   b. mucosa → submucosa → muscularis → serosa

   c. muscularis → serosa → mucosa → submucosa

   d. submucosa → mucosa → serosa → muscularis

29. Which cells secrete HCl and intrinsic factor?

   a. G cells

   b. mucous cells

   c. chief cells

   d. parietal cells

30. Which cells secrete pepsinogen?

   a. chief cells

   b. zymogenic cells

   c. pepsin cells

   d. A and B are correct

31. Gastric cells are found in the _____.

   a. stomach

   b. colon

   c. intestine

   d. mouth

Provide a medical term to complete a meaningful analogy.

32. Teeth are to dentes as canines are to _____.

33. Primary teeth are to _____ teeth as secondary teeth are to permanent teeth.

Select the best answer to each of the following questions.

34. Hematochezia refers to _____.

   a. bright red blood discharged from the rectum

   b. bloody stools

   c. a bloody colon

   d. hemorrhoids

35. Which term does not belong?

   a. dyspepsia

   b. colic

   c. flatulence

   d. truss

Match the sign or symptom with its correct definition.

_____ 36. anorexia

a. attack of abdominal pain caused by colonic spasms

_____ 37. halitosis

b. loss of appetite

_____ 38. colic

c. bad breath

_____ 39. melena

d. difficulty swallowing

_____ 40. dysphagia

e. black-colored stools

Match the sign or symptom with its correct definition.

_____ 41. gingivitis

a. extremely thin resulting from starvation

_____ 42. peritonitis

b. fatty stools

_____ 43. steatorrhea

c. inflammation of abdominal membrane

_____ 44. regurgitation

d. inflammation of the gums

_____ 45. emaciation

e. bringing up undigested food from the stomach and esophagus to the mouth

Match the diagnostic procedure with its description.

_____ 46. barium enema

a. endoscopic examination of the esophagus

_____ 47. barium swallow

b. introduction of barium sulfate into the large intestine through the anus for diagnostic purposes

_____ 48. cholecysto-gram

c. x-ray study of pharynx and esophagus after ingesting barium sulfate

_____ 49. cholangio-gram

d. x-ray of the gallbladder

_____ 50. esophago-scopy

e. radiograph of the bile ducts after dye introduction

Match the laboratory test with its description.

_____ 51. hepatitis virus studies

a. stool test for hidden blood

_____ 52. serum lipase

b. enzyme test used to assess liver damage

_____ 53. fecal occult blood test

c. test for detecting hidden blood in feces

_____ 54. guaiac test

d. test for antibodies to hepatitis virus

_____ 55. alanine amino-transferase (AST) test

e. test measuring pancreatic enzyme levels

Match the pathology with its key characteristics or description.

_____ 56. anorexia nervosa

a. inflammation of the pancreas

_____ 57. pancreatitis

b. lack of eating for fear of gaining weight

_____ 58. phenylke-tonuria

c. ill health resulting from an inadequate diet

_____ 59. primary malnutrition

d. severe malnutrition in children

_____ 60. marasmus

e. hereditary metabolic disorder with phenylalanine deficiency

Match the pathology with its key characteristics or description.

_____ 61. strangulated hernia

a. intestinal disease of gluten intolerance

_____ 62. diverticulitis

b. presence of diverticula

_____ 63. diverticulosis

c. inflammation of diverticula

_____ 64. celiac disease

d. alternating attacks of constipation and diarrhea

_____ 65. irritable bowel syndrome

e. protrusion of intestine interfering with blood flow and fecal passage

Match the pathology with its key characteristics or description.

_____ 66. cirrhosis

a. tooth decay or cavities

_____ 67. dental caries

b. pus-filled cavity

_____ 68. aphtha

c. chronic, scarred liver disease

_____ 69. peptic ulcer

d. white oral ulcer of unknown cause

_____ 70. abscess

e. sore on the upper GI tract membrane

Match the treatment with its description.

_____ 71. proton pump inhibitors

a. pressure-applying device to support hernias

_____ 72. lavage

b. insertion of a plug in the upper chest region to stop bleeding

_____ 73. truss

c. artificial opening from the colon to the exterior

_____ 74. colostomy

d. gastric secretion-suppressing drugs

_____ 75. epigastric tamponade

e. washing out of an organ

What is the term described by each of the following definitions?

76. swallowing _____

77. chewing _____

78. gums _____

79. belching, burping _____

Define the following abbreviations.

80. CHO _____

81. BMR _____

82. IBS _____

83. HAV _____

84. IBD _____

Unscramble the letters to form a medical term.

85. robmigyrob _____

86. nicehrolgic _____

87. tagiilno _____

88. sitthepia _____

89. stiloic _____

90. aheinr _____

Identify the correctly spelled term in each set.

_____ 91.   a. kwashiorkor   b. kwasiorkor
            c. kwashiorcor   d. kwasshiorkor

_____ 92.   a. esophagoscopy b. esofagoscopy
            c. esophigoscopy d. esophogoscopy

_____ 93.   a. Vallsalva maneuver
            b. Valsalva maneuver
            c. Valselve maneuver
            d. Velsalva maneuver

_____ 94.   a. accult   b. ocult
            c. occalt   d. occult

_____ 95.   a. nasea   b. nausa
            c. nauza   d. nausea

_____ 96.   a. flatulance   b. flatalence
            c. flatulence   d. flatullence

_____ 97.   a. dafecation   b. defecation
            c. defecetion   d. deffecation

_____ 98.   a. diarhea   b. diarea
            c. diarrhea   d. diarrhhea

Define the following terms.

99. hepatomegaly _____

100. appendectomy _____

101. antiemetic _____

102. emetic _____

103. gingivectomy _____

Using the following word parts, form a medical term for each definition. Each word part is used only once.

cec-	enter-	-itis
chol-	gastro-	-ology
-ectomy	gastro-	-pathy
-emia	hepat-	

104. stomach disease _____

105. inflammation of the cecum _____

106. surgical removal of the liver _____

107. presence of bile in the blood _____

108. study of the stomach and intestines

_____

LEVEL THREE: THINKING CRITICALLY

Provide a short answer to each of the following questions.

109. A patient has been losing weight and experiencing bouts of vomiting. A barium swallow test showed the presence of the barium swallow still in the stomach 12 hours after ingestion. Provide an explanation for this occurrence.

_____

_____

_____

110. A patient has been diagnosed with lactose intolerance. Her physician explains that she may still enjoy milk products if she ingests commercially prepared lactase drops whenever she eats foods containing lactose. Why would lactase drops alleviate her symptoms?

_____

_____

_____

KEY TERMS SPELLING TEST FROM CD-ROM

Use the CD-ROM to test yourself on the spelling of key terms from this chapter. Listen to the terms and write them on a separate sheet of paper. Use a medical dictionary to check your answers.

ANSWERS

WORD GROUPING

Definition	Word Part
an appendix	appendico-
abdomen, belly	celi-, celio-
alveolus (tooth socket), alveolar	alveoli-, alveolo-
anus and rectum	proct-, procto-
bile	A. bili-
	B. chol-, chole-, cholo-
bile duct, biliary passage	cholangi-, cholangio-
blind (closed), cecum	cec-, ceco-
cheek	bucco-
chemical compound containing -NH$_2$	amino-
chyle (milky fluid taken up by intestines)	chyl-, chyli-, chylo-
colon	col-, coli-, colo-
duodenum, duodenal	duoden-, duodeno-
eating or swallowing	-phagia
esophagus, esophageal	esoph-, esopho-
enzyme	-ase
glucose, sugar	gluco-, glyc-, glyco-
head	cephal-, cephalo-
heat	calori-
hernia	hernio-
ileum, ileal	ile-, ileo-
intestine	enter-, entero-
lip	cheil-, cheilo-
lipid, fat	lip-, lipo-
liver	hepat-, hepato-
milk	galact-, galacto-
mouth	stomat-, stomato-
mouth, oral	oro-
muscular opening, pylorus	pylor-, pyloro-
omentum (apron), epiploon (omentum)	epiplo-
palate	palato-
pancreas, pancreatic	pancre-, pancreo-
peritoneum	peritoneo-
pertaining to the jejunum	jejun-, jejuno-
pharynx, pharyngeal	pharyng-, pharyngo-
rectum, rectal	rect-, recto-
saliva, salivary	sial-, sialo-
sigmoid, S-shaped	sigmoid-, sigmoido-
starch	amyl-, amylo-
stomach, gastric	gastr-, gastro-
stone, calculus	lith-, litho-
sugar	sacchar-, sacchari-, saccharo-
tongue	A. gloss-, -glossa, glosso-
	B. lingu-, lingua-, lingui-, linguo-
tooth, dental	dent-, denti-, dento-
uvula	uvul-, uvulo-
vomiting, emesis	emet-, emeto-
worm, worm-like	vermi-

WORD BUILDING

Word Part	Meaning	Common or Known Word	Example Medical Term
amino-	chemical compound containing -NH$_2$	amino acid	amino acid
-ase	enzyme	lactase	maltase
bucco-	cheek	buccinator	buccal phase
calori-	heat	calorie	kilocalorie
cephal-, cephalo-	head	cephalic	cephalic phase
chol-, chole-, cholo-	bile	cholesterol	cholecystokinin
col-, coli-, colo-	colon	colon	colon
dent-, denti-, dento-	tooth, dental	dentist	dentition
duoden-, duodeno-	duodenum, duodenal	duodenum	duodenum
galact-, galacto-	milk	galactose	galactose
gastr-, gastro-	stomach, gastric	gastritis	gastric juice
gluco-, glyc-, glyco-	glucose, sugar	glucose	gluconeogenesis
hepat-, hepato-	liver	hepatitis	hepatocytes
hernio-	hernia	herniated	herniorrhaphy
lip-, lipo-	lipid, fat	liposuction	lipase
pancre-, pancreo-	pancreas, pancreatic	pancreas	pancreas
pharyng-, pharyngo-	pharynx, pharyngeal	pharyngitis	pharyngeal phase
proct-, procto-	anus and rectum	proctologist	proctologist
sacchar-, sacchari-, saccharo-	sugar	saccharine	monosaccharide

KEY TERM PRACTICE

Digestive System Preview

1. chemical; mechanical
2. alimentary canal

Oral Cavity

1. papilla; papillae
2. uvula; uvuli
3. below; tongue; sublingual

Teeth

1. a. incisors;
   b. cuspids (canines);
   c. bicuspids (premolars);
   d. molars
2. cementa

Esophagus

1. esophagus; esophagi
2. esophageal hiatus

Stomach

1. The four regions are cardia, fundus, body, and pylorus.
2. Intrinsic factor

Pancreas

1. pancreata
2. acinar

Peritoneal Membranes

1. peritoneum
2. lesser; greater

Liver and Gallbladder

1. a. gluconeogenesis;
   b. glycogenesis;
   c. glycogenolysis
2. common bile duct (CBD)
3. bile or gall

Small Intestine

1. a. duodenum, duodena;
   b. jejunum, jejuna;
   c. ileum, ilea
2. a. microvillus, microvilli;
   b. plica, plicae

Large Intestine

1. a. ascending colon
   b. transverse colon
   c. descending colon
   d. sigmoid colon

Gastrointestinal Activity

1. enzymes
2. Absorption
3. emesis

Nutrition

1. two; sugar; disaccharide
2. amino acids

Oral Cavity Disorders

1. thrush
2. herpes simplex virus 1 (HSV1)

Ulcers

1. ulcer
2. gastric; gastr-

Appendicitis

1. diarrhea
2. Appendicitis

Gallbladder Disorders

1. cholelithiasis
2. bile duct or biliary passage; cholangiogram

Pancreas Disorders

1. pancre-; inflammation; pancreatitis
2. anorexia

Eating, Nutritional, and Metabolic Disorders

1. Bulimia
2. primary malnutrition

Gastroesophageal Disorders

1. gastroesophageal reflux disease
2. esophageal varices

Hernias

1. hiatal hernia
2. hernia

Small Intestine Diseases

1. gastroenteritis; gastro-; enter-; -itis
2. steatorrhea

Large Intestine Disorders

1. peritoneo-; -itis; peritonitis
2. cryosurgery
3. diverticulum, diverticula

Colon Disorders

1. colitis; col-; -itis
2. colonoscopy

Liver Disorders

1. a. hepatitis A
   b. hepatitis B
   c. hepatitis C
   d. hepatitis D
   e. hepatitis E
   f. hepatitis G

CASE STUDY

1. b is the correct answer.
   - a is incorrect because *hemo-* refers to "blood" and *dialysis* refers to the "separation of substances in a fluid."
   - c is incorrect because no blood is being transfused, which involves the administration of blood from one person into the bloodstream of another person; Mr. Lynn's own blood is being removed, cleansed, and returned to him.
   - d is incorrect because although electrolyte balance is achieved through hemodialysis, the equilibrium is short-lived; Mr. Lynn would have to be on continuous dialysis to maintain that balance.

2. d is the correct answer.
   - a is incorrect because organic compounds contain carbon; sodium, potassium, phosphorus, and calcium are inorganic elements.
3. Mr. Lynn weighs 107.27 kg, which is calculated by dividing 236 lb. by 2.2 kg: $236 \div 2.2 = 107.27$.
4. Mr. Lynn's energy requirements are between 3218.10 and 3754.45 kcal. The energy parameters for Mr. Lynn are 30–35 kcal/kg, and his weight is 107.27 kg: $107.27 \times 30 = 3218.10$ for the lower limit and $107.27 \times 35 = 3754.45$ for the upper limit.

REAL WORLD REPORT

1. potassium, phosphorus, and average fluid gain—all are too high
2. 95.70 kg
3. 6.4 lb. (2.9 kg)
4. minerals or electrolytes
5. a simple carbohydrate with the chemical formula $C_6H_{12}O_6$; the body's primary fuel source

REVIEW AND APPLICATION: THREE-LEVEL LEARNING SYSTEM

Level One: Reviewing Facts and Terms Using Recall

1. a
2. b
3. d
4. b
5. d
6. c
7. c
8. a
9. c
10. d
11. b
12. a
13. c
14. b
15. a
16. b
17. b
18. c
19. a
20. d
21. c
22. a
23. d
24. b
25. b
26. a

Level Two: Reviewing Concepts

27. c
28. a
29. d
30. d
31. a
32. cuspids
33. deciduous
34. a
35. d
36. b
37. c
38. a
39. e
40. d
41. d
42. c
43. b
44. e
45. a
46. b
47. c
48. d
49. e
50. a
51. d
52. e
53. a
54. c
55. b
56. b
57. a
58. e
59. c
60. d
61. e
62. c
63. b
64. a
65. d
66. c
67. a
68. d
69. e
70. b
71. d
72. e
73. a
74. c
75. b
76. deglutition
77. mastication
78. gingivae
79. eructation
80. carbohydrate
81. basal metabolic rate
82. irritable bowel syndrome
83. hepatitis A virus
84. inflammatory bowel disease
85. borborygmi
86. cholinergic
87. ligation
88. hepatitis
89. colitis
90. hernia
91. a
92. a
93. b
94. d
95. d
96. c
97. b
98. c
99. enlargement of liver
100. removal of appendix
101. agent that prevents or relieves vomiting
102. agent that induces vomiting
103. excision of gum tissue
104. gastropathy
105. cecitis
106. hepatectomy
107. cholemia
108. gastroenterology

Level Three: Thinking Critically

109. The barium sulfate is not able to exit the stomach because of an obstruction, most likely at the pyloric sphincter. Thus, the stomach contents remain in the stomach. This would explain the vomiting; and because no nutrients are absorbed across the gastric mucosa, this provides an explanation for the weight loss as well.

110. The lactase drops supply the missing enzyme, lactase, which is necessary for the digestion of milk sugar. Hence, the patient may still eat milk products as long as she takes the required enzyme.

chapter 15

Urinary System

OBJECTIVES

After completing this chapter, you should be able to:

1. Identify the organs of the urinary system.
2. Cite the primary functions of each organ in the system.
3. Trace the pathway of urine through the system.
4. Define common signs, symptoms, and treatments of various urinary system diseases.
5. Explain clinical tests and diagnostic procedures related to the urinary system.
6. Describe anatomical and physiological alterations throughout the lifespan.
7. Define abbreviations related to the urinary system.
8. Define prefixes, suffixes, and roots of terms used for the urinary system.
9. Define terms used in medical reports involving the urinary system.
10. Correctly define, spell, and pronounce the chapter's medical terms.

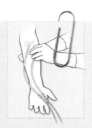

Professional Profile: Dialysis Nurse

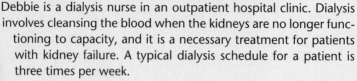

Debbie is a dialysis nurse in an outpatient hospital clinic. Dialysis involves cleansing the blood when the kidneys are no longer functioning to capacity, and it is a necessary treatment for patients with kidney failure. A typical dialysis schedule for a patient is three times per week.

To be a dialysis nurse, one must complete the requirements for the registered nurse (RN) degree, pass the required licensure examination, and then receive advanced training in urology, the study of the urogenital system. Dialysis nurses work closely with nephrologists, physicians specializing in kidney disorders. Patients receiving dialysis treatment are in various stages of renal distress, usually from the ravages of diseases like diabetes. The dialysis nurse must carefully monitor both the dialysis equipment and the patient who is receiving treatment because blood pressure and other vital signs fluctuate during the procedure.

Debbie consults with the doctor to analyze the patient's kidney function and the effectiveness of the dialysis treatment. She must gather the relevant information from a variety of tests. The patient's age, urinary output, weight, blood pressure, blood chemistry profiles, and urinalysis information are all important to the evaluation. Diagnostic reports often come from the radiologist's office.

A working knowledge of medical terminology that goes beyond the kidney is necessary. For example, diabetes, which affects a majority of dialysis patients, can involve almost every body system. The dialysis nurse must be able to communicate with other health-care professionals in various medical specialties about patient conditions.

Dialysis nurses educate patients about kidney anatomy and physiology, citing the importance of blood pressure monitoring, because the kidneys play an important role in regulating blood pressure. The role of nutrition is also important, so those working in a dialysis clinic need to be able to explain the importance of limiting protein intake when kidney function is compromised. Debbie also explains how kidney function can change with age and how it can be affected by various diseases and conditions that might arise as one gets older.

Patients on dialysis are generally quite sick, and the death rate is high as a result of renal failure. Once the kidneys begin to fail, other body systems follow suit. So dialysis nurses must be prepared to work with a patient group that is subject to both a high morbidity and a high mortality rate.

FACT **The kidneys receive about 25% of the blood pumped by the heart!**

FACT **Approximately 1666 L (440 gal.) of blood flow through the kidneys daily!**

FACT **Kidneys excrete 1–2 L (4.25–8.5 cups) of fluid per day!**

INTRODUCTION

The urinary system plays an important role in maintaining fluid and electrolyte balance while also ridding the body of physiological wastes, toxins, and drugs. Urine is a principal waste product, and its formation begins with blood. As blood circulates through the two kidneys, useful substances are separated from useless particles. The substances the body can use are returned to the bloodstream and the remainder becomes urine for excretion outside the body. Although the urinary system has coordinated activities with other body systems, the kidneys begin the job of urine formation, and the ureters, bladder, and urethra complete the job of urine elimination.

The genital and urinary organs are collectively known as the genitourinary system. Abnormalities of this system are usually the result of primary kidney (renal) abnormality or are secondary to a systemic disease, such as diabetes. Clinical and laboratory diagnostics are used to evaluate genitourinary pathology, which generally have demonstrative signs or symptoms. This chapter describes the basic anatomy and physiology of the urinary system and provides information relevant to disorders of the system.

MEDICAL TERM PARTS

WORD PARTS

Medical term prefixes, suffixes, and combining forms related to the urinary system are introduced in this section.

Word Parts	Meaning
azot-, azoto-	nitrogen, nitrogenous
calyc-	small cup, calyces
cortic-, cortico-	covering, renal cortex
cyst-, cysti, cysto-	urinary bladder
detrus-	force away, detrusor muscle
glomerul-, glomerulo-	glomerulus, small rounded mass
glyc-, glyco-	sweet, glucose
hem-, hemo-, hemato-	blood
hydr-, hydro-	water
juxta-	beside, near to; juxtamedullary nephron
ket-, keto-	presence of ketone group (chemical compound)
lith-, -lith, litho-	stone
meat-, meato-	meatus, opening
mict-	to pass urine
nephr-, nephro-	kidney
noct-, nocti-, nocto-, noctu-	night
olig-, oligo-	scanty, little
papillo-	nipple-like
-ptosis	drooping, sinking down
py-, pyo-	pus
pyel-, pyelo-	renal pelvis
prox-, proxim-, proximo-	nearest
ren-, reno-	kidney
scler-, sclero-	hardening
trigon-	triangular shape
ur-, uro-	urine, urinary
ureter-, utero-	urinary tube, urinary
urethr-, urethro-	urethra
-uria	condition of urine
urin-, urino-	urine
vas-, vasi-, vaso-	vessel

WORD ETYMOLOGY

Some words have Greek or Latin word roots but are not true word parts. This section lists those that are used as medical terms.

Word	Definition
albumen	egg white
fenestra	window
glomus	ball of yarn
vas	vessel

MEDICAL TERM PARTS USED AS PREFIXES

Prefix	Definition
calyc-	small cup, calyces
detrus-	force away, detrusor muscle
juxta-	beside, near to, juxtamedullary nephron
mict-	to pass urine
papillo-	nipple-like
trigon-	triangular shape

MEDICAL TERM PARTS USED AS SUFFIXES

Suffix	Definition
-ptosis	drooping, sinking down
-lith	stone
-uria	condition of urine

WORD GROUPING

Using the "Medical Term Parts" tables, identify the prefix, suffix, or combining form for each of the following definitions. The first one has been done as an example.

Definition	Word Part
sweet, glucose	glyc-, glyco-
beside, near to, juxtamedullary nephron	
blood	
condition of urine	
covering, renal cortex	
drooping, sinking down	
force away, detrusor muscle	

Definition	Word Part
glomerulus, small rounded mass	
hardening	
kidney	A.
	B.
meatus, opening	
nearest	
near to, beside	
night	
nipple-like	
nitrogen, nitrogenous	
pus	
presence of ketone group (chemical compound)	
renal pelvis	
scanty, little	
small cup, calyces	
stone	
to pass urine	
triangular shape	
urethra	
urinary bladder	
urinary tube, urinary	
urine	
urine, urinary	
vessel	
water	

WORD BUILDING

Word parts, introduced in the "Medical Term Parts" section, are listed in the following table. For this exercise, first supply the meaning of each word part, then use the word part to build a word you already know. The word you list under "Common or Known Word" does not have to be a medical term; a commonly used word is fine. Be sure, however, that the word correctly reflects the intended meaning. The first one has been done as an example.

Word Part	Meaning	Common or Known Word	Example Medical Term
prox-, proxim-, proximo-	nearest	proximity	proximal convoluted tubule
cortic-, cortico			cortex

Word Part	Meaning	Common or Known Word	Example Medical Term
cyst-, cysti, cysto-			cystitis
glyc-, glyco-			glycosuria
hem-, hemo-, hemato-			hematuria
hydr-, hydro-			hydronephritis
juxta-			juxtamedullary
lith-, -lith, litho-			lithotripsy
ren-, reno-			renin
scler-, sclero-			sclerosis
ur-, uro-			urine
ureter-, utero-			ureter
urethr-, urethro-			urethritis
urin-, urino-			urinary

ANATOMY AND PHYSIOLOGY

Structures of the Urinary System

- Bladder
- Kidneys
- Ureters
- Urethra

Urinary System Preview

The urinary system is the body's blood filtering plant, which consists of two kidneys, a pair of tubular ureters, a sac-like bladder, and a urethra (Fig. 15-1). The **kidneys** remove substances from blood to be excreted in the urine. These bean-shaped organs also regulate metabolic processes such as blood pressure. The tubular **ureters** transport urine from the kidneys to the bladder. Serving as a reservoir for urine, the **bladder** is a distensible (expandable) sac that stores the liquid before **micturition** (urination). The job of the **urethra** is to transport the urine outside the body.

The system functions to help regulate body fluids and blood composition by the processes of filtration, resorption, secretion, and excretion. The kidneys are key organs, which enable the body to retain what it needs by filtering substances from the blood. Through **filtration**, body fluid is passed through the kidneys, resulting in a filtrate. During **resorption**, water and solute molecules such as glucose, proteins, and sodium, are absorbed again from the filtrate as it enters the renal tubule. This process of being reabsorbed, is alternatively termed *reabsorption*. Furthermore, the kidneys are involved with secretion. **Secretion** refers to the process of producing a substance from the kidneys and then discharging it.

Filtration, resorption, and secretion ensure that the blood returning to the body contains the essential components. The remaining fluid that the body cannot use becomes urine, which is excreted. **Excretion** is the process whereby waste products are eliminated from the body.

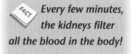

Every few minutes, the kidneys filter all the blood in the body!

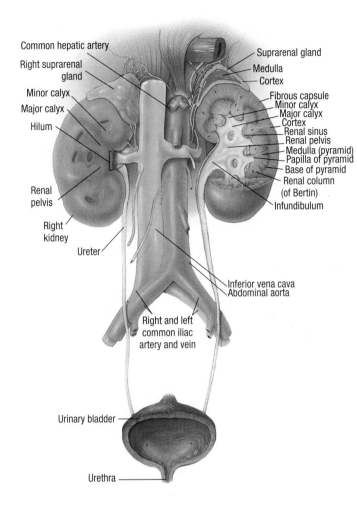

Common hepatic artery
Right suprarenal gland
Minor calyx
Major calyx
Hilum
Renal pelvis
Right kidney
Ureter

Suprarenal gland
Medulla
Cortex
Fibrous capsule
Minor calyx
Major calyx
Cortex
Renal sinus
Renal pelvis
Medulla (pyramid)
Papilla of pyramid
Base of pyramid
Renal column (of Bertin)
Infundibulum

Inferior vena cava
Abdominal aorta
Right and left common iliac artery and vein

Urinary bladder

Urethra

FIGURE 15-1
The urinary system helps regulate body fluids and blood composition by the processes of filtration, resorption, secretion, and excretion. The major structures of the system are the kidneys, ureters, bladder, and urethra. (Image provided by Anatomical Chart Co.)

Key Terms	Definitions
kidney	organ of waste removal
ureter (yoo REE tur)	tube that transports urine to the bladder
bladder	storage site for urine
micturition (mick choo RISH un)	the act of urinating
urethra (yoo REE thruh)	tube that transports urine outside the body
filtration	process by which water and solute molecules, depending on their size, pass through the renal membranes
resorption	process by which water and solutes are removed from the filtrate and returned to the body
secretion	release of materials
excretion	elimination of waste particles

Key Term Practice: Urinary System Preview

1. What are the four primary functions of the urinary system?

   a. _____

   b. _____

   c. _____

   d. _____

2. The _____ are the key organs of the system, which are primarily responsible for forming urine.

Kidneys

Nearly 1200 mL (5 cups) of blood flows through the kidneys every minute!

Situated **retroperitoneally** (behind the membrane lining the abdominal cavity) the two bean-shaped kidneys lie on either side of the vertebral column, between thoracic vertebra 12 (T12) and lumbar vertebra 3 (L3). The left kidney is slightly higher than the right kidney because of the placement of the liver within the cavity. Both fat and fascia (sheet of connective tissue) hold the kidneys firmly in place against the muscles of the back.

Kidneys are rich in vasculature (blood vessel arrangement), which is important for removing unnecessary components and retaining required molecules. Blood flow into and out of the kidneys begins with the **renal arteries**, arising from the abdominal aorta, and ends with the **renal veins**, exiting the kidneys.

Kidney anatomy is relatively complex. The primary components are the renal corpuscle, renal cortex, renal medulla, pyramids, papillae, columns, sinus, vasa recta, calyces, pelvis, hilum, and renal capsule (Fig. 15-2). Forming a fibrous sheath around the entire kidney and encircling the cortex is the **renal capsule**. The **cortex** is the outer portion of the kidney. **Medulla** means "inner," and it is the innermost part of the kidney. **Pyramids** are cone-shaped divisions in the medulla that contain the renal tubules. The apexes of the renal pyramids form the **papilla**, which empty formed urine into the calyces. Cortical renal **columns** are anatomic structures that dip into the medulla between the pyramids.

Sinuses are simply hollow chambers within the organ that serve as blood channels. The **vasa recta** is a specialized capillary loop, and the **calyces** are cup-shaped structures that drain into the renal pelvis. The **pelvis** is a funnel-shaped region at the superior ends of the ureters that serves as a reservoir for formed urine before it flows into the ureter. The **hilum**, marked by the renal artery, renal vein, and ureters, is the region where structures enter or exit the kidney. The **renal corpuscle** is a cluster of capillaries (**glomerulus**) and the sac-like **glomerular** (Bowman's) **capsule** that surrounds it. **Podocytes** are epithelial cells with foot-like processes that form the thin, membranous layer attached to the renal glomerulus.

Nephrons are the functional units of the kidney (Fig. 15-3). Each kidney contains approximately 1.25 million of these microscopic structures, and each nephron consists of a renal corpuscle and a renal tubule. The **renal tubule** is a coiled tube that leads away from the glomerular capsule and empties into the renal pelvis. The respective position of parts in the renal tubule are as follows: proximal convoluted tubule, descending limb of the loop of nephron, loop of nephron, ascending limb of loop of nephron, and the distal convoluted tubule. Another term for the loop of nephron is the loop of Henle. Two types of nephrons exist in the kidneys: cortical and juxtamedullary. Cortical nephrons are so named because their nephron loops are located within the cortex and do not dip into the medulla. Nephrons with corpuscles close to the medulla are termed juxtamedullary.

If the nephrons were lined up end to end, they would reach 50–75 miles (80–121 kilometers)!

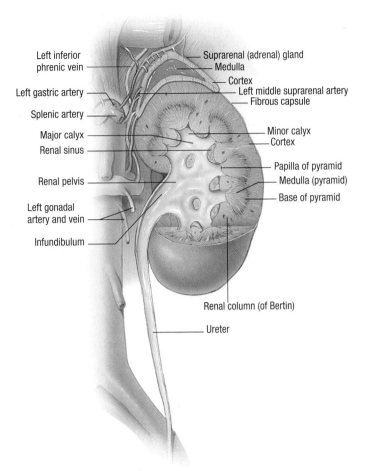

FIGURE 15-2
Cross section of the left kidney and adrenal gland. (Image provided by Anatomical Chart Co.)

Left inferior phrenic vein
Left gastric artery
Splenic artery
Major calyx
Renal sinus
Renal pelvis
Left gonadal artery and vein
Infundibulum

Suprarenal (adrenal) gland
Medulla
Cortex
Left middle suprarenal artery
Fibrous capsule
Minor calyx
Cortex
Papilla of pyramid
Medulla (pyramid)
Base of pyramid

Renal column (of Bertin)
Ureter

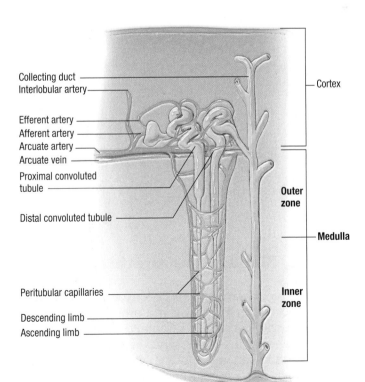

FIGURE 15-3
Nephrons are the functional units of the kidney. (Image provided by Anatomical Chart Co.)

Collecting duct
Interlobular artery
Efferent artery
Afferent artery
Arcuate artery
Arcuate vein
Proximal convoluted tubule
Distal convoluted tubule
Peritubular capillaries
Descending limb
Ascending limb

Cortex
Outer zone
Medulla
Inner zone

Key Terms	Definitions
retroperitoneally (ret roh perr i toh NEE ul ee)	at the back of the abdominal wall
renal (REE nul) **artery**	vessel that carries blood away from the heart into the kidney
renal (REE nul) **vein**	vessel that carries blood from the kidney toward the heart
renal (REE nul) **capsule**	outermost layer of the kidney
cortex (KOR tecks)	outer section of the kidney
medulla (me DUL uh)	inner section of the kidney
pyramid	cone-shaped division of the inner kidney layer
papilla (pap PIL uh)	small, nipple-like projection
column	pillar-shaped anatomic structure
sinuses	hollow spaces or cavities
vasa recta (VAY suh RECK tuh)	specialized capillary vessels next to the nephron loop
calyx (KAY licks)	cup-like structure(s)
pelvis	basin or basin-shaped cavity
hilum (HIGH lum)	area for the entrance and exit of vessels
renal corpuscle (REE nul KOR pus ul)	structure composed of the glomerulus and the surrounding glomerular capsule
glomerulus (gloh MERR yoo lus)	capillary cluster in the renal corpuscle
glomerular (gloh MERR yoo lur) **capsule**	sac surrounding the kidney glomerulus
podocyte (POHD oh site)	epithelial cell with foot-like processes that attaches to the capillary basement membrane of the renal glomerulus
nephron (NEF ron)	functional unit of the kidney
renal tubule (REE nul TEW bewl)	glandular kidney ducts involved in the formation of urine

Key Term Practice: Kidneys

1. The outer region of the kidney is termed the _____, and the innermost area is called the _____.

2. The functional unit of the kidney is the _____.

Ureters, Bladder, and Urethra

Ureters are tubular structures between each kidney and the bladder that transport formed urine by peristalsis. **Peristalsis** is a progression of rhythmic, wave-like contractions in smooth muscle that propels substances along the tube. A flap-like fold in the bladder, at the point where urine enters, serves as a valve to prevent urine backflow into the ureters.

The bladder is an organ located within the pelvic cavity, posterior to the symphysis pubis, which serves as a urine reservoir before micturition (Fig. 15-4). The symphysis pubis is on the anterior body surface at the juncture of the pubic bones, just inferior

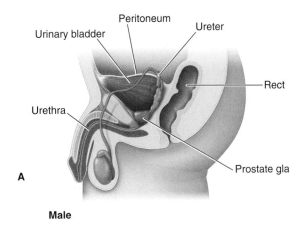

Male

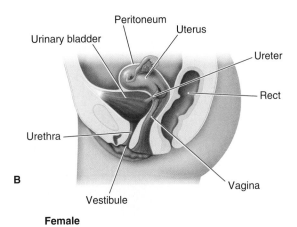

Female

FIGURE 15-4
The (**A**) male and
(**B**) female bladders.

to the hips. In males, the bladder is situated posteriorly against the rectum, and the prostate gland attaches to the bladder at the inferior angle. In females, the bladder contacts the walls of the uterus and vagina. This explains why pregnant women feel the urge to urinate more frequently than usual.

The membranous bladder is composed of the **detrusor,** a bundle of multidirectional, interlaced, smooth muscle fibers within the wall that enables the organ to stretch and contract (Fig. 15-5). **Rugae** (sing., ruga) are folds within the bladder's inner mucosa that allow the organ to expand while storing urine. The bladder's two entrances from the ureters and one exit to the urethra form a triangular region referred to as the **trigone.**

Parasympathetic nerve fibers from the autonomic nervous system stimulate the detrusor before micturition. When the bladder volume reaches 200–300 mL (6.6–10 oz.), stretch receptors initiate an impulse, and one feels an urge to urinate.

The last structure in the urinary system is the urethra. Layered with longitudinal smooth muscles, its purpose is to discharge urine outside the body. The urethra in females is considerably shorter than that in males. Female urethrae are 2.5–5 cm (1-2 in.) long, whereas male urethrae are 17.5–20 cm (7–8 in.) long. In males, the urethra is also part of the reproductive system. During male ejaculation, a sphincter closes the opening to the bladder, enabling the urethra to transport and propel only semen.

Urethral structures include the external urethral sphincter, the internal urethral sphincter, and the external urethral meatus. A **sphincter** is a circular muscle surrounding an orifice (opening). The external urethral sphincter is a band of voluntary skeletal muscle, whereas the internal urethral sphincter is composed of involuntary smooth muscle. The external sphincter is one that can be consciously controlled. The external urethral **meatus,** also called the external urethral **orifice,** is the opening to the outside. In males, the orifice is located at the tip of the penis, and in females, it is found between the labia minora of the external genitals.

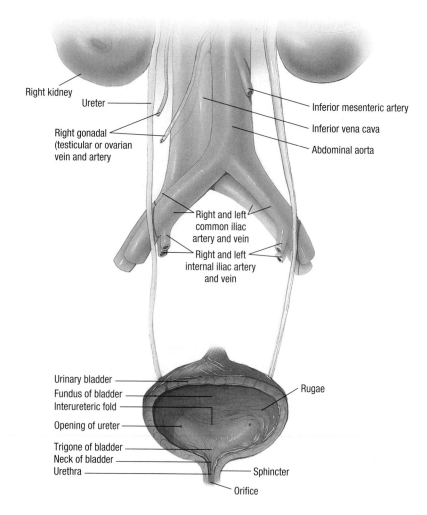

FIGURE 15-5
The urinary bladder.
(Image provided by
Anatomical Chart Co.)

Key Terms	Definitions
peristalsis (perr i STAL sis)	waves of smooth muscle contractions that propel substances through a structure, such as urine along the ureters
detrusor (dee TROO ser)	muscle making up the urinary bladder
rugae (ROO gee)	mucosal folds in an organ
trigone (TRYE gohn)	triangular region of the bladder marked by three openings: the two entrances of the ureters and the exit to the urethra
sphincter (SFINK tur)	muscular ring that contracts to close off an opening in the body
meatus (mee AY tus)	an opening or passageway
orifice (OR i fis)	an opening

Key Term Practice: Ureters, Bladder, and Urethra

1. What are the two medical terms that mean an opening? _____

2. The triangular area on the inner surface of the bladder marked by the openings to the ureters and urethra is termed the _____.

3. What are the singular and plural forms of the term meaning mucosal folds in the bladder?

   singular = _____

   plural = _____

Kidney Physiology and Urine Formation

Hormones, chemical messengers, are critical to kidney physiology. Three hormones associated with the kidney are erythropoietin, antidiuretic hormone, and aldosterone. Red blood cell formation is regulated by the release of the renal hormone, **erythropoietin**, into the blood.

Cells in the hypothalamus produce antidiuretic hormone, which is stored in the neurohypophysis (posterior pituitary gland). **Antidiuretic hormone** (ADH) targets the distal convoluted tubule and collecting tubule, where it promotes water resorption and thus causes water retention in the body. The hormone is released in response to decreasing blood or body fluid volume and decreasing blood pressure.

Aldosterone is a physiologically important steroid hormone produced by the adrenal cortex. Aldosterone controls salt and water balance in the kidney by stimulating sodium retention and water conservation. When aldosterone is pumped out, sodium is conserved. Wherever sodium goes, water follows; urine output is therefore decreased. To help you remember the function of aldosterone, think about sodium as being a component of salt. The letters *s, a, l,* and *t* are found in *aldosterone*.

Renin is an enzyme released from the **juxtaglomerular cells** (smooth muscle cells adjacent to the glomerulus) that regulates blood pressure through a complicated system called the renin-angiotensin mechanism. In this system, renin enables the conversion of angiotensinogen (a normal constituent of blood) to angiotensin, which ultimately affects systemic blood pressure.

The kidneys function as blood filters, forming concentrated or dilute urine. Urine contains about 95% water and 5% solids. Factors affecting urine volume include fluid intake, diet (particularly caffeine, which acts as a diuretic), environmental temperature, humidity, emotional state, respiratory rate, and body temperature. Metabolic wastes are the byproducts of cellular activities and are removed from the blood and eliminated in the urine through excretion. The kidneys are also responsible for activating vitamin D, which is essential for the absorption of calcium.

The first step of urine formation involves glomerular filtration, the process whereby water and dissolved substances are filtered out of the glomerular capillary plasma. Glomerular capillaries are highly permeable owing to the numerous **fenestrae** (openings). These substances then diffuse into the peritubular (around the tubules) capillaries. Tubular secretion is the final step. During this process, substances move out of the peritubular capillaries into the renal tubule.

Each part of the renal tubules plays a critical role in maintaining fluid balance, primarily through resorption. Most nutrients are reabsorbed at the proximal convoluted tubule, that segment of the tube closest to the glomerulus. At the loop itself, an extension of the proximal convoluted tubule, materials are transported across hairpin-shaped membranes. The job of the ascending limb is to reabsorb negative chloride ions (charged particles) and positive sodium ions. Sodium ions follow the chloride ions as a result of the attraction of opposite charges.

Within the collecting system of the kidney, the collecting duct reabsorbs water, and depending on the body's need, it either reabsorbs or secretes sodium, potassium, hydrogen, and bicarbonate ions. These ions are **electrolytes**, elements important for body functions. The duct then delivers urine to the renal calyx for export out of the kidney.

Key Terms	Definitions
hormone (HOR mohn)	chemical messenger found in the blood
erythropoietin (e rith roh POY e tin)	renal hormone necessary for the production of red blood cells
antidiuretic hormone (an tee DYE yoo ret ick HOR mohn)	hormone synthesized by the hypothalamus and secreted by the posterior pituitary that causes water retention, thereby elevating blood pressure
aldosterone (al DOS ter ohn)	hormone that stimulates the kidneys to retain water and sodium
renin (REE nin)	enzyme released by the juxtaglomerular cells when there is a drop in renal blood flow
juxtaglomerular (jucks tuh gloh MERR yoo lur) **cell**	smooth muscle cells found in the afferent and efferent arterioles adjacent to the glomerulus
fenestra (fe NES truh)	small opening
electrolyte (ee LECK troh lite)	soluble, inorganic ion (charged particles), such as sodium and chloride, found in body fluids

Key Term Practice: Kidney Physiology and Urine Formation

1. What are the singular and plural forms of the medical term meaning a small opening in the glomerular capillaries?

    singular = _____

    plural = _____

2. _____ is an enzyme released from the juxtaglomerular cells that is important for blood pressure regulation.

3. Renal _____ carry blood into the kidneys and renal _____ carry blood out of the kidneys.

THE CLINICAL DIMENSION

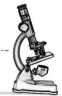

Pathology of the Urinary System

Alterations of renal and urinary tract function have profound systemic effects because this system is involved with cleansing the body's blood and creating urine from those products not needed by the body. Disease recognition is often made possible by examining the urine. Although there are several steps involved in diagnosing disorders of the urinary system, the first is usually a common urinalysis. Other disorders are accompanied by characteristic signs and symptoms that often manifest as back pain, difficulty urinating, discolored urine, and/or itching upon micturition. Some pathologies that can be determined by urinalysis are infection, kidney malfunction, diabetes, and liver disease. After initial investigation of the urine, the clinician may then order more complex clinical tests and diagnostic procedures to identify the underlying disease or condition. Once the pathology has been determined, appropriate treatments can be employed. This section describes various pathologies, along with their signs, symptoms, clinical tests, diagnostic procedures, and treatments, related to the urinary system.

Urinalysis

Urinalysis (UA) is the examination and analysis of urine. Physical, chemical, and microscopic characteristics of urine are determined by urinalysis. Physical measurements include the following: osmotic concentration, water content, color, odor, turbidity, and specific gravity. Osmotic concentration, also called **osmolarity**, refers to the total concentration of dissolved substances in a solution.

The normal color range for urine is pale yellow to amber; but color depends on diet, vitamin intake, and medications. The yellow urinary pigment, **urochrome**, affects the tint. Diet and medications can also significantly affect the color of urine. Urine has a slight odor, which depends on diet, nutritional status, diseases, and drug intake. **Turbidity** refers to the clarity of urine and is affected by suspended particles; normal urine is clear.

Specific gravity (sp. gr.) is the density of urine compared to water, which has a specific gravity of 1.000. It is measured using a hydrometer. Values for urine specific gravity range from 1.010 to 1.035. The value varies according to fluid intake and disease. Low specific gravity may be the result of increased fluid intake or severe renal damage, whereas a high specific gravity could be caused by decreased fluid intake, loss of fluids, uncontrolled diabetes mellitus, or severe anemia.

Chemical characteristics of urine are measures of pH, solutes, sediment, ketone bodies (byproducts of fat metabolism), glucose and protein levels, salts, and ions. Acidity and alkalinity are determined on the pH scale, which measures the concentration of free hydrogen ions (H^+). The scale ranges from 0 to 14; 0 indicates extremely acidic, 7 indicates neutral, and 14 indicates extremely basic or alkaline. The average pH value for urine is slightly acidic at 6.0; however, the normal range is 4.6–8.0. Values < 4.5 may be caused by high-protein diets or uncontrolled diabetes mellitus. Individuals who have a diet rich in vegetables or who have severe anemia may have urine pH values > 8.0.

A renal threshold for glucose exists, and glucose must reach a certain level in the blood before it is excreted; however, small amounts of glucose may be present in the urine after a big meal or when an individual is experiencing stress. Excreted glucose, termed **glycosuria** or **glucosuria**, is often an indication of disease, generally diabetes mellitus.

Large amounts of protein molecules are abnormal constituents of urine, yet a very small quantity may be present because diet and disease can affect urine protein levels. Patients with severe anemia usually excrete protein. Protein in the urine is known as **proteinuria**. When the primary protein is albumin, it is called **albuminuria.**

Microscopic tests are used to determine microbial counts, the presence of casts (protein clumps), crystals (precipitates), and other substances that are not visible to the naked eye. Normal urine is sterile, meaning no bacteria or other microorganisms are present. **Bacteriuria** is the presence of bacteria in the urine. The common bacterium *Escherichia coli* is frequently the culprit.

Key Terms	Definitions
urinalysis (yoor i NAL i sis)	examination of the urine
osmolarity (oz moh LAIR i tee)	total concentration of dissolved substances in a solution; osmotic concentration
urochrome (YOOR oh krome)	yellow pigment in the urine
turbidity (tur BID i tee)	refers to the clarity of a liquid
specific gravity	measure of the density of the urine compared to that of water
glycosuria (glye koh SOO ree uh)	glucose in the urine
glucosuria (gloo koh SOO ree uh)	glucose in the urine
proteinuria (proh tee NEW ree uh)	protein in the urine
albuminuria (al bew mi NEW ree uh)	protein in the urine
bacteriuria (back teer ee YOO ree uh)	presence of bacteria in the urine

Key Term Practice: Urinalysis

1. What are the two terms meaning glucose in the urine? _____

2. What are the two terms that mean protein in the urine? _____

General Kidney Disorders

Inflammation of the kidney may involve the nephron or another specific region. A general term used to describe inflammation of the nephrons is **nephritis. Interstitial nephritis** is an inflammation of renal intercellular connective tissue (interstitium) and tubules. Acute interstitial nephritis is frequently the result of drug-induced reactions, and chronic interstitial nephritis is caused by underlying kidney disease. The term **pyelitis** is used to describe generalized inflammation of the kidney pelvis and calyces.

Hydronephrosis is a condition characterized by dilation of the pelvis and calyces of one or both kidneys (Fig. 15-6). Its cause is generally an obstruction of the ureters, which creates an accumulation of urine in the renal collecting system and subsequent high pressure within the kidney. It may be a congenital disorder or may also result from neuromuscular problems, pregnancy, or some other unknown reason. Usually, the obstruction develops over weeks or months, although acute hydronephrosis also occurs. The obstruction can lead to infection or renal failure if not treated.

Nephroptosis is a movable or displaced kidney. **Renal ptosis** is kidney drop owing to loss of supporting adipose tissue. Wasting diseases, anorexia nervosa, and starvation, in which the fatty deposits surrounding the kidney are diminished, may cause it.

Kidney stones formed by the concentration of excessive calcium, mineral salts, cholesterol, or uric acid, are called **renal calculi** (Fig. 15-7). Their size and numbers vary. For example, a single stone may be the size of a grain of sand or large enough to fill the renal pelvis, called a staghorn calculus. The cause is unknown; however, there appears to be a hereditary tendency toward their development. Symptoms include flank (lumbar region) pain, **urgency** (sudden, compelling urge to urinate), and **hematuria** (blood in the urine). Hematuria is marked by a reddish hue in recently discharged urine. The diagnosis is made through kidney, ureter, bladder (KUB) radiographic studies; urinalysis; intravenous pyelogram (IVP); or intravenous urogram (IVU).

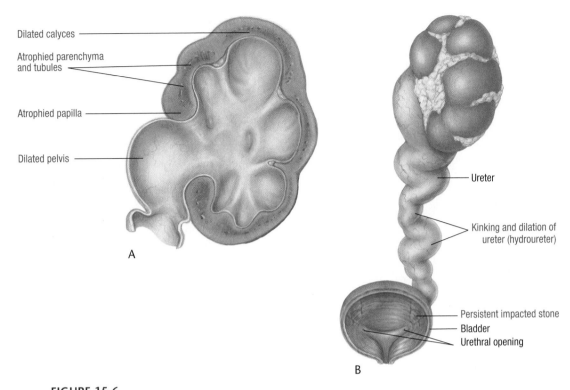

Dilated calyces

Atrophied parenchyma
and tubules

Atrophied papilla

Dilated pelvis

A

Ureter

Kinking and dilation of
ureter (hydroureter)

Persistent impacted stone
Bladder
Urethral opening

B

FIGURE 15-6
(**A**) Renal damage in hydronephrosis, in cross section. (**B**) Advanced renal hydronephrosis with associated affected structures. (Images provided by Anatomical Chart Co.)

In **KUB radiographic studies**, the patient is injected with a contrast medium that is taken up within the vascular kidneys, enabling kidney vessel functioning and obstructions to be visualized on a renogram. In addition to the KUB, the **intravenous pyelogram** provides radiographic images of the kidney pelvis and ureter. This procedure involves the injection of a contrast medium into a vein. As the material traverses the bloodstream, it will eventually enter the highly vascular kidneys, where the contrast material can be seen on an x-ray. Similarly, the **intravenous urogram** provides a radiograph of the entire urinary tract after infusion with a contrast dye.

Treatment of renal calculi may involve **extracorporeal shock wave lithotripsy** (ESWL), whereby a patient is submerged in water or the patient lies on top of a cushion while shock waves are delivered to the kidney region in an effort to crush the stones to allow for natural passage (Fig. 15-8). This is also known as **lithotripsy.**

Key Terms	Definitions
nephritis (ne FRYE tis)	inflammation of the nephrons, kidney inflammation
interstitial nephritis (in tur STISH ul ne FRYE tis)	inflammation of the renal intercellular interstitium and tubules
pyelitis (pye eh LYE tis)	inflammation of the kidney pelvis and calyces
hydronephrosis (high droh nuh FROH sis)	dilation of the renal pelvis and calyces of one or both kidneys
nephroptosis (NEF rop toh sis)	movable or displaced kidney

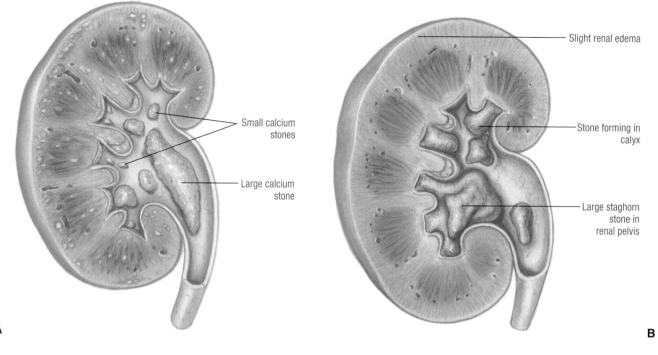

Small calcium
stones

Large calcium
stone

A

Slight renal edema

Stone forming in
calyx

Large staghorn
stone in
renal pelvis

B

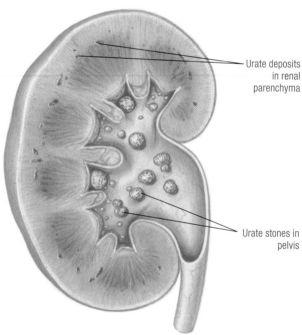

Urate deposits
in renal
parenchyma

Urate stones in
pelvis

C

FIGURE 15-7
Kidney stones are formed by the concentration of excess calcium, mineral salts, cholesterol, or uric
acid. (**A**) Calcium stones. (**B**) Staghorn stones. (**C**) Uric acid stones. (Images provided by
Anatomical Chart Co.)

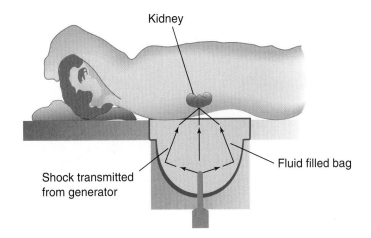

Kidney

Shock transmitted
from generator

Fluid filled bag

FIGURE 15-8
Extracorporeal shock
wave lithotripsy treats
renal calculi by deliv-
ering shock waves to
the kidney region in
an effort to crush the
stones and allow for
natural passage.

renal ptosis (REE nul TOH sis)	kidney drop resulting from loss of supporting adipose tissue
renal calculi (REE nul KAL kew lye)	kidney stones
urgency	pressing desire to empty the bladder
hematuria (hee muh TEW ree uh)	blood in the urine
KUB radiographic (RAY dee oh graf ick) **study**	an isotope (radioactive substance) is injected into the patient's blood and taken up by the urinary system and visualized through a renogram
intravenous pyelogram (in truh VEE nus PYE e loh gram)	procedure in which a contrasting material is injected into a vein to be excreted by the kidneys to permit x-ray visualization of the kidneys
intravenous urogram (in truh VEE nus YOOR oh gram)	radiograph of the urinary tract
extracorporeal (ecks truh kor POH ree ul) **shock wave lithotripsy** (lith oh TRIP see)	procedure in which shock waves are transmitted to the kidneys to break apart renal calculi; lithotripsy
lithotripsy (lith oh TRIP see)	procedure in which shock waves are transmitted to the kidneys to break apart renal calculi; extracorporeal shock wave lithotripsy

Key Term Practice: General Kidney Disorders

1. What is the medical term for kidney stones? _____

2. The word part *nephr-* means _____, and the word part *-itis* means _____; thus _____ is the medical term for inflammation of the nephrons, the functional units of the kidney.

Glomerular Disorders

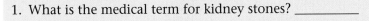

Inflammation of the glomeruli is termed **glomerulonephritis** (Fig. 15-9). Acute glomerulonephritis is characterized by hematuria and proteinuria. It is also called Bright disease. The sudden (acute) onset of glomerulonephritis typically occurs 1–2 weeks after a streptococcal bacterial infection. Although the bacteria do not invade the kidney, the antigen–antibody complexes (immune responses) become trapped in the glomerular capillaries, creating obstructions.

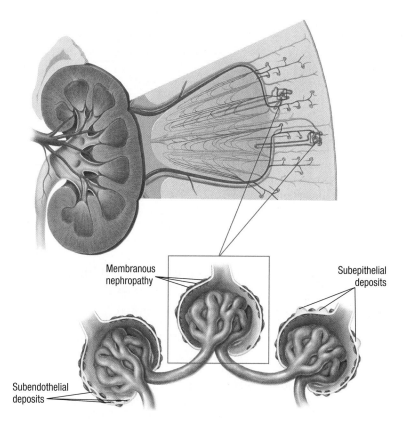

Membranous
nephropathy

Subepithelial
deposits

Subendothelial
deposits

FIGURE 15-9
Glomerulonephritis is
inflammation of the
glomeruli. (Image
provided by
Anatomical Chart Co.)

Diagnosis is usually made by patient history, physical examination, urinalysis, KUB, and possibly blood tests. Hematologic findings indicate an elevated blood urea nitrogen level and hypoalbuminemia. **Blood urea nitrogen** (BUN) is a diagnostic test performed to determine the amount of urea present in the blood. An increase in urea blood levels (uremia) indicates malfunctioning kidneys. Uremia can lead to unconsciousness or death. **Hypoalbuminemia** is low blood albumin (protein) concentration owing to albumin loss in the holes of damaged glomeruli. Available treatment consists of antibiotic therapy if infection persists and the administration of diuretics to promote **diuresis** (excessive urine excretion), thereby reducing edema and hypertension (high blood pressure).

Nephrotic syndrome, also called **nephrosis**, occurs as a result of another existing kidney disorder. It is characterized by proteinuria, hypoproteinemia, anasarca (generalized edema), hyperlipidemia, and normal blood pressure. The basement membrane of renal glomeruli is primarily affected. Nephrosis may become evident after glomerulonephritis. Pregnancy, kidney (renal) transplants, diabetes mellitus, infections, allergic reactions, or exposure to toxins may lead to the syndrome. **Renal transplantation** involves a kidney from a donor being placed into the patient (recipient). In a typical transplant case, the transplanted kidney is placed in the recipient's pelvic cavity, and the renal artery is sutured to the internal iliac artery. The renal artery and the renal vein of the donor kidney are connected to the recipient's renal artery and renal vein, and the lower end of the donor ureter is connected to the recipient's bladder (**ureterocystostomy**). The recipient's diseased kidney may or may not be removed. The transplanted kidney in the recipient, as well as the remaining kidney in the donor, will hypertrophy and function fully.

Tests of glomerular function evaluate the **glomerular filtration rate** (GFR), the speed of filtrate formation at the glomerulus. A clearance test can determine the GFR by monitoring plasma and renal concentrations of the protein creatinine. A creatinine **clearance test** is used as an index of the GFR. Creatinine, the end product of creatine metabolism, is excreted by the kidneys at a constant rate. This test can determine how well the glomeruli are functioning.

Chronic (developing and progressing slowly) glomerulonephritis begins asymptomatically and is not caused by an infection, although antigen–antibody immune complexes form. Disease progression leads to **oliguria** (scanty urine output), proteinuria, hematuria, and edema. Later stages are characterized by renal failure, hypertension, and **azotemia** (increased serum urea levels). Diagnosis protocols are the same as for acute glomerulonephritis. Treatment is aimed at controlling hypertension and **uremia**, an elevated protein level in blood.

Dialysis may also be an option. **Dialysis** is a procedure to filter the blood of unwanted substances that are normally removed by healthy kidneys. There are two types of dialysis: **hemodialysis** and **peritoneal dialysis** (PD). These methods replace kidney function. In both cases, a sem-permeable membrane cleanses the blood. Hemodialysis removes blood wastes by using an artificial kidney (**hemodialyzer**) (Fig. 15-10). Before dialysis treatment, an internal **fistula** (passage connecting an artery and a vein) is surgically built in an arm or leg for dialysis access. At the fistula site, blood passes from the body to a machine equipped with a semipermeable membrane for filtering; the cleansed blood is then returned to the body. This procedure is generally done at a hospital or clinic three times per week and usually takes 4–5 hours each session.

Peritoneal dialysis is performed using a special dialysate solution diffused across a peritoneal membrane that filters toxins. The dialysate enters the peritoneal cavity through a permanent catheter. Wastes diffuse into the fluid, which is then drained and replaced with new dialysis fluid. There are three types of peritoneal dialyses: continuous ambulatory peritoneal dialysis (CAPD), continuous cycling peritoneal dialysis (CCPD), and intermittent peritoneal dialysis (IPD).

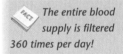
The entire blood supply is filtered 360 times per day!

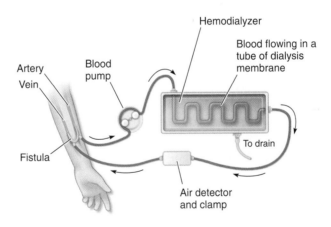

Hemodialyzer

Blood flowing in a tube of dialysis membrane

Artery
Vein
Blood pump

Fistula

To drain

Air detector and clamp

FIGURE 15-10
Hemodialysis cleans the blood for the kidneys.

Key Terms	Definitions
glomerulonephritis (gloh merr yoo loh nef RIGH tis)	inflammation of the glomeruli
blood urea (YOO ree uh) **nitrogen**	diagnostic test performed to determine the amount of urea present in the blood
hypoalbuminemia (high poh al bew min EE mee uh)	low blood albumin (protein) concentration
diuresis (dye yoo REE sis)	increased urine excretion
nephrotic (ne FROT ick) **syndrome**	degenerative renal lesions resulting from damage to the basement membrane of the glomeruli; nephrosis

nephrosis (ne FROH sis)	degenerative renal lesions resulting from damage to the basement membrane of the glomeruli; nephrotic syndrome
renal (REE nul) transplantation	a donor kidney is placed into a patient
ureterocystostomy (yoo ree tur oh sis TOS tuh mee)	surgical connection made between the ureter and the bladder
glomerular (gloh MERR yoo lur) filtration rate	the rate at which blood is filtered at the glomerulus
clearance test	test used to determine the glomerular filtration rate
oliguria (ol i GOO ree uh)	scanty urine production
azotemia (az oh TEE mee uh)	abnormal concentration of urea and nitrogenous substances in the blood
uremia (yoo REE mee uh)	excessive urea and nitrogenous wastes in the blood
dialysis (dye AL i sis)	artificial procedure used to replace normal kidney filtering
hemodialysis (hee moh dye AL i sis)	filtering of blood through an external machine that stands in for the kidneys
peritoneal dialysis (perr i toh NEE ul dye AL i sis)	filtration procedure using a dialysis solution in the peritoneal cavity to filter blood
hemodialyzer (hee moh DYE uh lye zur)	machine that acts as an artificial kidney during dialysis
fistula (fist YOO luh)	passage between and connecting structures

Key Term Practice: Glomerular Disorders

1. Another term for nephrotic syndrome is _____.

2. GFR is the abbreviation for _____.

3. Inflammation of the glomeruli is called _____.

Kidney Function Disorders

Renal failure is a significant decline in kidney function. Two types of renal failure exist: acute and chronic. Acute (sudden) renal failure (ARF) is characterized by a rapid decrease in kidney functioning and is usually triggered by an acute disease process. Conversely, chronic renal failure (CRF) is characterized by diminished kidney function that declines over months to years. The three stages of CRF are early, second, and third stage. The early stage is marked by renal impairment. Renal insufficiency (kidney function at 25%) characterizes the second stage, and the third stage is characterized by end-stage renal disease.

Renal failure may progress to **end-stage renal disease** (ESRD), which is also termed **end-stage renal failure** (ESRF). This is the final phase of kidney disease, occurring when < 10% of normal renal function remains. Complete absence of urine formation, **anuria,** is common. It is characterized by the inability of the kidneys to filter the body's blood because of progressive nephron destruction, a drop in glomerular filtration rate, and a rise in BUN. These changes lead to uremia, represented by toxic waste retention, azotemia, **hyperuricemia** (uric acid crystals in the blood), anorexia, nausea, vomiting, and pruritus (itching). An obvious physical manifestation is **uremic frost**, in which the skin appears powdery from urea and uric acid salt deposits excreted in sweat. The condition is fatal if not treated and involves dialysis and dietary management. In some cases, treatment may include administration of erythropoietin to increase red blood cell production and alleviate anemia.

Key Terms	Definitions
renal (REE nul) **failure**	malfunctioning kidneys
end-stage renal (REE nul) **disease**	final phase of kidney disease marked by the inability to filter the body's blood; end-stage renal failure
end-stage renal (REE nul) **failure**	final phase of kidney disease marked by the inability to filter the body's blood; end-stage renal disease
anuria (an YOO ree uh)	absence of urine output
hyperuricemia (high pur yoo ri SEE mee uh)	elevated uric acid levels in the blood
uremic (yoo REE mick) **frost**	skin appears powdery as a result of severe uremia

Key Term Practice: Kidney Function Disorders

1. _____ describes excessive urea and nitrogenous waste products in the blood.

2. _____ is a significant decline in kidney function, which can progress to _____, a condition identified as kidney functional capacity of less than 10%.

Diabetes

Two types of diabetes exist: diabetes insipidus and diabetes mellitus. **Diabetes insipidus** is an endocrine disorder caused by inadequate secretion of antidiuretic hormone from the posterior pituitary (neurohypophysis) or resistance of the kidney to the action of ADH. Its effects on the urinary system are exhibited as **polyuria** (excessive urination) because the nephrons are unable to absorb water back into the bloodstream. Thus the water increases urine volume. This creates compensatory **polydipsia**, excessive thirst.

Diabetes mellitus (DM) is a chronic disorder of carbohydrate metabolism caused by pancreatic dysfunction or improper insulin utilization. The associated **nephropathy** (kidney disease) is characterized by glycosuria (glucose in the urine), hyperglycemia (increased blood glucose concentrations), polyuria, and polydipsia. Complications include glomerulosclerosis, urinary retention, renal hypertension, proteinuria, and urinary tract infection. **Glomerulosclerosis** is described as hardening or scarring of the glomeruli. In **urinary retention**, the kidneys continue to make urine, but the urine remains in the bladder and is not excreted. Increased blood pressure as a result of kidney disease is termed **renal hypertension** (Fig. 15-11).

Key Terms	Term Practice
diabetes insipidus (dye uh BEE teez in SIP i dus)	disorder resulting from ADH deficiency
polyuria (pol ee YOO ree uh)	excessive urination
polydipsia (pol ee DIP see uh)	excessive thirst
diabetes mellitus (dye uh BEE teez mel EYE tus)	disorder of carbohydrate metabolism

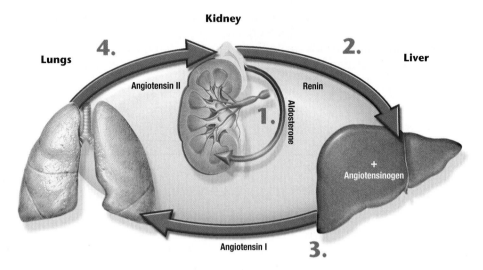

FIGURE 15-11
The mechanism of
renal hypertension.
(Image provided by
Anatomical Chart Co.)

Mechanism of renovascular hypertension
1. Renal artery stenosis causes reduction of blood flow to kidneys.
2. Kidneys secrete renin in response.
3. Renin combines with angiotensinogen in the liver to form angiotensin I.
4. In the lungs, angiotensin I is converted to angiotensin II, a vasoconstrictor.

nephropathy (ne FROP uth ee)	kidney disease
glomerulosclerosis (gloh merr yoo loh skle ROH sis)	fibrosis of the renal glomeruli
urinary (YOOR i nerr ee) **retention**	inability to discharge urine
renal hypertension (REE nul high pur TEN shun)	increased blood pressure owing to kidney disease

 Key Term Practice: Diabetes

1. The term _____ refers to hardening of the glomeruli.

2. The medical term used to describe the inability to discharge urine is _____.

Urinary Tract Infections

A bacterial infection of any part of the urinary system is termed a **urinary tract infection** (UTI). Routes of infection in the urinary tract are shown in Figure 15-12. Signs and symptoms include flank pain, urgency, intense burning while urinating (**dysuria**), hematuria, and **pyuria** (pus in urine). **Pyelonephritis**, an inflammation of the kidneys, renal pelvis, and associated connective tissue, is a common UTI (Fig. 15-13). Diagnosis is made through patient history, physical examination, and urinalysis from a **clean-catch urine specimen.** To obtain a clean-catch urine specimen, one urinates slightly to flush the external genitalia of resident bacterial flora, then a specimen cup is placed under the urine stream to collect a sample.

Three other common lower urinary tract disorders are cystitis, ureteritis, and urethritis (Fig. 15-14). **Cystitis** (urinary bladder inflammation), **ureteritis** (ureter inflammation), and **urethritis** (inflammation of the urethra) are generally caused by a microbial infection.

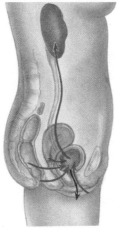
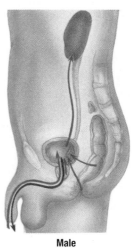

Female   **Male**

1. Ascending from bladder to kidney (reflux)

2. Ascending from urethra to bladder

3. Descending from bladder to urethra

4. From rectum, cervix, or prostate to bladder

5. From bowel to bladder

FIGURE 15-12
Routes of infection in the urinary tract. (Image provided by Anatomical Chart Co.)

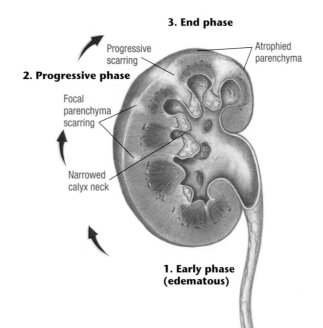

3. End phase

Progressive scarring

Atrophied parenchyma

2. Progressive phase

Focal parenchyma scarring

Narrowed calyx neck

1. Early phase (edematous)

FIGURE 15-13
Pyelonephritis—an inflammation of the kidneys, renal pelvis, and associated connective tissue—is a common urinary tract infection. (Image provided by Anatomical Chart Co.)

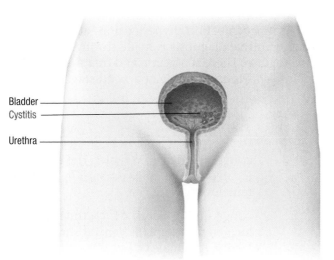
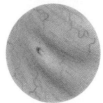

Bladder

Cystitis

Urethra

Normal wall

Acute cystitis

A   B

FIGURE 15-14
(**A**) Cystitis (urinary bladder inflammation) is generally caused by a microbial infection. (**B**) Comparison of the normal bladder wall and a bladder wall affected by acute cystitis, endoscopic view. (Images provided by Anatomical Chart Co.)

Key Terms	Definitions
urinary (YOOR i nerr ee) **tract infection**	infection of the kidneys, ureters, bladder, and/or urethra
dysuria (dis YOO ree uh)	painful, burning sensation while urinating
pyuria (pye YOOR ee uh)	pus in the urine
pyelonephritis (pye eh loh ne FRYE tis)	interstitial inflammation of the kidney
clean-catch urine specimen	urine sample obtained after urinating to flush the external genitalia
cystitis (sis TYE tis)	inflammation of the bladder
ureteritis (yoo ree ter EYE tis)	inflammation of the ureter
urethritis (yoo ree THRYE tis)	inflammation of the urethra

Key Term Practice: Urinary Tract Infections

1. The word part *pyel-* refers to _____, the word part *nephr-* means _____, and the word part *-itis* means _____; so _____ is the medical term for inflammation of the kidney.

2. A urine sample obtained after urinating to flush the external genitalia is referred to as a/an _____.

3. What is the medical term for inflammation of the urethra? _____

Inherited and Congenital Kidney Disorders

A congenital (existing at time of birth) defect in which the urethral opening is not positioned anatomically correctly is called **epispadias.** In males, the urethral opening is located on the dorsum of the penis instead of centrally within the glans penis. Epispadias rarely occurs in females and is marked by the urethral opening at the clitoris. **Hypospadias** in males is characterized by the urethral orifice at the ventral surface of the penis instead of the tip. In females, the urethral opening is located at the vagina. Stenosis (narrowing) of the prepuce (foreskin) on the penis is referred to as **phimosis.** The prepuce cannot be drawn back to uncover the penis, so it may interfere with normal urination.

Polycystic kidney disease is an inherited disease in which normal kidney tissue becomes replaced with grape-like cysts (Fig. 15-15). The cysts progressively develop in both kidneys. Signs and symptoms include flank pain, hematuria, proteinuria, polyuria, nocturia, urinary tract infection, hypertension, and calculi. These may not appear until adulthood. Definitive diagnosis is made through patient history, urinalysis, and intravenous pyelogram. There is no cure, and treatment options include dialysis and kidney transplant. This is an example of an end-stage renal disease.

Key Terms	Definitions
epispadias (ep i SPAY dee us)	congenital defect in which the urethral opening is located on the penis dorsum in males or clitoris in females
hypospadias (high poh SPAY dee us)	congenital defect in which the urethral opening is located on the penis ventral surface in males or vagina in females

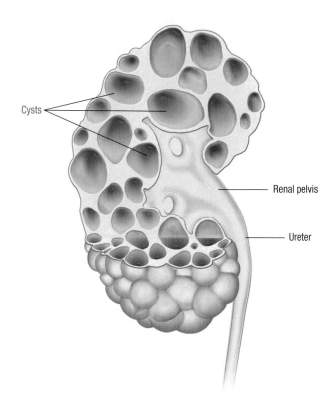

Cysts

Renal pelvis

Ureter

FIGURE 15-15
Polycystic kidney disease is an inherited disease in which the normal kidney tissue becomes replaced with grape-like cysts. The kidney shown in cross-section. (Image provided by Anatomical Chart Co.)

| **phimosis** (figh MOH sis) | stenosis of the penis prepuce |
| **polycystic** (pol ee SIS tick) **kidney disease** | inherited disorder characterized by deformed nephrons |

Key Term Practice: Inherited and Congenital Kidney Disorders

1. _____ is the medical term for the inherited kidney disorder characterized by deformed nephrons.

2. Identify two congenital defects of the urethral opening. _____

3. The term used to describe a narrowing of the penile foreskin is _____.

Cancer

Renal cell carcinoma, or kidney cancer (CA), can develop anywhere within the organ (Fig. 15-16). The cancer, which accounts for 2% of all cancers in adults, often metastasizes (spreads) to the bones and lungs. It affects males at twice the rate of females, typically appearing in the 6th or 7th decade of life, and cigarette smoking may cause it. Classic signs and symptoms include hematuria, weight loss, and flank pain. Diagnosis is made through laboratory tests, radiographic studies, renal biopsy, KUB, magnetic resonance imaging (MRI), ultrasonography, or computed tomography (CT) scan.

These diagnostic procedures enable the clinician to stage (identify disease progression of) the tumor. **Nephrectomy,** surgical removal of the kidney, is the preferred treatment because this type of cancer responds poorly to radiation and chemotherapy. An individual can function nearly normally with only one kidney provided the remaining kidney is healthy.

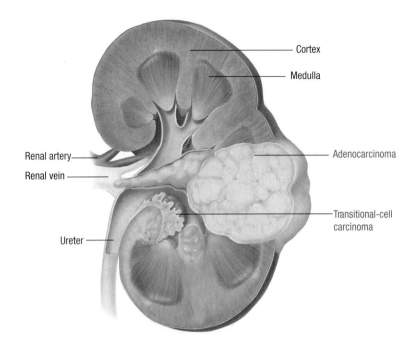

FIGURE 15-16
Renal cell carcinoma can develop anywhere within the kidney. Two common forms, adenocarcinoma and transitional cell carcinoma, are shown. (Image provided by Anatomical Chart Co.)

Wilms tumor is a rapidly developing kidney tumor in infants or children with an unknown cause. It may be treated with surgery, radiation, or chemotherapy.

Bladder cancer is malignant growth of cells in the urinary bladder (Fig. 15-17). The first sign is usually hematuria. Initial diagnosis is made by the history and physical examination, urinalysis, and x-rays; it is confirmed by biopsy using a **cystoscope** (cysto), an instrument for viewing the bladder. Treatment depends on the growth, size, and location of the tumor.

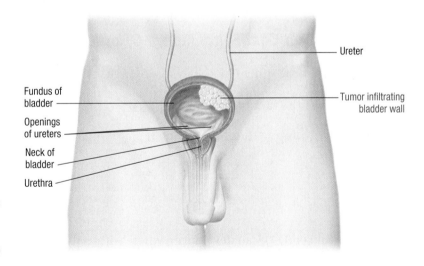

FIGURE 15-17
Bladder cancer is malignant growth of cells in the urinary bladder. (Image provided by Anatomical Chart Co.)

Key Terms	Definitions
renal (REE nul) **cell carcinoma** (kahr si NOH muh)	cancerous kidney tumor
nephrectomy (ne FRECK toh mee)	surgical removal of a kidney
Wilms (vilms) **tumor**	rapidly developing kidney tumor in children

bladder cancer	malignant cell growth in the urinary bladder
cystoscope (SIS toh skope)	medical instrument used for viewing the bladder and ureters

Key Term Practice: Cancer

1. Another term for kidney cancer is _____.

2. _____ tumor is a rapidly developing abnormal kidney growth in children.

Urinary Bladder Disorders

Interstitial cystitis (IC) is a chronic bladder condition in which the bladder connective tissue is inflamed. Signs and symptoms include urgency, frequency, and incontinence. **Frequency** describes the act of urinating often, and **incontinence** is the inability to consciously control urination. A disorder that affects children is **enuresis**, involuntary nighttime bedwetting.

Blockage of the bladder exit, termed **bladder neck obstruction** (BNO), is another disorder. BNO occurs as a result of disease or anatomic abnormality.

Neurogenic bladder describes neurologic deficits resulting in urinary bladder dysfunctions such as incontinence and retention.

Ruptured bladder results from any disruption of the bladder wall. Traumatic injuries are a common cause, and surgical treatment is necessary.

Key Terms	Definitions
interstitial cystitis (in tur STISH ul sis TYE tis)	chronic bladder condition in which the connective tissue is inflamed
frequency	urinating often
incontinence (in KON ti nunce)	inability to control urination
enuresis (en yoo REE sis)	involuntary nighttime bedwetting, particularly in children
bladder neck obstruction	blockage of the bladder outlet
neurogenic (new roh JEN ick) bladder	urinary bladder dysfunction resulting from impaired nervous system functioning
ruptured bladder	disruption of the bladder wall

Key Term Practice: Urinary Bladder Disorders

1. Involuntary nighttime bedwetting is called _____.

2. The inability to control urination is termed _____.

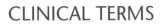

CLINICAL TERMS

Clinical Dimension	Term	Description
DISORDERS		
	bladder cancer	malignant cell growth in the urinary bladder
	bladder neck obstruction (BNO)	blockage of the bladder outlet
	cystitis	inflammation of the bladder
	dehydration	condition resulting from excessive water loss
	diabetes insipidus	disorder resulting from ADH deficiency
	diabetes mellitus (DM)	disorder of carbohydrate metabolism
	end-stage renal disease (ESRD)	final phase of kidney disease marked by the inability to filter the body's blood; end-stage renal failure
	end-stage renal failure (ESRF)	final phase of kidney disease marked by the inability to filter the body's blood; end-stage renal disease
	enuresis	involuntary nighttime bedwetting, particularly in children
	epispadias	congenital defect in which the urethral opening is located on the penis dorsum in males or clitoris in females
	glomerulonephritis	inflammation of the glomeruli
	glomerulosclerosis	fibrosis of the renal glomeruli
	hydronephrosis	dilation of the renal pelvis and calyces of one or both kidneys
	hypospadias	congenital defect in which the urethral opening is located on the penis ventral surface in males or vagina in females
	interstitial cystitis	chronic bladder condition in which the connective tissue is inflamed
	interstitial nephritis	inflammation of the renal intercellular interstitium and tubules
	nephritis	inflammation of the nephrons, kidney inflammation
	nephrolithiasis	presence of calculi in kidney or collecting system
	nephropathy	kidney disease
	nephroptosis	movable or displaced kidney
	nephrosis	degenerative lesions resulting from damage to the basement membrane of the glomeruli; nephrotic syndrome
	nephrotic syndrome	degenerative lesions resulting from damage to the basement membrane of the glomeruli; nephrosis
	neurogenic bladder	urinary bladder dysfunction owing to impaired nervous system functioning
	phimosis	stenosis of the penis prepuce

Clinical Dimension	Term	Description
	polycystic kidney disease	inherited disorder characterized by deformed nephrons
	pyelitis	inflammation of the kidney pelvis and calyces
	pyelonephritis	interstitial inflammation of the kidney
	renal calculi	kidney stones
	renal cell carcinoma	cancerous kidney tumor
	renal failure	malfunctioning kidneys
	renal hypertension	increased blood pressure resulting from kidney disease
	renal ptosis	kidney drop owing to loss of supporting adipose tissue
	ruptured bladder	disruption of the bladder wall
	suppression	complete stoppage of urine production
	uremia	elevated level of urea and nitrogenous wastes in the urine
	uremic syndrome	group of renal changes characterized by hyper-uricemia, polyuria, anuria, and nocturia
	ureteritis	inflammation of the ureter
	urethritis	inflammation of the urethra
	urinary tract infection (UTI)	infection of the kidneys, ureters, bladder, and/or urethra
	Wilms tumor	rapidly developing kidney tumor in children
SIGNS AND SYMPTOMS		
	albuminuria	protein in the urine
	anuria	absence of urine output
	azotemia	abnormal concentration of urea and nitrogenous substances in the blood
	azoturia	increased nitrogenous substances in the urine
	bacteriuria	presence of bacteria in the urine
	diuresis	increased urine excretion
	dysuria	pain, burning sensation while urinating
	frequency	urinating often
	glucosuria	glucose in the urine
	glycosuria	glucose in the urine
	hematuria	blood in the urine
	hyperuricemia	elevated uric acid levels in the blood
	hypoalbuminemia	low blood albumin (protein) concentration
	incontinence	inability to control urination
	nocturia	purposeful nighttime urination

Clinical Dimension	Term	Description
	oliguria	scanty urine output
	polydipsia	excessive thirst
	polyuria	excessive urination
	proteinuria	protein in the urine
	pyuria	pus in the urine
	uremic frost	skin appears powdery as a result of severe uremia
	urgency	pressing desire to empty the bladder
	urinary retention	inability to discharge urine
CLINICAL TESTS AND DIAGNOSTIC PROCEDURES		
	blood urea nitrogen (BUN)	diagnostic test performed to determine the amount of urea present in the blood
	cast	protein masses found in the urine
	clean-catch urine specimen	urine sample collected after urinating to flush the external genitalia
	clearance test	test used to determine the glomerular filtration rate
	cystometrogram	diagnostic study measuring urinary bladder pressure and capacity during gradual filling, using a cystometer, to evaluate urinary dysfunction and incontinence
	cystoscope	medical instrument used for viewing the bladder and ureters
	cystoscopy	procedure using a cystoscope
	glomerular filtration rate (GFR)	the rate at which blood is filtered at the glomerulus
	intravenous pyelogram (IVP)	procedure in which a contrasting material is injected into a vein to be excreted by the kidneys to permit x-ray evaluation of the kidneys
	intravenous urogram	radiograph of the urinary tract
	KUB radiographic studies	an isotope (radioactive substance) is injected into the patient's blood and taken up by the urinary system and visualized through a renogram
	panendoscope	instrument used to provide a wide-angle view of the bladder
	pH	measure of the acidity or alkalinity of urine
	renal biopsy	surgical extraction of kidney tissue
	retrograde pyelography	x-ray visualization of the renal collecting system after catheter introduction of a contrast medium into the ureters using a cystoscope
	specific gravity (sp. gr.)	measure of the density of urine compared to that of water
	urinalysis (UA)	examination of the urine
	voiding cystourethrogram (VCUG)	picture taken of the bladder while urinating

Clinical Dimension	Term	Description
TREATMENTS		
	cystectomy	surgical removal of the bladder
	dialysis	artificial procedure used to replace normal kidney filtering
	extracorporeal shock wave lithotripsy (ESWL)	procedure in which shock waves are transmitted to the kidney to break apart renal calculi; lithotripsy
	fistula	passage between and connecting structures
	hemodialysis	filtering of blood through an external machine that steps in for the kidneys
	hemodialyzer	machine that acts as an artificial kidney during dialysis
	lithotripsy	procedure in which shock waves are transmitted to the kidney to break apart renal calculi; extracorporeal shock wave lithotripsy
	nephrectomy	surgical removal of a kidney
	peritoneal dialysis (PD)	filtration procedure using a dialysis solution in the peritoneal cavity to filter blood
	pyelolithotomy	removal of a kidney stone from the renal pelvis
	pyelotomy	incision made in the renal pelvis
	renal transplantation	a donor kidney is placed into a patient
	ureterocystostomy	surgical connection made between the ureters and the bladder
	urinary catheterization	procedure in which a tube is placed through the urethra to assist in bladder emptying

Lifespan

Development of the renal system begins during the 3rd week of embryonic life. Excretory function of the system begins as early as the 6th week in utero; and urine formation, which occurs during the 3rd month of fetal life, contributes to the surrounding amniotic fluid. By the 5th month of fetal life, the collecting ducts are formed. Other portions of the system continue to develop throughout the remainder of the pregnancy.

Nephron number is fixed at birth, and recent research has correlated low nephron number to hypertension, thereby suggesting that this disease can be predicted at birth. Newborns typically will not urinate until 12–24 hours after birth. Infant urine is dilute with little urea because all the protein (from which urea is derived) is being used for growth processes. Immature kidneys are also less able to maintain fluid and electrolyte balance; therefore, infections, diarrhea, dehydration, or malnutrition can rapidly develop into a serious condition.

At birth, the infant's ureters are shorter than those found in an adult. The kidneys reach their full size during adolescence. Furthermore, between birth and adolescence, the kidneys increase in weight 10-fold.

Age affects the urinary system. Some changes go unnoticed, but others may impede normal physiological functioning. Beginning around age 20 years, the kidney cell numbers diminish so that by age 80 years, the kidney mass has declined by about one third. Fortunately, there is considerable organ reserve to compensate for this loss. As one ages, kidney function decreases owing to the decline in functional nephrons. Aged kidneys appear grainy and scarred as a result of increasing fibrous connective tissue on the renal capsule. Furthermore, there is a reduction in the glomerular filtration rate that can be attributed to glomeruli atrophy, replacement of normal tissue with connective tissue, or unraveling of the coils. Renal tubules may accumulate fat, affecting resorption and secretion. Medications and drugs also remain longer in the circulation as a result of diminished renal activity.

A reduced sensitivity to ADH, which leads to dehydration, also occurs as one ages, and there may be difficulty with the micturition reflex. Also, the ureters, bladder, and urethra lose elasticity with aging. Common disorders in the elderly include incontinence, urinary tract infections, renal calculi, and prostate disorders in the male. Prostate disorders in men can lead to urinary retention.

In the News: Hemolytic Uremic Syndrome

In 1993, approximately 700 people in the states of Washington, Nevada, and Idaho became ill after ingesting undercooked hamburgers prepared at a fast-food chain. Of those afflicted, four children died and numerous people were hospitalized with kidney disorders and bleeding. What the unsuspecting victims did not realize was that the meat was contaminated with *E. coli* O157:H7 bacteria, an extremely pathogenic germ.

The Centers for Disease Control and Prevention (CDC) report that 5–10% of children who become ill from the bacterium develop hemolytic uremic syndrome (HUS). Moreover, 90% of HUS cases develop in children under age 3 years. This disease is characterized by bloody diarrhea, hemolytic anemia with abnormally shaped erythrocytes, thrombocytopenia (decreased number of platelets), and azotemia. Blood vessel walls become damaged by the bacterium's toxin, and the highly vascular kidneys begin to malfunction. Sadly, 1 in 20 children will die as a result of multiple organ failure. Of the individuals who survive, 1 in 3 will sustain permanent kidney damage, and 1 in 10 will develop complications such as hypertension or recurring seizures.

Prevention is the key to thwarting HUS. Although the primary culprit is undercooked ground beef, other foods such as steaks, roasts, and unpasteurized fruit juices and milk may also be contaminated. To prevent possible illness, meats should be thoroughly cooked and unpasteurized milk and juice should be avoided.

COMMON ABBREVIATIONS

Abbreviation	Term
ADH	antidiuretic hormone
ARF	acute renal failure
CRF	chronic renal failure
BNO	bladder neck obstruction
BUN	blood urea nitrogen
CA	cancer
CAPD	continuous ambulatory peritoneal dialysis

Abbreviation	Term
CCPD	continuous cycling peritoneal dialysis
CDC	Centers for Disease Control and Prevention
CRF	chronic renal failure
CT	computerized tomography
cysto	cystoscopic examination
DM	diabetes mellitus
ESRD	end-stage renal disease
ESRF	end-stage renal failure
ESWL	extracorporeal shock wave lithotripsy
GFR	glomerular filtration rate
H^+	hydrogen ion
HUS	hemolytic uremic syndrome
IC	interstitial cystitis
IPD	intermittent peritoneal dialysis
IVP	intravenous pyelogram
IVU	intravenous urogram
KUB	kidney, ureter, and bladder
L	lumbar
MRI	magnetic resonance imaging
PD	peritoneal dialysis
RN	registered nurse
sp. gr.	specific gravity
T	thoracic
UA	urinalysis
UTI	urinary tract infection
VCUG	voiding cystourethrogram

Case Study

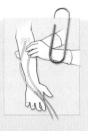

Mr. Green's primary-care physician sent him to the nephrologist. Mr. Green, age 65 years, who has insulin-dependent diabetes, lives alone. He has been retired for the past 15 years. The physician performed a cursory physical examination and took notes pertaining to Mr. Green's immediate history.

   While taking the medical history, the doctor discovered several key factors critical to making a diagnosis. For the past 2 weeks, Mr. Green has been complaining of a backache in the right lower flank. He stated that he had not been engaged in any physical activity and primarily sits and watches television all day. He had been taking aspirin to ease the pain; however, it did not work. He was not sure how much aspirin he had taken, but he thought it was perhaps four pills a day, although he was uncertain of the dosage. Mr. Green stated that he has been urinating more frequently than usual. Furthermore, he is experiencing pain and a burning sensation while urinating. Physical examination revealed the following information:

- Height: 5 ft. 10 in.
- Weight: 233 lb.
- Blood pressure: 160/120 mm Hg
- Temperature: 99°F
- Respiration rate: 26/min
- Pulse: 80 bpm

The nephrologist ordered an IVP and KUB study, and a blood glucose stick and urinalysis were performed. The results from the blood and urine tests were obtained immediately. The blood glucose test indicated a glucose concentration of 200 mg/dL. The urinalysis indicated the following:

Test	Test Result
color	red
pH	3.0
specific gravity	1.050
glucose	positive
protein	negative

The nephrologists made a diagnosis of uncontrolled diabetes mellitus and UTI. Antibiotic therapy and nutrition education were prescribed. No further action would be taken until the results of the IVP and KUB were known.

Case Study Questions

Select the best answer to each of the following questions.

1. **Mr. Green stated he had pain in the right lower flank. In medical language, this region is called the right _____ region.**

   a. umbilical
   b. cervical
   c. sacral
   d. lumbar

2. **The source of Mr. Green's pain is likely his _____.**

   a. latissimus dorsi muscle
   b. abdominal aorta
   c. right kidney
   d. spleen

3. **Painful, burning urination is a classic sign of _____.**

   a. a urinary tract infection (UTI)
   b. renal calculi
   c. ureters calculi
   d. renal carcinoma

4. **The urinalysis revealed a red color. This may indicate _____.**

   a. blood in the urine
   b. eating beets
   c. a bacterial infection
   d. a and c

5. **Normal urine pH is 4.6–8.0, but Mr. Green's urine had a pH of 3.0. This may indicate _____.**

   a. a normal result
   b. uncontrolled diabetes mellitus
   c. hemoglobin in the urine
   d. anemia

6. **Mr. Green's urine had a specific gravity of 1.050. A specific gravity above 1.035 is considered high. Among the causes of a high specific gravity is/are _____.**

   a. loss of fluids
   b. uncontrolled diabetes mellitus
   c. increased fluid intake
   d. a and b

7. Mr. Green tested positive for glucose in the urine. This condition is known as _____.
   a. hematuria
   b. oliguria
   c. anuria
   d. glucosuria

8. The IVP test was ordered because it could detect _____.
   a. a renal calculus
   b. a pulled muscle
   c. hematuria
   d. gout

REAL WORLD REPORT

Debbie received a copy of Mr. Green's KUB and IVP reports. She and the nephrologist evaluated the results.

UROLOGY EXAMINATION

Patient name:	John Green
Age:	65 years
Date:	November 15, 2004

KUB
The bowel gas pattern appears unremarkable. Multiple bladder calculi are noted.

IVP WITH TOMOGRAMS (SECTIONAL RADIOGRAPHS)
After injection of contrast there is prompt excretion of contrast by both kidneys. A large left renal cyst is noted. This was confirmed with ultrasound of the left kidney. Both ureters show evidence of obstructive uropathy. The bladder again shows multiple bladder calculi. Some of the calculi are probably in the bladder diverticula. A postvoid study shows a moderate amount of residual contrast in the bladder.

IMPRESSION
- Multiple bladder calculi
- Large left renal cyst

Dictated by: Sally Wright
This document has been reviewed and electronically approved

REAL WORLD REPORT QUESTIONS
The following exercises review the medical terms in the preceding medical report.
1. What are bladder calculi? _____
2. The tests revealed hematuria.
   a. The word part *hemat-* means _____
   b. The word part *-uria* means _____
   c. The term hematuria means _____
3. What word in the report technically translates as "disorder of the urinary tract"? _____

REVIEW AND APPLICATION: THREE-LEVEL LEARNING SYSTEM

LEVEL ONE: REVIEWING FACTS AND TERMS USING RECALL

Use the following terms to complete the statements. Each term is used only once.

a. glomerulus   b. nephron

c. urine   d. kidneys

e. excretion   f. filtration

g. cortex   h. retroperitoneal

i. hilum   j. glomerular capsule

k. rugae   l. erythropoietin

1. The hormone _____ is necessary for the production of red blood cells.

2. Podocytes in the _____ receive glomerular filtrate.

3. The _____ are mucosal folds in the urinary bladder.

4. _____ is the end product of kidney filtration.

5. The outer portion, or _____, forms the kidney shell.

6. The organs responsible for filtering the blood are the _____.

7. _____ is the process whereby metabolic wastes are removed from the blood.

8. The functional unit of the kidney is the _____.

9. Moving wastes outside the body is termed _____.

10. If an organ is situated _____, it means it is attached to the posterior wall of the abdominal body cavity.

11. The region called the _____ describes the point where vessels enter an organ.

12. The _____ filters water and dissolved substances from the plasma.

Select the best answer to each of the following questions.

13. The hollow chambers within the kidneys are called _____.
    a. vestibules
    b. sinuses
    c. hila
    d. capsules

14. The word part *nephr*- means _____, and the word part *-osis* means _____.
    a. kidney; condition of
    b. renin; pathology of
    c. urine; inflammation of
    d. nephron; condition of

15. Surgical removal of a kidney is termed _____.
    a. lithotomy
    b. lithotripsy
    c. nephrectomy
    d. pyelotomy

16. The _____ delivers urine to the outside.
    a. urinary tubule
    b. papillary duct
    c. ureter
    d. urethra

17. The structure connecting the kidney to the bladder is the _____.
    a. renal tubule
    b. papillary duct
    c. ureter
    d. urethra

18. Hormones affecting the kidney include all of the following *except* _____.
    a. adrenocorticotropic hormone (ACTH)
    b. antidiuretic hormone (ADH)
    c. aldosterone
    d. renin

19. The term used to describe rhythmic, wave-like contractions of smooth muscle is _____.

    a. wave summation

    b. segmentation

    c. filtration

    d. peristalsis

20. The muscle that makes up the bladder is the _____.

    a. extensor

    b. detrusor

    c. trigone

    d. sphincter

21. Sugar in the urine is aptly named _____.

    a. glycosuria

    b. glucosuria

    c. hypoglycemia

    d. a and b

22. The triangular region of the urinary bladder that is formed from the openings of the urethra and ureters is the _____.

    a. trapezium

    b. terminal

    c. trigone

    d. transitional epithelium

23. Renal failure often progresses to _____.

    a. end-stage renal disease (ESRD)

    b. end-stage renal failure (ESRF)

    c. acute glomerulonephritis

    d. a and b

24. The urethral _____ is a circular muscle surrounding the external urethral orifice.

    a. circularis

    b. sphincter

    c. muscularis

    d. serosa

25. A test of the physical, chemical, and microscopic composition of urine is termed _____.

    a. urinalysis

    b. turbidity

    c. urine probe

    d. osmolarity

Define the following word parts.

26. olig- _____

27. detrus- _____

28. -ptosis _____

29. -lith _____

30. -uria _____

LEVEL TWO: REVIEWING CONCEPTS

Select the best response to each of the following questions.

31. Kidneys and the urinary system perform the jobs of _____.

    a. filtration, dialysis, and resorption

    b. filtration, resorption, and secretion

    c. dialysis, resorption, and excretion

    d. secretion, dialysis, and excretion

32. Within the kidneys, erythropoietin and renin are _____.

    a. secreted

    b. excreted

    c. filtered

    d. removed

33. What is the correct order of structures within the nephron, beginning with the proximal convoluted tubule (PCT)?

    a. PCT → distal convoluted tubule → descending limb → loop of nephron → ascending limb

    b. PCT → loop of nephron → distal convoluted tubule → ascending limb → descending limb

c. PCT → ascending limb → loop of nephron → descending limb → distal convoluted tubule

d. PCT → descending limb → loop of nephron → ascending limb → distal convoluted tubule

34. Whenever an ion is reabsorbed in the convoluted tubule, this means that the particular ion will be _____.

   a. removed from the blood and excreted to the outside

   b. retained by the blood to be excreted to the outside

   c. retained in the blood to remain for use by the body

   d. removed from the blood to be excreted as urine

35. The secretion of antidiuretic hormone will _____ during times of dehydration, thereby _____ urine output to ensure water balance.

   a. increase; increasing

   b. decrease; decreasing

   c. decrease; increasing

   d. increase; decreasing

36. ADH targets the distal convoluted tubule to promote water _____.

   a. resorption

   b. secretion

   c. excretion

   d. filtration

37. Aldosterone, produced by the adrenal cortex, stimulates sodium _____.

   a. secretion

   b. excretion

   c. filtration

   d. retention

38. If sodium is retained in the body, _____ automatically is too.

   a. water

   b. hydrogen

   c. calcium

   d. vitamin D

39. Extracorporeal shock wave lithotripsy (ESWL) is used to destroy _____.

   a. renal calculi

   b. renal ptosis

   c. bacteriuria

   d. nephrons

40. A pyelogram is used to assess the _____.

   a. renal artery

   b. renal vein

   c. glomerulus

   d. renal pelvis

41. Bacteria often cause _____.

   a. calculi

   b. pyeloliths

   c. urinary tract infections (UTIs)

   d. bladder cancer

42. Females are more prone to urinary tract infections than males because _____.

   a. females usually sit to urinate, thus bacteria enter the urinary tract from an infected toilet seat

   b. males usually stand to urinate, thus there is relatively little risk of the penis being infected from a contaminated toilet seat

   c. after urinating, women must wipe, therefore contributing to infection

   d. the female urethra is shorter than the male urethra, thus enabling bacteria to enter the urinary tract more readily

43. The micturition reflex leads to the act of _____.

   a. urinating

   b. filtering

   c. childbirth

   d. swallowing

44. Physical characteristics of urine include all of the following *except* _____.

   a. color

   b. turbidity

   c. osmolarity

   d. pH

45. Increased levels of nitrogenous waste products, causing _____, results from kidney _____.

    a. hypoalbuminemia; disease

    b. hypospadias; nephritis

    c. uremia; failure

    d. proteinemia; failure

46. As one ages, kidney function declines as a result of _____.

    a. kidney ptosis

    b. a decrease in the number of functional nephrons

    c. increased sensitivity to ADH

    d. incontinence

47. The term that best describes a scanty urine output is _____.

    a. oliguria

    b. anuria

    c. dysuria

    d. polyuria

48. Inflammation of the kidney pelvis is termed _____.

    a. nephritis

    b. pyelitis

    c. polycystitis

    d. pyelonephritis

Match the following terms with the correct definition. Each term is used only once.

_____ 49. inflammation of the urethra   a. Wilms tumor

_____ 50. sugar in the urine   b. suppression

_____ 51. abnormal growth on the kidney in children   c. hematuria

_____ 52. inability to void urine because the kidneys fail to produce urine   d. phimosis

_____ 53. blood in the urine   e. enuresis

_____ 54. stenosis of prepuce   f. glycosuria

_____ 55. nighttime bedwetting, particularly in children   g. urethritis

Match the urinary system medical term with its correct characteristic or definition.

_____ 56. glomerulonephritis   a. progressing decline in kidney functioning

_____ 57. renal failure   b. excessive urination

_____ 58. polyuria   c. glomeruli inflammation

_____ 59. diabetes mellitus   d. pus in the urine

_____ 60. pyuria   e. disorder of glucose metabolism

Match the sign or symptom with its correct definition.

_____ 61. anuria   a. scanty urine output

_____ 62. hematuria   b. purposeful nighttime urination

_____ 63. oliguria   c. glucose in the urine

_____ 64. glucosuria   d. blood in the urine

_____ 65. nocturia   e. absence of urine output

Match the procedure or clinical test with its correct definition.

_____ 66. nephrectomy   a. shock wave therapy to crush kidney stones

_____ 67. urinalysis   b. examination of urine

_____ 68. dialysis   c. surgical removal of a kidney

_____ 69. lithotripsy   d. used to assess GFR

_____ 70. clearance test   e. blood cleansing by artificial means

Define the following abbreviations.

71. KUB _____

72. ESRD _____

73. IVP _____

74. UA _____

75. BUN _____

LEVEL THREE: THINKING CRITICALLY

Select the best answer to each of the following questions.

76. After urinating, Ginger noticed that her urine appeared to have sand-like particles in it. The debris could conceivably be _____.

   a. bacteria

   b. viruses

   c. sand

   d. renal calculi deposits

77. Your neighbor tells you that her doctor diagnosed her as having hematuria and a UTI. You ask about her urine, and she tells you that it was _____.

   a. red and clear

   b. yellow and clear

   c. red and turbid

   d. green and turbid

78. Kyley has been dieting and states that she has never felt better. She has noticed that she urinates only about once per day, though. The dietitian tells her that she needs to drink more fluids. Kyley needs to take in more liquids to _____.

   a. reduce her sodium sensitivity

   b. increase her sodium sensitivity

   c. gain fluids that are lost through urination

   d. avoid the risk of dehydration

Provide a short answer to each of the following questions.

79. Two college students, Kelsey and Marcy, are discussing a party they attended over the weekend. Kelsey said, "Whenever I drink a couple beers, I have to go to the bathroom at least five times that night. According to what I learned in my medical terminology class, I think I am secreting too much ADH." Marcy tells her she is all wrong because going to the bathroom so often after drinking a few beers is a clear indication that she is not secreting ADH. Who is correct and why?

   _____

   _____

   _____

80. Katie tells you that she has a pain in her right, lower back. She does not know why her back hurts because she has not done any strenuous activity. She slept comfortably but the pain began that morning while she was showering. What may be the source of this pain?

   _____

   _____

   _____

81. Sasha complains that she has had severe back pain for several days. She then states that the pain mysteriously disappeared after she urinated. Provide a plausible explanation for this phenomenon.

   _____

   _____

   _____

82. Some antihypertensive drugs, termed angiotensin-converting enzyme (ACE) inhibitors, are targeted at the kidneys. Why would a drug that is supposed to lower blood pressure target the kidneys?

   _____

   _____

   _____

83. You are a safe driver, always wear your seat belt, but are in a hurry to make it home for Thanksgiving break. The Wednesday before the holiday, you realize that you have been riding in the automobile for several hours, have drunk three cups of coffee, and have not stopped to urinate. All of a sudden, the car crashes. You arrive at the emergency room with no injuries except a ruptured bladder. Provide a plausible explanation for the ruptured bladder.

_____

_____

_____

84. Your doctor has asked for a routine urine sample. After her initial inspection, she notices an unusual color and odor. She asks if you have been megadosing on multivitamins and eating an overabundance of green, leafy vegetables. What may have prompted these questions?

_____

_____

_____

KEY TERMS SPELLING TEST FROM CD-ROM

Use the CD-ROM to test yourself on the spelling of key terms from this chapter. Listen to the terms and write them on a separate sheet of paper. Use a medical dictionary to check your answers.

ANSWERS

WORD GROUPING

Definition	Word Part
sweet, glucose	glyc-, glyco-
beside, near to, juxtamedullary nephron	juxta-
blood	hem-, hemo-, hemato-
condition of urine	-uria
covering, renal cortex	cortic-, cortico-
drooping, sinking down	-ptosis
force away, detrusor muscle	detrus-
glomerulus, small rounded mass	glomerul-, glomerulo-
hardening	scler-, sclero-
kidney	A. nephr-, nephro-
	B. ren-, reno-
meatus, opening	meat-, meato-
nearest	prox-, proxim-, proximo-
night	noct-, nocti-, nocto-, noctu-
nipple-like	papillo-
nitrogen, nitrogenous	azot-, azoto-
presence of ketone group (chemical compound)	ket-, keto-
pus	py-, pyo-
renal pelvis	pyel-, pyelo-
scanty, little	olig-, oligo-
small cup, calyces	calyc-
stone	lith-, litho-, -lith
to pass urine	mict-
triangular shape	trigon-
urethra	urethr-, urethro-
urinary bladder	cyst-, cysti-, cysto-
urinary tube, urinary	ureter-, utero-
urine	urin-, urino-
urine, urinary	ur-, uro-
vessel	vas-, vasi-, vaso-
water	hydr-, hydro-

WORD BUILDING

Word Part	Meaning	Common or Known Word	Example Medical Term
prox-, proxim-, proximo-	nearest	proximity	proximal convoluted tubule
cortic-, cortico-	covering, renal cortex	cortical	cortex
cyst-, cysti-, cysto-	urinary bladder	cystic	cystitis
glyc-, glyco-	sweet, glucose	glycogen	glycosuria
hem-, hemo-, hemato	blood	hemoglobin	hematuria
hydr-, hydro-	water	hydrogen	hydronephritis
juxta-	beside, near to, juxtamedullary nephron	juxtaposition	juxtamedullary
lith-, -lith, litho-	stone	lithograph	lithotripsy
ren-, reno-	kidney	renal	renin
scler-, sclero-	hardening	sclera	sclerosis
ur-, uro-	urine, urinary	urine	urine
ureter-, utero-	urinary tube, urinary	ureter	ureter
urethr-, urethro-	urethra	urethra	urethritis
urin-, urino-	urine	urine	urinary

KEY TERM PRACTICE

Urinary System Preview

1. a. filtration; b. resorption; c. secretion; d. excretion
2. kidneys

Kidneys

1. cortex; medulla
2. nephron

Ureters, Bladder, and Urethra

1. meatus; orifice
2. trigone
3. ruga; rugae

Kidney Physiology and Urine Formation

1. fenestra; fenestrae
2. renin
3. arteries; veins

Urinalysis

1. glycosuria; glucosuria
2. proteinuria; albuminuria

General Kidney Disorders

1. renal calculi
2. kidney; inflammation; nephritis

Glomerular Disorders

1. nephrosis
2. glomerular filtration rate
3. glomerulonephritis

Kidney Function Disorders

1. Uremia
2. Renal failure; end-stage renal disease (ESRD) or end-stage renal failure (ESRF)

Diabetes

1. glomerulosclerosis
2. urinary retention

Urinary Tract Infections

1. renal pelvis; kidney; inflammation; pyelonephritis
2. clean-catch urine specimen
3. urethritis

Inherited and Congenital Kidney Disorders

1. Polycystic kidney disease
2. epispadias; hypospadias
3. phimosis

Cancer

1. renal cell carcinoma
2. Wilms

Urinary Bladder Disorders

1. enuresis
2. incontinence

CASE STUDY

1. d is the correct answer.
   - a is incorrect because umbilical describes the anterior navel region.
   - b is incorrect because cervical describes the neck region.
   - c is incorrect because the lumbar describes the lower back or hip region.
2. c is the correct answer.
   - a is incorrect because he had not been engaged in any sort of physical activity that may have pulled or stretched his muscle.
   - b is incorrect because the abdominal aorta runs centrally throughout the abdominal cavity.
   - d is incorrect because the spleen is located in the left hypochondriac region, just above the left kidney.
3. a is the correct answer.
   - b is incorrect because burning during urination is a classic sign of bacterial infection not renal calculi.
   - c is incorrect because burning during urination is a classic sign of bacterial infection not ureter calculi.
   - d is incorrect because burning during urination is a classic sign of bacterial infection not renal carcinoma.
4. d is the correct answer.
   - b is incorrect because beets will cause the urine to have a reddish brown color.

5. b is the correct answer.
   - a is incorrect because the normal urine pH range is 4.6–8.0.
   - c is incorrect because the urine would appear red. Furthermore, when a high volume of blood is lost, it may result in anemia, which would elevate the pH.
   - d is incorrect because in anemic states, the pH is elevated.
6. d is the correct answer.
   - c is incorrect because increased fluids leads to a low specific gravity.
7. d is the correct answer.
   - a is incorrect because hematuria is the term for blood in the urine.
   - b is incorrect because oliguria is the term for scanty urine output.
   - c is incorrect because anuria is the term for absence of urination.
8. a is the correct answer.
   - b is incorrect because an IVP does not detect a pulled muscle. Soft tissue injuries are more appropriately diagnosed by other measures.
   - c is incorrect because an IVP does not detect hematuria, which would be determined through microscopic examination of the urine.
   - d is incorrect because an IVP does not detect gout, which is characterized by severe joint pain and uric acid crystals in the blood.

REAL WORLD REPORT

1. bladder stones
2. a. blood; b. urine; c. blood in the urine
3. Uropathy, a disorder involving the urinary tract.

REVIEW AND APPLICATION: THREE-LEVEL LEARNING SYSTEM

Level One: Reviewing Facts and Terms Using Recall

1. l
2. j
3. k
4. c
5. g
6. d
7. f
8. b
9. e
10. h
11. i
12. a
13. b
14. a
15. c
16. d
17. c
18. a
19. d
20. b
21. d
22. c
23. d
24. b
25. a
26. scanty, little
27. force away, detrusor muscle
28. drooping, sinking down
29. stone
30. condition of urine

Level Two: Reviewing Concepts

31. b
32. a
33. d
34. c
35. d
36. a
37. d
38. a
39. a
40. d
41. c
42. d
43. a
44. d
45. c
46. b
47. a
48. b
49. g
50. f
51. a
52. b
53. c
54. d
55. e
56. c
57. a
58. b
59. e
60. d
61. e
62. d
63. a
64. c
65. b
66. c
67. b
68. e
69. a
70. d
71. kidney, ureter, bladder
72. end stage renal disease
73. intravenous pyelogram
74. urinalysis
75. blood urea nitrogen

Level Three: Thinking Critically

76. d
77. c
78. d
79. ADH is secreted by the body to conserve water. Therefore, it is secreted during times of dehydration or when the body is lacking fluids. If Kelsey had been drinking a few beers, she obviously had plenty of fluid intake and would not be secreting ADH. Thus Marcy is correct: ADH secretion is suppressed when the body has plenty of circulating fluid.
80. Katie's pain is probably not muscle related if she has not been engaged in physical activity. Although she may have pulled a muscle by twisting or turning unnaturally, her pain may be the result of a kidney problem. Katie describes her pain at the location where the kidneys are found. Kidney pain frequently indicates an infection or kidney stones, called renal calculi.
81. Sasha may have been suffering from pain secondary to a kidney stone or renal calculus. She may have passed (excreted) the stone while urinating, thus the source of the pain was removed.

82. The kidneys play a role in raising blood pressure through the renin-angiotensin mechanism. ACE inhibitors target this mechanism. Renin, produced by the juxtaglomerular cells of the kidney, is important for blood pressure regulation. When blood pressure drops below a certain level, renin is released from the kidneys. Renin is essential for the conversion of angiotensinogen (a normal constituent of blood) to angiotensin 1. Angiotensin-converting enzymes in the lung capillaries are then required for the conversion of angiotensin 1 to angiotensin 2. The drugs known as ACE inhibitors block the release of these angiotensin-converting enzymes. If their release is blocked, blood pressure cannot increase; therefore, this limits the amount the kidneys can increase the pressure.

83. The accident occurred while the bladder was full. In a normal, seated position, the lap seat belt rests on the abdomen at the point of the urinary bladder. Because of the increased pressure on the full bladder, the lap belt was able to rupture the bladder. The lesson to be learned is to take frequent breaks while driving to empty the bladder and thus thwart the possibility of rupturing the bladder should you get in an accident.

84. Water-soluble vitamins are excreted in the urine. If you are megadosing on them, the body cannot make use of them all and will excrete the excesses. Vitamins in the urine have an unpleasant odor. Many plant pigments found in green, leafy vegetables are not broken down in the body and are frequently excreted in the urine, giving the urine a darker color. Although eating these vegetables is not detrimental to one's health, and in fact is beneficial, the urine will appear to have a deeper hue instead of the characteristic pale yellow color.

16

Reproductive Systems

OBJECTIVES

After completing this chapter, you should be able to:

1. Define the meaning of word parts relating to the reproductive systems.
2. Identify organs of the male and female reproductive systems.
3. Cite a function of each reproductive organ.
4. Describe available birth control methods and practices.
5. Define common signs, symptoms, and treatments of various reproductive system diseases.
6. Explain clinical tests and diagnostic procedures related to the reproductive systems.
7. Describe anatomical and physiological alterations throughout the lifespan.
8. Define abbreviations related to the reproductive systems.
9. Define terms used in medical reports involving the reproductive systems.
10. Correctly define, spell, and pronounce the chapter's medical terms.

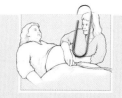

Professional Profile: Midwife

Martha is a midwife, with professional expertise in the area of gynecologic and reproductive health of women, including obstetrics, childbirth, and childcare. Most midwives practice in an obstetric and gynecology office under the supervision of a physician, with privileges extended to a variety of settings such as hospitals and birthing centers. Midwifery embraces the holistic (treating the mind and the body) approach to women's health care by emphasizing the interrelatedness among physical, mental, and social conditions surrounding a patient, instead of just the physical symptoms. For example, midwifery (MID wif ree or MID wif fur ee) views childbirth as a normal physiological process in which medical intervention should usually be limited.

Midwives have practiced since biblical times. In 1955, the first professional midwifery society, the American College of Nurse Midwives (ACNM), was established. The ACNM developed a national certification system during the 1970s: the certified nurse midwife (CNM). Beginning in the 1980s, midwives received legal authority (prescriptive licensure) to write prescriptions and were able to collect insurance reimbursements and practice in hospitals and clinics. Then, in 1985, the Institute of Medicine not only highly endorsed midwifery but also recommended its use. Today, midwives attend (oversee) approximately 10% of American births.

Although the CNM licensure is legal in all states, most require that a midwife have an agreement with a physician for consultation purposes. The focus is on maintaining wellness throughout life, so midwives are frequently the primary-care health provider for women. Research has shown that women are satisfied with and prefer care by midwives because of the strong patient–practitioner interaction. In addition, midwives recognize when cases are outside their scope of practice and necessitate referral.

For those interested in becoming a midwife, there are two career paths. One is the ACNM route, in which the individual is trained in nursing and midwifery; the other is the direct-entry track through the Midwifery Education Accreditation Council (MEAC), which is designed for individuals who do not have a nursing degree. Martha completed a university-affiliated nurse midwifery program that was accredited by the ACNM, which makes her an advanced practice nurse. Her program enabled her to receive a bachelor of science in nursing (BSN). After an additional 2 years of graduate study, Martha was certified in midwifery. Her program was rich in classroom study, clinical experience, and practice in both a hospital and a birthing center. To attain licensure, she then passed the national nursing boards along with the written CNM examination.

INTRODUCTION

Ova are the biggest human body cells and can be seen with the naked eye!

The reproductive system is responsible for the continuation of the human species, and it is the only body system that differs significantly between the sexes. Male sex cells called sperm and female sex cells known as ova (eggs) carry the genetic information that creates unique individuals. Internal and external structures, accessory glands and organs, and ova and sperm play interactive, interdependent roles in ensuring the process. Despite the necessity of the reproductive systems for propagating human life, men and women can function quite well when some reproductive organs must be removed for medical reasons. In addition to normal anatomy and physiology, the signs, symptoms, diagnostic tests and clinical procedures associated with reproductive pathology are considered in this chapter.

MEDICAL TERM PARTS

WORD PARTS

Medical term prefixes, suffixes, and combining forms related to the reproductive systems are introduced in this section.

Word Parts	Meaning
acr-, acro-	tip, end, head
andr-, andro-	male, masculine
arch-, arche-, archi-	beginning, first, original
balan-, balano-	glans penis
-cele	swelling, tumor, hernia
cervic-, cervico-	neck, cervix, cervical
colp-, colpo-, -colpos	vagina, vaginal
crypt-, crypto-	hidden, covered
embry-, embryo-	embryo
epididym-, epididymo-	epididymis
gam-, gamo-	sexual, generative
-genesis	origination, development
gyn-, gyne-, -gyne, gyneco-	female, woman
hyster-, hystero-	uterus
labio-	labial, lip
leio-, lio-	smooth
mamm-, mammo-	breast
mammill-, mammillo-	nipple
mast-, masto-	breast
meat-, meato-	meatus, opening
men-, meno-	menses, menstruation
metr-, metro-	uterus
olig-, oligo-	few, deficiency
oo-	egg, ovum
oophor-, oophoro-	ovary, ovarian
orch-, orchi-, orcho-, orchid-, orchido-	testis
ovari-, ovario-	ovary, ovarian
ovi-, ovo-	egg
pelvi-, pelvio-, pelvo-	pelvis
perineo-	perineum
proct-, procto-	rectum or anus
prostat-, prostato-	prostate gland

Word Parts	Meaning
salping-, salpingo-	uterine tube
sperm-, sperma-, spermi-, spermio-	sperm, semen, seed
spermat-, spermato-	spermatozoa, spermatic, seminal
-spermia	condition of spermatozoa or semen
uter-, utero-	uterus, uterine
vagin-, vagino-	vagina, vaginal

WORD ETYMOLOGY

Some words have Greek or Latin word roots but are not true word parts. This section lists those that are used as medical terms.

Word	Definition
genitalis	pertaining to reproductive organs
gyne	woman
kleitoris	clitoris
klimax	staircase
kryptos	hidden, concealed
mensis	month

MEDICAL TERM PARTS USED AS PREFIXES

Prefix	Definition
labio-	labial, lip
oo-	egg, ovum
perineo-	perineum

MEDICAL TERM PARTS USED AS SUFFIXES

Suffix	Definition
-cele	swelling, tumor, hernia
-colpos	vagina, vaginal
-genesis	origination, development
-gyne	female, woman
-spermia	condition of spermatozoa or semen

WORD GROUPING

Using the "Medical Term Parts" tables, identify the prefix, suffix, or combining form for each of the following definitions. The first one has been done as an example.

Definition	Word Part
male, masculine	andr-, andro-
beginning, first, original	
breast	A. B.
condition of spermatozoa or semen	
egg	
egg, ovum	
embryo	
epididymis	
female, woman	
few, deficiency	
glans penis	
hidden, covered	
labial, lip	
meatus, opening	
menses, menstruation	
neck, cervix, cervical	
nipple	
origination, development	
ovary, ovarian	A. B.
pelvis	
perineum	
prostate gland	
rectum or anus	
sexual, generative	
smooth	
sperm, semen, seed	
spermatozoa, spermatic, seminal	
swelling, tumor, hernia	
testis	
tip, end, head	
uterine tube	

Definition	Word Part
uterus	A. B.
uterus, uterine	
vagina, vaginal	A. B.

WORD BUILDING

Word parts, introduced in the "Medical Term Parts" section, are listed in the following table. For this exercise, first supply the meaning of each word part, then use the word part to build a word you already know. The word you list under "Common or Known Word" does not have to be a medical term; a commonly used word is fine. Be sure, however, that the word correctly reflects the intended meaning. The first one has been done as an example.

Word Part	Meaning	Common or Known Word	Example Medical Term
arch-, arche-, archi-	beginning, first, original	menarche	menarche
andr-, andro-			androgens
cervic-, cervico-			cervical cancer
crypt-, crypto-			cryptorchidism
embry-, embryo-			embryonic
gam-, gamo-			gamete
-genesis			oogenesis
gyn-, gyne-, -gyne, gyneco-			gynecomastia
hyster-, hystero-			hysterectomy
mamm-, mammo-			mammary gland
mammill-, mammillo-			mammilla
meat-, meato-			urethral meatus
men-, meno-			menopause
orch-, orchi-, orcho-, orchid-, orchido-			orchiectomy
ovari-, ovario-			ovarian
ovi-, ovo-			oviduct
pelvi-, pelvio-, pelvo-			pelvic examination
proct-, procto-			proctocele
prostat-, prostato-			prostatitis
sperm-, sperma-, spermi-, spermio-			spermiogenesis
spermat-, spermato-			spermatogenesis
uter-, utero-			uterus
vagin-, vagino-			vaginitis

Structures of the Reproductive Systems

- Male structures
  - Penis
  - Prostate
  - Scrotum
  - Testes
- Female structures
  - Mammary glands
  - Ovaries
  - Uterine tubes
  - Uterus
  - Vagina

Reproductive Systems Preview

Human **reproduction** is the process by which genetic material is sexually passed from one generation to the next via the formation of a new person. Numerous organs and associated structures enable **procreation** (production of offspring by reproduction). A general term used to describe an organ that produces **gametes** (reproductive cells) for procreation is **gonad**. Male gonads are testes, and female gonads are ovaries. The reproductive anatomy of each sex is described in this chapter.

Male reproductive structures include accessory glands and organs, ducts, and external genitalia (Fig. 16-1). Accessory glands and organs that secrete fluids and ducts that

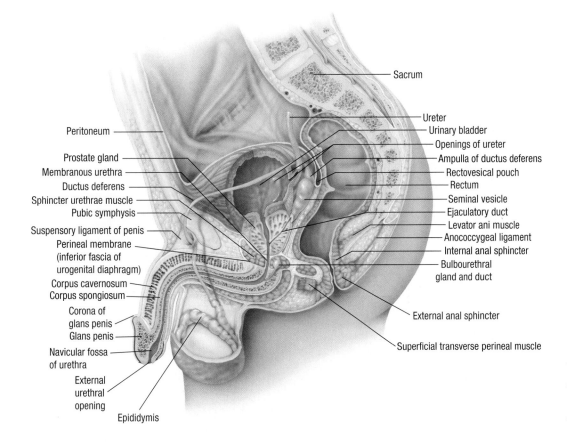

FIGURE 16-1

The male reproductive structures. (Image provided by Anatomical Chart Co.)

transport, receive, and store gametes accomplish the primary functions. The male gametes unite with the female's ova. The male external genitalia are the testes and penis. A major gland is the **prostate**, a round, fluid-secreting organ surrounding the urethra, just inferior to the bladder. **Testes** (sing., testis), also called **testicles**, are the paired glands situated within the scrotum that produce sperm and hormones; the **penis** is the external organ of copulation (sexual intercourse). The word *sperm* is synonymous with *spermatozoa*. The **scrotum** (scrotal sac) is a fleshy pouch hanging from the pelvic region that encloses the testes. The visible exterior ridge joining the two halves of the scrotum is called the **raphe**, derived from the Greek word for "seam." Hormones from the hypothalamus, adenohypophysis (anterior pituitary), and testes control male reproductive functions.

The primary purposes of the female reproductive system are to produce ova, secrete sex hormones, receive sperm from the male, nourish a developing embryo and fetus, deliver a baby, and nurse an infant. These functions are accomplished through the actions of several organs, including paired mammary glands, ovaries, and uterine tubes; the single uterus and vagina; and the external genitalia (Fig. 16-2).

The **mammary glands** (breasts) are milk-producing structures composed of a network of ducts and cavities leading to the nipple. The **ovaries** produce eggs and female sex hormones. Two narrow tubes that serve as a passageway from the ovaries to the uterus are termed **uterine tubes.** The **uterus** (womb) is the hollow muscular organ in the pelvic region in which a developing embryo and fetus is nourished before birth. An embryo is the early developmental stage that begins at conception and ends at the 8th week of gestation. From the 8th week until birth, the developing human is referred to as a fetus. In the absence of pregnancy, the uterine lining is shed monthly during menstruation. The **vagina** is a muscular tube connecting the uterus to the outside. Hormones from the hypothalamus, adenohypophysis, ovaries, and uterus control female reproductive functions.

The **perineum** is the region surrounding the urogenital and anal openings. In females, it is found between the **vulva** (external genitalia) and the anus; in males the perineum is between the scrotum and the anus.

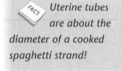

Uterine tubes are about the diameter of a cooked spaghetti strand!

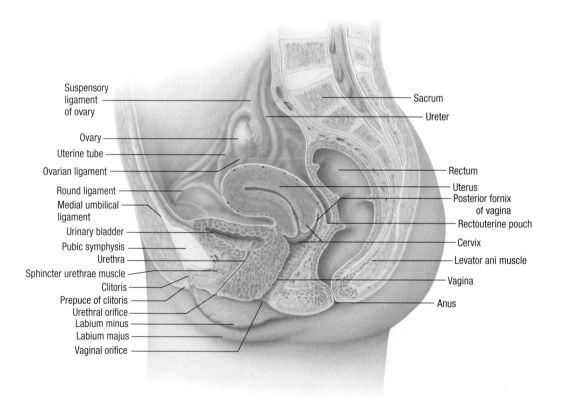

FIGURE 16-2

The female reproductive structures. (Image provided by Anatomical Chart Co.)

Key Terms	Definitions
reproduction	organisms giving rise to organisms of the same kind
procreation (proh kree AY shun)	producing offspring
gametes (GAM eets)	egg and sperm reproductive cells
gonad (GOH nad)	general term for ovary or testis
prostate (PROS tate)	organ surrounding the neck of the urinary bladder and beginning of the urethra and the largest auxiliary gland of the male reproductive system
testis; pl. testes (TES tis; TES teez)	male gonad(s) or reproductive gland(s); testicle(s)
testicles (TES ti kulz)	male gonads or reproductive glands; testes
penis	male organ of copulation and urination
scrotum (SKROH tum)	pouch containing the testes
raphe (RAY fee)	seam or ridge indicating the junction of symmetrical halves
mammary (MAM uh ree) **glands**	breasts
ovaries (OH vur eez)	pair of glandular organs that contain and release ova
uterine (YOO tur in) **tubes**	structures connecting the ovaries to the uterus; oviducts, fallopian tubes
uterus (YOO tur us)	womb or organ of gestation
vagina (vuh JYE nuh)	musculomembranous canal from the uterus to outside the body
perineum (perr i NEE um)	region between the anus and the scrotum in males and between the anus and the vulva in females
vulva (VUL vuh)	female external genitals

Key Term Practice: Reproductive Systems Preview

1. What are the singular and plural forms for the term that means egg and sperm reproductive cell?

   singular = _____

   plural = _____

2. What are the singular and plural forms for the term that means a male gonad?

   singular = _____

   plural = _____

3. What is the anatomic term for each of the following definitions?

   a. region between the urogenital openings and the anus _____

   b. collective term describing the female external genitalia _____

Male Internal Genitalia

Male reproductive structures are divided into internal and external genitalia. Male internal genitalia include the testis, epididymis, spermatic cord, ductus deferens (vas deferens), seminal vesicle, and prostate. Important structures and functions are described in this section.

The testes are a pair of oval-shaped structures located within the scrotum and have two primary functions: **spermatogenesis** (the formation of sperm cells) and hormone production (Fig. 16-3). Before the testes can be fully functional, they must drop from the pelvic cavity. A fibromuscular cord called the **gubernaculum** connects the fetal testis to the developing scrotum and guides the descent of each testicle to its permanent position.

The **tunica albuginea**, composed of membranous connective tissue, form septa that partition the testes into lobules, which contain tubules. The **seminiferous tubules** are approximately 800 tightly coiled structures, about 80 cm (32 in.) long, in which spermatogenesis occurs. The **rete testis** is a maze of tightly coiled passageways that are drained by the **efferent ductules**, which are the transport tubes for sperm. Because *efferent* means "away," these ducts carry sperm away from the body to the exterior.

Each testis contains a tightly coiled tube attached to the posterior border called the **epididymis.** The comma-shaped epididymides are nearly 7 m (23 ft.) in length. The

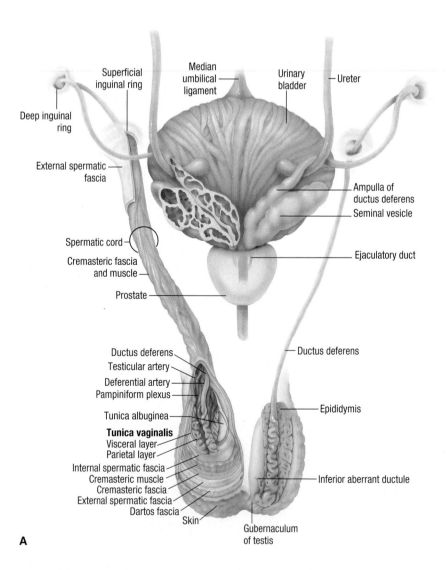

FIGURE 16-3

The testes and their relationship to the bladder and prostate, (A) posterior view and

A

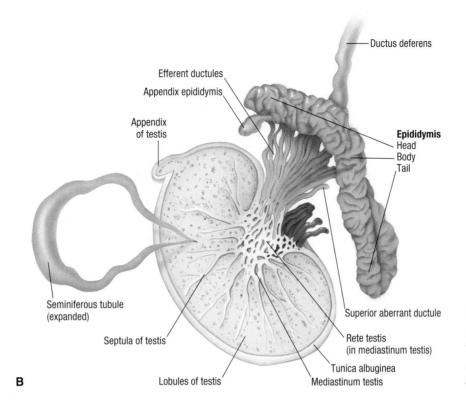

Ductus deferens

Efferent ductules

Appendix epididymis

Appendix of testis

Epididymis
Head
Body
Tail

Seminiferous tubule (expanded)

Septula of testis

Superior aberrant ductule

Rete testis (in mediastinum testis)

Tunica albuginea

Lobules of testis

Mediastinum testis

B

FIGURE 16-3
(Continued) (**B**) sagittal section. (Images provided by Anatomical Chart Co.)

functions of these tubes are monitoring and adjusting the composition of the fluid produced by the seminiferous tubules, serving as a recycling center for damaged sperm cells, and storing and protecting the maturing sperm.

The term *vas* means "a vessel or duct," and the **vas deferens** are a pair of ducts that carry sperm from the testes to the urethra during ejaculation. Another name for the vas deferens is the **ductus deferens.** This muscular structure is 41–46 cm (16–18 in.) long and begins at the tail of the epididymis. It serves as the connecting vessel between the epididymis and the ejaculatory duct. Sperm can remain in the vas deferens for more than 1 month. The **spermatic cord** travels through the inguinal canal to the testes and encloses the vas deferens, arteries, veins, lymphatics, and nerves in each testis.

The prostate, a gland about 4 cm (1.6 in.) in diameter, produces a slightly acidic solution called prostatic fluid. Other fluid-secreting glands, located at the base of the penis just inferior to the prostate, are the **bulbourethral glands,** which are also called Cowper glands. The name of these paired structures describes their location at the bulb of the urethra. The fluid they secrete serves to lubricate the tip of the penis just before the ejaculation of semen.

Semen is the thick, white fluid containing **spermatozoa,** the male reproductive gametes. Semen is also referred to as *ejaculate* because this is the fluid that is ejected from the penis during orgasm. The **seminal vesicles** are paired glands that secrete seminal fluid into the ejaculatory duct. This alkaline, viscous fluid contains fructose, prostaglandins, and fibrinogen. Fructose is needed for sperm energy production; prostaglandins aid sperm movement toward the egg and stimulate muscular contractions in the female reproductive organs after ejaculation into the vagina; and fibrinogen forms a temporary clot in the vagina, which protects the inner mass of sperm cells from the vagina's inhospitable environment. The alkalinity of the fluid neutralizes the secretions from the prostate gland and the acidic vagina. Fluid from the seminal vesicles is the last fluid to be expelled from the urethra during ejaculation. To summarize, the structures secreting seminal fluid substances are the testes, epididymides, prostate, bulbourethral glands, and seminal vesicles.

The union of the seminal vesicle duct and the vas deferens forms the **ejaculatory duct.** It is < 2 cm (1 in.) long and empties into the urethra. The duct pathway through the testes is as follows:

seminiferous tubules → rete testis → efferent ductules →

epididymides → vas deferens → ejaculatory duct → urethra

Key Terms	Definitions
spermatogenesis (spur muh toh JEN e sis)	production of spermatozoa
gubernaculum (gew bur NACK yoo lum)	fibrous cord in the inguinal canal that guides the testes in their descent outside the pelvic cavity
tunica albuginea (TEW ni kuh al bew JIN ee uh)	dense connective tissue in the testes
seminiferous tubules (sem i NIF ur us TEW bewlz)	tubules of the testes where sperm are manufactured
rete testis (REE tee TES tis)	network of blood vessels in the testes
efferent ductules (EF ur unt DUCK tewlz)	ducts that connect the rete testis with the epididymides
epididymis; pl. epididymides (ep i DID i mis; ep i DID i mi deez)	portion(s) of the seminal duct connected to the testis (testes) by the efferent ductules
vas deferens (VAS DEF uh renz)	portion between the epididymis and the ejaculatory duct; ductus deferens
ductus deferens (DUCK tus DEF uh renz)	portion between the epididymis and the ejaculatory duct; vas deferens
spermatic (spur MAT ick) **cord**	paired structure consisting of fascia and muscle that encloses the ductus deferens, blood vessels, nerves, and lymphatic vessels in each testis
bulbourethral (bul boh yoo REE thrul) **glands**	pair of glands located in the urogenital diaphragm, anterior to the prostate gland; Cowper glands
semen (SEE mun)	fluid of the male reproductive organs that contains spermatozoa
spermatozoon; pl. spermatozoa (spur muh toh ZOH un; spur muh toh ZOH uh)	mature sperm cell(s)
seminal vesicles (SEM i nul VES i kulz)	glands of the male reproductive tract that produce the majority of the volume of semen
ejaculatory (ee JACK yoo luh toh ree) **duct**	one of two ducts that pass within the prostate gland, connecting the ductus deferens with the prostatic urethra

Key Term Practice: Male Internal Genitalia

1. What are the singular and plural forms of the term that describes the portion of the seminal duct connected to each testis by the efferent ductules?

   singular = _____

   plural = _____

2. What are the singular and plural forms of the term that means mature sperm cell?

   singular = _____

   plural = _____

3. The word part _____ refers to "spermatozoa," and the word part _____ means "formation of;" therefore, the word _____ means the production of sperm cells.

Male External Genitalia

Male external genitalia include the scrotum, penis, and urethra. The temperature required for normal sperm formation is approximately 3°F below normal body temperature; hence sperm are produced in the scrotum, which is located outside the pelvic cavity where body heat is cooler. Contraction of the **cremaster** muscle, an extension of the internal oblique abdominal muscle covering the spermatic cord and testis, regulates testicle temperature by raising or lowering the scrotum, based on ambient temperature. The smooth muscle responsible for the appearance of the scrotum is the **dartos.** This muscle pulls the scrotal skin close to the testes for temperature regulation. The scrotal sac wrinkles when the muscle contracts, thereby reducing the surface area for heat loss. Males can be sterile, incapable of inducing pregnancy, if the temperature is too high to produce viable sperm. Both the dartos and cremaster muscles contract in response to cold temperature and sexual arousal.

In addition to urination, the penis is considered the organ of **coitus** (sexual intercourse or **copulation**). The **urethra** is the central tube within the penis and has two jobs: It carries urine from the bladder out of the body and transports semen during ejaculation. During ejaculation, a valve seals the urethral opening at the bladder so that only semen may be ejaculated from an erect penis. It is 18–20 cm (7–8 in.) long and runs through the center of the prostate gland.

Anatomic features of the penis consist of three regions and a prepuce (Fig. 16-4). The regions are divided into the root, body, and glans penis. The root is the portion that attaches the penis to the body wall. The majority of the structure is called the body or shaft and is composed of three columns of erectile tissue that run the length of the penis. Erectile tissue is capable of filling with blood under pressure to swell and become stiff, resulting in **erection.** The three columns are a pair of columns called the **corpora cavernosa** and a single column (which the urethra) called the **corpus spongiosum.** *Corpora* is the plural form of the word *corpus,* and the corpora cavernosa are two columns of tissues. Associate the *s* in *single* with the *s* in corpu*s s*pongiosum to remember that it is a single column of erectile tissue.

Surrounding the urethral **meatus** (opening) is the **glans penis**, the rounded tip. The last penile structure is the **prepuce,** or foreskin, the loose fold of skin covering the penis tip in uncircumcised males. **Circumcision** is a medical intervention in which the penile prepuce is removed. Circumcision is performed on many infants in the United States; however, this practice is continually debated.

Key Terms	*Definitions*
cremaster (kree MAS tur)	muscle controlling the spermatic cord and testes
dartos (DAHR tohs)	smooth muscle in the subcutaneous tissue of the scrotum

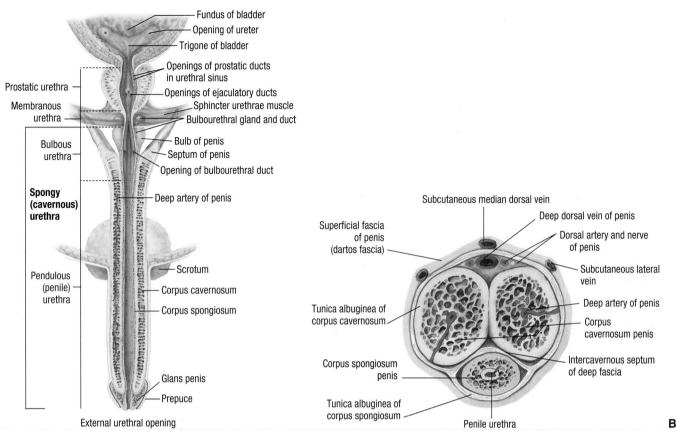

FIGURE 16-4
The penis, (**A**) sagittal section and (**B**) cross section. (Images provided by Anatomical Chart Co.)

coitus (KOH i tus)	act of sexual union; copulation
copulation (kop yoo LAY shun)	act of sexual union; coitus
urethra (yoo REE thruh)	canal through which urine and semen are discharged
erection	enlarged state of the penis erectile tissue, which is engorged with blood
corpora cavernosa (KOR poh ruh kav ur NOH sum)	two cylinders of erectile tissue in the penis
corpus spongiosum (KOR pus spon jee OH sum)	single cylinder of erectile tissue surrounding the urethra in the penis
meatus (mee AY tus)	opening
glans (GLANZ) **penis**	cone-shaped region at the distal end of the penis that is an expansion of the corpus spongiosum
prepuce (PREE pewce)	foreskin or fold of skin covering the glans penis in uncircumcised males
circumcision (sur kum SIZH un)	removal of the prepuce (foreskin) from the penis

Key Term Practice: Male External Genitalia

1. Identify the three columns of erectile tissue composing the penis.

  a. _____

  b. _____

  c. _____

2. What is the singular form for corpora cavernosa? _____

3. Provide the two terms for sexual intercourse. _____

Male Reproductive Hormones

Several hormones, chiefly androgens, are responsible for male reproductive functions. **Androgens** are steroid sex hormones that are responsible for the development of male sex organs and secondary sexual characteristics. **Secondary sexual characteristics** are those features that develop at puberty but are not directly concerned with reproduction. An example of a secondary sexual characteristic is the appearance of facial hair.

   Primary male hormones stimulate gamete development and sex hormone secretion. **Testosterone**, the principal androgen produced, maintains accessory organs and glands of reproduction. **Follicle-stimulating hormone** (FSH) is secreted by the adenohypophysis to stimulate spermatogenesis; and **luteinizing hormone** (LH), from the adenohypophysis, acts with FSH to stimulate testosterone secretion by the interstitial cells in the testes.

Key Terms	Definitions
androgens (AN droh jenz)	hormones promoting the development of male structures and secondary sex characteristics
secondary sexual characteristics	traits that develop at puberty but are not directly concerned with reproduction, such as voice, body hair distribution, and adipose tissue patterns
testosterone (tes TOS tur ohn)	hormone synthesized from cholesterol that is the principal hormone secreted by the testes
follicle- (FOL i kul) **stimulating hormone**	anterior pituitary hormone causing spermatogenesis in testes
luteinizing (LOO tee in eye zing) **hormone**	adenohypophysis hormone that stimulates testosterone secretion

Key Term Practice: Male Reproductive Hormones

1. The general term for the male sex hormones is _____.

2. Traits that develop at puberty but are not directly concerned with reproduction are termed _____.

Spermatogenesis

Spermatogenesis is the formation and development of spermatozoa in the testes and involves mitosis (somatic or nonsex cell division), meiosis (gamete cell division), and spermiogenesis. **Meiosis** is the step in gamete cell division in which the **diploid** (containing 46 chromosomes) sperm cell divides to become a **haploid** cell with 23 chromosomes. Haploid chromosome number is usually designated with the letter n, and the diploid chromosome number is represented by 2n. The father's sperm and the mother's ovum provide chromosomal pairs. Thus the father and mother each contribute 23 single chromosomes to make a fertilized egg with a total of 23 chromosome pairs or 46 single chromosomes.

Through various differential stages, a mature sperm capable of fertilizing a female egg is formed. These progressional stages are spermatogonium, spermatocyte, spermatid, and spermatozoon (Fig. 16-5). **Spermatogonia** are stem cells (cells that give rise to a lineage of cells) that form primary spermatocytes by mitosis. **Spermatocytes** are derived from spermatogonia; these cells are found in the seminiferous tubules and undergo meiosis. **Spermatids** are any of the four cells that are formed from a spermatocyte and develop into a mature male gamete called a spermatozoon. **Spermiogenesis** is the stage of spermatogenesis during which a spermatid is transformed into a spermatozoon.

Sperm are tadpole-shaped cells made in the seminiferous tubules of the testes. A physically mature spermatozoon has four different regions, aptly named the head, neck, middle piece, and tail (Fig. 16-6). The tail is actually a **flagellum** that propels the spermatozoon. The spermatozoon is the only cell in the human body possessing a flagellum. The flagellum's whip-like motion moves the sperm about 4 mm (0.15 in.) per minute. Fructose is absorbed from the surrounding fluid for the energy needed for movement.

FACT *Approximately 300 million sperm are produced daily in both testicles!*

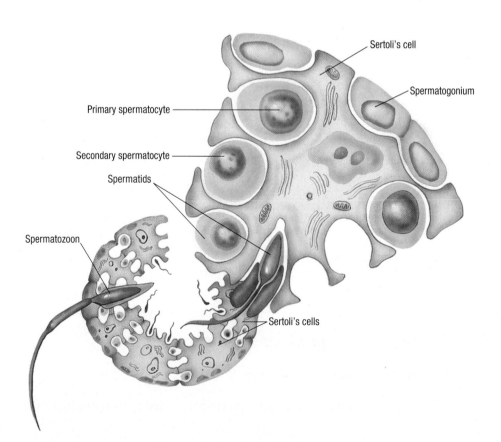

FIGURE 16-5
A sperm goes through differential stages as it matures: spermatogonium, spermatocyte, spermatid, and spermatozoon. (Image provided by Anatomical Chart Co.)

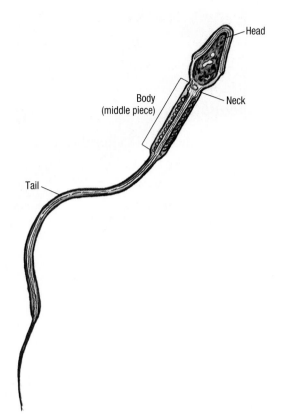

FIGURE 16-6
The mature sperm
has four regions.
(Image provided by
Anatomical Chart Co.)

Male **fertility**, the ability to reproduce, is influenced by sperm factors. For example, sperm number, shape, and motility are important considerations in the reproductive process. Not only must the sperm be perfectly shaped and quite capable of motility but there must be many of them for fertilization; too few sperm results in not enough being able to make the journey to the awaiting ovum. Once in the vagina, spermatozoa undergo an activation process called **capacitation** in which physical changes on the sperm coat permit penetration and fertilization of an egg.

Key Terms	Definitions
meiosis (migh OH sis)	cell division that results in half the number of chromosomes
diploid (DIP loid)	containing 23 pairs or 46 chromosomes
haploid (HAP loid)	containing 23 single chromosomes, characteristic of gametes
spermatogonium (spur muh toh GOH nee um)	primitive (original, undifferentiated) male germ cell
spermatocytes (spur MAT oh sites)	cells at the stage between spermatogonium and spermatid
spermatids (SPUR muh tidz)	sperm cells immediately before their final form
spermiogenesis (spur mee oh JEN e sis)	transformation of spermatids into spermatozoa
flagellum (fla JEL um)	tail on spermatozoon

fertility	ability to bring about fertilization; the union of male and female gametes
capacitation (kuh pas i TAY shun)	activation process allowing sperm to successfully fertilize an oocyte

Key Term Practice: Spermatogenesis

1. What is the sperm cell state immediately before the mature spermatozoon?

   _____

2. What are the singular and plural forms of the term that means the tail on spermatozoa?

   singular = _____

   plural = _____

Female Internal Genitalia

Structures of the female internal genitalia include the ovaries, uterine tubes, uterus, and vagina (Fig. 16-7). The ovaries are paired oval-shaped organs located near the lateral walls in the pelvic cavity. They function to secrete hormones and to produce and release **ova** (sing., ovum), reproductive cells. An **oocyte** is a developing female gamete just before completion and release. **Ovulation** refers to the ripening and release of an ovum from the ovary. Generally, one ovum is released from an ovary every month on an alternating pattern of one ovary one month, the other ovary the next.

Uterine tubes are two narrow structures associated with the ovaries to provide a conduit for ova to the uterus. Alternate names for uterine tubes are fallopian tubes and **oviducts.**

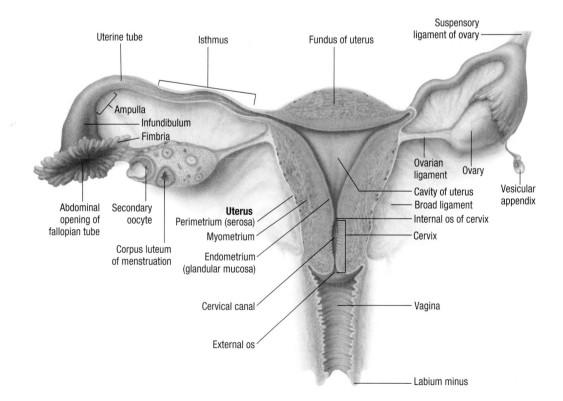

FIGURE 16-7
The ovaries, uterine tubes, uterus, and vagina. (Image provided by Anatomical Chart Co.)

Regions of the uterine tube are the ampulla, infundibulum, and isthmus. The **infundibulum** is the funnel-shaped opening of the oviduct encircling the top portion of the ovary. A gap exists between oviducts and ovaries, thus there is no physical connection. A fringed border of finger-like projections called **fimbriae** forms its outer margins to assist in capturing a recently released ovum and bringing it into the uterine tubes. The **ampulla** is the middle segment between the infundibulum and isthmus, and the **isthmus** connects to the uterus. Sweeping ciliary action and peristalsis facilitate ovum movement through the tubes toward the uterus. The oviducts are the normal site of fertilization by "upstream swimming" sperm, and the normal time for an ovum to reach the uterus is 3–4 days.

The uterus is a hollow, muscular organ located between the urinary bladder and the rectum. Its functions include serving as the site of implantation of a fertilized ovum, protecting and sustaining embryonic and fetal life, playing a role in parturition (childbirth), and serving as the source of menstrual flow in nonpregnant females.

The uterus has three layers. The outer perimetrium is an incomplete tissue layer that does not cover the **cervix**, the uterine portion dipping into the vagina. The middle muscular layer is called the myometrium, and the inner tissue that is shed during menstruation is termed the **endometrium.**

Anatomic features of the uterus are the body, fundus, cervix, and fornix. The main portion of the uterus is termed the body, and the **fundus** is the central, dome-shaped portion of the body. The **fornix** is the recessed portion between the vaginal wall and the cervix. Holding the uterus in place are several ligaments, called the broad, uterosacral, round, and lateral.

The vagina is a muscular canal, 7.6–9 cm (3–3.5 in.) long, located posterior to the urethra. It connects the uterine cervix to the outside. The hymen is a fold of mucous membrane covering the vaginal orifice. It ruptures from a variety of reasons, such as sexual intercourse or tampon use, and it is often absent, even in virgins. Functions of the vagina include receiving the penis during coitus, serving as a passageway for menstrual fluids, and acting as the "birth canal" for a fetus during childbirth.

Key Terms	Definitions
ovum (OH vum)	egg cell capable of developing into another human after fertilization
oocyte (OH oh site)	an egg cell immediately before maturation
ovulation (ov yoo LAY shun)	maturation and discharge of an ovum
oviduct (OH vi dukt)	tube that transports the ovum to the uterus; uterine tube, fallopian tube
infundibulum (in fun DIB yoo lum)	funnel-shaped passage at the superior aspect of the ovary
fimbriae (FIM bree ee)	fringe-like processes on the outer extremity of the infundibulum
ampulla (am PYOOL uh)	section of oviduct between the infundibulum and the isthmus
isthmus (IS mus)	constricted part (neck) of the oviduct connecting to the uterus
cervix (SUR vicks)	section of the uterus dipping into the vagina
endometrium (en doh MEE tree um)	mucous membrane lining the uterus

fundus (FUN dus)	dome-shaped region of the uterus farthest from the vaginal opening
fornix (FOR nicks)	cul-de-sac between the cervix and the vaginal wall

Key Term Practice: Female Internal Genitalia

1. The release of an oocyte from the ovary is termed _____.

2. What is the alternative term for uterine tubes and fallopian tubes? _____

3. What are the singular and plural forms of the term for the section of uterine tube between the infundibulum and the isthmus?

   singular = _____

   plural = _____

4. What are the singular and plural forms of the term that means a funnel-shaped passage on the superior portion of the ovary?

   singular = _____

   plural = _____

Female External Genitalia

Vulva, which literally means "wrapper," is the collective term used to describe the female external genitalia (Fig. 16-8). These genitals are the mons pubis, two pairs of fleshy folds called the labia majora and labia minora, the clitoris, the vestibule, the vaginal and urethral orifices, and the greater and lesser vestibular glands. The **mons pubis** is a subcutaneous pad of adipose tissue encasing the junction of the pubic bones in females. It is covered in pubic hair at puberty. The **labia majora** (sing., labium majus) are two thick outer folds of skin that surround the clitoris, the urethral opening, and the vagina. The **labia minora** (sing., labium minus) are two small folds of skin that lie immediately inside the labia majora and protect the vaginal and urethral openings. The **clitoris**, measuring about 2 cm (1 in.) in length, is highly sensitive erectile tissue richly supplied with sensory nerve endings at the front junction of the labia minora that responds to sexual stimulation.

The central space between the labia minora is the **vestibule.** The vaginal and urethral orifices are the openings to the vagina and urethra, respectively. Lubricating glands associated with the vestibule are the mucus-secreting glands known as the **lesser vestibular glands** (paraurethral glands or Skene glands) and **greater vestibular glands** (Bartholin glands). The greater vestibular glands have the same embryologic origin as the bulbourethral glands in the male.

Key Terms	Definitions
mons pubis (PEW bis)	eminence on the pubic bones
labia majora (LAY bee uh muh JOR uh)	outer folds of the female external genitals
labia minora (LAY bee uh muh NOR uh)	folds on the inner surface of the labia majora

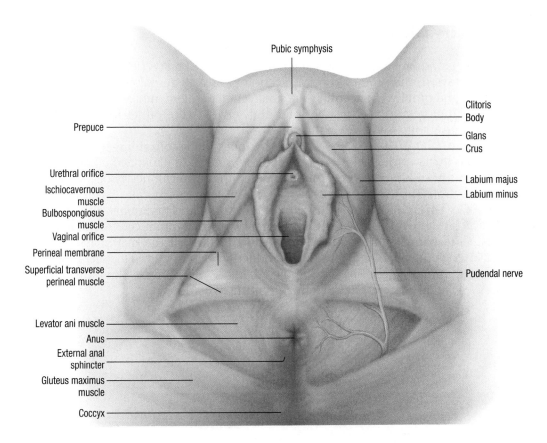

FIGURE 16-8
Female perineum.
(Image provided by
Anatomical Chart Co.)

clitoris (KLIT oh ris)	small, erectile organ at the junction of the labia minora
vestibule (VES ti bewl)	chamber
lesser vestibular (ves TIB yoo lur) **glands**	mucus-secreting glands of the vulva; paraurethral glands, Skene glands
greater vestibular (ves TIB yoo lur) **glands**	mucus-secreting glands opening into the vestibule; Bartholin glands

Key Term Practice: Female External Genitalia

1. What are the singular and plural forms of the term for the outer folds of the female external genitals?

   singular = _____

   plural = _____

2. What are the singular and plural forms of the term for the inner folds of the female external genitals?

   singular = _____

   plural = _____

3. The structure that is supplied with sensory nerve endings that respond to sexual stimulation and is located at the junction of the labia minora is termed the _____.

Mammary Glands

Mammary glands are modified sweat glands within the breasts (Fig. 16-9). Their function is **lactation**, the production and ejection of milk. External components include the areola and nipple. The **areola** is the small, circular pigmented area around the nipple. The nipple marks the breast center and serves as the outlet for the lactiferous (milk-secreting) ducts when breastfeeding.

The glandular tissue is separated into lobes that contain secretory lobules. Lactiferous ducts exiting the secretory lobules form 15–20 expanded chambers called lactiferous sinuses that converge on the nipple surface. Hormones associated with lactation are prolactin (PRL) and oxytocin (OT). **Prolactin** stimulates lactation by contracting lactiferous ducts and sinuses; **oxytocin** stimulates mammary milk ejection.

Breastfeeding involves nourishing an infant with milk produced by the mammary glands. **Colostrum**, or "first milk," is a yellowish fluid of the mammary glands secreted after giving birth and before the production of true milk. This secretion is rich in protein, immunoglobulins, fat-soluble vitamins, and minerals. Breastfeeding suppresses FSH and LH secretion, thereby inhibiting ovulation.

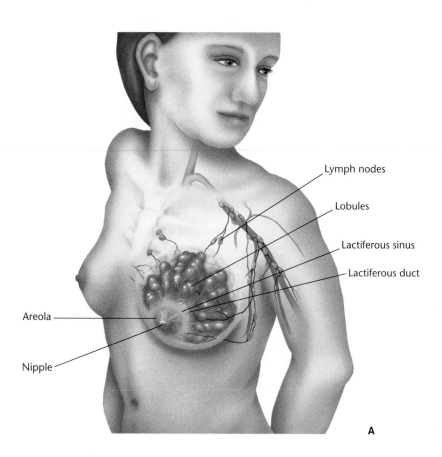

FIGURE 16-9
Mammary gland. (**A**)
Frontal view (Images
provided by
Anatomical Chart Co.)

Key Terms	Definitions
lactation (lack TAY shun)	milk formation and secretion
areola (ah REE oh luh)	pigmented ring surrounding the nipple
prolactin (proh LACK tin)	anterior pituitary hormone that stimulates lactation
oxytocin (ock si TOH sin)	hormone that stimulates uterine contraction and lactation

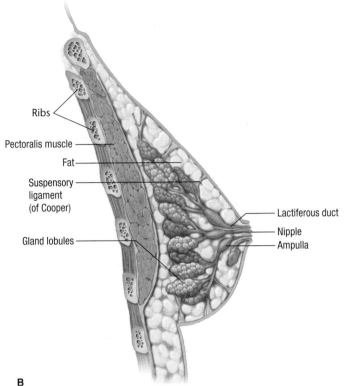

B

FIGURE 16-9
(Continued)
(B) Sagittal section.

colostrum (koh LOS trum)	first milk from a mother's breasts after she's given birth

Key Term Practice: Mammary Glands

1. What are the singular and plural forms of the term describing the pigmented ring surrounding the breast nipple?

   singular = _____

   plural = _____

2. Milk formation and secretion is termed _____.

Female Reproductive Hormones

The female reproductive hormones are estrogens, progestins, relaxin, FSH, inhibin, and LH. **Estrogens** are steroid hormones produced mainly in the ovaries and include estradiol, estrone, and estriol. **Progestins** are steroid hormones manufactured in the corpus luteum (yellow mass of tissue that forms in the ovary after ovulation); the principal progestin is the hormone progesterone. Estrogen supports ovum maturation and female secondary sexual characteristics, and **progesterone** prepares the uterus for embryo implantation and the mammary glands for lactation. **Relaxin** is a hormone produced by the corpus luteum and placenta (organ surrounding fetus) that relaxes the pelvic ligaments and pubic symphysis during pregnancy. Follicle-stimulating hormone stimulates oogenesis (ova formation) in females. The ovary secretes inhibin to halt the anterior pituitary gland's production of FSH. Luteinizing hormone, secreted by the pituitary gland, targets the ovary, causing it to produce ova and trigger ovulation.

Key Terms	Definitions
estrogens (ES troh jenz)	class of female steroid hormones
progestins (proh JES tinz)	generic term for several steroid hormones—principally progesterone, which prepares the uterus for pregnancy
progesterone (proh JES tur ohn)	steroid hormone essential for pregnancy and the menstrual cycle
relaxin (ree LACK sin)	hormone that causes relaxation of the pelvic ligaments and symphysis pubis during pregnancy

Key Term Practice: Female Reproductive Hormones

1. Estradiol, estrone, and estriol are members of a class of female steroid hormones called _____.

2. _____ is the steroid hormone that is essential for embryo implantation and pregnancy maintenance.

Oogenesis

Oogenesis is the process by which ova are formed in the ovaries (Fig. 16-10). Oogenesis begins with an **oogonium**, a stem cell in the ovaries that is formed before birth. A series of differential stages completes the transformation of an oogonium to an ovum. To begin, a daughter cell of an oogonium becomes a diploid **primary oocyte**, which differentiates into a haploid secondary oocyte. This **secondary oocyte** eventually divides into a mature haploid ovum, capable of fertilization by a sperm. The stages follow this sequence:

oogonium → primary oocyte → secondary oocyte → ovum

A sac within the ovary called a **follicle** holds the immature egg cells. Every month, follicles enlarge until one fluid-filled follicle outpaces the others, ruptures, and releases an ovum from an ovary. Ova are about the size of a grain of sand and can be seen without a microscope.

In the female, all mitotic divisions are complete before birth; therefore, a female infant is born with the maximum number of primary oocytes she will ever have. At birth, the infant has approximately 2 million oocytes that remain in a state of suspended development, but by puberty that number drops to about 400,000 or less.

Key Terms	Definitions
oogenesis (oh oh JEN e sis)	process of origin, growth, and formation of an ovum in preparation for fertilization
oogonium (oh oh GOH nee um)	a cell that gives rise to an oocyte
primary oocyte (OH oh site)	stage of cellular differentiation between the oogonium and the secondary oocyte
secondary oocyte (OH oh site)	cell derived from the primary oocyte that transforms into an ovum
follicle (FOL i kul)	bag or sac

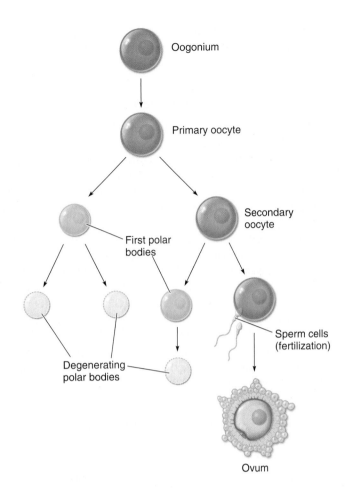

FIGURE 16-10
Oogenesis.

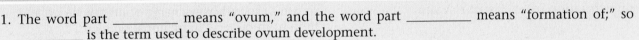

Key Term Practice: Oogenesis

1. The word part _____ means "ovum," and the word part _____ means "formation of;" so _____ is the term used to describe ovum development.

2. The cell of oogenesis formed immediately before the secondary oocyte stage is called a/an _____.

Uterine Cycle

The **uterine cycle** or **menstrual cycle** is the series of phases occurring in the uterus on a 28-day rotation. The phases are menses, proliferative, and secretory. **Menses** marks the beginning of the cycle and lasts until day 7. The Latin word *mensis* means "month," which is related to the English word *moon,* which has an approximately monthly cycle. During menses, the endometrial lining is sloughed (shed). This is commonly called **menstruation,** the monthly process of discharging blood and other matter from the uterus when the woman is not pregnant. The **proliferative phase** is the stage between the end of menses (day 8) and ovulation (day 14). Other terms include postmenstrual, estrogenic, and follicular phases. During the proliferative phase, the increase in blood estrogen causes a growth of small, spiraling arteries on the endometrial wall and an increase in endometrial water content. In essence, the body is preparing the uterus for implantation and nurturing of a developing embryo and fetus.

Day 14, ovulation, marks the release of an ovum. The **secretory phase** (days 15–28) occurs between ovulation and the onset of menses. It is also called the premenstrual, postovulatory, or luteal phase. During this phase, an increase in blood estrogen causes secretion from endometrial cells, an increase in water content of the endometrium, and a decrease in myometrium contractions. The cycle can be illustrated as follows:

Days

| 1 | → | 7 | | 8 | → | 13 | | 14 | | 15 | → | 28 |
| | menses | | | proliferative phase | | | | ovulation | | | secretory phase | |

Terms associated with the uterine cycle include menarche, female climacteric, and menopause. **Menarche** is the first menstrual cycle of a maturing female and typically occurs during puberty, some time between the ages of 8 and 17 years. Vaginal secretions change from alkaline to acidic with menarche. The transitional period leading to menopause is termed the **female climacteric. Menopause** is the diminishing and ultimate cessation of menstrual cycles. The average age of onset is between 45 and 50 years. The characteristic "hot flashes" result from an increase in gonadotropin hormone concentrations and a decrease in estrogen concentrations.

Hormone-replacement therapy (HRT) is used in postmenopausal women to reduce symptoms associated with menopause such as hot flashes, emotional fluctuations, and bone loss. The decision to treat with HRT is made after careful consideration and weighing the benefits versus the effects. Therapy is highly individualized and may require modification, but standard protocols suggest the administration of estrogen-only pills in women without a uterus and a combination estrogen–progesterone pill for women with an intact uterus. Hormone-replacement therapy is contraindicated in some females with estrogen-dependent tumors, history of blood clots, or some other medical condition precluding its use.

Key Terms	Definitions
uterine (YOO tur in) **cycle**	28-day cycle of menstruation; menstrual cycle
menstrual (MEN stroo ul) **cycle**	28-day cycle of menstruation; uterine cycle
menses (MEN seez)	recurrent monthly discharge of uterine blood and fluid from puberty to menopause; menstruation
menstruation (men stroo AY shun)	recurrent monthly discharge of uterine blood and fluid from puberty to menopause; menses
proliferative (proh LIF ur uh tiv) **phase**	stage of the uterine cycle between the end of menses and ovulation
secretory (se KREET uh ree) **phase**	days 15–28 postovulation
menarche (me NAHR kee)	point in puberty when menstruation first begins
female climacteric (klye MACK tur ick)	transitional period leading to menopause
menopause (MEN oh pawz)	physiologic cessation of menstruation
hormone-replacement therapy	treatment used to maintain female hormone levels after menopause

Key Term Practice: Uterine Cycle

1. Postmenstrual, estrogenic, and follicular phases are other terms for the _____ phase, the stage of the uterine cycle between the end of menses and ovulation.

2. The terms used to describe the recurrent 28-day rotation of uterine bloody discharge are _____ cycle and _____ cycle.

Sexual Intercourse

Coitus (sexual intercourse) is an act carried out for reproduction and/or pleasure. It involves the insertion of an erect penis into the vagina. **Arousal** is characterized by the parasympathetic ("breed-and-feed" division) nervous system outflow, resulting in erection of the penis and clitoris and increased secretion from sexual glands.

Intercourse occurs by the sexual response cycle: erection, lubrication, emission, ejaculation, orgasm, and detumescence. In males, erection is characterized by blood accumulating in the erectile tissues, causing the penis to swell and stiffen. Vaginal tissues becoming engorged with blood and creating swelling in those tissues characterize female erection. Male lubrication involves secretion from the bulbourethral glands; in females, the greater and lesser vestibular glands secrete mucus to reduce friction of moving parts during intercourse.

Although **emission** does not occur in females, in males it involves sympathetic stimulation in which subsequent peristaltic contractions push fluid and sperm into the internal prostatic urethra. The prostatic urethra is that segment running through the prostate. **Ejaculation** is the ejecting of semen from the penis during orgasm, thus it does not occur in the female. During ejaculation, ischiocavernosus and bulbospongiosus muscles rhythmically contract to force semen to the outside.

Orgasm (**climax**) is the culmination of sexual excitement characterized by intense psychological and physiological responses in both the male and the female. There is intense muscle tightening around the genitalia accompanied by pleasurable waves of tingling sensations throughout the body. In the female, the uterus, oviducts, and vagina contract rhythmically.

Detumescence is the gradual reduction of swelling as the blood exits erectile tissues. Erection subsides in the male; and in the female, blood leaves the vagina and clitoris and pleasant sensations diminish.

Key Terms	Definitions
arousal	sexual excitement
emission (ee MISH un)	seminal discharge into the internal prostatic urethra
ejaculation (ee jack yoo LAY shun)	sudden ejection of semen during orgasm
orgasm (OR gaz um)	period of greatest sexual intensity; climax
climax	period of greatest sexual intensity; orgasm
detumescence (dee tew MES unce)	subsidence after orgasm

Key Term Practice: Sexual Intercourse

1. _____ involves the discharge of semen into the prostatic urethra, and _____ is the expulsion of this semen from the penis.

2. _____ is characterized by diminished swelling in erectile organs after orgasm.

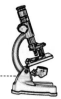

THE CLINICAL DIMENSION

Pathology of the Reproductive Systems

The reproductive system has considerable changes throughout life. One is usually well aware of this system; however, some serious pathologies can be hidden, displaying no signs or symptoms. Unlike with other systems, males and females may have different pathologic conditions because males and females do not contain the same reproductive organs. Some infectious diseases affect both males and females. This section considers birth control methods, sexually transmitted diseases, and a variety of pathologies.

Testicle and Penis Disorders

A congenital anomaly of the penis in which the urethra opens on the ventral surface is termed **hypospadias** (Fig. 16-11). In **epispadias**, another congenital condition, the urethral opening is located on the penis dorsum. Surgery is required to correct the abnormal locations.

Inflammation of the epididymis is known as **epididymitis.** It results from a urinary tract infection (UTI) or sexually transmitted disease. Common disease-causing agents are *Neisseria gonorrhoeae, Chlamydia trachomatis, Escherichia coli,* and members of the *Staphylococcus* and *Streptococcus* genera. Epididymitis is diagnosed by the history and physical examination, urinalysis indicating bacterial presence, and elevated white blood cell count. It is treated with antibiotics and analgesics. If left untreated, it can lead to sterility.

Hydrocele refers to an accumulation of serous fluid in the testis or within the spermatic cord; it often causes swelling of the scrotal sac (Fig. 16-12). Hydroceles that are present at birth generally resolve within 1 year. If the hydrocele persists after 1 year,

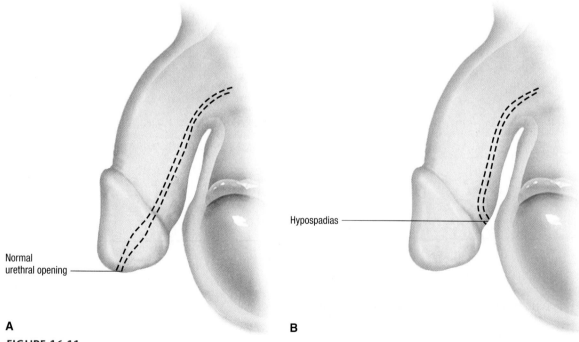

Normal urethral opening

Hypospadias

A

B

FIGURE 16-11

(A) The normal urethral opening. Two congenital disorders are (B) hypospadias and

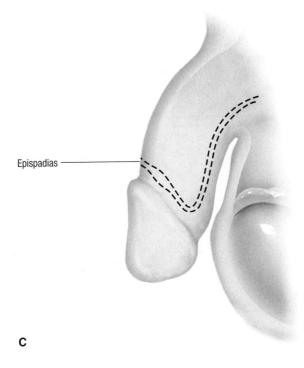

Epispadias

FIGURE 16-11
(Continued) (**C**) epispadias. (Images provided
by Anatomical Chart
Co.)

C

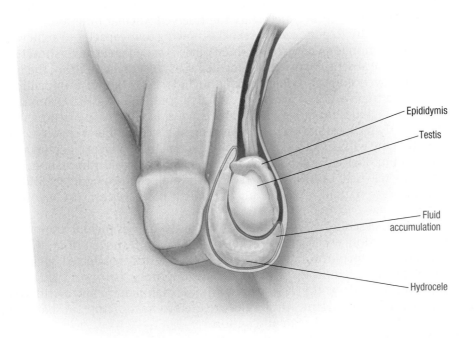

Epididymis

Testis

Fluid
accumulation

Hydrocele

FIGURE 16-12
Hydrocele.
(Image provided by
Anatomical Chart Co.)

surgical ligation is recommended. Hydroceles affecting adults result from the inability
of the scrotal tissue to absorb fluid; are caused by trauma, infection, or tumor; or are idiopathic in nature. The size of the enlargement ranges from slightly larger than the testis
to the size of a grapefruit. Diagnosis is confirmed by ultrasonography, and treatment involves aspirating the fluid and injecting a sclerosing agent to prevent recurrence.

Testicular torsion is a disorder in which the spermatic cord rotates, producing
ischemia of the testis (Fig. 16-13). Signs and symptoms include testicular pain and
swelling. The condition can affect males at any point in life but is most common in
newborns and adolescents. Onset is either spontaneous or may follow physical

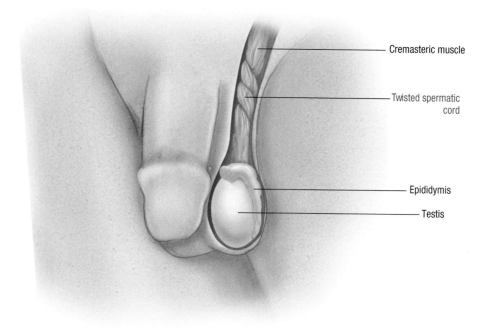

Cremasteric muscle

Twisted spermatic cord

Epididymis

Testis

FIGURE 16-13
Testicular torsion.
(Image provided by
Anatomical Chart Co.)

exertion or injury. An initial urinalysis is performed to rule out infection, and the diagnosis is confirmed by ultrasonography. Immediate treatment by manual manipulation or surgical fixation is necessary to preserve testicular function.

Male inability to perform the sexual act owing to incapacity to achieve or maintain a penile erection long enough for intercourse is called **erectile dysfunction**, or **impotence.** In the absence of disease or medications that affect erection, the most probable cause is psychological. Other reasons include nerve impulse impediment, fatigue, stress, and trauma. It is diagnosed through a complete physical examination and history that includes investigation of medicinal side effects. The treatments depend on the underlying cause and are aimed at causing a sustainable erection. Options include drug therapy with sildenafil citrate (one trade name is Viagra), penile implants, external vacuum devices, and penile injections. During sexual stimulation, nitric oxide is normally released, causing the erectile tissues to become engorged. **Sildenafil citrate** enhances the natural release of nitric oxide; it has no effect in the absence of sexual stimulation.

Orchitis describes inflammation of the testis. Causes include trauma and bacterial or viral infection, especially with rubeola virus, the pathogen of mumps. Severe cases result in atrophy of the affected testicle. If both testes are affected, it can lead to sterility. Signs and symptoms are swelling, tenderness, pain, and flu-like indicators. Diagnosis is made by the history and physical examination and a urinalysis that identifies the causative agent. Antibiotics are used to treat orchitis. A scrotal support may also be necessary to alleviate discomfort.

Testicular cancer, malignant growth in the testicles, has an unknown cause but is associated with **cryptorchidism** (failure of one or both of the testes to descend into the scrotum), inguinal hernia during childhood, and having had mumps (Fig. 16-14). Although rare (it accounts for 1% of all cancers in men), it is the most common type of cancer in men aged 20–35 years. Its primary sign and symptom is a painless testicular lump (Fig. 16-15). It is diagnosed by palpation and a biopsy confirming cancer. It is treated by orchiectomy of the infected testicle, followed by radiation and chemotherapy. The surgical removal of one testicle or both testes is termed an **orchiectomy** or **castration.**

Prompt treatment is necessary to prevent spread to the lymphatic system. Prognosis is good if diagnosed and treated early. Men should perform monthly testicular self-examinations (TSEs) to detect the presence of abnormal growths.

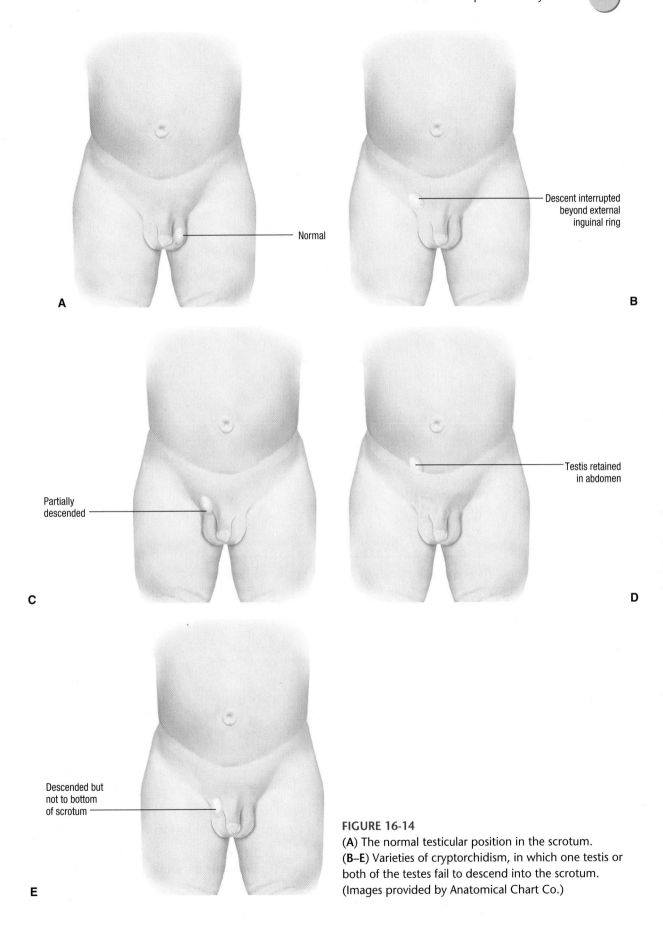

Normal

Descent interrupted
beyond external
inguinal ring

A

B

Partially
descended

Testis retained
in abdomen

C

D

Descended but
not to bottom
of scrotum

E

FIGURE 16-14
(**A**) The normal testicular position in the scrotum.
(**B–E**) Varieties of cryptorchidism, in which one testis or
both of the testes fail to descend into the scrotum.
(Images provided by Anatomical Chart Co.)

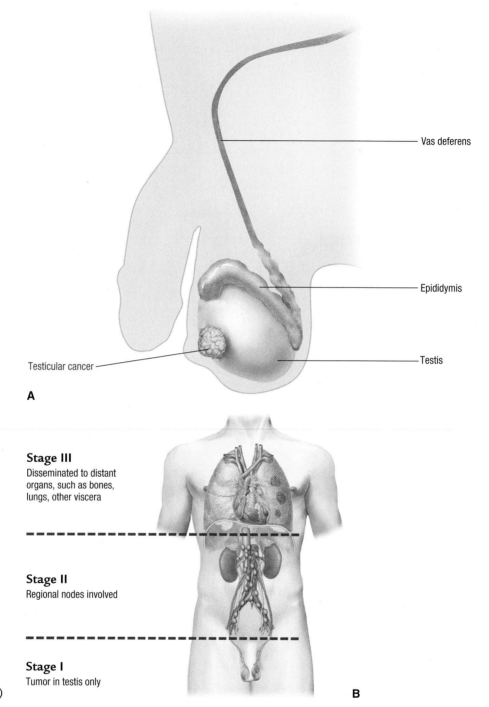

Vas deferens

Epididymis

Testis

Testicular cancer

A

Stage III
Disseminated to distant
organs, such as bones,
lungs, other viscera

Stage II
Regional nodes involved

Stage I
Tumor in testis only

B

FIGURE 16-15
(A) Testicular cancer.
(B) The stages of
testicular cancer.
(Images provided by
Anatomical Chart Co.)

Key Terms	Definitions
hypospadias (high poh SPAY dee us)	congenital disorder characterized by the penile urethral opening located on the ventral surface
epispadias (ep i SPAY dee us)	congenital disorder characterized by the penile urethral opening located on the dorsal surface
epididymitis (ep i did i MIGH tis)	inflammation of the epididymis
hydrocele (HIGH droh seel)	accumulation of fluid in the scrotal sac

testicular (tes TICK yoo lur) **torsion**	rotation of the spermatic cord that causes an interruption in the blood supply to the tissue
erectile (ee RECK tile) **dysfunction**	incapable of filling with blood under pressure to become stiff enough to perform sexual intercourse; impotence
impotence (IM puh tunce)	incapable of filling with blood under pressure to become stiff enough to perform sexual intercourse; erectile dysfunction
sildenafil citrate (sil DEN uh fil SIT rate)	drug used to treat male impotence; trade name Viagra
orchitis (or KIGH tis)	testis inflammation
testicular (tes TICK yoo lur) **cancer**	malignant cell growth in the testis
cryptorchidism (kript OR kid iz um)	failure of one or both of the testes to descend into the scrotum
orchiectomy (or kee ECK tuh mee)	surgical removal of one testicle or both testicles; castration
castration	surgical removal of one testicle or both testicles; orchiectomy

Key Term Practice: Testicle and Penis Disorders

1. The word part _____ refers to "the testis," and the word part *-itis* means _____; so the medical term for inflammation of the testes is _____.

2. The word part _____ refers to "the epididymis," and the word part *-itis* means _____; so _____ is the medical term for inflammation of the epididymis.

Prostate Disorders

Pathology of the prostate ranges from inflammation and hyperplasia to cancer. Inflammation of the prostate is termed **prostatitis** (Fig. 16-16). Its cause may be bacterial, viral, or unknown. Men may be asymptomatic or experience pain and burning while urinating (dysuria). Prostatitis primarily affects men over age 50 years. It is diagnosed by urinalysis and digital rectal examination. A **digital rectal examination** (DRE) is an evaluative procedure involving direct palpation of the prostate with the fingers (digits) through the rectum to examine for swelling or growths (Fig. 16-17). Treatment options include antimicrobics, analgesics, and increased fluid intake. Prognosis for the acute form is good. Chronic prostatitis leads to urinary tract infections, urethral obstruction, and urinary retention.

Benign prostatic hyperplasia (BPH), also known as **benign prostatic hypertrophy** (BPH), is a condition characterized by prostate hypertrophy (enlargement) and is common in men over age 50 years. Although the cause is not known, it is associated with age-related metabolic and endocrine changes. Signs and symptoms include difficulty with starting urination, inability to maintain a steady urine stream, urinary retention, and frequent urination. The anatomic location of the gland itself contributes to urinary system problems because the urethra runs through the gland's center. BPH is diagnosed by the history and physical examination, DRE, intravenous pyelogram (IVP)—a kidney function test—and cytoscopy. Treatments include prostate gland massage, catheterization, drug therapy with α-adrenergic blockers to relax the prostate

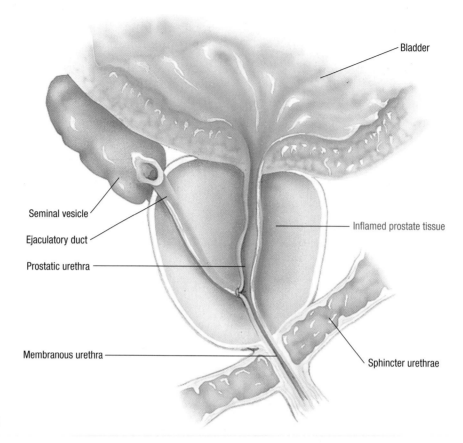

Bladder

Seminal vesicle

Ejaculatory duct

Prostatic urethra

Inflamed prostate tissue

Membranous urethra

Sphincter urethrae

FIGURE 16-16
Inflammation of the prostate is termed prostatitis. (Image provided by Anatomical Chart Co.)

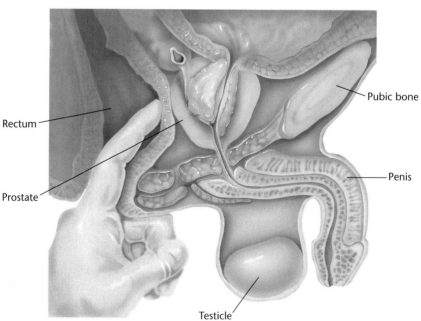

Pubic bone

Rectum

Prostate

Penis

Testicle

FIGURE 16-17
Digital rectal examination of the prostate. (Image provided by Anatomical Chart Co.)

muscles, surgery, and antibiotics to prevent the spread of infection. If the kidneys become involved, it can lead to pyelonephritis, hydronephrosis, and uremia.

Prostate cancer, malignant neoplasia in the prostate gland, is the leading cause of cancer death among men, and age 73 years is the average time of diagnosis (Fig. 16-18). If affects < 1% of the male population younger than age 50 years, 16% of men between the ages of 60 and 64 years, and 83% of men 65 years and older. Data from autopsies show that two thirds of men over age 80 years died *with* (not of) prostate cancer. Prostate cancer often metastasizes to the bones before it is diagnosed.

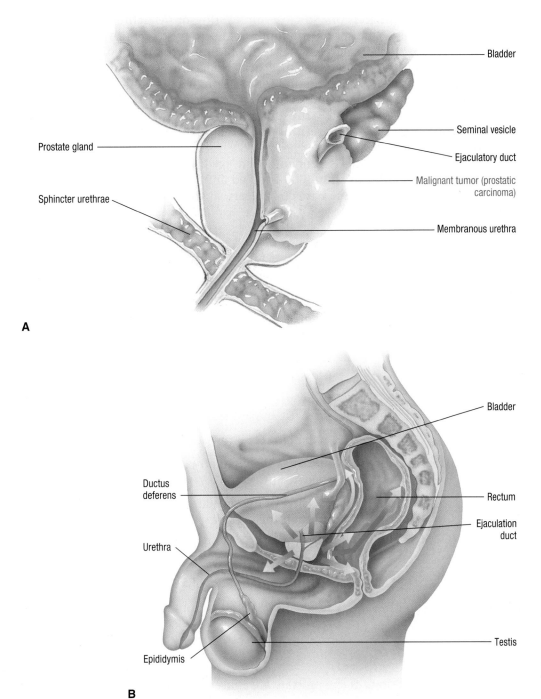

Prostate gland

Sphincter urethrae

Bladder

Seminal vesicle

Ejaculatory duct

Malignant tumor (prostatic carcinoma)

Membranous urethra

A

Ductus deferens

Urethra

Epididymis

Bladder

Rectum

Ejaculation duct

Testis

B

FIGURE 16-18
(**A**) Prostate cancer. (**B**) The pathway for metastasis of prostate cancer. (Images provided by Anatomical Chart Co.)

The cause of prostate cancer is unknown, but dietary fat is associated with onset and may dictate its aggressiveness. The cancer may also be linked to a genetic predisposition. Signs and symptoms, if present, are interrupted urine flow, difficulty starting or stopping urine stream, urinary retention, pain or burning while urinating, and hematuria (blood in the urine). The history and physical examination, DRE, ultrasound, and elevated prostate-specific antigen levels in the blood diagnose the cancer; a biopsy is used for confirmation. The **prostate-specific antigen** (PSA) **test** measures the serum level of this normal protein of the prostate. Increased levels occur with age, but greatly increased levels are associated with prostate cancer and some cases BPN.

Treatment depends on the disease stage. If the man is over age 60 years when the cancer is discovered, often no treatment is administered because he will probably outlive the disease progression, so close monitoring or "watchful waiting" is used. Other options include hormonal therapy, orchiectomy to reduce hormone levels, transurethral resection of the prostate, transurethral prostatectomy, prostatectomy, radiation, and chemotherapy. **Transurethral resection** (TUR) involves inserting a tubular instrument through the urethra for excision of a portion of the prostate to alleviate signs and symptoms of prostatitis. The surgical removal of part or all of the prostate (**prostatectomy**) through the urethral canal using a tubular instrument called a **resectoscope**, is termed **transurethral prostatectomy** (TURP). The prognosis is poor if the disease has metastasized.

Prostate cancer screening is prudent. Men aged 40 years and over should have yearly DREs, and PSA levels should be checked annually in men 50 years and older. Screenings may be discontinued at age 70 years, as the disease is not as aggressive at this point.

Key Terms	Definitions
prostatitis (pros tuh TYE tis)	prostate gland inflammation
digital rectal examination	manual examination of the prostate through the rectum
benign prostatic hyperplasia (pros TAT ick high pur PLAY zhuh)	noncancerous prostate enlargement; benign prostatic hypertrophy
benign prostatic hypertrophy (pros TAT ick high PUR truh fee)	noncancerous prostate enlargement; benign prostatic hyperplasia
prostate (PROS tate) **cancer**	malignant cell growth of the prostate gland
prostate- (PROS tate) **specific antigen** (AN ti jen) **test**	measures the circulating blood levels of prostate-specific antigen
transurethral resection (trans yoo REE thrul ree SECK shun)	excision of the prostate via a resectoscope passed through the urethra
prostatectomy (pros tuh TECK tuh mee)	excision of part or all of the prostate
resectoscope (ree SECK tuh skope)	endoscopic instrument for the transurethral removal of structures or parts of structures
transurethral prostatectomy (trans yoo REE thrul pros tuh TECK tuh mee)	surgical excision of all or part of the prostate using a resectoscope

Key Term Practice: Prostate Disorders

1. Which two synonymous medical conditions of the prostate are abbreviated BPH? _____

2. The word part _____ refers to "the prostate," the word part *-itis* means _____; so the medical term for inflammation of the prostate is _____.

Female Pelvic and Inflammatory Disorders

A fairly common disorder of the female reproductive system is **endometriosis**, a condition characterized by the presence of endometrial tissue in abnormal locations such as the uterine wall, ovaries, or extragenital sites (Fig. 16-19). The misplaced islands of endometrium imitate the menstrual cycle and cause pain at the locale. The underlying cause is not known. **Dysmenorrhea**, abdominal pain, cramping, and

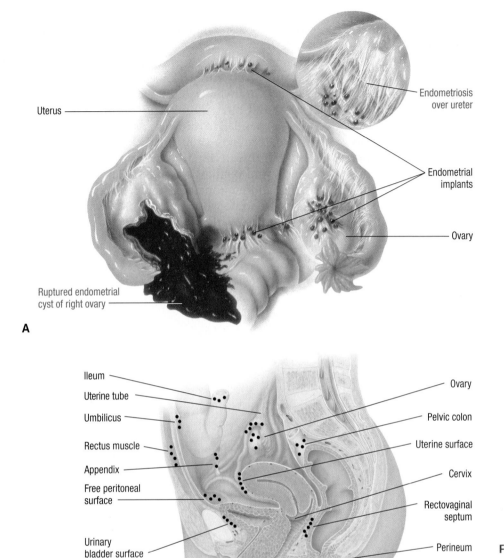

A

B

FIGURE 16-19
(**A**) Endometriosis.
(**B**) Common sites of endometriosis.
(Images provided by Anatomical Chart Co.)

difficult menstruation, is a hallmark of the condition. Heavy menses and pelvic pain during intercourse are also evident. The condition is diagnosed by pelvic examination and laparoscopy.

The **pelvic examination** is one method for assessing the internal pelvic organs and adnexa in both males and females. In general, **adnexa** mean appendages attached to structures. In gynecology, adnexa refer to the appendages of the uterus: the oviducts, ovaries, and ligaments holding the uterus in place. Four types of pelvic examinations are vaginal examination, bimanual palpation of the uterus, and rectovaginal examination in females and the bimanual palpation of the prostate and adnexa in males. The index and middle finger are inserted into the vagina in the vaginal examination; bimanual palpation of the uterus combines the vaginal examination with manual palpating on the external pelvic region to feel the uterus and adnexa. The rectovaginal examination is accomplished by inserting the middle finger into the rectum and the index finger into the vagina and applying pressure to the pelvic region with the other hand. In men, bimanual palpation of the prostate and adnexa involves inserting the index and middle fingers into the rectum while palpating the pelvic region with the other hand.

Treatment of endometriosis is necessary to prevent infertility, ectopic (outside uterus) pregnancy, and spontaneous abortion. Conservative measures involve hormone administration. Invasive action includes dilation and curettage, **hysterectomy** (surgical removal of the uterus), and bilateral salpingo-oophorectomy. The surgical treatment in which the cervix is expanded to allow access to the uterus with a curette to scrape away endometrial tissue is called a **dilation and curettage** (D&C). The medical term describing the excision of the uterine tube and ovary is **salpingo-oophorectomy**. Excision of both oviducts and ovaries is termed bilateral salpingo-oophorectomy (BSO). Pregnancy, nursing, and menopause often cause symptom remission.

An ovarian condition that afflict some women is ovarian cysts. **Ovarian cysts** are fluid-filled sacs forming on or near the ovaries (Fig. 16-20). Symptoms may not be pre-

Follicular cyst

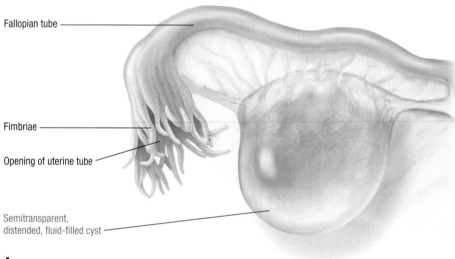

Fallopian tube

Fimbriae

Opening of uterine tube

Semitransparent,
distended, fluid-filled cyst

A

Dermoid cyst

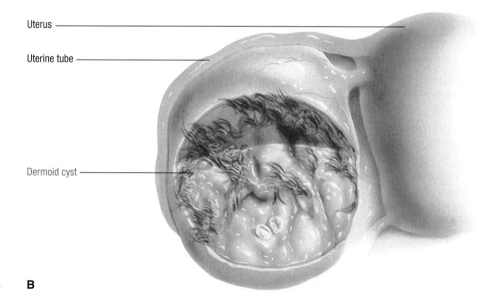

Uterus

Uterine tube

Dermoid cyst

FIGURE 16-20
Common ovarian cysts include
(A) follicular cysts and
(B) dermoid cysts.
(Images provided by Anatomical Chart Co.)

B

sent initially; however, with time the increased size may cause pain, swelling, and urinary retention if the bladder is affected. Two types exist: physiologic and neoplastic. Physiologic cysts do not affect ovarian function, but neoplastic cysts may be either benign or malignant. Ovarian cysts are diagnosed by ultrasonography and laparoscopy. If necessary, benign cysts may be drained, but generally no treatment is required. Neoplastic cysts are removed and appropriate follow-up treatment is given.

Pelvic inflammatory disease (PID) is inflammation of the female genital tract typified by abdominal pain, fever, and cervix tenderness (Fig. 16-21). It is caused by infection from a variety of microbes, most notably *Neisseria gonorrhoeae,* the causative agent of gonorrhea. It is more common in **nulliparous** (never having borne a child) women. Intrauterine device use also increases the risk. Signs and symptoms are fever, chills, malaise, foul-smelling vaginal discharge, and abdominal pain.

This pathology is diagnosed by painful vaginal examination, Gram stain to determine the causative agent, laparoscopy, and ultrasound to detect abnormalities. A **Gram stain** is a differential staining procedure that identifies bacteria as either Gram positive (G+) or Gram negative (G−) according to the dye absorbed by the cell membrane. Gram-positive organisms retain the blue color of crystal violet; G− microbes appear pink because they do not retain the crystal violet dye. It is important to know the Gram reaction so that appropriate antibiotics can be administered because some antibiotics target G+ organisms, others G− organisms, and still others cover both types. Aggressive antibiotic therapy and analgesics for pain relief are used to treat PID. Early therapeutic intervention is necessary to prevent peritonitis or widespread infection, especially septicemia (systemic blood infection).

Another disorder is **premenstrual syndrome** (PMS), a condition of unknown origin characterized by emotional and physical manifestations, including headache, fatigue, irritability, breast tenderness, and joint pain. It occurs only in ovulating women a few days before the onset of menstruation when estrogen levels peak, and it subsides when the menstrual period begins. It is diagnosed by physical examination and history that includes a record of symptoms matched to the menstrual cycle. Chronic depression must be ruled out. Therapy varies among individuals but is aimed at treating

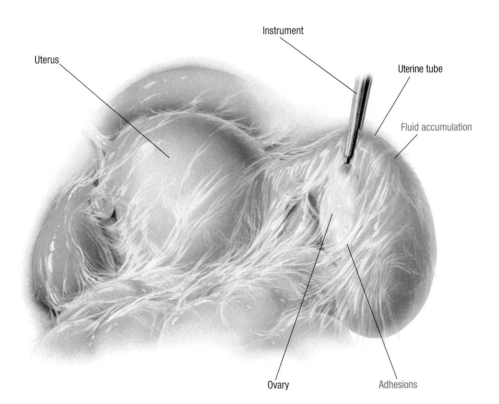

FIGURE 16-21
Adhesions resulting from pelvic inflammatory disease. (Image provided by Anatomical Chart Co.)

the signs and symptoms associated with bloating and depression that appears shortly before menstruation. Exercise, reduced sodium intake, analgesics, and diuretics are often prescribed. Drugs from the family of selective serotonin reuptake inhibitors may be prescribed to ease depression. As their name suggests, **selective serotonin reuptake inhibitors** (SSRIs) belong to a class of psychiatric medications that impede the reuse of the neurotransmitter serotonin, thereby causing elevated levels.

Premenstrual dysphoric disorder (PMDD) is a disorder similar to PMS; however, the signs and symptoms persist after the onset of menstruation. The term *dysphoric* means "physical discomfort," which is a key characteristic of PMDD. The cause may be an abnormal response to native ovarian hormones. It is diagnosed by the history and physical examination. Drugs such as leuprolide that interfere with gonadotropin-releasing hormone (GnRH) or SSRIs treat premenstrual dysphoric disorder.

Key Terms	Definitions
endometriosis (en doh mee tree OH sis)	endometrium is present and functioning outside the uterus
dysmenorrhea (dis men oh REE uh)	difficult and painful menstruation
pelvic (PEL vick) **examination**	manually palpating and examining the vagina, uterus, rectum, and accessory organs and structures
adnexum (ad NECK sum)	appendage(s) of the uterus, including the ovaries, oviducts, and uterine ligaments
hysterectomy (his tur ECK tuh mee)	surgical removal of the uterus
dilation and curettage (kewr e TAHZH)	gynecological procedure in which the cervix is widened and the uterus is scraped
salpingo-oophorectomy (sal pin goh-oh oh foh RECK toh mee)	removal of the uterine tube and ovary
ovarian (oh VAIR ee un) **cysts**	fluid-filled sacs on or near the ovaries
pelvic (PEL vick) **inflammatory disease**	inflammation of the reproductive organs that, if untreated, can cause infertility
nulliparous (nuh LIP uh rus)	having never given birth to a child
Gram stain	differential stain used to identify microbes according to the dye retained within the bacterial cell wall
premenstrual (pree MEN stroo ul) **syndrome**	group of symptoms experienced by some women in the days preceding menstruation
selective serotonin (seer oh TOH nin) **reuptake inhibitors**	psychiatric medications that increase the serotonin levels in the body to ease depression
premenstrual dysphoric (pree MEN stroo ul dis FOR ick) **disorder**	group of symptoms similar to PMS that persist after the onset of menstruation

Key Term Practice: Female Pelvic and Inflammatory Disorders

1. A gynecological procedure in which the cervix is widened and the uterus is scraped is called _____.

2. The condition in which endometrium appears outside the uterus is termed _____.

Female Cancers

Cancers affecting the female reproductive organs include breast, cervical, endometrial, labial or vulvar, ovarian, and vaginal. Although considered primarily a female cancer, breast cancer also affects men but to a much lesser extent.

Breast cancer, carcinoma of mammary tissue, occurs primarily in females, however, 1200 new cases are reported each year in American men. It involves a strong genetic predisposition. Other linked factors include exposure to high estrogen levels, having borne no children, and experiencing a late first pregnancy. Breast cancer usually develops as a single, small, hard, painless nodule (Fig. 16-22). The advanced stage is marked by skin dimpling and nipple discharge. Measures to detect the cancer as quickly as possible are key. These include regular mammograms and monthly breast self-examinations (BSEs). **Mammography**, radiographic examination of breast tissue, is used for the initial diagnosis. It may be performed with contrast dye injected into mammary ducts. It is recommended that a baseline mammogram be taken between ages 35 and 39 years; thereafter, regular mammograms are suggested as part of routine health care. The false-negative (the mammogram is interpreted as having no pathology when abnormality does exist) rate is approximately 10%. Thus management of a palpable anomaly must be based on clinical grounds. Confirmation of disease is provided by biopsy. Treatment includes surgery (lumpectomy or mastectomy), radiation, and chemotherapy..

The surgical removal of a breast is termed **mastectomy**, and reconstructive surgery generally follows the procedure. One such restorative procedure is the **trans–rectus abdominis musculocutaneous** (TRAM) **flap** in which a lower abdominal muscle is threaded under the abdominal and thoracic cavities to the mastectomy site. Nipple reconstruction can also be completed after TRAM flap surgery. Drug treatment is commonly done with tamoxifen, a member of a class of drugs known as selective estrogen receptor modulators. **Selective estrogen receptor modulators** (SERMs) function as native estrogen in some tissue but block its action in others. In this case, the SERM obstructs estrogen in the breast but preserves the hormone elsewhere in the body.

Malignant neoplasms of the cervix are called **cervical cancer.** It is associated with human papillomavirus (HPV) infection. In addition, cigarette smoking has also been implicated as a causative factor. Watery, bloody, foul-smelling vaginal discharge and bleeding between periods or after intercourse are the main signs. It is easily diagnosed with a **Pap smear** or **Pap test**, a procedure in which cells are exfoliated (scraped) from the cervix and viewed in stained smears (Fig. 16-23). The cells are then determined to be in five classes based on their characteristics. When abnormal cells are found, excision of a cone of cervix tissue, called a **conization**, is often performed. The cells can then be cultured or examined histologically. Surgery, radiation, cryosurgery, electrocoagulation, and laser ablation are common treatments. **Cryosurgery** involves the localized freezing of diseased tissues without significant harm to adjacent structures. The destruction or hardening of tissues with high-frequency currents that cause blood clumping is termed **electrocoagulation. Laser ablation** is the surgical removal of

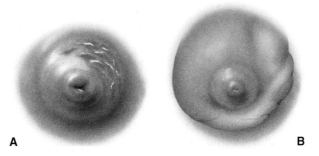

A

B

FIGURE 16-22

Type of breast cancer. (**A**) Paget disease. (**B**) Cystosarcoma phyllodes. (Sarcoma is cancer originating in connective tissue.) (Images provided by Anatomical Chart Co.)

Carcinoma in situ   **Squamous cell carcinoma**

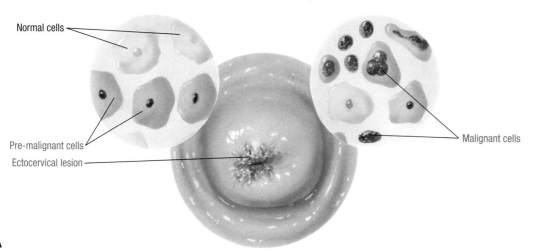

Normal cells

Pre-malignant cells

Ectocervical lesion

Malignant cells

A

Normal
- Large, surface type squamous cells
- Small, pyknotic nuclei

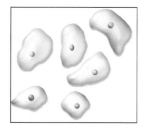

B1

Mild dysplasia
- Mild increase in nuclear:cytoplasmic ratio
- Hyperchromasia
- Abnormal chromatin pattern

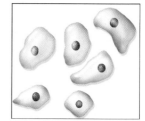

B2

Severe dysplasia, carcinoma in situ
- Basal type cells
- Very high nuclear:cytoplasmic ratio
- Marked hyperchromasia
- Abnormal chromatin

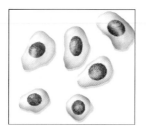

B3

Invasive carcinoma
- Marked pleomorphism
- Irregular nuclei
- Clumped chromatin
- Prominent nucleoli

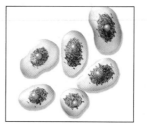

B4

FIGURE 16-23
(**A**) Cervical cancer.
(**B**) Pap smear diagnosis. (Images provided by Anatomical Chart Co.)

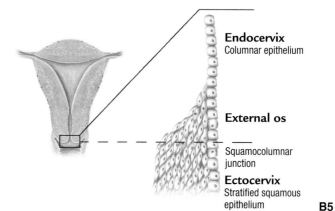

Endocervix
Columnar epithelium

External os

Squamocolumnar junction

Ectocervix
Stratified squamous epithelium

B5

tissue via a laser instrument that uses radiation of optical frequencies. The prognosis is excellent if treated in the early stages. A new vaccine is currently available to prevent HPV infection.

Carcinoma of the endometrium that develops from endometrial ulcers, usually occurring after menopause, is termed **endometrial cancer.** This cancer is associated with estrogen-replacement therapy (ERT), early menarche, late menopause, hypertension, diabetes mellitus, obesity, and use of tamoxifen (drug that inhibits the actions of estrogen). It occurs most often in women who have never been pregnant. Signs and symptoms are irregular menses, mucoid vaginal discharge, hyperplasia (excessive tissue formation), dysplasia (abnormal cell growth), and carcinoma in situ (CIS) in which anaplastic cells that do not behave like cancer replace normal cells. Diagnosis is made by the history and physical examination, pelvic examination, and biopsy (Fig. 16-24). A total hysterectomy with radiation is the usual treatment for endometrial cancer. The prognosis is good if the cancer is detected in the early stages.

Labial cancer or **vulvar cancer** is a cancer of unknown cause affecting the labia or vulva. The most common form is squamous cell carcinoma, which occurs principally in postmenopausal women. It is associated with pelvic infection and venereal warts. The first sign is a lump in the vulva that develops into a bleeding ulcer (Fig. 16-25). Labial and vulvar cancer is diagnosed by the history and physical examination, D&C, and biopsy for confirmation. Treatments include vulvectomy and radiation therapy. The 5-year survival rate is 60%.

Another form of cancer with an unknown origin is **ovarian cancer**, which is characterized by metastatic tumors found in one ovary or both ovaries (Fig. 16-26). Ovarian cancer is a leading cause of death from pathologies of the female reproductive system. A familial history of breast cancer or ovarian cancer increases the risk of disease. Signs

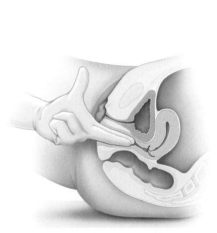

Vaginal examination

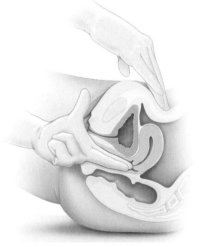

Bimanual palpation
of uterus

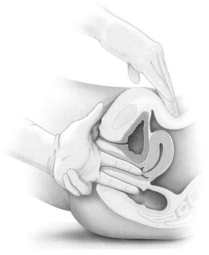

Rectovaginal examination

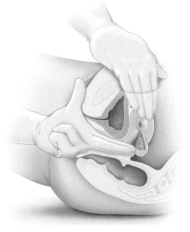

Bimanual palpation
of adnexa

FIGURE 16-24
A pelvic examination allows a health-care specialist to feel the interior of the vagina and the shape and surface of the uterus, vagina, rectum, internal supportive membranes, uterine tubes, and ovaries.

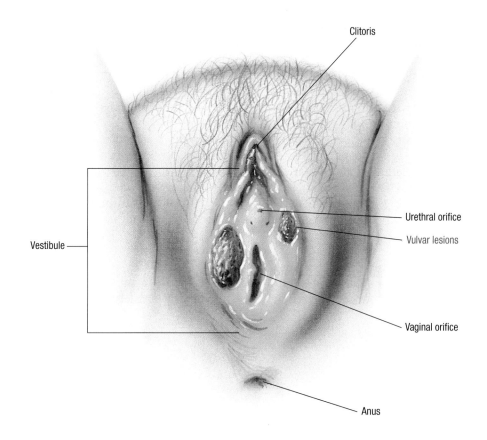

FIGURE 16-25
Carcinoma of the vulva. (Image provided by Anatomical Chart Co.)

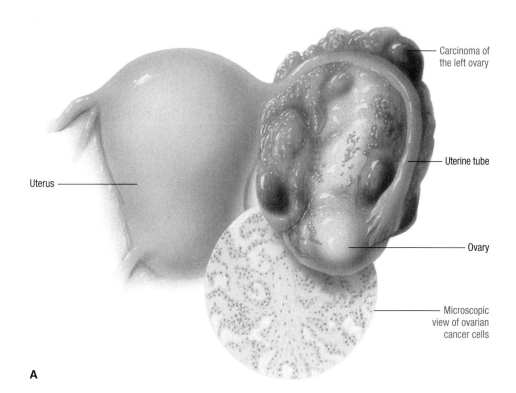

FIGURE 16-26
Ovarian cancer (**A**) and metastatic sites for ovarian cancer

A

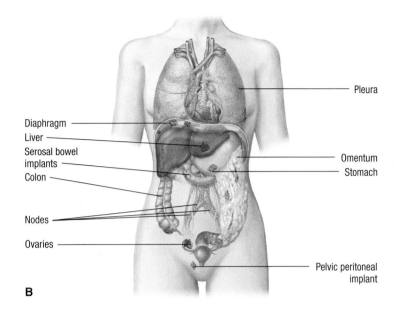

Pleura

Diaphragm

Liver

Serosal bowel implants

Colon

Omentum

Stomach

Nodes

Ovaries

Pelvic peritoneal implant

B

FIGURE 16-26
(Continued) **(B)**
(Images provided by Anatomical Chart Co.)

and symptoms may be absent. When present, they include lower abdominal pain, weight loss, ascites (abdominal fluid accumulation), and gastrointestinal disturbances. Transvaginal sonography and laparoscopy are used for diagnosis. **Transvaginal sonography** uses an ultrasonic probe that is inserted into the vagina. Echograms from the probe identify ovarian structures. **Laparoscopy**, a method of examining the peritoneal cavity using an endoscope equipped with biopsy forceps, confirms the diagnosis. Treatment measures consist of excision of only the diseased ovary if the female is still considering bearing children. Otherwise, a complete bilateral salpingo-oophorectomy or hysterectomy is performed. Surgical treatment is followed by radiation and chemotherapy. The fatality rate is high if it is not detected early.

Vaginal cancer is a rare cancer that is typically derived from squamous cell carcinoma. The adenocarcinoma type is associated with diethylstilbestrol (DES) use and occurs in daughters of women who were given this drug to prevent miscarriages. The main signs are bloody vaginal discharge and **leukorrhea**, a whitish mucopurulent vaginal discharge.

Key Terms	Definitions
breast cancer	carcinoma of the mammary tissue
mammography (ma MOG ruh fee)	x-ray examination of the breast
mastectomy (mas TECK tuh mee)	breast excision
trans–rectus abdominis musculocutaneous (trans–RECK tus ab DOM in nus mus kew loh kew TAY nee us) **flap**	surgical procedure to reconstruct the mammary region after mastectomy
selective estrogen receptor modulators	drugs that function as native estrogen in some tissue but blocks its action in others
cervical (SUR vi kul) **cancer**	malignant cells of the cervix
Pap smear	test used to detect precancerous or cancerous cells of the cervix; Pap test
Pap test	test used to detect precancerous or cancerous cells of the cervix; Pap smear

conization (kohn i ZAY shun)	excision of a cone of tissue, most notably from the cervix
cryosurgery (krye oh SUR juh ree)	surgery in which low temperatures are applied to tissues to seal or remove them
electrocoagulation (ee leck troh koh ag yoo LAY shun)	cauterizing tissue to stop bleeding
laser ablation (ab LAY shun)	removal of tissue with a laser
endometrial (en doh MEE tree ul) **cancer**	malignant cells of the uterine endometrium
labial (LAY bee ul) **cancer**	malignant cells of the folds surrounding the female genitalia; vulvar cancer
vulvar (VUL vur) **cancer**	malignant cells of the folds surrounding the female genitalia; labial cancer
ovarian (oh VAIR ee un) **cancer**	malignant tumor of the ovary or ovaries
transvaginal sonography (trans VAJ i nul suh NOG ruh fee)	procedure for obtaining echograms of the ovaries and ovarian structures
laparoscopy (lap uh ROS kuh pee)	examination of abdominal internal organs using a laparoscope
vaginal (VAJ i nul) **cancer**	malignant cells of the vagina
leukorrhea (lew koh REE uh)	thick discharge from the vagina

Key Term Practice: Female Cancers

1. What two terms describe malignant tumors in the folds surrounding the female genitalia?

   _____ _____

2. The word part _____ means "breast," and the word part -*ectomy* means _____; so the surgical removal of a breast is termed _____.

Female Benign Tumors

Leiomyomas and fibroids are the most common type of benign tumors of the female reproductive tract. **Leiomyomas** are composed of smooth muscle cells and occur in the uterus. A myoma is a benign neoplasm of muscular tissue. **Fibroids** are fibrous tumors found in the uterus (Fig. 16-27). They are also called **leiomyomas uteri.** Both types are stimulated by estrogen and occur only in premenopausal women. Females are often asymptomatic, but some experience pelvic pain, abnormal bleeding, and heavy menses. These benign tumors are identified during a pelvic examination or through ultrasound, laparoscopy, D&C, or biopsy. The medical management depends on the severity. Tumor removal is the most common form of treatment, but hysterectomy may be warranted.

Fibrocystic breast disease is a condition that affects women between 30 and 40 years of age and is characterized by fluid-filled, palpable breast cysts (Fig. 16-28). The primary sign is a cyst that fluctuates in size throughout the menstrual cycle. A persistent lump is often the only sign. It is diagnosed by mammography and biopsy. Treatments include wearing a support bra to ease discomfort and restricting caffeine and sodium intake, because these appear to influence the cysts' development.

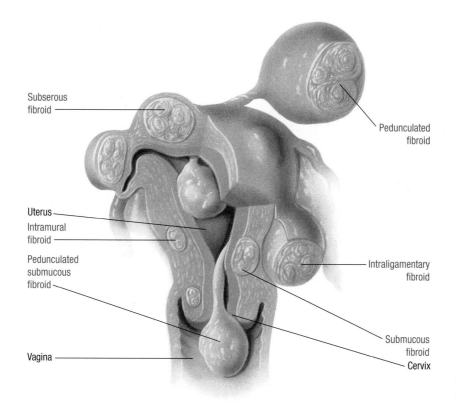

Subserous
fibroid

Pedunculated
fibroid

Uterus

Intramural
fibroid

Pedunculated
submucous
fibroid

Intraligamentary
fibroid

Vagina

Submucous
fibroid

Cervix

FIGURE 16-27
Uterine fibroids are benign tumors of the uterus. (Image provided by Anatomical Chart Co.)

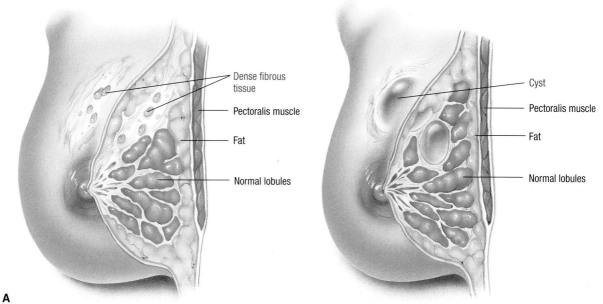

Dense fibrous
tissue

Pectoralis muscle

Fat

Normal lobules

Cyst

Pectoralis muscle

Fat

Normal lobules

A

B

FIGURE 16-28
Fibrocystic breast disease is characterized by fluid-filled, palpable breast cysts. (**A**) Fibrocystic changes. (**B**) Breast cyst.

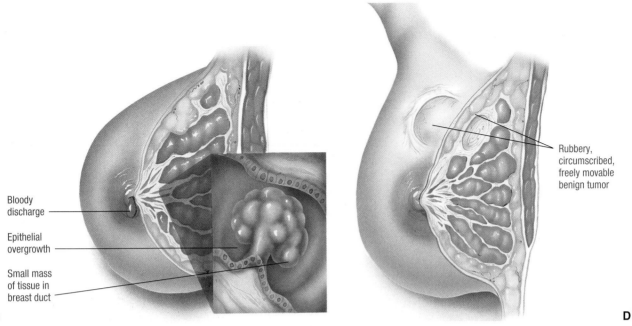

Bloody
discharge

Epithelial
overgrowth

Small mass
of tissue in
breast duct

Rubbery,
circumscribed,
freely movable
benign tumor

C

D

FIGURE 16-28
(Continued) (**C**) Intraductal papilloma. (**D**) Fibroadenoma. (Images provided by Anatomical Chart Co.)

Key Terms	Definitions
leiomyomas (lye oh migh OH muhz)	benign tumors of smooth muscle cells
fibroids (FIGH broidz)	benign fibrous tumors
leiomyomas uteri (lye oh migh OH muhz YOO tur eye)	fibrous tumors with smooth muscle cells in the uterus
fibrocystic (figh broh SIS tick) **breast disease**	unusual growth of fibrous tissue in the breast

Key Term Practice: Female Benign Tumors

1. A general term for benign tumors composed of smooth muscle cells is _____.

2. A benign fibrous tumor is termed a/an _____.

Reproductive Hernias

Hernias are conditions in which part of an internal organ projects abnormally through a body wall or cavity. Hernias are also called ruptures. Two types of hernias related to the reproductive system are cystoceles and rectoceles. A herniation of the urinary bladder into the vagina is termed a **cystocele.** It results from trauma or weakened pelvic muscles and ligaments. Pregnancy, labor, and aging are associated with cystocele development. Signs and symptoms include pelvic pressure, urinary frequency, urgency, and incontinence. It is diagnosed by the history and physical examination.

Treatment involves Kegel exercises, estrogen therapy to improve muscle tone, or colporrhaphy. With **Kegel exercises,** one voluntarily contracts the pelvic floor muscles to strengthen muscle tissue and also voluntarily starts and stops urine flow several times during micturition (urination). Practicing Kegel exercises can alleviate urinary leakage as a result of weakened pelvic floor muscles. Repairing the vagina by sutures is called **colporrhaphy**, and surgical repair that involves restructuring is known as **colpoplasty**.

A **proctocele** or **rectocele** is a protrusion of the rectum into the vagina caused by a weakened vaginal wall resulting from trauma, pregnancy, or childbirth. Fecal incontinence, flatulence, and difficulty evacuating the bowels are common signs. A complete history and physical examination are generally all that is necessary for the diagnosis. Treatment consists of a colpoplasty. When a simultaneous rectocele and cystocele operation is performed, it is referred to as an anterior and posterior (A&P) repair.

Key Terms	Definitions
cystocele (SIS toh seel)	hernia of the urinary bladder through the vaginal wall
Kegel exercises	alternate contraction and relaxation of the perineal muscles to increase the strength of the pelvic floor muscles to treat urinary incontinence
colporrhaphy (kol POR uh fee)	vaginal suture
colpoplasty (kol poh PLAS tee)	vaginal repair and restructure
proctocele (PROCK toh seel)	hernia of the rectum through the vaginal wall; rectocele
rectocele (RECK toh seel)	hernia of the rectum through the vaginal wall; proctocele

Key Term Practice: Reproductive Hernias

1. Vaginal repair and restructure is termed _____.

2. Which two terms mean a hernia of the rectum through the vaginal wall?

_____ _____

Infertility and Sterility

Two closely related terms with fine nuances of distinction are infertility and sterility, conditions affecting both males and females. The terms are frequently used interchangeably. **Infertility** is the diminished or absent ability of a couple to achieve pregnancy after 1 year of unprotected sex or the inability to carry a pregnancy to term. Female infertility is characterized by the inability to conceive. A common cause is failure to ovulate owing to adenohypophysis hyposecretion (low hormone output) and endometriosis. Male infertility is marked by the inability of sperm to fertilize an ovum. Other causes are structural anomalies, such as scar tissue and varicocele; sexually transmitted diseases; antisperm antibodies; and low sperm count. A **varicocele** is swelling in one testicle or both, usually the left one, caused by swelling of the testicular veins that drain the testes (Fig. 16-29). The distension of the testicular veins can lead to lowered sperm counts because the blood causes an increased temperature.

Forms of infertility are diagnosed by the history and physical examination, semen analysis, hormone level evaluation, and laparoscopy to rule out uterine or oviduct abnormalities. A **semen analysis** measures sperm count, motility, morphology (shape), and volume produced. Decreased sperm numbers and semen volume, abnormal sperm shape, and impaired movement are associated with infertility.

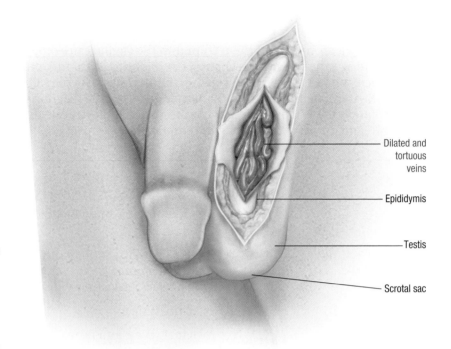

Dilated and tortuous veins

Epididymis

Testis

Scrotal sac

FIGURE 16-29
A varicocele is swelling in one testicle or both testicles, caused by distension of the testicular veins that drain the testes. (Image provided by Anatomical Chart Co.)

Sterility refers to the inability to conceive in the female or the incapability to induce conception in the male. Female sterility specifically is termed **infecundity** because the term *fecund* means "fertile." Male sterility may be associated with impotence, and a frequent cause of female sterility is blocked uterine tubes. Functional sterility refers to a sperm count below 50 million per milliliter of semen. Diagnosis is based on the history and physical examination. Treatment for both infertility and sterility, if available, depends on the underlying cause.

Sterility can also be medically induced. For example, the removal of reproductive organs or the administration of drugs that prevent adequate hormone secretion (known as chemical sterility) renders one sterile. It is interesting that nearly 90% of couples attempting pregnancy are able to do so within 1 year of regular, unprotected sex. Infertility is not as irreversible as sterility.

Key Terms	Definitions
infertility	inability of a couple to achieve pregnancy
varicocele (VAIR i koh seel)	swelling of the veins in the spermatic cord of the scrotum
semen (SEE mun) **analysis**	measures the volume of semen secreted and sperm number, morphology, and motility
sterility	total inability to reproduce
infecundity (in fe KUN di tee)	female sterility

Key Term Practice: Infertility and Sterility

1. Another medical term for female sterility is _____.

2. _____ is the inability of a couple to achieve pregnancy.

Infections

Pathologic states caused by microorganisms that can be acquired by means other than sexual intercourse are described in this section. **Candidiasis** is a fungal disease caused by *Candida albicans*. This is the same yeast infection that causes **vaginitis** (vaginal inflammation) (Fig. 16-30). Itching, burning, and leukorrhea are common signs and symptoms. Antibiotic use predisposes females to this infection, which is diagnosed by the clinical picture. Oral and cream antifungal medications are used to treat it. Individuals taking antibiotics are encouraged to eat yogurt daily to keep intestinal flora in balance, thereby thwarting possible yeast infections.

Hepatitis B (or serum hepatitis) is a chronic, sometimes fatal form of hepatitis transmitted by the hepatitis B virus (HBV). It is characterized by hepatomegaly, jaundice, fatigue, and abdominal pain. Modes of transmission include contact with blood,

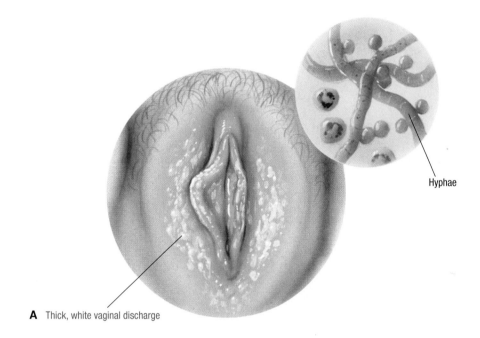

Hyphae

A Thick, white vaginal discharge

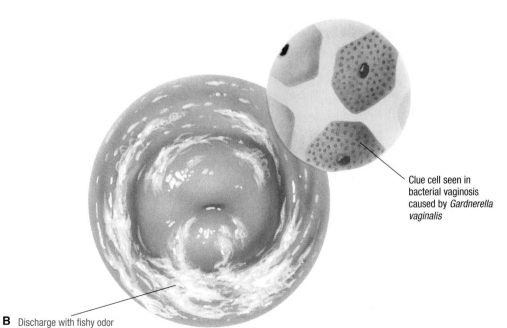

Clue cell seen in bacterial vaginosis caused by *Gardnerella vaginalis*

B Discharge with fishy odor

FIGURE 16-30
Vaginitis is the term for vaginal inflammation. (**A**) Candida infection. (**B**) Bacterial vaginosis. (Images provided by Anatomical Chart Co.)

semen, saliva, or vaginal secretions. The initial diagnosis is made by the history and physical examination and confirmed by the presence of hepatitis B antibodies. Because there is no cure, treatment is palliative. The Heptavax B vaccine is available for preventive measures.

Toxic shock syndrome (TSS) is an acute, potentially fatal systemic disease caused by *Staphylococcus aureus* that occurs in menstruating females who use tampons. TSS is characterized by widespread homeostatic imbalances as a reaction to toxins produced by the organism. Superabsorbent tampons have been implicated because the bacterial toxin increases in their presence while in the vagina. Common signs and symptoms are fever, rash, hypotension, gastrointestinal upset, and neuromuscular disturbances. It is diagnosed by physical examination, history of tampon use, and accompanying elevated liver enzymes. The condition is treated with antibiotics and fluids to increase blood pressure. It is recommended that tampons be changed every 8–10 hours to prevent TSS.

Key Terms	Definitions
candidiasis (kan di DYE uh sis)	vaginal yeast infection caused by *Candida albicans* fungus
vaginitis (vaj i NIGH tis)	vaginal inflammation
hepatitis (hep uh TYE tis) **B**	form of hepatitis caused by the hepatitis B virus that is spread through sexual contact or contact with infected body fluids; serum hepatitis
toxic shock syndrome	circulatory failure associated with tampon use and the growth of toxin-producing staphylococcal bacteria

Key Term Practice: Infections

1. The disease associated with tampon use that has systemic effects is _____.

2. _____ is a vaginal yeast infection caused by a fungus.

Sexually Transmitted Diseases

Sexually transmitted diseases (STDs), or **venereal diseases** (VDs), are contagious infections acquired during sexual intercourse. They are spread by contact with body fluids such as semen and vaginal secretions and by anal or oral sex. More than 20 STDs have been identified, and it is possible to have more than one simultaneously. Common VDs include chancroid, chlamydia, genital herpes, genital warts, gonorrhea, lymphogranuloma venereum, syphilis, and trichomoniasis (Fig. 16-31). The incidence of STDs is rising in the United States. Public health measures are aimed at education and prevention strategies.

An acute, localized venereal disease caused by *Haemophilus ducreyi* is termed **chancroid.** It is characterized by **chancres** (sores or ulcers at the point where the pathogen enters the body), lymph node enlargement, and suppuration (pus formation) that occur 7–10 days after sexual intercourse with an infected person. A Gram stain is done to confirm the causative organism. Treatment consists of antibiotic administration and sexual abstinence throughout the course of therapy.

Chlamydia is a bacterial infection caused by the bacterium *Chlamydia trachomatis.* In women, it is often a silent STD because females are frequently asymptomatic and may transmit the disease unknowingly. Symptoms appear in men within 1–3 weeks

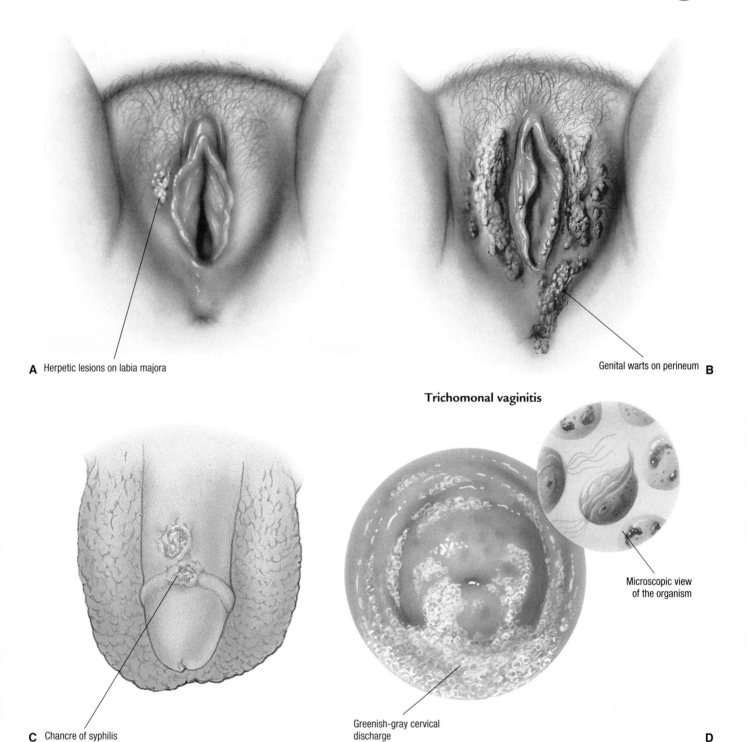

A Herpetic lesions on labia majora

Genital warts on perineum **B**

Trichomonal vaginitis

Microscopic view
of the organism

Greenish-gray cervical
discharge

C Chancre of syphilis

D

FIGURE 16-31
Sexually transmitted diseases. (**A**) Genital herpes. (**B**) Genital warts. (**C**) Chancre of syphilis. (**D**) Trichomoniasis. (Images provided by Anatomical Chart Co.)

after exposure about 75% of the time. It is the leading cause of PID in women. Signs and symptoms of chlamydia when apparent in females are thick vaginal discharge, genital burning and itching, abdominal pain, **dyspareunia** (painful sexual intercourse), nongonococcal urethritis, and lymphogranuloma venereum. Males experience penile discharge, genital burning and itching, urethritis, and scrotal swelling. Enlarged lymph nodes are noted in both sexes, as are possible lesions within the genitourinary tract. Newborns can contract chlamydia from infected mothers during the birthing process. Antigen-specific serologic studies and the Giemsa stain (which identifies blood particles) are used for diagnosis. Initial treatment involves antibiotic injections for both partners and following up with a course of oral antibiotics. Prompt treatment is necessary.

Another sexually transmitted infectious disease caused by *C. trachomatis* is **lymphogranuloma venereum** (LGV). Primary signs are genital ulceration and regional lymphadenitis, which are detected during a physical examination. Diagnosis is confirmed by identifying *C. trachomatis* as the causative agent. Antibiotics are used to treat the condition.

Vesicles on the genitals caused by the herpes simplex virus type 2 (HSV2) are called **genital herpes** or **herpes progenitalis.** The virus often remains in a latent state in the nervous system between flare-ups and has a tendency to recur at irregular intervals. The virus enters the body through interruptions in mucous membranes. Painful genital sores and blister-like lesions around and in genitals are common. The person may also experience flu-like symptoms. All infected people are contagious during outbreaks, and some individuals called "shedders" are contagious even when no symptoms or outward signs are present. In the United States, one out of every five individuals aged 12 years and over is infected with the virus. Diagnosis is made by presence of the characteristic lesions and a tissue culture identifying the virus. There is no cure, and the virus remains in certain nerve cells for life. Antiviral medications reduce the duration and frequency of outbreaks.

Genital herpes is associated with cervical cancer. Pregnant women can pass the virus unto her unborn children, particularly if her first episode occurs during pregnancy. If an outbreak that is not the first episode occurs during pregnancy, the risk of infection to the child during delivery is low. If an outbreak occurs during labor and delivery and the lesions are present in or near the birth canal, a cesarean section is performed. Therefore, infected pregnant women are advised against vaginal births.

Warts on the external genitalia, anus, vagina, and cervix characterize **genital warts.** They are caused by HPV and are spread via sexual contact. Diagnosis is confirmed by presence of warts and isolation of the virus. There is no cure, and they are also associated with the later development of cervical cancer.

Gonorrhea is a venereal disease caused by the bacterium *Neisseria gonorrhoeae.* The primary characteristic is mucopurulent inflammation of genital tract mucosa. Complications include septicemia, arthritis, PID, endocarditis, and meningitis. The signs and symptoms are similar to those of chlamydia. Most women with the condition are asymptomatic and may spread the disease unknowingly. Men develop dysuria. Gonorrhea can become a systemic infection. Eye infections can lead to blindness. Newborns can acquire this STD from infected mothers during the vaginal birthing process. Therefore, prophylactic erythromycin antibiotic salve is routinely applied to the eyes of all infants at birth. Gram stain is used to identify the causative agent. This disease is treated with antibiotics such as ceftriaxone, penicillin, and tetracycline. Untreated forms can also lead to blindness. The prognosis is good with treatment.

Syphilis, also known as **lues,** is a systemic infection caused by the *Treponema pallidum* spirochete. Lesions occur in any tissue or vascular body organ. It produces various clinical pictures and symptoms characteristic of other diseases. Painless, contagious local lesions called chancres appear on male and female genitalia. Syphilis has primary, secondary, and tertiary stages. During the primary stage, the microbe multiplies and spreads to the lymph nodes and bloodstream. The chancre disappears within 4–6 weeks with or without treatment. Primary lesions heal and a latent (secondary) period lasting from 1 to 40 years follows with subclinical or asymptomatic manifestations. The tertiary stage is marked by gumma invasion of vascular organs and the central nervous system, which can lead to blood vessel damage, blindness, emotional instability, hallucinations, and insanity. A **gumma** is a mass of rubber-like necrotic (dead) tissue. Another word for gumma is **syphiloma,** and the terms are interchangeable. During the tertiary stage, the individual is no longer infectious. Diagnosis is made by the *T. pallidum* immobilization (TPI) test, which detects a particular antibody in a patient with syphilis, and/or other serum antibody tests. It is critical to treat syphilis with penicillin G or an alternative antibiotic in the early stages to prevent irreversible damage.

An infection of the genitourinary tract with the flagellate protozoan *Trichomonas vaginalis* is termed **trichomoniasis.** Most cases are asymptomatic, allowing the disease to spread unknowingly. Signs and symptoms, when present, include urethritis, dysuria, and vaginitis with green-yellow discharge. Diagnosis is made by isolating the causative agent in the urine or through microscopic examination of vaginal secretions. Antiprotozoal drugs are administered to both partners until the infection is completely eradicated. Failure to complete the treatment regimen leads to "Ping-Pong" vaginitis because the infection goes back and forth between one infected partner and the other.

Acquired immunodeficiency syndrome (AIDS) is caused by human immunodeficiency virus (HIV) infection. Initially there are no symptoms; flu-like symptoms occur approximately 6 weeks after an infection and marks early illness. The asymptomatic period may last up to 10 years because the virus remains latent. HIV infects macrophages and CD4$^+$ lymphocytes of the immune system, thereby hampering the protective response and allowing for the development of other infections and cancer, notably Kaposi sarcoma. AIDS is actually an advanced HIV infection, which is transmitted via contact with HIV in blood, semen, and vaginal secretions. Another major mode of transmission is by needle sharing among HIV-infected drug users and from mother to infant at childbirth. Preventive measures include abstinence from sexual intercourse, condom use, and refraining from needle sharing. There is no cure, but life can be prolonged through pharmacological treatment with reverse transcriptase inhibitors and protease inhibitors used in combination.

Key Terms	Definitions
venereal (ve NEER ee ul) **disease**	diseases transmitted through sex acts; sexually transmitted diseases
chancroid (SHANK roid)	sexually transmitted disease characterized by painful, ragged ulcers at the infection site
chancres (SHANK urz)	skin lesions or ulcers at the point where the disease-causing organism enters the body
chlamydia (kla MID ee uh)	sexually transmitted disease caused by the bacterium *Chlamydia trachomatis*
dyspareunia (dis puh ROOH nee uh)	painful sexual intercourse
lymphogranuloma venereum (lim foh gran yoo LOH muh ve NEER ee um)	sexually transmitted bacterial disease caused by *Chlamydia trachomatis*
genital herpes (HUR peez)	sexually transmitted disease caused by the herpes simplex virus; herpes progenitalis
herpes progenitalis (HUR peez proh jen i TAY lis)	sexually transmitted disease caused by the herpes simplex virus; genital herpes
genital warts	warts on the genitalia or in the anus region caused by human papilloma virus
gonorrhea (gon uh REE uh)	sexually transmitted disease caused by *Neisseria gonorrhoeae*

syphilis (SIF i lis)	sexually transmitted disease caused by *Treponema pallidum*; lues
lues (LEW eez)	sexually transmitted disease caused by *Treponema pallidum*; syphilis
gumma (GUM uh)	rubbery tumor that occurs in the tertiary stage of syphilis; syphiloma
syphiloma (sif i LOH muh)	rubbery tumor that occurs in the tertiary stage of syphilis; gumma
trichomoniasis (trick oh moh NIGH uh sis)	sexually transmitted disease caused by the protozoan parasite *Trichomonas vaginalis*
acquired immunodeficiency (im yoo noh dee FISH un see) **syndrome**	disease caused by infection with the human immunodeficiency virus (HIV), a retrovirus that causes immune system failure

Key Term Practice: Sexually Transmitted Diseases

1. What is the advanced disease caused by infection with HIV?

   _____

2. As a class, sexually transmitted diseases are also known as _____.

3. Genital herpes and herpes _____ are the same condition.

Birth Control Methods

The deliberate limiting of the number of children born is known as birth control (BC). It usually involves some form of **contraceptive**, a measure used to prevent sperm from fertilizing an egg. Birth control strategies can be used by both sexes.

The current measures for males are condoms and vasectomy. **Condoms** are close-fitting physical barriers that cover the penis to prevent pregnancy or the spread of a sexually transmitted disease by capturing ejaculated semen. They are commonly called rubbers or prophylactics. A surgical operation that prevents sperm from being ejaculated is termed a **vasectomy** (Fig. 16-32). A vasectomy involves cutting and removing a 1-cm (0.39-in.) segment of the vas deferens from each testis. The ends are then retied, but it is impossible for spermatozoa to travel from the epididymis to the distal portions of the reproductive tract. Sperm that are produced then degenerate in the epididymides.

Female methods of birth control include female condoms, implants, injections, intrauterine devices, oral contraceptives, tubal ligation, and vaginal barriers. A **female condom** is a loose-fitting polyurethane sheath, much like a male condom, that is closed on one end with flexible rings at both ends. It is inserted into the vagina where the interior lines the vaginal walls, and the exterior covers the labia.

Norplant is the trade name for levonorgestrel implants, which are six time-released hormone capsules that resemble matchsticks that are placed subcutaneously in the brachial region every 6 months. **Depo-Provera** is the trade name for medroxyprogesterone acetate, an intramuscular hormone injection that is administered every 12 weeks to females. Both Norplant and Depo-Provera suppress ovulation and are 99% effective.

An **intrauterine device** (IUD) is a small plastic or metal loop or T that is inserted into the uterine cavity. Its mechanism of action remains unclear; however, its pres-

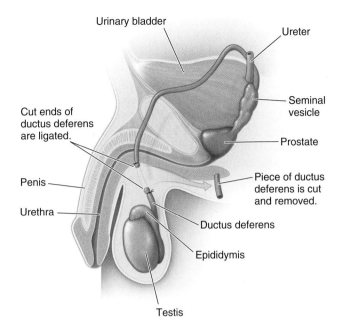

Urinary bladder

Ureter

Cut ends of
ductus deferens
are ligated.

Seminal
vesicle

Prostate

Penis

Piece of ductus
deferens is cut
and removed.

Urethra

Ductus deferens

Epididymis

Testis

FIGURE 16-32
Vasectomy is a surgi-
cal operation that
prevents sperm from
being ejaculated.

ence stimulates prostaglandin production that ultimately changes the chemical composition of uterine secretions and lowers the chances of fertilization and implantation. **Oral contraceptives** (OCTs), commonly called the pill, birth control pills (BCPs), or oral contraceptive pills (OCPs), are tablets taken daily to manipulate the female hormone cycle so that ovulation does not occur. They usually contain a combination of estrogen and progesterone. Oral contraceptives are known to reduce the risk of ovarian cysts and cancer, endometrial cancer, and benign breast disease, an added benefit. In women taking OCTs, there is less iron-deficiency anemia, rheumatoid arthritis, endometriosis, dysmenorrhea, and premenstrual syndrome symptoms.

A sterilization technique in which a woman's uterine tubes are surgically blocked or tied to prevent ova from entering the uterus is called a **tubal ligation** (Fig. 16-33). Ova are released, but cannot reach the uterus or incoming sperm. The oocytes degenerate and are absorbed by the body. **Vaginal barriers** are physical blockades that prevent sperm from entering the uterus. Examples include a **diaphragm**, a dome-shaped device placed inside the vagina at the entrance to the uterus and a similar device called

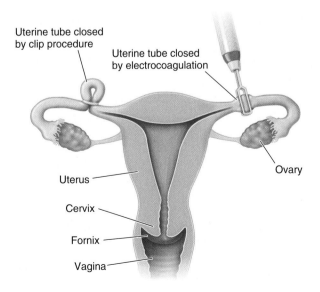

Uterine tube closed
by clip procedure

Uterine tube closed
by electrocoagulation

Uterus

Ovary

Cervix

Fornix

Vagina

FIGURE 16-33
Two different
procedures for tubal
ligation.

the **cervical cap.** This apparatus is placed inside the vagina and fitted tightly over the entrance to the cervix.

Another vaginal device is the pessary. A **pessary** is an appliance or medicine-containing suppository placed in the vagina for therapeutic purposes, vaginal or uterine support, or contraception.

Contraceptive measures that involve either or both sexes include abstinence, the rhythm method, and sterilization. **Abstinence** is refraining from penile–vaginal intercourse. The **rhythm method** is a form of contraception in which sexual intercourse is avoided on days that ovulation may be occurring or when a woman is most likely to conceive. A surgical procedure that prevents reproduction by total or partial removal of the reproductive organs is called **sterilization.** Removal of organs may render the person incapable of producing functional gametes or unable to sustain a pregnancy.

Key Terms	Definitions
contraceptive (kon truh SEP tiv)	agent that prevents conception or fertilization of oocyte by sperm
condoms	sheaths worn over the penis during copulation
vasectomy (vas ECK tuh mee)	surgical division of the ductus deferens used to produce male sterility
female condom	sheath worn inside the vagina during sexual intercourse
Norplant	six hormone capsules inserted subcutaneously in the brachial region of women to suppress ovulation
Depo-Provera	intramuscular hormone injection administered every 12 weeks to females to suppress ovulation
intrauterine (in truh YOO tur in) **device**	mechanical apparatus placed in the uterus to prevent embryo implantation
oral contraceptives (OR ul kon truh SEP tivs)	daily pills that manipulate the female hormonal cycle to prevent ovulation
tubal ligation (lye GAY shun)	surgical blocking of the uterine tubes
vaginal (VAJ i nul) **barrier**	physical blockade placed in the vagina to deny sperm entry into the uterus
diaphragm (DYE uh fram)	device worn at the uterine entrance during copulation to prevent conception
cervical (SUR vi kul) **cap**	tight-fitting device worn over the entrance to cervix
pessary (PES uh ree)	device or suppository containing medicine that is inserted into the vagina
abstinence	restraint from sexual intercourse
rhythm method	form of contraceptive in which coitus is avoided on ovulation days or when the occyte is still in the oviduct
sterilization	procedure that renders one incapable of procreating

Key Term Practice: Birth Control Methods

1. Which form of birth control is strictly male? _____

2. Identify the two birth control measures that involve no pharmacological agents, devices, or surgery.
   _____ _____

3. Surgical blocking of the oviducts is termed _____.

CLINICAL TERMS

Clinical Dimension	Term	Description
DISORDERS		
	acquired immunodeficiency syndrome (AIDS)	disease caused by infection with the human immunodeficiency virus (HIV), a retrovirus that causes immune system failure
	benign prostatic hyperplasia (BPH)	noncancerous prostate enlargement; benign prostatic hypertrophy
	benign prostatic hypertrophy (BPH)	noncancerous prostate enlargement; benign prostatic hyperplasia
	breast cancer	carcinoma of the mammary tissue
	candidiasis	vaginal yeast infection caused by the *Candida albicans* fungus
	cervical cancer	malignant cells of the cervix
	chancroid	sexually transmitted disease characterized by painful, ragged ulcers at the infection site
	chlamydia	sexually transmitted disease caused by the bacterium *Chlamydia trachomatis*
	cryptorchidism	failure of one or both of the testes to descend into the scrotum
	cystocele	hernia of the urinary bladder through the vaginal wall
	endometrial cancer	malignant cells of the uterine endometrium
	endometriosis	endometrium is present and functioning outside the uterus
	epididymitis	inflammation of the epididymis
	epispadias	congenital defect characterized by the penile urethral opening located on the dorsal surface
	erectile dysfunction	incapable of filling with blood under pressure to become stiff enough to perform sexual intercourse; impotence
	fibrocystic breast disease	unusual growth of fibrous tissue in the breast
	fibroids	benign fibrous tumors

Clinical Dimension	Term	Description
	genital herpes	sexually transmitted disease caused by the herpes simplex virus; herpes progenitalis
	genital warts	warts on the genitalia or in the anus region caused by the human papilloma virus (HPV)
	gonorrhea	sexually transmitted disease caused by *Neisseria gonorrhoeae*
	gynecomastia	enlarged breasts on a man
	hepatitis B	form of hepatitis caused by the hepatitis B virus that is spread through sexual contact; serum hepatitis
	hermaphroditism	having both male and female genitalia and secondary sexual characteristics; androgyny
	herpes progenitalis	sexually transmitted disease caused by the herpes simplex virus; genital herpes
	hydrocele	accumulation of fluid the scrotal sac
	hypospadias	congenital disorder characterized by the penile urethral opening located on the ventral surface
	impotence	incapable of filling with blood under pressure to become stiff enough to perform sexual intercourse; erectile dysfunction
	infecundity	female sterility
	infertility	inability of a couple to achieve pregnancy
	labial cancer	malignant cells of the folds surrounding the female genitalia; vulvar cancer
	leiomyomas	benign tumors of smooth muscle cells
	leiomyomas uteri	fibrous tumors of smooth muscle cells
	lues	sexually transmitted disease caused by *Treponema pallidum*; syphilis
	lymphogranuloma venereum (LGV)	sexually transmitted disease caused by *Chlamydia trachomatis*
	menorrhagia	excessive menstrual flow
	metrorrhagia	excessive bloody discharge between menstrual cycles
	ovarian cancer	malignant tumor of the ovary or ovaries
	ovarian cysts	fluid-filled sacs on or near the ovaries
	pelvic inflammatory disease (PID)	inflammation of the reproductive organs that, if untreated, can cause infertility
	phimosis	abnormal narrowing of the foreskin opening in uncircumcised males that prevents its retraction to uncover the glans penis
	precocious puberty	advanced reproductive development at an early age
	premenstrual dysphoric disorder (PMDD)	group of symptoms similar to premenstrual syndrome (PMS) that persist after the onset of menstruation

Clinical Dimension	Term	Description
	premenstrual syndrome (PMS)	group of symptoms experienced by some women in the days preceding menstruation
	priapism	persistent, painful penis erection in the absence of sexual interest
	proctocele	hernia of the rectum through the vaginal wall; rectocele
	prostate cancer	malignant cell growth of the prostate gland
	prostatitis	prostate gland inflammation
	rectocele	hernia of the rectum through the vaginal wall; proctocele
	serum hepatitis	form of hepatitis caused by the hepatitis B virus that is spread through sexual contact; hepatitis B
	sterile	incapable of becoming pregnant or incapable of inducing pregnancy
	sterility	total inability to reproduce
	syphilis	sexually transmitted disease caused by *Treponema pallidum*; lues
	testicular cancer	malignant cell growth in the testis
	testicular torsion	rotation of the spermatic cord that causes an interruption in the blood supply to the tissue
	toxic shock syndrome (TSS)	circulatory failure associated with tampon use and the growth of toxin-producing staphylococcal bacteria
	trichomoniasis	sexually transmitted disease caused by the protozoan parasite *Trichomonas vaginalis*
	uterine prolapse	distension of uterus into the vagina
	vaginal cancer	malignant cells of the vagina
	varicocele	swelling of the veins in the spermatic cord of the scrotum
	venereal diseases (VD)	diseases transmitted through sex acts; sexually transmitted diseases
	vulvar cancer	malignant cells of the folds surrounding the female genitalia; labial cancer
SIGNS AND SYMPTOMS		
	chancres	skin lesions or ulcers at the point where the disease-causing organism enters the body
	dysmenorrhea	difficult and painful menstruation
	dyspareunia	painful sexual intercourse
	gumma	rubbery tumor that occurs in the tertiary stage of syphilis; asyphiloma
	frigidity	lack of sexual response
	leukorrhea	thick discharge from the vagina
	libido	sexual desire

Clinical Dimension	Term	Description
	mastalgia	breast pain
	mittelschmerz	pain that occurs midway through the uterine cycle between menstrual periods
	oligospermia	low sperm count in the semen
	oophoritis	ovary inflammation
	orchitis	testis inflammation
	salpingitis	uterine tube inflammation
	smegma	cheesy secretion that collects around the clitoris in females or under the prepuce in males
	syphiloma	rubbery tumor that occurs in the tertiary stage of syphilis; gumma
	vaginitis	vaginal inflammation

CLINICAL TESTS AND DIAGNOSTIC PROCEDURES

Clinical Dimension	Term	Description
	culdocentesis	removal of intraperitoneal fluid through the vagina
	culdoscopy	examination with a culdoscope inserted in the vagina to view the pelvic cavity
	digital rectal examination (DRE)	manual examination of the prostate through the rectum
	female serum tests	evaluate levels of estrogen, estradiol, follicle-stimulating hormone, luteinizing hormone, progesterone, pregnanediol, and prolactin
	Gram stain	differential stain used to identify microbes according to the dye retained within the cell wall
	hysterosalpingography	x-ray examination of the uterus and the oviducts after the injection of radiopaque dye into their cavities
	laparoscopy	examination of abdominal internal organs using a laparoscope
	mammography	x-ray examination of the breast
	Pap smear	test used to detect precancerous or cancerous cells of the cervix; Pap test
	Pap test	test used to detect precancerous or cancerous cells of the cervix; Pap smear
	pelvic examination	manually palpating and examining the vagina, uterus, rectum, and accessory organs and structures
	prostate-specific antigen (PSA) test	measures the circulating blood levels of prostate-specific antigen
	resectoscope	endoscopic instrument for the transurethral removal of structures or parts of structures
	semen analysis	measures the volume of semen secreted and the sperm number, morphology, and motility
	serum α-fetoprotein (AFP) test	measures α-fetoprotein in the blood

Clinical Dimension	Term	Description
	serum test for testosterone	measures circulating levels of testosterone
	thermography	recording of the visual image of heat that breast tissue emits as infrared radiation
	transrectal ultrasonography	method of obtaining echograms through a probe inserted into the rectum
	transvaginal sonography	procedure for obtaining echograms of the ovaries and ovarian structures
	Treponema pallidum immobilization (TPI) test	determines the presence of antibodies to the *Treponema* spirochete
	ultrasonography	procedure using sound waves to produce an image for diagnostic purposes
	venereal disease research laboratory (VDRL) test	initial serological test done to identify syphilis
TREATMENTS		
	abstinence	restraint from sexual intercourse
	castration	surgical removal of one testicle or both testicles; orchiectomy
	cervical cap	tight-fitting contraceptive device worn over the entrance to the cervix
	chemotherapy	use of chemical agents (drugs) to treat disease
	circumcision	removal of the prepuce (foreskin) from the penis
	colpoplasty	vaginal repair and restructure
	colporrhaphy	vaginal suture
	condoms	sheaths worn over the penis during copulation
	conization	excision of a cone of tissue, most notably from the cervix
	contraceptive	agent that prevents conception or fertilization of the oocyte by sperm
	cryosurgery	surgery in which low temperatures are applied to tissues to seal or remove them
	Depo-Provera	intramuscular hormone injection administered every 12 weeks to females to suppress ovulation
	diaphragm	device worn at the uterine entrance during copulation to prevent conception
	dilation and curettage (D&C)	gynecological procedure in which the cervix is widened and the uterus is scraped
	electrocoagulation	cauterizing tissue to stop bleeding
	estrogen-replacement therapy (ERT)	treatment used for a variety of reasons to maintain female estrogen levels
	female condom	sheath worn inside the vagina during sexual intercourse

Clinical Dimension	Term	Description
	hormone-replacement therapy (HRT)	treatment used to maintain female hormone levels after menopause
	hysterectomy	surgical removal of the uterus
	intrauterine device (IUD)	mechanical apparatus placed in the uterus to prevent embryo implantation
	Kegel exercises	alternate contraction and relaxation of the perineal muscles to increase the strength of the pelvic floor muscles to treat urinary incontinence
	laser ablation	removal of tissue with a laser
	mastectomy	breast excision
	Norplant	six hormone capsule inserted subcutaneously in the brachial region of women to suppress ovulation
	oral contraceptives	daily pills that manipulate the female hormonal cycle to prevent ovulation
	orchiectomy	surgical removal of one testicle or both testicles; castration
	pessary	device or suppository containing medicine that is inserted into the vagina
	prostatectomy	excision of part or all of the prostate
	radiation	treatment of disease using ionizing radiation
	radical hysterectomy	removal of the uterus, upper vagina, and parametrium
	rhythm method	form of contraceptive in which coitus is avoided on ovulation days or when an oocyte is still in the oviduct
	salpingo-oophorectomy	removal of the uterine tube and ovary
	selective estrogen receptor modulators (SERMs)	drugs that function as native estrogen in some tissue but block its action in others
	selective serotonin reuptake inhibitors (SSRIs)	antidepressant medications that increase the body levels of serotonin
	sildenafil citrate	drug used to treat male impotence; trade name Viagra
	sterilization	procedure that renders one incapable of procreating
	trans–rectus abdominis musculocutaneous (TRAM) flap	surgical procedure to reconstruct the mammary region after mastectomy
	transurethral prostatectomy	surgical excision of all or part of the prostate using a resectoscope
	transurethral resection prostatectomy	excision of the prostate via a resectoscope passed through the urethra

Clinical Dimension	Term	Description
	tubal ligation	surgical blocking of the uterine tubes
	vaginal barriers	physical blockades placed in the vagina to deny sperm entry into the uterus
	vasectomy	surgical division of the ductus deferens used to produce male sterility

Lifespan

Reproductive system formation begins early in embryonic development. The gonads form from gonadal ridges in the mesoderm during the 5th week of gestation. Adjacent structures called mesonephric (Wolffian) ducts and paramesonephric (Müllerian) ducts respectively form male and female reproductive structures.

In regard to gender determination, male embryonic sex cells contain a large X chromosome and a smaller Y chromosome; two large X chromosomes represent females. The sex-determining region of the Y chromosome (SRY) initiates the male pattern of development during the 7th embryonic week. Developing Sertoli cells secrete a hormone, Müllerian-inhibiting substance (MIS), that halts the development of female reproductive structures. By week 8, interstitial cells begin secreting testosterone and stimulating male reproductive structures.

The female uterus, oviducts, and vagina are formed from the paramesonephric ducts. The gonads develop into ovaries in the absence of SRY.

Sexual differentiation occurs around the 8th week when some male embryonic testosterone is converted to dihydrotestosterone (DHT). Dihydrotestosterone promotes urethral, prostate, scrotum, and penis development. Female embryos lack DHT, thus the clitoris, labia minora, labia majora, and vestibule form.

Anatomic testicular and ovarian changes occur before birth. At 2 months before delivery, the testes of males descend toward the scrotum. Hormones and the gubernaculum guide this movement. In females, the ovaries move down into the pelvic cavity guided by the gubernaculum, which later divides to form the ovarian and uterine round ligaments.

The reproductive system remains in a latent state from birth until the onset of puberty. Puberty, which occurs some time between the ages of 10 and 15 years, is characterized by the development of secondary sexual characteristics in both sexes and the onset of menstruation in females. Hormones drive the psychological and physiological changes that occur.

Males and females differ significantly in terms of reproductive functional capacity. Women have a limited time of fertility between menarche and menopause. For 1–2 years after the onset of menses, ovulation occurs in only about 10% of the cycles. Thereafter, regular ovulatory cycles continue until menopause. It is currently thought that there is no male equivalent to menopause, but some research indicates men may actually experience something akin to menopause.

The aging female reproductive system experiences a great amount of change. Between ages 40 and 50 years, estrogen secretion decreases, leading to permanent menstrual cessation. Reproductive organs also atrophy, but there is no correlation between loss of reproductive function and sexual desire as libido (sexual drive) is maintained throughout life.

The aging male reproductive system has less profound changes than the female. Although testosterone production declines around age 55 years, males retain spermatogenesis ability until age 80 or 90 years. Sperm production in the aging male does have some consequences. For example, it takes 20–25 minutes for the sperm of young men to travel up the oviducts, but it takes 2.5 days for the sperm of men in their 70s to make this same journey. Prostatic hypertrophy is a common age-related condition often causing polyuria, nocturia, and postvoiding dribbling. Research suggests that nearly all elderly men will experience some enlargement of the prostate gland.

In the News: Mifepristone (RU-486) and Plan B

Use of the morning-after pill has been debated since its initial production. In December 2003, however, the dispute resurfaced when two advisory committees recommended to the U.S. Food and Drug Administration (FDA) that it should legalize over-the-counter (OTC) access to Plan B (levonorgestrel), an emergency contraceptive *similar* to mifepristone (RU-486). The FDA ignored the recommendations of the expert panels and has denied over-the-counter access to Plan B emergency contraception (EC).

Mifepristone (MIF pris tone), better known as RU-486, is an aborticant developed during the early 1980s in France, where it has been approved for use since 1988. Widespread testing of the drug has occurred in other countries outside the United States.

It is an effective postcoital contraceptive that binds to progesterone receptors, thereby inhibiting the ability of the uterus to sustain a pregnancy. A single 600-mg dose is an effective contraceptive after unprotected sex; therefore, RU-486 has been referred to as the "morning-after" pill.

Early clinical trials indicate mifepristone may be beneficial in the treatment of endometriosis, breast cancer, and other neoplasms containing glucocorticoids or progesterone receptors. To date, it is not approved for contraceptive use in the United States. It is approved, however, for treating patients with Cushing syndrome (condition caused by excessive adrenocortical hormone) who fail to respond to other therapeutic measures.

Plan B is a two-tablet EC; one tablet is taken as soon as possible and within 72 hours of intercourse, and the other tablet is taken 12 hours later. Plan B does not cause miscarriage; it actually prevents pregnancy by preventing ovulation or fertilization by altering tubal transport of the sperm or ova. If Plan B is accidentally taken during early pregnancy, it cannot terminate the pregnancy. Currently, a prescription is needed for Plan B. Whether or not Plan B will make it to the pharmacy store shelves as an over-the-counter medicine is yet to be determined.

COMMON ABBREVIATIONS

Abbreviation	Term
ACNM	American College of Nurse Midwives
AFP test	α-fetoprotein
AIDS	acquired immunodeficiency syndrome
A&P repair	anterior and posterior repair
BC	birth control
BCP	birth control pill
BPH	benign prostatic hyperplasia; benign prostatic hypertrophy

Abbreviation	Term
BSE	breast self-examination
BSN	bachelor of science in nursing
BSO	bilateral salpingo-oophorectomy
CIS	carcinoma in situ
CNM	certified nurse midwife
D&C	dilation and curettage
DES	diethylstilbestrol
DHT	dihydrotestosterone
DRE	digital rectal examination
EC	emergency contraception
ERT	estrogen-replacement therapy
FDA	Food and Drug Administration
FSH	Follicle-stimulating hormone
G−	Gram negative
GnRH	gonadotropin-releasing hormone
G+	Gram positive
HBV	hepatitis B virus
HIV	human immunodeficiency virus
HPV	human papilloma virus
HRT	hormone-replacement therapy
HSV-2	herpes simplex virus type 2
IUD	intrauterine device
IVP	intravenous pyelogram
LGV	lymphogranuloma venereum
LH	luteinizing hormone
MEAC	Midwifery Education Accreditation Council
MIS	Müllerian-inhibiting substance
n	haploid chromosome number
OCPs	oral contraceptive pills
OCT	oral contraceptive
OT	oxytocin
OTC	over-the-counter
PID	pelvic inflammatory disease
PMDD	premenstrual dysphoric disorder
PMS	premenstrual syndrome
PRL	prolactin
PSA	prostate-specific antigen
SERM	selective estrogen receptor modulator
SRY	sex-determining region of the Y chromosome
SSRI	selective serotonin reuptake inhibitor
STD	sexually transmitted disease

Abbreviation	Term
TPI test	*Treponema pallidum* immobilization test
TRAM flap	trans–rectus abdominis musculocutaneous flap
TSE	testicular self-examination
TSS	toxic shock syndrome
TUR	transurethral resection
TURP	transurethral prostatectomy
2n	diploid chromosome number
UTI	urinary tract infection
VD	venereal disease
VDRL test	venereal disease research laboratory test

Case Study

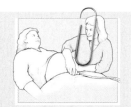

Carla Saschen is a 40-year-old nulliparous woman who arrived at Martha's office for a routine physical examination, including a complete pelvic and breast examination. Clinical information revealed a complaint of nipple discharge and pelvic pain. A right breast mass was discovered during mammary palpation. Ms Saschen uses an IUD. The pelvic examination was unremarkable. Mammograms and pelvis and transvaginal ultrasound studies were ordered.

The results of mammography studies indicated heterogeneously dense fibroglandular tissue dispersed to the superior lateral aspect of each breast. There was no definitive evidence of malignancy or microcalcification. Benign-appearing lymph nodes were also noted in the right axilla. The results of the ultrasound studies were not yet known.

Case Study Questions

Select the best answer to each of the following questions.

1. Nipple discharge is _____.

    a. normal
    b. abnormal in nulliparous women
    c. normal depending on day in menstrual cycle
    d. nothing to cause concern

2. The word *nulliparous* refers to _____.

    a. having borne no children
    b. having borne at least one child
    c. being premenopause
    d. having had a hysterectomy

3. Benign-appearing lymph nodes in right axilla refers to _____.

    a. noncancerous nodes in adjacent lymphatic structures

    b. cancer of lymph nodes
    c. noncancerous nodes in the hip region
    d. an inconclusive mammography

4. Why were pelvis and transvaginal ultrasound studies ordered?

    a. The source of the pelvic pain required further study.
    b. Nipple discharge is associated with pelvic pain.
    c. Mammography revealed abnormal endometrium.
    d. All of the above are correct.

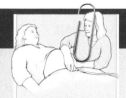

REAL WORLD REPORT

Martha's office received the medical report from the imaging department for Carla Saschen's pelvis and transvaginal ultrasound studies.

IMAGING DEPARTMENT

NAME:	Carla Saschen
AGE:	40 years
TEST:	Pelvis and transvaginal ultrasound
DATE ORDERED:	06/07/2003
ATTENDING:	J. R. Baum, MD
DOB:	05/22/1953
CLINICAL NOTES:	Pelvic pain; patient with IUD
EXAM DATE:	06/07/2003
REFERRING:	B. E. Rosen, DO

PELVIS AND TRANSVAGINAL ULTRASOUND

Real-time ultrasound evaluation of the pelvis was performed using both the transabdominal and the transvaginal approach. The patient's urinary bladder is not well distended, thus limiting transabdominal imaging.

Estimation of uterine size is approximately 9.5 × 4.5 × 6.8 cm. The intrauterine device is visualized within the endometrium. The endometrial lining measures 8–9 mm in thickness. There is no endometrial fluid. Incidental note is made of an 8-mm Nabothian cyst.

Both ovaries were visualized, with the right measuring 3.6 × 2.7 × 2.4 cm and the left 2.3 × 2.6 × 1.9 cm. There are bilateral adnexal cysts. The larger on the right measured 2.6 cm. That on the left measured 1.8 cm. There was no free pelvic fluid.

IMPRESSION

Bilateral adnexal cysts, the larger being on the right. Appropriate positioning of the intrauterine device within the endometrial canal.

DICTATED BY: S. K. Lowell, MD

REAL WORLD REPORT QUESTIONS

The following exercises review the medical terms in the preceding medical report. One eponymous term that may be new to you is Nabothian cyst. Nabothian (na BOH thee un) glands are mucous glands of the cervix.

1. Endometrial lining refers to the _____.

   a. outer layer of the uterus

   b. inner layer of the vagina

   c. middle layer of the vagina

   d. inner layer of the uterus

2. IUD is the abbreviation for

_____.

3. Identify the location of the 8-mm Nabothian cyst.

_____.

_____.

_____.

4. Explain what is meant by bilateral adnexal cysts.

_____.

_____.

_____.

REVIEW AND APPLICATION: THREE-LEVEL LEARNING SYSTEM

LEVEL ONE: REVIEWING FACTS AND TERMS USING RECALL

Select the best response to each of the following questions.

1. The term that means producing offspring is _____.

    a. procreation

    b. gametogenesis

    c. spermiogenesis

    d. oogenesis

2. _____ is a general term used to describe an ovary or testis.

    a. Gonad

    b. Gamete

    c. Ovum

    d. Reproduction

3. Identify the organ that is *not* part of the female reproductive system.

    a. uterine tube

    b. ovary

    c. prostate

    d. vagina

4. Which of the following features is associated with the testes?

    a. fimbriae

    b. median raphe

    c. infundibulum

    d. penis

5. The canal leading from the uterus to the exterior is the _____.

    a. urethra

    b. fallopian tube

    c. rectum

    d. vagina

6. Spermatozoa production is termed _____.

    a. fertility

    b. spermatogenesis

    c. spermatid

    d. flagellum

7. The _____ ductules connect the rete testis with the epididymis.

    a. tunica albuginea

    b. seminiferous

    c. ejaculatory

    d. efferent

8. The _____ is a network of blood vessels in the testicles.

    a. Sertoli cell

    b. seminiferous tubule

    c. rete testis

    d. spermatozoan

9. This structure serves as an exit for both urine and semen.

    a. ejaculatory duct

    b. prepuce

    c. urethra

    d. prostate gland

10. The opening at the tip of the penis is the _____.

    a. meatus

    b. glans penis

    c. prepuce

    d. hiatus

11. An alternate term for copulation is _____.

    a. erection

    b. ejaculation

    c. climax

    d. coitus

12. Hormones that promote male secondary sex characteristics are called _____.

    a. testosterone

    b. androgens

    c. gonadotropins

    d. estrogens

13. The transitional period leading to female menopause is _____.

    a. menarche

    b. menstruation

    c. detumescence

    d. female climacteric

14. Which of the following terms means activation process allowing sperm to successfully fertilize an oocyte?

    a. capacitation

    b. meiosis

    c. fertilization

    d. none of these

15. Surgical blocking of the oviducts is termed _____.

    a. vaginal barrier

    b. intrauterine device

    c. tubal ligation

    d. vasectomy

16. _____ is a hormone that causes pelvic relaxation.

    a. Progesterone

    b. Relaxin

    c. Progestin

    d. Estrogen

17. Vaginal inflammation is termed _____ from the word part _____, which refers to "the vagina" and the suffix -itis meaning "inflammation."

    a. oophoritis; oo-

    b. salpingitis; salping-

    c. vaginitis; vagin-

    d. orchitis; orch-

18. Orchitis is inflammation of the _____.

    a. ovary

    b. uterine tube

    c. prostate

    d. testis

19. Another term for a bag or sac is a/an _____.

    a. follicle

    b. secondary oocyte

    c. egg

    d. sperm

20. The constricted portion of the oviduct connecting it to the uterus is called the _____.

    a. fimbriae

    b. isthmus

    c. ampulla

    d. infundibulum

21. The passage that is closed at one end (cul-de-sac) between the cervix and the vaginal wall is termed the _____.

    a. fornix

    b. fundus

    c. uterine body

    d. follicle

22. Circumcision is the procedure in which the _____ is removed from the _____.

    a. foreskin; prepuce

    b. prepuce; foreskin

    c. prepuce; glans penis

    d. glans penis; prepuce

23. _____ is the cessation of menstrual cycles.

    a. Menarche

    b. Menses

    c. Menstruation

    d. Menopause

24. _____ is the onset of menstruation and marks the very first menstrual cycle occurring during puberty.

    a. Menarche

    b. Female climacteric

    c. Menopause

    d. Ovulation

25. Sexual intercourse is also known as _____.

    a. orgasm and climax

    b. coitus and climax

    c. coitus and copulation

    d. climax and arousal

26. The culmination of sexual excitement is termed _____.

    a. orgasm

    b. arousal

    c. lubrication

    d. A and B are correct

LEVEL TWO: REVIEWING CONCEPTS

Select the best response to each of the following questions.

27. Male glands include _____.

    a. bulbourethral and ejaculatory

    b. bulbourethral and seminal vesicles

    c. Cowper and spermatic

    d. ejaculatory and urethra

28. Female glands include _____.

    a. lesser vestibular and greater vestibular

    b. mons pubis and Skene

    c. clitoris and Bartholin

    d. greater vestibular and clitoris

Match the sign or symptom with its correct definition.

_____ 29. gumma   a. testes inflammation

_____ 30. dyspareunia   b. gumma as a result of syphilis

_____ 31. chancre   c. painful sexual intercourse

_____ 32. syphiloma   d. rubbery tumor associated with syphilis

_____ 33. orchitis   e. ulcer associated with syphilis

Match the medical term with its correct definition.

_____ 34. pessary   a. inflammation of the epididymis

_____ 35. leukorrhea   b. low sperm count

_____ 36. mastectomy   c. urethral opening located on the penile ventral surface

_____ 37. epididymitis   d. surgical removal of a breast

_____ 38. hypospadias   e. thick, white vaginal discharge

Match the clinical test or diagnostic procedure with its correct definition.

_____ 39. digital rectal examination   a. clinical test in which cells scraped from the cervix are cultured

_____ 40. Gram stain   b. x-ray examination of the breast tissue

_____ 41. transrectal ultrasono-graphy   c. manual examination of the prostate through the rectum

_____ 42. Pap test   d. differential staining technique used to identify bacteria

_____ 43. mammo-graphy   e. method of obtaining echograms through a probe inserted into the rectum

Match the disorder with its description.

_____ 44. fibroids   a. fibrous tumors composed of smooth muscle cells

_____ 45. vulvar cancer b. benign fibrous tumors

_____ 46. leiomyomas   c. inflammation of the female reproductive organs

_____ 47. pelvic inflammatory disease   d. fluid-filled sacs found on or near the ovaries

e. labial carcinoma

_____ 48. ovarian cysts

Match the disorder with its description.

_____ 49. infertility   a. erectile dysfunction

_____ 50. impotence   b. malignant cell growth in the prostate gland

_____ 51. prostate cancer   c. STD caused by *T. pallidum*

_____ 52. chancroid   d. involuntary reduction in reproductive ability

_____ 53. syphilis   e. STD caused by *H. ducreyi*

Match the treatment with its key description.

_____ 54. colporrhaphy   a. drug used to treat erectile dysfunction

_____ 55. hysterectomy   b. castration; surgical removal of the testicle(s)

_____ 56. sildenafil citrate   c. surgical removal of the uterus

_____ 57. orchiectomy   d. removal of part or all of the prostate gland

_____ 58. prostatectomy   e. vaginal suture

Match the birth control method with its definition.

_____ 59. oral contraceptives   a. tight-fitting device worn at the cervical entrance

_____ 60. diaphragm   b. device worn by the female at the uterine opening during coitus

_____ 61. cervical cap   c. the pill

_____ 62. sterilization   d. mechanical apparatus placed in the uterus

_____ 63. intrauterine device   e. procedure that makes one unable to carry on reproductive functions

Provide a medical term to complete a meaningful analogy.

64. Oviducts are to _____ as scrotal sac is to scrotum.

65. _____ glands are to breasts as _____ are to testes.

66. Orgasm is to _____ as _____ is to syphiloma.

67. Lues is to _____ as foreskin is to _____.

68. _____ glands are to paraurethral glands as Bartholin glands are to _____ glands.

Define the following terms.

69. areola _____

70. cryptorchidism _____

71. cystocele _____

72. conization _____

73. electrocoagulation _____

What is the term described by each of the following definitions?

74. agent that prevents conception _____

75. surgery in which low temperatures freeze tissue _____

76. STD caused by the herpes simplex virus _____

77. STD caused by *C. trachomatis* _____

78. cancer of unknown origin affecting the labia or vulva _____

Using the following word parts, form a medical term for each definition. Each word part is used only once.

-cele	-celeo
-ectomy	-itis
leio-	-myoma
ophor-	recto-
varico-	vagin-

79. inflammation of the vagina _____

80. benign tumor of the uterine smooth muscle _____

81. swelling of the veins in the scrotal spermatic cord _____

82. hernia of the rectum through the vaginal wall _____

83. removal of an ovary _____

Identify the correctly spelled term in each set.

84. _____
   a. colostrum
   b. colostrom
   c. collostrum
   d. collostrom

85. _____
   a. chanchre
   b. kanchre
   c. chankre
   d. chancre

86. _____
   a. yoorethra
   b. urithra
   c. urethra
   d. urrethra

87. _____
   a. perrineum
   b. perineum
   c. perinium
   d. perenium

88. _____
   a. ogenesis
   b. oogenesis
   c. oogenisis
   d. oogeneses

Unscramble the letters to form a medical term.

89. nipes _____

90. rutseu _____

91. creetino _____

92. tiiletyfr _____

93. sciitlro _____

Define the following abbreviations.

94. BPH _____

95. BSO _____

96. ERT _____

97. PID _____

98. D&C _____

LEVEL THREE: THINKING CRITICALLY

Provide a short answer to the following question.

99. A couple is having difficulty conceiving a child. Semen analysis reveals oligospermia. The fertility specialist suggests that the man wear boxer shorts instead of tight-fitting briefs. Provide a plausible explanation for this recommendation.

_____

_____

KEY TERMS SPELLING TEST FROM CD-ROM

Use the CD-ROM to test yourself on the spelling of key terms from this chapter. Listen to the terms and write them on a separate sheet of paper. Use a medical dictionary to check your answers.

ANSWERS

WORD GROUPING

Definition	Word Part
male, masculine	andr-, andro-
beginning, first, original	arach-, arche-, archi-
breast	A. mamm-, mammo-
	B. mast-, masto-
condition of spermatozoa or semen	-spermia
egg	ovi-, ovo-
egg, ovum	oo-
embryo	embry-, embryo-
epididymis	epididym-, epididymo-
female, woman	gyn-, gyne-, -gyne, gyneco-
few, deficiency	olig-, oligo-
glans penis	balan-, balano-
hidden, covered	crypt-, crypto-
labial, lip	labio-
meatus, opening	meat-, meato-
menses, menstruation	men-, meno-
neck, cervix, cervical	cervic-, cervico-
nipple	mammill-, mammillo-
origination, development	-genesis
ovary, ovarian	A. oophor-, oophoro-
	B. ovari-, ovario-
pelvis	pelvi-, pelvio-, pelvo-
perineum	perineo-
prostate gland	prostat-, prostato-
rectum or anus	proct-, procto-
sexual, generative	gam-, gamo-
smooth	leio-, lio-
sperm, semen, seed	sperm-, sperma-, spermi-, spermio-
spermatozoa, spermatic, seminal	spermat-, spermato-
swelling, tumor, hernia	-cele
testis	orch-, orchi-, orcho-, orchid-, orchido-
tip, end, head	acr-, acro-
uterine tube	salping-, salpingo-
uterus	A. hyster-, hystero-
	B. metr-, metro-
uterus, uterine	uter-, utero-
vagina, vaginal	A. colp-, colpo-, -colpos
	B. vagin-, vagino-

WORD BUILDING

Word Part	Meaning	Common or Known Word	Example Medical Term
arch-, archi-	beginning, first, original	menarche	menarche
andr-, andro-	male, masculine	androgynous	androgens
cervic-, cervico-	neck, cervix, cervical	cervical region	cervical cancer
crypt-, crypto-	hidden, covered	cryptic	cryptorchidism
embry-, embryo-	embryo	embryo	embryonic
gam-, gamo-	sexual, generative	gamete	gamete
-genesis	origination, development	histogenesis	oogenesis
gyn-, gyne-, -gyne, gyneco-	female, woman	gynecologist	gynecomastia
hyster-, hystero-	uterus	hysterectomy	hysterectomy
mamm-, mammo-	breast	mammogram	mammary gland
mammill-, mammillo-	nipple	mammilla	mammilla
meat-, meato-	meatus, opening	auditory meatus	urethral meatus
men-, meno-	menses, menstruation	menstruation	menopause
orch-, orchi-, orcho-, orchid-, orchido-	testis	orchitis	orchiectomy
ovari-, ovario-	ovary, ovarian	ovarian cancer	ovarian
ovi-, ovo-	egg	oviparous	oviduct
pelvi-, pelvio-, pelvo-	pelvis	pelvis	pelvic examination
proct-, procto-	rectum or anus	proctologist	proctocele
prostat-, prostato-	prostate gland	prostate	prostatitis
sperm-, sperma-, spermi-, spermio-	sperm, semen, seed	sperm	spermiogenesis
spermat-, spermato-	spermatozoa, spermatic, seminal	spermatic	spermatogenesis
uter-, utero-	uterus, uterine	uterus	uterus
vagin-, vagino-	vagina, vaginal	vagina	vaginitis

KEY TERM PRACTICE

Reproductive Systems Preview

1. gamete; gametes
2. testis; testes
3. a. perineum; b. vulva

Male Internal Genitalia

1. epididymis; epididymides
2. spermatozoan; spermatozoa
3. spermato-; -genesis; spermatogenesis

Male External Genitalia

1. a. corpus spongiosum; b and c. corpora cavernosa (a pair)
2. corpus cavernosum
3. coitus; copulation

Male Reproductive Hormones

1. androgens
2. secondary sexual characteristics

Spermatogenesis

1. spermatid
2. flagellum; flagella

Female Internal Genitalia

1. ovulation
2. oviduct
3. ampulla; ampullae
4. infundibulum; infundibula

Female External Genitalia

1. labium majus; labia majora
2. labium minus; labia minora
3. clitoris

Mammary Glands

1. areola; areolae
2. lactation

Female Reproductive Hormones

1. estrogens
2. Progesterone

Oogenesis

1. oo-; -genesis; oogenesis
2. primary oocyte

Uterine Cycle

1. proliferative
2. uterine; menstrual

Sexual Intercourse

1. Emission; ejaculation
2. Detumescence

Testicle and Penis Disorders

1. orch-; inflammation; orchitis
2. epididym-; inflammation; epididymitis

Prostate Disorders

1. benign prostatic hyperplasia; benign prostatic hypertrophy
2. prostat-; inflammation; prostatitis

Female Pelvic and Inflammatory Disorders

1. dilation and curettage (D&C)
2. endometriosis

Female Cancers

1. labial cancer; vulvar cancer
2. mast-; removal of; mastectomy

Female Benign Tumors

1. leiomyoma
2. fibroid

Reproductive Hernias

1. colpoplasty
2. proctocele; rectocele

Infertility and Sterility

1. infecundity
2. Infertility

Infections

1. toxic shock syndrome (TSS)
2. Candidiasis

Sexually Transmitted Diseases

1. acquired immunodeficiency syndrome (AIDS)
2. venereal diseases (VDs)
3. progenitalis

Birth Control Methods

1. vasectomy
2. abstinence; rhythm method
3. tubal ligation

CASE STUDY

1. b is the correct answer.
   - Answers a and c are incorrect because nipple discharge is not normal in women who are not breast feeding.
   - Answer d is incorrect because nipple discharge is an abnormal condition in nonlactating women. Thus further investigation is warranted.
2. a is the correct answer.
   - Answers b, c, and d are incorrect because these phrases do not define nulliparous.
3. a is the correct answer.
   - Answer b is incorrect because the lymph nodes are benign, or not a threat to life or long-term health.
   - Answer c is incorrect because the axilla refers to the armpit, not the hip region.
   - Answer d is incorrect because the mammogram provides a good subsequent reading, although the 10% false-positive rate for mammography must be considered.
4. a is the correct answer.
   - Answer b is incorrect because there is no known association with nipple discharge and pelvic pain. Furthermore, the purpose of these tests is to view pelvic and vaginal structures.
   - Answer c is incorrect because mammography is used to study breast tissue, not endometrial (uterine) tissue.
   - Answer d is incorrect because only a is correct.

REAL WORLD REPORT

1. d
2. intrauterine device
3. The cysts are found in the cervix because they are distensions of the mucous (Nabothian) glands of the uterine cervix.
4. Bilateral adnexal cysts are closed, abnormal sacs attached to both the right and the left ovaries. Adnexal means that they are adjoined to anatomic parts.

REVIEW AND APPLICATION: THREE-LEVEL LEARNING SYSTEM

Level One: Reviewing Facts and Terms Using Recall

1. a
2. a
3. c
4. b
5. d
6. b
7. d
8. c
9. c
10. a
11. d
12. b
13. d
14. a
15. c
16. b
17. c
18. d
19. a
20. b
21. a
22. c
23. d
24. a
25. c
26. a

Level Two: Reviewing Concepts

27. b
28. a
29. d
30. c
31. e
32. b
33. a
34. b
35. e
36. d
37. a
38. c
39. c
40. d
41. e
42. a
43. b
44. b
45. e
46. a
47. c
48. d
49. d
50. a
51. b
52. e
53. c
54. e
55. c
56. a
57. b
58. d
59. c
60. b
61. a
62. e
63. d
64. uterine tubes; fallopian tubes
65. Mammary; testicles
66. climax; gumma
67. syphilis; prepuce
68. lesser vestibular; greater vestibular
69. pigmented area surrounding nipple
70. failure of the testes to descend into scrotum
71. hernia of urinary bladder that protrudes through the vaginal wall
72. excision of a cone of cervix tissue for therapeutic or diagnostic purposes
73. cauterizing tissue to stop bleeding
74. contraceptive
75. cryosurgery
76. genital herpes or herpes progenitalis
77. chlamydia
78. labial cancer or vulvar cancer
79. vaginitis
80. leiomyoma
81. varicocele
82. rectocele
83. oophorectomy
84. a
85. d
86. c
87. b
88. b
89. penis
90. uterus
91. erection
92. fertility
93. clitoris
94. benign prostatic hyperplasia or benign prostatic hypertrophy
95. bilateral salpingo-oophorectomy
96. estrogen replacement therapy
97. pelvic inflammatory disease
98. dilate and curettage

Level Three: Thinking Critically

99. Normal sperm development requires that the temperature be approximately 3°F cooler than body temperature. Thus boxer shorts will allow the testicles to drop down farther from the pelvic region and allow the sperm to develop in a slightly cooler environment, away from the groin area.

chapter 17

Pregnancy, Human Development, and Child Health

OBJECTIVES

After completing this chapter, you should be able to:

1. Define the meaning of word parts relating to pregnancy, human development, and child health.

2. Define key terms significant to fertilization, gestation, and placentation.

3. Explain the process of identical and fraternal twinning.

4. Describe genes, chromosomes, inheritance, and mutations.

5. Define common signs, symptoms, and treatments of various pregnancy and human development disorders, and childhood diseases.

6. Explain clinical tests and diagnostic procedures related to pregnancy and childhood disorders.

7. Describe anatomical and physiological alterations throughout the lifespan.

8. Define abbreviations related to pregnancy, human development, and child health.

9. Define terms used in medical reports involving pregnancy, human development, and child health.

10. Correctly define, spell, and pronounce the chapter's medical terms.

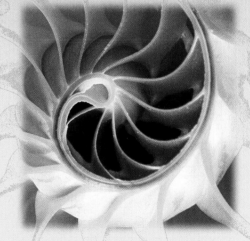

Professional Profile: Diagnostic Medical Sonographer

Mandy is a diagnostic medical sonographer (ultrasonographer). As an ultrasonographer, she is employed by a hospital to perform diagnostic testing on patients.

Sonography uses sound waves to generate images of internal body structures. To do this, a gel is spread across the skin surface and a transducer is moved across the area. The gel aids in the transmission of sound waves. During the scanning procedure, Mandy views the screen and looks for subtle clues that distinguish unhealthy tissue from normal tissue. She then selects which images will be shown to the physician.

Sonographers spend a great deal of time with patients explaining the procedure, recording the medical history, and setting up the equipment. Mandy's is a physically demanding job because she must stand all day while assisting with lifting and moving patients to the desired positions for the best pictures. Good communication skills are essential, especially because patients are usually apprehensive about the diagnostic procedure or the results that may be revealed.

Although Mandy is cross-trained to perform ultrasound on nearly every body area, including the abdomen, brain, and cardiovascular system, she most enjoys obstetric and gynecological sonography. Fetal health, growth, and status can be directly measured through ultrasonography.

Mandy was educated at a vocational school, where she earned an associate's degree from a program accredited by the Joint Review Committee on Education for Diagnostic Medical Sonography. Course work included classes in anatomy and physiology, basic physics, medical ethics, medical terminology, and patient care. Licensure is not required, but the hospital that employs her requires certification. To that end, she obtained registration through the American Registry of Diagnostic Medical Sonographers (ARDMS) by passing a general physics and instrumentation examination, along with a specialty examination in obstetrics/gynecology and abdominal viewing. She keeps her registration current by completing 30 hours of continuing education every 3 years.

INTRODUCTION

Life begins with the fertilization of an ovum, recently released from the ovary, by a sperm. Within 3 days, the fertilized egg, called a zygote, implants itself on the uterine wall.

From conception, marked by the beginning of pregnancy, to death, human beings constantly undergo changes. Human development is the progression in maturation from an embryonic stage to an adult phase, and life span development encompasses the prenatal stage through the gerontologic phase of life. This chapter focuses primarily on the stages of life beginning at fertilization and continuing to childhood. Along with a summary of human genetics and inheritance, the events of pregnancy, including the transformations of embryo, fetus, mother, and baby are described. Disorders of pregnancy, labor, delivery, neonates, and children are also discussed.

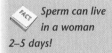

FACT
Sperm can live in a woman 2–5 days!

MEDICAL TERM PARTS

Word Parts	Meaning
allant-, allanto-	allantoic, allantois, an extraembryonic membrane
amnio-	amnion, amnionic
blast-, -blast, blasto-	formative cell, bud
case-, caseo-	resembling cheese
chori-, chorio-	chorion, outermost fetal membrane
embry-, embryo-	embryo, fetus, embryonic, fetal
encephal-, encephalo-	brain
episio-	vulva
gnath-, gnatho-	jaw
heter-, hetero-	different, unlike
hom-, homo-	common, like, same
kary-, karyo-	nucleus
lact-, lacti-, lacto-	milk
mening-, meningo-	meninx, meninges
mes-, meso-	middle
ped-, pedo-	child
phen-, pheno-	appearance
talo-	talus, ankle
terato-	malformed
troph-, tropho-	nutrition, nutritive, nourishment
zyg-, zygo-	joined

WORD ETYMOLOGY

Some words have Greek or Latin word roots but are not true word parts. This section lists those that are used as medical terms.

Word	Definition
caseus	cheese
fetus	offspring
gamos	marriage
gravid	pregnant
gravis	heavy
nates	buttocks
parturio	to be in labor
partus	childbirth

MEDICAL TERM PARTS USED AS PREFIXES

Prefix	Definition
amnio-	amnion, amnionic
episio-	vulva
talo-	talus, ankle
terato-	malformed

MEDICAL TERM PARTS USED AS SUFFIXES

Suffix	Definition
-blast	formative cell, bud

WORD GROUPING

Using the "Medical Term Parts" tables, identify the prefix, suffix, or combining form for each of the following definitions. The first one has been done as an example.

Definition	Word Part
resembling cheese	*case-, caseo-*
allantoic, allantois, an extraembryonic membrane	
amnion, amnionic	
appearance	
brain	
child	
chorion, outermost fetal membrane	
common, like, same	
different, unlike	
embryo, fetus, embryonic, fetal	
formative cell, bud	
jaw	
joined	
malformed	
meninx, meninges	
middle	
milk	
nucleus	
nutrition, nutritive, nourishment	
talus, ankle	
vulva	

WORD BUILDING

Word parts, introduced in the "Medical Term Parts" section, are listed in the following table. For this exercise, first supply the meaning of each word part, then use the word part to build a word you already know. The word you list under "Common or Known Word" does not have to be a medical term; a commonly used word is fine. Be sure, however, that the word correctly reflects the intended meaning. The first one has been done as an example.

Word Part	Meaning	Common or Known Word	Example Medical Term
allant-, allanto-	allantoic, allantois, an extraembryonic membrane	allantoin	allantois
amnio-			amniocentesis
blast-, -blast, blasto-			trophoblast
embry-, embryo-			embryology
episio-			episiotomy
heter-, hetero-			heterozygous
hom-, homo-			homozygous
mening-, meningo-			meningocele
mes-, meso-			mesoderm
ped-, pedo-			pediatrics
phen-, pheno-			phenotype
talo-			talipes equinovarus
zyg-, zygo-			zygote

ANATOMY AND PHYSIOLOGY

Structures of Pregnancy and Human Development

- Embryo
- Fetus
- Ovary
- Placenta
- Umbilical cord
- Uterine tubes
- Uterus
- Vagina
- Zygote

Pregnancy, Human Development, and Child Health Preview

Comprehension of human development requires a basic understanding of general terms such as fertilization, zygote, placenta, embryo, fetus, and gestation. **Fertilization** is the fusion of an ovum with a spermatozoon (Fig. 17-1). Once fertilized, the egg is referred to as a **zygote.** Ovaries are the sites of ova release, and the uterine tubes serve as the structures for fertilization. The zygote makes its way to the uterus, where implantation occurs; the placenta is formed to become the home of embryonic and fetal growth and development. The **placenta** is a vascular organ that develops inside the uterus to supply food and oxygen to the developing human through the **umbilical cord,** a structure consisting of two arteries and one vein.

Embryo is the term describing a human offspring in the early stages after conception to the end of the 8th week; thereafter, it is called a **fetus. Gestation** is the time spent in utero (in the womb). When the gestational phase is complete, the fetus is normally delivered by way of the vagina. After delivery, the new human is called an infant or baby.

Life expectancy is the average number of years a person born today can expect to live under current mortality conditions. For a male infant born in the United States today, the life expectancy is 74 years; for females, it is 80 years. **Life span** is the length of time that a member of a particular species can remain alive. One's life span is the extreme limit of human longevity. The human life span appears to be fixed at approximately 100 years; however, some have lived to be 120, and Jeanne Calment of France died in 1997 at the age of 122.

FACT *Fetus weight increases 3000 times between the 8th gestational week and birth!*

FACT *Sperm travel at a speed of 7.6 cm (3 in.) per hour!*

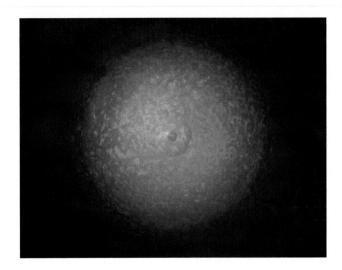

FIGURE 17-1
Fertilization is the fusion of an ovum with a spermatozoon, here seen seconds after the ovum was fertilized. (Reprinted with permission from LifeART image. © 2005 Lippincott Williams & Wilkins. All rights reserved.)

Key Terms	Definitions
fertilization	union of the male sperm and the female ovum
zygote (ZYE gote)	fertilized ovum
placenta (pluh SEN tuh)	organ of pregnancy on the wall of the uterus to which the embryo/fetus is attached by the umbilical cord
umbilical (um BIL i kul) **cord**	cylindrical structure containing the two umbilical arteries and one vein connecting the fetus with the placenta

embryo (EM bree oh)	product of conception from the moment of fertilization to end of the 8th gestational week
fetus (FEE tus)	unborn offspring beginning at week 9 after fertilization
gestation (jes TAY shun)	period of development from fertilization of the ovum until birth
life expectancy	the average number of years a person born today can expect to live
life span	the average duration of human life; longevity

Key Term Practice: Pregnancy and Human Development Preview

1. A fertilized egg is known as a/an _____.

2. After fertilization, the developing human is called a/an _____ until the 9th week of gestation.

Fertilization and Implantation

The union of male and female reproductive cells, **gametes**, forming a zygote is known as fertilization. Fertilization usually occurs in the uterine tube, where sperm penetration of the ovum is facilitated by hyaluronidase, an enzyme released from the sperm head (acrosome). The zona pellucida, a noncellular layer surrounding the ovum, contains a sperm receptor site called ZP3 that allows only one sperm to fertilize it, a process called **syngamy.**

The steps of fertilization can be summarized as follows:

sperm adheres to ovum → sperm acrosome releases hyaluronidase → sperm penetrates zona pellucida → sperm membrane fuses with ovum membrane → zygote is formed

The zygote contains 23 pairs of chromosomes and is genetically unique.

After zygote formation, cleavage occurs 30 hours to 3 days later. **Cleavage** is a period of early cell divisions of a zygote that form **blastomeres.** After 3 days of cleavage, the blastomeres form a solid ball of cells called a **morula.** Near the end of cleavage, the morula then develops into a **blastula** (blastocyst), a hollow ball of cells (Fig. 17-2).

The stage at which the blastula becomes imbedded in the lining of the uterus is termed **implantation.** It usually implants on the upper posterior uterine wall around the 5th day to the end of the 2nd week after fertilization. Proteolytic enzymes digest a hole in the endometrium for attachment. A structure known as a trophoblast forms to attach the blastula to the uterine wall. Primary germ layers—endoderm, ectoderm, and mesoderm—are then derived from the trophoblast through a process called **gastrulation.** These primary germ layers give rise to all other body tissues and organs by **histogenesis.**

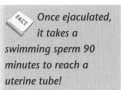 *Once ejaculated, it takes a swimming sperm 90 minutes to reach a uterine tube!*

Key Terms	Definitions
gametes (GAM eets)	male or female reproductive cells
syngamy (SIN guh mee)	joining together of gametes during fertilization
cleavage	early stage of development between fertilization and blastula when the embryo consists of a mass of dividing cells

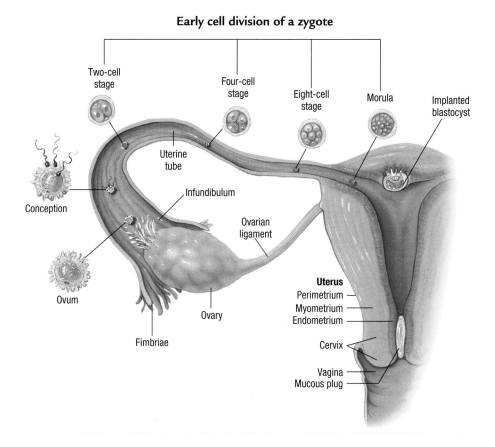

Early cell division of a zygote

FIGURE 17-2
The stages of cleavage are shown. (Image provided by Anatomical Chart Co.)

blastomeres (BLAS toh meerz)	cleavage cells, any cell into which the zygote divides
morula (MOR yoo luh)	cluster of blastomeres
blastula (BLAS tew luh)	hollow ball of cells formed near the end of cleavage; blastocyst
implantation	embedding of the embryo into the endometrium
gastrulation (gas troo LAY shun)	development of the embryonic germ layers
histogenesis (his toh JEN e sis)	formation of tissues from the primary germ layers

Key Term Practice: Fertilization and Implantation

1. The word part *histo-* means _____ and the word part _____ means "formation of;" thus _____ means the formation of tissues.

2. _____ is the development of embryonic germ layers.

Placentation and Gestation

Embryonic development is characterized by the formation of the placenta, extraembryonic membranes, and umbilical cord (Fig. 17-3). **Placentation** refers to the process of forming a placenta during pregnancy. The placenta, a structure about 16 cm (6 in.) in diameter and nearly 2 cm (1 in.) thick, serves as the organ of metabolic exchange between the mother and the fetus. At birth it weighs about 600 g (1.3 lb). Constituting nearly one-sixth the fetal weight, it is formed partly by maternal tissue and partially

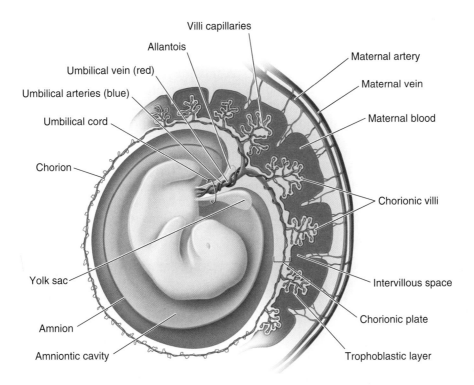

Villi capillaries
Allantois
Umbilical vein (red)
Umbilical arteries (blue)
Umbilical cord
Chorion
Yolk sac
Amnion
Amniontic cavity

Maternal artery
Maternal vein
Maternal blood
Chorionic villi
Intervillous space
Chorionic plate
Trophoblastic layer

FIGURE 17-3
The placenta serves as the organ of metabolic exchange between the mother and the fetus.

by embryonic tissue. Although blood does not flow between the layers, other substances are able to diffuse across the membrane.

Extraembryonic membranes play a role in placenta formation and the nurturing of the developing human. These include the yolk sac, amnion, allantois, and chorion. The yolk sac is a thin membrane that surrounds the embryo, forming blood cells, and giving rise to sex cells. A combination of mesoderm and ectoderm, the **amnion** is a fluid-filled sac that encircles the developing embryo/fetus and contains amnionic fluid. The word *amnionic* means "related to the amnion," but its synonym is amniotic, spelled with a *t* instead of an *n*. Both spellings are correct.

The allantois is a membranous sac derived from a combination of the endoderm and mesoderm that forms the umbilical blood vessels, and the **chorion** is a membrane consisting of a combination of mesoderm and trophoblast. Contacting the uterine wall, it has a dense concentration of blood vessels and becomes part of the placenta. Projections from its outer surface, **chorionic villi**, attach the embryo to the uterine wall. There is no mixing of maternal and fetal blood because the trophoblast layers separate the two.

The umbilical cord is a structure connecting the developing infant to the placenta. It consists of two umbilical arteries and one vein. It serves as the passageway for materials between the mother and the embryo/fetus.

During placentation and gestation, the developing human is most susceptible to injury from alcohol, cigarette smoking, drugs, ionizing radiation, lead, medications, mercury, and viruses. Substances such as these that cause **congenital** (evident at birth) malformations and defects are termed **teratogens. Teratology** is the study of abnormal development and congenital malformations caused by such agents.

A group of blood tests designed to identify teratogenic diseases in pregnant women and neonates is known as the **TORCH series.** TORCH is an acronym for toxoplasma (a protozoan), other disease-causing viruses (including hepatitis B virus, varicella, and group B β-hemolytic strep), rubella virus, cytomegalovirus (CMV), and herpes simplex virus type 2 (HSV2). All of these diseases can cross the placenta and infect the fetus.

Once formed, the placenta has endocrine functions and secretes hormones. Placental hormones include human chorionic gonadotropin (hCG), human placental

FACT *NNK, a derivative of nicotine, has been found in the urine of babies born to mothers who smoked during pregnancy!*

lactogen (hPL), estrogens, progesterone, and relaxin. **Human chorionic gonadotropin** maintains high estrogen and progesterone levels during the early weeks of pregnancy. Its level peaks 8–9 weeks after fertilization. The **human placental lactogen test** is a maternal blood examination useful for evaluating placental function. Low values indicate fetal distress or possible miscarriage. Estrogens, progesterone, and placental prolactin maintain pregnancy by acting on uterine tissue. **Relaxin** relaxes the symphysis pubis and assists in dilation of the cervix near the end of pregnancy.

Human growth depends on a nutritive environment during gestation. It is typically classified into trimesters, each 3 months in duration; 40 weeks serves as the gestational age of a full-term infant (Fig. 17-4). The first trimester is a period of embryologic and early fetal development. Cleavage, implantation, placentation, and embryogenesis occur during this period. At 4 weeks, the embryo is about the size of a pea. Organ formation begins by week 8, and the fetus develops recognizable arms and legs.

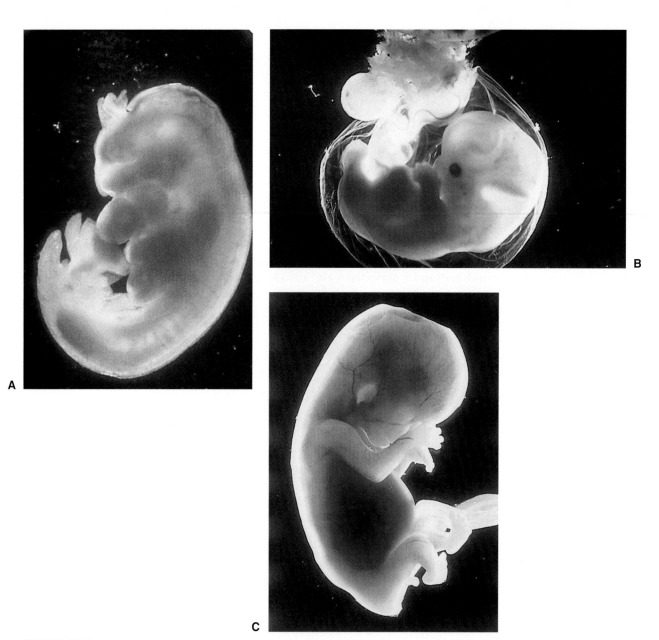

FIGURE 17-4
The human embryo at (**A**) 4 weeks, (**B**) 5 weeks, and (**C**) 6 weeks. (Reprinted with permission from Petit Format/Nestle/Science Source/Photo Researchers).

During the second trimester, organs and systems develop. By week 9, the fetus is the size of a strawberry. In this stage, the fetus begins to look distinctly human. Hair, eyebrows, and eyelashes develop, and lanugo (fine, fetal hair) covers the skin. The mother can feel fetal movements, and the heartbeat can be auscultated (heard through a stethoscope). The third trimester is characterized as a phase of rapid fetal growth. The fetus sleeps, wakes, engages in thumb sucking, and is easily startled during the period before birth.

> **FACT** *At birth, a baby's head is one quarter its body length; by adulthood, it is only one eighth!*

Key Terms	Definitions
placentation (plas en TAY shun)	formation and attachment of the placenta
amnion (AM nee on)	innermost fetal membrane forming a fluid-filled protective sac
chorion (KOH ree on)	outermost fetal membranes that form part of the placenta
chorionic villi (KOH ree on ick VIL eye)	projections from the chorion's outer surface
congenital (kun JEN i tul)	existing before or at birth, though not necessarily detected then
teratogens (TERR uh toh jenz)	agents that alter the normal development of a fetus, with results that are evident at birth or later
teratology (terr uh TOL uh jee)	scientific study of conditions caused by the interruption of normal human development
TORCH series	blood tests used to identify teratogenic diseases in pregnant women
human chorionic gonadotropin (KOH ree on ick goh nad oh TROH pin)	hormone originating in chorionic tissue
human placental lactogen (pluh SEN tul LACK toh jen) **test**	maternal blood test used to evaluate placental function
relaxin (ree LACK sin)	hormone secreted during pregnancy that causes pelvic relaxation

Key Term Practice: Placentation and Gestation

1. Projections from the outer surface of the chorion are termed _____.

2. The word part _____ means "malformed," and the word part _____ means "the study of;" therefore, the study of substances that cause congenital malformations is known as _____.

Fetal Circulation

There are circulatory differences between an unborn fetus and a fully developed birthed child. As the lifeline between mother and child, the umbilical cord contains two arteries and one vein. The arteries are extensions of the internal iliac arteries and carry fetal blood *to* the placenta, while the vein transports nutrients and oxygen-rich blood *from* the placenta to the fetus. In the adult, the proximal section of the umbilical arteries persists to supply blood to the urinary bladder. The umbilical vein eventually becomes the ligamentum teres, the round ligament at the caudal portion of the falciform ligament that holds the liver to the diaphragm.

In the fetal circulation, a vessel known as the **ductus venosus** connects the umbilical vein with the fetal inferior vena cava and shunts blood around the liver (Fig. 17-5). Blood in this location is high in oxygen and nutrients. Because the fetus does not breathe air, an opening in the interarterial septum (between the right and left atria) called the **foramen ovale** allows blood to bypass the fetal lungs. Foramen is the medical term for natural opening. Blood actually passes from the right atrium into the left atrium. After birth, this opening closes as a result of increasing pressure in the left atrium, but complete closure may take up to 1 year. In the adult heart, this structure persists as the **fossa ovalis.** (The medical term for "pit or depression" is *fossa.*)

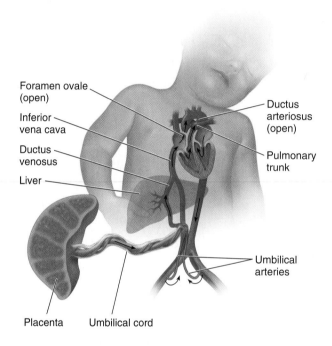

A Full-term fetus (before birth)

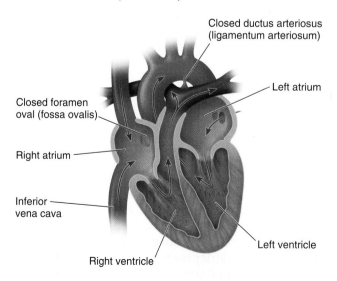

B After delivery

FIGURE 17-5
Fetal circulation at (**A**) term and (**B**) after delivery.

Another structure, the ductus arteriosus, allows fetal blood to move from the pulmonary trunk into the aorta. The **ductus arteriosus** connects the pulmonary artery with the descending thoracic aorta. After birth, it becomes the **ligamentum arteriosum**, the fibrous cord between the pulmonary trunk and the aorta. Prostaglandins effect its closure, which may take a couple months after birth to complete.

Key Terms	*Definitions*
ductus venosus (DUCK tus vee NOH sus)	venous channel in the embryonic liver that shunts blood from the left umbilical vein to the sinus venosus of heart
foramen ovale (foh RAY mun oh VAY lee)	fetal opening between the atria shunting blood from the right to the left atrium
fossa ovalis (FOS uh oh VAY lis)	oval depression in the interatrial septum that is a vestige of the foramen ovale
ductus arteriosus (DUCK tus ahr teer ee OH sus)	portion of the aortic arch forming a fetal shunt between the left pulmonary artery and the aorta
ligamentum arteriosum (lig uh MEN tum ahr teer ee OH sum)	fibrous cord between the pulmonary trunk and the aorta

Key Term Practice: Fetal Circulation

1. The fetal opening between the atria that shunts blood from the right atrium into the left atrium, thereby allowing blood to bypass fetal lungs, is termed _____.

2. The depression on the interarterial septum of an adult heart that serves as a remnant of the foramen ovale is called the _____.

Pregnancy

During pregnancy, the maternal systems undergo significant changes. For example, maternal respiratory rate and blood volume increase, and nutritional requirements multiply 10–30%. The mammary glands and the uterus enlarge. In addition, the maternal glomerular filtration rate increases by approximately 50%.

Gynecology (GYN) is the medical specialty concerned with female reproductive health. Many gynecologists also practice **obstetrics** (OB), the branch of medicine concerned with the care of women and their offspring during pregnancy, parturition, and puerperium. An **obstetrician** (OB) is a physician specializing in pregnancy, delivering babies, and the care of women after childbirth. The time period between the beginning of cervical dilation and the actual **parturition**, the act of giving birth to a baby, is called **labor.** The period of time immediately after parturition is termed **postpartum. Puerperium** is the time frame for complete involution of the uterus; it usually lasts about 42 days.

Remarkable skin changes occur throughout pregnancy. These include chloasma, linea nigra, and striae gravidarum. Hyperpigmentation occurring chiefly on the forehead, temples, and cheeks is termed **chloasma.** It is commonly referred to as the "mask of pregnancy." **Linea nigra** describes the dark, pigmented line extending medially from the pubis upward in pregnant women; and **striae gravidarum** is the medical term for stretch marks that occur during pregnancy on the abdomen, thighs, and breasts. (*Striae* refers to "line, and *gravid* means "pregnant.") Fetal and uterine growth are depicted in Figure 17-6.

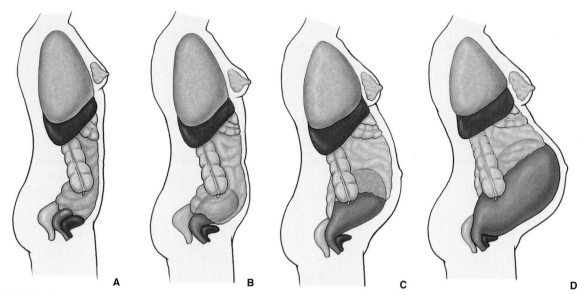

FIGURE 17-6

Uterine growth at (**A**) conception, (**B**) first trimester, (**C**) second trimester, and (**D**) third trimester. The uterus is red. (Images provided by Anatomical Chart Co.)

The formula used to calculate an infant's date of birth is known as **Nägele's rule**. The calculation involves subtracting 3 months from the beginning of the last normal menstrual period. Then 7 days are added to that date. For example, if the last menstrual period began on December 20, count back 3 months to September 20. Then add 7 days to determine September 27 as the expected delivery date. The **gestational age** is the age of the developing human computed from the 1st day of the last menstrual period to any point in time thereafter until birth.

A closely related term is the **gestation period**, which is the length of pregnancy. The average length of human gestation is 10 lunar months, 280 days, or 40 weeks. (A lunar month is 28 days.) This is calculated from the onset of the last menstrual period and varies between 250 and 310 days.

Various signs indicate fetal presence and pregnancy. A diagnostic maneuver used to palpate a floating fetus by tapping against the uterus through the vagina is called **ballottement**. The fetus will "bounce" within the amniotic fluid with the impact felt by the palpating fingers or hand. **Braxton Hicks contractions** are irregular and painless uterine contractions that occur with increasing frequency throughout pregnancy. The **Chadwick sign** is the characteristic blue-violet color of the cervix and vagina around the 6th week of pregnancy. This results from increased blood flow to the pregnant uterus. A softening of the cervix, considered to be evidence of pregnancy, is the **Goodell sign**. The cervix continues to soften or "ripen" as pregnancy progresses, appearing "mushy" just before birth. The **Hegar sign** is the softening of the lower segment of uterus that occurs about the 6th week of pregnancy. **Quickening** is the first feeling of fetal movements by the pregnant woman, occurring during the 4th–5th month of pregnancy.

Key Terms	Definitions
obstetrics (ob STET ricks)	relating to childbirth
obstetrician (ob ste TRISH un)	physician who practices obstetrics
parturition (pahr tew RISH un)	process of giving birth; childbirth
labor	series of processes whereby the fetus is expelled during parturition

postpartum (pohst PAHR tum)	period after childbirth
puerperium (pew ur PEER ee um)	period of about 42 days after childbirth in which the uterus returns to its natural shape
chloasma (kloh AZ muh)	dark coloration on the facial skin caused by pregnancy-induced hormonal changes
linea nigra (LIN ee uh NIGH gruh)	dark line extending up the center of the abdomen of a pregnant woman
striae gravidarum (STRYE ee grav i DAHR um)	stretch marks seen in pregnancy
Nägele's (NAY guh leez) rule	formula used to calculate the infant's predicted delivery date
gestational (jes TAY shun ul) age	age of the developing embryo/fetus computed from the 1st day of the last menstrual cycle to any point in time
gestation (jes TAY shun) period	length of pregnancy
ballottement (ba LOT munt)	diagnostic maneuver used to palpate a floating fetus
Braxton Hicks (BRACKS tun HICKS) contractions	irregular and painless uterine contractions that are different from the contractions of labor
Chadwick sign	blue-violet color of the cervix and vagina, indicative of pregnancy
Goodell sign	softening of the cervix, indicative of pregnancy
Hegar (HAY gar) sign	softening of the lower portion of the uterus occurring at about week 6 of pregnancy
quickening	fetal movements felt by the mother

Key Term Practice: Pregnancy

1. The medical term for delivering or birthing a baby is _____.

2. A/an _____ is a physician who practices obstetrics.

Labor and Delivery

Medical terms associated with labor and delivery are numerous. Those describing the cervix or uterus include effacement, incompetent cervix, and lightening. **Effacement** describes the gradual flattening of the cervix during labor; an **incompetent cervix** is a condition in which the cervix dilates prematurely before the fetus reaches full term. If not sutured until full-term pregnancy is achieved, incompetent cervix results in **spontaneous abortion**, an unexpected, premature expulsion of an embryo or fetus. This physiologically induced ejection is also known as a **miscarriage. Lightening** refers to the sinking or dropping of the fetus into the pelvic inlet with an accompanying descent of the uterus. Lightening occurs during late pregnancy when the fetal head begins to descend into the mother's pelvis, resulting in a lessening of pressure on the diaphragm during the last weeks before delivery.

The exact mechanism that triggers the events of labor are not known; however, there is a surge of oxytocin (OT) that stimulates the contractions before, during, and after birth (for delivery of the placenta). The synthetically produced drug called

Pitocin is artificial oxytocin and is often given to induce labor. In the medical vernacular it may be referred to as "vitamin P."

There are four stages of labor: dilation, expulsion, placental delivery, and postdelivery (Fig.17-7). The first stage begins with contractions and cervical dilation. **Contractions** are the tightening of uterine muscles that occur at increasingly frequent intervals immediately before childbirth. Dilation of the cervix to about 10 cm (4 in.) occurs in the first stage of labor and is characterized by rupture of the amniochorionic membrane. This is more commonly known as having one's "water break." The average duration of this stage is 8 hours. During the second stage, or expulsion stage, contractions reach their maximum intensity and eventually push the baby out of the womb. Within 1 hour after parturition, placenta delivery (stage three) occurs when the organ separates from the uterine wall and is discharged through the vagina. This is often referred to as "afterbirth." The fourth stage occurs 1–2 hours after delivery, when uterine tone returns.

The normal birth position is termed **vertex**, in which the fetus is positioned upside down with the head toward the cervix and birth canal. If the fetus does not rotate as normally occurs and presents feet or buttocks first, it is a **breech** birth. An **episiotomy**,

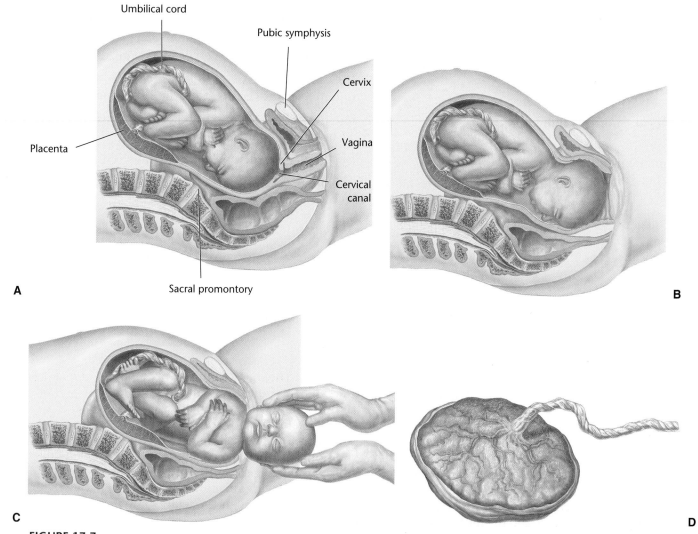

FIGURE 17-7
The stages of labor and birth. (**A**) Full term before labor. (**B**) The first stage is dilation. (**C**) The second stage is expulsion. (**D**) The third stage is placental. The fourth stage is after delivery when the uterine tone returns to normal. (Images provided by Anatomical Chart Co.)

a surgical incision of the vulva to prevent undue laceration at delivery time, may be performed before a vaginal birth. The incision enlarges the vaginal opening to prevent tearing. Another term for episiotomy is vaginoperineotomy, a descriptive term denoting an incision in the vaginal and perineal regions.

Infants may be delivered via the natural route of the vagina or by a surgical procedure termed a cesarean section. Radiographic measurements of the female pelvic inlet and outlet, called **pelvimetry**, determine the feasibility of vaginally birthing a child. A **cesarean section** (C-section) is delivery of a fetus through an abdominal and uterine incision. It is performed when the fetus's head is too large to fit through the pelvic girdle, when there is hemorrhage owing to abruptio placentae or placenta previa, with a breech or shoulder presentation, or when there is fetal and/or maternal distress (Fig. 17-8).

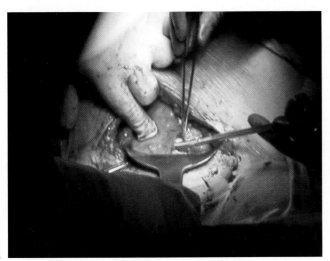
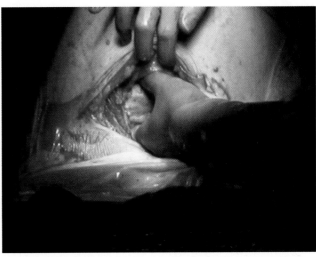

A   B

FIGURE 17-8
Cesarean section. (**A**) Incision through the abdominal region. (**B**) Removal of the fetus from the uterus. (Image courtesy of Laura and Michael Wahl.)

Sometimes during a vaginal birth, it may be necessary to use **obstetric forceps**, a large, double-bladed instrument that interlocks around the fetal head to facilitate delivery during a difficult labor. **Vaginal birth after cesarean** (VBAC) is the phrase that describes the birth of a child through the vaginal canal when the mother's pervious child was delivered by cesarean section.

At birth, the infant is covered with a cheesy-appearing substance referred to as **vernix caseosa**. The term is derived from the word part *caseo-*, which means "resembling cheese." Immediately after birth, the condition of a newborn baby is assessed in five areas: heart rate, breathing, skin color, muscle tone, and reflex response. This **Apgar score** or **Apgar rating** is a quantitative estimate of the condition of the neonate (newborn) at 1 and 5 minutes after birth. Points are assigned to the quality of the five assessment areas, and each category receives a score ranging from 0 (poor) to 2 (excellent). The Apgar score is the total sum of the five assessment points; thus 10 is the maximum rating.

As the infant adjusts to life outside the womb, a number of changes take place. For example, the neonate loses weight within the first 48 hours as fluid shifts occur. The branch of medicine dealing with growth and development of children from birth through adolescence is **pediatrics**. The focus of pediatrics is on care, treatment, and prevention of diseases, injuries, and defects. The word part *ped-* means "child," thus a physician who specializes in pediatrics is a **pediatrician**.

An infant has about 1 qt. (.95 L) of blood!

Key Terms	Definitions
effacement (e FACE munt)	gradual flattening of the cervix during labor
incompetent cervix (in KOM puh tunt SUR vicks)	premature dilation of the cervix
spontaneous abortion	sudden, unplanned expulsion of the fetus from the uterus before it is viable; miscarriage
miscarriage	sudden, unplanned expulsion of the fetus from the uterus before it is viable; spontaneous abortion
lightening	movement of the fetus into the pelvis
contractions	shortening of the uterine muscle fibers
vertex (VUR tecks)	fetus positioned so the crown of the head presents in the cervix and the vaginal canal
breech	fetus positioned so the buttocks and/or feet present in the cervix and vaginal canal
episiotomy (e piz ee OT oh mee)	surgical incision in the perineum to enlarge the opening and facilitate childbirth; vaginoperineotomy
pelvimetry (pel VIM i tree)	radiographic measurement of the female pelvic inlet and outlet to determine feasibility of vaginally birthing a child
cesarean (se ZAIR ee un) **section**	operation to deliver a baby by cutting through the mother's abdomen and uterus
obstetric forceps (ob STET rick FOR seps)	instrument resembling tongs used for grasping the fetus's head
vaginal (VAJ i nul) **birth after cesarean** (se ZAIR ee un) **(VBAC)**	vaginal delivery of a baby when the previous birth was via cesarean section
vernix caseosa (VUR nicks kay see OH suh)	cheesy-appearing deposit on the surface of the fetus
Apgar score	score assessing the condition of the newborn baby; Apgar rating
Apgar rating	score assessing the condition of the newborn baby; Apgar score
pediatrics (pee dee AT ricks)	branch of medicine dealing with the care and development of children and with the prevention and treatment of children's diseases
pediatrician (pee dee uh TRISH un)	physician specializing in the care and development of children and in the prevention and treatment of children's diseases

Key Term Practice: Labor, and Delivery

1. The word part _____ means "vulva" and the word part _____ refers to "incision;" so the surgical incision in the perineum to enlarge the opening and facilitate childbirth is termed _____.

2. A normal birth presentation is termed _____, and a birth in which any part except the head presents in the cervix is called _____.

Lactation

After parturition, nourishment is delivered to a breastfed newborn by lactation. **Lactation** is the period during which milk is secreted and ejected by the mammary glands. Hormones influence this event, which is controlled by a positive-feedback mechanism. As the infant suckles at the breast, the action causes secretion known as milk "let down," which in turn causes more infant suckling. Managing this positive-feedback loop requires hormones. Prolactin (PRL), estrogens, and progesterone control milk secretion, and oxytocin causes milk ejection.

The yellowish fluid rich in antibodies and minerals secreted by a mother's breasts after giving birth and before the production of true milk is known as **colostrum**. This "first milk" is produced during the first 2–3 days postpartum; thereafter, breast milk is produced. Colostrum contains less fat than breast milk and is richer in immunoglobulins. Colostrum also acts as a laxative, assisting in meconium expulsion. **Meconium** is the dark, greenish colored feces that collect in the intestines of an unborn baby. This first fecal discharge is composed of epithelial cells, bile, and lanugo hairs. The pasty material is expelled 3–4 days after birth. If any meconium is detected in the amniotic fluid, it is an indication of fetus distress.

A colostrum-like milk secretion sometimes occurs in the mammary glands of newborn infants of either sex 3–4 days after birth, and lasts 1–2 weeks. It is sometimes referred to as "witch's milk" and is the result of endocrine stimulation from the mother before birth.

Key Terms	Definitions
lactation (lack TAY shun)	formation and secretion of breast milk
colostrum (koh LOS trum)	first milk expressed from the mother's breasts after childbirth
meconium (mee KOH nee um)	dark greenish feces released from a baby shortly after birth

Key Term Practice: Lactation

1. _____ is the secretion and ejection of breast milk, derived from the word part _____, which means "milk."

2. The first milk produced by lactating breasts is termed _____.

Artificial Fertilization and Multiple Births

Couples who have been unsuccessful in conceiving a child may choose in vitro fertilization. **In vitro fertilization** is union of an ovum by sperm outside the body when normal conception is not achievable. *In vitro* in Latin means literally "in glass," referring in this case to laboratory tools. A female's ovum is retrieved from the uterine tube and placed in a small circular dish with male sperm obtained from ejaculate. The cells are cultured and then returned to the uterus for implantation. This artificial culturing medium mimics the natural process, but the zygote must be implanted into a human uterus to nurture a developing embryo and sustain life. Fertilization occurs in an artificial environment, thus popularizing the phrase "test tube baby;" however, this is inaccurate because the process actually occurs in a Petri dish. Conversely, fertilization that occurs within the body is termed **in vivo fertilization**, from the Latin phrase that means "in a living being."

Women opting for this method are injected with pregnancy hormones before zygote introduction so that the uterus is prepared to nurture a developing fetus. Once implanted, the body recognizes the pregnancy and naturally produces the necessary hormones.

Twins, triplets, quadruplets, and quintuplets describe giving birth to more than one child in a single pregnancy. Multiple births result when there is more than one fertilized ovum, a separation of blastomeres in early cleavage, or a division of blastula before gastrulation. Identical (maternal) twins are **monozygotic twins**, a term used to describe two individuals derived from a single (mono) fertilized egg (zygote). Monozygous twins are always the same gender. The splitting of the zygote divides into two inner cell masses during the blastocyst stage. The twins have the same genetic code and usually share the same placenta.

Fraternal (nonidentical) twins are **dizygotic twins**, which means they developed from two (di) separately fertilized ova. Two placentas are present with dizygotic twins, and they look no more alike than any other two siblings born at different times. Therefore, they can be the same or opposite sex. Although the reason is not known, naturally occurring multiple births occur at a fairly predictable exponential rate. For example, twins are born at a rate of 1 per 89 births, triplets occur in 1 per 89^2 births, quadruplets at 1 per 89^3 births, and quintuplets at a rate of 1 per 89^4 births.

FACT *In the United States, 1 in 90 pregnancies leads to twins!*

Key Terms	Definitions
in vitro (VEE troh) **fertilization**	fertilization of an ovum by sperm outside the body when normal conception is not achievable
in vivo (VEE voh) **fertilization**	fertilization occurring inside a living organism
monozygotic (mon oh zye GOT ick) **twins**	developed from a single fertilized egg; maternal twins, identical twins
dizygotic (dye zye GOT ick) **twins**	developed from two fertilized ova; fraternal twins, twins

Key Term Practice: Artificial Fertilization and Multiple Births

1. Fraternal twins are also called _____ twins.

2. What type of twinning results in two genetically identical individuals?

_____

Developmental Stages

Life after birth proceeds through various phases. A newborn infant is termed a **neonate**, and remains such until the end of the first 4 weeks of life. During this period, metabolism and oxygen consumption increase.

At birth, the first breath must be quite forceful because the infant's lungs are fluid-filled and collapsed. The traditional spank on the bottom initiates the breath by making the newborn angry; however, a recently discovered master gene may actually initiate the first breath. Stored fat is used as the primary energy source for the first few days after birth. Wastes are also eliminated. During this time, the kidneys excrete relatively dilute urine. Furthermore, the neonate has a limited ability to regulate body temperature, so it typically fluctuates.

The end of the first 4 weeks of life up to 1 year is designated **infancy.** Muscle coordination develops, and the head is still disproportionately large—approximately one fourth the total body height. The infant birth weight doubles during the first 4 months, and it triples by 1 year.

Infancy is distinguished by several benchmarks. By the end of the 2nd month, the infant is able to follow a moving object with his or her eyes. At 6 months, deciduous (first) teeth may appear, and by 12–18 months, the spinal lumbar curvature appears.

Childhood is denoted as the time between infancy and puberty. Although myriad changes occur during this period, two of the most profound are the establishment of bladder control and the development of the nervous system.

The period from puberty to adulthood is **adolescence.** The onset of puberty is marked by increased production of gonadotropin releasing hormone (GnRH), increased circulating levels of follicle stimulating hormone (FSH) and luteinizing hormone (LH), and increased sensitivity of ovarian and testicular cells to FSH and LH. At puberty, the reproductive organs are functional. Females generally begin menstruation by age 12, and males complete their rapid growth stage by age 14. **Adulthood** is the era between adolescence and old age. The process of aging, termed **senescence**, ends with death. Senescence describes all the postmaturational changes that an individual undergoes.

Key Terms	Definitions
neonate (NEE oh nate)	newborn infant, specifically from birth through the 28th day of life
infancy	baby period or the 2nd–12th months of life
childhood	period of life between infancy and adolescence
adolescence	period of life from puberty to maturity
adulthood	period of life after adolescence
senescence (se NES unce)	state of aging

Key Term Practice: Developmental Stages

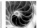

1. _____ is the term for a newborn, derived from the word part _____ meaning "new."

2. _____ describes the aging process.

Genes and Chromosomes

Cell divisions occur during meiosis and mitosis. During **meiosis**, the nucleus divides into four nuclei, each of which contains half the usual number of chromosomes. Meiosis produces gametes with half the normal somatic chromosome complement and occurs during spermatogenesis and oogenesis. The process by which a cell divides into two daughter cells, each of which has the same number of chromosomes as the original cell, is called **mitosis.**

We are who we are because of the passage of genetic material in the form of deoxyribonucleic acid (DNA) from one generation to the next, called inheritance. The **genotype** is the genetic makeup of an individual, and the **phenotype** is the outward physical manifestation of the organism. Phenotypes are expressed as external appearances, such as auburn hair or hazel eyes, and are displayed through the interaction between the genotype and the environment.

Genes are basic units that combine to create a genotype. Genes are portions of DNA molecules and consist of a specific sequence that occupies a specific **locus**

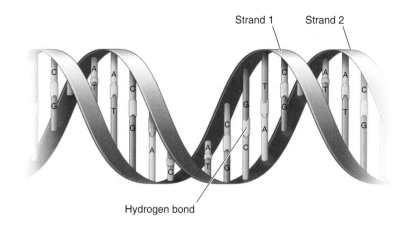

FIGURE 17-9
Components of DNA are adenine (A), cytosine (C), guanine (G), and thymine (T).

(particular site) on a specific chromosome. One can think of genes as determining the structure and function of the body. Components of DNA are adenine (A), cytosine (C), guanine (G), and thymine (T), known as the four-letter alphabet of the genetic code of life (Fig. 17-9).

A **chromosome** is a rod-shaped structure, resembling an asymmetrical *X*, located in a cell's nucleus; as a group, they carry the genes that determine not only sex but all the characteristics an individual inherits from his or her parents (Fig. 17-10). The word part *chromo-* means "colored;" and when stained, chromosomes appear tinted. **Somatic cells** are the cells of the body except the gametes (sex cells). Human somatic cells each contain 46 chromosomes, or 23 pairs. That is, each cell except the gametes contains 23 chromosomes from each parent for a total of 46.

Gametes, or sex cells, are specialized male or female cells that contain half the normal number of chromosomes, meaning each gamete contains a total of 23 chromosomes. One gamete unites with a gamete of the opposite sex in sexual reproduction. Independent assortment, whereby the genetic code is uniquely created, occurs during meiosis and ensures that each offspring will be genetically distinctive. Thus each gamete has a unique set of 23 chromosomes. A photomicrograph (mapping) of an entire set of

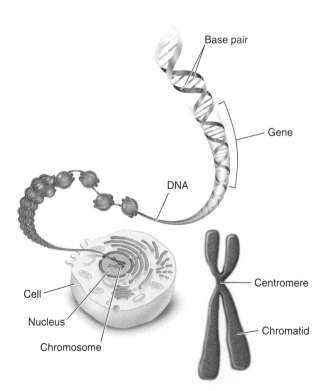

FIGURE 17-10
A chromosome is a rod-shaped structure carrying the genes that determine sex and the characteristics an individual inherits.

a cell's chromosomes arranged according to size and classification is called a **karyotype** (Fig. 17-11). Karyotypes are useful for obtaining genetic information, particularly for counseling purposes.

The entire set of chromosomes in a human cell that are inherited from the parents is termed the **genome.** The human genome consists of 22 pairs of homologous (sharing a similarity) chromosomes and one pair of sex chromosomes, X and Y. **Homologous** chromosomes are pairs of similar chromosomes with one member of each pair derived from the mother and the other from the father. Human females have 23 pairs of homologous chromosomes, but human males have only 22 pairs of homologous chromosomes and one pair of dissimilar chromosomes. Sex chromosomes are the pair that determines an individual's gender. Males are designated XY because their pair of sex chromosomes consist of one X chromosome and one Y chromosome;

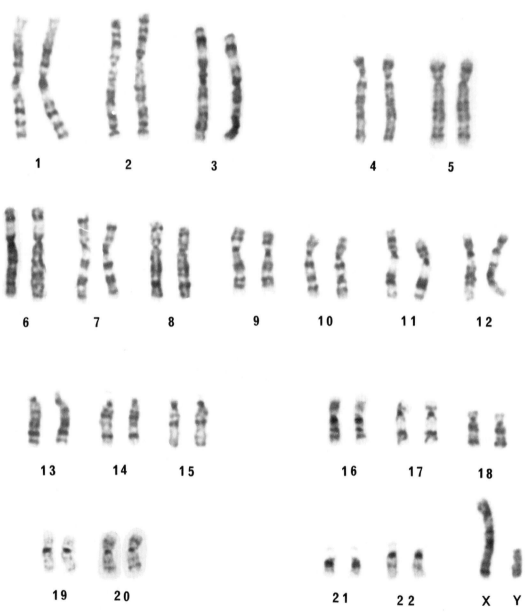

FIGURE 17-11

A karyotype is a photomicrograph of the entire set of a cell's chromosomes arranged according to size and classification. This image shows the karyotype of a normal male. (Reprinted with permission from McClatchey KD. Clinical laboratory medicine. 2nd ed. Philadelphia: Lippincott Williams & Wilkins, 2002.)

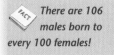

There are 106 males born to every 100 females!

females are XX because they have two X chromosomes. The Y chromosome of the male sperm determines the sex of an offspring, and this chromosome is slightly smaller than the X chromosome. With respect to mature sperm cells, 50% possess an X chromosome and 50%, a Y chromosome. It is interesting that sperm containing a Y chromosome swim faster than sperm with an X chromosome, perhaps because there is not the extra weight of an X chromosome.

Key Terms	Definitions
meiosis (migh OH sis)	nuclear cell division in the formation of gametes
mitosis (migh TOH sis)	nuclear and cytoplasmic cellular division that produces two identical daughter cells
genotype (JEE noh tipe)	genetic constitution of an organism resulting from the combination of chromosomes from its parents
phenotype (FEE noh tipe)	visible expression of the genotype
genes	hereditary factors made of DNA
locus (LOH kus)	position of gene on a chromosome
chromosome (KROH muh sohm)	deeply staining body that carries hereditary factors (genes)—in humans, 46 chromosomes are found in each cell except the sex cells, which carry half or 23
somatic (soh MAT ick) **cells**	all body cells except a mature ovum or sperm
karyotype (KAIR ee oh tipe)	number, form, and size of the chromosomes from a cell's nucleus arranged as a chromosome photomicrograph according to a standard classification
genome (JEE nome)	complete set of genes carried by an individual
homologous (hoh MOL uh gus) **chromosomes**	pair of similar chromosomes, with one member of each pair derived from the mother and one from the father

Key Term Practice: Genes and Chromosomes

1. A chromosomal mapping useful for genetic counseling purposes is termed a _____.

2. The outward appearance of an individual, such as blond hair and blue eyes, is known as the _____.

Inheritance

An elementary understanding of gene and chromosome interaction is fundamental to understanding inheritance and genetic disorders. The characteristics and qualities transmitted from parent to offspring is known as **inheritance.** An **allele** is a variant form of a gene that affects the same characteristic. An **autosome** is a chromosome other than the X or Y sex chromosome. **Homozygous** refers to having two copies of the same allele. When an individual has a pair of identical alleles he or she is homozygous for that gene or genetic trait. For example, individuals with the an allele pair of dd, DD, mm, or MM are homozygous for that gene. If the alleles of a particular gene are different, the pair is **heterozygous.** When an individual is heterozygous for a particular gene, his or her phenotype is determined by the nature of the interaction of those alleles.

Heterozygous allele pairs are designated by a capital letter for one allele and a lowercase letter for the other, as in Dd and Mm.

Other terms related to genetics are dominant, recessive, incomplete dominance, and codominance. **Dominant genes** or alleles control a particular trait, and their effects appear in the offspring's phenotype. Dominant genes inhibit the expression of recessive genes. A gene or allele that is not expressed in the heterozygous condition is termed a **recessive gene.** The effects of recessive genes do not appear in the offspring because the dominant gene masks them. Dominant genes are designated by a capital letter and recessive genes are given a lowercase letter. For any given allele pair, an individual can be homozygous dominant (DD, AA, MM), homozygous recessive (dd, aa, mm), or heterozygous (Dd, Aa, and Mm).

In **incomplete dominance**, neither allele is dominant over the other. For some traits, when one allele is inherited from the mother and a different allele is inherited from the father, the individual's genotype is a blend of the parents' phenotypes. For example, if a person inherited an allele for red hair and another for green hair (if this were possible), the person would have yellow hair, a blend of the effects of the two alleles. Some diseases, such as sickle-cell anemia, are expressed through incomplete dominance for red blood cell shape, but codominance determines the hemoglobin.

For some traits, individuals who are heterozygous exhibit the characteristics of both alleles, referred to as **codominance.** With codominant genes, each allele has an equal effect in making the characteristic it controls appear in the individual. For example, using the red and green hair example, the person would have patches of red hair and patches of green hair. Codominant genes determine the human ABO blood types.

As the name implies, **sex-linked traits** (also called X-linked traits) are related to genes located on the X chromosome that determine particular characteristics. Males express more recessive sex-linked traits than females because they have only one X chromosome. The Y chromosome contains less genes than the X chromosome; thus males do not have a second allele for traits carried on either chromosome. Red-green color blindness is an example of a sex-linked trait.

Another type of inheritance that pertains to the sex cells is holandric inheritance. The transmission of genes located on a segment of the Y chromosome for which there is no matching region on the X chromosome is known as **holandric inheritance.** These genetic traits are carried on the Y chromosome and therefore can be inherited only by males.

Mutations occurring at the genetic level often result in genetic disease. **Mutations** are random changes in a gene or chromosome that result in a new trait. They result from changes in the nucleotide sequences of DNA. A mutation can be a source of beneficial genetic variation, have neutral effects, or demonstrate harmful outcomes.

Genetic diseases are categorized into three main groups on the basis of the timing of the gene's expression. The first classification includes disorders with effects that occur during embryonic or fetal development. The newborn exhibits characteristics of the disease. Conditions that affect metabolic processes and that are expressed postpartum make up the second group. An example of a postpartum effect is seen in phenylketonuria (PKU), an inborn error of metabolism in which the body lacks the enzyme to metabolize phenylalanine. It is detected at birth; and if left untreated, PKU results in developmental deficiency, seizures, and tumors. Group three is reserved for conditions that have effects expressed during adolescence or adulthood. Examples include hypercholesterolemia and diabetes mellitus.

Key Terms	Definitions
inheritance	transmission of genetically controlled characteristics from parent to offspring
allele (a LEEL)	one of a pair of genes having the same location on homologous chromosomes

autosome (AW toh sohm)	any chromosome other than the X and Y chromosomes
homozygous (hoh moh ZYE gus)	having two like alleles for a particular gene
heterozygous (het ur oh ZYE gus)	having dissimilar alleles for a particular gene
dominant genes	genes that are expressed even in the presence of other alleles.
recessive (ree SES iv) **gene**	allele that is not expressed in the presence of a dominant allele
incomplete dominance	genes that result in distinctly different phenotypes from the parents
codominance	both dominant and recessive phenotypes are expressed
sex-linked traits	applied to genes located on the X chromosome and to characteristics that may occur in either sex conditioned by such genes
holandric (hol AN drick) **inheritance**	pertaining to genes carried by the Y chromosome
mutation	change in the genetic material, usually in a single gene

Key Term Practice: Inheritance

1. Traits carried on the X chromosome are termed _____ traits.

2. A/An _____ is a change in genetic material, usually in a single gene.

THE CLINICAL DIMENSION

Pathology of Pregnancy, Human Development, and Child Health

Pathology associated with pregnancy, human development, and childhood is the result of various factors, some of which are not known or fully understood. Abnormal conditions include disorders of pregnancy, congenital disorders, prematurity and affiliated consequences, syndromes, and infectious childhood diseases.

Pregnancy Conditions

The common tool used to confirm pregnancy tests **human chorionic gonadotropin** in **maternal serum or urine.** In-home pregnancy kits test for the presence of hCG in the urine. This hormone is not found in the urine of nonpregnant females, and serum levels are negligible. Maternal urine levels rise to around 500,000 international units (IU) within 24 h of pregnancy. Although fairly accurate, in-home urine tests are not as reliable as blood serum tests for detecting pregnancy.

Gestational diabetes (GD) is a condition in which pregnant women develop the inability to appropriately metabolize carbohydrates, resulting in hyperglycemia. Polyuria (excessive urination), polydipsia (excessive thirst), and polyphagia (frequent eating), the classic signs of diabetes mellitus, are frequently absent with GD, and women are often asymptomatic. Thus pregnant women are routinely screened. A common test evaluating circulating blood glucose levels is the **2-hour postprandial glucose test.** (The term *postprandial* means "occurring after a meal.") About 2 hours after ingesting a concentrated glucose solution, the glucose level of maternal blood is tested. Normal values are between 70 and 140 mg/dL; elevated levels indicate possible diabetes.

Risk factors for gestational diabetes include a history of birthing babies over 10 lb, obesity, maternal age over 30 years, family history of diabetes, and previous stillbirths. Although the condition resolves after parturition, women with GD are at increased risk of developing diabetes mellitus type 2 later in life.

A transformation of all or part of the placenta into grape-like cysts is termed **hydatidiform mole.** This relatively rare mass or tumor occurs at the beginning of a pregnancy. It is also known as molar pregnancy, derived from the word *molar* meaning "mass." Signs and symptoms include nausea, bleeding, anemia, unusually large uterus for gestational period, absence of fetal heart sounds, edema, and hypertension. An ultrasound demonstrating no fetal skeleton and elevated hCG levels are used for diagnosis. Uterine evacuation and dilation and curettage are treatments. **Dilation and curettage** (D&C) involves the physical scraping of the uterine cavity wall to eliminate extraneous tissue. The extracted tissue is examined for malignant cells. The woman is closely monitored for 1 year and advised against pregnancy during this time. When hCG levels and uterine tissue returns to normal, pregnancy may be attempted. In some cases, hysterectomy is necessary.

A malignant tumor of a pregnant uterus that appears after pregnancy or abortion is termed a **choriocarcinoma.** It requires surgical excision and chemotherapy. A benign tumor of the placenta composed of fetal blood vessels, connective tissue, and trophoblast is termed **chorioangioma.** It is usually of no clinical significant and expels with the placenta after childbirth.

In an extrauterine pregnancy, called **ectopic pregnancy,** an impregnated ovum develops at an abnormal location outside the uterine cavity. Ectopic pregnancies are never viable and must be surgically removed. The risk increases in women who douche regularly and in those with pelvic inflammatory disease (PID). Nearly 95% of ectopic pregnancies occur in the uterine tube.

Abruptio placentae is the separation of placenta from the uterine wall prematurely before delivery. It usually occurs around month 5. Bleeding can lead to anemia, shock, or kidney failure. Fetal mortality rate is high. Another disorder is **placenta previa,** a condition in which the placenta is positioned over the opening of the cervix into the vagina. It occurs when implantation is near the cervix instead of the upper two-thirds portion of the uterine wall. Ultrasound confirms the diagnosis. Women with placenta previa remain on total bedrest until the fetus reaches a size for successful cesarean delivery.

Eclampsia, a disease occurring in the latter half of pregnancy, is characterized by acute hypertension (high blood pressure), proteinuria (protein in the urine), edema (swelling), sodium retention, convulsions, and sometimes coma. **Preeclampsia** is toxemia occurring in the latter half of pregnancy characterized by acute hypertension, edema, abnormal weight gain, and proteinuria, but without convulsions or coma. It occurs after the 20th week of gestation or in the presence of trophoblastic disease. **Toxemia of pregnancy** is a pathologic condition occurring in the latter half of pregnancy manifested by eclampsia or preeclampsia. The maternal cardiovascular system is affected. Signs include chronic hypertension and proteinuria. Emergency C-section may be ordered to save the life of the mother and/or fetus. The cause of each of these conditions is pregnancy.

Pregnancy termination occurs when an embryo or fetus is removed from the womb before its independent survival is possible or when its end is brought about at an early stage. **Abortion** is the medical term describing expulsion of an embryo or fetus before its ability to live on its own outside the uterus. Artificially induced abortions are performed by D&C, vacuum aspiration (suction), and stimulation of uterine contractions. When a woman gives birth to a dead fetus around the 28th week of pregnancy, the term **stillbirth** is applied.

Key Terms	Definitions
human chorionic gonadotropin (KOH ree on ick goh nad oh TROH pin) **in maternal serum or urine**	test that measures the level of hCG in the serum or blood—increased hCG values indicate pregnancy
gestational diabetes (jes TAY shun ul dye uh BEE teez)	faulty carbohydrate metabolism that occurs only during pregnancy
2-hour postprandial (pohst PRAN dee ul) **glucose test**	determines blood glucose levels 2 hours after drinking a sugar solution
hydatidiform (high da TID i form) **mole**	mass or tumor of unknown origin forming within the uterus at the beginning of pregnancy
dilation and curettage (kewr e TAHZH)	surgical procedure involving expansion of the cervix and scraping of the uterus
choriocarcinoma (koh ree oh kahr si NOH muh)	malignant tumor of the pregnant uterus
chorioangioma (koh ree oh an jee OH muh)	benign tumor of the placenta
ectopic (eck TOP ick) **pregnancy**	development of the fertilized egg outside the womb
abruptio placentae (ab RUP tee oh pla SEN tee)	premature separation of the placenta from the uterine wall
placenta previa (pluh SEN tuh PREE vee uh)	placenta positioned at the opening of the uterine cervix in the vagina
eclampsia (ek LAMP see uh)	illness occurring during the later stages of pregnancy characterized by high blood pressure, convulsions, and sometimes coma
preeclampsia (pree ek LAMP see uh)	toxemia occurring in the later stages of pregnancy, similar to eclampsia but is not marked by convulsions or coma
toxemia (tock SEE mee uh) **of pregnancy**	condition characterized by hypertension, swelling, and proteinuria—the late stage of preeclampsia and eclampsia
abortion	to bring to expel an embryo or fetus before pregnancy completion
stillbirth	birth of a dead fetus

Key Term Practice: Pregnancy Conditions

1. _____ is the final stage of preeclampsia and has profound cardiovascular effects.

2. Toxemia occurring during the later stages of pregnancy that is similar to eclampsia but is not marked by convulsions or coma is termed _____.

Autosomal Recessive Diseases

Albinism is a congenital lack of normal pigmentation characterized by absence of melanin (dark pigment) in the hair, skin, and eyes. It results from defective metabolism of tyrosine, the precursor molecule to melanin. It is associated with several congenital ocular abnormalities and visual defects.

A common fatal genetic disease, characterized by dysfunction of exocrine glands, is **cystic fibrosis** (CF). Cystic fibrosis manifests as a disease primarily of the respiratory and digestive system as thick mucus clogs glandular ducts because of impaired chloride ion transport. The gene for CF is found on chromosome 7. Research suggests that carriers (individuals with the gene for the trait but who are not affected by the disorder) are protected against cholera. Genetic counseling is indicated for couples who are carriers or who have a family history of CF.

Severe combined immune deficiency (SCID) is a congenital disorder characterized by severe lymphocyte deficit and plasma cell absence. It is inherited as an X-linked (sex-linked) or autosomal recessive defect in which the lymphocytes fail to develop as a result of deaminase (an enzyme that breaks down amino acids) deficiency. Consequently, cellular and humoral immunity is poor, and the risk of infections increases because of the hampered immune response. This disorder is treated with bone marrow stem cell transplants from a human leukocyte antigen–(HLA) matched donor. If detected early enough, SCID may be curable. Unfortunately, because screening for SCID is not routine, the disease is frequently well advanced by the time it is diagnosed. In progressive cases, the child must live life in a sterile environment (plastic bubble) and typically dies young.

Phenylketonuria is an autosomal recessive metabolic disorder in which there is a deficiency of phenylalanine hydroxylase, an enzyme necessary for the metabolism of the amino acid phenylalanine to another important amino acid, tyrosine. This results in an accumulation of phenylalanine in the blood, tissues, and urine, impairing early neuronal development. Untreated forms lead to mental retardation, eczema (skin inflammation with itching), fair hair, and seizures. Newborns are automatically screened by the **Guthrie test**, which detects the presence of phenylalanine in the blood. Treatment includes a dietary monitoring of phenylalanine. Thus protein intake is restricted because this amino acid is a naturally occurring component. Because diet sodas often contain phenylalanine, a warning for individuals with PKU appears on the label.

A genetic disease characterized by an abnormal lipid accumulation in the brain and nerves that leads to tissue damage is **Tay-Sachs disease.** It principally affects individuals of eastern European Jewish heritage. Tay-Sachs disease is caused by a deficiency of, or defect in, the enzyme hexosaminidase A. It results in loss of sight and other brain functions. Signs and symptoms appear within the first 3–6 months of age and include abnormal startle reaction, decreased axial muscle tone, and blindness. There is no cure. Death occurs at 3–5 years of age.

Key Terms	*Definitions*
albinism (AL bi niz um)	hereditary absence of melanin pigment
cystic fibrosis (SIS tick figh BROH sis)	hereditary disease of infancy affecting various glands
severe combined immune deficiency	autosomal recessive congenital disorder marked by deficient immune system and response
phenylketonuria (fen il kee toh NEW ree uh)	genetic disease in which the body lacks the enzyme to metabolize phenylalanine
Guthrie test	determines the level of phenylalanine in the serum of a neonate to detect PKU

Tay-Sachs (SACKS) **disease**	genetic disease marked by accumulation of lipids in nervous tissue affecting people of eastern European Jewish ancestry

 ## Key Term Practice: Autosomal Recessive Diseases

1. Which genetic disease results in the absence of the enzyme that metabolizes phenylalanine?

   _____

2. Which genetic disease is characterized by an accumulation of lipids in the nervous system and affects individuals of eastern European Jewish descent.

   _____

Congenital Syndromes

A **syndrome** is a group of signs and symptoms that when considered together are characteristic of or indicate a specific disease or other disorder. Many syndromes are endocrine diseases but are described here because they are genetic disorders that are present at birth.

Several tests exist to detect congenital disease, including α-fetoprotein serum test, amniocentesis, and chorionic villus sampling. The α-fetoprotein **serum test** is used to identify possible congenital defects. Normal adult levels are below 40 ng/mL. α-Fetoprotein peaks between the 16th and 18th gestational week, and elevated levels occur in women carrying fetuses with Down syndrome, anencephaly, and spina bifida.

An **amniocentesis** is a test performed between the 15th and 18th gestational week to determine chromosomal abnormalities and the health, sex, and genetic constitution of a fetus by withdrawing fetal cells in the amniotic fluid through a needle inserted into the womb of the mother (Fig. 17-12). The amniotic sac is punctured through the abdominal wall with a trocar (also spelled trochar) and cannula. A **trocar** is a sharp-pointed surgical instrument fitted with a hollow **cannula** (artificial tube of various sizes) used to puncture a body cavity and withdraw fluid. Analysis of amniotic fluid is often used to look for Tay-Sachs disease, hemophilia, sickle-cell anemia, and Down syndrome.

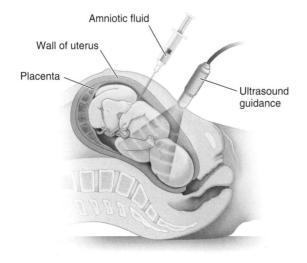

Amniotic fluid

Wall of uterus

Placenta

Ultrasound guidance

FIGURE 17-12
Amniocentesis is a test performed by withdrawing fetal cells from the amniotic fluid through a needle inserted into the womb of the mother.

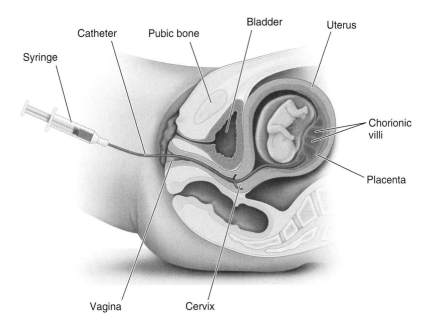

Syringe

Catheter

Pubic bone

Bladder

Uterus

Chorionic villi

Placenta

Vagina

Cervix

FIGURE 17-13
Perform a chorionic villus sampling by withdrawing cells from the villi of the chorion through a needle inserted into the vagina. This test is performed sooner than an amniocentesis, and the results are obtained faster than an amniocentesis.

Another invasive procedure is **chorionic villus sampling** (CVS) or **chorionic villus biopsy** (CVB), a prenatal test for birth defects carried out by examining cells from the villi of the chorion, which has the same DNA as the fetus (Fig. 17-13). The tiny outgrowths (villi) are withdrawn through a needle inserted into the vagina under guided ultrasound for chromosomal analysis. This test can be performed sooner than an amniocentesis (as soon as the 2nd month of pregnancy), and the results are obtained faster than an amniocentesis. With CVS, there is danger that the amniotic sac will not seal and fluid leakage will occur, resulting in loss of pregnancy. The CVS test is also linked to causing limb abnormalities in the newborn.

Cri-du-chat syndrome, or cat's cry syndrome, is a syndrome of congenital defects including laryngeal anomaly associated with cat-like cry in humans, brachycephaly, epicanthus, hypertelorism, micrognathia, hypotonia (decreased muscle tone), strabismus, and severe mental retardation. **Brachycephaly** refers to a short, broad, nearly spherical head. The medial and downward fold of skin from the upper eyelid causing covering of the inner canthus (angle formed by eyelid junction) and caruncle (small red nodule on medial aspect of eyes) is called an **epicanthus.** An epicanthic fold partially covers the part of the eye nearest the nose. Excessive width between two organs or body parts is known as **hypertelorism. Micrognathia** means small jaws, a condition exhibited with some congenital disorders. **Strabismus** is an eye abnormality in which the visual axes do not meet at the desired objective point. It is caused by deletion of the short arm of one of the number 5 chromosomes. The clinical picture, the presence of the characteristic cat-like cry, and a karyotype study demonstrating chromosomal abnormality lead to the diagnosis. The only treatment is supportive.

Down syndrome results from a chromosomal disorder. The trait is caused by trisomy of chromosome 21. Trisomy refers to the fact there is a triplet instead of a pair of chromosomes. Signs and symptoms include mild to severe mental retardation, multiple structure defects, and characteristic facial features such as small head with flat skull back, eye slant, low-set ears, simian line (horizontal crease) across the palm, and short stubby fingers. It is also associated with heart defects. It occurs more often in babies borne to women over age 35 years, and a mother's chance of producing a trisomic child increases dramatically just before menopause. Severe forms are diagnosed at birth, while milder forms appear later. It can also be detected in utero using CVS, CVB, or amniocentesis. The presence of white dots on the iris and a karyotype confirm the diagnosis. There is no cure. A multifaceted approach is employed to enhance the quality of life and maximize motor skills and mental development. The life expectancy has improved because of surgical interventions for heart defects.

A syndrome caused by a triplet of chromosome 18 is **Edwards syndrome**, or trisomy 18. It results from a mistake in meiosis called nondisjunction. Mental retardation, abnormal skull shape, low-set and malformed ears, small mandible, cardiac defects, short sternum, diaphragmatic or inguinal hernia, Meckel diverticulum (remains of embryonic yolk sac persist in the ileum), abnormal flexion of fingers, and dermatoglyphic (configurations of characteristic ridge patterns on fingertips forming fingerprints) anomalies characterize this fatal chromosomal disorder. There is no cure and death occurs within 2–3 years.

Klinefelter syndrome is a chromosomal anomaly in which the individual has a chromosome count of 47 caused by an extra X chromosome (XXY sex chromosomes). The syndrome is characterized by a constellation of abnormal conditions, including hypogonadism (small gamete-producing structures), gynecomastia (breast presence in males), **eunuchoidism** (prepuberal testicular characteristics), elevated gonadotropins (sex hormones), and decreased testicular size with a normal penis. The person afflicted with Klinefelter syndrome is considered to be a male.

Individuals with the syndrome are generally tall and thin and are infertile as a result of to azoospermia. The noninherited disease results from nondisjunction (failure to separate) of the chromosomes during gamete formation. History and physical examination provide the initial diagnosis. Semen analysis indicating lack of sperm production, serum studies demonstrating decreased gonadotropin levels, and a karyotype confirming the presence of an extra X chromosome provide conclusive evidence for the disorder. Treatment includes long-term hormone therapy begun at puberty and continued throughout life to maintain other normal physiologic development and sexual function. Currently, no treatment exists to restore sperm production.

Turner syndrome is an inherited chromosomal disorder with a chromosome count of 45 occurring in females and resulting in nondevelopment of the gonads (designated XO). The cause is nondisjunction of the X chromosome during gametogenesis. The absence or abnormality of one of the two X chromosomes results in an underdeveloped uterus, vagina, and breasts and in infertility. Other signs include short stature; webbed neck; chest and spine deformities; skin, face, ear, and eye abnormalities; cardiac anomalies; lymphedema in the hands and feet; sexual infantilism; amenorrhea; and increased urinary gonadotropin levels. It is diagnosed by a karyotype demonstrating only one X chromosome instead of two. There is no treatment to restore fertility, but hormone therapy is prescribed to reduce other physiologic signs and symptoms.

Key Terms	*Definitions*
syndrome	group of symptoms and signs that, when considered together, are known or presumed to characterize a disease
α-fetoprotein (fee toh PROH teen) **serum test**	a marker for certain congenital defects
amniocentesis (am nee oh sen TEE sis)	prenatal diagnostic test in which amniotic fluid is evaluated
trocar (TROH kahr)	sharply pointed steel rod sheathed with a cannula used to extract fluid from a body cavity; trochar
cannula (KAN yoo luh)	cylindrical tube
chorionic villus (koh ree ON ick VIL us) **sampling**	prenatal test used to detect birth defects by analyzing cells of the chorion; chorionic villus biopsy
chorionic villus (koh ree ON ick VIL us) **biopsy**	prenatal test used to detect birth defects by analyzing cells of the chorion; chorionic villus sampling

cri-du-chat (kree–due–shah) **syndrome**	congenital defect with a characteristic cat-like cry; cat's cry syndrome
brachycephaly (brack ee SEF uh lee)	shortness of the head
epicanthus (ep i KAN thus)	skin fold from the eyelid that partially covers the eye part nearest the nose
hypertelorism (high pur TEL ur iz um)	excessive width between two organs or body parts
micrognathia (migh kroh NATH ee uh)	small jaws
strabismus (stra BIZ mus)	eye abnormality that results in an inability to focus on the desired object
Down syndrome	congenital syndrome characterized by mild to severe mental retardation that occurs from a tripling of chromosome 21; trisomy 21
Edwards syndrome	congenital syndrome characterized by several physical anomalies from a tripling of chromosome 18; trisomy 18
Klinefelter syndrome	congenital syndrome characterized by male phenotype with an extra X chromosome, XXY
eunuchoidism (YOO nuh koid iz um)	lacking fully developed male sexual organs or characteristics
Turner syndrome	chromosomal disorder occurring in females resulting in nondevelopment or absence of reproductive organs, XO

Key Term Practice: Congenital Syndromes

1. What syndrome is characterized by each of the following genotypes?

   a. XXY _____

   b. XO _____

2. Provide an alternate medical term for each of the following syndromes.

   a. trisomy 18 _____

   b. trisomy 21 _____

Nongenetic Syndromes

Two nongenetic syndromes are fetal alcohol and Reye. **Fetal alcohol syndrome** (FAS) is a condition that affects infants born to women who drank excessive amounts of alcohol during pregnancy. Various birth defects, including facial abnormalities and learning difficulties, are observed in offspring of mothers with extreme alcohol consumption while pregnant. Other common signs are small size for gestational age (SGA), microcephaly, and mental retardation. The physical examination and a history of maternal alcohol abuse confirm the diagnosis. Treatment is supportive, ensuring adequate nutrition. Because no safe levels of alcohol intake in pregnant women have been established, pregnant females are advised to consume no alcohol during gestation.

An acute illness of childhood of unknown cause, which usually follows a respiratory, gastrointestinal, or varicella (chickenpox) infection, is **Reye syndrome.** Fever, vomiting, and disturbances of consciousness that can progress to coma characterize the syndrome. Aspirin use during bouts of respiratory, gastrointestinal, or viral infection has been associated with its development. Fatty infiltrates of liver and kidneys occur, along with swelling of those organs. Convulsions are common. This rare and serious disease, generally affecting children under 16 years, is often fatal as a result of brain edema. The history, physical examination, and elevated serum ammonia levels are used to diagnose it. Treatment includes hospitalization for medical management, surveillance, and rapid intervention. Because aspirin has been implicated with the onset of Reye syndrome, it is recommended that children not receive aspirin.

Key Terms	Definitions
fetal alcohol syndrome	pattern of malformation found among children of mothers who abused alcohol while pregnant
Reye syndrome	serious childhood infection of unknown cause that follows a respiratory or varicella infection and results in encephalopathy

Key Term Practice: Nongenetic Syndromes

1. The syndrome that affects children of mothers who consumed large quantities of alcohol while pregnant is _____.

2. _____ is an acquired encephalopathy of unknown cause that affects children after a bout of chickenpox or respiratory infection.

Congenital Bone Disorders

Congenital disorders affecting osseous (bone) tissue are cleft palate, hip dysplasia, and talipes equinovarus. A congenital defect caused by fusion failure of embryonic facial bones that results in a fissure through the palate is termed **cleft palate.** Mild to severe forms exist in which the division extends through both the hard and the soft palate into the nose, often resulting in cleft lip. **Cleft lip** (harelip) is a congenital opening in the upper lip resulting from incomplete union of the maxillary and median nasal processes (Fig. 17-14). Cleft palate is a multifactorial genetic disorder affecting 1 in 10,000 births. Surgical repair as soon as possible is the best treatment.

Congenital hip dysplasia (CHD) is a birth defect of the hip joint characterized by instability of the articulation at the femoral head or total hip dislocation. Signs include asymmetric folds in the thigh of a newborn with limited abduction of the affected leg. A shortened femur is evident when the knees are flexed. The cause is unknown, but the abnormality is obvious before or shortly after birth. It is possibly caused by ligament shortening that occurs from the maternal secretion of relaxin. Congenital hip dysplasia is more common in females and babies born breech. A positive Ortolani sign, a physical assessment maneuver that detects hip dysplasia, initially

Cleft lip

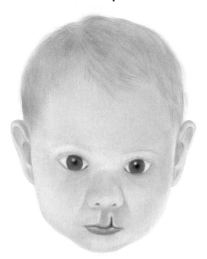

FIGURE 17-14
Cleft lip is a congenital opening in the upper lip resulting from incomplete union of maxillary and median nasal processes. (Image provided by Anatomical Chart Co.)

diagnoses it (Fig. 17-15). Physical examination and x-rays confirm the diagnosis. It is treated by manipulation of the femoral head into the acetabulum. The joint may require splinting, casting, a Pavlik harness to limit mobility, or surgery.

Talipes is the medical term for clubfoot, and **talipes equinovarus** is the most common form of foot deformity. It is characterized by fixed plantar flexion and an inward turning of the foot. Its cause is thought to be fetal position while in utero, but genetic factors have been implicated. Treatment options include casting, splinting, and orthopedic surgery if necessary.

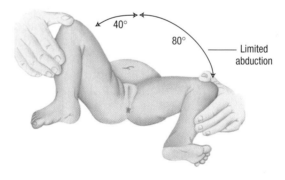

FIGURE 17-15
A physical maneuver that detects hip dysplasia. (Image provided by Anatomical Chart Co.)

Key Terms	Definitions
cleft palate	congenital fissure along the midline of the roof of the mouth
cleft lip	congenital cleft in the upper lip resulting from cleft palate; harelip
congenital (kun JEN i tul) **hip dysplasia** (dis PLAY zhuh)	defect of the hip joint that is present at birth
talipes (TAL i peez)	congenital foot deformity; clubfoot
talipes equinovarus (TAL i peez ee kwye noh VAY rus)	congenital foot deformity in which the foot is twisted and turned inward

Key Term Practice: Congenital Bone Disorders

1. A congenital fissure along the midline of the roof of the mouth is known as _____.

2. The medical term for clubfoot is _____.

Congenital Cardiac Disorders

Atrial septal defect (ASD) is an abnormal opening between the left and the right atrium that causes left to right blood shunting. If the hole is small, the signs and symptoms are fatigue, dyspnea, and infections. A large breach is marked by cyanosis (blue coloration owing to lack of oxygen), dyspnea (shortness of breath), and syncope (fainting). A murmur (blowing or roaring sound) can be heard with the stethoscope. Atrial septal defect is associated with prematurity and patent ductus arteriosus. Surgery is needed to correct the condition.

Patent ductus arteriosis (PDA) is a congenital anomaly in which the fetal ductus arteriosus persists after birth. The ductus arteriosis is a fetal structure that directs blood from the left pulmonary artery to the aorta. Its failure to close permits oxygenated blood to recirculate to the lungs. A murmur with thrills (vibrations) when palpated confirms the diagnosis. Treatment consists of the administration of antiprostaglandin drugs to close the opening or surgery to correct the condition. It is common in premature infants.

Narrowing of the aorta that causes partial blood flow obstruction is termed **coarctation of aorta.** The condition results in increased left ventricular pressure and decreased blood pressure distal to the constriction. Signs and symptoms may not be evident until adolescence. When present, they include left ventricular failure, pulmonary edema, cyanosis, dyspnea, and tachycardia (increased heart rate). Surgical treatment is aimed at creating a clear passage within the aorta.

The term *tetralogy* refers to "four related items." **Tetralogy of Fallot** is a congenital heart defect with a combination of four abnormalities. The first is pulmonary stenosis, or tightening of the pulmonary valve. Right ventricular hypertrophy, which is caused by increased pressure in the right ventricle, is the second. Ventricular septal defect, an abnormal opening between the ventricles, is the third aberration; and an overriding aorta is the fourth. The overriding aorta is a displacement of the aorta so that it crosses (overrides) the ventricular septum and receives both venous and arterial blood. Infants born with the condition exhibit cyanosis because the atrial blood is not fully oxygenated; thus they appear blue. Hypoxia (low oxygen levels), tachycardia, tachypnea, and dyspnea are also present. It is diagnosed by the history and physical examination demonstrating finger and toe clubbing, delayed growth, and other signs common to the separate conditions. Surgical treatment is necessary.

The reversal of the aorta and pulmonary artery that results in two closed-loop systems in the newborn is termed **transposition of great arteries.** In this condition, the aorta originates from the right (instead of the left) ventricle and the pulmonary artery originates from the left (instead of the right) ventricle. Neonates are cyanotic and have tachypnea. Heart failure ensues unless surgical measures are immediately initiated to correct the anomalies.

A congenital defect of the cardiac septum between the ventricles characterized by an abnormal opening that allows blood to shunt from the higher pressure left ventricle to the lower pressure right ventricle is known as **ventricular septal defect.** It is heard as a murmur with a stethoscope. Signs include increased heart and respiratory rates and failure to gain weight. Surgery is necessary to correct the flaw.

Key Terms	Definitions
atrial septal defect	abnormal opening between the atria
patent ductus arteriosis (DUCK tus ahr teer ee OH sus)	presence of ductus arteriosis after birth that causes oxygenated blood to recirculate to the lungs
coarctation (koh ark TAY shun) **of aorta** (ay OR tuh)	narrowing of the aorta causing blood flow obstruction
tetralogy (te TRAL uh jee) **of Fallot** (fah LOH)	congenital heart defect with four abnormalities
transposition of great arteries	rotation of the aorta and the pulmonary artery resulting in two closed-loop systems
ventricular (ven TRICK yoo lur) **septal defect**	abnormal opening between the left and the right ventricle

Key Term Practice: Congenital Cardiac Disorders

1. What is the congenital heart defect characterized by four cardiac anomalies.

   _____

2. An abnormal opening between the right atrium and the left atrium is termed _____.

Congenital Nervous System Disorders

Pathology of the nervous system tends to be profound. A tragic condition in which a fetus or infant lacks the cerebrum, cerebellum, and flat bones of the skull is called **anencephaly.** Because these critical structures are absent, the fetus usually dies before birth, during the birth process, or shortly after parturition. It results from a failure of the cephalic neural tube to close during the 2nd or 3rd week of prenatal development. There is a familial occurrence pattern, and the condition is more common in females. Ultrasound and increased α-fetoprotein (AFP) levels diagnose anencephaly before birth. There is no treatment.

Another congenital nervous system disorder is cerebral palsy. **Cerebral palsy** (CP) is a group of congenital, usually nonprogressive, diseases characterized by major bilateral motor dysfunction. Cerebral palsy is noticed shortly after birth or during early childhood. The major signs are difficulty suckling or swallowing. Three primary forms, spastic CP, dyskinetic CP, and ataxic CP, exist. Recurrent, continuous spasms (rapid muscle contractions), toe walking, and scissor gait (crossing one foot over the other) are common markings of **spastic cerebral palsy.** Involuntary, jerky movements and difficulty with fine motor coordination characterize **dyskinetic cerebral palsy.** Individuals may also have trouble speaking. **Ataxic cerebral palsy** is typified by uncoordinated action of voluntary muscle groups, particularly those involved with walking or reaching for an object. Poor balance is also noted. Some CP patients exhibit signs of all three types. Cerebral palsy is caused by inadequate blood or oxygen supply to the brain during fetal development, during the birth process, or in early childhood up to about 9 years of age. The condition is more common in premature infants and male babies. It is diagnosed by the clinical picture and accompanying neurologic examination. There is no cure, so treatment is aimed at achieving maximum function. Palliative measures, muscle relaxants, and anticonvulsive drugs may be warranted.

Duchenne muscular dystrophy (MD) is progressive degeneration and weakening of skeletal muscles with an onset shortly after birth or some time before age 5 years.

Muscles of the upper respiratory and pelvic areas are primarily involved, often resulting in death before maturity. Fat replaces atrophied muscle tissue; lordosis (inward curving of the lower spine) and spinal deformities are common. Disease progression results in total muscle contractures, debilitation, and immobility. It is an X-linked genetic disease, thus generally affecting only males. Nearly one third of cases have no familial history, suggesting the disease persists by newly acquired mutations. It is diagnosed by the presence of characteristic signs and symptoms. Muscle biopsy and elevated creatine kinase (CK)—an enzyme in muscles—levels confirm the diagnosis. There is no cure. Physical therapy, occupational therapy, and orthopedic appliances assist in helping the individual achieve maximum functioning capacity. Individuals with Duchenne MD are generally wheelchair bound by the time they are 12 years of age. Death results from cardiac or respiratory failure. The average survival rate is 10–15 years after disease onset.

Hydrocephalus is distension of the cerebral ventricles with cerebrospinal fluid (CSF). (The term *hydrocephalus* literally means "water on the brain.") It is caused by an obstruction in the subarachnoid space that prevents CSF from circulating or being properly absorbed. The abnormal increase in CSF around the brain results in infant head enlargement because the bones of the skull are still not fused. In addition to head enlargement, other signs and symptoms are bulging fontanelles, high-pitched crying, and abnormal leg muscle tone. Hydrocephalus is caused by fetal head trauma, blood clot, prematurity, and infection. The outward appearance and clinical picture lead to the initial diagnosis, which is confirmed by computed tomography (CT) or magnetic resonance imaging (MRI) scans. Treatment involves the placement of shunts to drain the excess fluid. Shunt catheters are positioned to empty either into the peritoneal cavity (ventriculoperitoneal shunt) or the right atrium (ventriculoatrial shunt) (Fig. 17-16).

Erythroblastosis fetalis (hemolytic disease of the newborn) is a serious blood disease of fetuses and neonates in which the antibodies produced by Rh⁻ mothers destroys the red blood cells of an Rh⁺ fetus. It can occur only in fetuses and infants with a positive blood Rh factor who are borne to females with Rh⁻ negative blood who have previously given birth to an Rh⁺ child. The blood of the fetus contains an antigen that is lacking in the mother's blood, thereby stimulating maternal antibody formation

FIGURE 17-16
Shunt placements for the correction of hydrocephalus. (**A**) A ventriculoperitoneal shunt drains excess fluid from the lateral ventricle into the peritoneal cavity. (**B**) A ventriculoatrial shunt drains into the right atrium of the heart, where the excess fluid is pumped into the bloodstream.

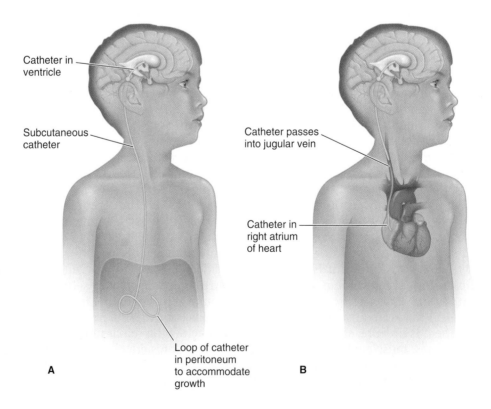

Catheter in ventricle

Subcutaneous catheter

Catheter passes into jugular vein

Catheter in right atrium of heart

Loop of catheter in peritoneum to accommodate growth

A

B

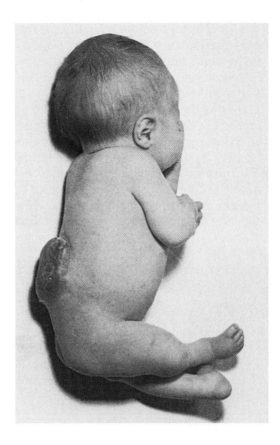

FIGURE 17-17
Spina bifida is a congenital defect in the closure of the vertebral canal characterized by hernial protrusion of the spinal cord meninges. (Reprinted with permission from O'Doherty N. Atlas of the newborn. Philadelphia: Lippincott, 1979.)

against the infant's erythrocytes, and these maternal antibodies cross the placenta to enter the fetus's blood. A complication of erythroblastosis fetalis is **kernicterus**, which is bilirubin pigmentation of the gray matter of the central nervous system (CNS) accompanied by degeneration of nerve cells in neonates. Kernicterus causes neurologic defects or death.

A congenital defect in the closure of the vertebral canal with hernial protrusion of spinal cord meninges is known as **spina bifida** (Fig. 17-17). It results from incomplete closure of the neural tube, and partial or total paralysis of the lower body is common. The herniated (protruding) portion contains cerebrospinal fluid and sometimes nervous tissue. It occurs primarily in the lumbosacral region. It is diagnosed by amniocentesis revealing an elevated AFP level.

Spina bifida is associated with maternal exposure to ionizing radiation during embryonic and fetal life. Prenatal ultrasonography is useful for diagnosing purposes. Visual inspection and x-ray examination postpartum may reveal the disease. If the individual is asymptomatic, it may never be discovered. The asymptomatic form is termed spina bifida occulta (hidden), and the only obvious sign may be a tuft of hair located on the skin overlying the defect. Some forms are treated by surgery.

The protrusion of the meninges through a defect in the skull or vertebra to form a CSF-filled cyst is termed **meningocele.** Skin overlying the region of defect may be tender. The cause is unknown but may be influenced by genetic and environmental factors. It is diagnosed by physical examination and confirmed by radiographic studies. Surgery within 48 hours is recommended to treat the deformity.

Spina bifida with protrusion of meningeal sac that contains spinal cord tissue is termed **myelomeningocele.** It is also known as spina bifida cystica. Neurologic deficits depend on the spinal cord level of involvement. Myelomeningocele results from neural tube closure failure. Although the cause is not identified, it may have a genetic component. Neurosurgery is performed within 24 hours of birth. Many of these individuals never develop bowel or urinary control or the ability to walk. Death usually results within 2 years.

A congenital disorder affecting the intestinal tract with an underlying nervous system component is Hirschsprung disease. **Hirschsprung disease**, also called **congenital aganglionic megacolon**, is often a familial disorder characterized by the inability to defecate as a result of ganglion cell absence in a given segment of colon or rectum. The accumulation of feces causes colon enlargement, signified by the term *megacolon*. The first sign is the failure of meconium to be discharged. Other indications are a distended abdomen, failure to thrive, constipation, and vomiting. Hirschsprung disease affects more males than females, and the risk increases with Down syndrome. It is diagnosed by history and physical examination and an x-ray of the bowel. Tissue biopsy confirms the absence of ganglionic cells. Treatment is surgical removal of the affected bowel portion and then resectioning the functional bowel together. A colostomy (temporary opening made in the abdomen to function as an anus) is necessary while the resectioned bowel heals. Untreated forms lead to growth retardation.

Key Terms	Definitions
anencephaly (an en SEF uh lee)	absence of all or part of the brain and part of the skull at birth or before birth
cerebral palsy (SERR e brul/se REE brul PAWL zee)	neurologic condition caused by brain damage around the time of birth, marked by lack of muscle control
spastic cerebral palsy (SPAS tick SERR e brul/se REE brul PAWL zee)	cerebral palsy marked by recurrent, continuous spasms and scissor-like gait
dyskinetic cerebral palsy (dis ki NET ick SERR e brul/se REE brul PAWL zee)	cerebral palsy marked by recurrent, slow, worm-like position changes of the fingers, toes, hands, or feet
ataxic cerebral palsy (a TACK sick SERR e brul/se REE brul PAWL zee)	cerebral palsy marked by uncoordinated action of voluntary muscle groups
Duchenne (doo SHAYNZ) **muscular dystrophy** (DIS truh fee)	X-linked degenerative disease attacking muscles of the upper respiratory and pelvic areas
hydrocephalus (high droh SEF uh lus)	enclosed accumulation of CSF around the brain, causing bulging infant fontanelles
erythroblastosis fetalis (e rith roh blas TOH sis fee TAY lis)	blood disease in which maternal antibodies attack the developing red blood cells of the fetus
kernicterus (kur NICK tur us)	bilirubin pigmentation of CNS gray matter as a consequence of erythroblastosis fetalis
spina bifida (SPYE nuh BIH fih duh)	congenital condition characterized by the spinal cord or meninges protruding through a cleft in the spinal column
meningocele (me NING goh seel)	protrusion of the meninges through an interruption in the skull or backbone forming a cyst
myelomeningocele (migh e loh me NING soh seel)	spina bifida with bulging of the meningeal sac that contains spinal cord tissue; spina bifida cystica
Hirschsprung (HIRSH sprung) **disease**	congenital defect in which a section of the intestine lacks nerve cells that enable peristalsis; aganglionic megacolon
congenital aganglionic megacolon (kun JEN i tul ay gang glee ON ick MEG uh koh lun)	congenital defect in which a section of the intestine lacks nerve cells that enable peristalsis; Hirschsprung disease

Key Term Practice: Congenital Nervous System Disorders

1. The word part *an-* means _____ and the word part _____ refers to "the brain"; thus _____ is absence of the brain.

2. The word part _____ means "water"; the word part *cephal-* means _____; thus _____ is fluid accumulation on the brain causing the head to bulge.

Premature Infant

An infant born before the 37th gestational week is termed a **premature infant.** Within a health-care setting, these infants are often referred to as "preemies." Signs of prematurity include low birth weight and underdeveloped or incomplete organ systems. Low birth weight is designated as a weight between 0.34 and 2.4 kg (12 oz. and 5.5 lb), like the infant shown in Figure 17-18. There is a medical difference between babies born small and premature infants. Small for gestational age infants are not premature, but rather designated as low-birth-weight infants.

Premature infants are at a high risk because they are unable to swallow or suck, and infections occur owing to an immature immune system. Causes include maternal trauma, multiple fetuses, hypertension, maternal infection, or bicornuate (two-horned) uterus. Treatment depends on gestational age. Premature infants often have several co-existing conditions, and the treatment of each depends on the underlying cause. Airway management and pulmonary function need to be established. Supplemental oxygen flow that is required to sustain life often causes ROP, a condition that can lead to blindness. Known measures to prevent premature births include adequate nutrition intake, appropriate prenatal care, no smoking or alcohol use, and addressing other known risk factors.

Infant respiratory distress syndrome (IRDS) is a disease of unknown cause occurring in the first few days of life in a premature infant. It is characterized by respiratory distress, cyanosis, alveoli collapse, and loss of pulmonary surfactant. Abnormal hyaline membrane lines alveoli and alveolar ducts when the disease persists longer than a few hours. Thus it is also known as hyaline membrane disease. Signs and symptoms include nasal flaring, grunting respirations, and ineffective gas exchange. It is diagnosed by the heightened respiratory rate, which is a compensatory mechanism to increase gas exchange, and blood gas studies indicating the potential for poor tissue oxygenation. Chest radiographic studies demonstrate the presence of hyaline membranes. Treatment involves restoring respiratory function as soon as possible, surfactant (lipoprotein that decreases surface tension to prevent alveoli from sticking together) aerosol infusion, or surfactant delivery through an endotracheal tube to the pulmonary structures. Infants treated for IRDS are predisposed to developing bronchopulmonary dysplasia. Prevention is the best measure. When a premature birth is eminent, the mother may be injected with a corticosteroid to stimulate the surfactant-synthesizing system.

Another disorder affecting premature infants is **bronchopulmonary dysplasia** (BPD), a dose-related consequence of oxygen therapy in newborns with IRDS. It manifests as a chronic lung disease. Signs are overinflated lungs and lobular emphysema that are revealed on chest x-rays. Other signs and symptoms include dyspnea, tachypnea (rapid breathing rate), wheezing, cyanosis, sternal retractions, and cracking sounds heard through auscultation. The oxygen pressure delivered to the young lungs to sustain life irreversibly damages the structures. Abnormal arterial blood gases (ABGs), lung scarring, and decreased lung oxygen levels with increased lung carbon dioxide levels confirm the diagnosis. Supportive treatment is given as new alveoli continue to develop

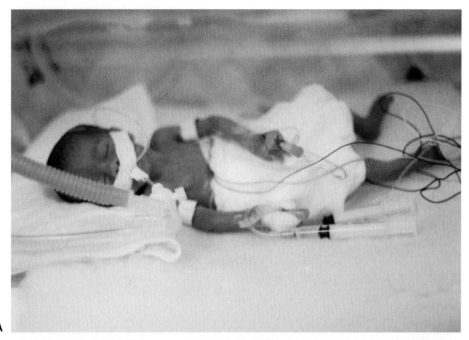

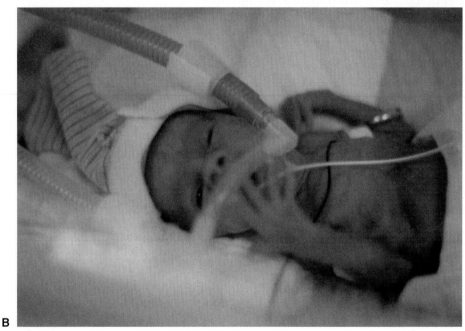

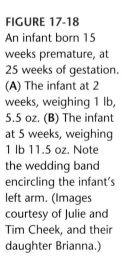

FIGURE 17-18
An infant born 15 weeks premature, at 25 weeks of gestation. (**A**) The infant at 2 weeks, weighing 1 lb, 5.5 oz. (**B**) The infant at 5 weeks, weighing 1 lb 11.5 oz. Note the wedding band encircling the infant's left arm. (Images courtesy of Julie and Tim Cheek, and their daughter Brianna.)

until about age 8 years. Bronchodilators, nutrition, anti-inflammatory drugs, theophylline (vasodilator and smooth muscle relaxant that opens bronchial airways), anticholinergic drugs, and diuretics are given. Diuretics decrease fluid accumulation, thereby lessening the incidence of pulmonary hypertension. Nutritional demands increase because the infant expends a great deal of energy in the process of breathing. There are no preventive measures, but the infant should be weaned as early as possible from mechanical ventilation.

Premature infants placed on auxiliary breathing therapy are at risk of developing an oxygen-induced disease of the eye blood vessels termed **retinopathy of prematurity** (ROP), or **retrolental fibroplasia.** Retrolental is the term describing something located behind the lens of the eye. There are no obvious signs or symptoms, but retinal-screening studies should be initiated in these infants beginning at 4–6 weeks. Because retinal vessels develop around the 28th gestational week, premature infants born before this critical time are at the highest risk of developing ROP. The lower the birth weight and the more premature the infant is, the greater the possibility. Careful monitoring of oxygen delivery is essential. Oxygen-saturation levels and titration concentrations should be adjusted to achieve the best possible outcome. Artificial lighting also increases the risk in premature infants. Ophthalmoscopic evaluation or scleral depression (procedure in which an instrument is slid behind the eyeball to view the retina) is used for diagnosis. Mild forms are self-limiting and the condition resolves with no further treatment. In other situations, laser therapy may be used to cauterize abnormal vasculature. Severe cases result in blindness.

Necrotizing enterocolitis (NEC) is a condition a premature infant develops when the intestinal tract becomes functional. It is characterized by an inflammation of the small intestine and colon. Signs and symptoms include feeding intolerance, distended abdomen, diarrhea, bloody stool, bile-colored vomit, and decreased or absent bowel sounds. Although the cause is unknown, it is thought to be the result of an abnormal defense response that allows normal gastrointestinal flora to invade the intestinal mucosa. Blood shunts away from the alimentary canal causing vasoconstriction. Normal mucus production also diminishes, exposing the intestinal lumen.

Predisposing risk factors consist of oral feeding of high-calorie formula, catheters, and IRDS. Feeding pattern changes, inability to maintain normal body temperature, abdominal distension, increased white blood cell count, and bloody stools are indicators of NEC. Radiographic studies confirm the diagnosis. Treatment is immediate and aggressive. The infant receives nothing by mouth (abbreviated NPO for non per os), gastric contents are emptied via nasogastric (NG) tube, and intravenous (IV) fluids with antibiotics are administered. Drinking breast milk confers some immunity. Close monitoring is essential because many infants die from NEC.

Key Terms	Definitions
premature infant	infant born before the 37th gestational week
infant respiratory (RES pi ruh tohr ee) **distress syndrome**	disease of the pulmonary system affecting premature infants within the first few days of life
bronchopulmonary dysplasia (brong koh PUL moh nair ee dis PLAY zhuh)	disorder that results from oxygen therapy delivered to infants with IRDS
retinopathy (ret i NOP uh thee) **of prematurity**	eye disease caused by oxygen administration in premature infants; retrolental fibroplasias
retrolental fibroplasia (ret roh LEN tul figh broh PLAY zhuh)	eye disease caused by oxygen administration in premature infants; retinopathy of prematurity
necrotizing enterocolitis (NECK roh tize ing en tur oh koh LYE tis)	condition of unknown cause involving small intestine and colon inflammation that occurs in premature infants

Key Term Practice: Premature Infant

1. _____ and _____ are two medical terms for the eye disease caused by oxygen administration in premature infants.

2. An infant born before the 37th gestational week is termed a/an _____ infant.

Infectious Diseases of Childhood

Infectious diseases are caused by a microbial agent, such as a bacterium or virus, and can be passed from one person to another. Typical infectious diseases of childhood include chickenpox (varicella), diphtheria, measles (rubeola), mumps (epidemic parotitis), whooping cough (pertussis), German measles or 3-day measles (rubella), and tetanus. Viral-born infections are chickenpox, measles, mumps, and rubella; bacteria cause diphtheria, pertussis, and tetanus. Fortunately, **vaccines**, inoculations that produce immunity, exist for these diseases that otherwise would cause illness.

The varicella-zoster virus (VZV) is a herpesvirus that causes chickenpox, which is also known as **varicella.** Varicella is a highly contagious viral disease that causes an acute infection in unvaccinated children and young adults. The contagion is spread by respiratory droplets or from contact with fluid from skin lesions. The virus has an incubation period of 2–3 weeks. **Incubation** refers to the development of an infection inside the body to the point at which the first signs of disease become apparent. A person is contagious 1–2 days before the appearance of the characteristic lesions to approximately 6 days after final eruptions. Signs are cutaneous (skin) lesions that begin as red macules (small, pigmented spot), transform to papules (small, hard, round bumps), and eventually become fluid-filled vesicles (sacs). The vesicles eventually crust and heal with no or slight scarring. Intense pruritus (itching) is a common symptom. The disease resolves in about 2 weeks, and then the person has lifetime immunity. It is diagnosed by the presence of macules and a history of virus exposure.

Treatment is supportive. Anti-viral medications can lessen the severity of symptoms if the disease is discovered in the very early stages. Presently, a vaccine, Varivax, is available. A single injection is given to children aged 1–12 years old; adolescents and adults receive the injection and a followup booster 4–8 weeks later. Duration of vaccine protection is currently not known because the vaccine is relatively new, and it is too soon to determine the long-lasting effects.

A serious infectious disease caused by the bacterium *Corynebacterium diphtheriae* that attacks the membranes of the throat and releases a toxin that damages the heart and nervous system is **diphtheria.** It is characterized by local inflammation and formation of a false membrane notably in the pharyngeal region. Absorption of the diphtheria toxin has deleterious effects on the heart and peripheral nerves. The incubation period is 2–5 days, and the patient is contagious for 2–4 weeks. If antibiotic therapy is initiated, the person is contagious only during the first few days. Signs and symptoms are sore throat, dysphagia (difficulty swallowing), cough, fever, swollen cervical lymph nodes, and halitosis (foul-smelling breath). Presence of the pseudomembrane on the pharyngeal arch and throat provide the initial diagnosis. Microbial studies identifying the causative agent confirm the diagnosis.

Treatment consists of administering diphtheria antitoxin, a serum containing antibodies that specifically neutralize the diphtheria toxin. Diphtheria toxoid, a detoxified toxin, is given as a vaccine to produce active immunity against diphtheria. The toxoid does not cause serum sensitivity.

Rubeola, or measles, is an acute, infectious viral disease characterized by fine, dusty, rose-red maculopapular skin eruptions. Symptoms include a high temperature, sore throat, and bright red rash of small spots that spread, covering the entire body. The incubation period is 2 weeks. Then coryza (severe nasal congestion), cough, conjunctivitis, and Koplik spots appear. **Koplik spots** are tiny, gray-white areas on a bright red base occurring on the parotid gland. Fever, chills, and the emergence of tiny rose-red eruptions mark days 3 and 4 of the infection. The rash gradually fades within 3–4 days, conferring lifetime immunity. Vaccines are readily available. The clinical picture and history of exposure lead to the diagnosis.

Care is supportive. High-risk or nonimmunized persons can be injected with the measles immunoglobulin up to 5 days after exposure.

Mumps, also called **epidemic parotitis,** is an acute, communicable (contagious) viral disease characterized by fever and inflamed parotid salivary glands. Other organ tissues, notably the testes, pancreas, ovaries, and meninges, are often involved. Males have testicular tenderness. The virus is contracted via droplet nuclei (small drops of liquid) in the air. It has an incubation period of 14–21 days; the patient is contagious for 1–7 days before swelling and up to 9 days past the characteristic signs. Lifelong immunity is conferred through active infection or vaccination. It is diagnosed by history and physical examination. Treatment is supportive. Immunization within 48 hours of disease exposure is another treatment option.

A highly infectious bacterial disease that causes violent coughing spasms is termed **pertussis,** or whooping cough. (The term *tussis* means "cough.") This disease of the respiratory systems is caused by *Bordetella pertussis* and is characterized by an explosive paroxysmal (sudden attack) cough followed by a sharp, shrill inhalation. The ending inhalation makes a "whooping" sound. It is spread by direct or indirect contact with nasopharyngeal secretions (droplet nuclei) of an infected person. Diagnosis is based on the characteristic cough and the presence of *B. pertussis* in bacterial studies. Pertussis is treated with erythromycin antibiotic and palliative (alleviating pain and symptoms without eliminating cause) care. A vaccine is available.

Another acute, viral, contagious disease characterized by fever, pale pink rash and cervical lymphadenitis is termed **rubella.** Other terms for this condition are epidemic roseola, German measles, and 3-day measles. It is associated with fetal abnormalities when maternal infection occurs during pregnancy. The reddish pink rash appears first on the face, and the person is contagious 1 week before eruption until 1 week after the rash appearance. The incubation period after exposure is 14–21 days. Active infection confers lifetime immunity. The clinical picture, history, and physical examination make the initial diagnosis. Diagnosis is confirmed by virology studies indicating rubella virus presence. Rubella is treated symptomatically. Vaccines are also available to prevent primary infection.

An acute infectious disease that is usually contracted through a penetrating wound is called **tetanus.** Tetanus is characterized by extreme body stiffness, painful muscular spasms and contractions, especially around the neck and jaw providing the foundation for the common term for the illness, "lockjaw." Generalized involuntary contractions or convulsions without loss of consciousness are also common. The disease results from the exotoxin produced by the anaerobic bacterium, *Clostridium tetani,* which interferes with the reflex arc of the nervous system. Infection occurs from wound contamination. Puncture wounds are the most common source because they are void of bacterial-killing oxygen. The incubation period is 3–21 days; however, the onset of disease is usually within 8 days after infection. The history, physical examination, and clinical picture are enough to provide a diagnosis.

Treatments include supportive care, muscle relaxants, and prompt wound cleaning with hydrogen peroxide. Vaccines containing tetanus antitoxin are available and boosters are administered every 10 years. A nonimmunized person can be given tetanus immunoglobulin (TIG) within 72 hours of injury. The mortality rate is about 35%, thus immunization is important.

Through a rigorous immunization program, people have become resistant to particular diseases. **Immunizations** and **vaccinations** are synonymous terms describing vaccines (inoculations, shots, or serums) given to protect against certain diseases by stimulating an immune response through the activation of antibodies. The antibodies formed from the stimulation confer immunity against particular infectious agents. Childhood diseases that are prevented through immunizations include pneumonia, influenza, hepatitis B, *Hepatitis influenzae* type B, polio, measles, mumps, rubella, diphtheria, tetanus, pertussis, and varicella. The vaccination schedule changes frequently, and updated schedules are available through the Centers for Disease Control and Prevention (CDC) and the American Academy of Pediatrics (AAP). An example vaccine schedule is given in Table 17-1.

TABLE 17-1 Vaccine Dosage Schedule

Vaccine	Dose				
	First	**Second**	**Third**	**Fourth**	**Fifth**
diphtheria, tetanus, pertussis (DTP)	2 months	4 months	6 months	15–18 months	4–6 years
hepatitis B	at birth	2–4 months	6–18 months		
influenza	yearly for children aged 2–23 months				
H. influenzae type B	2 months	4 months	6 months	12 or 15 months	
measles, mumps, rubella (MMR)	12 or 15 months	4–6 years			
polio	2 months	4 months	6 months	4–6 years	
pneumococcal	2 months	4 months	6 months	12 months	
varicella	after 12 months				

Key Terms	*Definitions*
vaccines (VACK seenz)	preparation administered to stimulate the immune system to produce antibodies against a disease
varicella (vair i SEL uh)	infectious disease caused by the varicella-zoster virus (VZV); chickenpox
incubation	phase of an infectious disease from the time of infection to the appearance of symptoms
diphtheria (dif THEER ee uh)	acute, infectious disease caused by *Corynebacterium diphtheria*
rubeola (roo BEE oh luh)	very contagious, acute viral disease characterized by fever and a red rash of small spots; measles
Koplik spots	small gray-white areas on a red background occurring on the parotid duct gland that are characteristic of measles
epidemic parotitis (ep i DEM ick pair oh TYE tis)	acute, contagious disease that causes fever and swelling of the salivary glands; mumps
pertussis (pur TUS is)	infectious respiratory bacterial disease caused by *Bordetella pertussis*; whooping cough
rubella (roo BEL uh)	highly contagious viral disease that causes swelling of the lymph glands and a skin rash
tetanus (TET uh nus)	infectious disease contracted through a penetrating wound caused by *C. tetani*; lockjaw
immunizations	vaccines that render immunity; vaccinations
vaccinations	vaccines that render immunity; immunizations

Key Term Practice: Infectious Diseases of Childhood

1. What is the medical term for the childhood disease caused by *Bordetella pertussis*?

   _____

2. What is the medical term for chickenpox?

   _____

3. _____ are chemical agents used to induce immunity.

CLINICAL TERMS

Clinical Dimension	Term	Description
DISORDERS		
	abruptio placentae	premature separation of the placenta from the uterine wall
	albinism	hereditary absence of melanin pigment
	anencephaly	absence of all or part of the brain and part of the skull at birth or before birth
	ataxic cerebral palsy	cerebral palsy marked by uncoordinated action of voluntary muscle groups
	atrial septal defect	abnormal opening between the atria
	bronchopulmonary dysplasia	disorder that results from oxygen therapy delivered to infants with IRDS
	cat's cry syndrome	congenital defect with a characteristic cat-like cry; cri-du-chat syndrome
	cerebral palsy (CP)	neurologic condition caused by brain damage around the time of birth, marked by lack of muscle control
	chorioangioma	benign tumor of the placenta
	choriocarcinoma	malignant tumor of the pregnant uterus
	cleft lip	congenital cleft in the upper lip, resulting from cleft palate; harelip
	cleft palate	congenital fissure along the midline of the roof of the mouth
	coarctation of aorta	narrowing of the aorta causing blood flow obstruction
	congenital aganglionic megacolon	congenital defect in which a section of the intestine lacks nerve cells that enable peristalsis; Hirschsprung disease
	congenital hip dysplasia (CHD)	defect of the hip joint that is present at birth

Clinical Dimension	Term	Description
	cri-du-chat syndrome	congenital defect with a characteristic cat-like cry; cat's cry syndrome
	cystic fibrosis (CF)	hereditary disease of infancy affecting various glands
	diphtheria	acute, infectious disease caused by *Corynebacterium diphtheria*
	Down syndrome	congenital syndrome characterized by mild to severe mental retardation that occurs from a tripling of chromosome 21; trisomy 21
	Duchenne muscular dystrophy	X-linked degenerative disease attacking muscles of the upper respiratory and pelvic areas
	dyskinetic cerebral palsy	cerebral palsy marked by recurrent, slow, worm-like position changes of the fingers, toes, hands, or feet
	eclampsia	illness occurring during the later stages of pregnancy characterized by high blood pressure, convulsions, and sometimes coma
	ectopic pregnancy	development of the fertilized egg outside the uterus
	Edwards syndrome	congenital syndrome characterized by several physical anomalies from a tripling of chromosome 18; trisomy 18
	epidemic parotitis	acute, contagious disease that causes fever and swelling of the salivary glands; mumps
	erythroblastosis fetalis	blood disease in which maternal antibodies attack the developing red blood cells of the fetus
	eunuchoidism	lacking fully developed male sexual organs or characteristics
	fetal alcohol syndrome (FAS)	pattern of malformation found among children of mothers who abused alcohol while pregnant
	galactosemia	genetic disorder resulting in the absence of galactase, an enzyme necessary for the breakdown of galactose
	gestational diabetes (GD)	faulty carbohydrate metabolism that occurs only during pregnancy
	harelip	cleft in the upper lip, resulting from cleft palate; cleft lip
	Hirschsprung disease	congenital defect in which a section of the intestine lacks nerve cells that enable peristalsis; a congenital aganglionic megacolon

Clinical Dimension	Term	Description
	hydatidiform mole	mass or tumor of unknown origin forming with the uterus at the beginning of pregnancy
	hydrocephalus	enclosed accumulation of CSF around the brain, causing bulging infant fontanelles
	incompetent cervix	premature dilation of the cervix
	infant respiratory distress syndrome (IRDS)	disease of the pulmonary system affecting premature infants within the first few days of life
	kernicterus	bilirubin pigmentation of CNS gray matter as a consequence of erythroblastosis fetalis
	Klinefelter syndrome	congenital syndrome characterized by male phenotype with an extra X chromosome, XXY
	meningocele	protrusion of the meninges through an interruption in the skull or backbone forming a cyst
	myelomeningocele	spina bifida with bulging of the meningeal sac that contains spinal cord tissue; spina bifida cystica
	necrotizing enterocolitis (NE)	condition of unknown cause involving small intestine and colon inflammation that occurs in premature infants
	patent ductus arteriosis (PDA)	presence of ductus arteriosis after birth that causes oxygenated blood to recirculate to the lungs
	pertussis	infectious respiratory bacterial disease caused by *Bordetella pertussis*; whooping cough
	phenylketonuria (PKU)	genetic disease in which the body lacks the enzyme to metabolize phenylalanine
	placenta previa	placenta positioned at the opening of the uterine cervix in the vagina
	preeclampsia	toxemia occurring in the later stages of pregnancy, similar to eclampsia but it is not marked by convulsions or coma
	premature infant	infant born before the 37th gestational week
	retinopathy of prematurity (ROP)	eye disease caused by oxygen administration in premature infants; retrolental fibroplasia
	retrolental fibroplasias	eye disease caused by oxygen administration in premature infants; retinopathy of prematurity
	Reye syndrome	serious childhood infection of unknown cause that follows a respiratory or varicella infection and results in encephalopathy

Clinical Dimension	Term	Description
	rubella	highly contagious viral disease that causes swelling of the lymph glands and a skin rash
	rubeola	very contagious, acute viral disease characterized by fever and a red rash of small spots; measles
	severe combined immune deficiency (SCID)	autosomal recessive congenital disorder marked by deficient immune system and response
	spastic cerebral palsy	cerebral palsy marked by recurrent, continuous spasms and scissor-like gait
	spina bifida	congenital condition characterized by the spinal cord or meninges protruding through a cleft in the spinal column
	syndrome	group of symptoms and signs that, when considered together, are known or presumed to characterize a disease
	talipes	congenital foot deformity; clubfoot
	talipes equinovarus	congenital foot deformity in which the foot is twisted and turned inward
	Tay-Sachs disease	genetic disease marked by accumulation of lipids in nervous tissue affecting people of eastern European Jewish ancestry
	tetanus	infectious disease contracted through a penetrating wound caused by *C. tetani*; lockjaw
	tetralogy of Fallot	congenital heart defect with four abnormalities
	toxemia of pregnancy	condition characterized by hypertension, swelling, and proteinuria—the late stage of preeclampsia and eclampsia
	transposition of great arteries	rotation of the aorta and the pulmonary artery, resulting in two closed-loop systems
	Turner syndrome	chromosomal disorder occurring in females resulting in nondevelopment or absence of reproductive organs, XO
	varicella	infectious disease caused by the varicella-zoster virus (VZV); chickenpox
	ventricular septal defect	abnormal opening between the left and the right ventricle
SIGNS AND SYMPTOMS		
	brachycephaly	shortness of the head
	Braxton Hicks contractions	irregular and painless uterine contractions that are different from the contractions of labor

Clinical Dimension	Term Description
Chadwick sign	blue-violet color of the cervix and vagina, indicative of pregnancy
chloasma	dark coloration on the facial skin caused by pregnancy-induced hormonal changes
effacement	gradual flattening of the cervix during labor
epicanthus	skin fold from the eyelid that partially covers the eye part nearest the nose
Goodell sign	softening of the cervix, indicative of pregnancy
Hegar sign	softening of the lower portion of the uterus occurring at about week 6 of pregnancy
hypertelorism	excessive width between two organs or body parts
Koplik spots	small gray-white areas on a red background occurring on the parotid duct gland that are characteristic of measles
lightening	movement of the fetus into the pelvis
linea nigra	dark line extending up the center of the abdomen of a pregnant woman
micrognathia	small jaws
miscarriage	sudden, unplanned expulsion of the fetus from the uterus before it is viable; spontaneous abortion
spontaneous abortion	sudden, unplanned expulsion of the fetus from the uterus before it is viable; miscarriage
stillbirth	birth of a dead fetus
strabismus	eye abnormality that results in an inability to focus on the desired object
striae gravidarum	stretch marks seen in pregnancy
quickening	fetal movements felt by the mother

CLINICAL TESTS AND DIAGNOSTIC PROCEDURES

α-fetoprotein serum test	a marker for certain congenital defects
amniocentesis	prenatal diagnostic test in which amniotic fluid is evaluated
ballottement	diagnostic maneuver used to palpate a floating fetus
bilirubin test	determines the level of bilirubin (a liver pigment) to detect jaundice and erythrocyte hemolysis by the mother's Rh antibodies
blood test	determines blood type and Rh factor

Clinical Dimension	Term	Description
	chorionic villus biopsy (CVB)	prenatal test used to detect birth defects by analyzing cells of the chorion; chorionic villus sampling
	chorionic villus sampling (CVS)	prenatal test used to detect birth defects by analyzing cells of the chorion; chorionic villus biopsy
	contraction stress test (CST)	determines the ability of the fetus to tolerate the stress of labor—oxytocin is delivered through an intravenous line to stimulate uterine contractions; oxytocin challenge test
	creatinine test	determines fetal maturity—creatinine is a product of creatine metabolism
	external fetal monitoring (EFM) test	monitoring devices are on placed on the mother's external abdomen to measure fetal heart rate and the force of the uterine contractions
	fetal cell sorting	fetal cells are separated from maternal cells using a fluorescence-activated cell sorter and interpreted by a genetic counselor
	galactose-1-phosphate test	assess the level of galactose-1-phosphate in the hemoglobin—decreased values indicate galactosemia
	Guthrie test	determines the level of phenylalanine in the serum of a neonate to detect PKU
	human chorionic gonadotropin in maternal serum or urine	test that measures the level of hCG in the urine or blood—increased hCG values indicate pregnancy
	human placental lactogen (hPL) test	evaluates placental function—hPL is a hormone secreted by the placenta that enters maternal circulation and disappears from circulation after delivery or when the placenta is not functioning normally
	internal fetal monitoring test	monitors fetal heart rate and uterine contractions by an electrode attached to the fetal scalp avia a catheter in the uterus
	lecithin to sphingomyelin (L:S) ratio	determines fetal lung maturity—when fetal lungs are mature, the ratio is 2:1 and levels below 2:1 indicate fetal immaturity
	nipple stimulation test	determines the fetus's ability to withstand normal labor—the mother strokes her nipples causing the natural release of oxytocin, which is much less stressful on the mother and fetus than the contractions stress test
	oxytocin challenge test	determines the ability of the fetus to tolerate the stress of labor—oxytocin is delivered through an intravenous line to stimulate uterine contractions; contraction stress test
	pelvimetry	radiographic measurement of the female pelvic inlet and outlet to determine feasibility of vaginally birthing a child

Clinical Dimension	Term	Description
	TORCH series	group of blood tests designed to identify teratogenic diseases in pregnant women and neonates
	2-hour postprandial glucose test	determines blood glucose levels 2 hours after drinking a sugar solution
	ultrasound	imaging technique using high-frequency sound waves that reflect off internal body parts to create images, especially of the fetus in the womb
TREATMENTS		
	abortion	to expel an embryo or fetus before pregnancy completion
	dilation and curettage (D&C)	procedure involving the expansion of the cervix and scraping of the uterus
	immunizations	vaccines that render immunity; vaccinations
	in vitro fertilization	fertilization of an ovum by sperm outside the body when normal conception is not achievable
	in vivo fertilization	fertilization occurring inside a living organism
	vaccines	preparation administered to stimulate the immune system to produce antibodies against a disease
	vaccinations	vaccines that render immunity; immunizations

Lifespan

Physiological and anatomic changes throughout the lifespan were reviewed in earlier sections in this chapter. Numerous tests have been developed to chart developmental progress. One such assessment is the Denver Developmental Screening Test (DDST), which is a standardized screening tool that assesses the developmental progress of children from birth through adolescence. Psychologists and pediatricians use the test to evaluate gross motor skills, language proficiency, fine motor coordination, and social interactions. Statistical analyses are applied to identify patterns of developmental deficits.

Development phases are marked by periods of anatomic growth and structures not evident at birth. During the fetal stage, organs are established, but immature; and the primary germ layers quickly grow.

Prenatal development includes the formation of all body systems. The integumentary system is complete by the 7th gestational month; epiphyseal cartilages are formed by month 8; and muscle formation is nearly complete by month 6, although both muscle mass and control increase throughout postnatal development. The nervous system is complete by month 6, but myelination and CNS formation continue throughout the postnatal development. The endocrine and digestive systems are in place by the 7th gestational month, but the sense organs and complete respiratory system structures are not completed until nearly the 9th gestational month. Nephron formation (urinary system) and testicle descent (reproductive system) are completed toward the end of the 8th month of gestation. The reproductive system may not be fully functional until puberty. At delivery, the head is disproportionately large and remains so for quite some time after birth.

General effects of aging are numerous and involve every body system. For example, nervous system changes include glaucoma and cataracts. Musculoskeletal effects are evidenced by a loss of skeletal muscle strength and shaggy-appearing bone margins, called lipping. The circulatory system loses efficiency, atherosclerosis becomes more apparent, skin is less elastic, and nephron numbers decline nearly 50% between the ages of 30 and 75 years.

In the News: Fetus in Fetu

It is a curiosity: A fetus is found within the abdominal cavity of another living person. Cases of fetus in fetu generally capture the attention of the international news media because of the condition's bizarre nature. Fetus in fetu is an unusual condition in which a small, imperfectly formed fetal mass is contained within the abdomen of a normally developed fetus, and remains during life as a nonliving being. First described in the late 18th century, this rare pathologic state has been reported approximately 80 times in the professional literature and is sensationalized by the press. It is estimated to occur in 1 out of every 500,000 deliveries.

The cause is not known but appears as a twin inside the body of its partner. Two leading theories propose that it either results from an anomaly during embryogenesis in a monochorionic twin pregnancy in which one malformed twin lies within the body of the other twin or it could be an unusual, highly organized teratoma. A teratoma is a neoplasm of embryologic tissue that contains three primary germ layers. It occurs more commonly in males, who usually present with an abdominal mass by the 1st year of age, although cases have been reported in teenagers and adults. CT studies reveal its presence, typically located in the retroperitoneum. In some instances, the discovered mass has weighed as much as 2 kg (4.4 lb), and one was 30 cm (11.8 in.) in length! Descriptions are varied: extremities well developed with hair covering the entire body; bone, cartilage, teeth, fat, and muscles found in masses of tissue. It is seemingly an abortive attempt of identical twinning in which one fetus is drawn into the abdominal cavity of the other.

Patients present with localized pain. Signs and symptoms include abdominal distension, vomiting, feeding difficulty, and dyspnea related to mass size. The fetus in fetu mass size can increase, causing hemorrhage. Intra-abdominal fetus in fetu is self-contained in a sac with no major vascular connections to the host. In cases of delayed reporting, the fetus in fetu is attached to significant vessels and appears to grow with the host. CT scans confirm the presence of a vertebral column, a distinguishing feature of the condition. Chromosomal analyses are normal and identical to the host. Surgical excision of the mass is recommended because of the potential for impaired renal function and malignancy.

COMMON ABBREVIATIONS

Abbreviation	Term
A	adenine
AAP	American Academy of Pediatrics
ABG	arterial blood gas
AFP	α-fetoprotein
ARDMS	American Registry of Diagnostic Medical Sonographers

Abbreviation	Term
ASD	atrial septal defect
BPD	bronchopulmonary dysplasia
C	cytosine
CDC	Centers for Disease Control and Prevention
CHD	congenital hip dysplasia
CF	cystic fibrosis
CK	creatine kinase
CNS	central nervous system
CP	cerebral palsy
C-section	Cesarean section
CSF	cerebrospinal fluid
CMV	cytomegalovirus
CT	computed tomography
CVB	chorionic villus biopsy
CVS	chorionic villus sampling
D&C	dilation and curettage
DDST	Denver Developmental Screening Test
DNA	deoxyribonucleic acid
DTP	diphtheria-tetanus-pertussis
EDC	estimated date of confinement
EFM	external fetal monitoring
FAS	fetal alcohol syndrome
FHR	fetal heart rate
FSH	follicle-stimulating hormone
G	guanine
GD	gestational diabetes
GnRH	gonadotropin-releasing hormone
GYN	gynecology
hCG	human chorionic gonadotropin
HLA	human leukocyte antigen
hPL	human placental lactogen
HSV-II	herpes simplex virus type II
IRDS	infant respiratory distress syndrome
IV	intravenous
LH	luteinizing hormone
LMP	last menstrual period
L:S	lecithin to sphingomyelin ratio
MD	muscular dystrophy
MMR	measles, mumps, rubella
MRI	magnetic resonance imaging
NEC	necrotizing enterocolitis

Abbreviation	Term
NG	nasogastric
NPO	non per os; nothing by mouth
OB	obstetrician; obstetrics
OT	oxytocin
PDA	patent ductus arteriosus
PG US	pregnancy ultrasound
PID	pelvic inflammatory disease
PKU	phenylketonuria
PRL	prolactin
ROP	retinopathy of prematurity
SCID	severe combined immune deficiency
SGA	small for gestational age
T	thymine
TIG	tetanus immune globulin
TORCH series	Toxoplasma, Other disease-causing viruses, Rubella virus, Cytomegalovirus, Herpes simplex virus type II
VBAC	vaginal birth after Cesarean section
VZV	varicella-zoster virus

Case Study

Sabine Bauer is a 22-year-old female who presented in the OB/GYN office for prenatal care. Her last menstrual period (LMP) was February 14, 2004. Her appoint date was July 2, 2004. Pregnancy ultrasound revealed a single fetus in the vertex position. The fetal heart rate (FHR) was 147 beats per minute. The anteriorly located placenta was low lying, suggesting a probable placenta previa. Diagnostic ultrasound demonstrated a fetal spine, 4-chamber heart, cord insertion, stomach, three-vessel cord, kidneys, and bladder. All were unremarkable. Estimated menstrual age was 20 weeks and 5 days. Estimated date of confinement (EDC), or the day the baby was due, was November 21, 2004. A small choroid plexus cyst measuring 6 by 4 mm was noted. The obstetrician recommended follow-up ultrasound for the low-lying placenta and choroid plexus cyst.

Case Study Questions

Select the best answer to each of the following questions.

1. Ms Bauer's LMP was February 14, 2004. This means that _____.

   a. she had been bleeding for about 5 months

   b. February 14, 2004 was the first day of her menstrual cycle

   c. February 14, 2004 was the last day of her menstrual cycle

   d. the baby was due on February 14, 2004

2. The vertex position is _____.

   a. a normal finding

   b. an abnormal finding

   c. indicates a breech birth

   d. indicates that the baby will be born feet first

3. Placenta previa is best described as a condition in which the _____.

a. placenta is implanted in the lower portion of the uterus, extending toward the cervix

b. placenta is implanted in the upper portion of the uterus, extending toward the cervix.

c. uterus is bicornuate.

d. placenta contains more than one fetus.

4. The ultrasound test confirmed the presence of a three-vessel cord. This refers to _____.

a. the spinal cord that contains nerves, arteries, and veins

b. an umbilical cord with two arteries and one vein

c. an umbilical cord with one artery and two veins

d. a spermatic cord that contains ductus deferens, blood vessels, and lymphatic vessels

5. How did the obstetrician arrive at November 21st as the EDC?

a. the Braxton Hicks formula was used

b. the Goodell sign was applied

c. the Chadwick sign was applied

d. Nägele's rule was used

REAL WORLD REPORT

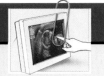

Mandy performed the pregnancy ultrasound (PG US) on Sabine Bauer. The ultrasound report follows.

IMAGING DEPARTMENT

NAME:	Sabine Bauer	DOB:	02/02/1981
AGE:	22 years		
DATEORD:	08/27/2004	EXAM DATE:	08/27/2004
TEST:	PG US	ORDPHYS:	K. K. Miner, MD

CLINICAL INFORMATION: Followup for possible placenta previa and possible choroid plexus cyst.

PREGNANCY ULTRASOUND

Multiple ultrasonographic scans of the lower abdomen and pelvis were obtained and compared with previous examination of July 1, 2004. There is a single intrauterine pregnancy in cephalic presentation. The placenta lies anteriorly in unremarkable position. The previously described low-lying position of the placenta is no longer present on this examination.

Fetal cardiac and somatic motion were visible during the examination. An adequate amount of amniotic fluid is demonstrated.

There is a moderate dilatation of the lateral ventricles, which was not observed on the previous examination. The previously described choroid plexus cyst cannot be positively identifiable on this examination.

The fetal measurement is consistent with a 28-week 4-day menstrual age.

IMPRESSION

1. A single intrauterine pregnancy in cephalic presentation. Anterior placenta is noted; the placental position is unremarkable on this examination.

2. There is mild to moderate dilatation of the lateral ventricles, which was not observed on the previous study.

3. Sonogram reveals ultrasonographic menstrual age of 28 weeks, 4 days.

4. A repeat ultrasonographic examination in several weeks for reevaluation of the intracranial structures is recommended.

REAL WORLD REPORT QUESTIONS

The following exercises review the medical terms in the preceding medical report.

1. Define single intrauterine pregnancy.

    _____

2. Amniotic fluid refers to fluid _____.

    a. contained in amniotic sac surrounding fetus

    b. contained in uterus that surrounds fetus

    c. produced by choroid plexus

    d. secreted by mammary glands

3. Define cephalic presentation.

    _____

4. The medical report used the terms intrauterine and intracranial. Define the following word parts.

    a. *intra-* _____

    b. uter- _____

    c. crani- _____

REVIEW AND APPLICATION: THREE-LEVEL LEARNING SYSTEM

LEVEL ONE: REVIEWING FACTS AND TERMS USING RECALL

Select the best response to each of the following questions.

1. The organ in which a fetus develops is a/an _____.

   a. embryo

   b. placenta

   c. zygote

   d. chorion

2. _____ is the number of years a particular individual can live.

   a. Life span

   b. Life expectancy

   c. Senescence

   d. Life inheritance

3. An unborn offspring at gestational week 9 is termed a/an _____.

   a. zygote

   b. embryo

   c. fetus

   d. ovum

4. The period of time spent developing in the womb is called _____.

   a. fertilization

   b. development

   c. growing

   d. gestation

5. Male and female reproductive cells are _____.

   a. gametes

   b. blastomeres

   c. trophoblasts

   d. blastocysts

6. The endoderm, ectoderm, and mesoderm make up _____.

   a. the uterine wall

   b. the primary germ layers

   c. layers of the amnion

   d. the secondary germ layers

7. Embryonic germ layers are formed through this process.

   a. histogenesis

   b. oogenesis

   c. spermatogenesis

   d. gastrulation

8. A group of congenital, usually nonprogressive diseases, characterized by major bilateral motor dysfunction, is known as _____.

   a. Down syndrome

   b. cerebral palsy

   c. hydrocephalus

   d. varicella

9. _____ describes shortness of the head.

   a. Micrognathia

   b. Patent ductus arteriosis

   c. Kernicterus

   d. Brachycephaly

10. Agents that cause birth defects are termed _____.

    a. congenital producers

    b. congenital enhancers

    c. teratogens

    d. mutations.

11. Which term means existing before or at birth?

    a. teratogen

    b. congenital

    c. placental

    d. gestation

12. The _____ is the outermost fetal membrane.

    a. chorion

    b. yolk sac

    c. amnion

    d. allantois

13. The _____ is the innermost fetal membrane.

    a. chorion

    b. yolk sac

    c. amnion

    d. allantois

14. A physician specializing in pediatrics is a/an _____.

    a. podiatrist

    b. obstetrician

    c. pediatrician

    d. B and C are correct

15. The period of life between puberty and adulthood is _____.

    a. senescence

    b. infancy

    c. childhood

    d. adolescence

16. The term _____ means both alleles of a pair of genes are alike.

    a. homozygous

    b. heterozygous

    c. autosome

    d. recessive

17. The complete set of genes on all the chromosomes is referred to as the _____.

    a. karyotype

    b. alleles

    c. genome

    d. genotype

18. Both dominant and recessive phenotypes are expressed with _____.

    a. incomplete dominance

    b. codominance

    c. homozygous chromosomes

    d. somatic cells

19. _____ is reduction division, and _____ creates two identical daughter cells.

    a. Meiosis; mitosis

    b. Mitosis; meiosis

    c. Mutation; meiosis

    d. Mitosis; mutation

20. The joining of gametes at fertilization is known as _____.

    a. implantation

    b. cleavage

    c. syngamy

    d. parturition.

LEVEL TWO: REVIEWING CONCEPTS

Select the best response to each of the following questions.

21. Which is the correct order of blastocyst development?

    a. blastomere → morula → blastocyst

    b. morula → blastocyst → blastomere

    c. blastula → morula → blastocyst

    d. blastocyst → blastomere → morula

22. A _____ is a solid ball of cells, and a _____ is a hollow ball of cells.

    a. blastocyst; blastula

    b. morula; blastomere

    c. morula; blastocyst

    d. blastomere; blastocyst

23. Which lists the developmental stages in order of youngest to oldest?

    a. infancy → neonatal period → adolescence → adulthood

    b. neonatal period → infancy → childhood → adulthood

    c. infancy → adolescence → childhood → adulthood

    d. childhood → infancy → adolescence → neonatal period

24. The genotype of a male child is _____.

25. The genotype of a female child is _____.

26. Name the two structures that enable blood to avoid the nonfunctioning fetal lungs.

    _____

Provide a medical term to complete a meaningful analogy.

27. Chorionic villus biopsy is to _____ as miscarriage is to _____.

28. Congenital aganglionic megacolon is to _____ as measles is to _____.

Match the sign with its definition.

_____ 29. lightening

_____ 30. epicanthus

_____ 31. hypertelorism

_____ 32. strabismus

_____ 33. effacement

    a. skinfold that partially covers the part of the eye nearest the nose

    b. excessive width between two organs

    c. inability of the eye to focus on the desired object

    d. gradual flattening of the cervix during labor

    e. dropping of the fetus into the pelvis

Match the test with its description.

_____ 34. hCG test

_____ 35. amniocentesis

_____ 36. 2-h postprandial glucose test

_____ 37. TORCH series

_____ 38. chorionic villus sampling

    a. blood test to identify teratogenic diseases in pregnant women

    b. laboratory test to determine blood sugar levels

    c. measures level of hCG in the blood or urine to detect pregnancy

    d. prenatal test evaluating extensions of the chorion

    e. prenatal test evaluating fluid in the placenta

Match the test with its description.

_____ 39. ballottement

_____ 40. Guthrie test

_____ 41. hPL test

_____ 42. α-fetoprotein serum test

_____ 43. pelvimetry

    a. blood test performed on the mother to evaluate placental function

    b. diagnostic maneuver to palpate a floating fetus

    c. blood test used to detect phenylalanine

    d. x-ray study to determine feasibility of a vaginal delivery

    e. fetal protein test to detect fetal disorders

Match the term with its definition

_____ 44. quickening

_____ 45. Chadwick sign

_____ 46. Hegar sign

    a. blue-violet color of the cervix and vagina during pregnancy

    b. birth of a dead fetus

_____ 47. Goodell sign

_____ 48. stillbirth

c. softening of the cervix, which indicates pregnancy

d. softening of the lower uterus at week 6 of pregnancy

e. fetal movements felt by the mother

Match the pregnancy condition with its definition.

_____ 49. abruptio placentae

_____ 50. miscarriage

_____ 51. chorioan-gioma

_____ 52. eclampsia

_____ 53. choriocarci-noma

a. malignant tumor of the pregnant uterus

b. benign tumor of the placenta

c. premature separation of the placenta from the uterus

d. illness of late pregnancy characterized by hypertension and convulsions

e. physiological expulsion of the fetus

Match the disorder with its description.

_____ 54. severe combined immune deficiency (SCID)

_____ 55. cystic fibrosis (CF)

_____ 56. patent ductus arteriosus (PDA)

_____ 57. spina bifida

_____ 58. tetanus

a. hereditary disease affecting the exocrine glands

b. presence of ductus arteriosus after birth

c. congenital disorder marked by a deficient immune system

d. infectious disease contracted through a deep, penetrating wound

e. congenital disorder in which the spinal cord protrudes through a cleft in the spinal column

Match the disease with its description.

_____ 59. mumps

_____ 60. rubella

_____ 61. diphtheria

_____ 62. measles

_____ 63. varicella

a. chickenpox; caused by VZV

b. disease caused by *C. diphtheria*

c. viral disease characterized by a red rash of small spots

d. disease affecting the salivary glands

e. viral disease of the lymph glands

Define the following terms.

64. vertex _____

65. vernix caseosa _____

66. incompetent cervix _____

67. spontaneous abortion _____

68. implantation _____

69. meningocele _____

What is the term described by each of the following definitions?

70. formation and attachment of the placenta _____

71. study of malformations caused by agents that bring about birth defects _____

72. hormone that causes relaxation of the pelvis _____

73. score/rating assessing the condition of the neonate _____

74. branch of medicine dealing with the care of children _____

75. spina bifida with a bulging meningeal sac _____

Identify the correctly spelled term in each set.

_____76.   a. allele   b. allelle
              c. alelle   d. aleal

_____77.   a. genotype   b. genotipe
              c. jenotype   d. genetype

_____78.   a. purperium   b. peurperium
              c. puerperium d. purpurium

_____79.   a. jestation   b. gestetion
              c. gestasion   d. gestation

_____80.   a. line nigrea   b. linea nigra
              c. linea nigera d. linee niger

Unscramble the letters to form a medical term.

81. teemtallbont _____

82. pietocc _____

83. robtaoin _____

84. sinbimal _____

85. nicerutresk _____

Using the following word parts, form a medical term for each definition. Each word part is used only once.

amnio-   -cele   centesis   embryo-

embryo-   -logy   meningo-   -pathy

86. embryonic or congenital defect resulting in faulty development _____

87. study of the embryo and its development _____

88. procedure for withdrawing amniotic fluid for analysis _____

89. protrusion of the meninges through the skull or vertebra form a CSF-filled cyst _____

Define the following abbreviations.

90. DTP _____

91. BPD _____

92. hCG _____

93. EDC _____

94. SGA _____

95. PKU _____

What is the alternate spelling of each of the following terms?

96. trocar _____

97. amniotic _____

LEVEL THREE: THINKING CRITICALLY

Provide a short answer to the following questions.

98. Is it possible for fraternal twins to have two different biologic fathers? Explain your answer.

_____

_____

_____

99. Identify one similarity between an organism floating in outer space and an organism floating in utero.

_____

_____

_____

100. Calculate the birth date of an infant whose mother's last menstrual period (LMP) was March 17.

_____

KEY TERMS SPELLING TEST FROM CD-ROM

Use the CD-ROM to test yourself on the spelling of key terms from this chapter. Listen to the terms and write them on a separate sheet of paper. Use a medical dictionary to check your answers.

ANSWERS

WORD GROUPING

Definition	Word Part
resembling cheese	case-, caseo-
allantoic, allantois, an extraembryonic membrane	allant-, allanto-
amnion, amnionic	amnio-
appearance	phen-, pheno-
brain	encephal-, encephalo-
child	ped-, pedo-
chorion, outermost fetal membrane	chori-, chorio-
common, like, same	hom-, homo-
different, unlike	heter-, hetero-
embryo, fetus, embryonic, fetal	embry-, embryo-
formative cell, bud	blast-, -blast, blasto-
jaw	gnath-, gnatho-
joined	zyg-, zygo-
malformed	terato-
meninx, meninges	mening-, meningo-
middle	mes-, meso-
milk	lact-, lacti-, lacto-
nucleus	kary-, karyo-
nutrition, nutritive, nourishment	troph-, tropho-
talus, ankle	talo-
vulva	episio-

WORD BUILDING

Word Part	Meaning	Common or Known Word	Example Medical Term
alant-, allanto-	allantoic, allantois, an extraembryonic membrane	allantoin	allantois
amnio-	amnion, amnionic	amniotic fluid	amniocentesis
blast-, -blast, blasto-	formative cell, bud	blastocyst	trophoblast
embry-, embryo-	embryo, fetus, embryonic, fetal	embryo	embryology
episio-	vulva	episiotomy	episiotomy
heter-, hetero-	different, unlike	heterosexual	heterozygous
hom-, homo-	common, like, same	homosexual	homozygous
mening-, meningo-	meninx, meninges	meninges	meningocele
mes-, meso-	middle	mesosphere	mesoderm
ped-, pedo-	child	pedophile	pediatrics
phen-, pheno-	appearance	phenomenon	phenotype
talo-	talus, ankle	talon	talipes equinovarus
zyg-, zygo-	joined	zygomatic arch	zygote

KEY TERM PRACTICE

Pregnancy, Human Development, and Child Health Preview
1. zygote
2. embryo

Fertilization and Implantation
1. tissue; -genesis; histogenesis
2. Gastrulation

Placentation and Gestation
1. chorionic villi
2. terato-; -ology; teratology

Fetal Circulation
1. foramen ovale
2. fossa ovalis

Pregnancy
1. parturition
2. obstetrician

Labor and Delivery
1. episio-; -otomy; episiotomy
2. vertex; breech

Lactation
1. Lactation; lact-
2. colostrum

Artificial Fertilization and Multiple Births
1. dizygotic or nonidentical
2. monozygotic

Developmental Stages
1. Neonate; neo-
2. Senescence

Genes and Chromosomes
1. karyotype
2. phenotype

Inheritance
1. sex-linked
2. mutation

Pregnancy Conditions
1. Toxemia of pregnancy
2. preeclampsia

Autosomal Recessive Diseases
1. phenylketonuria (PKU)
2. Tay-Sachs disease

Congenital Syndromes
1. a. Klinefelter syndrome; b. Turner syndrome
2. a. Edwards syndrome; b. Down syndrome

Nongenetic Syndromes
1. fetal alcohol syndrome (FAS)
2. Reye syndrome

Congenital Bone Disorders
1. cleft palate
2. talipes

Congenital Cardiac Disorders
1. tetralogy of Fallot
2. atrial septal defect

Congenital Nervous System Disorders
1. without; encephal-; anencephaly
2. hydro-; head; hydrocephalus

Premature Infant
1. Retinopathy of prematurity (ROP); retrolental fibroplasia
2. premature

Infectious Diseases of Childhood
1. pertussis
2. varicella
3. Vaccines

CASE STUDY

1. b is the correct answer.
   - a is incorrect because the ultrasound indicated a fairly normal pregnancy; there was no indication of spotting or bleeding, and LMP refers to the 1st day of the last menstrual period.
   - c is incorrect because LMP refers to the 1st day of the last menstrual period, not the last day.
   - d is incorrect because the baby's due date was November 21, 2004, as indicated in the report.
2. a is the correct answer.
   - b is incorrect because the vertex (head-first) position is a normal finding.
   - c is incorrect because the vertex position is normal; breech birth means the fetus is positioned with feet or buttocks first, which is abnormal.
   - d is incorrect because feet first indicates a breech birth, the reverse of the normal vertex position.
3. a is the correct answer.
   - b is incorrect because placenta previa is a condition in which implantation occurs in the lower, not the upper, portion of the uterus.
   - c is incorrect because a bicornuate uterus refers to a uterus with two horns, something not indicated in the report and not the definition of placenta previa.
   - d is incorrect because the report revealed a single fetus, and placenta previa relates to abnormal implantation in the uterus.

4. b is the correct answer.
   - a is incorrect because spinal cord structures are not described as a three-vessel cord. Moreover, there are more than three nerves, arteries, and veins contained within the spinal cord.
   - c is incorrect because the fetal umbilical cord contains two arteries and one vein, not one artery and two veins; anything else is an abnormal finding.
   - d is incorrect because the report relates to the umbilical cord; furthermore, there are more than three ductus deferens, blood vessels, and lymphatic vessels.
5. d is the correct answer.
   - a is incorrect because Braxton Hicks refers to contractions not a formula.
   - b is incorrect because the Goodell sign is a softening of the cervix, which indicates pregnancy; it is not a formula used to determine expected delivery date.
   - c is incorrect because the Chadwick sign is the characteristic blue-violet color of the cervix and vagina around the 6th week of pregnancy; it is not a formula used to determine infant arrival date.

REAL WORLD REPORT

1. there is one fetus contained within the uterus/womb.
2. a
3. the fetus is in the vertex position with the head pointing downward toward the cervix.
4. a. within, inside; b. uterus, uterine; c. cranium, head

REVIEW AND APPLICATION: THREE-LEVEL LEARNING SYSTEM

Level One: Reviewing Facts and Terms Using Recall

1. b
2. a
3. c
4. d
5. a
6. b
7. d
8. b
9. d
10. c
11. b
12. a
13. c
14. c
15. d
16. a
17. c
18. b
19. a
20. c

Level Two: Reviewing Concepts

21. a
22. c
23. b
24. XY
25. XX
26. foramen ovale; ductus arteriosus
27. chorionic villus sampling; spontaneous abortion
28. Hirschsprung disease; rubeola
29. e
30. a
31. b
32. c
33. d
34. c

35. e
36. b
37. a
38. d
39. b
40. c
41. a
42. e
43. d
44. e
45. a
46. d
47. c
48. b
49. c
50. e
51. b
52. d
53. a
54. c
55. a
56. b
57. e
58. d
59. d
60. e
61. b
62. c
63. a
64. crown of fetus's head is presenting in the cervix
65. cheesy appearing deposit on the skin of the fetus
66. premature dilation of the cervix
67. natural, physiologic-induced termination of a pregnancy
68. embedding of an embryo into or on the endometrial lining
69. protrusion of the meninges through an interruption in the skull or backbone, forming a cyst
70. placentation
71. teratology

72. relaxin
73. Apgar score or Apgar rating
74. pediatrics
75. myelomeningocele
76. a
77. a
78. c
79. d
80. b
81. ballottement
82. ectopic
83. abortion
84. albinism
85. kernicterus
86. embryopathy
87. embryology
88. amniocentesis
89. meningocele
90. diphtheria-tetanus-pertussis
91. bronchopulmonary dysplasia
92. human chorionic gonadotropin
93. estimated date of confinement
94. small for gestational age
95. phenylketonuria
96. trochar
97. amnionic

Level Three: Thinking Critically

98. Yes, fraternal twins could have different biologic fathers. Fraternal twins result from the fertilization of two separate female eggs. If two oocytes were released and fertilized by sperm from two separate men, fraternal twins with different biologic fathers could result.
99. Life in utero and life in space are both characterized by a sense of weightlessness, and both are marked by a connection: The baby has an umbilical cord connecting it to the uterus and an astronaut has a tether connecting him or her to the spacecraft.
100. December 24

chapter 18

Mental Disorders

OBJECTIVES

After completing this chapter, you should be able to:

1. Define the meaning of word parts relative to mental disorders.
2. Explain the function of neurotransmitters in normal and abnormal brain physiology.
3. Describe the role of each type of mental health professional.
4. Identify the significance of the *ICD-9-CM* and *DSM-IV-TR* publications in regard to mental disorders.
5. Characterize various mental disorders.
6. Explain different signs, symptoms, and treatments of various mental disorders.
7. Describe clinical tests, scales, and diagnostic procedures related to mental disorders.
8. Summarize mental disorders throughout the lifespan.
9. Define abbreviations related to mental disorders.
10. Define terms used in medical reports involving mental disorders.
11. Correctly define, spell, and pronounce the chapter's medical terms.

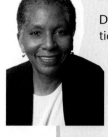

Professional Profile: Clinical Psychologist

Dr. Elizabeth Christopher is a clinical psychologist in private practice, who also provides therapy for residents in several long-term care facilities. During her career, she has also taught psychology in higher education and has worked with children in a private school, providing counseling and consulting with teachers and parents. Although some psychologists prefer working with a specific population, Elizabeth believes working with individuals of various ages is more rewarding and interesting. She practices from an eclectic perspective, using a variety of interventions based on the client's diagnosis.

From a historical perspective, psychologists have been providing psychotherapy to clients since Sigmund Freud, who was the first person to engage in the "talking cure." Early American psychologists focused on individual differences in people and adapting to the environment in which one lives. The behavioral movement in psychology provided therapists with a structured plan to help people change their behavior, using reinforcement and punishment. Cognitive therapists focus on how a person's thinking affects their behavior. For example, many depressed people think their life is terrible. A cognitive therapist helps a person examine his or her life more logically, explore more productive behaviors, and eventually feel less depressed.

Elizabeth completed her doctoral degree in clinical psychology, which took about 4 years after undergraduate schooling. This process included coursework, taking major examinations, writing a dissertation, and completing an internship. She needed to complete a sufficient number of internship hours before she could take the written portion of her licensing examination. After passing the written portion, Elizabeth was required to complete another examination administered orally by the state. Her specialty areas include family and individual therapy, geriatrics, and substance abuse. Before she can renew her license every 2 years, she must complete 24 hours of continuing education.

> **FACT** One in five children has a diagnosable mental, emotional, or behavioral disorder; however, 70% do not receive treatment.

> **FACT** Nearly 15% of adults with a mental illness also have a co-occurring substance-abuse disorder.

INTRODUCTION

> **FACT** More than 54 million Americans have a mental disorder yearly, but fewer than 8 million seek treatment.

Mental disorders are psychiatric conditions that affect brain function and often lead to abnormal behavior. There may be impaired intellectual function, including memory, orientation, and judgment. Mental disorders are associated with impairment in social functioning. They are distinguishable from neurologic disorders, which are disturbances in the structure or function of the central nervous system (CNS) and result from developmental abnormality, disease, injury, or toxicity.

Mental illness is a broad term used to describe pathology of the mind with the inference of underlying brain dysfunction. It includes brain disease, with behavioral symptoms, and diseases of the mind, evidenced by abnormal behavior. Examples of brain diseases are paresis and alcoholism; hysteria is an example of a mind disease.

To appreciate the current classification system for mental disorders, a historical perspective is necessary. Impaired mental function may be secondary to some physical disorder. Various classifications of disorders have existed for over two millennia. Whether the information was to be used in clinical, educational, research, or statistical settings often determined the schema used.

Until relatively recently, there was a need for comprehensive, acceptable taxonomy of mental disorders. Detailed descriptions and definitions that could be used accurately to diagnose disorders were essential. An official nomenclature (system of names assigned to terms in the mental health field) for applicability to a variety of settings requiring uniform medical terminology was established. The end products to date are the *Diagnostic and Statistical Manual of Mental Disorders, Fourth Edition, Text Revision* (*DSM-IV-TR*) and *International Statistical Classification of Diseases and Related Health Problems, Ninth Edition, Clinical Modification* (*ICD-9-CM*). The *ICD-9-CM* provides standardized diagnostic codes for mental disorders, and the *DSM-IV-TR* gives descriptions and terms and serves as the standard for clinicians by offering guidelines for various mental disorders. *DSM-IV-TR* revisions were facilitated by the growing body of research and the necessity for consistent nomenclature that could be used by clinicians and researchers alike.

Authors of both volumes worked closely together to develop mutually beneficial texts. Codes and terms in both are compatible; thus congruency exists between the manuals. The official coding system of mental disorders in the *DSM-IV-TR* and the *ICD-9-CM* are identical. This has aided considerably in terms of studying, diagnosing, treating, and communicating about mental disorders. Mental conditions and related medical terms from these two sources are highlighted in this chapter.

MEDICAL TERM PARTS

WORD PARTS

Medical term prefixes, suffixes, and combining forms related to mental disorders are introduced in this section.

Word Parts	Meaning
ap-, aph-, apo-	away, separated, deprived
cata-	down
hypn-, hypno-	sleep, hypnosis
hyster-, hystero-	hysteria
-lalia	condition involving speech
log-, -logia, logo-	word, speech
-mania	obsession, compulsion
morph-, morpho-	form, shape
narco-	stupor, narcosis
neur-, neuri-, neuro-	nerve, nerve tissue
-phil, -phile	affinity for, craving for
-phobia	fear or dread
-phoria	tendency
-phrenia	mental disorder
psych-, psyche-, psycho-	mind, mental, psychologic
schiz-, schizo-	split, cleft
somat-, somato-	somatic, body
somn-, somno-	sleep
thym-, thymi-, -thymia, thymo-	mind, soul, emotions

WORD ETYMOLOGY

Some words have Greek or Latin word roots but are not true word parts. This section lists those that are used as medical terms.

Word	Definition
iatreia	medical treatment
limos	hunger
orexis	appetite
psyche	soul
psychikos	psychic
somnus	sleep

MEDICAL TERM PARTS USED AS PREFIXES

Prefix	Definition
cata-	down
narco-	stupor, narcosis

MEDICAL TERM PARTS USED AS SUFFIXES

Suffix	Definition
-lalia	condition involving speech
-logia	word, speech
-mania	obsession, compulsion
-phil, -phile	affinity for, craving for
-phobia	fear or dread
-phoria	tendency
-phrenia	mental disorder
-thymia	mind, soul, emotions

WORD GROUPING

Using the "Medical Term Parts" tables, identify the prefix, suffix, or combining form for each of the following definitions. The first one has been done as an example.

Definition	Word Part
down	cata-
affinity for, craving for	
away, separated, deprived	
condition involving speech	
fear or dread	
form, shape	

Definition	Word Part
hysteria	
mental disorder	
mind, mental, psychologic	
mind, soul, emotions	
nerve, nerve tissue	
obsession, compulsion	
sleep	
sleep, hypnosis	
somatic, body	
split, cleft	
stupor, narcosis	
tendency	
word, speech	

WORD BUILDING

Word parts, introduced in the "Medical Term Parts" section, are listed in the following table. For this exercise, first supply the meaning of each word part, then use the word part to build a word you already know. The word you list under "Common or Known Word" does not have to be a medical term; a commonly used word is fine. Be sure, however, that the word correctly reflects the intended meaning. The first one has been done as an example.

Word Part	Meaning	Common or Known Word	Example Medical Term
ap-, aph-, apo-	away, separated, deprived	apathy	apathy
cata-			catatonic
hypn-, hypno-			hypnosis
hyster-, hystero-			hysteria
log-, -logia, logo-			logospasms
-mania			hypermania
morph-, morpho-			dysmorphophobia
narco-			narcolepsy
neur-, neuri-, neuro-			neurosis
-phil, -phile			pedophile
-phobia			agoraphobia
-phrenia			schizophrenia
psych-, psyche-, psycho-			psychology
schiz-, schizo-			schizophrenia
somat-, somato-			somatoform
thym-, thymi-, -thymia, thymo-			dysthymia

FUNDAMENTALS

Mental Disorders Preview

The brain is the controlling center of the CNS. It is the foundation for personality, intellect, thinking, and behavior while also serving as the source for maintaining vital life systems and normal physiologic function.

Relative to mental functions, the **psyche** refers to the subjective aspects of the mind, self, and soul. The mind is the intellectual entity, the self is individual consciousness, and the soul is the seat of feeling. These components are functional entities serving to adjust the body to the needs or demands of the environment. The word part *psyche-* means "mind, mental, or psychological." Psyche is often used interchangeably with **mind**, which means the conscious, subconscious, and unconscious considered together. The mind stores knowledge and memories.

Cognition refers to the conscious faculty or process of acquiring knowledge by using reasoning, intuition, and perception; the **consciousness** is the part of the mind that is aware of feelings, thoughts, and surroundings. The emotional feeling, tone, and mood attached to a thought is termed **affect.** Subjective aspects of affection are deemed affect.

Underlying brain physiology involves the role of neurotransmitters. **Neurotransmitters** are chemical messengers that carry messages between different nerve cells, called **neurons.** Neurons are the basic functional units of the nervous system. The chemical agents are produced by neuron endings to react with receptors on neighboring cells to produce a response (Fig. 18-1). The neurotransmitter is released by a presynaptic cell, crosses the synapse (gap), and stimulates or inhibits the postsynaptic cell. One or several neurotransmitters may be released at any given time. These neurotransmitters are important in causing of disorders resulting from neurobiologic mechanisms. In fact, problems with neurotransmitters may contribute to mental disorders. Clinically important neurotransmitters are dopamine, epinephrine, γ-aminobutyric acid (GABA), norepinephrine, and serotonin.

Neuroimaging techniques can provide pictures of brain regions involved with certain pathologies. **Organic brain disease** is impaired functioning associated with recognizable, structural changes in the brain. Organic brain diseases have a known or presumed physical/physiological cause. Other brain dysfunction cannot be determined by viewing its anatomy.

In the study of mental disorders, clarification between two important terms—neurosis and psychosis—is required. A **neurosis** is a psychological or behavioral disorder with anxiety as the primary characteristic, whereas a **psychosis** is both a mental and a behavioral disorder causing gross distortion of reality, disorganized affective response, and the inability to cope with ordinary demands of everyday life. Both neurotic and psychotic disorders can produce profound impairment in social functioning, and a person with a neurosis may be unable to perform daily activities.

The key and critical difference between a neurosis and a psychosis relates to something known as "reality testing." People with neurotic disorders can use their five senses to judge what is real and what is not. They may be completely disabled by the neurotic disorder, but their senses are functioning normally. Psychotic disorders always involve significant impairment in reality testing whereby the individual cannot trust his or her five senses to provide accurate information regarding the world. Thus a person with a psychotic disorder experiences either hallucinations (perceptions of nonexisting stimuli) or delusions (false beliefs). A psychosis always involves hallucinations and/or delusions. Also most affective disorders do not fall into the psychotic category. Most cases of depression or mania are not psychotic (although they may be).

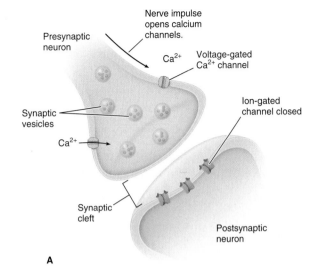

Nerve impulse opens calcium channels.

Presynaptic neuron

Ca²⁺

Voltage-gated Ca²⁺ channel

Ion-gated channel closed

Synaptic vesicles

Ca²⁺

Synaptic cleft

Postsynaptic neuron

A

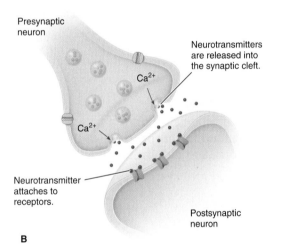

Presynaptic neuron

Neurotransmitters are released into the synaptic cleft.

Ca²⁺

Ca²⁺

Neurotransmitter attaches to receptors.

Postsynaptic neuron

B

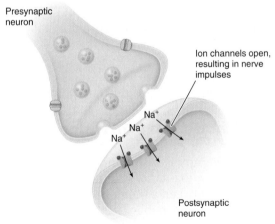

Presynaptic neuron

Ion channels open, resulting in nerve impulses

Na⁺

Na⁺

Na⁺

Postsynaptic neuron

C

FIGURE 18-1
Neurotransmitters are chemical messengers that carry messages between different nerve cells to produce a response.

Key Terms	Definitions
psyche (SIGH kee)	subjective aspects of the mind, self, and soul
mind	center of consciousness that generates thoughts feelings, ideas, and perceptions
cognition (kog NISH un)	conscious faculty or process of knowing, including understanding and reasoning
consciousness	general awareness and responsiveness to the environment
affect	feeling, sentiment, passion, or mood attached to a thought
neurotransmitters (new roh trans MIT urz)	chemical messengers of the nervous system
neurons (NEW ronz)	nerve cells with a body, axon, and dendrites that transmit impulses
organic brain disease	disease with a definite structural alteration
neurosis (new ROH sis)	mild psychiatric disorder characterized by anxiety
psychosis (sigh KOH sis)	psychiatric disorder characterized by incoherence, delusions, and hallucinations

Key Term Practice: Mental Disorders

1. What are the singular and plural forms for the term that means a mild psychiatric disorder characterized by incoherence, delusions, and hallucinations?

   singular = _____

   plural = _____

2. What are the singular and plural forms for the term that means a mild, psychiatric disorder characterized by anxiety?

   singular = _____

   plural = _____

Mental Health Professionals

Psychotherapy is treatment of mental disorders by psychological means such as verbal or nonverbal communication with patients. It involves the use of interpersonal exchange between a therapist and a client in the hope of ultimately producing cognitive, affect, and behavioral change. No chemical or physical measures are used. **Counseling** is a therapeutic relationship in which a trained professional assists a person in solving and adjusting to problems and situations through dialogue and activities. Advice, opinion, and instruction are given to aid in the transition. Types include genetic, marital, and pastoral counseling. Psychologists, psychiatrists, and social workers licensed in the field often do counseling.

There are several educational paths for achieving a license to practice therapy. Psychologists must complete a doctoral degree before they can take the licensing examination in their state to practice psychotherapy. Counselors and social workers need to complete only a master's degree to become licensed. Depending on the level of their license, some counselors and social workers may be limited in the types of disorders that they can treat and diagnoses they can make. For example, in Ohio, license levels include professional counselor (PC), professional clinical counselor (PCC), licensed social worker (LSW), licensed independent social worker (LISW), and psychologist; other states may use similar or different titles.

School counselors and school psychologists are also licensed professionals in most states. They must complete a master's degree and take a licensing examination. School counselors work directly with children, individually or in groups. School psychologists provide assessment services and consult with parents and teachers to develop plans to help children succeed academically and socially.

Professionals enter the field of mental health from a variety of backgrounds. **Counselors** are professionals who help others with personal, social, or psychological problems, whereas **psychoanalysts** practice a method developed by Sigmund Freud for the exploration and synthesis of patterns in emotional thinking and development for the treatment of a wide variety of emotional disorders. Freudian psychoanalysis is rarely practiced in the United States today and has been replaced with more effective and fast-acting forms of psychotherapy.

The medical science and specialty that deals with the origins, diagnosis, prevention, and treatment of mental and emotional disorders is termed **psychiatry**, and physicians with postgraduate training in psychiatry are called **psychiatrists**. **Psychology** is the science that studies the functions of the mind, including sensation, perception, memory, thought, learning, and behavior; professionals with a state-issued license are termed **psychologists**. Psychologists generally hold doctorate degrees, such as a PhD, and are usually licensed to provide therapeutic services and/or work in academic settings. Unlike psychiatrists, most psychologists do not have prescriptive powers; thus they cannot prescribe medications. However, a few states have allowed psychologists who pass a pharmacology examination to write prescriptions for medications. Quite often, psychologists and psychiatrists work in concert to treat mental illness. **Social workers** are professionals who provide help to people in need of social services.

About half of primary-care physician visits are the result of conditions caused or exacerbated by mental or emotional problems.

Key Terms	Definitions
psychotherapy (sigh koh THERR uh pee)	treatment of mental disease by psychological methods
counseling	assistance with personal or psychological matters given by a professional
counselors	professionals who give advice on personal, social, health, or psychological problems
psychoanalysts (sigh koh AN uh lists)	professionals trained in a specific therapeutic mode called psychoanalysis
psychiatry (sigh KIGH uh tree)	medical specialty concerned with the diagnosis and treatment of mental and behavioral disorders
psychiatrists (sigh KIGH uh trists)	physicians trained in the diagnosis, treatment, and prevention of psychiatric disorders
psychology (sigh KOL uh jee)	study of the human mind and mental states
psychologists (sigh KOL uh jists)	professionals who study and/or treat human behavior, mental states, and experiences
social workers	trained professionals in the social work field

Key Term Practice: Mental Health Professionals

1. A _____ practices psychiatry; a psychologist practices _____.

2. The word part *psycho-* refers to _____, and the treatment of mental disease by psychological methods is termed _____.

THE CLINICAL DIMENSION

Pathology Related to Mental Disorders

 During the 1970s, Judd Marmor led a successful drive to have homosexuality removed from the DSM.

This section provides a description of tests and scales and signs and symptoms of various disorders, diagnostic procedures, and treatments pertaining to mental disease. An overview of general pathology presents a sense of the magnitude of mind conditions while demonstrating that they are not trivial considerations. Pathological conditions are presented according to *DSM-IV-TR* headings.

Using the *DSM-IV-TR*

Disorders in the *DSM-IV-TR* are categorized as mild, moderate, severe, in partial remission, in full remission, and prior history. These categorizations are called **severity and course specifiers.** Mild refers to few or no symptoms with minor impairment, and moderate means that there are symptoms and functional impairment. Severe describes symptoms with marked impairment in social or occupational functioning. When some signs and symptoms remain for a condition that had previously met the criteria for a condition, the individual is said to be in partial remission. Full remission connotes that there are no longer any signs or symptoms, but it is still clinically relevant to document the disorder. The category prior history states that an individual was previously diagnosed with a disorder but is now recovered.

In addition to the severity and course specifiers, the *DSM-IV-TR* contains a multiaxial classification system for comprehensive patient evaluation. The **multiaxial assessment** evaluates an individual on five axes; each refers to a separate domain (Fig. 18-2; Table 18-1). This tool assists the clinician in deriving a treatment plan and predicting an outcome. It also allows clinicians to note primary and secondary diagnoses and report them in clinical notes. The diagnostic codes are obtained from the *DSM-IV-TR* and/or the *ICD-9-CM*.

Axis I is for reporting the mental disorder as identified according to the criteria for the particular condition. Axis I is the most important in terms of clinical diagnosis. Personality disorders and mental retardation are not recorded in this section because they are reported in axis II. Prominent maladaptive personality and defense mechanisms are also noted in axis II. Axis II is an indicator of personality disorder, which can make a significant difference in the length and type of treatment sought.

General medical conditions that could be relevant to understanding or managing the mental disorder are recorded in axis III. Axis III is an indicator to possible medical problems that could make a difference in the direction of treatment and in the type of medical providers needed to provide the best treatment. Psychosocial and environmental problems, such as a negative life event or a familial or interpersonal stress, are documented in axis IV. Axis IV helps specify the psychosocial/environmental factors that affect the client, which also affects the direction of and people involved with treatment.

Multiaxial Evaluation Report Form

AXIS I: **Clinical Disorders**
Other Conditions That May Be a Focus of Clinical Attention

Diagnostic code   DSM-IV name

___ ___ ___.___ ___   _____

___ ___ ___.___ ___   _____

___ ___ ___.___ ___   _____

AXIS II: **Personality Disorders**
Mental Retardation

Diagnostic code   DSM-IV name

___ ___ ___.___ ___   _____

___ ___ ___.___ ___   _____

AXIS III: **General Medical Conditions**

ICD-9-CM code   ICD-9-CM name

___ ___ ___.___ ___   _____

___ ___ ___.___ ___   _____

___ ___ ___.___ ___   _____

AXIS IV: **Psychosocial and Environmental Problems**

Check:
___ Problems with primary support group   Specify: _____
___ Problems related to the social environment   Specify: _____
___ Educational problems   Specify: _____
___ Occupational problems   Specify: _____
___ Housing problems   Specify: _____
___ Economic problems   Specify: _____
___ Problems with access to health care services   Specify: _____
___ Problems related to interaction with the
       legal system/crime   Specify: _____
___ Other psychosocial and environmental problems Specify: _____

AXIS V: **Global Assessment of Functioning Scale**

Score: ___ ___ ___
Time frame: _____

FIGURE 18-2
The Multiaxial Evaluation Report Form. (Reprinted with permission from the *Diagnostic and Statistical Manual of Mental Disorders* © 2000. American Psychiatric Association.)

TABLE 18-1 Domains of the Multiaxial Assessment

Axis	Domain
axis I	clinical disorders, other conditions that may be a focus of clinical attention
axis II	personality disorders, mental retardation
axis III	general medical conditions
axis IV	psychosocial and environmental problems
axis V	global assessment of functioning (GAF)

Axis V is for reporting the clinician's assessment of the client's overall level of functioning. The global assessment of functioning (GAF) scale is used to make this judgment (Fig. 18-3). The GAF is also used to provide a psychobehavioral snapshot of where the person is now and compare it to the client's peak functioning over the past several years. This reveals how the dysfunctions from axes I to IV have affected the client. The vast majority of insurance companies require the information from these scales before approving treatments for the insured.

Global Assessment of Functioning (GAF) Scale

Code

100 | 91	Superior functioning in a wide range of activities, life's problems never seen to get out of hand, is sought out by others because of his or her many positive qualities. No symptoms.
90 | 81	Absent or minimal symptoms, good functioning in all areas, interested and involved in a wide range of activities, socially effective, generally satisfied with life, no more than everyday problems or concerns.
80 | 71	If symptoms are present, they are transient and expectable reactions to psychosocial stressors; no more than slight impairment in social, occupational, or school functioning.
70 | 61	Some mild symptoms OR some difficulty in social, occupational, or school functioning, but generally functioning pretty well, has some meaningful interpersonal relationships.
60 | 51	Moderate symptoms, OR moderate difficulty in social, occupational, or school functioning.
50 | 41	Serious symptoms OR any serious impairment in social, occupational, or school functioning.
40 | 31	Some impairment in reality testing or communication OR major impairment in several areas, such as work or school, family relations, judgment, thinking, or mood.
30 | 21	Behavior is considerably influenced by delusions or hallucinations OR serious impairment in communication or judgment OR inability to function in almost all areas.
20 | 11	Some danger of hurting self or others OR occasionally fails to maintain minimal personal hygiene OR gross impairment in communication
10 | 1	Persistent danger of severely hurting self or others OR persistent inability to maintain minimal personal hygiene OR serious suicidal act with clear expectation of death.
0	Inadequate information.

FIGURE 18-3
The Global Assessment of Functioning Scale. (Reprinted with permission from the *Diagnostic and Statistical Manual of Mental Disorders* © 2000. American Psychiatric Association.)

The *DSM-IV-TR* classification scheme was developed to group the various mental disorders. The 18 categories and subcategories follow.

1. Disorders usually first diagnosed in infancy, childhood, or adolescence
   A. Mental retardation
   B. Learning disorders
   C. Motor skills disorder

    D. Communication disorders

    E. Pervasive developmental disorders

    F. Attention-deficit and disruptive-behavior disorders

    G. Feeding and eating disorders of infancy or early childhood

    H. Tic disorders

    I. Elimination disorders

    J. Other disorders of infancy, childhood, or adolescence

2. Delirium, dementia, and amnestic and other cognitive disorders

    A. Delirium

    B. Dementia

    C. Amnestic disorders

    D. Other cognitive disorders

3. Mental disorders caused by a general medical condition not elsewhere classified

4. Substance-related disorders

    A. Alcohol-related disorders

    B. Amphetamine (or amphetamine-like) related disorders

    C. Caffeine-related disorders

    D. Cannabis-related disorders

    E. Cocaine-related disorders

    F. Hallucinogen-related disorders

    G. Inhalant-related disorders

    H. Opioid-related disorders

    I. Sedative-, hypnotic-, or anxiolytic-related disorders

    J. Polysubstance-related disorder

    K. Other (or unknown) substance-related disorders

5. Schizophrenia and other psychotic disorders

6. Mood disorders

    A. Depressive disorders

    B. Bipolar disorders

7. Anxiety disorders

8. Somatoform disorders

9. Factitious disorders

10. Dissociative disorders

11. Sexual and gender-identity disorders

    A. Sexual dysfunctions

    B. Paraphilias

    C. Gender-identity disorders

12. Eating disorders

13. Sleep disorders

    A. Primary sleep disorders

    B. Sleep disorders related to another mental disorder

    C. Other sleep disorders

14. Impulse-control disorders not elsewhere classified

15. Adjustment disorders

16. Personality disorders

17. Other conditions that may be a focus of clinical attention
    A. Psychological factors affecting medical conditions
    B. Other medication-induced disorders
    C. Relational problems
    D. Problems related to abuse or neglect
    E. Additional conditions that may be a focus of clinical attention
18. Additional codes

Key Terms	Definitions
severity and course specifiers	qualifiers regarding specific conditions
multiaxial assessment	five coordinates used to assess a mental disorder

Key Term Practice: Using the DSM-IV-TR

1. The five coordinates used to assess a mental disorder within the *DSM-IV-TR* are collectively termed _____.

2. Qualifiers—such as mild, moderate, severe, in partial remission, in full remission, and prior history—regarding specific conditions in the *DSM-IV-TR* are known as _____.

Clinical Tests and Scales

Tests have been designed to measure the ability to learn facts and skills and to apply this aptitude. An **intelligence quotient** (IQ) is a numerical rating used to designate a person's mental astuteness, insight, and acumen. It is based on performance on a standardized mental test. Table 18-2 lists IQ scores with their representative descriptions.

One of the most common scales used in the United States is the **Stanford-Binet intelligence scale** (Stanford-Binet intelligence test). This scale consists of a series of questions designed to assess intelligence and cognitive abilities in children and adults. The test is administered by a clinically trained examiner and interpreted by a trained

TABLE 18-2 IQ Scores and Descriptions

Score	Description
< 20	profound retardation
20–35	severe retardation
35–50	moderate retardation
50–70	mild retardation
70–90	dull normal
90–110	normal
110–125	superior
125–140	very superior
≥ 140	genius

professional, usually a psychologist. The raw scores are based on the number of items answered by the test taker and are then converted into a standard age score. This score, which corresponds to a particular age group, is similar to the numerical rating used in the intelligence quotient. Thus the answers provided indicate the mental age of the test taker. An adult version, normalized against adult age levels, also exists.

Another measuring tool is the **Wechsler intelligence scale**, which is a standardized test for measuring psychological, personality, or behavioral characteristics. Developed by psychologist David Wechsler, the scales are continually revised and updated and are used to measure general intelligence in preschool children (Wechsler Preschool and primary scale of intelligence), children (Wechsler intelligence scale for children), and adults (Wechsler adult intelligence scale).

The **Rorschach test** is a psychological test in which a person describes what he or she sees on a series of 10 standardized inkblots of various designs and colors, like the one in Figure 18-4. The responses indicate personality patterns, special interests, originality of thought, deviations of affect, and neurotic and psychotic tendencies. A trained professional scoring the test can also determine attitudes, emotions, and personality. This test is also called the inkblot test.

The **thematic apperception test** (TAT) is a projective psychological test using a set of pictures that suggest life situations from which the person constructs a story. *Apperception* means the "comprehension or assimilation of something in terms of previous experiences." The tool is designed to recall attitudes, emotions, sentiments, and conflicts of personality that are then interpreted by a psychologist.

The **Minnesota Multiphase Personality Inventory** (MMPI) is an empirical scale of an individual's personality based primarily on responses to a questionnaire. The 567 true–false statements are coded on four validity and 10 personality scales. The administration format is either individually or as a group. The MMPI is used widely in recruitment and mental health screening.

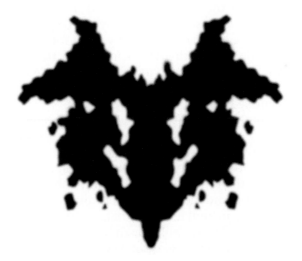

FIGURE 18-4
The Rorschach test is also called the inkblot test. Responses to the inkblots can indicate attitudes, emotions, and personality.

Key Terms	Definitions
intelligence quotient	numerical rating used to designate a person's intelligence
Stanford-Binet intelligence scale	intelligence test commonly given to children and adults
Wechsler intelligence scale	individually administered IQ test for preschoolers, children, and adults

Rorschach (ROHR shahk) test	test of personality or mental state based on the person's interpretation of standard inkblots; inkblot test
thematic apperception test	test for exploring aspects of the personality in which the person is shown pictures of people in various situations and asked to describe what is happening
Minnesota Multiphase Personality Inventory	standardized test that uses true–false questions to assess the person's psychological and social adjustment

Key Term Practice: Clinical Tests and Scales

1. List two tests commonly used to assess intelligence.

_____

2. What is the alternate name for the inkblot test?

_____

Disorders Usually First Diagnosed in Infancy, Childhood, or Adolescence

Although the disorders discussed in this section first appear during infancy, childhood, or adolescence, they may not be properly diagnosed until adulthood. Thus categorizing a mental disorder by age is for convenience's sake only because there are no clear lines of distinction demarcating the various mental disorders. Disorders of infancy, childhood, and adolescence include mental retardation, learning disorders, logospasm (stuttering), autistic disorder, attention-deficit/hyperactivity disorder, and Tourette disorder.

Mental retardation is subnormal intellectual function that is present at birth or during early life. The limitations of the disorder depend on the severity of the condition. In general, mental retardation limits the capacity to learn and to function independently. Primary mental retardation may be the result of familial or hereditary factors with no known brain **lesion** (physical change) or prenatal cause. Secondary mental retardation results from brain tissue anomalies or a chromosomal disorder; prenatal, maternal, or postnatally acquired infections; intoxication, trauma, or prematurity; disorders of growth, nutrition, or metabolism; degenerative diseases, tumor, or major psychiatric disorders. They can also be associated with psychosocial/environmental deprivation. Any condition that interrupts or compromises blood, oxygen, or nutrient supply to the brain can result in neurologic damage and subsequent mental retardation.

Mental retardation is classified as mild, moderate, severe, or profound. With the exception of Down syndrome, there may be no outward physical manifestations. Impaired intellectual and social growth is often the first indication. Delayed motor and communication skills lead to further evaluation. Observation of behaviors and confirmation of intellectual capacity using standardized tests of intelligence provide the initial diagnosis. Limitations in two of the following areas are necessary for diagnostic purposes: communication, home living, self-care, social and interpersonal skills, self-direction, and health and safety. Usually more than one test is used to confirm the diagnosis. Underlying causes that respond to therapy are treated. Other treatment measures include providing occupational therapy (OT), physical therapy (PT), and psychotherapy to ensure the highest quality of life and establish as much cognitive function as possible.

Formerly known as academic skills disorders, **learning disorders** (LDs) are any defect or disturbance in a child's ability to acquire skills in reading, writing, or arithmetic. Learning disorders are often complicated by behavioral disturbances resulting from feelings of inadequacy. The child may have normal to above normal intelligence and adequate educational opportunities, yet is hindered from learning basic skills or information at the same rate as most people of the same age. Learning disorders have an unknown cause, but cognitive processing abnormalities have been implicated. Language barriers, lack of opportunity, poor teaching, inadequate schooling, and environmental and nutritional factors must be ruled out in the preliminary diagnosis. If the problem still persists, LD is assumed to be present. Treatment involves designing individual educational plans (IEPs) complete with specially formulated teaching techniques. Currently, one-on-one instruction appears to be the best method. Educational psychology has advanced research in this realm.

Communication disorders are characterized by the ineffective use of words to convey ideas or information. Stuttering, or **logospasm**, is a kind of communication disorder demonstrated by the inability to enunciate a phonetic segment not more than one syllable in length without repeating it, straining unnaturally, or both. It is characterized by frequent repetitions or prolongations of sounds or syllables, impeding the speech pattern. The typical age of onset is between 2 and 7 years. Its cause is unknown, but may have a genetic component because there appears to be a familial trend. Stuttering occurs more frequently in males. Anxiety and nervousness seem to be major factors in the persistence of logospasm.

A feeling of apprehension, uncertainty, or tension stemming from anticipation of an imagined or real event is known as **anxiety.** Tachycardia (rapid heart rate), palpitations (heart fluttering), sweating, disturbed breathing, gastrointestinal distress, trembling, weakness, and perhaps paralysis accompany anxiety. After hearing difficulties have been ruled out, the diagnosis is based on observed pattern of speech cadence disturbance. Speech therapy and not drawing attention to the speaker's disorder while talking are treatments.

Pervasive developmental disorders are characterized by severe, persistent, and all-encompassing impairment in several areas of development, including social, communication, and behavior. Autistic disorder is an example of a pervasive developmental disorder. **Autistic disorder** is a form of behavior and thinking observed in young children in which the child seems to concentrate on herself or himself without regard to other environmental influences. Other names for the disorder are early infantile autism, childhood autism, and Kanner autism. Manifestations are obvious within the first 3 years of life. Language usage, reaction to stimuli, interpretation of the world, and formation of relationships are not fully established and follow unusual patterns.

Signs and symptoms include excessive shyness, aloofness, withdrawal, introspection, and possible seizures. Proper communication and age-appropriate activities are not displayed. Autistic children often engage in obsessive behaviors with a preoccupation with objects and memorizing lists or facts. Children with autism perform nonfunctional rituals and are easily upset by trivial environmental changes. Four primary symptoms are key characteristics of the disorder: language deficits, cognitive impairment, repetitive movements and body rocking, and social isolation. The cause is unknown, but an organically based CNS dysfunction has been implicated. It occurs more commonly in males. Behavior observation, notably the four primary characteristics, leads to the diagnosis.

Cognitive behavior therapy (CBT) that includes the child and family is prescribed to promote adaptive responses and skills to encourage self-sufficiency in the individual. **Cognitive behavior therapy** is a form of treatment combining traditional cognitive therapy techniques with methods taken from behavior therapy. The result is an intervention that seeks to change cognitions with the goal of behavioral change. **Behavior**

therapy uses behavior-modification techniques in which a person's desirable responses are positively reinforced while undesirable behaviors are negatively rewarded.

Attention-deficit/hyperactivity disorder (ADHD) is a type of attention-deficit and disruptive behavior disorder characterized by a persistent pattern of inattention and/or increased activity and impulsivity that is frequently displayed. It is manifested at home, school, and in social situations with an onset before age 7 years. Children are often impatient, unable to do seat work in the classroom, and avoid situations requiring attentive behavior. The cause is unknown, but a familial pattern exists. It is diagnosed by behavior observation and impaired function that directly results from the behavior. Behavior therapy that rewards appropriate behavior to establish desired acts while extinguishing undesirable or inappropriate behavior is beneficial. Amphetamine drugs such as methylphenidate (Ritalin), dextroamphetamine (Dexedrine), and amphetamine-dextroamphetamine (Adderall) may be prescribed.

A condition found under the topic of feeding and eating disorders of infancy or early childhood is pica. **Pica** is a desire for strange food or other substances of no nutritional value. (It may also occur during pregnancy as a result of emotional distress or malnutrition.) Examples of nonnutritive substances include clay, dirt, sand, and hair, but the ingested material typically varies with age. Eating material of no nutritious worth on a persistent basis for at least 1 month fulfills the criterion for pica diagnosis. The disorder appears to last for several months and then remits with no treatment.

Tic disorders are habitual, irresistible, repetitive movements that the person feels compelled to do. A **tic** is a sudden, rapid, recurrent, nonrhythmic, stereotyped involuntary motor movement or vocalization. These motions can be voluntarily suppressed for only brief moments. Examples include throat clearing, excessive eye blinking, sniffing, or lip pursing. The movements are more pronounced when the person is under stress. There is no known cause.

Tourette disorder is a type of tic disorder characterized by multiple motor tics and one or more vocal tics. It is also known as Gilles de la Tourette disease. The disorder generally begins in late childhood and adolescence, but may start as early as 2 years old. Additional features include **echolalia** (purposeless, involuntary repetition of words spoken by another person), obscene utterances, and other compulsive acts that are present for more than 1 year. Vocal tics may include clicks, grunts, or snorts. Obsessive–compulsive behavior and attention-deficit disorder may accompany this lifelong condition. The cause is unknown and the disorder affects more males than females. Observation confirms the diagnosis. Patients administered haloperidol (Haldol) have shown some improvement.

> **FACT** ADHD affects 3–5% of school-age children in the United States.

Key Terms	Definitions
mental retardation	below normal intellectual function
lesion (LEE zhun)	structural change
learning disorder	any defect or disturbance in a child's ability to acquire skills in reading, writing, or arithmetic
logospasm (LOG oh spazm)	stuttering, or saying something haltingly and repeating sounds when attempting to pronounce them
anxiety (ang ZYE i tee)	overwhelming sense of apprehension
autistic (aw TIS tick) **disorder**	disturbance in psychological development that is marked my mental introversion and concentration on self or one object

cognitive behavior therapy	treatment whose goal is to change problem actions, manners, and cognition through conditioning, learning, and cognitive restructuring
behavior therapy	treatment that uses behavior-modification techniques in which a person's desirable responses are positively reinforced while undesirable behaviors are negatively rewarded
attention-deficit/hyperactivity disorder	condition characterized by hyperactivity, inability to concentrate, and impulsive or inappropriate behavior
pica (PYE kuh)	craving to eat substances that provide no nutritional value
tic	spasmodic muscular contraction or vocalization
Tourette disorder	condition typified by multiple twitches, involuntary vocal grunts, and obscene speech
echolalia (eck oh LAY lee uh)	speech disorder characterized by an involuntary repetition of the same word or words spoken by another person

Key Term Practice: Disorders Usually First Diagnosed in Infancy, Childhood, or Adolescence

1. Abnormal cravings to eat substances containing no health benefit is termed _____

2. _____ disorder is characterized by multiple twitches, involuntary grunts, and indecent language.

3. A structural change in the brain that may cause a disorder is termed a/an _____.

Delirium, Dementia, and Amnestic and Other Cognitive Disorders

Delirium, dementia, and amnestic and other cognitive disorders are marked by a pronounced deficit in cognition caused by organic disease, medical conditions, chemical substances, or a combination thereof. **Delirium** is a disordered mental state of acute onset and transient nature. It is characterized by confusion, disorientation, illusions, and delusions. A **delusion** is a belief maintained in the face of incontrovertible evidence to the contrary. Fever, poisoning, metabolic disorders, or brain injury can cause it. Treatment involves addressing the underlying pathology along with pharmacological or behavioral therapy as appropriate.

Dementia is the progressive deterioration of intellectual functions, reasoning, and memory. Although these functions wane, other brain functions are often retained. The result of organic brain disease, it is characterized by confusion, disorientation, **apathy** (total indifference or absence of interest), and stupor. Depending on the cause, the onset may be insidious (gradual) or sudden.

Dementia of the Alzheimer type (Alzheimer disease; AD) is a progressive dementia with diffuse cerebral cortical atrophy, sulci and ventricle enlargement, and microscopic snarls of protein called neurofibrillary tangles. It results in memory impairment and dementia manifested as confusion, visual–spatial disorientation, hampered judgment, delusions, and possible hallucinations. **Hallucinations** are sensory experiences of something not actually existing in the external world. These alterations in perception could be auditory (hearing nonexisting voices) or visual (seeing objects that are not there).

Alzheimer disease makes up 70% of all dementia cases. The onset is usually during late middle life, and death ensues within 5–10 years. It currently ranks as the fourth leading cause of death in the United States. Nearly all persons with Down syndrome who live past age 40 years develop AD. Risk factors include advancing age, history of head injury, and not maintaining mental stimulation throughout life. A familial history is noted in 10% of all cases and is linked to gene mutations. Treatment involves ruling out all other organic brain disorders. Magnetic resonance imaging (MRI) and computed tomography (CT) scans reveal widened sulci, enlarged ventricles, and brain atrophy. The diagnosis can be confirmed only at autopsy by pathological studies that demonstrate neurofibrillary tangles and clumps of protein called amyloid deposits that cause senile plaques. It is one of the most overdiagnosed and misdiagnosed disorders because of overlapping signs and symptoms and its similarity to other dementias.

Vascular dementia, formerly called multi-infarct dementia, is a step-like decline in intellectual functions with focal neurologic signs produced as the result of multiple infarctions (areas of tissue death owing to lack of oxygen) of the cerebral hemispheres. In addition to cognitive deficits, there is evidence of cerebrovascular disease. The onset is usually insidious. Signs and symptoms include apathy, disregard for personal hygiene, disorientation, depression, anxiety, restlessness, and sleeplessness.

Depression is characterized by persistent extreme sadness, melancholy, or dejection that is unrealistic and out of proportion to the cause. The symptoms progress as the disease advances. The cause is ischemia (decreased blood flow) to brain tissue resulting in neuron necrosis (death of nerve cells). The history and physical examination, along with arteriograms and vascular studies confirming occlusion, provide the diagnosis. The goal of pharmacological treatment is to increase blood flow to the brain. Endarterectomy, excision of deposits in the arteries, restores blood flow.

 Depression increases the risk of developing cardiovascular disease.

Key Terms	Definitions
delirium (de LIRR ee um)	state marked by extreme restlessness, confusion, and perhaps hallucinations
delusion (de LEW zhun)	false conviction held before strong contradictory evidence; false belief
dementia (de MEN shuh)	deterioration or loss of intellectual faculties, reasoning power, memory, and will
apathy (AP uh thee)	lack of feeling or emotion
dementia (de MEN shuh) **of the Alzheimer type**	degenerative brain disorder that causes dementia, especially late in life; Alzheimer disease
hallucinations (huh lew si NAY shuns)	perceptions of things with no basis in reality
vascular dementia (VAS kew lur de MEN shuh)	cognitive impairment caused by inadequate blood supply to the brain because of blocked blood vessels
depression	state of profound sadness

Key Term Practice: Delirium, Dementia, and Amnestic and Other Cognitive Disorders

1. Cognitive impairment that results from multiple brain infarctions is known as _____.

2. Characteristics of this disease include neurofibrillary tangles, senile plaques, and dementia._____

Substance-Related Disorders

Substance-related disorders are associated with drug abuse, medication side effects, and toxin exposure. **Alcohol abuse** or **alcoholism** is excessive use of alcoholic drinks to the extent that they interfere with health, interpersonal relations, or occupation. It is characterized by an increasing adaptation to the effects of alcohol such that increased amounts are required to achieve the same results. The abuse can lead to medical diseases such as cirrhosis, pancreatitis, and peripheral neuropathy, as well as psychiatric disorders.

A neurologic disorder caused by thiamine deficiency that is often seen in chronic alcoholics is Wernicke-Korsakoff syndrome. Formerly called Korsakoff's psychosis, **Wernicke-Korsakoff syndrome** is characterized by necrosis of brain tissue, confusion, ataxia (inability to coordinate muscle movements), and memory impairment. Alcohol withdrawal is often accompanied by **delirium tremens** (DT), a form of delirium induced by the removal of alcohol after a prolonged period of intoxication. Wakefulness, tremor, hallucinations, delusions, fever, dilated pupils, sweating, and tachycardia characterize it. These also occur with barbiturate removal.

Alcohol is absorbed by the gastrointestinal tract, and the CNS concentration is directly proportional to blood alcohol concentration. Furthermore, the alcohol metabolism rate in the liver is constant. Thus the liver metabolizes 10–15 mL of alcohol every hour. That is the equivalent to one 12-oz, beer, 6-oz. glass of wine, or 1-oz. of 86-proof liquor per hour.

The onset of alcohol abuse is insidious or perpetrated by an event. Signs and symptoms include anxiety, depression, insomnia, impotence (inability to perform sexual act), behavioral disorders, **amnesia** (memory loss or impairment), and hypertension. Alcohol abuse increases the risk of gastrointestinal cancers. It is diagnosed by the history and physical examination that includes a questionnaire regarding frequency of alcohol use. Laboratory findings are also indicators. The γ-glutamyltransferase (GGT) blood analysis is a sensitive test that detects blood alcohol levels.

Treatment involves rehabilitation programs and abstinence. Membership in Alcoholics Anonymous (AA) offers a successful treatment option. AA is a fellowship of people formerly addicted to alcohol who support one another to overcome their addiction.

Besides alcohol, prescription medications, such as benzodiazepines and various pain killers, are popular choices among addicts for drug abuse. In recent years, oxycodone (OxyContin), a CNS depressant that relieves pain, has become so popular among abusers that many pharmacies no longer keep it on site. Opiates are also commonly abused. Furthermore, there is an ongoing debate about the addictive properties of caffeine and the likelihood of caffeine addiction.

> FACT *Depression and anxiety each affect 12 million Americans annually.*

Key Terms	Definitions
alcohol abuse	excessive use of alcohol creating an addiction to drinking alcoholic beverages; alcoholism
alcoholism (AL kuh hol iz um)	excessive use of alcohol creating an addiction to drinking alcoholic beverages; alcohol abuse
Wernicke-Korsakoff syndrome	form of brain damage occurring in long-term alcoholics from thiamine deficiency
delirium tremens (de LIRR ee um TREE munz)	agitation, tremors, and hallucinations that are caused by alcohol withdrawal
amnesia (am NEE zhuh)	memory loss or impairment

Key Term Practice: Substance-Related Disorders

1. Two medical terms describing excessive use of alcohol that creates an addiction are _____ and _____.

2. The term for agitation, tremors, and hallucinations caused by alcohol withdrawal is _____.

Schizophrenia and Other Psychotic Disorders

> **FACT** Nobel Prize winner John Nash has schizophrenia.

Schizophrenia is a group of psychotic disorders that typically begins during adolescence or in young adulthood. It is characterized by hallucinations and/or delusions. Associated affective, behavioral, and intellectual disturbances occur in various degrees and combinations. The disorder is marked by withdrawal tendencies, ambivalence, inappropriate mood responses, unpredictable disturbances in thought patterns, and often hallucinations and delusions. Types of schizophrenia include paranoid, disorganized, catatonic, undifferentiated, and residual.

Paranoid-type schizophrenia is characterized by delusions of persecution and/or grandeur, hallucinations, and hostility. **Disorganized-type schizophrenia**, also known as hebephrenic, is marked by incoherent, scattered delusions, dull feelings, social impairment, poor functioning and adaptation, and disorganized mannerisms. Disturbances in motor behavior, stupor, rigidity, excitement, and frenzied motor activity are characteristics of **catatonic-type schizophrenia. Undifferentiated-type schizophrenia** is typified by disorganized behavior, incoherence, delusions, hallucinations, and mixed symptomology. **Residual-type schizophrenia** is described as having at least one schizophrenic episode but currently without symptoms. Illogical thinking and odd behavior are still present.

The cause of schizophrenia is thought to be malfunctioning of neuronal systems that use dopamine, serotonin, glutamate, and GABA as neurotransmitters. There may be an underlying genetic component in which a brain lesion is present in early life but does not manifest until adolescence or adulthood. Current theories focus on a genetic predisposition along with a possible prenatal viral infection.

> **FACT** Suicide is the 11th leading cause of death in the United States.

Schizophrenics display abnormal perceptions and content of thought. Schizophrenia is not "split personality," as popularly thought; that pathology is known as dissociative identity disorder. Schizophrenia is the most prevalent psychosis in America, affecting 2 million people (1% of the population). Approximately 25% of individuals with schizophrenia require custodial or institutional care, and 10% commit suicide. The gradual onset is usually before age 40 years with an obvious precipitating cause.

> **FACT** Suicide is the 8th leading cause of death for males, and the 19th leading cause of death for females— 30,622 people commit suicide in the United States each year.

Signs and symptoms include prodromal (indicating onset of disease) signs of confusion, odd behavior, disinterest in school or work, shortened attention span, memory deficits, diminished decision-making ability, **alogia** (inability to speak), **anhedonia** (chronic absence of pleasure in acts that were once normally pleasurable), **abulia** (abnormal inability to make a decision), delusions, auditory hallucinations, social withdrawal, and disorganized thinking.

Neurophysiologic studies indicating generalized limbic lobe and prefrontal cortex abnormalities and a small thalamus indicate schizophrenia. Brain imaging studies are inconsistent. Other tests that may assist in the diagnosis include the Rorschach test, TAT, and the MMPI-2; however, the Rorschach test and TAT are rarely used today.

Schizophrenia is treated with intense psychotherapy, cognitive behavioral therapy, and antipsychotic drugs. Inconsistent results have been achieved with cognitive behavior therapy. **Antipsychotic drugs**, also known as neuroleptic drugs, are a functional category of chemical agents helpful in the treatment of psychoses and ameliorating thought disorders. Atypical antipsychotics are a newer class of drugs exerting their action via serotonergic blockade (stopping the actions of serotonin). Antipsychotics also counteract or alleviate the symptoms of some neuroses. These drugs include clozapine, olanzapine, quetiapine, and risperidone. Drugs shorten the episodes of acute psychosis, limit the need for institutional care, and reduce the risk of relapse. Unfortunately, patients frequently stop taking their medications, and it is estimated that only half of people with schizophrenia are receiving medical treatment or supervision at any given time.

    Tardive dyskinesia (TD) is a condition characterized by involuntary movements of the tongue, facial muscles, limbs, and trunk that results from long-term treatment of schizophrenia with phenothiazine tranquilizers and similar drugs.

Key Terms	Definitions
schizophrenia (skit soh FREE nee uh)	psychotic disorder with a mixture of signs and symptoms characterized by withdrawal, hallucinations, and delusions
paranoid-type schizophrenia (skit soh FREE nee uh)	disorder marked by delusions and hallucinations
disorganized-type schizophrenia (skit soh FREE nee uh)	disorder marked by inappropriate affect, giggling, and inappropriate mannerisms; hebephrenic
catatonic- (kat uh TON ick) **type schizophrenia** (skit soh FREE nee uh)	disorder marked by motor disturbances, stupor, and rigidity
undifferentiated-type schizophrenia (skit soh FREE nee uh)	disorder marked by mixed symptomology, including disorganized behavior
residual-type schizophrenia (skit soh FREE nee uh)	disorder marked by at least one schizophrenic episode but presently without disorder symptoms
alogia (uh LOH jee uh)	inability to speak owing to mental deficiency or an episode of dementia
anhedonia (an hee DOH nee uh)	overall chronic absence of enjoyment in acts that used to be enjoyable
abulia (uh BOO lee uh)	abnormal inability to make a decision
antipsychotic (an tee sigh KOT ick) **drugs**	chemical agents used to treat schizophrenia
tardive dyskinesia (TAHR div dis ki NEE zhuh)	condition characterized by spasms of the tongue and facial muscles resulting from long-term use of drugs that treat schizophrenia

Key Term Practice: Schizophrenia and Other Psychotic Disorders

1. The condition characterized by spasms of the tongue and facial muscles that results from long-term use of drugs that treat schizophrenia is termed _____.

2. Catatonic, disorganized, paranoid, residual, and undifferentiated are various types of a condition called _____.

Mood Disorders

Mood is a state of mind. **Mood disorders** are affects that disrupt all other aspects of life. Examples include depressive and bipolar disorders.

Major depressive disorder is a mental condition characterized by sustained depressive mood; anhedonia; sleep and appetite disturbances; and feelings of worthlessness, guilt, and hopelessness. The individual often experiences a deep, persistent sadness. Approximately 20 million Americans are affected yearly. About 10% of men and 25% of women will experience it at some point in their lives; and 15–30% of those afflicted commit suicide.

Risk factors for major depressive disorder include alcohol abuse, chronic physical illness, stress, social isolation, history of physical or sexual abuse, and family history of depression. The cause is an electrochemical malfunction of the limbic system resulting in metabolic disturbances of dopamine and serotonin. In addition, glial cell (supportive neuron) numbers are diminished in individuals with a familial history. The diagnosis is based on a depressed mood and marked reduction or interest in pleasurable activities lasting at least 2 weeks. Furthermore, three or more of the following must also be present: weight loss or gain, increased or decreased sleep, increased or decreased level of psychomotor activity, fatigue, feelings of guilt or worthlessness, diminished ability to concentrate, and recurring thoughts of suicide or death.

Antidepressants, drugs used to prevent or reduce depression, are used to treat it. These drugs include tricyclic antidepressants, selective serotonin reuptake inhibitors (SSRIs), monamine oxidase (MAO) inhibitors, and protriptyline. Cognitive psychotherapy is another form of treatment.

Electroconvulsive shock therapy and transcranial magnetic stimulation have demonstrated value in cases that do not respond to the other therapy options. Passing an electric current through the brain produces convulsions and seizures known as **electroconvulsive therapy** (ECT). It is particularly useful in the treatment of depressive and severe psychiatric disorders. It is also known as electroshock therapy and electroconvulsive shock therapy. The response rate for ECT is about 80%. In **transcranial magnetic stimulation** (TMS), a magnetic current is passed through the brain. The exact mechanism is not known, but the effects are similar to those of ECT. The stimulation entices neurochemical change.

Another mood disorder, **dysthymic disorder,** is a chronically depressed mood that occurs for most of the day, more days than not, for at least 2 years. During the depressed state, at least two of the following symptoms must be present for diagnosis: poor appetite or overeating, insomnia or hypersomnia, low energy or fatigue, low self-esteem, poor concentration or difficulty making decisions, and feelings of hopelessness. Psychotherapy and antidepressants are courses of treatment.

Bipolar disorder is an affective disorder characterized by alternating periods of euphoria (mania) and depression. **Euphoria** is an exaggerated sense of physical and emotional well-being that is usually not appropriate to the situation. Rapid speaking, fleeting ideas, insomnia, excessive energy, impaired judgment, delusions, and even hallucinations may mark the manic episodes. Indifference (flat affect), sadness, withdrawal, loss of appetite, and sleep disturbances characterize the depressive aspect. The cause is unknown but thought to be the result of neurotransmitter alterations. The risk is greater among family members with the disorder. The history, physical examination, and psychological evaluation provide the diagnosis. The drug **lithium carbonate** is given for the manic phase, and antidepressants are administered for the depressive phase. Psychotherapy also provides benefit.

The main symptom of a seasonal pattern disorder is the onset and remission of major depressive episodes at characteristic times of the year. Most begin in fall or winter and remit in the spring. **Seasonal affective disorder** (SAD) is a seasonal pattern mood disorder occurring and resolving at the same time over a period of years. It frequently occurs in the winter and is characterized by morning hypersomnia, decreased energy, increased appetite, weight gain, and carbohydrate craving. The symptoms dissipate

FACT *Suicide was the 3rd leading cause of death among people aged 15–24 years and the 6th leading cause of death for 5–14 year olds in the United States.*

FACT *It is estimated that as many as 1 in 33 children and 1 in 8 adolescents may have depression in the United States.*

with the onset of spring. The incidence is greater in women than men. Its cause is suggested to be increased melatonin secretion by the pineal gland because the disorder is more prevalent at higher latitudes and in areas of shortened sunlight hours. The hormone melatonin is released in response to darkness and suppressed by light. Exposure to artificial sunlight has shown some therapeutic merit.

Key Terms	Definitions
mood disorders	ailments characterized by emotional disturbances that disrupt other aspects of life
major depressive disorder	psychological illness marked by sustained unhappiness and hopelessness with suicidal tendencies
antidepressants (an tee dee PRES unts)	drugs used in the treatment, alleviation, or prevention of depression
electroconvulsive therapy	passage of a small electric current through the brain to treat mental disorders
transcranial magnetic stimulation	passage of a magnetic current through the brain to treat mental disorders
dysthymic (dis THIGH mick) **disorder**	depressed mood for most of the day, for more days than not, for at least 2 years
bipolar (bye POH lur) **disorder**	disorder characterized by extreme mood swings between euphoria and severe depression
euphoria (yoo FOH ree uh)	exaggerated feeling of elation
lithium carbonate (LITH ee um KAHR buh nate)	drug used to treat bipolar disorders
seasonal affective disorder	depression associated with the onset of winter and thought to be caused by decreasing amounts of daylight

Key Term Practice: Mood Disorders

1. The disorder characterized by mood swings from euphoria to depression is known as _____.

2. _____ is characterized by feelings of unhappiness in the winter that resolve in the spring.

Anxiety Disorders

Anxiety disorders are a group of interrelated mental illnesses involving anxious and apprehensive reactions to stress. Panic disorder, phobias, obsessive–compulsive disorder, post-traumatic stress disorder, and generalized anxiety disorder are common types.

Panic disorder is characterized by repeated panic attacks. A panic attack is a sudden, overpowering feeling of fear or anxiety that prevents functioning. An attack is often triggered by a past or present source of anxiety. The extreme anxiety attack leads to total inaction or unreasonable acts. These recurrent attacks occur unpredictably. Signs include dyspnea (shortness of breath), dizziness, tingling, and anxiousness. The cause of panic disorders remains an enigma. Recent data have suggested that genetics appears to be a factor in many cases. This disorder affects 2–5% of the American population and is twice as common among women as men. Treatments are psychotherapy, behavioral therapy, hypnosis, and medication. **Hypnosis** is an artificially induced trancelike state of enhanced relaxation. There is no evidence of a shifting electroencephalogram (EEG) or consciousness. While in this state, the person is highly susceptible to suggestions, is oblivious to all else, and responds readily to commands and questions from the hypnotist. The scientific validity of hypnosis has been debated for two centuries and appears to run a cycle of acceptance and rejection.

Phobias are disproportionate, obsessive, persistent, and unrealistic fears of situations or objects. Specific types are named using a combining form expressing the object that inspires the fear (Fig. 18-5). For example, the word part *aqua-* refers to "water;" thus the word *aquaphobia* is "fear of water." Many people who have phobias realize the irrationality of their fears but are powerless to prevent it.

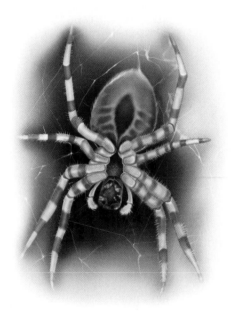

FIGURE 18-5
Arachnophobia is a disproportionate, obsessive, persistent, and unrealistic fear of spiders.

Phobias are produced by the interaction of two factors: genetic predisposition and classical conditioning. There is clear evidence that phobias may be the result of inherited temperament traits or some other factor that is yet unknown. It is also now accepted that phobias are conditioned early in life, either vicariously or through direct experience. The phobic stimulus is a conditioned stimulus that elicits CNS arousal and subsequent avoidance behavior. The history, physical examination, and oral evaluation lead to the diagnosis. Treatments are highly individualized and may include psychotherapy, behavioral therapy, hypnosis, and pharmaceutics. Table 18-3 lists selected phobias and their descriptions.

Obsessive–compulsive disorder (OCD) is an anxiety disorder characterized by intrusive, unwanted thoughts, which produce a rapid increase in anxiety. The anxiety leads the person to perform ritualistic behaviors (compulsions) in an attempt to reduce the anxiety. In OCD, the person cannot control his or her anxiety and is dominated by the repetitive impulses. The acts then become organized rituals such as hand washing and excessive neatness. This condition affects 2–3% of Americans. Some theorize it is a response to severe stress, but others purport genetic factors, frontal lobe abnormality, or neurotransmitter dysfunction. There is strong evidence pointing to the pre-frontal cortex as the primary neurologic structure involved in

TABLE 18-3   Phobias

Term	Description
acrophobia	fear of heights
agoraphobia	fear of open spaces
ailurophobia	fear of cats
androphobia	fear of men
arachnophobia	fear of spiders
claustrophobia	fear of confined space
cynophobia	fear of dogs
gamophobia	fear of marriage
gehydrophobia	fear of crossing a bridge
gynephobia	fear of women
hedonophobia	fear of pleasure
hemophobia	fear of blood
hypnophobia	fear of sleep
laliophobia	fear of stuttering
ochlophobia	fear of crowds
ophidiophobia	fear of snakes
pathophobia	fear of disease
phobophobia	fear of developing a phobia
pyrophobia	fear of fire
taphophobia	fear of being buried alive
triskaidekaphobia	fear of the number 13
xenophobia	fear of strangers
zoophobia	fear of animals

OCD. The history and physical examination confirm the diagnosis. A similar disorder, obsessive–compulsive personality disorder (OCPD), is characterized by perfectionism and rigidity.

Psychotherapy, hypnosis, stress reduction, relaxation techniques, biofeedback, exercise, and anxiolytics are treatments that may help. **Biofeedback** is a training technique that enables an individual to gain some voluntary control over autonomic body functions. Individuals using biofeedback techniques can learn to influence desired physiological responses such as lowering blood pressure, alleviating headache symptoms, or achieving conscious management over normally involuntary body physiology. **Anxiolytic** drugs, which act on GABA-receptor sites and generally do not cause excessive sedation, are sometimes prescribed. Common drugs of this type are benzodiazepines and diazepam. However, the gold standard of treatment for OCD is called exposure and response prevention (ERP). ERP is a form of cognitive therapy that involves exposing the OCD sufferer to the very thing that produces anxiety (such as germs or body fluids) and *not* allowing him or her to reduce the ensuing anxiety with any form of compulsive behavior. Research has found that with repeated exposures, the incidence of intrusive, obsessive thoughts decline.

Post-traumatic stress disorder (PTSD) is characterized by a group of symptoms that are displayed after a psychologically traumatic event. Signs and symptoms include numbed responsiveness to stimuli, cognitive dysfunction, and dysphoria that appear either within a short time of the event or may have a delayed onset. The condition of not feeling well or being ill at ease is termed **dysphoria.** People with dysphoria feel acutely hopeless, uncomfortable, and unhappy. The disorder may spontaneously resolve within 6 months. Post-traumatic stress disorder is common among combat veterans and survivors of major physical trauma. Intrusive, recurring flashbacks to the event give evidence for diagnosis. Counseling, behavior therapy, and drugs for anxiety and depression are therapeutic measures.

Another type of anxiety disorder is **generalized anxiety disorder** (GAD), a condition classified as chronic, repeated episodes of anxiety in which fear and dread accompany autonomic changes such as diarrhea, hypertension (high blood pressure), and muscle tension. The most prevalent type of anxiety disorder, it affects more females than males, and occurs primarily in individuals aged 20–25 years. It is diagnosed by observation of the signs and symptoms. Treatment options consist of psychotherapy, hypnosis, relaxation techniques, biofeedback, physical exercise, and administration of anxiolytic drugs. Physical manifestations are treated symptomatically.

Key Terms	Definitions
anxiety (ang ZYE i tee) **disorders**	group of disorders characterized by nervousness or agitation in response to anticipation of a future event
panic disorder	disorder in which person suffers repeated panic attacks that come on suddenly and are overwhelming and uncontrollable
hypnosis (hip NOH sis)	sleep-like condition that is artificially induced
phobias (FOH bee uhz)	irrational, powerful fears
obsessive–compulsive disorder	psychiatric disorder characterized by excessive unreasonable thoughts and irresistible impulsive behavior
biofeedback	technique for controlling automatic body functions
anxiolytic (ANG see oh lit ick)	drug that relieves anxiety
post-traumatic stress disorder	psychological condition affecting people who have suffered severe emotional trauma causing sleep disturbances, flashbacks, anxiety, tiredness, and depression
dysphoria (dis FOH ree uh)	exaggerated state of unhappiness
generalized anxiety (ang ZYE i tee) **disorder**	chronic, repeated episodes of nervousness, agitation, and feelings that something negative is going to happen

Key Term Practice: Anxiety Disorders

1. An irrational fear is called a/an _____.

2. _____ is a psychological condition affecting people who have witnessed or suffered a horrific event.

Somatoform Disorders

Somatoform disorders are a group of disorders in which physical symptoms suggest a disorder but in which no demonstrable organic dysfunction can be found or no known physiologic mechanism is evident. *Soma* refers to "body;" therefore, these disorders with physiological signs and symptoms are the result of psychological processes. An alternate term is **psychosomatic disorder.** There is strong evidence linking psychological factors to the physiological mechanisms. Psychotherapy and medications to manage pain may offer benefit for somatoform disorders if no underlying pathology is discovered.

Somatization disorder is characterized by the displacement of emotional conflicts onto the body. This results in various physical symptoms. Patients present with a complicated medical history and physical symptoms related to various organ systems. No organic foundation can be discovered. The onset is typically before age 30 years. Pain is felt in four or more body functions. Pain in the gastrointestinal (GI), reproductive, and neurologic systems is also noted. It is diagnosed by the presence of four pain symptoms, two GI symptoms, one sexual symptom, and one pseudoneurologic symptom. The individual never experiences a symptom-free period lasting longer than 1 year. Treatment involves ruling out any underlying pathology and then treating the remaining symptoms appropriately.

Conversion disorder is a defense mechanism in which an unconscious emotional conflict is transformed into a physical disability. The affected part may have symbolic meaning pertinent to the nature of the conflict. Physical signs and symptoms occur instead of anxiety. Symptoms may include blindness, deafness, paralysis, blurred vision, or numbness. Because no pathology can be determined, the disorder is treated symptomatically.

Pain disorder is severe and long-lasting pain resulting from psychological and physiological factors. The pain interferes with life activities, social functioning, and work. It often leads to depression. Diagnostic studies may reveal a pathologic condition, such as neuropathy or osteoporosis. After treating the underlying cause, pain medications and therapy may be beneficial.

Hypochondriasis is a chronic condition characterized by a morbid concern for one's physical or mental health. The person believes he or she is suffering from some grave, bodily disease even though there are no pathologic findings. The delusion is that one is suffering from a disease that does not exist. The person frequently searches the body for signs of pathology. For example, normal bumps and moles are immediately assumed to be symptomatic of cancer. It is also known as **hypochondria.** Many researchers now believe that hypochondriasis may be a form of OCD, and it responds well to ERP therapy.

Body dysmorphic disorder is a somatoform characterized by preoccupation with some imagined defect in appearance. It is also known as **dysmorphophobia,** which describes the condition as a morbid fear of being deformed.

Briquet syndrome and hysteria are disorders with somatoform symptoms that do not meet the criteria for any of the specific disorders. **Briquet syndrome** is a chronic, fluctuating mental disorder characterized by frequent complaints of physical illness involving multiple organ systems simultaneously. It is more common in females than males. **Hysteria** is an alteration or loss of physical functioning simulating a physical disease but is instead an expression of a psychological conflict. The impaired function may be mental, sensory, motor, or visceral. It is generally cured by psychotherapy alone.

Key Terms	Definitions
somatoform (soh muh TOH form) **disorders**	disorders in which physiological alterations result from psychological functions
psychosomatic (sigh koh soh MAT ick) **disorder**	pathology resulting from the interrelationship between the mind and the body with symptoms of psychic and emotional origin
somatization (soh muh ti ZAY shun) **disorder**	disorder in which emotional conflicts are projected onto the body and revealed as pathological states
conversion disorder	condition marked by appearance of physical symptoms without physical cause but in the presence of psychological conflict
pain disorder	severe mental distress resulting from an underlying pathological condition
hypochondriasis (high poh kon DRYE uh sis)	preoccupation with health and bodily sensations accompanied by the conviction of having a serious disease without supportive evidence; hypochondria
hypochondria (high poh KON dree uh)	preoccupation with health and bodily sensations accompanied by the conviction of having a serious disease without supportive evidence; hypochondriasis
body dysmorphic (dis MOR fick) **disorder**	disorder in a normal-appearing person characterized by an abnormal fear of being deformed; dysmorphophobia
dysmorphophobia (dis mor foh FOH bee uh)	disorder in a normal-appearing person characterized by an abnormal fear of being deformed; dysmorphic disorder
Briquet syndrome	disorder marked by complaints of physical illness of several body systems all at once with no underlying pathology
hysteria	an emotionally unstable state that results from a traumatic experience

Key Term Practice: Somatoform Disorders

1. Which two terms mean a mental disorder characterized by a preoccupation with bodily functions and the interpretation of normal sensations as physical ailments? _____

2. The word part *hyster-* refers to _____; and the word _____ describes an emotionally unstable state as a result of a traumatic event.

Factitious Disorders

Physical and psychological signs and symptoms that are intentionally produced or feigned to gain attention and play the sick role are called **factitious disorders.** Two examples of factitious disorders are Münchhausen syndrome and Münchhausen syndrome by proxy. The syndrome is named after Baron K. F. H. von Münchhausen, a German soldier and proverbial teller of exaggerated tales.

Münchhausen syndrome is a personality disorder in which a patient presents with false symptoms or simulates acute illness, the extent to which depends on the person's medical knowledge base. Individuals are eager to undergo examinations, hospitalizations, diagnostic procedures, and therapeutic manipulations. When no underlying cause can be revealed, they often leave a health-care facility without notice and seek attention at another institution.

Münchhausen syndrome by proxy is a form of Münchhausen syndrome in which symptomology is projected onto a child by a caregiver, usually the mother. The term *proxy* means "a person is acting as a substitute for somebody else." In this case, because of the child's supposed illness, the mother or caregiver gains the sympathy. It is considered a form of child maltreatment or abuse because often the clinical signs are induced or artificially stimulated by the caregiver. For example, emetic agents may be given to the child to induce unwarranted vomiting. The person may tamper with the child's medical specimens to create a need for further medical care. This leads to medical interventions and investigations. Occasionally, children are placed in danger as a result. Serious health consequences and death have been reported. The disorder is also known as **factitious illness by proxy.**

The cause of both factitious disorders is not known. It is thought to be a form of attention-seeking behavior. A history of repeated hospitalizations, no underlying pathology, symptoms that do not match laboratory findings, and recurrent fabricated stories provide the diagnosis. The treatment is psychotherapy.

Key Terms	Definitions
factitious (fack TISH us) **disorder**	disorder brought about by contrived and unnatural means
Münchhausen (MUN chow zun) **syndrome**	disorder in which a person pretends to have an illness to undergo testing or treatment or be admitted to a hospital
Münchhausen (MUN chow zun) **syndrome by proxy**	disorder in which a caregiver harms a child, falsifies medical records, and/or tampers with laboratory specimens to create a situation requiring medical attention; factitious illness by proxy
factitious (fack TISH us) **illness by proxy**	disorder in which a caregiver harms a child, falsifies medical records, and/or tampers with laboratory specimens to create a situation requiring medical attention; Münchhausen syndrome by proxy

Key Term Practice: Factitious Disorders

1. Conditions brought about by contrived or unnatural means are termed _____ disorders.

2. The factitious disorder that is characterized by a person pretending to be sick to gain attention and hospital admission is termed _____.

Dissociative Disorders

Dissociative disorders are characterized by the sudden, transient, or chronic alteration in usual integrated functions of consciousness, memory, identity, or perception. Forms include dissociative amnesia, dissociative fugue, dissociative identity disorder, and depersonalization disorder. Intense psychotherapy is the treatment for all forms.

Dissociative amnesia (formerly psychogenic amnesia) is the inability to recall important personal information that goes beyond normal forgetfulness. The memory impairment is usually reversible. It can appear in any age group with the main symptom being a retrospective memory gap. Acute forms occur in response to natural disaster or severe trauma.

Dissociative fugue (formerly psychogenic fugue) is the unexpected travel away from home or one's usual place of daily activities accompanied by the inability to recall some or all of one's past. **Fugue** is a condition in which a person suddenly abandons a present activity or lifestyle and begins a new or different one for a period of time, often in a different city. Amnesia during the fugue period is reported, although earlier events are remembered and habits and skills are unaffected.

Dissociative identity disorder (formerly multiple personality disorder) is the presence of two or more distinct identities or personality states that control one's behavior. The individual is unable to recall important personal information and memory gaps are common. Severe physical and sexual abuse during childhood have been linked to the disorder.

Depersonalization disorder is persistent or recurrent experiences of feelings of detachment. Individuals report feeling like being in a dream state. Social and occupational functioning are impaired.

Key Terms	Definitions
dissociative disorder	disorder characterized by the sudden, transient, or chronic alteration in usual integrated functions of consciousness, memory, identity, or perception
dissociative amnesia (am NEE zhuh)	inability to recall important personal information that goes beyond normal forgetfulness
dissociative fugue (fewg)	unexpected travel away from home or one's usual place of daily activities accompanied by the inability to recall some or all of one's past
fugue (fewg)	condition in which a person suddenly abandons a present activity or lifestyle and begins a new or different one for a period of time, often in a different city
dissociative identity disorder	the presence of two or more distinct identities or personality states that control one's behavior
depersonalization disorder	persistent or recurrent experiences of feelings of detachment

Key Term Practice: Dissociative Disorders

1. _____ refers to a condition in which a person suddenly abandons a present activity or lifestyle and begins a new or different one for a period of time, often in a different city.

2. _____ disorders are characterized by the sudden, transient, or chronic alteration in usual integrated functions of consciousness, memory, identity, or perception

Sexual and Gender-Identity Disorders

Sexual and gender-identity disorders involve sexual dysfunctions, paraphilias, gender-identify disorders, and other sexual disorders. **Sexual dysfunctions** are characterized by a disturbance in the sexual-response cycle or by pain associated with sexual intercourse. Sexual dysfunctions are a group of behavioral and psychophysiologic disorders with variability in sexual functioning. Sexual activity, desire, arousal, and orgasm can be affected and are often a source of great distress and interpersonal difficulty. Psychotherapy and counseling are common forms of treatment.

Paraphilias are sexual deviations such as exhibitionism, fetishism, and pedophilia. These behaviors are a marked contrast with generally accepted forms of sexual activities. A sexual perversion (a turning aside from the normal course) in which pleasure is obtained by exposing the genitalia is termed **exhibitionism.** **Fetishism** is characterized by using an inanimate object (fetish) or nonsexual body part to arouse erotic feelings. For example, the person may **masturbate** (manipulate genitalia to produce orgasm) while smelling or fondling an item. It is diagnosed as a disorder if the behavior recurs over 6 months and impairs social and occupational functioning.

Pedophilia is abnormal sexual attraction to children by adults. The disorder usually begins in adolescence. Clinically, the sexual activity must be with a prepubescent child (age 13 years or younger). Furthermore, the pedophile must be at least 16 years of age and at least 5 years older than the child. Sexual desire fluctuates with the pedophile's stress level. Twice as many males as females are afflicted. If the behavior recurs over 6 months, it is diagnosed as pedophilia. Treatment for paraphilias requires various forms of intense therapy.

Gender-identity disorders are mental disorders in children, adolescents, and adults characterized by a strong and enduring cross-gender identification. Throughout life, the individual identifies with and desires to be the other sex. Clinically significant impairment in functioning in the genetically assigned sex is apparent. Individuals often play the role of the other sex. It is also known as **transsexualism.** A transsexual is a person whose chromosomes, gonads, and other body markings are of one sex, but the individual identifies psychically with the other. Persons may routinely live and dress as a member of the opposite sex. The cause is unknown. It is diagnosed on the basis of two criteria that must both be present: There must be strong and persistent evidence of cross-gender identification and there must be constant discomfort about one's assigned sex. A history of transsexual behaviors, along with a stated desire to live as the opposite sex, often leads to sex reassignment operations and hormonal therapy.

Key Terms	Definitions
sexual dysfunction	disturbances in sexual desire and in the response cycle
paraphilias (pair uh FIL ee uhz)	sexual divergences from normally accepted behaviors
exhibitionism (eck si BISH un iz um)	disorder causing a compulsion to show one's genitals in public
fetishism (FET ish iz um)	the use of an object (fetish) to produce sexual arousal
masturbate	to give oneself sexual pleasure by stroking the genitals to achieve orgasm

pedophilia (pee doh FIL ee uh)	abnormal fondness of children by adults for sexual purposes
gender-identity disorders	disorders characterized by a person identifying with, and wanting to become, a member of the opposite sex; transsexualism
transsexualism (trans SECK shoo ul iz um)	disorder characterized by a person identifying with, and wanting to become, a member of the opposite sex; gender–identity disorder

Key Term Practice: Sexual and Gender-Identity Disorders

1. The use of objects to produce sexual arousal is called _____.

2. The general term _____ describes disorders of sexual divergence from normally accepted behaviors.

Eating Disorders

Eating disorders are characterized by disturbances in eating behavior. Examples include anorexia nervosa and bulimia nervosa. Although obesity is a health condition of clinical significance, it is not associated with a psychological or behavioral syndrome; thus, it does not appear in *DSM-IV-TR*; however, it is included in the *ICD-9-CM*.

Anorexia nervosa is a disorder of unknown cause characterized by a profound food aversion for fear of gaining weight and by an abnormal perception of body size and shape. The condition leads to emaciation, nutritional deficiencies, and even death. It is more common in women than in men. Individuals are afraid of becoming obese. The distorted body image is accompanied by hyperactivity and, in women, by amenorrhea (absence of menstrual periods) as a result of low fat reserves.

Binge eating (uncontrolled rapid ingestion over short periods) and inappropriate compensatory measures to prevent weight gain characterize **bulimia nervosa.** The insatiable appetite and excessive food intake is followed by self-induced vomiting, diuretic or laxative use, fasting, and vigorous exercise to avoid gaining additional pounds. Feelings of guilt, depression, and self-disgust are typical.

Anorexia nervosa and bulimia nervosa are diagnosed by the complete history of the behavior and physical examination. Psychotherapy or counseling is the primary treatment method.

FACT *Anorexia nervosa and bulimia nervosa affects millions of Americans yearly, 85–90% of whom are teens and young adult women.*

Key Terms	Definitions
anorexia nervosa (an oh RECK see uh nur VOH suh)	eating disorder characterized by extreme fear of becoming overweight that leads to dieting to the point of illness and sometimes death
bulimia nervosa (bew LIM ee uh nur VOH suh)	eating disorder characterized by bouts of overeating that are followed by undereating, laxative use, or vomiting

Key Term Practice: Eating Disorders

1. List two disorders characterized by eating behavior disturbances.

Sleep Disorders

Sleep disorders are listed in the *DSM-IV-TR* because they can produce significant impairment in cognitive, affective, and behavioral states, and thus negatively affect social functioning. Many cause profound alterations in daily physical and psychological functioning.

Sleep disorders are grouped by **dyssomnias**, abnormalities in the amount, quality, or timing of sleep, and **parasomnias**, abnormal behavioral or physiological events associated with sleep, sleep stages, or sleep–wake transitions. Examples of parasomnias are sleepwalking with no recollection of event, seizures that cause one to awaken, and nightmares with vivid recall. Parasomnias are organically, psychologically, or drug induced. Treatment is aimed at removing hindrances for sleepwalkers to prevent injury. Drugs such as diazepam (Valium) may be prescribed.

The average length of daily sleep for adults is 6–8 hours; children and adolescents require more. Sleep disorders are evaluated and assessed by **polysomnography**, the simultaneous and continuous monitoring of relevant normal and abnormal physiologic activity during sleep. The instrument measures rapid eye movements (REMs)—the symmetrical, quick scanning movements of the eyes— that occur frequently during sleep in clusters for 5–60 minutes and are associated with dreaming. The non-REM sleep cycle is divided into four stages. Stage 1 is transition and accounts for 5% of sleep; stage 2 is deeper and occupies about 50% of sleep; stages 3 and 4 are characterized as slow-wave deep sleep that makes up 10–20% of the sleeping regimen.

Primary insomnia is characterized by sleeplessness and the inability to sleep in the absence of external impediments. The cause may be pain, thyroid disorder, alcohol and caffeine ingestion, amphetamine use, anxiety, fear, or stress. Diagnosis is confirmed if the condition has continued for more than 1 month and interferes with normal functioning. Treatment consists of ruling out any possible underlying pathology, creating a favorable sleep environment, removing stimuli, instituting a regular bedtime, engaging in stress-relief activities, and exercising.

Narcolepsy is a disorder of the sleep mechanism closely related, or perhaps identical, to REM sleep. It is characterized by bouts of drowsiness during the day, **cataplexy** (temporary paralysis of cranial and somatic musculature), attacks of muscular strength loss, sleep paralysis, and vivid hypnagogic hallucinations. **Hypnagogic hallucinations** are images seen or imagined with the onset of sleep. For no apparent reason, the person is plunged into REM sleep from a waking state. Narcolepsy, also known as **paroxysmal sleep**, occurs from a few seconds to 30 minutes. The onset is usually before age 25 years. Nocturnal sleep is often disrupted. Data suggest a strong genetic role in its cause. It is diagnosed by a history of repeated episodes. Treatment includes napping, establishing a routine bedtime, and administering low doses of amphetamines.

Breathing-related sleep disorders are characterized by sleep disruption that leads to excessive sleepiness and interfere with activities of daily living. **Sleep apnea**, intermittent breathing cessation of short duration during sleep, is an example of a breathing-related sleep disorder. Snorting and gasping are common after periods of breathlessness. The frequent awakening results in daytime tiredness. The condition occurs more commonly in men than in women. Causes include obesity, hypertension, airway obstruction, and alcohol ingestion. Sleep history, daytime sleepiness, sleep laboratory studies, and accounts of others witnessing the event provide a diagnosis. Any underlying pathology should be treated.

If the condition persists, weight loss, continuous positive airway pressure (CPAP) therapy, uvulopalatopharyngoplasty (UPPP), and drugs such as protriptyline hydrochloride are treatment options. **Protriptyline**, an antidepressant, is used in the treatment of sleep apnea; the psychostimulant modafinil (Provigil) has recently gained approval to treat the condition. **Continuous positive airway pressure** is a type of respiratory therapy in which airway pressure is maintained above atmospheric pressure throughout the respiratory cycle. This form of treatment forces the airways to remain open. **Uvulopalatopharyngoplasty** is a surgical procedure to remove portions of the uvula (V-shaped fleshy extension hanging above the tongue at the throat entrance), soft palate (back portion of the roof of the mouth), and posterior pharyngeal mucosa (lining of the back of the throat) to open the airway and create an obstructive-free passage. It is also known as palatopharyngoplasty. The surgical resection of unnecessary palatal and oropharyngeal tissue improves signs and symptoms of snoring from all causes.

Key Terms	Definitions
dyssomnias (dis SOM nee uhz)	disorders of the sleep mechanisms
parasomnias (pair uh SOM nee uhz)	disorders characterized by behavioral or physiological events associated with sleep
polysomnography (pol ee som NOG ruh fee)	monitoring of the physiological activities that occur during sleep
primary insomnia (in SOM nee uh)	inability to fall asleep or sleep long enough to feel rested over a period of 1 month
narcolepsy (NAHR koh lep see)	condition characterized by frequent, brief, uncontrollable bouts of deep sleep; paroxysmal sleep
cataplexy (KAT uh pleck see)	sudden loss of muscle power after a strong emotional stimulus
hypnagogic (hip nuh GOJ ick) **hallucination**	perceptions of something with no basis in reality during the period of drowsiness just before sleep
paroxysmal (pair ock SIZ mul) **sleep**	condition characterized by frequent, brief, uncontrollable bouts of deep sleep; narcolepsy
sleep apnea (AP nee uh)	temporary cessation of breathing that occurs while a person sleeps
protriptyline (proh TRIP tuh leen)	antidepressant used for sleep apnea
continuous positive airway pressure	respiratory therapy that maintains the air passages at a greater pressure than atmospheric pressure by means of mechanical support to assist with the breathing cycle
uvulopalatopharyngoplasty (yoo vew loh pal uh toh fuh RIN goh plas tee)	surgical resection of unnecessary tissues of the soft palate and oropharyngeal region; palatopharyngoplasty

Key Term Practice: Sleep Disorders

1. The medical term for disorders of the sleep mechanisms is _____.

2. _____ is characterized by a temporary pause of breathing during sleep.

Personality Disorders

Personality disorders are a group of disorders designated by pathologic trends in character. They are manifested by lifelong patterns of abnormal behavior or actions, rather than psychotic or neurotic disturbances. Impaired judgment, affect, impulse control, and interpersonal functioning mark personality disorders. This section discusses 5 of the 10 identified personality disorders.

Paranoid personality disorder is characterized by the tendency to be hypersensitive, rigid, extremely self-important, and jealous. The person projects hostile feelings, is suspicious of and mistrusts others, and is quick to blame others or attribute evil motives to them. This often interferes with the ability to maintain healthy interpersonal relationships because the actions of others are misinterpreted as harmful, demeaning, or threatening.

The **schizoid personality disorder** is characterized as extremely shy and introverted. Traits include social withdrawal, emotional coldness or aloofness, and indifference to others. People with this type of personality disorder have difficulty expressing anger.

A refusal to accept the obligations and restraints imposed by society is characteristic of **antisocial personality disorder.** There is a pervasive pattern of behavior with disregard for and violation of the rights and safety of others. The onset is before age 15 years. Early childhood signs include chronic lying, stealing, fighting, and truancy; adolescent signs are unusually early or aggressive sexual behavior, excessive drinking, and illicit drug use. Excessive alcohol consumption and illicit drug use may persist into adulthood. Guilt is not expressed, and these individuals frequently do not learn from their mistakes. This is a common diagnosis applied to serial killers.

The **histrionic personality disorder** is characterized by exaggerated, dramatic gestures, attitudes, speech, and facial expressions. Attention-seeking behavior and demands for approval and reassurance that begin in childhood and endure in adulthood. People with this disorder need to be the center of attention.

A pervasive pattern in adulthood of self-centeredness, self-importance, lack of empathy for others, sense of entitlement, and viewing others as objects to meet one's need characterize **narcissistic personality disorder.** The disorder is named for Narcissus, a beautiful youth in Greek mythology who falls in love with his own reflection in a pool.

The cause of personality disorders is unknown, although biological, social, and environmental factors have been implicated. Treatment is psychotherapy and family education to promote the best environment to achieve desired outcomes.

Key Terms	*Definitions*
personality disorders	psychiatric disorders in attitude or behavior that cause difficulty in getting along with others or succeeding in the workplace or social situations
paranoid personality disorder	disorder marked by being unreasonably suspicious of other people and their thoughts and/or motives
schizoid (SKIZ oid) **personality disorder**	disorder marked by detachment and unresponsiveness
antisocial personality disorder	disorder marked by being inconsiderate of the needs of others

histrionic (his tree ON ick) **personality disorder**	disorder marked by overdramatic reactions or behaviors
narcissistic (nahr si SIS tick) **personality disorder**	disorder marked by excessive self-admiration and self-centeredness

Key Term Practice: Personality Disorders

1. Psychiatric conditions in attitude or behavior that cause difficulties in getting along with others are termed _____ disorders.

2. Which personality disorder is characterized by excessive self-centered behavior? _____

CLINICAL TERMS

Clinical Dimension	Term	Description
DISORDERS		
	alcohol abuse	excessive use of alcohol creating an addiction to drinking alcoholic beverages; alcoholism
	alcoholism	excessive use of alcohol creating an addiction to drinking alcoholic beverages; alcohol abuse
	anorexia nervosa	eating disorder characterized by extreme fear of becoming overweight that leads to dieting to the point of illness and sometimes death
	antisocial personality disorder	disorder marked by being inconsiderate of the needs of others
	anxiety disorders	group of disorders characterized by nervousness or agitation in response to anticipation of a future event
	attention-deficit/ hyperactivity disorder (ADHD)	condition characterized by hyperactivity, inability to concentrate, and impulsive or inappropriate behavior
	autistic disorder	disturbance in psychological development that is marked by mental introversion and concentration on self or one object
	bipolar disorder	disorder characterized by extreme mood swings between euphoria and severe depression
	body dysmorphic disorder	disorder in a normal-appearing person characterized by an abnormal fear of being deformed; dysmorphophobia
	Briquet syndrome	disorder marked by complaints of physical illness of several body systems all at once with no underlying pathology
	bulimia nervosa	eating disorder characterized by bouts of overeating followed by undereating, laxative use, or vomiting

Clinical Dimension	Term	Description
	catatonic-type schizophrenia	disorder marked by motor disturbances, stupor, and rigidity
	conversion disorder	condition marked by the appearance of physical symptoms without physical cause but in the presence of psychological conflict
	delirium	state marked by extreme restlessness, confusion, and perhaps hallucinations
	dementia	deterioration or loss of intellectual faculties, reasoning power, memory, and will
	dementia of the Alzheimer type	degenerative brain disorder that causes dementia, especially late in life; Alzheimer disease
	depersonalization disorder	persistent or recurrent experiences of feelings of detachment
	disorganized-type schizophrenia	disorder marked by inappropriate affect, giggling, and inappropriate mannerism; hebephrenic
	dissociative amnesia	inability to recall important personal information that goes beyond normal forgetfulness
	dissociative disorders	disorders characterized by the sudden, transient, or chronic alteration in usual integrated functions of consciousness, memory, identity, or perception
	dissociative fugue	unexpected travel away from home or one's usual place of daily activities accompanied by the inability to recall some or all of one's past
	dissociative identity disorder	the presence of two or more distinct identities or personality states that control one's behavior
	dysmorphophobia	disorder in a normal-appearing person characterized by an abnormal fear of being deformed; body dysmorphic disorder
	dyssomnias	disorders of sleep the mechanisms
	dysthymic disorder	depressed mood for most of the day, for more days than not, for at least 2 years
	exhibitionism	disorder causing a compulsion to show one's genitals in public
	factitious disorder	disorder brought about by contrived and unnatural means
	factitious illness by proxy	disorder in which a caregiver harms a child, falsifies medical records, and/or tampers with laboratory specimens to create a situation requiring medical attention; Münchhausen syndrome by proxy
	fetishism	the use of an object (fetish) to produce sexual arousal
	fugue	condition in which a person suddenly abandons a present activity or lifestyle and begins a new or different one for a period of time, often in a different city

Clinical Dimension	Term	Description
	gender-identity disorders	disorders characterized by a person identifying with, and wanting to become, a member of the opposite sex; transsexualism
	generalized anxiety disorder	chronic, repeated episodes of nervousness, agitation, and feelings that something negative is going to happen
	hebephrenic	disorder marked by inappropriate affect, giggling, and inappropriate mannerisms; disorganized-type schizophrenia
	histrionic personality disorder	disorder marked by overdramatic reactions or behaviors
	hypochondria	preoccupation with health and bodily sensations accompanied by the conviction of having a serious disease without supportive evidence; hypochondriasis
	hypochondriasis	preoccupation with health and bodily sensations accompanied by the conviction of having a serious disease without supportive evidence; hypochondria
	hysteria	an emotionally unstable state that results from a traumatic experience
	learning disorder (LD)	any defect or disturbance in a child's ability to acquire skills in reading, writing, or arithmetic
	logospasm	stuttering, or saying something haltingly and repeating sounds when attempting to pronounce them
	major depressive disorder	psychological illness marked by sustained unhappiness and hopelessness with suicidal tendencies
	mental retardation	below normal intellectual function
	mood disorders	aliments characterized by emotional disturbances that interfere with other aspects of life
	Münchhausen syndrome	disorder in which a person pretends to have an illness to undergo testing or treatment or be admitted to a hospital
	Münchhausen syndrome by proxy	disorder in which a caregiver harms a child, falsifies medical records, and/or tampers with laboratory specimens to create a situation requiring medical attention; factitious illness by proxy
	narcissistic personality disorder	disorder marked by excessive self-admiration and self-centeredness
	narcolepsy	condition characterized by frequent, brief, uncontrollable bouts of deep sleep; paroxysmal sleep
	obsessive–compulsive disorder (OCD)	psychiatric disorder characterized by excessive, unreasonable thoughts and irresistible, impulsive behavior
	obsessive–compulsive personality disorder (OCPD)	condition similar to OCD that is characterized by perfectionism and rigidity

Clinical Dimension	Term	Description
	pain disorder	severe mental distress resulting from an underlying pathological condition
	panic disorder	disorder in which a person suffers repeated panic attacks that come on suddenly and are overwhelming and uncontrollable
	paranoid personality disorder	disorder marked by being unreasonably suspicious of other people and their thoughts and/or motives
	paranoid-type schizophrenia	disorder marked by delusions and hallucinations
	paraphilias	sexual divergences from normally accepted behaviors
	parasomnias	disorders characterized by behavioral or physiological events associated with sleep
	paroxysmal sleep	condition characterized by frequent, brief, uncontrollable bouts of deep sleep; narcolepsy
	pedophilia	abnormal fondness of children by adults for sexual purposes
	personality disorders	psychiatric disorders in attitude or behavior that cause difficulty in getting along with others or succeeding in the workplace or social situations
	phobias	irrational, powerful fears
	pica	craving to eat substances that provide no nutritional value
	post-traumatic stress disorder (PTSD)	psychological condition affecting people who have suffered severe emotional trauma causing sleep disturbances, flashbacks, anxiety, tiredness, and depression
	primary insomnia	inability to fall asleep or sleep long enough to feel rested over a period of 1 month
	psychosomatic disorder	pathology resulting from the interrelationship between the mind and the body with symptoms of psychic and emotional origin
	residual-type schizophrenia	disorder marked by at least one schizophrenic episode but presently without disorder symptoms
	schizoid personality disorder	disorder marked by detachment and unresponsiveness
	schizophrenia	psychotic disorder with a mixture of signs and symptoms characterized by withdrawal, hallucinations, and delusions
	seasonal affective disorder (SAD)	depression associated with the onset of winter and thought to be caused by decreasing amounts of daylight
	sexual dysfunctions	disturbances in sexual desire and in the response cycle
	sleep apnea	temporary cessation of breathing that occurs while a person sleeps

Clinical Dimension	Term	Description
	somatization disorders	disorders in which physiological alternations result from psychological functions
	somatoform disorder	disorder in which emotional conflicts are projected onto the body and revealed as pathological states
	tardive dyskinesia	condition characterized by spasms of the tongue and facial muscles, resulting from long-term use of drugs that treat schizophrenia
	tic	spasmodic muscular contraction or vocalization
	Tourette disorder	condition typified by multiple twitches, involuntary vocal grunts, and obscene speech
	transsexualism	disorder characterized by a person identifying with, and wanting to become, a member of the opposite sex; gender-identity disorder
	undifferentiated-type schizophrenia	disorder marked by mixed symptomology including disorganized behavior
	vascular dementia	cognitive impairment caused by inadequate blood supply to the brain because of blocked blood vessels
	Wernicke-Korsakoff syndrome	form of brain damage occurring in long-term alcoholics from thiamine deficiency
SIGNS AND SYMPTOMS		
	abulia	abnormal inability to make a decision
	alogia	inability to speak owing to mental deficiency or an episode of dementia
	amnesia	memory loss or impairment
	anhedonia	overall chronic absence of enjoyment in acts that used to be enjoyable
	apathy	lack of feeling or emotion
	anxiety	overwhelming sense of apprehension
	cataplexy	sudden loss of muscle power after a strong emotional stimulus
	clang association	psychic (conscious) sounds resulting from word associations
	delirium tremens (DT)	agitation, tremors, and hallucinations that are caused by alcohol withdrawal
	delusion	false conviction held before strong contradictory evidence; false belief
	denial	condition in which confrontation of problems are avoided by acting as though they did not exist
	depression	state of profound sadness
	dysphoria	exaggerated state of unhappiness
	echolalia	speech disorder characterized by an involuntary repetition of the same word or words spoken by another person

Clinical Dimension	Term	Description
	euphoria	exaggerated feeling of elation
	grief	deep distress caused by bereavement
	hallucinations	perceptions of things with no basis in reality
	hedonia	abnormal happiness
	hedonism	belief that every act is motivated to attain pleasure
	hypnagogic hallucination	perceptions of something with no basis in reality during the period of drowsiness just before sleep
	labile	unstable
	malinger	to pretend incapacitation or illness
	mutism	inability or refusal to speak
	repression	excluding distressing thoughts or memories from the consciousness
	sublimation	to divert an unacceptable feeling or idea to one that is considered more socially acceptable
	suppression	to intentionally exclude a thought or feeling from consciousness
CLINICAL TESTS AND DIAGNOSTIC PROCEDURES		
	intelligence quotient (IQ)	numerical rating used to designate a person's aptitude
	Minnesota Multiphase Personality Inventory (MMPI)	standardized test that uses true–false questions to assess the person's psychological and social adjustment
	multiaxial assessment	five coordinates used to assess a mental disorder
	polysomnography	monitoring of the physiological activities that occur during sleep
	Rorschach test	test of personality or mental state that is based on the person's interpretation of standard inkblots; inkblot test
	severity and course specifiers	qualifiers regarding specific conditions
	Stanford-Binet intelligence scale	intelligence test commonly given to children and adults
	thematic apperception test (TAT)	test for exploring aspects of the personality in which the person is shown pictures of people in various situations and asked to describe what is happening
	Wechsler intelligence	individually administered IQ test for preschoolers, children, and adults
TREATMENTS		
	antidepressants	drugs used in the treatment, alleviation, or prevention of depression
	antipsychotic drugs	chemical agents used to treat schizophrenia
	anxiolytic	drug that relieves anxiety

Clinical Dimension	Term	Description
	behavior therapy	treatment that uses behavior-modification techniques in which a person's desirable responses are positively reinforced while undesirable behaviors are negatively rewarded
	biofeedback	technique for controlling automatic body functions
	cognitive behavior therapy (CBT)	treatment whose goal is to change problem actions, manners, and cognitions through conditioning, learning, and cognitive restructuring
	continuous positive airway pressure (CPAP)	respiratory therapy that maintains the air passages at a greater pressure than atmospheric pressure by means of mechanical support to assist with the breathing cycle
	counseling	assistance with personal or psychological matters given by a professional
	electroconvulsive therapy (ECT)	passage of a small electric current through the brain to treat mental disorders
	exposure and response prevention (ERP)	form of cognitive therapy that involves exposing the person to the very thing that produces anxiety and not allowing him or her to reduce the anxiety by any from of compulsive behavior
	γ-glutamyltransferase (GGT) blood analysis	sensitive test that detects blood alcohol levels
	hypnosis	sleep-like condition that is artificially
	lithium carbonate	drug used to treat bipolar disorders
	palatopharyngoplasty	surgical resection of unnecessary tissues of the soft palate and oropharyngeal region; uvulopalatopharyngoplasty
	protriptyline	antidepressant used for sleep apnea
	transcranial magnetic stimulation (TMS)	passage of a magnetic current through brain to treatmental disorders
	uvulopalatopharyngo-plasty (UPPP)	surgical resection of unnecessary tissues of the soft palate and oropharyngeal region; palatopharyngoplasty

A to Z *Lifespan*

Mental disorders can strike at any point in life. Those evident at birth are often readily identified; others may be present at birth but may not manifest until early childhood, adolescence, or adulthood. Recent research suggests that exposure to stress during puberty may cause physical changes that alter behavior and brain chemistry.

According to research in the United States, late-life depression affects approximately 6 million adults; however, only 10% will receive treatment. At least 10–20% of widows or widowers develop clinically significant depression within 1 year of the death of a spouse. Older Americans are more likely to commit suicide than any other age group, albeit they constitute only 13% of the U.S. population. In 2000, individuals aged 65 years and older accounted for 20% of all suicides.

Research suggests that several factors contribute to the development of mental disorders. There may be a genetic predisposition for mental illness or prenatal and perinatal factors may also contribute, either solely or in conjunction with other issues. Viral infections and nutritional deficiencies occurring at a specific stage of development and growth may influence mental disorder development. Neuroanatomic alterations, neurotransmitter abnormalities, and neurochemical dysregulation at a later phase of life may cause mental illness. For example, dementias primarily affect the population over age 50 years, unless there is an underlying pathologic condition that precipitates an earlier onset. A great variability exists among and between the various disorders. Much is still to be learned in this medical field, especially in terms of understanding the causes, preventing, and treating mental diseases.

In the News: Alzheimer Disease Present Physically but Not Psychologically

Degenerated brain cells and β-amyloid (abnormal protein) create the core of senile plaques and neurofibrillary tangles that occur in Alzheimer disease. In fact, these are the hallmarks of diagnosing the disease postmortem. An interesting finding was made recently about these plaques and tangles in the brains of 19 nuns who demonstrated no outward manifestation of the disease.

The Nun Study is a longitudinal study conducted by David Snowdon at the University of Kentucky. More than 600 members of the School Sisters of Notre Dame religious congregation have donated their bodies to science. Annually, these sisters undergo cognitive and physical examinations and blood work, and all convent and medical records are examined. This group has become the largest brain donor group in the world so that Alzheimer disease could be studied.

At the autopsy of Sister Mary, aged 101 years, the researchers uncovered plaques and tangles that would be expected in someone who in life showed signs of advanced Alzheimer disease. Sister Mary, however, was mentally and spiritually active, kept up with current affairs, and exhibited clear reasoning and thinking. Researchers noted 18 other nuns with similar medical profiles also exhibited brain pathology indicative of Alzheimer disease.

Dr. Snowden found that the nuns who showed Alzheimer signs only in their brains also had minimal stroke evidence. Nuns whose brains demonstrated both strokes and the changes of Alzheimer disease showed symptoms of dementia in 93% of cases. Although the reason is not clear, it is surmised that good nutrition, exercise, aspirin intake, and remaining mentally active may help in preventing stroke, thereby staving off this form of dementia.

COMMON ABBREVIATIONS

Abbreviation	Term
AA	Alcoholics Anonymous
AD	Alzheimer disease
AD/HD	attention-deficit/hyperactivity disorder
CBT	cognitive behavior therapy
CNS	central nervous system
CPAP	continuous positive airway pressure

Abbreviation	Term
CT	computed tomography
DSM-IV-TR	*Diagnostic and Statistical Manual of Mental Disorders, Fourth Edition, Text Revision*
DT	delirium tremens
ECT	electroconvulsive therapy
EEG	electroencephalogram
ERP	exposure and response prevention
GABA	γ-aminobutyric acid
GAF	global assessment of functioning
GAD	generalized anxiety disorder
GGT	γ-glutamyltransferase
GI	gastrointestinal
ICD-9-CM	*International Statistical Classification of Diseases and Related Health Problems, Ninth Edition, Clinical Modification*
IEP	individual educational plan
IQ	intelligence quotient
LD	learning disorder
LISW	licensed independent social worker
LSW	licensed social worker
MAO	monamine oxidase
MMPI	Minnesota Multiphase Personality Inventory
MRI	magnetic resonance imaging
OCD	obsessive–compulsive disorder
OCDP	obsessive–compulsive personality disorder
OT	occupational therapy
PC	professional counselor
PCC	professional clinical counselor
PT	physical therapy
PTSD	post-traumatic stress disorder
REM	rapid eye movement
SAD	seasonal affective disorder
SSRI	selective serotonin reuptake inhibitor
TAT	thematic apperception test
TD	tardive dyskinesia
TMS	transcranial magnetic stimulation
UPPP	uvulopalatopharyngoplasty

Case Study

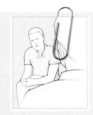

Elizabeth began treating John Johnson, aged 54 years. During the initial therapy session, John noted that he was recently divorced but had been separated from his wife for 18 months. He had been living in a small apartment and seeing his children on weekends. Since the court date to finalize the divorce 1 month earlier, he reported not sleeping well or eating much, and described himself as feeling depressed most of the day every day. He was not eating because he felt nauseous and reported frequent upset stomachs. He said he had lost about 10 lb.

At work, his fellow computer programmers expressed concern because they noticed him staring at his computer monitor for long periods of time. He described himself as being unable to concentrate at work for the last couple weeks. He was surprised that he felt that way and is not certain if it is related to his divorce—because he had been separated from his wife for so long—or to a recent fight he had with his 16-year-old son, who no longer wants to visit him on weekends. John also mentioned that he did not feel like golfing with his friends and that he tended to spend a lot of time alone. He had never felt this way before in his life and decided he might need some help.

John admitted when asked that he had thought about suicide but had not thought about how or when he might kill himself.

Case Study Questions

Select the best answer to each of the following questions.

1. **John was probably suffering from _____.**
   a. attention-deficit/hyperactivity disorder (ADHD)
   b. dysthymic disorder
   c. major depressive disorder
   d. anorexia nervosa

2. **John's recurrent thoughts of suicide are _____.**
   a. typical with major depression
   b. highly abnormal
   c. not worth paying attention to
   d. signs that he is ready to die

3. **The psychosocial stressors that may have contributed to John's depression include _____.**
   a. gastroenteritis
   b. the size of his apartment
   c. the fight he had with his son
   d. no exercise

4. **Part of a treatment plan for John might be _____.**
   a. a referral to a psychiatrist
   b. referral to a family physician
   c. joint therapy with his son
   d. any of the above

REAL WORLD REPORT

Elizabeth conducted a multiaxial evaluation to obtain an assessment of John's overall condition in five areas. This allowed her to create and develop a treatment plan.

MULTIAXIAL EVALUATION REPORT FORM

AXIS I: CLINICAL DISORDERS—OTHER CONDITIONS THAT MAY BE A FOCUS OF CLINICAL ATTENTION

Diagnostic Code	*DSM-IV* Name
296-22	major depressive disorder, single episode, moderate

AXIS II: PERSONALITY DISORDERS—MENTAL RETARDATION

Diagnostic Code	*DSM-IV* Name
none	

AXIS III: GENERAL MEDICAL CONDITIONS

ICD-9-CM Code	*ICD-9-CM* Name
558-9	gastroenteritis, acute

AXIS IV: PSYCHOSOCIAL AND ENVIRONMENTAL PROBLEMS

X Problems with primary support group   Specify: <u>divorce; conflict with child</u>
X Occupational problems   Specify: <u>difficulty concentrating & completing projects</u>

AXIS V: GLOBAL ASSESSMENT OF FUNCTIONING SCALE

Score: 55
Time frame: past 2 weeks

REAL WORLD REPORT QUESTIONS

The following exercises review the medical terms in the preceding medical report.

1. What is the DSM diagnostic code?

   _____

2. What is the DSM axis I diagnostic name for John's mental disorder?

   _____

3. The report includes John's general medical condition.

   a. The ICD-9-CM code is _____.

   b. The ICD-9-CM name is _____.

4. List John's specific psychosocial and environmental problems.

   _____

REVIEW AND APPLICATION: THREE-LEVEL LEARNING SYSTEM

LEVEL ONE: REVIEWING FACTS AND TERMS USING RECALL

Select the best response to each of the following questions.

1. Conditions that affect brain function are termed _____.

   a. mental disorders

   b. mental psychoses

   c. mental neuroses

   d. cognition psychoses

2. Chemical messengers called _____ transmit impulses.

   a. drugs

   b. enzymes

   c. neurotransmitters

   d. blood

3. A disease with a definite morphologic change in the brain tissue is known as _____.

   a. cognitive decline

   b. organic brain disease

   c. neuropathy

   d. mental disorder

4. Individuals with doctorate degrees licensed to practice psychology are _____.

   a. psychiatrists

   b. social workers

   c. hypnotists

   d. psychologists

5. One's _____ involves feelings, sensations, and passion.

   a. affect

   b. neurons

   c. psychiatry

   d. consciousness

6. General wakefulness and responsiveness to the environment is termed _____.

   a. mind

   b. affect

   c. consciousness

   d. psyche

7. Five coordinates used to assess mental disorders are part of the _____.

   a. intelligence quotient

   b. multiaxial assessment

   c. severity and course specifiers

   d. signs and symptoms

8. _____ are qualifiers regarding specific conditions.

   a. Biofeedback techniques

   b. Dementia

   c. Stanford-Binet tests

   d. Severity and course specifiers

9. Trained professionals working with economically, physically, mentally, or socially disadvantaged people are called _____.

   a. alcoholics

   b. bulimics

   c. social workers

   d. schizophrenics

10. _____ are professionals who give advice on personal, social, health, or psychological problems.

   a. Psychics

   b. Counselors

   c. Somnographers

   d. Narcoleptics

LEVEL TWO: REVIEWING CONCEPTS

Select the best response to each of the following questions.

11. A client wishes to receive therapy from an individual trained in Freudian psychology. A _____ is the professional most likely to be skilled in this realm.

    a. psychoanalyst

    b. counselor

    c. social worker

    d. neurosurgeon

12. Courtney acts as though her diagnosed cancer did not exist. This is a classic example of _____.

    a. depression

    b. grief

    c. anxiety

    d. denial

13. Brian engages in behaviors that are self-serving, and he has total disregard for any other person. This is an example of _____.

    a. obsessive-compulsive disorder (OCD)

    b. panic disorder

    c. narcissistic personality disorder

    d. panic disorder

14. Ryan has tried nearly every form of therapy to treat his major depressive disorder. As a last resort, his psychiatrist recommended _____, treatment that uses electricity to induce convulsions.

    a. biofeedback

    b. electroshock

    c. psychotherapy

    d. hypnosis

Provide a medical term to complete a meaningful analogy.

15. Stuttering is to _____ as body dysmorphic disorder is to _____.

16. _____ is to factitious illness by proxy as _____ is to gender identity disorder.

Match the sign or symptom with its definition.

_____ 17. amnesia

_____ 18. dysphoria

_____ 19. euphoria

_____ 20. delusion

_____ 21. abulia

a. state of unhappiness

b. feeling of elation

c. abnormal inability to make a decision

d. memory loss

e. exhibiting false beliefs

Match the term with its definition.

_____ 22. hedonia

_____ 23. echolalia

_____ 24. hysteria

_____ 25. alogia

_____ 26. anxiety

a. emotionally unstable state resulting from a traumatic experience

b. overwhelming sense of apprehension

c. inability to speak that results from dementia or mental deficiency

d. echoing the words of others

e. abnormal happiness

Match the disorder with its description.

_____ 27. autistic disorder

_____ 28. mental retardation

_____ 29. vascular dementia

_____ 30. schizophrenia

a. disorder characterized by inescapable thoughts and excessive ritualistic behaviors

b. disorder characterized by withdrawal, hallucinations, and delusions

c. below normal intellectual function

d. disturbance in psychological development that impairs language, interpretation, and interpersonal relationships

_____ 31. obsessive–compulsive disorder (OCD)   e. cognitive impairment resulting from ischemia

Match the disorder with its key description.

_____ 32. somatoform disorder   a. disorder characterized by the person identifying with and wanting to become a member of the opposite sex

_____ 33. conversion disorder   b. psychosomatic disorder or physical condition caused by psychological function

_____ 34. Briquet syndrome   c. condition in which the person has uncontrollable bouts of deep sleep

_____ 35. gender-identity disorder   d. physical illness of several body systems without underlying pathology

_____ 36. narcolepsy   e. appearance of physical symptoms without a physical cause in the presence of psychological conflict

Match the disorder with its description.

_____ 37. antisocial personality disorder   a. disorder causing a compulsion to display one's genitals in public

_____ 38. exhibitionism   b. disorder marked by being unreasonably suspicious of others and their motives

_____ 39. histrionic personality disorder   c. disorder marked by detachment and unresponsiveness

_____ 40. paranoid personality disorder   d. disorder marked by overdramatic reactions or behaviors

_____ 41. schizoid personality disorder   e. disorder marked by being inconsiderate of others

Match the treatment with its definition.

_____ 42. biofeedback   a. treatment goal is to change problem actions

_____ 43. behavior therapy   b. technique for controlling automatic body functions

_____ 44. hypnosis   c. treatment of mental disorders by psychological methods

_____ 45. antipsychotic drugs   d. chemical agents used to treat schizophrenia

_____ 46. psychotherapy   e. artificially induced sleep-like state used to invoke behavioral change

Using the following word parts, form a medical term for each definition. Each word part is used only once.

gyne-   -phobia
patho-   -phobia
phobo-   -phobia
pyro-   -phobia
zoo-   -phobia

47. fear of developing a phobia _____

48. fear of fire _____

49. fear of animals _____

50. fear of women _____

51. fear of disease _____

Define the following terms.

52. counseling _____

53. apathy _____

54. tic _____

55. mood disorders _____

56. masturbate _____

What is the term described by each of the following definitions?

57. disorder brought about by contrived or unnatural means _____

58. to pretend incapacitation or illness _____

59. state marked by extreme restlessness, confusion, and hallucinations _____

60. spasms of the tongue and facial muscles after withdrawal from tranquilizers _____

61. group of disorders characterized by nervousness in response to an anticipated future event _____

Identify the correctly spelled term in each set.

62. _____

    a. sychosomatic

    b. psychosommatic

    c. psykosomatic

    d. psychosomatic

63. _____

    a. kataplexy

    b. cateplexy

    c. cataplexy

    d. cataplechsi

64. _____

    a. hypochondria

    b. hypokondria

    c. hyphchondrea

    d. hypechondria

65. _____

    a. pysychiatry

    b. psychiatry

    c. psychoiatry

    d. physchiatry

66. _____

    a. hallucination

    b. hallucinnation

    c. hallusination

    d. hallusincation

Unscramble the letters to form a medical term.

67. timsaatziona _____

68. caip _____

69. abailu _____

70. gotonniic _____

71. echyps _____

Define the following abbreviations.

72. CPAP _____

73. UPPP _____

74. ADHD _____

75. IQ _____

76. TAT _____

LEVEL THREE: THINKING CRITICALLY

Provide a short answer to the following question.

77. A patient has arm paralysis for which no known physiological disturbance can be found. This is an example of _____.

KEY TERMS SPELLING TEST FROM CD-ROM

Use the CD-ROM to test yourself on the spelling of key terms from this chapter. Listen to the terms and write them on a separate sheet of paper. Use a medical dictionary to check your answers.

ANSWERS

WORD GROUPING

Definition	Word Part
down	cata-
affinity for, craving for	-phil, -phile
away, separated, deprived	ap-, aph-, apo-
condition involving speech	-lalia
fear or dread	-phobia
form, shape	morph-, morpho-
hysteria	hyster-, hystero-
mental disorder	-phrenia
mind, mental, psychologic	psych-, psyche-, psycho-
mind, soul, emotions	thym-, thymi-, -thymia, thymo-
nerve, nerve tissue	neur-, neuri-, neuro-
obsession, compulsion	-mania
sleep	somn-, somno-
sleep, hypnosis	hypn-, hypno-
somatic, body	somat-, somato-
split, cleft	schiz-, schizo-
stupor, narcosis	narco-
tendency	-phoria
word, speech	log-, -logia, logo-

WORD BUILDING

Word Part	Meaning	Common or Known Word	Example Medical Term
ap-, aph-, apo-	away, separated, deprived	apathy	apathy
cata-	down	catacomb	catatonic
hypn-, hypno-	sleep, hypnosis	hypnotic	hypnosis
hyster-, hystero-	hysteria	hysteric	hysteria
log-, -logia, logo-	word, speech	logogram	logospasms
-mania	obsession, compulsion	mania	hypermania
morph-, morpho-	form, shape	morphology	dysmorphophobia
narco-	stupor, narcosis	narcotic	narcolepsy
neur-, neuri-, neuro-	nerve, nerve tissue	neuron	neurosis
-phil, -phile	affinity for, craving for	bibliophile	pedophile
-phobia	fear or dread	claustrophobia	agoraphobia
-phrenia	mental disorder	schizophrenia	schizophrenia
psych-, psyche-, psycho-	mind, mental, psychologic	psychiatrist	psychology
schiz-, schizo-	split, cleft	schizophrenia	schizophrenia
somat-, somato-	somatic, body	somatotype	somatoform
thym-, thymi-, -thymia, thymo-	mind, soul, emotions	thymic	dysthymia

KEY TERM PRACTICE

Mental Disorders Preview
1. psychosis; psychoses
2. neurosis; neuroses

Mental Health Professionals
1. psychiatrist; psychology
2. mind, mental, psychological; psychotherapy

Using the *DSM-IV-TR*
1. multiaxial assessment
2. severity and course specifiers

Clinical Tests and Scales
1. Stanford-Binet intelligence scale; Wechsler intelligence scale
2. Rorschach test

Disorders Usually First Diagnosed in Infancy, Childhood, or Adolescence
1. pica
2. Tourette
3. lesion

Delirium, Dementia, and Amnestic and Other Cognitive Disorders
1. vascular dementia
2. Alzheimer disease (AD) or dementia of the Alzheimer type

Substance-Related Disorders
1. alcohol abuse; alcoholism
2. delirium tremens (DT)

Schizophrenia and Other Psychotic Disorders
1. tardive dyskinesia
2. schizophrenia

Mood Disorders
1. bipolar disorder
2. Seasonal affective disorder (SAD)

Anxiety Disorders
1. phobia
2. Post-traumatic stress disorder (PTSD)

Somatoform Disorders
1. hypochondria; hypochondriasis
2. hysteria; hysteria

Factitious Disorders
1. factitious
2. Münchhausen syndrome

Dissociative Disorders
1. Fugue
2. Dissociative

Sexual and Gender Identity Disorders
1. fetishism
2. paraphilia

Eating Disorders
1. anorexia nervosa; bulimia nervosa

Sleep Disorders
1. dyssomnias
2. Sleep apnea

Personality Disorders
1. personality
2. narcissistic personality disorder

CASE STUDY

1. c is the correct answer.
   - a is incorrect because his lack of attention at work is a new behavior, and if he had ADHD, he would have had attention problems his whole life.
   - b is incorrect because dysthymic disorder occurs for a period of at least 2 years.
   - d is incorrect because John's weight loss is probably the result of his stomach problems and his depression.
2. a is the correct answer.
   - b is incorrect because most people with depression have at least considered suicide as an option.
   - c is incorrect because any thoughts of suicide should be addressed.
   - d is incorrect because someone who is serious about suicide has a method and a plan to carry it out.
3. c is the correct answer.
   - a is incorrect because gastroenteritis is a physical issue.
   - b is incorrect because John did not mention that he felt uncomfortable in his apartment.
   - d is incorrect because lack of exercise is a physical issue.
4. d is the correct answer.

REAL WORLD REPORT

1. 296.22
2. major depression disorder, single episode, moderate
3. a. 558.9; b. gastroenteritis acute
4. divorce, conflict with child, difficulty concentrating and completing projects

REVIEW AND APPLICATION: THREE-LEVEL LEARNING SYSTEM

Level One: Reviewing Facts and Terms Using Recall

1. a
2. c
3. b
4. d
5. a
6. c
7. b
8. d
9. c
10. b

Level Two: Reviewing Concepts

11. a
12. d
13. c
14. b
15. logospasm; dysmorphophobia
16. Münchhausen syndrome by proxy; transsexualism
17. d
18. a
19. b
20. e
21. c
22. e
23. d
24. a
25. c
26. b
27. d
28. c
29. e
30. b
31. a
32. b
33. e
34. d
35. a
36. c
37. e
38. a
39. d
40. b
41. c
42. b
43. a
44. e
45. d
46. c
47. phobophobia
48. pyrophobia
49. zoophobia
50. gynephobia
51. pathophobia
52. assistance with personal or psychological matters given by a professional
53. total indifference or absence of interest
54. spasmodic vocalization or muscular contraction
55. emotions that disrupt other aspects of life
56. to give oneself sexual pleasure by stroking the genitals to achieve orgasm
57. factitious disorder
58. Münchhausen syndrome
59. delirium
60. tardive dyskinesia
61. anxiety disorders
62. d
63. c
64. a
65. b
66. a
67. somatization
68. pica
69. abulia
70. cognition
71. psyche
72. continuous positive airway pressure
73. uvulopalatopharyngoplasty
74. attention-deficit/hyperactivity disorder
75. intelligence quotient
76. thematic apperception test

Level Three: Thinking Critically

77. hysteria

chapter 19

Pharmacology

OBJECTIVES

After completing this chapter, you should be able to:

1. Define the meaning of word parts relative to pharmacology.
2. Explain general principles of pharmacology.
3. Define basic pharmacological terms.
4. Describe the relationship between normal physiology and drug metabolism.
5. Identify drug treatments according to their classification.
6. Explain the necessity of altering dosage levels throughout the lifespan.
7. Define abbreviations related to pharmacology.
8. Define terms used in medical reports involving pharmacology.
9. Correctly define, spell, and pronounce the chapter's medical terms.

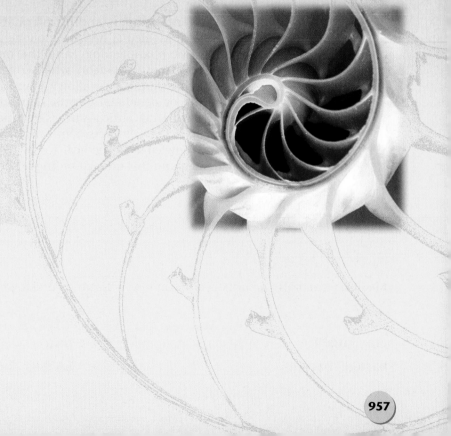

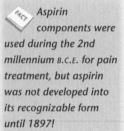

Professional Profile: Registered Pharmacist

Carl is a registered pharmacist (RPh) working in a hospital pharmacy. The hospital venue provides ample opportunity to be involved in drug-therapy decision making through interaction among physicians, nurses, dietitians, and patients.

Understanding drug classes is critical for knowing clinical effects, drug compositions, and physical and chemical properties. Hospital pharmacists do a considerable amount of drug compounding, which involves mixing ingredients to form tablets, capsules, ointments, and solutions. Regular evaluation of drug use patterns and outcomes for hospital patients is another aspect of the job. A monthly report summarizes the general use of each drug and the name of the prescribing physicians.

Carl graduated with a bachelor of science degree in pharmacy 15 years ago. The pharmacy program is 5 years of study. The first 2 years are spent taking prepharmacy courses like general biology and chemistry, anatomy and physiology, and organic chemistry. Medical terminology was not a required course for Carl, but it would have helped considerably in his anatomy and physiology and dispensing courses. During the 3rd and 4th years, Carl studied pharmaceutics, pharmaceutical chemistry, biochemical pharmacology, and pharmacy administration. The 5th year was an internship in which he worked under the direction of a licensed pharmacist. After graduation, he passed the state licensing examination and began work immediately.

As in all medical professions, it is important to keep accurate, confidential records of drugs dispensed. This is a rewarding field requiring scientific aptitude, good communications skills, and a desire to help others. Pharmacy also requires close attention to detail because filling prescriptions directly affects the lives of others.

Aspirin components were used during the 2nd millennium B.C.E. for pain treatment, but aspirin was not developed into its recognizable form until 1897!

INTRODUCTION

Approximately 80 billion aspirin tablets are taken yearly in the United States!

A fundamental understanding of pharmacology begins with learning medical terminology. Medicinal items, supplements, and terms inundate everyday life. Basic principles of pharmacology and the mechanisms of drug action are important considerations for any person, whether he or she works in the health-care field or not. Something as simple as swallowing an aspirin from the medicine cabinet can have devastating or beneficial effects, depending on the individual. Previous chapters mentioned pharmaceutic agents as treatments for pathologic conditions. This chapter focuses on a few key facts about and classification of common pharmaceutics. A working knowledge of medical terms helps in comprehending newly encountered drug names; and this understanding is beneficial to everyone.

MEDICAL TERM PARTS

WORD PARTS

Medical term prefixes, suffixes, and combining forms related to pharmacology are introduced in this section.

Word Parts	Meaning
alge-, algesi	pain
bacteri-, bacterio-	bacteria, bacterial

Word Parts	Meaning
chrys-, chryso-	gold
-cide	killer, killing
emet-, emeto-	vomiting
-esthesia, esthesio-	sense, sense perception
iatro-	physicians, medicine, treatment
ino-	muscle fiber
lingu-, lingua-, lingui, linguo-	tongue, lingual
pharmaco-	drug
rect-, recto-	rectum, rectal
-stat	substance that keeps something from changing
top-, topo-	local
tox-, toxi-, toxico-, toxo-	poison, toxin

WORD ETYMOLOGY

Some words have Greek or Latin word roots but are not true word parts. This section lists those that are used as medical terms.

Word	Definition
algos	a pain
iatros	physician
pharmakon	medicine

MEDICAL TERM PARTS USED AS PREFIXES

Prefix	Definition
iatro-	physicians, medicine, treatment
ino-	muscle fiber
pharmaco-	drug

MEDICAL TERM PARTS USED AS SUFFIXES

Suffix	Definition
-cide	killer, killing
-stat	substance that keeps something from changing

WORD GROUPING

Using the "Medical Term Parts" tables, identify the prefix, suffix, or combining form for each of the following definitions. The first one has been done as an example.

Definition	Word Part
tongue, lingual	lingu-, lingua-, lingui, linguo-
bacteria, bacterial	
drug	
gold	
killer, killing	
local	
muscle fiber	
pain	
physicians, medicine, treatment	
poison, toxin	
rectum, rectal	
sense, sense perception	
substance that keeps something from changing	
vomiting	

WORD BUILDING

Word parts, introduced in the "Medical Term Parts" section, are listed in the following table. For this exercise, first supply the meaning of each word part, then use the word part to build a word you already know. The word you list under "Common or Known Word" does not have to be a medical term; a commonly used word is fine. Be sure, however, that the word correctly reflects the intended meaning. The first one has been done as an example.

Word Part	Meaning	Common or Known Word	Example Medical Term
bacteri-, bacterio-	bacteria, bacterial	bacteria	bacteria
alge-, algesi			analgesia
-cide			bactericidal
-esthesia, esthesio-			anesthesia
iatro-			iatrogenic
lingu-, lingua-, lingui, linguo-			sublingual
pharmaco-			pharmacology
rect-, recto-			rectal
-stat			bacteriostatic
top-, topo-			topical
tox-, toxi-, toxico-, toxo-			toxicology

FUNDAMENTALS

Pharmacology Preview

The scope of health care is expanding, particularly with the arsenal of medicines currently available, and it is important to distinguish among the various terms related to this area of medicine. **Pharmacology** is the science and study of drugs, including the sources, chemistry, properties, nature, and actions of those drugs. Sources of drugs include plants, minerals, animals, bacteria, and laboratories for synthetically produced agents. A **pharmacologist** is a person who studies and practices pharmacology.

Pharmacotherapy, or chemotherapy, is the treatment of disease by means of drugs. The branch of pharmacology dealing with active substances found in plants and animal sources of crude (unrefined) drugs is termed **pharmacognosy. Toxicology** is the study of poisons, including their source, chemical composition, action on the body, and antidotes. The momentum for pharmacognosy is amazing as new plants and their medicinal merits are discovered. Furthermore, the nature of the human condition drives drug development so that disease can be prevented, treated, or eradicated.

Comparable to pharmacology, **pharmacy** is the science or profession of **dispensing** (preparing and distributing) drugs used as medical treatments. It is also the place where drugs for treating disorders are dispensed and sold. A **prescription** (Rx) is a written order issued by a qualified, licensed practitioner that authorizes a pharmacist to supply medication for a particular patient. The abbreviation *Rx* is derived from the Latin for "recipe" and literally means "take recipe." Prescription drugs can be dispensed only with the order from a licensed professional, such as a physician, and in some states nurse practitioners, psychologists, and optometrists. Over-the-counter (OTC) drugs require no prescription.

The person trained and licensed to dispense medicinal drugs and advise on their use is a **pharmacist**. The drugs distributed are known by two similar-sounding terms: **pharmaceuticals** or **pharmaceutics**.

Most instructional abbreviations commonly encountered on prescription and drug notes are derived from Latin terms. Table 19-1 explains each abbreviation.

A **generic** is the scientific name for a drug that does not carry a brand name or trademark. A brand name or trade drug name is usually the trademark of a manufacturer for a particular product. As a proper noun, brand names or trade drug names typically begin with capital letters. The chemical name indicates the description of the drug's chemical action or drug classification. For example, Tagamet is the trade name, cimetidine is the generic name, and H_2-histamine-receptor blocker is the classification.

This chapter focuses on the various classifications of drugs, their primary mechanism of action or function, and examples of commonly prescribed drugs. The fundamental principles of pharmacology are explained to teach medical terms associated with drugs and prescription orders.

Key Terms	Definitions
pharmacology (fahr muh KOL uh jee)	science of the nature and properties of drugs, particularly their actions
pharmacologist (fahr muh KOL uh jist)	one who studies pharmacology
pharmacotherapy (fahr muh koh THERR uh pee)	treatment of disease by drugs
pharmacognosy (fahr muh KOG nuh see)	science of crude natural drugs
toxicology (tock si KOL uh jee)	science of the nature and effects of poisons, their detection, and treatments
pharmacy	art and science of preparing and dispensing drugs; apothecary

TABLE 19-1 Prescription Order Abbreviations

Abbreviation	Term	Definition
$\bar{A}$	ante	before
aa	—	of each
ac	ante cibos	before meals
ad lib	ad libitum	as desired
agit	agitate	shake, stir
AM	ante meridiem	before noon; morning
Aq	aqua	water
Aq dest.	aqua destillata	distilled water
bid	bis in die	twice a day
c	cum	with
cap(s)	—	capsule, capsules
cc	—	cubic centimeter
cm	—	centimeter
D5W, D_5W	—	dextrose 5% in water
DAW	—	dispense as written
dc, D/C	—	discontinue
dil	dilutus	dilute, dissolve
disp	—	dispense
dr	—	dram
DS	—	double strength
elix	—	elixir
ext	—	extract
g	—	gram
gr	—	grain
gt	gutta	drop
gtt	guttae	drops
h, hr	—	hour
hs	hora somni	at bedtime
IA	—	intra-arterial
ID	—	infecting dose
IM	—	intramuscular
IV	—	intravenous
IVPB	—	IV piggyback
kg	—	kilogram
L	—	liter
lb.	—	pound
mEq, meq	—	milliequivalent
mg	—	milligram
mL	—	milliliter

TABLE 19-1 Prescription Order Abbreviations (*continued*)

Abbreviation	Term	Definition
no	—	number
non rep	—	do not repeat
NPO	non per os	nothing by mouth
OD	oculus dexter	right eye
oint, ung	—	ointment
OS	oculus sinister	left eye
OTC	—	over-the-counter
OU	oculus uterque	both eyes
oz.	—	ounce
p, p̄	post	after
pc	post cibos	after meals
PM	post meridiem	afternoon
PO, po	per os	by mouth
PR	per rectum	per rectum
prn	pro re nata	as needed
q	quodque	every
qam	—	every morning
qh	quaque hora	every hour
q2h, q3h	—	every 2 hours, every 3 hours
qhs	quaque hora somni	every night at bedtime
qid	quarter in die	four times a day
qs	quantum satis	sufficient quantity
R	—	rectal
rept, repet	—	may be repeated
Rx	recipe	take, prescription
s	sine	without
SC, SQ	—	subcutaneous
Sig, S	signa	label
sos	si opus sit	if needed
ss	semis	one-half
stat	statim	at once, immediately
sup, supp	—	suppository
tab	—	tablet
tbsp, T	—	tablespoon (15 mL)
tid	ter in die	three times a day
tinct	tinctura	tincture
tsp	—	teaspoon (5 mL)
TO	—	telephone order
VO	—	verbal order

dispensing	preparing and distributing medicines
prescription	order of written instructions designating the preparation and use of medication, therapy, or a medical device
pharmacist (FAHR muh sist)	one who practices pharmacy
pharmaceuticals (fahr muh SUE ti kulz)	medicinal drugs; pharmaceutics
pharmaceutics (fahr muh SUE ticks)	medicinal drugs; pharmaceuticals
generic (je NERR ick)	scientific name for a drug whose name is not registered or protected by trademark

Key Term Practice: Pharmacology Preview

1. An order of written instructions prescribing a medicine is called a/an _____.

2. The scientific name of a drug is termed the _____ name.

3. The word part _____ means "drug," and the word part *-logy* means _____; so _____ means the study of drugs.

Basic Pharmacologic Terms

The actions of drugs on the body and the body's reaction to drugs are the center of pharmacology. **Drugs** are any substances other than food or water that are taken for medicinal purposes. **Pharmacodynamics** is the study of drug actions on the body. For the most part, drugs interact with cell receptors, which mediate the actions of drugs. Individual reactivity to drugs is highly variable. **Pharmacokinetics** pertains to the effects of the body on drugs. It involves drug absorption, distribution, metabolism, and elimination.

Pharmacodynamics and pharmacokinetics are critical to realizing the drug's efficacy and potency. **Efficacy** is the maximum response of a drug, regardless of dose, and **potency** is the pharmacologic strength of that drug. The **lethal dose** is designated as LD, which is the amount likely to cause death, and the **effective dose** (ED) is the dose required to produce desired effects.

Dosage levels can be described in terms of their effectiveness. For example, the **curative dose** (CD) is the individual amount of medication needed to cure disease or correct deficiency, whereas the **loading dose** is a single, large dose of a drug initially given to achieve therapeutic level more quickly than repeated small doses would. The **maintenance dose** refers to the systematic dosage of medication required to maintain protection against exacerbation (increase in disease severity or symptoms).

For drugs to be effective, they must be readily accessible to the target tissue. **Bioavailability** is the degree to which a drug becomes available to target tissues after administration. Blood plasma delivers the drug to the tissues. Bioavailability is regarded as the amount of drug that reaches the systemic circulation by any route of administration. It is measured against the intravenous route, which is stipulated to have 100% bioavailability.

A primary factor to consider in bioavailability is first-pass metabolism or first-pass effect. **First-pass metabolism** is the initial barrier a medicine encounters, or where it is filtered. It involves intestinal and hepatic (liver) degradation and alteration of an oral drug after absorption, which removes some of the agent's active substances from the blood before it enters the general circulation. The liver metabolizes drugs on their way from the gastrointestinal (GI) tract to the body's systemic circulation. After passing through the liver, the drug must still contain enough compound (be biologically available) to be effective once it reaches its target tissue.

Key Terms	Definitions
drugs	natural or artificial substances used to treat or prevent illness
pharmacodynamics (fahr muh koh dye NAM icks)	drug actions on the body
pharmacokinetics (fahr muh koh ki NET icks)	effects of the body on a drug
efficacy (EF i kuh see)	ability of a drug to produce desired results
potency (POH tun see)	strength, or the dose or concentration required to bring about 50% of the drug's maximal effect
lethal dose	amount of drug that will cause death
effective dose	amount of drug that will produce desired effects
curative (KEW ruh tiv) **dose**	amount of drug required to cure disease or correct a deficiency
loading dose	single, large dose of a drug given at the onset of therapy to achieve a therapeutic level quickly
maintenance dose	amount of drug needed to keep the drug concentration at a desired level
bioavailability (bye oh uh vale uh BIL i tee)	amount of drug that is absorbed, obtainable, and delivered to the target tissue
first-pass metabolism	drug metabolism in the liver or intestines before reaching the general circulation; first-pass effect

Key Term Practice: Basic Pharmacologic Terms

1. The _____ is the amount of drug that will cause death.

2. The body's actions on the drug is termed _____; the action of the drug on the body is known as _____.

Drug Reactions, Regulations, and References

Before a drug can be marketed, it undergoes rigorous research, tests, and development. During the design stage, many effects are learned about the particular agent. However, despite scrupulous testing, a drug could still unfavorably affect a person. This undesirable response is known as an **adverse drug reaction** (ADR) or **adverse drug event** (ADE). Medical drugs and surgical treatments can also produce **iatrogenic** results, which are inadvertent, adverse responses induced by the treatment itself. A **side effect** is the result of a drug that is in addition to, or an extension of, the desired effect. It usually connotes an undesirable effect but is technically the expanded application of the drug's normal actions. For instance, excessive bleeding that occurs after administration of an anticoagulant demonstrates a side effect that is an extension of the desired treatment, although it is not desired. In other cases, a side effect could be an unrelated, undesirable result that occurs from drug administration. The development of Cushing disease after steroid treatment is an example of a negative side effect.

During drug testing, the agent is compared to an inert substance known as a **placebo,** which contains no active ingredients. Placebos are given to patients participating in clinical trials to compare to and assess the performance of the actual new drug. The placebo effect is a sense of benefit felt by a patient that arises solely from the knowledge that treatment has been given.

A drug **contraindication** is any special symptom, condition, or circumstance that makes the treatment improper, inadvisable, or undesirable. Contraindications are often seen with a drug interaction, whereby the effect of one drug is modified (usually negatively) by another drug given simultaneously or when a condition, such as pregnancy, renders a particular treatment imprudent. **Potentiation** means that the pharmacologic response of administering two or more drugs is greater than the sum of each acting separately. Thus giving two particular drugs simultaneously has greater benefit than giving either one or the other.

Terms directly related to the patient are addiction, compliance, palliative, and prophylactic. **Addiction** is a state of physiological or psychological dependence on a drug, and **compliance** refers to the patient's willingness to conform to treatment and/or a prescribed regimen. A prescribed recommended program of medication, diet, exercise, or other measures intended to improve health or fitness or stabilize a medical condition is termed **regimen**. A **palliative** is a medicine that treats symptoms only. The goal of palliative care is the relief of mental and physical pain when no cure is available. Last, a **prophylactic** is a drug that prevents the development of a disease or condition.

In the United States, the manufacture, distribution, and use of medications are regulated by the government. This guarantees that all drug preparations with the same name are of equal safety, strength, quality, and purity. The safety of food and drugs in the United States is ensured by the Food and Drug Administration (FDA), a part of the U.S. Department of Health and Human Services. This agency is responsible for enforcing the Food, Drug, and Cosmetic Act (FDCA), which regulates the quality, purity, potency, effectiveness, safety, labeling, and packaging of food, drug, and cosmetic products. Another act, the Controlled Substances Act, governs the prescribing, manufacturing, and dispensing of controlled substances, which are assigned to five schedules. **Controlled substances** or **schedule drugs**, are pharmacologic agents subject to the Controlled Substances Act. Substances are assigned to one of five schedules, numbered I to V, according to their potential for or evidence of abuse, potential for psychic or physiologic dependence, contribution to a public health risk, harmful pharmacologic effect, or role as a precursor of other controlled substances. Table 19-2 lists the drug schedules with examples.

The Controlled Substances Act requires prescribers and dispensers to register with the Drug Enforcement Agency (DEA), pay a fee, receive a personal registration number (DEA number) that accompanies all prescriptions, and keep a record of all controlled drugs prescribed and dispensed. The DEA enforces the Controlled Substances Act.

Uniform drug formulations, or standards, have been established to control the manufacture of like drugs from various pharmaceutic companies. Therefore, in the United States, a drug will have equal strength, quality, and purity regardless of place or manufacturer. The standard for preparing and dispensing drugs is outlined in the *United States Pharmacopeia* (*USP*), an authorized publication that serves as the national formulary. A **pharmacopeia** is a book or database that lists drugs used in medical practice and describes their composition, preparation, use, dosages, effects, and side effects. The federal government recognizes this listing as the official standard for all drugs dispensed in the United States. Over-the-counter medicines, such as vitamins and minerals that conform to these standards are stamped *USP* on the label.

Drug references are available in many forms. The *Physicians' Desk Reference* (*PDR*) is published yearly and lists patient information approved by the FDA. This large book describes the efficacy, adverse effects, pharmacology, and proper use of drugs. The vast majority of the information is the same as that found in pharmaceutic inserts or circulars contained in drug packaging. Manufacturers pay to be listed in the text, which is divided into six sections.

A drug **formulary** is a reference book containing formulas for the compounding of medicinal preparations. It also lists pharmaceutic products with details of their use and properties. Hospitals, medical offices, and insurance companies frequently refer to formularies.

FACT *In 2000, approximately 1.2% of the American population reported using heroin at least once.*

FACT *In 1874, chemist C. R. Alder Wright first synthesized heroin from morphine!*

TABLE 19-2   Drug Schedules

Schedule	Potential for Abuse	Description	Examples
I	high	• no current accepted medical use	heroin, marijuana, LSD, various amphetamines
II	high	• current accepted medical use • abuse leads to psychologic or physical dependence • no telephone orders • cannot be refilled	cocaine, codeine, Demerol, Dilaudid, morphine; certain Cannibis, amphetamines, barbiturates
III	medium—less than I or II	• current accepted medical use • moderate to low potential for physical dependence • can be refilled • 5 refill maximum • no prescription filled after 6 months of original prescription date	opium, Vicodin, Tylenol with codeine; other narcotic, amphetamine, barbiturates
IV	low—less than III	• current accepted medical use • limited potential for dependence • can be refilled • 5 refill maximum • no prescription filled after 6 months of original prescription date	Darvocet, Equanil, Librium, Valium, other barbiturates
V	less than IV	• current accepted medical use • limited dependence possible • can be refilled as authorized on the prescription by the prescribing practitioner • some may not require a prescription	Donnagel-PG, Lomotil, Robitussin A-C

Key Terms	Definitions
adverse drug reaction	undesirable response to a drug; adverse drug event
adverse drug event	undesirable response to a drug; adverse drug reaction
iatrogenic (eye at roh JEN ick)	induced inadvertently by medical treatment, procedure, or physician activity
side effect	an extension or secondary effect of a drug's action
placebo (pluh SEE boh)	substance with no medicinal ingredients, yet the person may derive therapeutic effects
contraindication (kon truh in di KAY shun)	symptom, indication, or condition in which a remedy or method of treatment is inadvisable

potentiation (poh ten shee AY shun)	the effect of the combination of two drugs resulting in an action greater than the total effect of each used separately; synergism
addiction	psychological and physiological dependence on a substance
compliance	readiness to conform to a treatment
regimen (REJ i mun)	treatment plan directed at improving health
palliative (PAL ee uh tiv)	relieving or soothing symptoms but not curing the disorder
prophylactic (proh fi LACK tick)	measure to prevent the development of a condition
controlled substances	drugs requiring a prescription; schedule drugs
schedule drugs	drugs requiring a prescription; controlled substances
pharmacopeia (fahr muh koh PEE uh)	book containing dosages and descriptions of selected medicinal substances
formulary (FOR mew lerr ee)	detailed collection of formulas for medicinal preparations

Key Term Practice: Drug Reactions, Regulations, and References

1. _____ results when two drugs taken together are more beneficial than if each were administered separately.

2. Drugs that have a high potential for abuse and can be legally obtained only by prescription are called _____ or _____.

3. A/an _____ effect occurs when the treatment itself causes patient harm and is derived from the word part _____, meaning "physicians, medicine, or treatment."

Routes of Administration

Physically introducing something into the body is termed administration. Several routes for administering drugs exist, and each differs in terms of bioavailability, the fraction of unchanged drug reaching systemic circulation (Fig. 19-1). A drug is administered directly into a vein with the **intravenous** (IV) **route.** This method allows for rapid delivery and 100% bioavailability. The **buccal route** is an administration between the cheeks and gum. Absorption occurs directly into the bloodstream, and first-pass metabolism is avoided. With **inhalation**, the drug is directly delivered to respiratory tissues and bioavailability ranges from 5% to 100%. The drug must be in an aerosol or gas phase (about 2 μg), and it is rapidly absorbed as a result of the large surface area covered by the alveoli. **Parenteral** administration refers to the introduction of a drug outside the intestines, by subcutaneous, intravenous, intramuscular, or intrasternal injection. Nutrient solutions containing carbohydrates, proteins, lipids, vitamins, and minerals, are often delivered parenterally directly into a vein, bypassing the intestines. **Intramuscular** (IM) **route** refers to the drug being injected into a muscle, which allows for administration of large doses. This type of administration offers long-term effects with high bioavailability because it avoids first-pass metabolism.

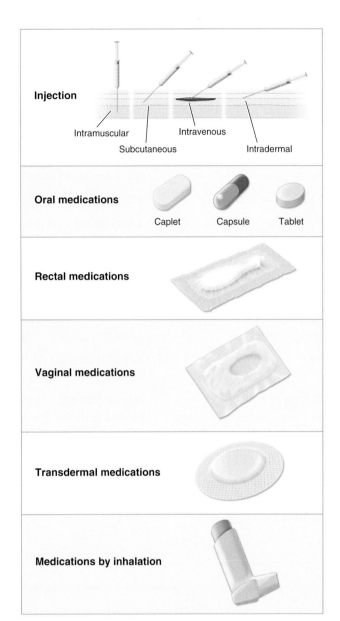

FIGURE 19-1
Several routes for administering drugs exist, and each differs in terms of the fraction of drug reaching systemic circulation.

The most common, yet complicated, route is the **oral route.** Although it is convenient, the bioavailability is altered by first-pass metabolism. *Per os* means "by mouth," and it is often charted as PO; *non per os* (NPO) means "nothing by mouth." With **rectal** administration, the drug is delivered by suppository with 30% to near 100% bioavailability, and there is less first-pass metabolism. The **vaginal** route is another method for drug delivery via a medicated suppository called a pessary (PES uh ree). An intermediate route is **subcutaneous** (SC), whereby the drug is delivered beneath the skin via hypodermic needle. There is a slower absorption rate than with IM administration, and the drug must be given in smaller dosages.

Sublingual delivery is beneath the tongue. There is immediate absorption and bioavailability with no first-pass metabolism. The **topical route** provides easy administration because the drug is applied to the body surface. The effect is local (limited to site) and absorption into circulation is slow. **Intradermal** (intracutaneous) administration involves drug delivery within the dermis. Last, **transdermal** administration occurs when a drug patch is applied to the skin to achieve systemic effects with long-term delivery.

Key Terms	Definitions
intravenous route	administering a drug into a vein
buccal (BUCK ul) **route**	administering a drug between the gum and cheek
inhalation route	substance in gas or vapor form is inspired
parenteral (puh REN tur ul) **route**	administering a drug outside the intestines by subcutaneous, intravenous, intramuscular, or intrasternal injection
intramuscular (in truh MUS kew lur) **route**	administering a drug within a muscle
oral route	administering a drug by mouth
rectal (RECK tul) **route**	administering a drug through the rectum
vaginal (VAJ i nul) **route**	administering a drug into the vagina using a medicated suppository
subcutaneous (sub kew TAY nee us) **route**	administering a drug beneath the skin
sublingual (sub LING gwul) **route**	administering a drug beneath the tongue
topical (TOP i kul) **route**	administering a drug directly to body surface being treated
intradermal (in truh DUR mul) **route**	administering a drug within the dermis; intracutaneous
transdermal (trans DUR mul) **route**	administering a drug through the skin via an adhesive patch

Key Term Practice: Routes of Administration

1. List the 13 routes of drug administration.

a. _____

b. _____

c. _____

d. _____

e. _____

f. _____

g. _____

h. _____

i. _____

j. _____

k. _____

l. _____

m. _____

THE CLINICAL DIMENSION

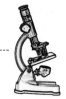

Pathology Related to Pharmacology

This section gives general features of drug classes for the sake of association. Mechanisms of action, functions, or purposes are provided, along with examples of drugs for treating specific disorders or body systems.

Autonomic Nervous System Drugs

Drugs acting on the autonomic nervous system interfere with the actions of neurotransmitters. The classifications of autonomic nervous system agents include agonists, antagonists, cholinergics, and andrenergics.

A drug that triggers a response by binding to specific receptors is termed an **agonist.** Alternately, an **antagonist** is a drug that nullifies, impedes, or opposes the effect of another substance.

Cholinergic fibers release the neurotransmitter acetylcholine (ACH) and are activated by it. **Cholinergic drugs** resemble ACH in either the way they work or the effect they have. The word part *choline-, -choline* is common to both acetyl*choline* and *choline*rgic and refers to a specific biochemical. Cholinergic agonists act on ACH, and antagonists obstruct the action of ACH.

Adrenergic drugs simulate the effects of epinephrine and norepinephrine, neurotransmitters released from the adrenal gland. Adrenergic agonists mimic the effects of epinephrine and norepinephrine and behave like those native compounds. Adrenergic antagonists reduce the effectiveness of epinephrine and norepinephrine.

Key Terms	Definitions
agonist (AG on ist)	drug that combines with receptors to initiate drug action
antagonist (an TAG uh nist)	drug that neutralizes or impedes the action of another substance
cholinergic (koh lin UR jick) **drugs**	drugs that act like acetylcholine
adrenergic (ad re NUR jick) **drugs**	drugs with characteristics of epinephrine and norepinephrine

Key Term Practice: Autonomic Nervous System Drugs

1. Drugs that act like the neurotransmitter acetylcholine are called _____ drugs.

2. _____ drugs have characteristics of epinephrine and norepinephrine from the adrenal gland.

Central Nervous System Drugs

Central nervous system (CNS) drugs affect the brain and spinal cord. Various classes exist. Anxiolytic and hypnotic drugs treat anxiety and other disorders and belong to drug classes known as barbiturates and benzodiazepines because they suppress nervous system activity. **Barbiturates** are CNS depressants that suppress respiratory functions, produce sedation and hypnosis, and can cause coma and death. Likewise, **benzodiazepines** are anxiolytic, hypnotic, anticonvulsant, and act as muscle relaxers. Drugs that prevent or reduce the severity of convulsive seizures, such as epileptic events, are called **anticonvulsants.**

Several **antidepressants**, drugs used to prevent or reduce depression, are currently available. **Selective serotonin reuptake inhibitors** (SSRIs) block the reuptake of the neurotransmitter serotonin, thereby allowing increased levels to remain in the circulation. The heightened amounts then positively affect mood.

Tricyclics and **heterocyclics** and are used to treat depression by blocking the reuptake of norepinephrine and serotonin. **Monoamine oxidase inhibitors** (MAOIs) increase the levels of norepinephrine, serotonin, and dopamine by inhibiting their degradation. These antidepressant drugs work by blocking the breakdown of monoamines by monoamine oxidase in the brain, thus allowing monoamines to build up.

Psychotropic drugs are agents that can alter psychic function, behavior, or experience. **Typical antipsychotics** block dopamine receptors. **Atypical antipsychotics** block dopamine and serotonin receptors. **Lithium** is used to treat bipolar disorder; its mechanism of action is unknown.

Epilepsy is a chronic disorder in which the brain neurons discharge sporadically causing seizures. The seizure type determines the therapy. **Antiepileptic drugs** treat partial and generalized seizures with and without convulsions.

Parkinson disease (PD) results from a loss of dopamine-containing neurons in the substantia nigra portion of the brain. Because dopamine cannot cross the blood–brain barrier (BBB), a precursor (substance that leads to another more stable compound) molecule to dopamine, such as **levodopa** (L-dopa), is needed. Levodopa is a natural substance that converts to dopamine in the brain after crossing the BBB. Dopamine agonists, such as selegiline, stimulate dopamine receptors. Anticholinergics are also used because they reduce the effectiveness of cholinergic neurons in the basal ganglia of the brain.

Narcotics are drugs that dull the senses, especially those derived from opium. Opiates act on specific CNS receptors to reduce pain perception. In therapeutic doses, narcotics diminish sensibility, relieve pain and discomfort, and produce sleep. In large doses, they cause stupor, coma, and convulsions. Opium, morphine, and codeine are classified as narcotics.

Opium is a brownish, gummy extract from the unripe seed pods of the opium poppy that contains highly addictive, narcotic alkaloid substances such as morphine and codeine. **Morphine** is the most active alkaloid of opium and is used as a narcotic **analgesic** (pain reliever). Analgesics alleviate pain without loss of consciousness. **Codeine** is an alkaloid of opium resembling morphine in action but is weaker. Codeine is used as an analgesic; **antitussive**, or cough suppressant; and **antidiarrheal**, a drug used to relieve diarrhea by either absorbing excess fluid or by slowing intestinal motility, thereby allowing more time for water reabsorption.

Opioid agonists cause analgesia, respiratory depression, smooth muscle spasms, and pinpoint pupils. Opioid antagonists have no effect when given alone, so they are administered after an agonist to reverse effects. They are typically given in cases of narcotic overdose as an antidote.

In 1853 hypodermic needle syringes with a point fine enough to pierce the skin were invented—their first use was intravenous morphine injection!

Key Terms	Definitions
barbiturates (bahr BITCH oo rates)	hypnotic and sedative drugs that depress higher brain centers
benzodiazepines (ben zoh dye AZ uh peenz)	antianxiety, hypnotic, anticonvulsant, and skeletal-muscle relaxant drugs
anticonvulsants (an tee kun VUL sunts)	drugs that treat, prevent, or arrest seizures
antidepressants (an tee de PRES unts)	drugs used to treat or prevent symptoms of persistent feelings of hopelessness

selective serotonin (serr oh TOH nin) **reuptake inhibitors**	drugs that block the reuptake of serotonin, causing increased levels to remain in circulation
tricyclics (try SICK licks)	drugs that block the reuptake of norepinephrine and serotonin
heterocyclics (het ur oh SICK licks)	drugs that block the reuptake of norepinephrine and serotonin
monoamine oxidase (mon oh AM een OCK si dace) **inhibitors**	drugs that block monoamine oxidase, thereby leading to an accumulation of amines on which this enzyme normally acts
psychotropic (sigh koh TROP ick) **drugs**	drugs that affect the mind and are used to treat psychiatric disorders
typical antipsychotics (an tee sigh KOT icks)	drugs that block dopamine receptors
atypical antipsychotics (an tee sigh KOT icks)	drugs that block dopamine and serotonin receptors
lithium (LITH ee um)	drug treatment for bipolar disorder
antiepileptic (an tee ep i LEP tick) **drugs**	agents that suppress or control epileptic seizures
levodopa (lee voh DOH puh)	natural substance that stimulates production of dopamine in brain; antiparkinson drug
narcotics	drugs that deaden the senses
opium	narcotic derived from the white poppy
morphine	narcotic analgesic
analgesic (an al JEE zick)	pain reliever
codeine (KOH deen)	drug that acts as an analgesic, antitussive, and antidiarrheal
antitussive (an tee TUS iv)	an agent that reduces the amount and severity of coughing
antidiarrheal (an tee dye uh REE ul)	an agent that prevents or reduces diarrhea

Key Term Practice: Central Nervous System Drugs

1. List two classes of anxiolytic and hypnotic drugs that suppress nervous system activity.

_____

2. Which drug class blocks receptors of only serotonin?

_____

3. What drugs are therapeutic for epilepsy?

_____

4. Opium, morphine, and codeine belong to a class of drugs called _____.

Anesthetics

Anesthetics are drugs that act on the central nervous system and cause insensibility to touch, pain, or other stimulation. An agent that induces sedation is termed a **sedative**. Sedatives have soothing or tranquilizing effects and produce drowsiness. **Tranquilizers** reduce anxiety and tension to calm a person without decreasing consciousness.

Local anesthetics typically relieve pain at the site of administration by blocking sodium channels and obstructing nerve conduction. **General anesthetics** produce drug-induced **anesthesia**, the absence of perception. There is a total loss of sensation and consciousness in the whole body.

The branch of medicine that deals with the study and use of anesthetic substances is **anesthesiology**, and a doctor or other qualified person who administers anesthesia is known as an **anesthesiologist** or **anesthetist**. Physicians specializing in anesthesiology are generally called anesthesiologists, while nurses with specialized training in anesthesiology are known as nurse anesthetists. To **anesthetize** a person is to induce anesthesia. General anesthesia is often called "putting people under" or "putting people asleep" before a surgical procedure. The mechanism of action of general anesthetics remains mostly unknown. General anesthesia is induced through inhaled and IV routes.

Key Terms	Definitions
anesthetics (an es THET icks)	drugs that cause insensibility to touch, pain, or other stimulation
sedative (SED uh tiv)	drugs that calm an anxious patient and produce drowsiness
tranquilizers (TRAN kwi lye zurz)	agents that produce a calming effect without inducing sleep
local anesthetics (an es THET icks)	drugs that cause loss of sensation at the site of administration
general anesthetics (an es THET icks)	drugs that produce loss of sensation in the whole body along with unconsciousness
anesthesia (an es THEEZH uh)	complete loss of sensation
anesthesiology (an es THEEZ ee ol uh jee)	art and science of delivering local and general anesthetics to produce sensation loss
anesthesiologist (an es theez ee OL uh jist)	physician specializing in anesthesiology who administers anesthesia
anesthetist (an ES the tist)	person who administers anesthetics
anesthetize (an ES thi tize)	to place a patient under the influence of an anesthetic

Key Term Practice: Anesthetics

1. A total loss of sensation is termed _____.

2. _____ are drugs that cause a loss of sensation at the site of administration.

3. The medical science dealing with anesthetics and anesthesia is known as _____.

Blood Drugs

Pharmacologic agents used to treat blood disorders vary in their target actions. **Antiplatelet drugs** inhibit thrombocyte aggregation (clumping), thereby prolonging bleeding; **anticoagulant drugs** interfere with hemostasis (blood clotting). **Antithrombotic drugs** reduce or prevent blood thrombi (clots), and **thrombolytic drugs** lyse (break apart) already formed thrombi. **Fibrinolytics** are drugs used to enhance the production of plasmin, a natural enzyme that dissolves clots. All these types of drugs are beneficial in the treatment of pulmonary embolism and deep vein thromboses (DVTs).

Anemia drugs treat reduced erythrocyte counts, low hemoglobin levels, or hematocrit disorders by targeting the underlying cause. Erythropoietin (epoetin alpha) is used to stimulate red blood cell production. Folic acid and vitamin B_{12} are used to treat vitamin-deficiency anemia, and iron is used to treat iron-deficiency anemia.

Lipid-lowering drugs, **antihyperlipidemics**, are used to treat increased lipoprotein levels. Classifications include statin drugs and others that increase lipase activity. Lipase is the enzyme that breaks down lipids (fats). Statin drugs inhibit an enzyme that controls cholesterol synthesis. Lipase activity enhancers increase lipoprotein lipase activity to break down lipids.

Key Terms	Definitions
antiplatelet drugs	agents that inhibit thrombocyte clumping
anticoagulant (an tee koh AG yoo lunt) **drugs**	agents that inhibit blood clotting
antithrombotic (an tee throm BOT ick) **drugs**	clot reducers or preventers
thrombolytic (throm boh LIT ick) **drugs**	agents that dissolve a thrombus (blood clot)
fibrinolytics (figh brin OH lit icks)	agents that trigger the body to produce fibrin, a natural clot-dissolving enzyme
anemia (uh NEE mee uh) **drugs**	agents used to treat reduced erythrocytes, hemoglobin, or hematocrit
antihyperlipidemics (an tee high pur lip I DEM icks)	drugs that lower blood cholesterol levels

Key Term Practice: Blood Drugs

1. Drugs that dissolve already-formed blood clots are called _____ drugs.

2. _____ drugs interfere with hemostasis.

Cardiovascular System Drugs

Cardiovascular drugs treat heart contraction disorders, hypertension (high blood pressure), heart failure, and arrhythmias (irregularity in the normal rhythm of heartbeat). Drugs that affect the force of cardiac contraction are termed **inotropics**. **Cardiac glycosides**, such as **digitalis**, are inotropics that improve heart muscle contraction to treat heart failure. **Sympathomimetic drugs** cause physiological changes similar to those produced by the sympathetic nervous system and increase heart contraction without changing blood pressure. (The word part *-mimetic* means "mimicry.") The sympathetic nervous system is involved in the "fight-or-flight" response.

Medications used to lower blood pressure are termed **antihypertensive** drugs. **Diuretics** increase urine output, thereby decreasing total fluid volume and blood pressure. Angiotensin-converting enzyme (ACE) inhibitors operate within the kidneys to block the synthesis of angiotensin II (AGII), which increases blood pressure. Another drug class, AGII receptor antagonists, interfere with the binding of AGII with its receptor. Blood pressure will not increase if the AGII signal is absent. **Calcium channel blockers** inhibit the entrance of calcium ions into heart cells to treat angina pectoris, arrhythmias, and sometimes hypertension. **Nitrates** are vasodilators (vessel relaxers) used to treat angina pectoris. **Alpha blockers** dilate arteries and veins to lower blood pressure, and **beta blockers** decrease blood pressure by preventing sympathetic stimulation of the heart. Heart failure is also treated using ACE inhibitors to reduce workload, diuretics to reduce fluid accumulation, and glycosides to enhance muscle contractility.

Targeting different aspects of cardiac physiology, primarily using blocking agents, treats heart arrhythmias. Sodium channel blockers block sodium entry into cell. Beta blockers are also used; however, their mechanism of action is unknown for treating arrhythmias. Potassium channel blockers prolong repolarization (restoration of the resting state) in heart. Calcium channel blockers slow conduction through the atrioventricular node in heart.

Key Terms	Definitions
inotropics (in oh TROP icks)	drugs that affect the force of cardiac muscle contraction
cardiac glycosides (GLYE koh sides)	drugs for treating cardiac contractility disorders
digitalis (dij i TAL us)	drug that increases the heart's contraction force
sympathomimetic (sim puh thoh mi MET ick) **drugs**	drugs that stimulate the sympathetic nervous system
antihypertensive (an tee high pur TEN siv)	drug that lowers blood pressure
diuretics (dye yoo RET icks)	agents that increase urine flow
calcium channel blockers	drugs that inhibit calcium ion flow into the heart tissue to widen the arteries and treat some cardiac conditions
nitrates (NIGH trates)	drugs used to treat angina pectoris
alpha blockers	drugs that dilate vessels to lower blood pressure
beta blockers	drugs that prevent sympathetic stimulation of the heart to lower blood pressure

Key Term Practice: Cardiovascular System Drugs

1. Drugs that affect cardiac contraction are termed _____, derived from the word part _____, meaning "muscle fiber."

2. The class of cardiac drugs that mimic the effect of the sympathetic nervous system is termed _____.

Respiratory System and Allergy Drugs

Histamine antagonists block histamine, a mediator of inflammation and part of the allergic response. Because of this action, histamine antagonists are called antihistamines. **Antihistamines** are capable of preventing, counteracting, or diminishing the effects of histamine such as sneezing and itching. They also reduce the rate of acid secretions in the stomach by blocking cell receptors for histamine. **Decongestants** reduce or relieve nasal congestion and swelling.

Beta agonists cause bronchodilation and are used as **bronchodilators**, agents that dilate the bronchial tree, in aerosol sprays. Bronchodilators treat asthma. Leukotriene modifiers cause bronchoconstriction for prophylactic treatment of chronic asthma. Cromolyn is used for the prophylactic treatment of asthma, but its mechanism of action is not known. Cholinergic antagonists block parasympathetic bronchoconstriction and are used to treat chronic obstructive pulmonary disease (COPD).

An agent that stimulates the production and secretion of phlegm to be liquefied and coughed up is termed an **expectorant. Mucolytics** are agents that dissolve mucus to facilitate ease of expectorating.

Key Terms	Definitions
antihistamines	drugs that block histamine receptors to prevent allergic effects
decongestants	agents that reduce or relieve nasal congestion
bronchodilators (bronk oh dye LAY turz)	drugs that widen and relax lung passages
expectorant (eck SPECK toh runt)	a medicine that promotes phlegm production and thinning to be coughed up and out
mucolytics (mew koh LIT icks)	agents that dissolve or liquefy mucus so that it can be coughed out

Key Term Practice: Respiratory System and Allergy Drugs

1. _____ are drugs that block cell receptors for histamine.

2. An agent that dissolves mucus is termed a/an _____.

Endocrine System Drugs

Drugs used to treat endocrine disorders replace hormones or impede hormonal action or secretion. **Adrenocortical hormones** are derived from the adrenal cortex and include glucocorticoids and mineralocorticoids. Glucocorticoids promote protein catabolism and gluconeogenesis (formation of glucose) and have anti-inflammatory properties. Mineralocorticoids are involved with sodium and water balance. Estrogen is used as a hormone-replacement therapy or as a component of oral contraceptives.

Sex steroids are the sex hormones—estrogens, antiestrogens, progestins, antiprogestins, androgens, and antiandrogens. Selective estrogen-receptor modulators (SERMs) are estrogen agonists used to prevent postmenopausal osteoporosis. Estrogen enhances calcium retention in bones and is beneficial for the treatment of osteoporosis in postmenopausal women. Calcitonin increases calcium deposition in bones and inhibits bone break down by osteoclasts. Antiestrogens stimulate ovarian function to treat infertility or are used in the treatment of breast cancer. Progestins are used in oral contraceptives to suppress ovulation. Antiprogestins are used to terminate pregnancy.

Androgens are used as hormone-replacement therapy for the treatment of testicular deficiency. Antiandrogens are used to treat excessive hair growth in women and prostate cancer in men. Thyroid treatments are aimed at replacing thyroid hormone or suppressing thyroid function. Thyroid hormones are used to treat hypothyroid conditions. Thyroid downers inhibit thyroid hormone synthesis and are used to treat hyperthyroid conditions.

Diabetes is a major pancreatic disorder treated by endocrine-system drugs. The goal of diabetes treatment is to lower circulating levels of blood glucose. Insulin can be injected to assist in lowering blood glucose levels. Oral hypoglycemics also decrease glucose levels.

Key Terms	Definitions
adrenocortical (a dree noh KOR ti kul) **hormones**	steroid hormones from the cortex of the adrenal gland
sex steroids (STERR oidz)	primary sex hormones

Key Term Practice: Endocrine System Drugs

1. Hormones derived from the adrenal cortex are termed _____ hormones.

Gastrointestinal System Drugs

Drugs treating the gastrointestinal system are divided into two categories: agents for upper-GI conditions and those for lower-GI conditions. Drugs that coat the mucosa, reduce acid secretion, or increase the rate of gastric emptying treat upper-GI conditions. Drugs targeting lower intestinal disorders treat diarrhea, constipation, and obesity.

Upper-GI drugs include antacids, antagonists, coaters, inhibitors, reducers, and effectors. An **antacid** is a drug that reduces or neutralizes stomach acid to relieve symptoms of indigestion and reflux esophagitis (heartburn). Histamine-receptor antagonists prevent histamine-induced acid release. Mucosa coaters form a protective coating on the GI mucosa, and acid inhibitors block hydrogen and potassium ions and enzymes in the stomach to reduce acid secretion. Acid reducers are prostaglandin analogues that increase bicarbonate ions and mucin release while decreasing acid secretion. A gastric-emptying effector increases the rate of gastric emptying.

Lower-GI drugs include bulk-forming agents, diarrhea and constipation treatments, and chemotherapeutics for treating other disorders. Bulk-forming agents absorb water and soften feces and can be used to treat diarrhea. Diarrhea treatments are drugs that cause constipation, whereas constipation drugs are stimulants that increase motility and increase water and electrolytes in stools. **Laxatives** promote bowel movement and defecation and are used to treat constipation or to evacuate the GI tract before surgery or radiographic examination. Lipase inhibitors reduce fat absorption and are a promising treatment for obesity.

An **emetic** is an agent used to induce vomiting, especially in cases of poisoning. Agents that suppress vomiting are called **antiemetics,** and drugs that suppress nausea are termed **antinauseants.** These agents act on the centers in the brain that control vomiting.

Key Terms	Definitions
antacid	drug that neutralizes or reduces stomach acid
laxatives	drugs that relieve constipation or evacuate the bowel
emetic (e MET ick)	an agent that induces vomiting
antiemetics (an tee e MET icks)	agents that prevent or relieve vomiting
antinauseants (an tee NAW zee unts)	agents that prevent or alleviate nausea

Key Term Practice: Gastrointestinal System Drugs

1. _____ are drugs that neutralize or reduce stomach acid.

2. The word part _____ means "against," and the word part *emet*- means _____; therefore, an _____ is an agent that prevents vomiting.

Immunosuppressive Drugs

Immunosuppressive drugs inhibit the immune response to prevent rejection of transplanted organs or to thwart autoimmune disorders. **Cyclosporine** inhibits antibody and cell-mediated immune responses and enhances tissue transplants, and **cytotoxins** kill proliferating cells. Monoclonal antibodies block T lymphocyte activation to impede the immune response.

    Corticosteroids are drugs used to reduce inflammation, control allergic disorders, and prevent tissue rejection. These synthetic drugs are identical to natural corticosteroid hormone derived from the adrenal gland. Gold therapy, **chrysotherapy**, is the use of gold compounds in the treatment of disease, notably the autoimmune disease rheumatoid arthritis.

Key Terms	Definitions
immunosuppressive (im yoo noh suh PRES iv) **drugs**	agents that dampen the immune response
cyclosporine (sigh kloh SPOR een)	drug used to inhibit organ transplant rejection
cytotoxins (sigh toh TOCK sins)	agents that kill cells
corticosteroids (kor ti koh STEER oidz)	synthetic drugs that are identical to natural corticosteroid derived from the adrenal gland, used to suppress the immune response
chrysotherapy (kris oh THERR uh pee)	using gold compounds to treat disease

Key Term Practice: Immunosuppressive Drugs

1. Drugs that hamper the immune response are termed _____ drugs.

2. _____ enhances tissue transplants by inhibiting cell-mediated immunity.

3. The word part _____ refers to "gold," and the use of gold compounds to treat disease is termed _____.

Antimicrobial Drugs

Antimicrobial agents are chemotherapeutic drugs that act on microorganisms (microbes) by inhibiting, suppressing, or preventing their growth. Each class of antimicrobic is designed to act against a microbe by a specific mechanism. They are effective against bacteria, viruses, fungi, protozoa, helminths, and mycobacteria.

Antibiotics are agents that work specifically against bacteria and provide no therapeutic measures against the other microbes. Antibacterial medications can be either bacteriostatic or bactericidal. **Bacteriostatic** agents hinder or arrest bacterial growth, whereas **bactericidal** drugs destroy bacteria. (The word part -*stat* refers to a "substance that keeps something from changing;" the word part -*cide* means "killer.") Notice the nuances in spelling: bacterio*static* has a combining *o*, but bactericidal does not.

An **antiseptic** is a topical agent that prevents or reduces bacterial growth to inhibit the development of infection in cuts, scratches, or surgical incisions. Another topically applied agent, an **astringent**, shrinks blood vessels and draws skin tissue together. Astringents are used to absorb lesion secretions and lessen skin sensitivity.

The proper administration of antibiotics, requires that the organism be identified and its Gram reaction known. However, this is often not done; and in some cases, time does not permit thorough testing. Thus physicians prescribe according to the clinical picture and experience. A **Gram** (G) **reaction** is a differential staining method used for bacterial identification (Fig. 19-2). It is useful for indicating cell wall differences for antimicrobial therapy.

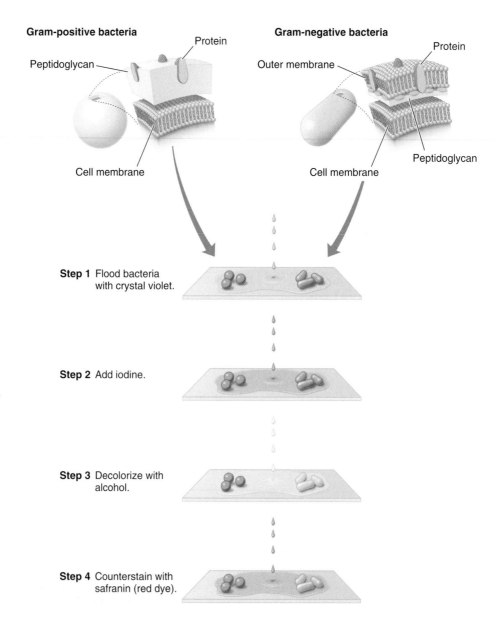

FIGURE 19-2
Gram-positive bacteria appear purple because they retain the dye. Gram-negative bacteria are pink because the cells are decolorized by alcohol. The differences in the Gram reaction are the result of variations in the bacterial cell walls, which become evident after the staining procedure.

Some drugs are more effective against Gram-positive (G+) organisms, others work better against Gram-negative (G−) microbes, and still others can be prescribed for both. **Broad-spectrum antibiotics** offer benefit against a wide variety of G+ and G− microbes. Broad-spectrum antibiotics are beneficial when a new infection in addition to a preexisting one, called a **superinfection**, exists. Prescribing an antibiotic for conditions that are not bacterial in origin (for example, against viruses) or prescribing the wrong antibiotic causes unwarranted problems and leads to microbial resistance.

Antimycobacterial drugs are effective against *Mycobacterium* species, characterized as G+ aerobic bacilli (air-requiring, rod-shaped microbes), which cause leprosy and tuberculosis. (Note the spelling of the term and avoid the temptation to write the nonsensical term "microbacterium" or the incorrectly spelled term "micobacterium.")

Key Terms	Definitions
antimicrobial (an tee migh KROH bee ul) **agents**	drugs that destroy, inhibit, or prevent microbial growth
antibiotics (an tee bye OT icks)	drugs used to fight bacterial infections
bacteriostatic (back teer oh STAT ick)	hindering bacterial growth
bactericidal (back teer i SIGH dul)	killing or destroying bacteria
antiseptic (an ti SEP tick)	agent that stops or inhibits bacterial growth
astringent (uh STRIN jent)	agent that shrinks or puckers tissues
Gram reaction	use of the Gram stain to identify bacteria
broad-spectrum antibiotics (an tee bye OT icks)	agents that are effective against both G+ and G− microorganisms
superinfection	infection in addition to a preexisting one or a second or subsequent infection
antimycobacterial (an tee migh koh back TEER ee ul) **drugs**	an agent effective against *Mycobacterium* species

Key Term Practice: Antimicrobial Drugs

1. Drugs that are effective against microorganisms are known collectively as _____ agents.

2. Drugs that are aimed at both G+ and G− organisms are called _____.

Antiviral Drugs

Antiviral drugs react against viruses. They weaken, are antagonistic to, or destroy these minute particles that live as parasites in organisms. Drugs discussed in this section treat human immunodeficiency virus (HIV), influenza, herpes, and respiratory syncytial virus (RSV).

HIV is a retrovirus that destroys the body's immune system. Acquired immunodeficiency syndrome (AIDS) is the disease that results from the absent or diminished immune response. HIV replicates using enzymes called reverse transcriptase and protease. **Reverse-transcriptase inhibitors (RTIs)** hamper reverse transcriptase and serve as one method for targeting the virus for eradication. **Protease inhibitors** interfere with viral protein processing, preventing new viral particle formation.

Influenza (flu) is a viral illness that produces a fever, sore throat, runny nose, headache, dry cough, and muscle pain. The function of influenza drugs is to lessen the severity of the symptoms. **Neuraminidase inhibitors** block the release of the influenza virus from infected cells.

Herpes is a viral infection that causes small, painful blisters and inflammation, most commonly at the junction of the skin and mucous membrane in the mouth, nose, or genitals. A herpes virus is also responsible for causing chickenpox. The function of antiherpes drugs is to lessen the severity of symptoms.

RSV causes an often serious respiratory infection in infants and children. Antiviral drugs targeted against RSV are aimed at lessening the severity of the symptoms of the infection.

Key Terms	Definitions
antiviral (an tee VYE rul) **drugs**	agents that act against viruses
reverse-transcriptase (tran SKRIP tace) **inhibitors**	agents that block the enzyme reverse transcriptase to eradicate viruses that use it for replication
protease (PROH tee ace) **inhibitors**	agents that block the enzyme protease to eradicate viruses that use it for replication
neuraminidase (newr a MIN i dace) **inhibitors**	agents that block the release of influenza virus from infected cells

Key Term Practice: Antiviral Drugs

1. Drugs acting against viruses are called _____ drugs.

Antifungal, Antiprotozoal, and Antihelminthic Drugs

Fungal infections most commonly occur on the skin, hair, and nails and to a lesser extent in the mouth, gastrointestinal tract, and in the perianal region. At times, systemic fungal infections do result. Fungi are organisms without chlorophyll that reproduce by spores and live by absorbing nutrients from organic matter. Their membranes contain ergosterol, a sterol (component of fat) that is the target of antifungal drugs. **Antifungal drugs** suppress or destroy fungi.

Protozoa are single-celled organisms, such as amoebae, that move and feed on organic compounds of nitrogen and carbon. **Antiprotozoal drugs** treat African sleeping sickness (an infection transmitted by the tsetse fly), amebiasis (diarrhea), trypanosomiasis (Chagas disease), dysentery, giardiasis (diarrhea), leishmaniasis, trichomoniasis (genital infection), malaria, *pneumocystic* infections, and toxoplasmosis.

Various parasitic worms such as flatworms, tapeworms, roundworms, or flukes are helminths. **Antihelminthic drugs** act against helminths.

Key Terms	Definitions
antifungal (an tee FUNG gul) **drugs**	agents that prevent or reduce the growth of fungi
antiprotozoal (an tee proh tuh ZOH ul) **drugs**	agents that are effective against protozoa infections
antihelminthic (an tee hel MIN thick) **drugs**	agents that target parasitic worms

Key Term Practice: Antifungal, Antiprotozoal, and Antihelminthic Drugs

1. _____ drugs target fungi and prevent or reduce their growth.

2. Agents that act against protozoa are termed _____ drugs.

3. _____ drugs target parasitic worms.

Cancer Drugs

Treatment of cancer generally involves the administration of several drugs used in combination to obtain synergistic effects. The goal of therapy is to eradicate cancer cells using **cytotoxic drugs.** Unfortunately, other cells in addition to cancer cells are killed, and numerous side effects occur with anticancer therapies. Classifications include alkylating agents, antimetabolites, immunomodulating agents, and colony-stimulating factors. An **alkylate** is used to treat certain types of malignancies. Antimetabolites compete for binding sites of enzymes or are incorporated into DNA or RNA. Immunomodulating agents enhance immune function. Colony-stimulating factors (CSFs) stimulate new cell growth after cytotoxic treatments.

Key Terms	Definitions
cytotoxic (sigh toh TOCK sick) **drugs**	agents that kill cells
alkylate (AL ki late)	drug used to treat malignances

Key Term Practice: Cancer Drugs

1. The word part *cyto-* means _____, and the word part *toxi-* means _____; thus _____ agents kill cells.

Nonsteroidal Anti-Inflammatory Drugs

Nonsteroidal anti-inflammatory drugs (NSAIDs) inhibit the synthesis of prostaglandin, a mediator of inflammation. All are analgesic and anti-inflammatory; some are **antipyretic** (fever reducing) and antithrombotic. Examples of NSAIDs are aspirin, acetaminophen (Tylenol), ibuprofen (Advil and Motrin), and naproxen (Aleve). The chemical name for **aspirin** is acetylsalicylic acid, thus it is commonly abbreviated ASA. Aspirin also inhibits cyclooxygenase (COX), an enzyme necessary for prostaglandin synthesis. COX2 inhibitors are NSAIDs that have therapeutic merit in treating rheumatoid arthritis and osteoarthritis. **Acetaminophen** has both analgesic and antipyretic properties.

> **FACT** In 1981, English physician Sir John Vane won the Nobel Prize for medicine after discovering in 1971 that aspirin works by inhibiting prostaglandin synthesis!

Key Terms	Definitions
nonsteroidal (non sterr OID ul) **anti-inflammatory drugs**	agents that relieve pain and inflammation
antipyretic (an tee pye RET ick)	fever reducer

| aspirin | drug that relieves pain and inflammation, reduces fever, and decreases the risk of blood clots |
| acetaminophen (as et uh MEE noh fen) | drug that relieves pain and reduces fever |

Key Term Practice: Nonsteroidal Anti-Inflammatory Drugs

1. Acetylsalicylic acid is the chemical name for _____.

2. Ibuprofen and naproxen are examples of _____.

CLINICAL TERMS

Term	Description
acetaminophen	drug that relieves pain and reduces fever
adrenergic drugs	drugs with characteristics of epinephrine and norepinephrine
adrenocortical hormones	steroid hormones from the cortex of the adrenal gland
agonist	drug that combines with receptors to initiate drug action
alkylate	drug used to treat malignancies
alpha blockers	drugs that dilate vessels to lower blood pressure
analgesic	pain reliever
anemia drugs	agents used to treat reduced erythrocytes, hemoglobin, or hematocrit
anesthetics	drugs that cause insensibility to touch, pain, or other stimulation
antacid	drug that neutralizes or reduces stomach acid
antagonist	drug that neutralizes or impedes the action of another substance
antibiotics	drugs used to fight bacterial infections
anticoagulant drugs	agents that inhibit blood clotting
anticonvulsants	drugs that treat, prevent, or arrest seizures
antidepressants	drugs used to treat or prevent symptoms of persistent feelings of hopelessness
antidiarrheal	an agent that prevents or reduces diarrhea
antiemetics	agents that prevent or relieves vomiting
antiepileptic drugs	agents that suppress or control epileptic seizures
antifungal drugs	agents that prevent or reduce the growth of fungi
antihelminthic drugs	agents that target parasitic worms

Term	Description
antihistamines	drugs that block histamine receptors to prevent allergic effects
antihyperlipidemics	drugs that lower blood cholesterol levels
antihypertensive	drug that lowers blood pressure
antimicrobial agents	drugs that destroy, inhibit, or prevent microbial growth
antimycobacterial drugs	agents effective against *Mycobacterium* species
antinauseants	agents that prevent or alleviate nausea
antiplatelet drugs	agents that inhibit thrombocyte clumping
antiprotozoal drugs	agents that are effective against protozoa infections
antipyretic	fever reducer
antiseptic	agent that stops or inhibits bacterial growth
antithrombotic drugs	clot reducers or preventers
antitussive	an agent that reduces the amount and severity of coughing
antiviral drugs	agents that act against viruses
aspirin	drug that relieves pain and inflammation, reduces fever, and decreases the risk of blood clots
astringent	agent that shrinks or puckers tissues
atypical antipsychotics	drugs that block dopamine and serotonin receptors
bactericidal	killing or destroying bacteria
bacteriostatic	hindering bacterial growth
barbiturates	hypnotic and sedative drugs that depress higher brain centers
benzodiazepines	antianxiety, hypnotic, anticonvulsant, and skeletal-muscle relaxant drugs
beta blockers	drugs that prevent sympathetic stimulation of the heart to lower blood pressure
broad-spectrum antibiotics	agents that are effective against both G+ and G− microorganisms
bronchodilators	drugs that widen and relax lung passages
calcium channel blockers	drugs that inhibit calcium ion flow into the heart tissue to widen arteries and treat some cardiac conditions
cardiac glycosides	drugs for treating cardiac contractility disorders
cholinergic drugs	drugs that act like acetylcholine
chrysotherapy	using gold compounds to treat disease
codeine	drug that acts as an analgesic, antitussive, and antidiarrheal

Term	Description
corticosteroids	synthetic drugs that are identical to natural corticosteroid derived from the adrenal gland, used to suppress the immune response
cyclosporine	drug used to inhibit organ transplant rejection
cytotoxic drugs	agents that kill cells
cytotoxins	agents that kill cells
decongestants	agents that reduce or relieve nasal congestion
digitalis	drug that increases heart contraction force
diuretics	agents that increase urine flow
emetic	an agent that induces vomiting
expectorant	a medicine that promotes phlegm production and thinning to be coughed up and out
fibrinolytics	agents that trigger the body to produce fibrin, a natural clot-dissolving enzyme
general anesthetics	drugs that produce loss of sensation in the whole body along with unconsciousness
heterocyclics	drugs that block the reuptake of norepinephrine and serotonin
immunosuppressive drugs	agents that dampen the immune response
inotropics	drugs that affect the force of cardiac muscle contraction
laxatives	drugs that relieve constipation or evacuate the bowel
levodopa (L-dopa)	natural substance that stimulates production of dopamine in the brain; antiparkinson drug
local anesthetics	drugs that causes loss of sensation at the site of administration
lithium	drug treatment for bipolar disorder
monoamine oxidase inhibitors (MAOIs)	drugs that block monoamine oxidase, thereby leading to an accumulation of amines on which this enzyme normally acts
morphine	narcotic analgesic
mucolytics	agents that dissolve or liquefy mucus so that it can be coughed out
narcotics	drugs that deaden the senses
neuraminidase inhibitors	agents that block the release of influenza virus from infected cells
nitrates	drugs used to treat angina pectoris
nonsteroidal anti-inflammatory drugs (NSAIDs)	agents that relieve pain and inflammation
opium	narcotic derived from the white poppy

Term	Description
protease inhibitors	agents that block the enzyme protease to eradicate viruses that use it for replication
psychotropic drugs	drugs that affect the mind and are used to treat psychiatric disorders
reverse-transcriptase inhibitors (RTIs)	agents that block the enzyme reverse transcriptase to eradicate viruses that use it for replication
sedative	drug that calms an anxious patient and produces drowsiness
selective serotonin reuptake inhibitors (SSRIs)	drugs that block the reuptake of serotonin, causing increased levels to remain in circulation
sex steroids	primary sex hormones
sympathomimetic drugs	drugs that stimulate the sympathetic nervous system
thrombolytic drugs	agents that dissolve a thrombus (blood clot)
tranquilizers	agents that produce a calming effect without inducing sleep
tricyclics	drugs that block the reuptake of norepinephrine and serotonin
typical antipsychotics	drugs that block dopamine receptors

Lifespan

The effects of drugs vary considerably among and between fetuses, newborns, infants, children, adults, and older adults. Pharmacokinetics also can be quite different in a pregnant or lactating woman than in other women. Most drugs administered to a pregnant female can cross the placenta and expose the embryo and fetus to their effects. Specific drugs are contraindicated during pregnancy owing to their potential as a teratogen (agent that causes birth defects). Drugs can also pass through breast milk. Furthermore, endocrine function during pregnancy may alter the effects of the drugs on the woman.

The first year of life marks the time in which the greatest drug variance can be found in a person. Unique factors in the neonate account for drug absorption variability. Gastric function, such as acid secretion and gastric emptying, fluctuates during the first few days of life, thus must be taken into consideration. Drug metabolism and excretion is also low in the neonate. Distribution volume of drugs changes as the infant develops.

The growing child presents further challenge because much of what is known about various drugs in children has been obtained through clinical experience and reporting, not by clinical tests because of the ethical issues involved in exposing children to unknown health risks to advance science. The body of evidence is growing, and pediatric charts are available for drug dosages.

Regardless of one's age, the mere process of growing older affects pharmacologic reaction. Drug responses are altered in the presence of other medical disorders, the general health of the individual, compliance, and dietary factors. There appears to be no age-associated decline in drug absorption; however, drug distribution does change as a result of reduced lean body mass and water composition and an increase in fat. Liver metabolism of drugs does not show a consistent decline to all agents. The decline in kidney weight and hepatic blood flow in older adults aged 60–80 years also affects drug pharmacokinetics. A high incidence of adverse drug reactions in the elderly occurs because these patients take an average of seven different prescriptions. Computer databanks are assisting in gathering critical information pertaining to drug interactions, pharmacokinetics, and pharmacodynamics throughout the lifespan.

In the News: Fen-Phen

The miracle drug for weight loss once appeared to be Fen-Phen. That is, until several cases of fatal and nonfatal pulmonary hypertension and valvular disorders were reported in women with no known risk factors for these conditions.

Fenfluramine is a drug closely related to amphetamine that affects brain levels of serotonin. Serotonin appears to be related to appetite and food intake. Fenfluramine was introduced in Europe more than 10 years ago as a drug to control appetite and food intake (anorexigenic effect) through its effects on serotonin. Its isomer (a chemical with the same number of atoms, but different chemical structure), dexfenfluramine (fen) was found to be twice as potent as fenfluramine. Controlled clinical trials demonstrated its effectiveness for controlling weight loss in patients for at least a year. Fen was then marketed in the United States and became a popular drug for rapid weight loss.

Later, life-threatening and fatal adverse effects were reported. It was difficult to determine the actual cause because dexfenfluramine was usually taken in conjunction with another amphetamine-like anorexiant, phentermine (phen), often called Fen-Phen.

Despite FDA approval and documented effects of other drugs, this is a clear case demonstrating the implications of drug interactions. Consequently, dexfenfluramine has been withdrawn from the market, and the courts have been flooded with lawsuits. Currently, the new replacement miracle cure for weight loss appears to be Phen-Pro, which consists of a combination of phentermine and fluoxetine (Prozac).

COMMON ABBREVIATIONS

Abbreviation	Term
ACE inhibitors	angiotensin-converting enzyme inhibitors
ACH	acetylcholine
ADE	adverse drug event
ADR	adverse drug reaction
AG II	angiotensin II
AIDS	acquired immunodeficiency syndrome
ASA	acetylsalicylic acid
BBB	blood–brain barrier

Abbreviation	Term
CD	curative dose
CNS	central nervous system
COPD	chronic obstructive pulmonary disease
COX	cyclooxygenase
CSFs	colony stimulating factors
DEA	Drug Enforcement Agency
DVT	deep vein thrombosis
ED	effective dose
FDA	Food and Drug Administration
FDCA	Food, Drug, and Cosmetic Act
fen	dexfenfluramine
G−	Gram negative
G+	Gram positive
GI	gastrointestinal
G reaction	Gram reaction
HIV	human immunodeficiency virus
IM	intramuscular
IV	intravenous
LD	lethal dose
L-dopa	levodopa
MAOIs	monoamine oxidase inhibitors
NPO	*non per os* (nothing by mouth)
NSAIDs	nonsteroidal anti-inflammatory drugs
OTC	over-the-counter
PD	Parkinson disease
PDR	*Physicians' Desk Reference*
phen	phentermine
PM	polymyositis
POS	physician's order sheet
RPh	registered pharmacist
RSV	respiratory syncytial virus
RTIs	reverse transcriptase inhibitors
Rx	prescription
SC	subcutaneous
SERMs	selective estrogen receptor modulators
SSRI	selective serotonin reuptake inhibitors
USP	*United States Pharmacopeia*

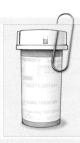

Case Study

Carl was working on a specific case with Dr. Wien, a rheumatologist, to best manage pharmacologic treatment for a patient. Wendell Jensen, a 34-year-old female, was diagnosed with polymyositis (PM) and mixed connective tissue disease. Raynaud's phenomenon initially led her to seek medical care when she began noticing that her fingertips were dark and her hands were frequently cold. She has difficulty walking up stairs and raising her arms. Mrs. Jensen made an appointment because she was feeling extremely weak and tired and thought perhaps she had a respiratory infection. Mrs. Jensen currently takes medicines on a daily basis. Her pharmaceutic agents are the following:

- methotrexate, 2.5 mg every day
- prednisone, 5 mg every other day
- diltiazem (Cardizem), 30 mg every day
- cimetidine (Tagamet), 400 mg bid
- azathioprine (Imuran), 50 mg every day

Case Study Questions

Select the best answer to each of the following questions.

1. **Polymyositis is an autoimmune disorder. Methotrexate, prednisone, and azathioprine are immunosuppressants. Immunosuppressants are best described as drugs that _____.**
   a. impede or hamper the immune response
   b. enhance the immune response
   c. alter cardiovascular function
   d. enhance tissue rejection

2. **Cardizem is classified as a calcium-channel blocker. Calcium-channel blockers _____.**
   a. are drugs that widen the arteries to slow the heart and treat heart conditions
   b. are diuretics
   c. are ACE inhibitors
   d. increase urinary output

3. **Cimetidine is used in the treatment of upper-GI conditions. This particular drug is a histamine-receptor antagonist, which _____.**
   a. increases histamine-induced acid release

   b. has no effect on acid
   c. blocks histamine-induced acid release
   d. treats diarrhea

4. **Cardizem, Imuran, and Tagamet are _____.**
   a. chemical names
   b. brand or trade names
   c. generic names
   d. formularies

5. **Cimetidine is prescribed at 400 mg bid. This means that Mrs. Jensen should take 400 mg _____.**
   a. once a day
   b. twice a day
   c. every other day
   d. every day

REAL WORLD REPORT

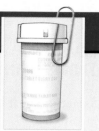

In the hospital, a physician's order sheet (POS), or chart order, is used. Carl relies on this document, which contains much of the same information as an outpatient prescription, but the duration of therapy or number of doses is often not listed. The POS contains the following information: patient's name, date of birth, name and strength of medication, dose, route and frequency of administration, date, time ordered, initials, and the physician's signature. Mrs. Jensen's report, which was received in the hospital pharmacy, follows.

CENTRAL HOSPITAL: PHYSICIAN'S ORDER SHEET

NAME: Wendell Jensen
DATE OF BIRTH: August 3, 1969
DATE: December 28, 2003

Time/Initials		Med, IV, Treatment	Dose	Route
1	1400/SKR	methotrexate	5 mg every day	oral
2	1400/SKR	prednisone	5 mg every other day	oral
3	1630/AMW	ampicillin	250 mg IV q6h × 7 days	IV
4	1700/JBN	diltiazem (Cardizem)	30 mg every day	oral
5	1700/JBN	esomeprazole magnesium (Nexium)	40 mg qam	oral
6	1700/JBN	folic acid	1 mg every day pc	oral

Physician Signature: *Dr. Wien*

REAL WORLD REPORT QUESTIONS

The following exercises review the medical terms in the preceding medical report.

1. How often was each of the following drugs administered?

   a. drug 5 _____

   b. drug 6 _____

   c. drug 3 _____

2. Ampicillin was one of the prescribed drugs.

   a. How was it administered? _____

   b. How long was the drug to be given?

   _____

3. What are the trade name for drugs 4 and 5?

   a. 4 _____

   b. 5 _____

4. Identify the meaning of pc with respect to drug 6.

   _____

REVIEW AND APPLICATION: THREE-LEVEL LEARNING SYSTEM

LEVEL ONE: REVIEWING FACTS AND TERMS USING RECALL

Select the best response to each of the following questions.

1. The science of the nature and properties of drugs is called _____.

    a. toxicology

    b. pharmacy

    c. apothecary

    d. pharmacology

2. The science of crude natural drugs is termed _____.

    a. pharmacy

    b. pharmacology

    c. pharmacognosy

    d. toxicology

3. A natural or artificial substance other than food used to treat or prevent illness is a/an _____.

    a. drug

    b. toxin

    c. loading dose

    d. agonist

4. A/an _____ is a drug that binds to a receptor to nullify the effects of an agonist.

    a. effector

    b. antagonist

    c. maintenance dose

    d. formulary

5. _____ is the ability of a drug to produce desired results.

    a. Loading dose

    b. Lethal dose

    c. Efficacy

    d. Bioavailability

6. Which term means the amount of drug absorbed and obtainable for use at the target tissue?

    a. first-pass effect

    b. bioavailability

    c. antagonist

    d. therapeutic index

7. Drug metabolism in the liver is known as _____.

    a. first-pass effect

    b. first-pass metabolism

    c. bioavailability

    d. a and b are correct

8. A/an _____ is a treatment plan for improving health.

    a. regimen

    b. compliance

    c. schedule

    d. formulary

9. An undesirable response to a drug is a/an _____.

    a. adverse drug reaction

    b. standard

    c. formulary

    d. addiction

10. A reference book of medicinal preparations is known as a/an _____.

    a. palliative

    b. apothecary

    c. formulary

    d. regimen

11. The _____ is the national formulary of the United States.

    a. DEA

    b. *U.S. Pharmacopeia*

19 —— Pharmacology **993**

c. FDCA

d. *PDR*

LEVEL TWO: REVIEWING CONCEPTS

Select the best response to each of the following questions.

12. A drug that calms an anxious patient and produces drowsiness is termed a/an _____.

   a. anesthetic

   b. diuretic

   c. agonist

   d. sedative

13. _____ are agents that directly affect bacteria.

   a. Antivirals

   b. Antibiotics

   c. Antimicrobics

   d. Antifungals

14. Drugs effective against *Mycobacterium* species are termed _____.

   a. antivirals

   b. antihelminthics

   c. antimycobacterials

   d. antifungals

15. _____ is a drug that hinders bacterial growth, and a/an _____ destroys bacteria.

   a. Bactericidal; bacteriostatic

   b. Antibiotic; bacteriostatic

   c. Antimicrobial; antibiotic

   d. Bacteriostatic; bactericidal

16. Which class of drugs improves heart muscle contraction?

   a. cardiac glycosides

   b. antihypertensives

   c. calcium channel blockers

   d. diuretics

17. While taking an antibiotic for a urinary tract infection, a patient comes down with a secondary respiratory infection. This is an example of a/an _____.

   a. superinfection.

   b. Gram reaction.

   c. bactericide.

   d. contraindication.

Provide a medical term to complete a meaningful analogy.

18. First-pass effect is to _____ as pharmaceutics are to _____.

19. Adverse drug reaction is to _____ as synergism is to _____.

Match the definition with its correct term.

_____ 20. effective dose
   a. amount of drug required to cure a disease or correct a deficiency

_____ 21. curative dose
   b. amount of drug that will produce the desired effects

_____ 22. lethal dose
   c. amount of drug needed to keep its concentration at a desired level

_____ 23. loading dose
   d. amount of drug that will cause death

_____ 24. maintenance dose
   e. single, large dose of drug given at the onset of therapy

Match the definition or action with its drug type.

_____ 25. digitalis
   a. drug that lowers blood pressure

_____ 26. antihypertensive
   b. drug that increases the force of cardiac contraction

_____ 27. diuretic
   c. drug that lowers blood cholesterol levels

_____ 28. nitrate   d. drug that treats angina pectoris

_____ 29. antihyper-lipidemic   e. drug that increases urine output

Match the term with its definition.

_____ 30. contraindication   a. one who practices pharmacy

_____ 31. expectorant   b. preparing and distributing medicines

_____ 32. pharmacist   c. symptom or condition for which the treatment is inadvisable

_____ 33. dispensing   d. drug that widens the respiratory passages

_____ 34. bronchodilator   e. medicine that promotes phlegm production to be coughed out

Match the definition with its correct term.

_____ 35. mucolytic   a. drug that inhibits organ transplant rejection

_____ 36. cytotoxic drug   b. agent that induces vomiting

_____ 37. emetic   c. agent that nondiscriminately kills cells

_____ 38. antipyretic   d. agent that liquefies mucus

_____ 39. cyclosporine   e. fever-reducing drug

Match the drug classification with its pharmacologic agents.

_____ 40. blood drugs   a. glucocorticoids, antiandrogens, estrogens

_____ 41. cardiovascular drugs   b. antiplatelet drugs, thrombolytics, anticoagulants

_____ 42. lipid-lowering drugs   c. glycosides, diuretics, vasodilators, ACE inhibitors

_____ 43. cancer drugs   d. lovastatin, bile acid-binding resins, lipase enhancers

_____ 44. endocrine system drugs   e. colony-stimulating factors and antimetabolites

Match the pharmacologic agents with their drug classification.

_____ 45. allergy and respiratory drugs   a. aspirin, acetaminophen, ibuprofen

_____ 46. GI drugs   b. estrogen, calcitonin, and SERMs

_____ 47. NSAIDs and analgesics   c. cyclosporine, monoclonal antibodies, cytotoxins

_____ 48. immunosuppressive drugs   d. acid inhibitors, histamine receptor antagonists, mucosa coaters

_____ 49. osteoporosis drugs   e. histamine-receptor antagonists, antihistamines, beta agonists

Using the following word parts, form a medical term for each definition. Each word part is used only once.

-cutaneous   -muscular
-dermal   pharmaco-
intra-   sub-
-lingual   sub-
-logy   trans-

50. study of drugs _____

51. across the skin _____

52. beneath the tongue _____

53. within the muscle _____

54. beneath the skin _____

What term is described by each of the following definitions?

55. strength; dose required to bring about drug's maximum effect _____

56. science of the nature and effects of poisons, their detection, and treatments _____

57. compound that binds to a cell receptor exerting an effect _____

58. readiness to conform to a treatment _____

59. general term for a person who administers anesthetics _____

Define the following terms.

60. pharmacologist _____

61. pharmacotherapy _____

62. placebo _____

Identify the correctly spelled term in each set.

_____ 63.   a. iatrogeneic   b. iatrogenic
            c. itrogenic   d. iatragenic

_____ 64.   a. palliative   b. paliative
            c. pallative   d. pallitive

_____ 65.   a. pharmicopeia   b. pharmacopeea
            c. pharmacopeia   d. pharmakopia

_____ 66.   a. anesthetecs   b. anasthetics
            c. enesthetics   d. anesthetics

_____ 67.   a. analgesic   b. anelgesic
            c. analgesick   d. anallgesic

Unscramble the letters to form a medical term.

68. ticnoddai _____

69. exitvaal _____

70. senthazitee _____

71. acceffiy _____

72. aaoocghlmpry _____

Define the following abbreviations.

73. NPO _____

74. NSAIDs _____

75. ACE inhibitors _____

76. bid _____

77. pc _____

LEVEL THREE: THINKING CRITICALLY

Provide a short answer to each of the following questions.

78. A patient seeks medical attention for the common cold, which is caused by a virus. The physician prescribes the antibiotic amoxicillin. Is this an appropriate therapy? Explain.

_____

_____

_____

79. A friend has been taking spironolactone, a diuretic, for over 2 weeks and notices that she has been urinating more frequently than usual. Is this a normal or an abnormal response? Explain.

_____

_____

_____

80. Using common abbreviations for chart orders, write a prescription indicating 500 milligrams of aspirin to be used every 5 hours as needed.

_____

_____

_____

KEY TERMS SPELLING TEST FROM CD-ROM

Use the CD-ROM to test yourself on the spelling of key terms from this chapter. Listen to the terms and write them on a separate sheet of paper. Use a medical dictionary to check your answers.

ANSWERS

ANSWERS TO WORD GROUPING EXERCISE

Definition	Word Part
tongue, lingual	lingu-, lingua-, lingui, linguo-
bacteria, bacterial	bacteri-, bacterio-
drug	pharmaco-
gold	chrys-, chryso-
killer, killing	-cide
local	top-, topo-
muscle fiber	ino-
pain	alge-, algesi-
physicians, medicine, treatment	iatro-
poison, toxin	tox-, toxi-, toxico-, toxo-
rectum, rectal	rect-, recto-
sense, sense perception	-esthesia, esthesio-
substance that keeps something from changing	-stat
vomiting	emet-, emeto-

ANSWERS TO WORD BUILDING EXERCISE

Word Part	Meaning	Common or Known Word	Example Medical Term
bacteri-, bacterio-	bacteria, bacterial	bacteria	bacteria
alge-, algesi	pain	analgesic	analgesia
-cide	killer, killing	suicide	bactericidal
-esthesia, esthesio-	sense, sense perception	anesthesia	anesthesia
iatro-	physicians, medicine, treatment	iatrogenic	iatrogenic
lingu-, lingua-, lingui, linguo-	tongue, lingual	linguist	sublingual
pharmaco-	drug	pharmacy	pharmacology
rect-, recto-	rectum, rectal	rectum	rectal
-stat	substance that keeps something from changing	electrostatic	bacteriostatic
top-, topo-	local	topical	topical
tox-, toxi-, toxico-, toxo-	poison, toxin	toxic	toxicology

KEY TERM PRACTICE

Pharmacology Preview
1. prescription (Rx)
2. generic
3. pharmaco-; field of study; pharmacology

Basic Pharmacologic Terms
1. lethal dose (LD)
2. pharmacokinetics; pharmacodynamics

Drug Reactions, Regulations, and References
1. Potentiation
2. controlled substances; schedule drugs
3. iatrogenic; iatro-

Routes of Administration
1. a. bucca; b. inhalation; c. intramuscular (IM); d. intravenous (IV); e. oral; f. rectal; g. subcutaneous; h. sublingual; i. topical; j. transdermal; k. vaginal; l. parenteral; m. intradermal (intracutaneous)

Autonomic Nervous System Drugs
1. cholinergic
2. Adrenergic

Central Nervous System Drugs
1. barbiturates; benzodiazepines
2. selective serotonin reuptake inhibitors (SSRIs)
3. antiepileptic drugs
4. narcotics

Anesthetics
1. anesthesia
2. Local anesthetics
3. anesthesiology

Blood Drugs
1. thrombolytic
2. Anticoagulants

Cardiovascular System Drugs
1. inotropic; ino-
2. sympathomimetic drugs

Respiratory System and Allergy Drugs
1. Antihistamines
2. mucolytic

Endocrine System Drugs
1. adrenocortical

Gastrointestinal System Drugs
1. Antacids
2. anti-; vomiting; antiemetic

Immunosuppressive Drugs
1. immunosuppressive
2. Cyclosporine
3. chryso-; chrysotherapy

Antimicrobial Drugs
1. antimicrobial
2. broad-spectrum antibiotics

Antiviral Drugs
1. antiviral

Antifungal, Antiprotozoal, and Antihelminthic Drugs
1. Antifungal
2. antiprotozoal
3. Antihelminthic

Cancer Drugs
1. cell, poison; cytotoxic

Nonsteroidal Anti-Inflammatory Drugs
1. aspirin
2. nonsteroidal anti-inflammatory drugs (NSAIDs)

CASE STUDY

1. a is the correct answer.
   - b is incorrect because immunosuppressants do not enhance the immune system.
   - c is incorrect because immunosuppressants do not alter cardiac function.
   - d is incorrect because immunosuppressants do not enhance tissue rejection.
2. a is the correct answer.
   - b is incorrect because diuretics are not calcium channel blockers, although they are used in the treatment of some heart conditions.
   - c is incorrect because ACE inhibitors are not calcium channel blockers, although they are used in the treatment of some heart conditions.
   - d is incorrect because calcium-channel blockers are not used to increase urinary output.
3. c is the correct answer.
   - a is incorrect because histamine-receptor antagonists reduce acid release.
   - b is incorrect because histamine-receptor antagonists reduce acid release.
   - d is incorrect because cimetidine is used to treat upper-GI conditions, and diarrhea treatments target the lower GI tract not the upper GI tract.
4. b is the correct answer.
   - a is incorrect because chemical names would indicate the drugs' chemical constituency.
   - c is incorrect because the generic names for these drugs are diltiazem, azathioprine, and cimetidine.
   - d is incorrect because formularies are reference books containing lists of pharmaceutic products with their descriptions and prescribing information.
5. b is the correct answer.
   - a, c, and d are incorrect by definition.

REAL WORLD REPORT

1. a. every morning; b. every day; c. every 6 h
2. a. intravenously (IV); b. every 6 h for 7 days.
3. a. Cardizem; b. Nexium
4. after meals

REVIEW AND APPLICATION: THREE-LEVEL LEARNING SYSTEM

Level One: Reviewing Facts and Terms Using Recall

1. d
2. c
3. a
4. b
5. c
6. b
7. d
8. a
9. a
10. c
11. b

Level Two: Reviewing Concepts

12. d
13. b
14. c
15. d
16. a
17. a
18. first-pass metabolism; pharmaceuticals
19. adverse drug event; potentiation
20. b
21. a
22. d
23. e
24. c
25. b
26. a
27. e
28. d
29. c
30. c
31. e
32. a
33. b
34. d
35. d
36. c
37. b
38. e
39. a
40. b
41. c
42. d
43. e
44. a
45. e
46. d
47. a
48. c
49. b
50. pharmacology
51. transdermal
52. sublingual
53. intramuscular
54. subcutaneous
55. potency
56. toxicology
57. agonist
58. compliance
59. anesthetist
60. person who studies pharmacology
61. treatment of disease by drugs
62. substance with no medicinal ingredient
63. b
64. a
65. c
66. d
67. a
68. addiction
69. laxative
70. anesthetize
71. efficacy
72. pharmacology
73. nothing by mouth; non per os
74. nonsteroidal anti-inflammatory drugs
75. angiotensin converting enzyme inhibitors
76. twice per day; bis in die
77. after meals; post cibos

Level Three: Thinking Critically

78. This is an inappropriate prescription therapy because amoxicillin is an antibiotic and is effective only against bacterial infections. The physician should either prescribe an antiviral medication or nothing at all if the symptoms began more than 30 h earlier.
79. Spironolactone is a diuretic, which is an agent that causes increased urinary output. Thus this is a normal response.
80. ASA 500 mg q5h prn

Index

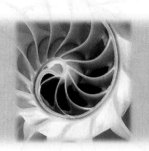

Page numbers followed by *f* and *t* indicate figures (illustrations) and tables, respectively.